NMS *Medicine*

NMS *Medicine*

7th EDITION

Editor

Susan D. Wolfsthal, MD

Celeste L. Woodward Professor in Humanitarian and Ethical Medical Practice
Associate Chair for Education, Residency Program Director
Department of Medicine
University of Maryland School of Medicine
Baltimore, Maryland

 Wolters Kluwer | Lippincott Williams & Wilkins
Health
Philadelphia · Baltimore · New York · London
Buenos Aires · Hong Kong · Sydney · Tokyo

Acquisitions Editor: Susan Rhyner
Product Manager: Sirkka Howes
Marketing Manager: Joy Fisher-Williams
Manufacturing Coordinator: Margie Orzech
Designer: Holly Reid McLaughlin
Compositor: Aptara, Inc.

Seventh Edition

Copyright © 2012, 2008, 2005, 2001, 1997, 1994, 1990 Lippincott Williams & Wilkins, a Wolters Kluwer business.

351 West Camden Street   Two Commerce Square
Baltimore, MD 21201   2001 Market Street
                                Philadelphia, PA 19103

Printed in China

9 8 7 6 5 4 3 2 1

Library of Congress Cataloging-in-Publication Data

NMS medicine / editor, Susan Wolfsthal. – 7th ed.
    p. ; cm. – (National medical series for independent study)
  Includes bibliographical references and index.
    ISBN 978-1-60831-581-9 (pbk. : alk. paper)
  1. Internal medicine–Outlines, syllabi, etc. 2. Internal medicine–Examinations, questions, etc. I. Wolfsthal, Susan D. II. Series: National medical series for independent study.
    [DNLM: 1. Internal Medicine–Examination Questions. 2. Internal Medicine–Outlines. WB 18.2]
    RC59.M44 2012
    616.0076–dc22

                                    2011004402

DISCLAIMER

Care has been taken to confirm the accuracy of the information present and to describe generally accepted practices. However, the authors, editors, and publisher are not responsible for errors or omissions or for any consequences from application of the information in this book and make no warranty, expressed or implied, with respect to the currency, completeness, or accuracy of the contents of the publication. Application of this information in a particular situation remains the professional responsibility of the practitioner; the clinical treatments described and recommended may not be considered absolute and universal recommendations.

The authors, editors, and publisher have exerted every effort to ensure that drug selection and dosage set forth in this text are in accordance with the current recommendations and practice at the time of publication. However, in view of ongoing research, changes in government regulations, and the constant flow of information relating to drug therapy and drug reactions, the reader is urged to check the package insert for each drug for any change in indications and dosage and for added warnings and precautions. This is particularly important when the recommended agent is a new or infrequently employed drug.

Some drugs and medical devices presented in this publication have Food and Drug Administration (FDA) clearance for limited use in restricted research settings. It is the responsibility of the health care provider to ascertain the FDA status of each drug or device planned for use in his or her clinical practice.

To purchase additional copies of this book, call our customer service department at (800) 638-3030 or fax orders to (301) 223-2320. International customers should call (301) 223-2300.

Visit Lippincott Williams & Wilkins on the Internet: http://www.lww.com. Lippincott Williams & Wilkins customer service representatives are available from 8:30 am to 6:00 pm, EST.

To my family, who always supports me with their love and patience, including my husband, Bill, my daughters, Rebecca and Jennifer, and my son-in-law, Yoni. A special thank you to my mentors, who been a source of inspiration and have encouraged me throughout my career in medical education at the University of Maryland.

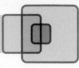

Contributors

Tareq Abou-Khamis, MD
Fellow, Division of Rheumatology and
    Clinical Immunology,
    Department of Medicine
University of Maryland Medical Center
Baltimore, Maryland

Temilolu Aje, MD
Chief Resident 2009–2010
Clinical Instructor
Department of Medicine
University of Maryland School of Medicine
Baltimore, Maryland

Michael Benitez, MD
Professor
Division of Cardiology,
    Department of Medicine
University of Maryland School of Medicine
Baltimore, Maryland

Mary E. Bollinger, DO
Associate Professor
Department of Pediatrics
Division of Pediatric Pulmonology
    and Allergy
University of Maryland School of Medicine
Baltimore, Maryland

Majid E. Cina, MD
Assistant Professor of Medicine
Division of General Internal Medicine,
    Department of Medicine
University of Maryland School of Medicine
Baltimore, Maryland

Marcia Driscoll, MD
Clinical Associate Professor
Department of Dermatology
University of Maryland School of Medicine
Baltimore, Maryland

Corinne Erickson, MD
Resident, Department of Dermatology
University of Maryland Medical Center
Baltimore, Maryland

Emily Fairchild, MD
Assistant Professor of Medicine
Division of General Internal Medicine,
    Department of Medicine
University of Maryland School of Medicine
Baltimore, Maryland

Raymond Flores, MD
Associate Professor
Division of Rheumatology and Clinical
    Immunology, Department of Medicine
University of Maryland School of Medicine
Baltimore, Maryland

Neda Frayha, MD
Chief Resident 2008–2009
Assistant Professor of Medicine
Division of General Internal Medicine,
    Department of Medicine
University of Maryland School of Medicine
Baltimore, Maryland

Esteban Gallego, MD
Chief Resident 2010–2011
Department of Medicine
University of Maryland School of Medicine
Baltimore, Maryland

Victoria Giffi, MD
Chief Resident 2010–2011
Department of Medicine
University of Maryland School of Medicine
Baltimore, Maryland

Bruce Greenwald, MD
Professor
Division of Gastroenterology and Hepatology,
    Department of Medicine
University of Maryland School of Medicine
Baltimore, Maryland

Robert Habicht, MD
Assistant Professor of Medicine and Pediatrics
Division of General Internal Medicine,
    Department of Medicine
Division of Education, Department of Pediatrics
University of Maryland School of Medicine
Baltimore, Maryland

Donna Hanes, MD
Clinical Associate Professor
Division of Nephrology, Department of Medicine
University of Maryland School of Medicine
Baltimore, Maryland

Janaki Kuruppu, MD
Assistant Professor
Division of Infectious Diseases,
    Department of Medicine
University of Maryland School of Medicine
Baltimore, Maryland

Elizabeth Lamos, MD
Chief Resident 2009–2010
Clinical Instructor
Department of Medicine
University of Maryland School of Medicine
Baltimore, Maryland

Ralph Lebron, MD
Chief Resident 2009–2010
Clinical Instructor
Department of Medicine
University of Maryland School of Medicine
Baltimore, Maryland

Thomas Macharia, MD
Chief Resident 2010–2011
Department of Medicine
University of Maryland School of Medicine
Baltimore, Maryland

Kristi Moore, MD
Chief Resident 2008–2009
Clinical Instructor of Medicine
Department of Medicine, Mercy Medical Center
University of Maryland School of Medicine
Baltimore, Maryland

Devang Patel, MD
Assistant Professor
Division of Infectious Diseases,
    Department of Medicine
University of Maryland School of Medicine
Baltimore, Maryland

Neil Porter, MD
Associate Professor
Department of Neurology
University of Maryland School of Medicine
Baltimore, Maryland

Darryn Potosky, MD
Visiting Instructor
Division of Gastroenterology and Hepatology,
    Department of Medicine
University of Maryland School of Medicine
Baltimore, Maryland

Norman Retener, MD
Chief Resident 2008–2009
Assistant Professor of Medicine
Division of General Internal Medicine,
    Department of Medicine
University of Maryland School of Medicine
Baltimore, Maryland

Janell A. Sherr, MD
Chief Resident in Medicine-Pediatrics
    2010–2011
Department of Medicine and
    Department of Pediatrics
University of Maryland Medical Center
Baltimore, Maryland

Leann Silhan, MD
Chief Resident 2009–2010
Fellow, Division of Pulmonary and
    Critical Care Medicine
Department of Medicine
University of Maryland Medical Center
Baltimore, Maryland

Katherine Tkaczuk, MD
Professor
Department of Medicine, Division of
    Hematology and Oncology
University of Maryland School of Medicine
Baltimore, Maryland

Arul Thomas, MD
Chief Resident 2010–2011
Department of Medicine
University of Maryland School of Medicine
Baltimore, Maryland

Nevins Todd, MD
Assistant Professor
Division of Pulmonary and Critical Care
    Medicine, Department of Medicine
University of Maryland School of Medicine
Baltimore, Maryland

Leroy Vaughan, MD
Chief Resident 2009–2010
Clinical Instructor
Department of Medicine
University of Maryland
    School of Medicine
Baltimore, Maryland

Ann Zimrin, MD
Associate Professor
Division of Hematology and Oncology,
    Department of Medicine
University of Maryland School of Medicine
Baltimore, Maryland

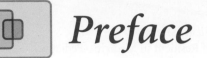# *Preface*

The first exposure to clinical medicine during medical school is an eye-opening experience—a time when the student brings together the vast amount of information learned in the basic sciences and merges that with actual patient care. It is a glorious time for learning, and the amount that needs to be absorbed grows exponentially with time. It is with these first steps into clinical medicine that the young student begins to comprehend the importance of being a lifelong learner. We absorb basic concepts and build upon them, modify what we know as new advances are discovered, and continually add to our knowledge for the rest of our lives as physicians.

Through this comprehensive review of internal medicine, we sought to capture the essential concepts and key elements of our specialty by focusing on general internal medicine and the numerous medical subspecialties. Although internal medicine is constantly evolving, there are basic principles and thought processes that remain the essence of our specialty. Learning the facts is only the beginning. Medical students must develop their skills in deductive reasoning and synthesize these facts, weighing the pros and cons of the evaluation and management choices for their patients.

As we did in the sixth edition, *NMS Medicine* was not only written by specialists in the field, but also coauthored by chief residents and senior internal medicine residents at the University of Maryland. Since the chiefs and senior residents are much closer to the medical students in terms of their training and experience, they bring a fresh and relevant approach to this material. We welcome them as authors of this text not only for their input, but also because we enjoy mentoring our young colleagues and providing them with an opportunity to advance their scholarly activities and academic careers.

This edition is completely updated, including the chapters, case studies, and comprehensive questions. You will find a significant amount of material online, including additional content, tables, and illustrations. The 🖱 icon signals to the reader where to find these supplemental online resources. Also available online is a comprehensive exam consisting of 150 board-style review questions with answers and explanations. In addition to medical students, we anticipate that this book will be useful for residents and practicing physicians learning or reviewing the essential principles, concepts, and information in internal medicine

We encourage you to use the material presented as the first step to advancing your understanding and knowledge of these topics in more depth, either by studying the larger and more classic textbooks of internal medicine or, more importantly, by reading the primary source literature. The process of being a lifelong learner begins here. We hope that you accept this challenge, are excited by the field of internal medicine, and share in our enthusiasm for our chosen profession. We wish you well in your studies and your career path.

Susan D. Wolfsthal, MD

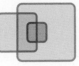

Contents

13 Dermatologic Disorders 601

CORINNE ERICKSON and MARCIA DRISCOLL

Case Studies in Clinical Decision Making 639

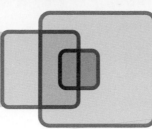

chapter 1

The Internist's Approach to Patient Care

MAJID E. CINA · SUSAN D. WOLFSTHAL

I THE INTERNIST'S APPROACH TO PATIENT CARE

A **The internist as physician** Internal medicine is a broad and comprehensive field that encompasses pathophysiology, clinical practice, and various procedures. Internists utilize their cognitive skills, gravitating toward general medicine and subspecialties such as nephrology, endocrinology, or infectious diseases. Some internists are more procedure oriented and practice subspecialties such as cardiology or gastroenterology, and others gravitate toward caring for patients with multiorgan failure, practicing pulmonary medicine and critical care. Most internists care for patients in the ambulatory setting, some only care for inpatients, whereas others care for patients in both settings.

For medical students who are just starting their clinical rotations, it may seem a daunting task to master internal medicine. Each student must find his or her center within this field and establish his or her career goals. With focus, clinical exposure, and lifelong learning, the student can expect a rewarding and successful career in internal medicine.

B **Principles of internal medicine** Certain principles are common among all internists. Although many are shared with clinicians in other specialties, internists are most likely to espouse these. In general, internists engage in the following:

1. Approach patient care in a comprehensive fashion with emphasis on the patient as a whole entity.

2. Use deductive reasoning to establish a comprehensive differential diagnosis and plan of care.

3. Use an evidence-based approach to evaluation, treatment, and preventive care.

4. Use a biopsychosocial model of care.

5. Provide continuity of care in a medical home model.

6. May care for a diverse group of patients or focus on certain populations, diseases, and age groups.

II VARIOUS ROLES OF THE INTERNIST

A **Primary Care**

1. A primary care practitioner or general internist is the backbone of our health care system. General internists care for the largest group of patients, who range from adolescents to the very elderly. General internists provide comprehensive care to their patients, focusing on preventive care, wellness, and maintenance of health. They see patients for acute or urgent issues and provide long-term care over many decades. They also perform consultations, such as perioperative risk assessment for their patients. Few other physicians have such a sustained and continuous relationship with their patients.

2. Patients often turn to their general internists with questions. They ask their doctor to validate what subspecialists have recommended. They also turn to their general internists for

psychiatric and social concerns, seeking their advice and counsel. There is no aspect of patient care in the physician–patient relationship that is not within the realm of the internist's responsibility.

B Hospital Medicine

1. Hospitalists are physicians who primarily or exclusively care for inpatients. The vast majority of physicians practicing hospital medicine are general internists. Internists who practice hospital medicine manage adults with acute care needs, focusing on issues that can be resolved during the patient's hospitalization but also continuing to address the patient's long-term needs by global patient assessment.

2. Hospitalists coordinate care with their patients' primary care providers. Effective communication is essential to success during transition of care from the outpatient setting to the inpatient setting and vice versa. While care of hospitalized patients affords fewer opportunities for sustained or longitudinal relationships with patients, internists in this role may quickly establish rapport with and impact behavior in patients, as patients may be more willing to make lifestyle changes while hospitalized for severe illness.

C Subspecialty Care

1. Training in internal medicine provides the student with the broadest choices for a future career in subspecialty care. Within internal medicine, physicians can subspecialize in fields in which they may care for the total needs of their patients. This approach is typical for nephrologists, oncologists, and infectious disease specialists. Others may focus on a particular system and have the patient's general internist care for their other needs. These subspecialists may include cardiologists, gastroenterologists, pulmonologists, or allergists. All of these subspecialists have patients who are part of their core practice and others for whom they serve as a consultant.

2. Some subspecialties of internal medicine allow physicians to do procedures as part of their clinical practice. In some subspecialties, such as invasive cardiology, electrophysiology, and gastroenterology, internists can spend the majority of their practice doing invasive procedures. Subspecialists in endocrinology, hepatology, and nephrology may do a select number of procedures, such as biopsies or catheter insertions. Critical care physicians perform a variety of procedures, such as thorocenteses and insertion of chest tubes and central venous catheters, among others.

3. These fields afford the practitioner enormous flexibility in terms of practice types. Most care for patients in the ambulatory setting, whereas some may be solely focused on caring for patients in the hospital. There also is a broad spectrum of inpatient settings, ranging from caring for patients on general medicine services as a consultant to providing care to patients in critical care settings, whether in coronary or medical intensive care units. In studying the chapters in this text, the student will come to understand the type of diseases each subspecialist may encounter in his or her practice.

III PREVENTIVE HEALTH AND SCREENING

A General Principles

1. A major focus of the internist's care of patients is to screen for common diseases and risk factors that have the potential to affect the patient's health in the years to come. The challenge lies in ensuring that one screens for diseases that have a reasonable prevalence in the population and that are amenable to treatments that prolong and improve the quality of life.

2. As determined by the World Health Organization (WHO), screening tests should have the following properties:
   a. **Sensitivity:** The screening test should have a high probability of being correct and be effective in detecting a disease in those who have the disease.
   b. **Specificity:** The screening test should have sufficient specificity such that negative test results are obtained in patients who are free of the disease.
   c. **Positive predictive value:** The screening test should have adequate positive predictive value so that patients who have the disease obtain a positive test result.

    d. Negative predictive value: The screening test should have adequate negative predictive value so that patients who are free of the disease obtain a negative test result.

    e. Acceptability: The screening test should be acceptable to patients in terms of access, discomfort, side effects, or other potential adverse outcomes.

3. Several prominent organizations have developed clinical guidelines for screening for various diseases. Since these guidelines change frequently, internists modify their approach every few years. Up-to-date guidelines and recommendations from the U.S. Preventive Services Task Force (USPSTF) can be accessed at http://www.ahrq.gov/clinic/uspstfix.htm. This organization is very strict in their interpretation of screening tests that meet the WHO criteria and do not recommend routine screening in asymptomatic individuals unless a positive benefit has been proven. The internist must weigh the opinions of the USPSTF and other organizations with the patient's personal and family history, as well the patient's concerns about his or health and well-being. The following is presented as the current guidelines for the most prevalent diseases seen in adults.

B Screening for Malignancy

1. Guidelines for cancer screening are detailed in Table 1–1 as advised by the USPSTF.

2. The following supplements are currently *not* recommended by the USPSTF: aspirin and nonsteroidal medications to prevent colon cancer and vitamin supplements to prevent cancer and cardiovascular disease.

3. Routine screening for the following cancers in *asymptomatic* individuals is currently *not* recommended by the USPSTF: screening for bladder cancer; breast cancer with genetic testing; lung cancer with chest x-ray, cytology, or computed tomography (CT) scanning; ovarian cancer with CA-125; and routine screening for testicular and pancreatic cancer.

C Screening for and Prevention of Common Diseases in Adults Recommendations for pregnant individuals are not included in these recommendations.

1. **Abdominal aortic aneurysm:** Screening with a single abdominal sonogram is recommended for men 65–75 years of age who have ever smoked.

2. **Cardiovascular disease:** Aspirin is recommended for men age 45–79 years when the potential benefit due to a reduction in myocardial infarctions outweighs the potential harm due to an increase in gastrointestinal hemorrhage. The USPSTF recommends the use of aspirin for women age 55–79 years when the potential benefit of a reduction in ischemic strokes outweighs the potential harm due to an increase in gastrointestinal hemorrhage.

3. **Hypertension:** All individuals 18 years and older should be screened for hypertension.

4. **Dyslipidemia:** The USPSTF strongly recommends screening men aged 35 years and older for lipid disorders, and recommends screening men aged 20–35 years for lipid disorders if they are at increased risk for coronary heart disease. They strongly recommend screening women aged 45 years and older for lipid disorders if they are at increased risk for coronary heart disease, and recommend screening women aged 20–45 years for lipid disorders if they are at increased risk for coronary heart disease.

5. **Infectious diseases:** The USPSTF strongly recommends that clinicians screen for human immunodeficiency virus (HIV) in all adolescents and adults at increased risk for HIV infection and for syphilis infection in persons at increased risk. They also recommend screening for chlamydial infection for all sexually active nonpregnant women aged 24 years and younger and for older nonpregnant women who are at increased risk. High-intensity behavioral counseling to prevent sexually transmitted infections (STIs) is recommended for all sexually active adolescents and for adults at increased risk for STIs.

6. **Diabetes:** The USPSTF recommends screening for diabetes in patients with sustained blood pressure greater than 135/80 mm Hg. Screening is recommended by the American Diabetes Association in individuals with a body mass index (BMI) of 25 or greater; with one or more risk factors for diabetes (positive family history, hypertension, dyslipidemia); or who are over the age of 45 years. Screening may be done with a fasting blood glucose or hemoglobin A1c (HbA1c) determination.

7. **Osteoporosis:** The USPSTF recommends screening all women aged 65 years or older and screening all women aged 60–64 years with increased risk, such as women who weigh less than 70 kg or

TABLE 1–1	Screening Guidelines for the Early Detection of Cancer in Average-Risk Asymptomatic People		
Cancer Site	**Population**	**Test or Procedure**	**Frequency**
Breast	Women, age 20+	Breast self-examination	Beginning in their early 20s, women should be told about the benefits and limitations of breast self-examination (BSE). The importance of prompt reporting of any new breast symptoms to a health professional should be emphasized. Women who choose to do BSE should receive instruction and have their technique reviewed on the occasion of a periodic health examination. It is acceptable for women to choose not to do BSE or to do BSE irregularly.
		Clinical breast examination	For women in their 20s and 30s, it is recommended that clinical breast examination (CBE) be part of a periodic health examination, preferably at least every 3 years. Asymptomatic women aged 40 and older should continue to receive a clinical breast examination as part of a periodic health examination, preferably annually.
		Mammography	Begin annual mammography at age 40.*
Colorectal[†]	Men and women, age 50+	*Tests that find polyps and cancer:*	
		Flexible sigmoidoscopy,[‡] or	Every 5 years, starting at age 50
		Colonoscopy, or	Every 10 years, starting at age 50
		Double-contrast barium enema (DCBE),[‡] or	Every 5 years, starting at age 50
		Tests that mainly find cancer:	
		Fecal occult blood test (FOBT) with ≥50% test sensitivity for cancer, or fecal immunochemical test (FIT) with ≥50% test sensitivity for cancer,[‡,§] or	Annually, starting at age 50
		Stool DNA test (sDNA)[‡]	Interval uncertain, starting at age 50
Prostate	Men, age 50+	Prostate-specific antigen test (PSA) with or without digital rectal exam (DRE)	Asymptomatic men who have at least a 10-year life expectancy should have an opportunity to make an informed decision with their health care provider about screening for prostate cancer after receiving information about the uncertainties, risks, and potential benefits associated with screening. Men at average risk should receive this information beginning at age 50. Men at higher risk, including African American men and men with a first-degree relative (father or brother) diagnosed with prostate cancer before age 65, should receive this information beginning at age 45. Men at appreciably higher risk (multiple family members diagnosed with prostate cancer before age 65) should receive this information beginning at age 40.

TABLE 1–1	Screening Guidelines for the Early Detection of Cancer in Average-Risk Asymptomatic People (Continued)		
Cancer Site	**Population**	**Test or Procedure**	**Frequency**
Cervix	Women, age 18+	Pap test	Cervical cancer screening should begin approximately 3 years after a woman begins having vaginal intercourse, but no later than 21 years of age. Screening should be done every year with conventional Pap tests or every two years using liquid-based Pap tests. At or after age 30, women who have had three normal test results in a row may get screened every 2–3 to years with cervical cytology (either conventional or liquid-based Pap test) alone, or every 3 years with an HPV DNA test plus cervical cytology. Women 70 years of age and older who have had three or more normal Pap tests and no abnormal Pap tests in the last 10 years and women who have had a total hysterectomy may choose to stop cervical cancer screening.
Endometrial	Women, at menopause		At the time of menopause, women at average risk should be informed about risks and symptoms of endometrial cancer and strongly encouraged to report any unexpected bleeding or spotting to their physicians.
Cancer-related checkup	Men and women, age 20+		On the occasion of a periodic health examination, the cancer-related checkup should include examination for cancers of the thyroid, testicles, ovaries, lymph nodes, oral cavity, and skin, as well as health counseling about tobacco, sun exposure, diet and nutrition, risk factors, sexual practices, and environmental and occupational exposures.

*Beginning at age 40 years, annual clinical breast examination should be performed prior to mammography.
†Individuals with a personal or family history of colorectal cancer or adenomas, inflammatory bowel disease, or high-risk genetic syndromes should continue to follow the most recent recommendations for individuals at increased or high risk.
‡Colonoscopy should be done if test results are positive.
§For FOBT or FIT used as a screening test, the take-home multiple sample method should be used. A FOBT or FIT done during a digital rectal exam in the doctor's office is not adequate for screening.
American Cancer Society. *Cancer Facts & Figures 2010*. Atlanta, GA: American Cancer Society; 2010.

women of white or Asian ancestry. The screening test of choice is dual-energy x-ray absorptiometry (DEXA).

8. While various specialty organizations recommend additional screening for disease states, the USPSTF finds insufficient evidence to recommend *for or against* screening the general population for thyroid disease, glaucoma, impaired visual acuity, or nontraditional coronary artery disease (CAD) risk factors such as elevated C-reactive protein or homocysteine levels. The USPSTF does not comment on screening for vitamin D deficiency. Despite the lack of strong evidence-based guidelines, many internists will screen for these entities based on expert opinion or emerging evidence.

9. The USPSTF does *not* recommend screening for the following conditions in *asymptomatic* individuals: carotid artery stenosis; chronic obstructive pulmonary disease; coronary artery disease with electrocardiogram (EKG), stress testing, or CT scan for coronary calcium; peripheral arterial disease; viral hepatitis; syphilis; dementia; or hemochromatosis.

D **Immunizations**

1. The following immunizations are recommended by the Centers for Disease Control and Prevention (CDC). The most up-to-date recommendations can be accessed at http://www.cdc.gov/vaccines/recs/schedules/adult-schedule.htm. Some vaccinations are contraindicated in immunocompromised individuals or during pregnancy, such as vaccinations for varicella zoster and measles, mumps, and rubella.

 a. **Tetanus, diphtheria, pertussis (Td/Tdap):** Once every 10 years with a one-time substitution of Tdap for Td booster. Td every 10 years over the age of 65 years.

    b. Human papilloma virus (HPV): three doses age 19–26 years (if not sooner).

    c. Varicella: two doses (if no immunity documented).

    d. Zoster: one dose at age 60 years.

    e. Measles, mumps, rubella: one or two doses up to age 50 years if no immunity documented; after age 50 years, one dose depending on occupation and lifestyle.

    f. Influenza: one dose annually.

    g. Pneumococcal disease: one to two doses up to age 65 years, depending on risk factors; one dose for all individuals over age 65 years.

    h. Hepatitis A: two doses depending on occupation and lifestyle.

    i. Hepatitis B: three doses depending on occupation and lifestyle.

    j. Meningococcal disease: one or two doses depending on risk factors and for all individuals living in close quarters, such as military personnel and college students.

E Wellness and the Approach to a Healthy Lifestyle

1. **Timing:** The internist and patient should discuss wellness at least annually or when merited by certain conditions, such as hypertension, obesity, or hyperlipidemia, and should encourage patients to take an active role in their health.

2. **Exercise and diet:** Patients should be advised to exercise at least 30 minutes each day, including vigorous walking or other activity. Portion control and maintaining a BMI in the normal range (<25) with a heart-healthy diet (low fat and sodium) should be encouraged. Additional restrictions may be needed depending on other medical conditions, such as diabetes or renal disease.

3. **Smoking, alcohol, and substance abuse:** The USPSTF recommends asking all adults about tobacco and alcohol use. Patients should be strongly encouraged to stop smoking or not to start smoking. Various techniques can be employed, including deciding on a quit date and using nicotine substitutes (gum, patches, and sprays). Screening for excessive alcohol consumption should be done and counseling offered as needed.

4. **Depression:** The USPSTF recommends screening for depression, especially when staff-assisted care supports are in place to assure accurate diagnosis, effective treatment, and follow-up.

5. **Domestic violence:** The physician should be alert to the potential for domestic violence between partners. Patients complaining of depression, difficulty sleeping, or vague abdominal or pelvic pain symptoms should be screened more closely for domestic violence by inquiring whether the patient feels safe in the relationship or has been physically injured or threatened or forced to have sexual activities that make the patient feel uncomfortable.

6. While various specialty organizations recommend additional lifestyle screening and while many of these may seem wise and intuitive, the USPSTF finds insufficient evidence to recommend *for or against* screening the general population for illicit substance use, physical inactivity, or sun overexposure. Despite the lack of evidence *for or against* screening in these areas, internists should address these areas, as potential for benefit exists and risk of harm through screening is low.

IV SPECIAL POPULATIONS

A Geriatrics

1. **General concepts**

    a. Geriatric medicine is a subspecialty of medicine focusing on the care of the elderly. Geriatricians are internists who devoted training specific to this population. However, most internists provide care for the elderly, as elderly patients have more chronic illness and require more frequent access to care than young patients.

    b. The U.S. Census Bureau estimates that the number of very old persons (age 85 years or older) will double every 20 years.

2. **Fall prevention**

    a. Age is associated with instability, frailty, and falls. From one fourth to one half of all elderly patients experience at least one fall annually. Falls increase the risk for function- and life-threatening trauma, including hip fracture and cerebral hemorrhage.

    b. Elderly patients with slow gait, difficulty performing tandem walk, decreased visual acuity, or small calf circumference are at higher risk for falls. Fall risk may be reduced by referral to a physical therapist for mobility exercises, home safety evaluation, and provision of assist devices such as a rolling walker and grab bars in the bathroom.

    c. In elderly patients who are at risk for or experience falls, screening for and treating osteoporosis, visual disturbance, or neuromuscular diseases may be beneficial. In such patients, use of anticoagulant therapy such as warfarin should be carefully reassessed to weigh the risk of hemorrhage with fall against expected clinical benefit.

3. Immobility and pressure sores

    a. Elderly patients are at greatest risk for muscular atrophy and difficulty returning to a functional state after prolonged immobility, such as during hospitalization. Immobility also suppresses antidiuretic hormone secretion and can lead to orthostasis, further impeding mobility.

    b. Immobility increases risk for pressure-induced skin ulceration, especially of the heels, trochanter, sacrum, and iliac crest. Pressure ulcers are staged based on severity.

        (1) Stage I features nonblanching erythema without skin breakdown.

        (2) Stage II includes superficial ulceration with partial-thickness skin loss.

        (3) Stage III is full-thickness skin loss with exposure of the dermis.

        (4) Stage IV is loss of tissue to muscle, tendon, or bone.

4. Urinary incontinence

    a. Urinary incontinence is extremely common in the elderly, especially in women, but it is not a normal consequence of aging.

    b. Urge incontinence is the most common form and often occurs with detrusor hyperreflexia due to progressive loss of communication between the frontal lobes and micturition center in the brainstem. Treatment involves behavioral therapy in which the patient progressively delays voiding until micturition occurs at a comfortable interval. Medical therapy includes antimuscarinic agents such as oxybutynin or tolterodine, although anticholinergic side effects may limit their usefulness.

    c. Stress incontinence usually occurs because of a hypermobile urethra, which allows for urine loss during periods of increased intra-abdominal pressure. Treatment includes perineal muscle contractions (Kegel exercises) and topical estrogen therapy.

    d. Overflow incontinence is commonly associated with prostate hypertrophy and urethral outlet obstruction, with high postvoid residual urine volume. First-line therapy for prostatic hypertrophy is an alpha-receptor antagonist. Another mechanism is detrusor areflexia due to anticholinergic medications, diabetic neuropathy, multiple sclerosis, or sacral cord or pelvic nerve dysfunction.

5. Erectile dysfunction

    a. Penile erection requires cyclic guanosine monophosphate (cGMP)–mediated smooth muscle relaxation, which increases flow to the penile tissue through the helicine artery. Engorgement compresses outflow venules and sustains the erection.

    b. Normal aging diminishes capacity for penile erection, but progression to a level of sexual dissatisfaction occurs more often in men with diabetic neuropathy and vasculopathy, men who have undergone pelvic surgeries, men who take beta-blockers, methyldopa, or thiazide diuretics, and men with low androgen levels.

    c. Treatment could include discontinuing offending medications or prescribing sildenafil, tadalafil, or vardenafil, which inhibit phosphodiesterase type V, the enzyme that breaks down cGMP.

6. Medication use in the elderly

    a. Because of changes in lifestyle, physiology, and more common multiple-drug use (polypharmacy), the elderly are prone to medication-related complications.

        (1) Reduced adherence is common and results from complicated medication regimens, dementia, or financial difficulty.

        (2) Drug–drug interactions are more likely in the setting of polypharmacy. Interactions may also be present with nonprescription medications or supplements.

        (3) Side effects from medication may be more difficult to ascertain and less well tolerated in the elderly. Delirium, imbalance, and syncope may be the direct result of medication intolerance.

(4) Paradoxical response to medication may occur, such as increased agitation with use of benzodiazepines or insomnia with use of nonselective antihistamines.

b. When prescribing medication for elderly patients, attention to the following principles may reduce adverse events.

(1) "Start low, go slow," with use of the lowest initial starting doses and gradual uptitration to effect. Equilibration of medication effect takes three to four half-lives and may take longer in elderly patients with renal or hepatic dysfunction.

(2) Make one medication change at a time whenever possible, as the cause of new symptoms that could be attributed to adverse reactions would be difficult to ascertain with multiple changes.

(3) Frequently review the whole regimen with the patient and a family member, with careful attention to potential drug–drug interactions. Reduce or eliminate medication that may be unnecessary or of limited benefit. Elderly patients may have multiple illnesses, and each medication in a complicated regimen may be technically indicated based on disease-specific guidelines, but in some instances removal of "indicated" therapy may be beneficial to reduce polypharmacy.

(4) Provide clear instructions, ideally in written format with large text, with clearly delineated medication names, doses, schedule, and indication. When making changes, provide a complete, updated list.

(5) Assess adherence to therapy via multiple means, including asking that patients bring in pill bottles, inquiring of the patient's pharmacy about the frequency of refill requests, gathering information from family or friends, and/or testing blood levels of certain medications. Determine the cause of nonadherence and address it, whether by counseling about importance, addressing side effects, or substituting for a less expensive alternative.

B Pregnancy

1. General concepts

   a. Many of the disease states associated with pregnancy, such as hypertension, diabetes, or thyroid disease, are illnesses familiar to the internist. However, care of pregnant patients with chronic medical conditions should occur in conjunction with input from an obstetric specialist. If possible, collaboration between the internist and the obstetrician begins when the patient first contemplates becoming pregnant.

   b. Some medical conditions can regress or exacerbate during pregnancy or the immediate postpartum period. For example, autoimmune conditions may regress during pregnancy or appear for the first time or flare postpartum.

   c. Therapy should focus on the well-being of both mother and fetus, especially medication prescription and surgical interventions.

2. Medications in pregnancy.

   a. The U.S. Food and Drug Administration (FDA) classifies all medications for safety in pregnancy using a standard category scale. Because risk for harm is high, internists should consult a medication reference or the patient's obstetrician before giving new medication to the pregnant patient.

   (1) Category A medications showed no risk in controlled studies.

   (2) Category B medications are not known to cause fetal harm in humans.

   (3) Category C medications may be harmful based on animal studies, and controlled human studies are lacking, but potential benefit may warrant use despite potential risks.

   (4) Category D medications are known to cause fetal harm in humans, but potential benefit may warrant use despite risks.

   (5) Category X medications are contraindicated in pregnancy based on strong evidence for fetal harm in humans.

   b. Several medications commonly prescribed in adults are dangerous to fetal health and should be avoided during pregnancy.

   (1) Warfarin increases fetal deformities, especially in the first trimester. Pregnant patients who require anticoagulation should use unfractionated or low–molecular-weight heparin.

   (2) Angiotensin-converting-enzyme (ACE) inhibitors and angiotensin-receptor blockers are contraindicated in pregnancy because of risk of fetal renal dysgenesis. Pregnant patients with hypertension should be treated with methyldopa or nifedipine, with other classes used in severe hypertension uncontrolled on these agents.

    c. The dose of some medications needs to be adjusted as pregnancy progresses. This is true for patients receiving thyroid supplementation for hypothyroidism. Thyroid function tests must be closely monitored and often necessitate an increase in the patient's daily dose of thyroid replacement.

    d. Other medications may need to be adjusted because the standard target of treatment is stricter in the pregnant patient. Individuals with diabetes and hypertension must have much tighter control during the time the patient is contemplating having a child and throughout her pregnancy.

C · Dying Patient and Palliative Care

1. General concepts

    a. Much of the internist's focus is on preventive care and treatment of chronic diseases. However, at some point, there are no further treatments that one can offer to a patient, and the focus of care shifts to alleviating pain and suffering at the end of life.

    b. The main concepts in palliative and end-of-life care include ensuring that the patient's wishes are honored, managing symptoms, communicating bad news, negotiating treatment priorities, dealing with legal issues, and using hospice services.

2. Advance directives. Optimally, patients should create several legal documents while they have the cognitive ability to do so. These documents include a living will or advance directives that detail patients' wishes for care should they have a terminal illness or be unable to make their own decisions. Patients make choices as to whether they would want to be resuscitated or receive intravenous fluids, enteral feedings, and other measures that may or may not prolong their condition. Patients designate a power of attorney or health care agent, who is aware of the patient's wishes and is legally empowered to act on behalf of the patient in making all health care decisions. Internists often have this discussion when patients are in mid-adult life so that the legal matters have been addressed long in advance of a medical crisis.

3. Hospice care

    a. Hospice organizations have become a standard part of health care delivery at the end of life. Services are provided either in the home or in a nursing home–type facility. Although most patients take advantage of hospice services during the last few weeks of life, they are eligible for hospice care when their life expectancy is 6 months or less. The earlier patients are referred for hospice care, the sooner they can benefit from the humane care provided by the extraordinary approach of these caregivers.

    b. An interdisciplinary group of individuals, including physicians, nurses, aides, mental health providers, social workers, clergy, and legal advisors, work in close partnership to provide the patient and family with support during this difficult time. Many insurance providers, including Medicare, offer special benefits for patients in need of palliative and end-of-life care.

4. Managing symptoms at the end of life

    a. Pain. The management of pain is one of the most difficult and undertreated symptoms at the end of life. Optimal control often involves a multidisciplinary approach of internists, anesthesiologists, surgeons, radiation oncologists, psychotherapists, and pain specialists. Pain is what patients fear most.

        (1) Assessment: A comprehensive assessment of the patient's type and level of pain is essential. The physician should determine the location, quality, severity, pace of progression, modifying or alleviating factors, and treatments already prescribed. Using a scale from 0 to 10, where 10 is the worst pain ever experienced, can be helpful in tracking the patient's response to treatment or identifying exacerbation over baseline symptoms. Pain is considered the "fifth vital sign" and should be included in the assessment of any patient.

        (2) Types of pain: There are generally two types of pain due to different mechanisms.

            (a) Somatic pain can be due to direct stimulation of nociceptive receptors, such as deep somatic or visceral pain. Pain due to diseases of muscle, bone, or soft tissue is called somatic pain, whereas pain due to lung, bowel, or cardiac disease is designated as **visceral pain.** The pain is often deep and unrelenting.

(b) Neuropathic pain is due to direct nerve damage and is often peripheral in nature. The patient may note paresthesias, or a burning or sharp sensation.

(3) Treatment

(a) Three basic concepts should guide the administration of analgesia.

(i) The initial analgesic prescribed should be one that provides **basal or continuous analgesia.** This drug should have a long enough half-life or be given frequently enough so that the patient does not have pain before the next dose is due. A long-acting analgesic should provide the basal relief needed.

(ii) In addition, the patient should be given an **analgesic for breakthrough pain.** This is usually a short-acting analgesic.

(iii) The physician must ensure a **dynamic approach to pain management.** Because the patient's symptoms may change over time due to a variety of factors or as the disease progresses, the regimen may need to be modified. Common problems that can arise during the patient's course are excess breakthrough pain, poorly tolerated side effect, such as constipation, mental confusion or slowed breathing, or reaching maximum doses and thus necessitating the use of adjuvant medications to enhance the analgesic effect. If the patient has excessive breakthrough pain, the physician may increase the dose of the basal analgesic or of the breakthrough medication. The addition of stool softeners and stimulant laxatives at the initiation of a pain regimen often prevents constipation. Changes in mental status or slowed breathing due to analgesics may be diminished by reducing the dose and using adjuvant pain. Adjuvant medications may also be helpful as the patient reaches the maximum doses of pain medications.

(b) The World Health Organization has developed a three-step model for assessing and treating pain. They stress the importance of administering pain medication promptly, advancing up the Pain Relief Ladder in a stepwise fashion, using adjuvant medication to calm anxiety and enhance the effect of analgesics, and administering medications by the clock as opposed to on demand. By giving medications by the clock, patients are less likely to experience heightened pain prior to receiving the next dose. The various levels provide suggestions for types and categories of analgesia that may be prescribed. The ultimate goal is for the patient to be pain free from the cancer or other ailment. Initially, these medications are administered via oral or transdermal route. As the patient's condition deteriorates or if the patient is unable to swallow, subcutaneous and sublingual administration can be done.

(i) **Mild pain (stage 1).** Nonopioid medications with or without adjuvant medications can be used at this stage. Examples include acetaminophen or nonsteroidal anti-inflammatory drugs (NSAID) such as aspirin, naproxen, or ibuprofen.

(ii) **Moderate pain (stage 2).** Opioids can be used at this stage for mild-to-moderate pain along with nonopioids. Opioids in this category include tramadol, codeine, and dihydrocodone.

(iii) **Severe pain (stage 3).** Opioids for moderate to severe pain, along with nonopioids, can be used. Stronger opioids in this category include morphine, fentanyl, oxycodone, and hydromorphone.

(iv) **Adjuvant treatments** can help reduce dose escalation of opioid medications and reduce anxiety and can be used in any of the stages listed previously. Examples of adjuvant treatments include antidepressant medications, anticonvulsants, steroids, muscle relaxants, psychological therapy, acupuncture, hydrotherapy, and exercise.

(v) **Other treatments.** Surgical intervention and ablation of targeted nerves may provide further pain relief. Use of transcutaneous nerve stimulators (TENS) may be useful in some circumstances.

b. Dyspnea. Shortness of breath in the dying patient can result from a variety of entities, including progression of lung disease or a direct result of cancer, such as masses, pleural effusions, and infiltrates. Pneumonia and other infections, congestive heart failure, and pulmonary embolism, among others, may all cause unrelenting shortness of breath. Treatment is geared toward identifying the underlying cause, if reversible, and making the patient as comfortable as possible. Supplemental oxygen may be helpful, and diuretics may be used to treat pulmonary edema. Opioids and benzodiazepines are the mainstay to relieve the discomfort and anxiety associated with dyspnea.

c. **Nausea and constipation.** Nausea and vomiting may be caused by gastrointestinal illness (e.g., obstruction, infection, or carcinomatosis), medications (e.g., opioids, chemotherapy, or radiation), central nervous system problems (e.g., increased intracranial pressure, metastases, or infection), or metabolic problems (e.g., hypercalcemia, renal or liver failure). The clinician must target therapy toward the underlying cause. Constipation may be caused by several of these entities or be a direct result of opioid pain medications. Common medications used to treat nausea and vomiting include dopamine antagonists (prochlorperazine, promethazine), serotonin antagonists (ondansetron), glucocorticoids, and benzodiazepines. To avoid constipation related to opioid use, patients should be concomitantly given stool softeners and/or laxatives.

d. **Delirium.** This is a common symptom at end of life and may be related to a broad range of metabolic and systemic disorders, including hypercalcemia, hypoxia, dehydration, liver or renal failure, electrolyte disturbance, medication side effects, infection, and constipation. Patients with delirium can either be agitated or somnolent, or may fluctuate between the two states. After excluding reversible causes, one of the most important approaches is to keep the patient orientated by keeping family and friends close, removing noisy or bright stimuli, and providing constant quiet reminders of the date, time, and surroundings. The use of neuroleptic agents (haloperidol, risperidone) and sedatives (benzodiazepines) may be useful in the management of delirium.

V   PERIOPERATIVE MEDICINE

A Cardiovascular risk reduction

1. **Cardiac risk assessment.** As a joint venture, in 2007 the American College of Cardiology and American Heart Association published guidelines for preoperative assessment of patients. The goal of the recommended stepwise approach is to reduce perioperative adverse cardiovascular events. Patients evaluated by an internist before surgery should undergo a complete history and physical examination. Additional preoperative cardiac testing or treatment depends on findings therein.

   a. **Emergency surgery.** Patients who require emergency surgery should proceed to surgery without obtaining diagnostic tests that would delay surgery.

   b. **High-risk conditions**
      (1) **Myocardial infarction.** Patients with recent myocardial infarction should not have elective surgery for 1 month.
      (2) **Active cardiac conditions.** Patients with severe ischemia, decompensated heart failure, significant dysrhythmias, or severe valvular heart disease should have these issues treated before elective surgery.

   c. **Low-risk surgeries.** In the absence of an active cardiac condition, patients with planned endoscopy, superficial procedure, or ambulatory same-day surgery should proceed to surgery without cardiac stress testing.

   d. **Activity tolerance.** Patients planned for higher-risk surgery may proceed to surgery if history suggests tolerance to moderate physical activity. Patients who may achieve greater than or equal to four metabolic equivalents of physical activity—such as climbing a full flight of stairs or washing dishes—without angina or angina-equivalent symptoms may proceed to surgery without cardiac stress testing.

   e. **Clinical risk factors.** Additional clinical risk factors cumulatively predict adverse perioperative outcomes. Among patients planned for higher-risk surgery who have poor activity tolerance, patients with two or more risk factors could be considered for preoperative cardiac stress testing, and patients with four or more risk factors should be considered for stress testing.
      (1) **High-risk surgery.** Intrathoracic, intra-abdominal, and peripheral vascular surgeries portend a higher risk of adverse cardiovascular events.
      (2) **Coronary artery disease.** Patients with previous coronary events or significant atherosclerosis more frequently suffer perioperative cardiac complications, even in the absence of active symptoms.

(3) **Congestive heart failure.** Although compensated heart failure is not a contraindication to surgery, it does predict perioperative complications.

(4) **Ischemic stroke.** Patients with prior history of ischemic stroke are at significantly increased risk of suffering perioperative stroke or acute coronary syndrome.

(5) **Diabetes mellitus.** Diabetic patients are at significantly increased risk of cardiovascular events, especially patients requiring insulin to treat the condition.

(6) **Chronic kidney disease.** Patients with advanced kidney disease are at increased risk for vascular events, especially when the serum creatinine chronically exceeds 2 mg/dL.

2. **Perioperative beta-blocker therapy.** Patients already on beta-blocker therapy should continue taking the medication during surgery. Patients with two or more clinical risk factors may benefit from initiation of beta blocker therapy before surgery, with titration to a resting heart rate of <65 bpm.

3. **Perioperative statins.** Patients already on statin therapy should continue taking the medication during surgery. Patients with one or more clinical risk factors may benefit from initiation of statin therapy before surgery.

B Bleeding risk

1. **Antiplatelet therapy.** Aspirin and clopidogrel increase bleeding risk. However, in patients at very high risk for cardiovascular ischemic events, the antiplatelet medication's benefit may outweigh the surgical bleeding risk. If deciding to discontinue antiplatelet therapy, the patient should cease use at least 7 days before surgery, since these agents irreversibly inhibit platelet function.

2. **Nonsteroidal anti-inflammatory drugs (NSAIDs).** NSAIDs reversibly inhibit platelet function and should be discontinued at least 3 days before surgery. Selective cyclooxygenase-2 inhibitors may be safely continued perioperatively unless there is risk for renal dysfunction.

3. **Anticoagulants.** Warfarin should be discontinued at least 3 days before surgery. Patients at very high risk for thrombosis should have "bridge therapy"—with intravenous unfractionated heparin, a low–molecular-weight heparin product, or the synthetic antithrombin III inhibitor fondaparinux—to minimize duration of anticoagulant absence.

C Other Medication Adjustments

1. **Diuretics.** Diuretic therapy should be held to reduce the risk for perioperative hypovolemia, especially if the patient will not be taking food or water for a prolonged period.

2. **Diabetes medications**
   a. **Sulfonylurea** medications increase the risk for perioperative hypoglycemia, which is associated with adverse cardiovascular events. These medications should be discontinued before surgery.
   b. **Metformin** increases the risk for lactic acidosis and should be discontinued before surgery.
   c. **Thiazolidinediones** such as rosiglitazone and pioglitazone are unlikely to induce hypoglycemia and have very prolonged activity. They can be safely continued in the perioperative period.
   d. **Basal insulin** such as glargine or detemir should be given at the usual or a slightly reduced dose before surgery. Patients with type 1 diabetes should not discontinue use of basal insulin.
   e. **Medium-action insulin** such as NPH should be given at a significantly reduced dose before surgery.
   f. **Short-action insulin** such as aspart, lispro, or glulisine should not be given immediately before surgery except to correct for severe preoperative hyperglycemia.

3. **Glucocorticoids.** Patients on chronic glucocorticoid therapy should continue the medication on the day of surgery. Patients planned for major surgery may benefit from an increased dose of glucocorticoid to reduce the incidence of intraoperative hypotension, which may result from suppression of endogenous cortisol release that would normally occur during surgery.

4. **Herbal medications.** Herbal therapies may cause hemodynamic instability (ephedra, ginseng, ma huang), hypoglycemia (ginseng), immunosuppression (echinacea, when taken for more than 8 weeks), abnormal bleeding (garlic, ginkgo, ginseng), or prolongation of anesthesia (kava, St. John's wort, valerian). All such therapy should be discontinued 1–2 weeks before surgery.

Study Questions

A 42-year-old woman presents for a routine health visit to her general internist. She has well-controlled hypertension, exercises regularly, and has regular menses. Her family history is remarkable for her father, who was diagnosed with colon cancer at age 51 years. Her physical examination, including breast and rectal examinations, are normal.

1. What screening test for colon cancer would you recommend to her?
   - [A] Stool cards to check for occult blood
   - [B] Colonoscopy
   - [C] CT scan colonography
   - [D] Fecal DNA testing
   - [E] Screening would not be indicated in this age group.

2. Which of the following is the best screening test for breast cancer in this patient?
   - [A] Breast self-examination
   - [B] Annual breast examination by a physician
   - [C] Breast sonography
   - [D] Screening mammogram
   - [E] Breast magnetic resonance imaging (MRI)

A 17-year-old female presents to your office complaining of abdominal pain. She describes the pain as dull, diffuse, and not related to meals or bowel movements. She denies any nausea, vomiting, or alcohol use. Recently she has noticed a small amount of vaginal discharge and some urinary burning. She is sexually active and endorses the use of condoms. She denies fever, chills, or any other systemic symptoms. On examination, she is withdrawn and makes little eye contact. She weighs 108 pounds and is 5′″5″, giving her a BMI of 18.0. Her examination is otherwise normal, including a benign abdominal examination. On pelvic examination, she has normal anatomy with a normal-appearing cervix. A small amount of white discharge is present. No tenderness or masses are appreciated. The wet prep and KOH smear demonstrate no bacteria or yeast. DNA probe testing for *Neisseria gonorrhoeae* and polymerase chain reaction (PCR) testing for *Chlamydia trachomatis* were negative. Urinalysis shows no white cells or bacteria.

3. What diagnostic entities should be considered as a cause of her abdominal pain?
   - [A] Depression and sexual abuse
   - [B] Urinary tract infection
   - [C] Bacterial vaginosis or yeast infection
   - [D] Diverticulitis
   - [E] Pancreatitis

A 75-year-old man is diagnosed with non–small cell lung cancer. He has extensive metastases with severe pain in his right femur and a large pleural effusion. The effusion causes him pleurisy with each inspiration along with shortness of breath. He coughs constantly, with occasional hemoptysis. He is a long-time smoker and was aware of his symptoms for several months before seeking medical attention. After consultation with a pulmonologist and oncologist, it is determined that he is not candidate for chemotherapy. Radiation is suggested to alleviate the pain from the metastasis in his right femur. Despite escalating doses of short-acting narcotic medication, he continues to have unrelenting pain in his chest and leg.

4. At this point, what would be the best plan to help alleviate his pain?
   - [A] Increase the dose of short-acting (3- to 4-hour) narcotic to the maximum dose.
   - [B] Discontinue short-acting narcotic and instead administer a long-acting (12-hour) narcotic.
   - [C] Administer a long-acting (12-hour) narcotic around the clock with a short acting narcotic for breakthrough pain.
   - [D] Order additional radiation therapy to the leg.
   - [E] Add an antidepressant medication to the short-acting narcotic medication.

A 91-year-old man presents to the office for follow-up after hospitalization. He was discharged 5 days ago with a diagnosis of pneumonia. His medical history includes atrial fibrillation. He had routinely been taking metoprolol and warfarin. In addition, he was discharged home with several new medications, including moxifloxacin for pneumonia, codeine for cough, and terazosin for a "prostate problem." He complains of nose bleeds and dizziness but denies pain, dyspnea, vomiting, or diarrhea. He is accompanied to the office by his daughter, who notes that he has been more sleepy and confused than usual. Temperature is 98°F, blood pressure is 100/60 mm Hg, pulse is 70/min and irregularly irregular, and respiratory rate is 14/min. The patient is sleepy but arousable. The nasal turbinates reveal no active bleeding, but there are multiple ecchymoses on the arms and legs. Lungs are clear to auscultation and resonant to percussion. Skin turgor is normal. Gait is appropriate, and the patient is speaking clearly. Electrocardiogram shows atrial fibrillation with no ST-segment abnormality.

5. Which of the following best explains the patient's epistaxis and ecchymoses, dizziness and hypotension, and lethargy and confusion?

   A Recurrent pneumonia, with sepsis syndrome and disseminated intravascular coagulopathy
   B Adverse effects of new medications, with drug–drug interactions and side effects
   C Cerebrovascular accident
   D Myocardial infarction with cardiogenic shock
   E Hypovolemia and renal failure

6. What is the likely diagnosis for which the patient was prescribed terazosin?

   A Erectile dysfunction as a result of normal aging
   B Hypertension, which was worsened by acute infection
   C Stress incontinence from prostatitis and frequent coughing
   D Urge incontinence from prostate cancer with brain metastasis
   E Overflow incontinence from prostatic hypertrophy or the anticholinergic effect of codeine

A 28-year-old woman presents to the office for continued treatment of hypertension. She also relates a desire to become pregnant and seeks advice for appropriate care. The patient currently takes lisinopril, a prenatal multivitamin, and folic acid. Blood pressure is 130/85 mm Hg. A urinalysis from last month reveals 1+ proteinuria.

7. What is the most appropriate treatment for this patient's hypertension?

   A Continue lisinopril alone.
   B Change to an angiotensin-receptor blocker (ARB).
   C Change to nifedipine or methyldopa.
   D Continue lisinopril and add hydrochlorothiazide.
   E Discontinue antihypertensives.

A 56-year-old man is hospitalized under the care of a vascular surgeon for claudication and severe peripheral arterial disease. You are asked to see the patient as a medical consultant to assess perioperative risk for planned femoral-popliteal bypass graft surgery. The patient reports a history of hypertension, smoking, diabetes mellitus type 1, and a stroke 5 years ago. He denies a history of heart or kidney disease. His medications include aspirin, clopidogrel, amlodipine, benazepril, and insulin. He reports inability to walk long distances due to calf pain, but he is able to perform household chores, including doing laundry and dish washing, without discomfort. He denies chest discomfort, dyspnea, or edema. Blood pressure is 150/80 mm Hg, and pulse is 80/min. Examination is normal except for a cool left leg with absent pedal pulses. Serum creatinine and glucose levels are normal. Electrocardiogram reveals normal sinus rhythm without abnormality.

8. Which of the following is the most appropriate recommendation?

   A Proceed to surgery without further testing and consider adding atenolol and simvastatin.
   B Proceed to surgery without further testing and discontinue insulin when the patient is NPO.
   C Request a cardiac stress test before operating.
   D Discontinue aspirin and clopidogrel and wait 7–10 days before operating.
   E Abandon surgical intervention, as the patient's perioperative risk is too high to justify the procedure.

Answers and Explanations

1. The answer is B [III B, Table 1–1]. Given that the patient has a first-degree relative with colon cancer, she should undergo a screening colonoscopy 10 years prior to the age of diagnosis of the relative's colon cancer. The use of three stool cards for occult blood would not be sufficient. Although one might detect occult bleeding, one needs to identify any polyps or other premalignant lesions in this high-risk individual. CT scan colonography or fecal DNA testing are not recommended as routine screening tests for colon cancer. Without a positive family history of colon cancer, initial screening is recommended at age 50 years.

2. The answer is D [III B, Table 1–1]. Although the initial screening for breast cancer includes both self-examination and a thorough examination by a physician, these are insufficient by themselves for a woman over the age of 40 years. Guidelines for mammography have changed in recent years and vary as to whether a woman in her 40s should have mammography every 1 or 2 years, or whether screening should be conducted at all. Most would recommend performing a mammogram every 2 years in women in their 40s. Women with first-degree relatives with breast cancer should begin screening 5 years prior to the age of the relative at the time of diagnosis of breast cancer and continue with annual examinations. Breast sonography and MRI are not appropriate screening tests for breast cancer in asymptomatic patients with no abnormalities on physical examination or who are not otherwise at high risk for breast cancer.

3. The answer is A [III E 5]. Patients who are victims of sexual abuse or domestic violence often do not directly tell their physician that this is occurring. They may feel insecure and threatened in their environment or relationship and can see no way to remove themselves from the situation. Patients may complain of vague abdominal or musculoskeletal pain, headaches, fatigue, or malaise. Often there are genitourinary symptoms, such as pain, dysuria or vaginal discharge. They may appear depressed. The physician must be alert to the possibility of such a patient at risk and inquire as to whether she feels safe at home and if anyone is hurting her. Screening for symptoms of depression should be done. In addition, her low BMI is concerning for anorexia and possible bulimia. Further history should be elicited to evaluate for these entities. Her negative urinalysis rules out a urinary tract infection. Similarly, the negative vaginal smears demonstrate no bacterial vaginosis or yeast infection. It would be very unusual for an adolescent to develop diverticulitis. In addition, she has no localizing abdominal pain to the left lower quadrant or fever. Her symptoms are not consistent with pancreatitis, in which the pain is severe, located in the epigastrum, and usually associated with nausea and vomiting.

4. The answer is C [IV C 4 a (3)]. This patient has terminal lung cancer metastatic to bone and pleural cavity. At this point, the physician's focus is on palliating his severe and unrelenting pain and making the patient pain-free. Optimal treatment includes the use of a 12-hour narcotic medication that is given around the clock, that is, whether the patient asks for the medication or not. Any breakthrough pain is then treated with short-acting narcotic medications. If the breakthrough episodes are frequent, then the dose of the long-acting medication should be increased until the patient has relief. Additional radiation therapy to bony lesions would likely provide limited benefit. Antidepressant medications, although helpful, are also unlikely to provide sufficient relief in this situation.

5. The answer is B [IV A 6 a]. The patient's moxifloxacin may be potentiating the warfarin effect and leading to bleeding and bruising. Hypotension may be the synergistic antihypertensive effects of both alpha-blockade (terazosin) and beta-blockade (metoprolol). Codeine may be causing fatigue and confusion as a direct side effect. This explanation is more plausible than recurrent pneumonia or sepsis syndrome, given the normal lung exam and absence of fever. Cerebrovascular accident is possible but less likely with a normal neurologic examination. There are no symptoms of myocardial infarction, including absence of pain or electrocardiogram findings. Hypovolemia is less likely, given absence of diarrhea, vomiting, or fever, and with normal skin turgor.

6. The answer is E [IV A 4, IV A 5]. The patient was told he may have a prostate problem. Terazosin is an alpha-receptor antagonist, which may relieve urinary obstruction related to prostatic hypertrophy, a condition associated with overflow incontinence. Erectile dysfunction is common in the elderly, but appropriate therapy would be a phosphodiesterase type V inhibitor such as sildenafil. Terazosin does reduce blood pressure, but the patient reported having been given this medication for a prostate problem. Stress incontinence may occur with vigorous coughing, but prostatitis would not explain the symptom, and terazosin would not be appropriate therapy. Urge incontinence is more frequent in younger patients and is best treated with anticholinergic medications.

7. The answer is C [IV B 2 b]. In patients who are pregnant or who plan pregnancy, ACE inhibitors and ARB medications are contraindicated because of their teratogenic effect. Despite the presence of proteinuria and probable glomerular injury, the potential for fetal harm outweighs the renoprotective benefit of these medications in the short term. First-line therapy for hypertension in pregnancy is methyldopa and/or nifedipine. Adding hydrochlorothiazide would not be indicated, as the blood pressure is acceptable. Discontinuation of antihypertensive medications would lead to uncontrolled hypertension, which may increase proteinuria and the risk for renal injury.

8. The answer is A [V A]. The patient has several risk factors for adverse perioperative events, including planned high-risk surgery, insulin-requiring diabetes, and history of stroke. However, he has fair exercise tolerance, as he is able to perform household chores of greater than four metabolic equivalents of activity, and the clinical picture does not suggest active ischemia or heart failure. Therefore, the patient should proceed to surgery without stress testing. A beta-blocker may reduce perioperative risk in this patient with two or more clinical risk factors, especially given the high blood pressure. A statin medication may reduce perioperative risk in this patient with one or more clinical risk factors, especially given the history of peripheral arterial disease. Insulin should not be discontinued in a patient with type 1 diabetes. Aspirin and clopidogrel do increase perioperative bleeding risk but are strongly indicated, given the severe peripheral arterial disease. Surgical risk is moderately high, but there are no absolute contraindications to surgery, which may improve this patient's quality of life.

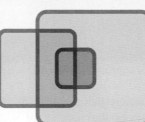

chapter 2

Cardiovascular Diseases

NORMAN RETENER · TEMILOLU AJE · MICHAEL BENITEZ

I   CONGESTIVE HEART FAILURE

A **Definition**   Congestive heart failure (CHF) is the inability of the heart, working at normal or elevated filling pressure, to pump enough blood to meet the oxygen requirements of the body tissues. CHF should never be considered a diagnosis. Rather, it is a syndrome resulting from many diseases that interfere with cardiac function. In acting as a muscular pump, the heart does only two things: It contracts (systole) and it relaxes (diastole). Therefore, heart failure can result from only two broad abnormalities—systolic dysfunction and diastolic dysfunction.

B **Etiology**

1. **Systolic dysfunction.** Systole is governed by three cardiac properties: **contractility**—the ability of myocardium to generate force; **afterload**—the force against which the heart must contract; and **preload**—the sarcomere stretch before contraction.

   a. **Decreased contractility.** Most cases of CHF occur when an insult to the myocardium reduces its ability to generate force, thereby reducing its contractility.

      (1) **Myocardial infarction (MI).** In MI, a portion of the myocardium undergoes necrosis and can no longer generate force, resulting in weakening of the ventricle. If extensive areas of the myocardium are infarcted, CHF results.

      (2) **Valvular heart disease** results in stenosis or regurgitation of the cardiac valves, which places a **pressure** or **volume overload,** respectively, on the ventricles. Initially, compensatory mechanisms [see I B 1 c] accommodate these overloads and maintain normal cardiac output at acceptable filling pressures. However, eventually these mechanisms fail and heart failure ensues.

      (3) **Hypertension.** Hypertension may contribute to either systolic or diastolic dysfunction.

      (4) **Cardiomyopathies** are diseases that directly injure the myocardium.

         (a) **Toxic.** Substances directly toxic to the myocardium (e.g., ethanol and catecholamines) may damage its force-generating ability. Prolonged exposure to these agents may lead to the development of CHF.

         (b) **Idiopathic.** When the contractile function of the myocardium fails in the absence of a known etiology, a viral cause often is implied but frequently cannot be proven. Other clinical presentations, including peripartum cardiomyopathy, are of unknown etiology.

         (c) **Infiltrative.** Infiltration of the myocardium by a variety of substances (e.g., amyloid) may reduce contractility.

   b. **Increased afterload.** Increasing the afterload makes it harder for the ventricular muscle fibers to shorten, thereby reducing cardiac output. Afterload can be quantified by calculating the systolic force on the myocardium using the Laplace equation for stress:

   $$\text{stress} = (\text{pressure} \times \text{radius})/(2 \times \text{thickness})$$

   Thus, disease states that increase either the systolic pressure (hypertension, aortic stenosis) or chamber radius (dilated cardiomyopathy, valvular regurgitation) increase afterload unless the wall thickness increases proportionately.

   c. **Compensatory mechanisms** develop in response to the ventricular pressure and volume overload that accompany decreased contractility.

(1) **The Frank–Starling mechanism** is activated when reduced ventricular emptying results in more volume retained in the ventricles at the end of systole, which leads to a greater volume at the end of diastole. Increased end-diastolic volume increases sarcomere stretch (preload), which increases the number of systolic actin–myosin cross-bridges that develop. The greater number of cross-bridges increases the strength of contraction.

(2) **Cardiac hypertrophy** provides additional muscle mass to bear the burden of various overloads.

(3) **Adrenergic stimulation** by endogenous catecholamines increases the inotropic state.

2. **Diastolic dysfunction.** Diastole is governed by **active** and **passive** properties. Active relaxation occurs early in diastole as calcium is pumped out of the myocardium, resulting in the near cessation of actin–myosin cross-bridge interaction. Passive filling occurs as the mitral valve opens, allowing the blood stored in the atria to fill the ventricles.

   a. **Abnormalities in active relaxation.** Active relaxation is impaired when there is delay in calcium reuptake at the beginning of diastole.

   b. **Abnormalities of passive filling.** Passive relaxation is impaired when the myocardium is stiffer than normal. Stiffness is defined as a change in pressure (ΔP) per unit change in volume (ΔV), or $\Delta P/\Delta V$. When stiffness is increased, any change in volume requires or causes a greater increase in pressure. Thus, to fill the heart to an adequate volume, high filling pressure occurs, which in turn leads to pulmonary and systemic congestion. Increased passive stiffness of the ventricles occurs when concentric hypertrophy causes the chamber wall to be thicker than normal, as might occur in hypertension or when the myocardium is infiltrated by abnormal substances such as amyloid.

3. **The neurohumoral hypothesis of heart failure.** Heart failure leads to the persistent activation of many neurohumoral systems and hormones, including the renin–angiotensin–aldosterone system, the adrenergic nervous system, inflammatory cytokines, endothelin, and vasopressin. Although once thought of as compensatory, persistent overactivation of these agents is cardiotoxic, in turn leading to a progressive decline in cardiac function. Thus, blockade of these systems should be beneficial in treating CHF.

C **Types of Heart Failure**

1. **High-output failure** is characterized by cardiac output that may be several times higher than normal but still is not adequate to maintain tissue perfusion needs or, if adequate, is maintained with a higher-than-normal filling pressure. A classic example of high-output failure is **chronic severe anemia,** which causes reduced oxygen-carrying capacity. In chronic severe anemia, the following occur:

   a. Compensation is provided by increased forward cardiac output, which is facilitated by cardiac enlargement, decreased total peripheral resistance, and increased venous return to the heart. This causes a volume overload of ventricles.

   b. Eventually the demands on the heart lead to cardiac failure; cardiac output, although high, still is not adequate to meet the circulatory demands placed on the heart by the anemia. Some other causes of high-output failure include arteriovenous fistula, beriberi, and thyrotoxicosis.

2. **Left-sided failure** indicates that the left ventricle is the failing chamber. A disease that primarily affects the left ventricle (e.g., MI) may reduce its contractile force, whereas the right ventricle continues to pump normally. Thus, left ventricular failure can occur without right ventricular failure.

3. **Right-sided failure** indicates that the right ventricle has failed, either as a result of left ventricular failure or in isolation from the left ventricle.

   a. The **most common cause** of right ventricular failure is **left ventricular failure.** When left ventricular failure occurs, the filling pressure in the left ventricle becomes elevated, increasing the workload of the right ventricle (the chamber responsible for filling the left ventricle). Thus overtaxed, the right ventricle eventually fails also.

   b. The right ventricle also may fail in isolation from the left ventricle. In the presence of **chronic obstructive pulmonary disease (COPD),** increased pulmonary vascular resistance develops as a result of architectural changes in the lungs. The higher pulmonary vascular resistance produces a pressure overload on the right ventricle, which leads to increased right ventricular work and eventual failure. Pulmonary embolism and primary pulmonary hypertension are some other causes of right-sided failure.

D **Clinical features**

1. **Symptoms**
   a. **Dyspnea** is the most frequently encountered symptom of CHF.
      (1) The feeling of breathlessness is caused by **vascular congestion,** which reduces pulmonary oxygenation. In addition, the vascular congestion diminishes lung compliance, increasing the work of breathing, thus adding to the feeling of breathlessness.
      (2) Dyspnea also results from **reduced cardiac output to the periphery,** which triggers the symptom through neurohumoral mechanisms. In the early stages of CHF, dyspnea occurs only with exertion. As heart failure progresses, the amount of exertion required to produce dyspnea becomes progressively less until dyspnea may occur at rest.
   b. **Orthopnea** refers to dyspnea that occurs in the recumbent position and is relieved by elevation of the head. Orthopnea results from volume pooling in the central vasculature during recumbency, which leads to increased cardiac volume and, in turn, to increased left ventricular filling pressure, pulmonary congestion, and the feeling of dyspnea. The physician may gauge the degree of orthopnea by noting the number of pillows the patient uses to sleep. However, it should be recognized that many patients sleep on more than one pillow out of habit, not because of breathlessness. **Nocturnal cough,** which has the same pathophysiology as orthopnea, may occur together with, or instead of, nocturnal dyspnea.
   c. **Paroxysmal nocturnal dyspnea** is the occurrence of sudden dyspnea that awakens the patient from sleep. Like orthopnea, it occurs during recumbency as a result of pooling in the central vasculature, which increases left ventricular filling pressure. Paroxysmal nocturnal dyspnea may occur in the orthopneic patient who inadvertently slips off the pillows used to elevate the upper body. Usually, the patient awakens from sleep and feels the need to sit upright or to go to an open window for increased ventilation. The symptom usually subsides after the patient has been in the upright position for 5–20 minutes.
   d. **Nocturia** develops in CHF as a result of increased renal blood flow when the patient is recumbent and asleep.
      (1) **During the day,** when the skeletal muscles are active, limited cardiac output is shifted away from the kidney toward the skeletal musculature. The kidney interprets this reduction in blood flow as **hypovolemia** and becomes sodium avid via activation of the **renin–angiotensin system.**
      (2) **At night,** when the patient is at rest, cardiac output is shifted toward the kidney, and diuresis ensues.
   e. **Edema.** There are many causes of peripheral edema, several of which are noncardiac. **Cardiac edema** occurs when the systemic hydrostatic venous pressure is greater than the systemic oncotic venous pressure. Thus, cardiac edema is a sign of **right-sided failure;** it occurs because of the increased systemic venous pressure that results from right ventricular dysfunction.

2. **Physical signs**
   a. **Tachycardia.** Increased heart rate occurs in heart failure due to increased release of catecholamines as a compensatory mechanism for maintaining cardiac output in the presence of decreased stroke volume. Catecholamines increase both the force and the rate of cardiac contraction. However, in chronic heart failure, adrenergic downregulation occurs, and heart rates greater than 100 bpm in the absence of arrhythmia are distinctly unusual.
   b. **Pulmonary rales.** The increased left-ventricular filling pressure associated with CHF is referred to the left atrium and the pulmonary veins. The increased hydrostatic pressure produces transudation of fluid into the alveoli. As air circulates through the alveoli, crackling sounds (rales) are produced. Note that there are multiple causes of pulmonary rales; the mere presence of rales does not necessarily indicate CHF.
   c. **Cardiac enlargement.** As the failing heart relies more and more on the Frank–Starling mechanism, it dilates and may develop eccentric hypertrophy. In the presence of cardiac enlargement, the point of maximal impulse (PMI) of the left ventricle is shifted downward and to the left. This shift is detected during a physical examination with the patient lying supine.

   d. Fourth heart sound (S_4). Patients in sinus rhythm and heart failure often have an S_4 (atrial gallop). The S_4 is produced as left atrial systole propels volume into the left ventricle. In CHF, the left ventricle is noncompliant, and the S_4 probably results from the reverberation of the blood ejected into the left ventricle. In elderly patients, however, an S_4 may indicate reduced compliance of a stiff left ventricle as a result of aging rather than heart failure. The S_4 also may be heard over the right ventricle in right ventricular failure.

   e. Third heart sound (S_3). An S_3 (**ventricular gallop**), which occurs early in diastole, probably is the most **reliable sign of left heart failure** revealed during physical examination. The S_3 occurs during rapid filling of the left ventricle. Increased left atrial pressure (which propels the blood forward with increased force) and noncompliance of the left ventricle are two important factors in the production of this extra sound. Although an S_3 is a reliable sign of heart failure in individuals older than age 40 years, a similar sound is a normal finding in young, healthy athletes.

   f. Neck vein distention. The neck veins can be considered manometers attached to the right atrium and, as such, reflect right atrial pressure [detection of central venous pressure is described online (Online Figure 2–1)].

   g. Hepatic enlargement. Elevated central venous pressure can lead to hepatic congestion, in turn causing hepatomegaly. On occasion, rapid hepatic enlargement may also cause liver tenderness.

   h. Edema. Lower-extremity and presacral edema occur in right-sided failure as increased venous pressure results in transudation of fluid into these areas. For edema to be attributable to CHF, distended neck veins indicative of elevated right-sided filling pressure also should be present.

   i. Ascites. Transudation of fluid into the **peritoneal space** also may occur as a result of increased systemic venous pressure. When ascites is caused by CHF, the neck veins typically are elevated and the liver is distended from passive congestion.

E Diagnosis. Management of CHF must focus on the cause of the heart failure, not simply on relieving the symptoms. Although a careful history and physical examination are the most important tools available in arriving at a diagnosis, in many cases a diagnosis may not be reached. In these instances, the following studies often are helpful:

1. The **electrocardiogram (ECG)** frequently is nonspecific. However, the presence of Q waves helps confirm that MI has been the cause of the CHF.

2. The **chest radiograph** is useful in demonstrating cardiac chamber enlargement and in documenting congestion in the lungs.

3. The **echocardiogram** is essential in identifying chamber enlargement and in quantifying left ventricular function and valvular function. The most commonly used descriptor of ventricular function is the **ejection fraction.** Ejection fractions between 55% and 75% are normal.

4. **Doppler interrogation** measures the direction and velocity of blood flow. This technique is useful for detecting blood flow moving in an abnormal direction, which is characteristic of valvular regurgitation and intracardiac shunts. In addition, Doppler interrogation can detect and quantify valvular stenoses by measuring how much velocity is necessary to maintain constant blood flow through a stenotic valve.

5. **Radionuclide ventriculography,** or **multiple gate acquisition (MUGA),** is a noninvasive nuclear medicine procedure that precisely quantitates left and right ventricular systolic function.

6. During **cardiac catheterization,** intracardiac pressures, chamber size, valvular stenosis, valvular regurgitation, and coronary anatomy can be evaluated. Given the current accuracy of echocardiography, catheterization is performed principally for the evaluation of ischemia.

F Therapy

1. **Etiologic therapy.** It is important, when possible, to direct treatment at the etiologic agent of CHF. For example, if aortic stenosis is the cause, aortic valve replacement is the most effective therapy.

2. **Systolic heart failure**

   a. Therapy has been shown to enhance survival and delay progression of the disease. Compensation for development of heart failure by increasing the neurohormones responsible for increasing cardiac contractility and heart rate can improve symptoms of heart failure in the short term. However, chronic stimulation leads to cardiac remodeling and decompensation [see I B 3]. Blockade of these agents have been shown to reverse remodeling, improve mortality, and delay the progression of heart failure.

  (1) **Renin–angiotensin system blockade.** Angiotensin-converting-enzyme (ACE) inhibitors have been shown to have a mortality benefit. Because many vasodilators have failed to improve survival despite reducing afterload, properties of ACE inhibitors other than vasodilation are thought to be operative, namely reversal of remodeling. In patients who develop coughing due to ACE inhibitors, angiotensin-receptor blockers (ARBs) may be substituted with similar efficacy. Additional blockade of the renin–angiotensin system using spironolactone or eplerenone to block the final product of this system, aldosterone, is also beneficial in selected patients.

  (2) **β-Blocking agents.** Because stimulation of the β-receptor increases the force of cardiac contraction, β-agonists have been used in the therapy of end-stage CHF [see I F 2 b (3) (b)]. Paradoxically, cautious use of β-receptor antagonists has also been effective in reversing the same syndrome. The mechanism of action for this class of agents in the treatment of heart failure stems from protection of the heart from the toxic effects of prolonged exposure to the high levels of circulating catecholamines.

  (3) **Hydralazine and nitrates.** The combination of hydralazine and nitrates used in class II and III heart failure has also been shown to improve mortality by decreasing preload and afterload and improving cardiac output. However, the mortality benefit with ACE inhibitors is greater.

 b. **Symptomatic therapy.** Although not shown to improve mortality, many drugs can improve the symptoms and morbidity of heart failure.

  (1) **Reducing afterload.** Agents that cause arteriolar dilation reduce impedance of the outflow of blood from the left ventricle. By diminishing resistance to ejection, these agents cause cardiac output to rise because the left ventricle can eject more completely against a lower afterload. The net effect is increased cardiac output without a serious fall in blood pressure, leading to symptomatic improvement. Several vasodilators are used in the treatment of CHF to reduce afterload, including ACE inhibitors, nitrates, and hydralazine.

  (2) **Reducing preload and left ventricular filling pressure.** The increased preload resulting from volume retention in the ventricles is a compensatory mechanism that helps increase forward cardiac output by use of the Frank–Starling mechanism; however, an excessive increase in preload is associated with increased left ventricular and right ventricular filling pressures, which is responsible for symptoms of pulmonary and systemic congestion. Judicious reduction in filling pressures without excessive reduction in preload is indicated in the therapy of CHF.

   (a) Diuretics reduce renal tubular absorption of sodium and water and increase the clearance of these substances from the body. The result is a reduction in central volume and in cardiac filling pressure.

   (b) Vasodilators, which increase the capacity of the systemic venous system, transfer central volume to the periphery, thus reducing central preload and filling pressure. Nitrates and ACE inhibitors are effective preload-reducing vasodilators.

  (3) **Increasing the contractile state.** Contractile dysfunction is the most common mechanism that produces heart failure; therefore, increasing the contractile state may result in symptomatic improvement.

   (a) Cardiac glycosides (e.g., digoxin) increase the contractile state by impeding the Na^+/K^+-ATPase–controlled intracellular pump. This results in the net influx of calcium into the myocardium, which increases contractile strength.

   (b) β-Adrenergic agonists (catecholamines, e.g., dobutamine) increase contractile function by increasing the production of cyclic adenosine monophosphate (cAMP), which results in greater myocardial calcium release. They are administered as a continuous infusion in end-stage heart failure as a temporizing measure.

   (c) Phosphodiesterase inhibitors (e.g., milrinone) increase contractile function by inhibiting the breakdown of cAMP. Similar to β-adrenergic agonists, they are also administered as a continuous intravenous infusion in end-stage heart failure for short-term use.

3. **Diastolic heart failure.** Unlike systolic heart failure, no medical treatment is available that reduces mortality in diastolic heart failure. Treatment is aimed at symptomatic relief.

    a. **Diuretics.** Diuretics are the mainstay of treatment. By reducing ventricular volume they lower ventricular pressure and reduce the symptoms of congestion. The dosing must be carefully regulated, however, as reduced ventricular volume also lowers stroke volume and cardiac output. The optimum range would be one that prevents excess dyspnea and hepatic congestion but allows for adequate cardiac output.

    b. **Induction of bradycardia.** Slowing the heart rate increases the time available for ventricular filling. β-Blockers and nondihydropyridine calcium channel blockers (verapamil and diltiazem) are used to cause relative bradycardia.

    c. **Relief of ischemia.** In patients with coronary disease, ischemia impairs the active relaxation phase of diastole by impairing calcium reuptake by the sarcoplasmic reticulum. Thus, standard therapy for angina is also effective in improving diastolic dysfunction. [See III A 5 a (4).]

    d. **Maintenance of sinus rhythm.** The normal atrial "kick" afforded by atrial contraction improves the efficiency of ventricular filling that is lost in atrial fibrillation. Thus, every effort should be made to maintain sinus rhythm [see II].

4. **Nonpharmacologic therapy**

    a. **Cardiac resynchronization.** Many patients with advanced heart failure develop electrical conduction disturbances, including left-bundle-branch block, which delays the impulse signaling contraction from reaching the left ventricle. This delay results in dyssynchronous contraction of the ventricles, which may reduce contractile efficiency. Active pacing of the left ventricle to resynchronize contraction in patients with conduction delays may improve functional capacity and quality of life and decreases mortality.

    b. **Physical conditioning.** Patients with CHF who participate in regular physical training tend to experience an improvement in their subjective quality of life. Exercise tolerance may improve as a training effect, and training does not appear to be harmful.

    c. **Cardiac transplantation** may offer an improved quality of life to selected patients in whom control of CHF is not possible and prognosis is poor. Currently, approximately 75% of patients undergoing cardiac transplantation achieve a 5-year survival rate. The paucity of cardiac donors is the primary factor limiting the use of this therapy. Left ventricular assist devices (LVADs) may provide a bridge to transplantation.

5. **Pulmonary edema** is the most extreme example of CHF, in which profound transudation of fluid into the pulmonary alveoli occurs because of a high left ventricular filling pressure. The result is impaired oxygenation and, if untreated, death. The goal of therapy is to improve oxygenation, to reduce left ventricular filling pressure, and to increase forward cardiac output.

    a. **Oxygen** should be administered by facemask because patients in pulmonary edema are so dyspneic that they breathe primarily through their mouths.

    b. **Diuretics.** Furosemide is likely the most commonly used medication in the treatment of acute pulmonary edema. This rapid-acting loop diuretic promotes an immediate diuresis in most cases.

    c. **Morphine sulfate.** This opioid reduces patient anxiety and acts as a venodilator, reducing preload in the volume-overloaded heart.

    d. **Other vasodilators.** Nitroglycerin (administered sublingually or intravenously) or nitroprusside (administered intravenously) is often effective in treating pulmonary edema when other therapies fail. Nesiritide, an analog of B-type natriuretic hormone that causes venous and arteriolar vasodilation, may also be beneficial. However, the potent vasodilating ability of these drugs requires that blood pressure be monitored constantly during administration to avoid hypotension.

    e. **Intravenous positive inotropic agents** (dobutamine, milrinone) may be used if peripheral perfusion is compromised. They increase contractility and reduce afterload, leading to improvement in cardiac output. These medications should be reserved for acute decompensation unresponsive to other measures and should be administered for the shortest possible duration.

    f. **Intubation and positive-pressure ventilation.** If the patient's oxygenation does not improve rapidly with the previously noted therapies, intubation or positive-pressure ventilation may be necessary to provide mechanical ventilation and improve oxygenation.

g. **Invasive hemodynamic monitoring.** Most cases of pulmonary edema resolve quickly, making hemodynamic monitoring unnecessary. In cases of refractory pulmonary edema, knowledge of intracardiac filling pressure may be useful in guiding therapy. Hemodynamic monitoring via Swan–Ganz catheterization provides this information so that optimal filling pressure and cardiac output may be obtained.

II   CARDIAC ARRHYTHMIAS

A **Introduction**   Bradyarrhythmias result from inadequate sinus nodal impulse generation or from blocked impulse propagation and usually are not cause for concern unless syncope or presyncope develops. Sustained atrial tachyarrhythmias usually permit adequate cardiac output and are less dangerous than sustained ventricular arrhythmias, which often cause collapse or death.

B **Atrial tachyarrhythmias**   The atrial tachyarrhythmias can be classified into two subcategories: those that produce a regular cardiac rhythm and those that produce an irregular cardiac rhythm. In general, atrial tachyarrhythmias do not interfere with interventricular or intraventricular conduction of the cardiac impulse, and therefore the QRS complex (which is generated from the ventricles) remains narrow in form. Occasionally, however, atrial arrhythmias cause aberrant ventricular conduction with a wide QRS complex, which may mimic arrhythmias of ventricular origin.

1. **Regular atrial tachycardias**
   a. **Sinus tachycardia.** Sinus tachycardia represents an increase in the sinus rate (>100 bpm) and is usually secondary to some other disease process. In general, the physician should treat the condition that is causing the sinus tachycardia, not the tachycardia itself. However, in some patients, such as those with coronary artery disease, sinus tachycardia must be controlled to prevent myocardial ischemia. In this instance, β-blocking agents or calcium antagonists (either verapamil or diltiazem) may be effective in controlling heart rate.
   b. **Supraventricular tachycardia (SVT).** The most common form of SVT is atrioventricular (AV) nodal reentrant tachycardia (AVNRT).
      (1) **ECG identification.** In SVT, the ECG shows regular, narrow QRS complexes without identifiable P waves at a rate of 150–200 bpm (Figure 2–2A).
      (2) **Therapy.** AVNRT is due to reentry within the compact AV node. Therapies that slow conduction or increase refractoriness usually succeed.
         (a) **Mechanical maneuvers** such as **carotid sinus massage** and the **Valsalva maneuver** are often effective in terminating the arrhythmia by increasing vagal tone. Patients with recurrent symptoms can be taught to perform the Valsalva maneuver as a means of managing their arrhythmia.
         (b) **Medical therapy. Intravenous (IV) adenosine** is the medical treatment of choice. Less commonly used agents include **verapamil** and **β-blockers.**
   c. **Atrial flutter** usually occurs in patients with antecedent heart disease, including coronary artery disease, pericarditis, valvular heart disease, and cardiomyopathy. Atrial flutter is characterized

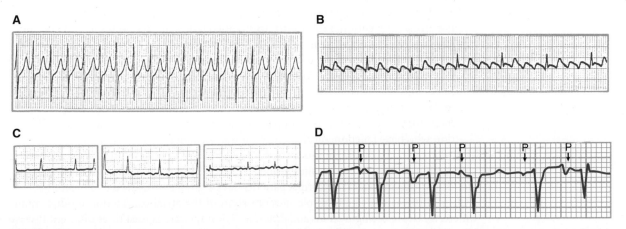

FIGURE 2–2   Atrial tachycardias: **A.** Supraventricular tachycardia. **B.** Atrial flutter. **C.** Atrial fibrillation. **D.** Multifocal atrial tachycardia.

by an atrial rate of 220–400 bpm and is usually conducted to the ventricle with block so that the ventricular rate is a fraction of the atrial rate. Occasionally, atrial flutter may be conducted irregularly. Treatment is the same as for regular atrial flutter.

(1) ECG identification. As shown in Figure 2–2B, this arrhythmia produces a classic sawtooth pattern on the ECG. In this example, there is 4:1 AV block with an atrial rate of 300 bpm and a ventricular rate of 75 bpm.

(2) Therapy

(a) Medications such as β-blockers, digoxin, or verapamil may be used to control the ventricular response, which, in turn, helps maintain hemodynamic stability. Once the ventricular rate has slowed as a result of increased AV block (3:1 or 4:1 conduction), **antiarrhythmic drugs** such as **ibutilide** or **direct current (DC) electrical cardioversion** can be employed to restore normal sinus rhythm.

(b) Radiofrequency catheter ablation is highly effective and should be considered for treatment of recurrent atrial flutter.

(c) As in all arrhythmias, **DC cardioversion** is necessary if the arrhythmia results in hemodynamic instability.

2. Irregular atrial tachycardias

a. Atrial fibrillation. Atrial fibrillation is an **irregularly irregular** arrhythmia in which there is no ordered contraction of the atria but, rather, multiple discoordinate wavefronts of depolarization that send a large number of irregular impulses to depolarize the AV node. The irregular impulses produce an irregular ventricular response, the rate of which depends on the number of impulses that are conducted through the AV node. Selected causes of atrial fibrillation include stress, fever, excessive alcohol intake, pericarditis, myocardial infarction, pulmonary embolism, mitral valve disease, thyrotoxicosis, and idiopathic atrial fibrillation.

(1) ECG identification. An example of atrial fibrillation is shown in Figure 2–2C.

(2) Therapy

(a) If patients with atrial fibrillation are hemodynamically unstable or demonstrate an increase in angina pectoris or worsening of CHF, immediate DC synchronous cardioversion is indicated.

(b) In hemodynamically stable patients, the physician should control the ventricular response to the atrial fibrillation by administering β-blockers, nondihydropyridine calcium channel blockers, or digoxin.

(c) In the absence of a contraindication, **systemic anticoagulation** should be instituted with unfractionated or low–molecular-weight heparin (LMWH).

(d) Cardioversion can be considered immediately after a transesophageal echocardiogram, provided no intracardiac thrombus is visualized, or after 4–6 weeks of adequate oral anticoagulation with warfarin.

(e) Long-term anticoagulation with oral warfarin should be considered in patients at increased risk of thromboembolism. Risks for thromboembolism include advanced age, hypertension, diabetes, congestive heart failure, and a history of prior embolism. For stroke prevention, rate control with anticoagulation has been shown to be superior to rhythm control. Antiarrhythmic drugs such as amiodarone may be useful for control of symptoms referable to atrial fibrillation.

(f) If patients do not respond to more conservative therapy, **catheter ablation** of the AV node with pacemaker placement can be considered. This does not obviate the need for anticoagulation. Catheter-based pulmonary vein isolation is an effective treatment that may be considered in patients with recurrent symptomatic atrial fibrillation who have failed medical attempts at maintenance of sinus rhythm.

b. Multifocal atrial tachycardia. In this arrhythmia, there is synchronous atrial contraction, but the contraction arises from many sites in the atria, not from the sinus node. In the majority of cases of multifocal atrial tachycardia, patients have significant medical comorbidities.

(1) ECG identification. The multiple sites of origin of the atrial contraction produce many different P-wave configurations and different R-R intervals. At least three different P-wave morphologies are required to make this diagnosis (Figure 2–2D).

(2) **Therapy.** Treatment is directed primarily at managing medical comorbidities. If these measures fail, β-blockers or nondihydropyridine calcium channel blockers may be useful in controlling the heart rate.

C **Bradyarrhythmias** occur when sinus node impulse generation is slowed or when normal sinus node impulses cannot be conducted to the ventricles because of AV nodal block or ventricular conducting system disease. In general, bradyarrhythmias are a cause for concern only when patients have become symptomatic with presyncope or syncope from the reduced cardiac output that the low heart rate produces. Medications such as β-blockers, nondihydropyridine calcium channel blockers, and digoxin may contribute to bradyarrhythmias.

1. **Sinus bradycardia**
   a. Sinus bradycardia may be a physiologic and normal response to cardiovascular conditioning, as in trained athletes. In such cases, the arrhythmia is obviously a normal finding and requires no therapy. However, extreme sinus bradycardia (<35 bpm) as a result of sinus node dysfunction may cause symptoms.
   b. **Therapy. Atropine** may be useful in temporarily increasing the sinus rate. **Withdrawal of offending medications** may be necessary.

2. **Sinus pauses.** This bradyarrhythmia is caused by the failure of the sinus node to generate an impulse on time. Such pauses may last for several seconds and induce syncope. Definitive therapy requires pacemaker implantation.

3. **AV block.** In AV block, some of the impulses generated from the sinus node are not conducted to the ventricles.
   a. **Types of AV block** (Figure 2–3)
      (1) **First-degree AV block.** Every atrial beat is conducted to the ventricle, but the P-R interval exceeds 0.20 seconds and remains constant (Figure 2–3A). This is most commonly due to a delay in the AV node. Treatment is rarely necessary.
      (2) **Second-degree AV block:**
         (a) **Mobitz type I (Wenckebach) block.** There is a progressive prolongation in the P-R interval until a P wave is not conducted (Figure 2–3B). This type of block usually occurs at the level of the AV node. It rarely produces symptoms.
         (b) **Mobitz type II block.** There is no prolongation of the P-R interval before the dropped beat (Figure 2–3C). Mobitz II atrioventricular block reflects disease within the His-Purkinje system, below the AV node, and requires treatment with a permanent pacemaker because of the high risk of progression to complete heart block. It may be difficult in 2:1 AV block to determine whether the mechanism is Mobitz 1 or Mobitz II. Invasive electrophysiologic studies are sometimes necessary in this case.

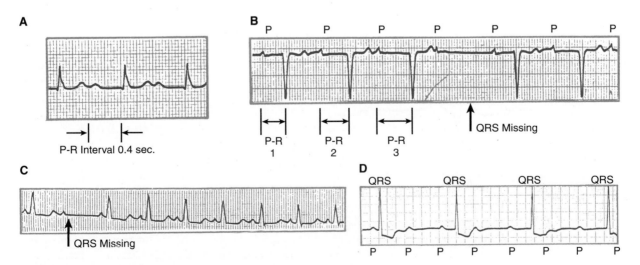

FIGURE 2–3 AV blocks. **A.** First-degree AV block. **B.** Type II AV block, Mobitz I. **C.** Type II AV block, Mobitz II. **D.** Third-degree/complete AV block.

(3) Third-degree/complete heart block. No impulses are conducted from the atria to the ventricles (Figure 2–3D), and heart rate becomes dependent on spontaneous ventricular depolarizations. Severe symptomatic bradycardia characterized by a heart rate of 25–40 bpm is seen.

b. Therapy. Atropine and isoproterenol are effective in temporarily increasing the ventricular response for block occurring at the AV node. Conduction block below the level of the AV node requires insertion of either a temporary or a permanent **cardiac pacemaker.**

D **Ventricular tachyarrhythmias**

1. **Types of ventricular arrhythmias** (Figure 2–4)
   a. **Premature ventricular contraction (PVC).** In this arrhythmia, heart beats arise directly from the ventricles, bypassing the specialized cardiac His-Purkinje conduction system.
      (1) ECG identification
         (a) Because the His-Purkinje system is bypassed, the **QRS configuration** is typically **widened** and **bizarre** in appearance.
         (b) PVCs usually do not affect atrial depolarization, which proceeds normally and in dissociation with the PVC. Thus, the next sinus beat occurs at the same time it would have occurred if no PVC had been present. Accordingly, a **full compensatory pause** usually follows a PVC (Figure 2–4A). The normally occurring P wave is usually buried in the PVC–QRS complex.
      (2) Therapy. Most isolated PVCs are benign and should not be treated.
   b. **Ventricular tachycardia** is a regular rhythm that occurs paroxysmally and exceeds 120 bpm. **AV dissociation,** which causes the ventricular arrhythmia to proceed independent of the normal atrial rhythm, is the hallmark of the arrhythmia. During ventricular tachycardia, cardiac relaxation is impaired. This factor, together with loss of AV synchrony (i.e., loss of the atrial "kick") and loss of the electrical coordination of the contraction by the His-Purkinje system, usually leads to severely reduced cardiac output, producing hypotension. **Sustained ventricular tachycardia is usually a life-threatening arrhythmia that degenerates into ventricular fibrillation and death if untreated.**
      (1) Physical examination. In many cases of ventricular tachycardia, severe decompensation precludes performance of a detailed physical examination.
         (a) If patients are relatively stable, physical diagnosis may demonstrate intermittent cannon 'a' waves in the jugular venous pulse. When atrial and ventricular contractions are dissociated, atrial contraction may intermittently occur when the mitral and tricuspid valves have already been closed by ventricular contraction. In this instance, a large retrograde venous pulse is seen in the jugular vein.
         (b) Variability in intensity of the S_1 results from variability in the degree of mitral and tricuspid valvular excursion at the time of ventricular contraction in patients with atrioventricular dissociation.

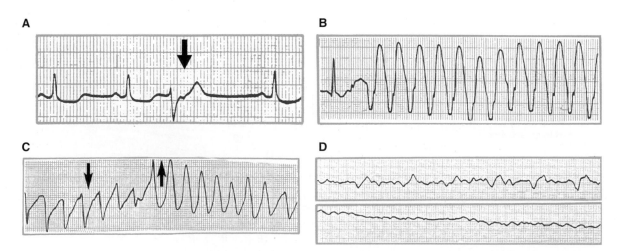

FIGURE 2–4   Ventricular arrhythmias. **A.** Premature ventricular contraction. **B.** Monomorphic ventricular tachycardia. **C.** Polymorphic ventricular tachycardia (torsades de pointes). **D.** Ventricular fibrillation.

(2) **ECG identification** (Figure 2–4B, C)

(a) **The QRS complex is widened and bizarre in appearance** because the arrhythmia does not use the specialized conducting system of the heart. Because the ventricles are operating independently of the atria, there is **no constant relationship between the P wave and the QRS complex.**

(b) The QRS complex may be **monomorphic** (i.e., of one shape), as shown in Figure 2–4B, or it may be **polymorphic,** as shown in Figure 2–4C. When the axis of a polymorphic arrhythmia appears to revolve about a central point the arrhythmia is termed **torsades de pointes. This is most often associated with a prolonged QT interval preceding the arrhythmia.**

(3) **Therapy**

(a) In hemodynamically unstable patients, **DC cardioversion** is urgently required.

(b) Stable patients with monomorphic ventricular tachycardia may be treated with IV **amiodarone.**

(c) Polymorphic ventricular tachycardia requires defibrillation. Common causes include electrolyte abnormalities, congenital long-QT disease, and drugs that prolong the QT interval. Treatment with IV magnesium may help prevent recurrence.

c. **Ventricular fibrillation** is characterized by a lack of ordered contraction of the ventricles. There is no effective cardiac output. **Ventricular fibrillation results in death unless conversion to an effective rhythm can be accomplished.** The physician should begin cardiac resuscitation, including mechanical ventilation, cardiac compression, and drug and electrical therapy immediately (Figure 2–4D).

2. **Prevention and treatment of ventricular arrhythmias.** 🖰 Online Table 2–1 lists the current classification and some of the side effects of drugs currently available for long-term prevention of ventricular arrhythmias. Implantable cardioverter-defibrillators (ICDs) are the best means of prevention of sudden death in patients who have had prior cardiac arrest or sustained ventricular tachycardia. These devices may also be indicated for prevention of a first event in selected patients, such as those with severely depressed systolic function and prior infarction. Drug therapy may be used to reduce the incidence of symptomatic ventricular arrhythmias but is not as effective in reducing sudden cardiac death as ICDs.

III · ISCHEMIC HEART DISEASE

A **Atherosclerotic coronary artery disease (ASCAD)**

1. **Definition.** ASCAD is the focal narrowing of the coronary arteries as a result of a **plaque** composed of the following:

a. **Lipids** (cholesterol esters and crystals), which are deposited at the center of the plaque and accumulate within macrophages

b. **Intimal secretory smooth muscle cells,** which proliferate

c. A **fibrous cap** made of connective tissue

2. **Incidence and risk factors.** Currently in the United States, the overall incidence of death as a result of ASCAD is 0.5 in 1000 and decreasing. However, ASCAD differs in frequency in subpopulations with the following risk factors:

a. **Age.** The incidence of ASCAD increases progressively with age. The risk of death is 1.5 in 1000 individuals at age 50 years.

b. **Gender.** ASCAD is more prevalent in men than in women. This difference is most marked in premenopausal women compared with men of similar age. By the time men reach the age of 50 years, they are affected five times more often than women of the same age. This difference declines as age increases.

c. **Serum cholesterol.** The incidence of ASCAD increases with increasing total serum cholesterol levels (🖰 Online Figure 2–5).

(1) Total serum cholesterol is carried in the blood by **low-density lipoprotein (LDL), very low density lipoprotein (VLDL),** and **high-density lipoprotein (HDL).**

(a) The higher the percentage of total cholesterol carried by LDL in relation to HDL, the higher is the risk of ASCAD. High levels of HDL seem to be protective.

(b) Total cholesterol level should be less than 200 mg/dL.

    (i) The LDL cholesterol level should be less than 130 mg/dL; in patients with known coronary disease, it should be less than 100 mg/dL. In high-risk patients, the target LDL is <70 mg/dL.

    (ii) The HDL cholesterol level should exceed 40 mg/dL.

(2) Several types of hyperlipidemia exist, and many are associated with an increased incidence of coronary artery disease. Online Table 2–2 presents an overview of the hyperlipidemias.

    d. Smoking. Compared with nonsmokers, cigarette smokers are 60% more likely to develop ASCAD when other risk factors are controlled for statistically. Smoking increases carbon monoxide levels in the blood, which may, in turn, damage the coronary endothelium. Smoking also increases platelet adhesiveness and thus the likelihood of thrombotic coronary occlusion.

    e. Hypertension. The higher the systolic or diastolic blood pressure, the more likely is the development of ASCAD. This likelihood is apparent in both men and women and becomes more pronounced with advancing age.

    f. Diabetes mellitus is associated with a 50% increase in the incidence of ASCAD in men and a 100% increase in women. In light of this, diabetes mellitus should be considered an ASCAD equivalent.

    g. Family history. A family history of premature heart disease is considered to be present when coronary artery disease has occurred in a first-degree male relative age 55 years or younger or a female first-degree relative of age 65 years or younger. A familial predisposition to coronary artery disease exists in part due to inheritance of the foregoing risk factors (except smoking). However, family history is the only risk factor in about one third of individuals with ASCAD.

3. Pathogenesis (Online Figures 2–6 and 2–7)

4. Pathophysiology of ischemia

    a. Supply–demand relationship. As wall stress and heart rate increase (e.g., with exercise), myocardial oxygen consumption rises. Autoregulated increases in coronary blood flow normally meet this increased demand. However, if demand exceeds supply, ischemia results. The product of heart rate and left ventricular systolic pressure or wall stress roughly approximate the oxygen needs of the myocardium [see I B 1 b].

    (1) **Increased demand.** In patients with ASCAD, stenosis of the coronary artery prevents the increase in coronary blood flow needed to compensate for an increased demand, resulting in an oxygen demand that exceeds the oxygen supply. **Myocardial ischemia** is the result of this imbalance.

    (2) **Reduced supply.** Atherosclerotic stenosis was once viewed as a fixed obstruction to coronary blood flow. In fact, the diseased area of the coronary artery often remains dynamic, and the effective lumen of the artery undergoes constant change. Changes are produced by vasoconstriction of the coronary artery, by production and degradation of local thrombi at the site of stenosis, and by progressive enlargement of the atherosclerotic plaque. Acute changes in lumen diameter may reduce the supply of coronary blood flow and thus produce ischemia without an increase in demand.

    b. Myocardial infarction (MI). The necrosis of myocardial tissue occurs as a result of prolonged ischemia. The rapidity and extent of the infarction process are determined by the extent of reduction of blood flow to the area. In some cases, **collateral flow** from other coronary arteries may supply enough blood flow to prevent infarction despite a total coronary occlusion.

    (1) **ST-segment elevation myocardial infarction (STEMI)** is associated with occlusion of a coronary artery by a **thrombus.** Coronary blood flow may be restored pharmacologically by lysis of the thrombus with agents such as **tissue plasminogen activator (tPA)** or mechanically, by balloon angioplasty and stenting to relieve pain, reestablish myocardial contractile function, and reduce myocardial damage [see III A 5 b (4) (b) (ii)].

    (2) **Non-STEMI (NSTEMI)** is due to severe coronary artery obstruction without total occlusion.

5. **Clinical consequences.** Atherosclerotic plaques may produce stable angina or an **acute coronary syndrome (ACS)** (unstable angina, NSTEMI, or STEMI).
   a. **Angina pectoris** is chest pain or pressure produced by myocardial ischemia.
      (1) **Characteristic features**
         (a) **Relation to exertion.** Exertion increases myocardial oxygen demand beyond the supply capabilities of diseased coronary arteries, producing ischemia. Other factors that increase myocardial oxygen demand (e.g., emotional upset, a meal, or the peripheral vasoconstriction caused by walking in cold weather) also may precipitate angina.
         (b) **Quality of pain.** Although many patients perceive angina as **chest pain,** others report a feeling of **pressure** in the chest area or complain of a **burning** sensation. In some patients, **exertional dyspnea** may represent an anginal equivalent.
         (c) **Radiation of pain.** Radiation of anginal pain to the left arm is well known. Pain also may radiate to the right arm, jaw, teeth, or throat. Occasionally, these may be the only sites of pain, and the chest is free of discomfort, or the chest discomfort, when present, may not radiate at all.
         (d) **Progression of ischemia and duration of symptoms.** Whatever the anginal symptom quality for a given patient, repeated episodes of ischemia usually reproduce that same quality. The symptom complex usually begins at a low intensity, increases over 2–3 minutes, and lasts a total of less than 15 minutes. Episodes longer than 30 minutes suggest that MI may have occurred.
      (2) **Types of ischemic episodes**
         (a) **Chronic stable angina** is angina that recurs under similar circumstances with a similar frequency and duration.
         (b) **Unstable angina (UA)** is a term applied to angina when a change in status occurs (e.g., new-onset angina; angina of increasing severity, duration, or frequency; or angina occurring at rest for the first time). It indicates progression of disease or plaque rupture and may be an immediate precursor of MI.
            (i) **Rest angina.** Angina at rest is particularly worrisome because it implies that decreased supply, rather than increased demand, is causing the angina. This concept in turn suggests that arterial occlusion and possible infarction may be imminent.
            (ii) **New-onset angina.** In cases of new-onset angina, it is difficult to generalize about clinical outcome. New-onset angina that progresses in frequency, severity, or duration over 1 or 2 months is worrisome. Conversely, some cases of new-onset angina may simply be the first episode in what becomes a chronic stable anginal pattern.
         (c) **Variant (Prinzmetal's) angina**
            (i) The **hallmark** of variant angina is the appearance of transient **ST-segment elevation** on the ECG during the angina attack. The ST-segment elevation represents **transmural ischemia** produced by a sudden reduction in coronary blood flow.
            (ii) The reduction in flow results from **transient coronary spasm,** which may or may not be associated with a fixed atherosclerotic lesion. The spasm produces total but transient coronary occlusion.
            (iii) Variant angina usually occurs at rest (often at night), and episodes frequently are complicated by complex ventricular arrhythmias.
      (3) **Diagnosis.** When a patient exhibits chest pain characteristic of angina, the diagnosis can be suspected strongly on the basis of patient history alone. The suspicion that coronary disease is present is heightened by the presence of one or more coronary risk factors.
         (a) **Physical examination.** Patients experiencing an episode of angina are usually uncomfortable and anxious. Blood pressure and pulse rate are increased in most cases.
         (b) **Resting electrocardiography.** The ECG taken in the absence of pain in patients with angina pectoris with no history of MI is normal in 50% of cases. Every effort should be made to obtain an ECG while the patient is experiencing chest pain.
            (i) The presence of **new horizontal** or **downsloping ST segments** on the ECG is highly suggestive of myocardial ischemia. **New T-wave inversion** also may occur, but this finding alone without ST-segment depression is less specific.
            (ii) During variant angina, ST elevations are present, and based upon the ECG, acute ST elevation myocardial infarction cannot be excluded. Rapid relief of pain and

ST elevation with nitroglycerin and angiographic absence of coronary athero-sclerosis support the diagnosis of coronary vasospasm.

(c) **Stress electrocardiography.** Recording the ECG during exercise substantially increases the sensitivity and specificity of electrocardiography. In addition, a formal exercise test permits quantification of the patient's exercise tolerance and observation of the effects of exercise on the patient's symptoms, heart rate, and blood pressure.

    (i) The appearance of horizontal or downsloping ST-segment depression of 1 mm or more during exercise has a sensitivity of approximately 70% and a specificity of 90% for the detection of coronary disease.

    (ii) The ST criteria for positivity are less accurate in women than in men. An abnormal ST segment on a resting ECG, as seen in **left-bundle-branch block, left ventricular hypertrophy,** or the use of **digoxin** by the patient **all reduce the accuracy of this test.**

(d) **Stress scintigraphy,** when used in combination with the stress ECG, has yielded increased sensitivity (80%) and specificity (92%) over the standard stress ECG alone. Therefore, it is a particularly useful diagnostic tool when the standard stress ECG is expected to be of low yield (e.g., in women and in patients with bundle-branch block) and in patients in whom a previous stress ECG has produced equivocal results.

    (i) **Method.** When the radioactive isotope **thallium 201** (^{201}TI) or the technetium-based isonitrile **sestamibi** is injected into the peripheral venous blood, the myocardial distribution of the substance is affected by blood flow and ischemia, with areas of less blood flow and ischemia taking up less ^{201}TI or sestamibi than areas of normal blood flow. With exercise, blood flow increases, but in patients with coronary artery disease, those parts of the myocardium supplied by diseased coronary arteries and areas of MI take up less ^{201}TI or sestamibi than normal areas, as shown in the scintigram (Online Figure 2–8). In patients who are unable to exercise, infusion of dobutamine (to increase oxygen demand) or dipyridamole or adenosine (to cause coronary vasodilation) are used to alter coronary flow.

(e) **Stress echocardiography.** Two-dimensional echocardiography can detect regional ischemia by identifying areas of wall motion abnormalities that occur with stress and are not present at rest. This regional dysfunction indicates that the area involved is not receiving adequate blood flow. The sensitivity is similar to that of radionucleotide imaging.

(f) **Cardiac catheterization with coronary arteriography** allows for direct visualization of the coronary arteries by selective injection of radiographic contrast material. This procedure is the **most sensitive and specific test commonly used for coronary artery disease.**

    (i) **Risk.** Unlike the previously mentioned tests, cardiac catheterization is an invasive procedure that carries a small but finite risk. The overall risk of mortality during coronary arteriography is approximately 0.2%.

    (ii) **Applications.** Cardiac catheterization should be reserved for cases in which the diagnosis is uncertain after noninvasive testing, when more information is needed to help determine whether medical or surgical therapy is most appropriate for the patient's coronary disease, or when intervention is necessary, as in patients with acute STEMI or UA. If surgery is contemplated, the arteriograms obtained at catheterization guide the surgeon's placement of the bypass grafts.

(g) **Cardiac computed tomography (CT).** An emerging and potentially powerful tool for detecting coronary artery disease is cardiac CT. The role of this modality has not yet been clearly established.

(4) **Therapy.** Treatment of angina pectoris is directed either at reducing myocardial oxygen demand to compensate for impaired flow through diseased coronary arteries or at increasing myocardial oxygen supply (i.e., blood flow).

(a) **Nitrates.** This class of drugs produces venodilation and, to a lesser extent, arteriolar vasodilation. They may increase coronary blood flow and decrease myocardial oxygen demand by decreasing preload and afterload.

(b) β-Adrenergic blocking agents. β-Adrenergic receptor stimulation results in an increase in heart rate and in the force of myocardial contraction. Both events increase myocardial oxygen demand. β-Blockers counteract these effects and **reduce myocardial oxygen demand.**

(c) Calcium channel blockers. Calcium regulates the contraction of smooth muscle, which is present in the walls of the coronary and peripheral arteries. Calcium channel blockers are particularly **effective in preventing the coronary spasm that causes variant angina.** They are also useful in treating cases of typical angina, in which they **act as coronary and peripheral arterial vasodilators.** The nondihydropyridine calcium channel blockers diltiazem and verapamil also reduce heart rate, and all calcium channel blockers may decrease blood pressure.

(d) Percutaneous coronary intervention (PCI). Removing or reducing the obstructive coronary atherosclerotic lesion can alleviate the angina.

   (i) During angioplasty, a small balloon is inserted into a femoral or brachial artery and guided to the obstruction of the affected coronary artery. The balloon is inflated, dilating the stenosis and reducing the obstruction.

   (ii) The initial success rate of simple balloon angioplasty approaches 90%, although there is a 33% restenosis rate after 6 months, making it necessary to repeat the procedure in some patients. Placement of small wire **stents** reduces the rate of restenosis and now accompanies the majority of angioplasties. Today some stents are coated with sirolimus or paclitaxel, which reduces the restenosis rate to approximately 5%. Procedural coadministration of abciximab, a IIb–IIIa platelet receptor antibody, or eptifibatide, a IIb–IIIa receptor antagonist, also enhances short- and long-term patency. The use of a thienopyridine, such as clopidogrel, is essential after stenting to prevent acute thrombosis.

(e) Coronary artery bypass grafting (CABG). CABG extends survival in patients with severe left main coronary artery disease or patients with severe three-vessel disease and depressed left ventricular function. There is continued debate regarding the role of CABG versus multivessel PCI in patients with severe multivessel disease and normal left ventricular function. CABG may be preferable in diabetic patients with multivessel disease that includes the left anterior descending artery.

(f) Refractory angina. Several new therapies have emerged for treatment of refractory angina, including transmyocardial laser revascularization, enhanced extracorporeal counter pulsation, and the medication ranolazine, which enhances myocardial glucose uptake and metabolism. These can be considered in patients who continue to experience angina despite maximal treatment on conventional medical therapy and revascularization.

b. Myocardial infarction (MI) occurs when the myocardium is deprived of its blood supply (and therefore oxygen) for a significant amount of time.

(1) Pathogenesis. An abrupt change in the atherosclerotic plaque seems to be one of the events precipitating an MI. Plaque rupture attracts platelets that trigger thrombus formation, leading to severe stenosis or total occlusion of the vessel.

(2) Symptoms. The patient usually experiences **severe, oppressive chest pain** or **pressure** that persists for more than 30 minutes and is unrelieved by nitroglycerin. The pain radiates in a pattern similar to that of angina pectoris.

(a) Frequently, **nausea, vomiting, diaphoresis,** and **shortness of breath** accompany the pain.

(b) An unusually large number of infarctions occur **between 6 A.M. and 10 A.M.,** when catecholamine levels increase on awakening.

(3) Diagnosis

(a) Physical examination. The patient experiencing MI is in obvious pain, is quite apprehensive, and often appears ashen. If the infarction is extensive, hypotension and tachycardia may be present. There also may be signs of CHF (e.g., elevation of the neck veins, pulmonary rales, and a cardiac gallop rhythm). The new murmur of mitral regurgitation may be present.

(b) Electrocardiography. The ECG is diagnostic in approximately 85% of cases. The remaining 15% of patients may experience MI without manifesting clear-cut evidence on the ECG.

  (i) STEMI is demonstrated by ST-segment elevation in those leads reflecting the area of the MI. As the ST segments fall, Q waves appear, and the T waves become inverted (🔲 Online Figure 2–9).

  (ii) NSTEMI will have less specific findings, such as ST depression or T-wave inversion.

(c) Cardiac enzyme studies

  (i) As myocardial necrosis occurs, the myocardium releases **creatine kinase (CK), including the MB isoform,** and **troponins,** thereby increasing serum concentrations of these enzymes.

  (ii) CK and troponin elevation appear 3 hours after infarction. CK and CK-MB usually return to baseline within 2 days, but troponin may remain elevated for up to 10 days following MI.

(4) Therapy

(a) Initial medical therapy. For patients presenting with either an STEMI or NSTEMI, several medical therapies should be initiated, providing there are no contraindications.

  (i) **Aspirin** should be given immediately to block platelet aggregation.

  (ii) **Oxygen** should be delivered to ensure adequate oxygenation of tissues.

  (iii) **Nitroglycerin** can alleviate pain by vasodilation, which increases blood flow, thereby decreasing oxygen demand and coronary vasospasm.

  (iv) **Heparin** should be started intravenously to decrease further clot formation. IV heparin is preferred for STEMI, when an early intervention is planned, as it can easily be turned off. LMWH may be preferable in NSTEMI, when intervention can be delayed, as there is no need for dose adjustment, and the mortality risk may be slightly lower.

  (v) **β-Blockers reduce** ventricular arrhythmias and the risk of reinfarction and decrease the workload and oxygen demand of the heart. They should be used with caution in patients with severe CHF, bradyarrhythmias, or bronchospasm.

(b) STEMI. In STEMI, persistent thrombotic occlusion is present in the majority of patients, leading to necrosis of myocardial tissue that is not being perfused. Mortality and morbidity are decreased with the establishment of early reperfusion of the occluded vessels, restoring blood flow to the myocardium.

  (i) **PCI.** If the patient presents within 12 hours of symptom onset and is able to undergo PCI within 90 minutes of presentation or is in cardiogenic shock, PCI is the preferred method of treatment for an STEMI as it offers the best chance for reperfusion and has improved outcomes compared to fibrinolysis.

  (ii) **Fibrinolysis.** If PCI is not readily available, fibrinolysis to dissolve the thrombus and promote reperfusion should be considered. Fibrinolytic agents (streptokinase, tPA, and urokinase) should be administered within 30 minutes of presentation. There is a significant risk of bleeding with thrombolytic therapy, and contraindications need to be ruled out before administration.

(c) UA/NSTEMI. In NSTEMI or UA, there is severe coronary obstruction usually without total occlusion of the coronary artery, and thus treatment is focused on stabilizing the plaque and treating residual ischemia.

  (i) **PCI.** Immediate PCI is not indicated in most patients. Angiography and possible PCI are performed after stabilization in high-risk patients, patients who continue to have pain despite anti-ischemic therapy, or in low-risk patients with evidence of ischemia on noninvasive stress testing.

  (ii) **Additional antiplatelet agents** are administered with aspirin and have been shown to decrease the mortality and morbidity associated with UA/NSTEMI. **Clopidogrel** further inhibits platelet activity by blocking adenosine diphosphate (ADP) receptors and preventing aggregation. A loading dose should be given, followed by daily oral dosing. **Glycoprotein IIb/IIIa inhibitors** such as eptifibatide, tirofiban, or abciximab prevent the final pathway of platelet aggregation and are administered via IV infusion.

(iii) **Bivalirudin is a synthetic direct thrombin inhibitor.** Bivalirudin is noninferior to heparin in the treatment of acute coronary syndromes and as an adjunct to PCI in the catheterization laboratory. Some studies have demonstrated a lower bleeding risk in comparison with heparin and thus it may be safely used in patients with a history of heparin-induced thrombocytopenia.

(d) **Long-term secondary prevention therapy.** In addition to modifying risk factors through smoking cessation and control of hypertension, diabetes, and hyperlipidemia, several classes of medications have been shown to have a mortality benefit when used post-MI.

(i) **Aspirin.** Long-term aspirin therapy increases the likelihood of patency of the affected arteries. If patients have an aspirin allergy, clopidogrel may be substituted.

(ii) **β-Blockers.** Long-term mortality benefit is likely due to a combination of an antiarrhythmic effect and neurohormonal modulation.

(iii) **3-Hydroxy-3-methylglutaryl coenzyme A (HMG-CoA) reductase inhibitors (statins).** Decreasing LDL is essential in lowering the risk of coronary heart disease. Statin therapy also has an anti-inflammatory effect that benefits mortality independent of lipid reduction.

(iv) Inhibition of the renin–angiotensin–aldosterone system with **ACE inhibitors** or **ARBs** prevents remodeling and decreases the risk of ischemic events and should be used in patients with anterior MI or systolic dysfunction.

(v) **Clopidogrel** added to aspirin improves outcomes after hospitalization in patients with NSTEMI, regardless of in-hospital treatment approach.

(e) **Automated implantable cardioverter-defibrillator (AICD).** Patients with prior **MI** and a left ventricular ejection fraction (LVEF) of ≤40% or patients who have survived resuscitation after cardiac collapse not associated with acute infarction should be evaluated by a cardiac electrophysiologist. Such patients may be candidates for insertion of an AICD. AICDs monitor the heart rhythm and defibrillate the heart if a lethal rhythm is detected. Patients who receive frequent shocks may be candidates for the addition of antiarrhythmic drugs or catheter-based ablation.

(5) **Prognosis.** Following an MI, a patient's prognosis is largely determined by pump function and residual ischemic burden.

(a) **Pump function.** LV function should be assessed following an MI by left ventriculography, multiple gated acquisition scan (MUGA), or echocardiogram. Prognosis is markedly worse for patients with an LVEF of ≤40%.

(b) **Residual ischemic risk.** All patients who have an MI should be evaluated by cardiac catheterization or stress testing to determine the risk of recurrent ischemia or infarction.

(6) **Complications.** An MI can occur with little clinical consequence; indeed, many are silent. The complications of MI, however, produce clinically significant events.

(a) **Arrhythmias.** A patient having an acute MI is subject to acute, **lethal ventricular arrhythmias** (i.e., ventricular tachycardia or ventricular fibrillation), as well as **less serious atrial arrhythmias** (e.g., atrial fibrillation, atrial flutter). The risk for a lethal arrhythmia is greatest within the first 48 hours, requiring close monitoring.

(b) **Acute conduction system abnormalities.** The specialized conducting system of the heart is itself myocardium, which may become ischemic or infarcted during an MI. This may lead to bradyarrhythmias, heart block, or both.

(i) **Inferior MI** usually occurs when the right coronary artery is diseased. Because this artery supplies the sinoatrial node (SA) node in 55% of patients and the AV node in 85% of patients, **sinus bradycardia** and varying degrees of **AV nodal block** can occur. Heart block occurring during inferior infarction is almost always transient.

(ii) **Anterior MI** usually occurs from occlusion of the anterior descending coronary artery, which supplies the interventricular septum. Because the bundle branches course through the septum, acute **right- or left-bundle-branch block** may occur during anterior MIs. **Complete heart block** also may occur due to dysfunction of both bundle branches or the bundle of His.

      (c) Pump failure. When 30% of the myocardium is infarcted from one or more MIs, CHF is likely to ensue. If more than 40% of the myocardium becomes infarcted, **cardiogenic shock** is likely to develop.

      (d) Mitral regurgitation. The **papillary muscles,** which are projections of the myocardium, tether the mitral valve. Dysfunction or infarction of the papillary muscles together with ventricular dilation may lead to systolic prolapsing of the mitral valve into the left atrium, causing varying degrees of mitral regurgitation. This may lead to a precipitous rise in the left ventricular filling pressure that is transmitted to the lungs, resulting in pulmonary edema.

      (e) Ventricular septal defect. The interventricular septum may become infarcted in either anterior or inferior MI, leading to rupture of the septum. This occurs in approximately 2% of patients, usually 2–5 days after infarction.

      (f) Cardiac rupture. MI of the free wall may lead to eventual perforation of the heart. This complication, which results in overwhelming **cardiac tamponade,** is nearly always fatal. Rarely, rupture may be contained by adherent pericardium, forming a pseudoaneurysm. Surgical correction is necessary.

      (g) Left ventricular aneurysm. The infarcted zone of the myocardium may bulge and heal with fibrous connective tissue, forming an aneurysm. Left ventricular aneurysms may produce cardiac failure and angina, and they also may be the source of severe left ventricular arrhythmias and systemic emboli.

    (7) Treatment of complications

  c. Sudden death

B **Nonatherosclerotic coronary artery disease**

IV   VALVULAR HEART DISEASE

A **Aortic stenosis**

  1. Etiology

    a. Congenital aortic stenosis usually is detected in pediatric patients but occasionally becomes apparent in early adulthood.

    b. Senile calcific aortic stenosis occurs when scarring and calcification of a tricuspid aortic valve lead to orifice narrowing in the sixth, seventh, and eighth decades of life. Although once considered a "degenerative" idiopathic disease, it is now clear that the pathology leading up to severe aortic stenosis is due to proliferative and inflammatory changes leading to calcification, similar to the development of the plaque in ASCAD.

    c. Bicuspid aortic valve is a common congenital cardiac abnormality. The flow characteristics of the bicuspid valve are more turbulent than those of the normal valve, leading to valve injury, calcification, and stenosis in the fourth and fifth decades of life.

    d. Rheumatic aortic stenosis never occurs alone and is always associated with mitral valve disease.

  2. Pathophysiology. Aortic valve stenosis produces a pressure overload on the left ventricle due to the greater pressure that must be generated to force blood past the stenotic valve. This commonly leads to compensatory left ventricular hypertrophy.

  3. Clinical features

    a. Symptoms. Asymptomatic patients with aortic stenosis are at little risk for sudden death. However, this risk increases dramatically when symptoms develop.

      (1) Angina occurs in 35%–50% of patients with aortic stenosis.

        (a) Fifty percent of patients who develop this symptom die within 5 years of its onset unless aortic valve replacement is performed.

        (b) Although the exact mechanism of angina is unknown, current data suggest that coronary blood flow reserve is impaired in the severely hypertrophied left ventricle. Impairment of the coronary blood flow reserve limits oxygen delivery to the myocardium and produces angina during exercise.

      (2) Syncope occurs during exercise when total peripheral resistance falls due to local autoregulatory mechanisms [see IX B, C 1 b (2) (b)]. When aortic stenosis is present, cardiac output across the stenotic aortic valve cannot increase during exercise. Because total peripheral resistance falls, blood pressure must also fall, and syncope occurs.

   (a) **Other causes** of syncope in aortic stenosis include a reflex vasodepressor response to high intraventricular pressure, **atrial** or **ventricular arrhythmias,** and **heart block** as a result of conduction system calcification.

   (b) After syncope occurs in patients with aortic stenosis, expected survival is 2–3 years without valve replacement.

(3) Heart failure. Fifty percent of patients who develop heart failure die within 1–2 years of presentation if the stenosis is not corrected. Heart failure occurs because the afterload placed on the myocardium becomes excessive and both contractile dysfunction and diastolic muscle dysfunction occur when the myocardium is exposed to a prolonged, severe pressure overload.

b. Physical signs

(1) Delayed carotid upstroke. In the presence of aortic stenosis, the carotid upstroke typically is delayed in timing and reduced in volume (pulsus parvus et tardus). This finding is the most reliable physical sign in gauging the severity of the disease.

(2) Systolic ejection murmur. A harsh, late-peaking systolic ejection murmur is heard in the aortic area and is transmitted to the carotid arteries. The murmur also may be reflected to the mitral area, producing the false impression that mitral regurgitation also is present **(Gallavardin's phenomenon).**

(3) Soft, single S_2. Because the aortic valve is stenotic, its motion is severely impaired. The reduction in motion of the valve causes the **aortic component (A_2)** of the S_2 to be absent. Thus, the only component of the S_2 that is heard is the **pulmonic component (P_2),** which is normally soft.

(4) S_4. An S_4 usually is heard as a result of the reduced left ventricular compliance that occurs in left ventricular hypertrophy.

(5) Sustained, forceful apex beat. The point of maximal cardiac impulse usually is not displaced unless heart failure has occurred. However, the impulse is sustained and forceful throughout systole.

4. Laboratory diagnosis

   a. Electrocardiography. The ECG usually shows evidence of left ventricular hypertrophy.

   b. Echocardiography can rule out significant aortic stenosis if valve motion is shown to be normal. However, Doppler examination of the aortic outflow tract during echocardiography can accurately measure the pressure gradient across the aortic valve and can be used to calculate the valve area.

   c. Cardiac catheterization. Diagnosis and evaluation of the severity of aortic stenosis may be confirmed by cardiac catheterization, during which the pressure gradient across the valve is measured and the degree of stenosis is calculated.

5. Therapy

   a. Palliative therapy

   (1) Medical therapy has no definitive role in the treatment of aortic stenosis, but **diuretics** may temporarily relieve the symptoms of volume overload until mechanical relief of the obstruction is performed.

   (2) Insertion and inflation of a large balloon in the aortic valve orifice **(balloon valvuloplasty)** may produce a temporary moderate improvement in the amount of obstruction and the patient's symptoms. It is usually considered a bridge to more definite therapy, and it does not reduce expected mortality without such therapy.

   b. High-risk patients. There are few options for patients with severe symptomatic aortic stenosis who are not considered candidates for traditional valve replacement surgery.

   (1) Percutaneous valve replacement. In this procedure, a stent-based bioprosthetic valve is expanded in the aortic valve position via a catheter, crushing the native valve and leaving the new prosthesis in its place. This procedure is investigational, but promising.

   (2) Apicoaortic surgery (aortic valve bypass). This procedure involves connecting a tube graft with an interposed bioprosthetic valve between the apex of the left ventricle and the descending thoracic aorta, thus bypassing the defective valve.

c. **Curative therapy** requires **aortic valve replacement,** which may be performed using a preserved human homograft valve, a bioprosthetic heterograft valve, a mechanical valve, or a pulmonary autograft.

   (1) **Homograft valves.** The hemodynamic flow pattern is excellent, and patients with homograft valves do not require anticoagulation therapy. Availability of these valves is limited because most suitable donors are also acceptable for whole-heart donation in cardiac transplantation.

   (2) **Heterograft valves.** Patients with heterograft valves do not require anticoagulation therapy, but the durability of the valve is limited, and deterioration after 10 years is common.

   (3) **Mechanical valves.** Patients with mechanical valves do require anticoagulation therapy. However, these valves are more durable than bioprostheses.

   (4) **Autograft (Ross procedure).** In this procedure, the patient's normal pulmonary valve is transplanted into the aortic position, where it has excellent durability and longevity. A homograft is then inserted into the pulmonary position, where low pressure enhances homograft longevity. In practiced hands, the results of this procedure are excellent.

B Mitral stenosis

1. **Etiology.** Almost all cases of mitral stenosis in adults are **secondary to rheumatic heart disease.** Most cases occur in women.

2. **Pathophysiology**

   a. Mitral valve stenosis impedes left ventricular filling, thereby increasing left atrial pressure as a pressure gradient develops across the mitral valve. Elevated left atrial pressure is referred to the lungs, where it produces **pulmonary congestion.** As the stenosis becomes more severe, it may significantly reduce forward cardiac output.

   b. Because the right ventricle is responsible for filling the left ventricle, the burden of propelling blood across the stenotic mitral valve is borne by the right ventricle. The overload on the right ventricle may be increased further when secondary pulmonary vasoconstriction occurs. Thus, the right ventricle must generate enough force both to overcome the resistance offered by the stenotic valve and to propel blood through constricted pulmonary arteries. Consequently, pulmonary arterial pressure may increase to three to five times normal, eventually resulting in **right ventricular failure.**

3. **Clinical features**

   a. **Symptoms**

      (1) **Left-sided failure. Dyspnea on exertion, orthopnea,** and **paroxysmal nocturnal dyspnea** occur as a result of reduced left ventricular output and increased left atrial pressure. In mitral stenosis, the symptoms of left ventricular failure usually are not attributable to left ventricular dysfunction but, rather, to the mitral stenosis itself.

      (2) **Right-sided failure.** When pulmonary hypertension occurs, the right ventricle may fail, producing **edema, ascites, anorexia,** and **fatigue.**

      (3) **Hemoptysis.** The high left atrial pressure produced in mitral stenosis may lead to rupture of small bronchial veins, producing hemoptysis.

      (4) **Systemic embolism.** Stagnation of blood in the enlarged left atrium and left atrial appendage occurs in mitral stenosis, particularly if atrial fibrillation is present. Under these circumstances, a thrombus may form in the left atrium and can become a source of systemic embolism.

      (5) **Hoarseness** may occur in mitral stenosis as the enlarged left atrium impinges on the left recurrent laryngeal nerve (Ortner's syndrome).

   b. **Physical signs**

      (1) **Atrial fibrillation.** Frequently, an irregularly irregular cardiac rhythm indicative of atrial fibrillation is present.

      (2) **Pulmonary rales.** Bilateral pulmonary rales occur secondary to elevated left atrial and pulmonary venous pressures.

      (3) **Increased intensity of the S_1.** The S_1 usually increases in intensity because the transmitral gradient limits spontaneous diastolic mitral valve closure. Thus, the mitral valve remains open until ventricular systole closes it forcibly, resulting in an increase in S_1 intensity.

Late in the course of the disease, the valve may become so stenotic that it no longer opens or closes, reducing the intensity of S_1.

    (4) Increased intensity of the P_2 component of the S_2. The P_2 component of the S_2 is usually increased in intensity if pulmonary hypertension has developed.

    (5) Opening snap. An **opening snap is heard following the S_2** as the stenotic valve is forced open in diastole by the high left atrial filling pressure. The higher the pressure, the sooner does the mitral valve open. Thus, a short interval (<0.10 second in duration) indicates relatively high left atrial pressure and severe stenosis.

    (6) Diastolic rumble. The murmur of mitral stenosis is a low-pitched apical rumble, which begins after the opening snap. If the patient is in sinus rhythm, atrial systole produces a presystolic accentuation of this murmur.

    (7) Sternal lift. Enlargement of the right ventricle as a result of pulmonary hypertension produces a systolic lift of the sternum.

    (8) Other symptoms. Neck vein distention, edema, hepatic enlargement, and **ascites** may be present if right ventricular failure occurs.

  4. Laboratory diagnosis

    a. Electrocardiography. The ECG may show atrial fibrillation, as well as signs of left atrial enlargement and right ventricular hypertrophy.

    b. Chest radiography

      (1) Straightening of the left heart border and a double density along the right heart border (formed by the right and left atria) occur as a result of left atrial enlargement.

      (2) Signs of pulmonary venous hypertension, including an increase in pulmonary vascular markings and **Kerley's lines,** are likely to be present.

      (3) When **pulmonary hypertension** leads to right ventricular enlargement, the lateral view shows a **loss of the retrosternal airspace.**

    c. Echocardiography usually provides excellent images of the mitral valve.

      (1) The echocardiogram shows reduction in the excursion of the valve leaflets and thickening of the valve. Two-dimensional echocardiography can be used to visualize and measure the residual mitral valve orifice. Invariably, left atrial enlargement is present.

      (2) Doppler examination of the mitral valve may also help to quantify the severity of the stenosis.

  5. Therapy

    a. Medical therapy is reserved for patients with mild-to-moderate symptoms of left-sided failure.

      (1) Diuretics. The mainstay of treatment, these agents are used to **control pulmonary congestion** and to **limit dyspnea and orthopnea.**

      (2) Digitalis. Because left ventricular muscle function usually is normal in mitral stenosis, the use of digitalis is of little benefit to patients in sinus rhythm. In patients in **atrial fibrillation,** however, digitalis is used to slow ventricular rate. A rapid ventricular rate in mitral stenosis shortens diastole, thereby reducing left ventricular filling, which, in turn, further increases left atrial pressure and reduces cardiac output. **β-Blockers** and **diltiazem** or **verapamil** may be added to digoxin if further heart rate control is necessary.

      (3) Anticoagulants. Patients with mitral stenosis and coexistent atrial fibrillation have a **high incidence of systemic embolism.** In such patients, anticoagulation therapy (e.g., with **warfarin**) usually is indicated.

    b. Balloon valvuloplasty. Unlike balloon valvuloplasty for aortic stenosis, balloon valvuloplasty for mitral stenosis can offer effective long-term improvement.

      (1) Valvuloplasty for mitral stenosis produces a commissurotomy similar to that produced at open heart surgery. During balloon mitral valvuloplasty, transseptal catheterization of the interatrial septum is performed, allowing passage of the balloon catheter from the right atrium to the left atrium. From the left atrium, the balloon catheter is advanced to the mitral valve and is inflated.

      (2) Echocardiography is essential in predicting immediate and long-term success. Factors influencing the feasibility and success of valvuloplasty include the degrees of mitral regurgitation, valvular thickening, calcification, mobility, and subvalvular involvement.

c. **Surgical therapy** is effective in relieving the symptoms of mitral stenosis and in prolonging life in symptomatic patients. Surgery should be performed prior to the development of pulmonary hypertension, which increases surgical risk. However, if pulmonary hypertension is present and surgery is successful, pulmonary hypertension usually regresses postoperatively.

C **Aortic regurgitation (or aortic insufficiency)**

1. **Etiology**
   a. **Idiopathic aortic root dilation.** Aortic root dilation, a common cause of aortic regurgitation, occurs more frequently in patients with hypertension but correlates best with increasing age. It is also seen more frequently in patients with bicuspid aortic valves.
   b. **Rheumatic heart disease.** Aortic insufficiency usually is present to some degree in most cases of rheumatic heart disease. Mitral stenosis usually predominates, but occasionally aortic insufficiency is the most severe manifestation of rheumatic heart disease.
   c. **Infective endocarditis.** Infection of the aortic valve may lead to **perforation or partial destruction of one or more aortic leaflets,** producing aortic insufficiency.
   d. **Marfan syndrome** may produce aortic insufficiency in two ways.
      (1) **Proximal root dilation.** The extreme expansion of the proximal aortic root seen in Marfan syndrome may produce aortic insufficiency.
      (2) **Aortic root dissection.** The advanced cystic medial necrosis present in Marfan syndrome may lead to an intimal tear and dissection of the aorta. If the dissection involves the proximal aortic root, the supporting structures of the aortic valve are disrupted, and the valve is rendered incompetent.
   e. **Aortic dissection.** Any cause of aortic dissection other than Marfan syndrome may lead to aortic insufficiency.
   f. **Syphilis** may produce **aortitis,** which may extend to the aortic valve and produce aortic incompetence.
   g. **Collagen vascular disease.** Systemic lupus erythematosus (SLE) and ankylosing spondylitis may cause aortic insufficiency.

2. **Pathophysiology**
   a. A portion of the left ventricular stroke volume ejected during systole regurgitates into the left ventricle during diastole. If no compensation occurs, left ventricular forward output decreases. However, chronic regurgitation of blood into the left ventricle produces eccentric cardiac hypertrophy and an increase in end-diastolic volume. The stroke volume (end-diastolic volume minus end-systolic volume) therefore increases, helping to compensate for the volume that is regurgitated. The increase in total stroke volume leads to an increase in pulse pressure and increased systolic pressure. The additional development of concentric hypertrophy compensates this second type of overload. **The additional volume and pressure that the left ventricle must generate eventually lead to left ventricular dysfunction and CHF.**
   b. An additional pathophysiologic consequence of aortic insufficiency is a **reduction in systemic diastolic blood pressure.**

3. **Clinical features**
   a. **Symptoms**
      (1) **Left ventricular failure**
         (a) **Chronic aortic insufficiency** may cause left ventricular dysfunction, leading to symptoms of **dyspnea, orthopnea,** and **paroxysmal nocturnal dyspnea.**
         (b) In **acute aortic insufficiency,** normal muscle function may coexist with heart failure. In this circumstance, reduced forward output and elevated left ventricular filling pressure occur prior to **compensatory left ventricular enlargement.**
      (2) **Syncope.** Reduction in diastolic systemic arterial pressure produces a reduction in mean arterial pressure. If the mean arterial pressure is reduced significantly, cerebral perfusion is compromised, and syncope may occur.
      (3) **Angina** occurs less commonly in aortic insufficiency than in aortic stenosis. The cause of angina in aortic insufficiency is **reduced coronary blood flow.** Coronary blood flow occurs primarily in diastole and is driven by the aortic diastolic blood pressure. This driving pressure is reduced in aortic insufficiency, in turn reducing coronary blood flow.

b. Physical signs

    (1) Left ventricular impulse. The PMI is **hyperdynamic** and is **displaced downward and to the left** as a result of left ventricular enlargement.

    (2) Diastolic murmur. The murmur of aortic insufficiency is a **high-pitched, diastolic blowing murmur** heard along the left sternal border. Often the murmur is heard best when the patient is sitting up and leaning forward.

    (3) Austin Flint murmur. A **low-pitched diastolic rumble** similar to that heard in mitral stenosis may be present in patients with aortic insufficiency. The Austin Flint murmur **usually indicates moderate-to-severe insufficiency.** The murmur is believed to be caused by reverberation of the regurgitant flow against the mitral valve, although the exact mechanism is unclear.

    (4) Total stroke volume and, consequently, **pulse pressure increase** in chronic aortic insufficiency. The increased stroke volume and pulse pressure lead to many physical signs, some of which are included in the following.

        (a) Corrigan's pulse. The carotid pulse has a rapid rise and full upstroke with a rapid fall in diastole.

        (b) Hill's sign refers to a disproportionate increase of systolic blood pressure (i.e., >30 mm Hg) when measured in the leg as compared with the systolic blood pressure measured in the arm. This sign suggests severe aortic insufficiency.

        (c) Pistol-shot femoral pulses. Auscultation over the femoral arteries reveals a pulse that sounds like a pistol shot.

        (d) Duroziez's sign. A stethoscope is placed over the femoral artery with enough pressure to produce a systolic bruit. The concomitant occurrence of a diastolic bruit constitutes Duroziez's sign.

        (e) de Musset's sign refers to a bobbing movement of the head caused by the increased stroke volume and pulse pressure.

        (f) Quincke's pulse is systolic blushing and diastolic blanching of the nail bed when gentle pressure is placed on the nail.

    (5) Acute aortic insufficiency. The preceding signs are usually absent in *acute* aortic insufficiency because compensatory increases in end-diastolic volume and stroke volume have not yet occurred. In fact, the clinical picture of acute severe aortic insufficiency is remarkably bland. The apical impulse is not enlarged. S_1 is soft because increased left ventricular end-diastolic pressure closes the mitral valve before systole. This finding marks a poor prognosis for patients treated without valve replacement.

4. Diagnosis

    a. Electrocardiography. The ECG usually shows left ventricular hypertrophy. In endocarditis, a prolonged PR interval may indicate abscess formation involving the conduction system.

    b. Chest radiography. Unless the aortic insufficiency is mild or acute, **cardiac enlargement** is usually present, and often the proximal aorta is dilated. The absence of cardiac enlargement is evidence against the diagnosis of severe chronic aortic insufficiency.

    c. Echocardiography. Evidence of an enlarged left ventricular cavity is usually present in aortic insufficiency. Frequently, diastolic vibration of the mitral valve is present, produced by the regurgitant flow striking the valve. Doppler examination of the aortic outflow tract reveals abnormal diastolic flow from the aorta to the left ventricle, which may be analyzed quantitatively.

    d. Cardiac catheterization. Aortography may be performed at the time of cardiac catheterization. This is useful if noninvasive testing is not diagnostic or discordant with clinical findings.

5. Therapy. If aortic insufficiency is severe, eventual **aortic valve replacement** is necessary.

    a. Timing of surgery is difficult, however, because the lesion may be tolerated for several years. Careful follow-up is required to detect early signs of decompensation; at this time, valve replacement is advisable. In most cases, valve replacement should be performed before the left ventricular echocardiographic end-systolic dimension exceeds 55 mm and the ejection fraction falls below 55%.

    b. For those who do not yet meet the criteria for surgery, **vasodilator therapy** with dihydropyridine calcium channel blockers or ACE inhibitors can improve hemodynamics and may delay onset of left ventricular dysfunction and the need for surgery.

D **Mitral regurgitation (or mitral insufficiency)**

1. **Etiology**
   a. **Mitral valve prolapse is** characterized by redundant mitral valve leaflets or chordae that permit systolic prolapse of the mitral valve into the left atrium with resultant mitral regurgitation.
      (1) This syndrome usually is benign, but in some cases it may be associated with significant mitral regurgitation. Additional complications include atypical chest pain, cardiac arrhythmias, and an increased risk of endocarditis. Most clinically important sequelae occur in those patients whose mitral valves are clearly thickened and echocardiographically abnormal.
      (2) A midsystolic click and a late systolic murmur typically are heard on physical examination.
   b. **Coronary artery disease** may lead to ischemia or infarction of the papillary muscles to which the mitral valve is tethered, thereby producing mitral incompetence.
   c. **Rheumatic heart disease.** Scarring and retraction of the mitral leaflets as a result of rheumatic heart disease cause mitral regurgitation.
   d. **Ruptured chordae tendineae.** Spontaneous rupture of the chordae tendineae may occur in otherwise healthy individuals. Chordal rupture permits prolapse of a portion of a mitral valve leaflet into the left atrium, rendering the valve incompetent.
   e. **Infective endocarditis.** Infection of the mitral valve may cause its destruction with subsequent regurgitation.

2. **Pathophysiology.** Mitral regurgitation permits a portion of the left ventricular stroke volume to be pumped backward into the left atrium instead of forward into the aorta, resulting in **increased left atrial pressure and decreased forward cardiac output.** Preload is increased by the volume overload, and afterload is initially decreased as the left ventricle empties a portion of its contents into the relatively (i.e., compared with the aorta) low-pressure left atrium. This augments ejection performance and helps compensate for the regurgitation.
   a. Initially, compliance of the left atrium is low, and the regurgitant volume produces high left atrial pressure with resultant congestive symptoms.
   b. With time, the left atrial compliance and volume increase, allowing accommodation of the regurgitant volume at more physiologic filling pressures.
   c. The development of left ventricular eccentric cardiac hypertrophy restores forward stroke volume.
   d. After a prolonged period of compensation, left ventricular muscle dysfunction eventually occurs, resulting in a fall in ejection fraction from supranormal to normal or even subnormal values.

3. **Clinical features**
   a. **Symptoms.** Characteristics include those of left ventricular failure (i.e., **dyspnea, orthopnea, and paroxysmal nocturnal dyspnea**).
      (1) If mitral regurgitation is severe and chronic, **pulmonary hypertension** and **symptoms of right-sided failure** also may occur.
      (2) Patients in atrial fibrillation may experience **symptoms of systemic embolization.** The risk of embolization appears to be less in patients with mitral regurgitation than in those with mitral stenosis, although this is debatable.
   b. **Physical signs**
      (1) **Left ventricular impulse.** As with aortic regurgitation, the PMI is hyperdynamic and displaced downward and to the left.
      (2) **Murmur.** The murmur of mitral regurgitation is a holosystolic apical murmur that radiates to the axilla. It does not vary in intensity with variation in R-R interval.
      (3) An S_3 usually is heard in mitral regurgitation and may occur even in the absence of overt heart failure. The S_3 is caused by the rapid filling of the left ventricle by the large volume of blood accumulated in the left atrium during systole.

4. **Diagnosis**
   a. **Electrocardiography.** The ECG shows signs of left ventricular hypertrophy and left atrial enlargement.

    b. Chest radiography shows cardiac enlargement. Vascular congestion indicates heart failure.

    c. Echocardiography

        (1) In cases of a **ruptured chorda** or **mitral valve prolapse,** the mitral valve can be seen extending into the left atrium during systole.

        (2) When the mitral valve has been damaged by **endocarditis,** vegetations on the mitral leaflets frequently are demonstrated. Transesophageal echocardiography is better than transthoracic echocardiography for detecting vegetations.

        (3) Regardless of the cause of the mitral regurgitation, **left atrial** and **left ventricular enlargement occur** if the condition is both chronic and severe.

        (4) Doppler examination reveals abnormal systolic flow from the left ventricle into the left atrium. Quantitative Doppler techniques can accurately assess the regurgitant orifice area and the regurgitant volume, both of which are important in determining severity.

    d. Cardiac catheterization. Right-heart catheterization yields a **pulmonary capillary wedge tracing** that often displays a **large v-wave** representative of the systolic volume overload on the left atrium. **Left ventriculography** demonstrates systolic regurgitation of contrast material into the left atrium.

5. Therapy

    a. Medical treatment. The goal of medical therapy is to relieve symptoms by increasing forward cardiac output and reducing pulmonary venous hypertension.

        (1) Digitalis. When atrial fibrillation occurs, digitalis is useful in controlling heart rate. In chronic mitral regurgitation with muscle dysfunction, this agent may be useful in increasing the inotropic state. In cases of acute mitral regurgitation when no inotropic deficit exists, it is not indicated.

        (2) Diuretics are used to reduce central volume overload, which in turn reduces pulmonary venous hypertension and congestion.

        (3) Vasodilators. Arteriolar vasodilators are **particularly useful** in managing acute mitral regurgitation. These agents **reduce resistance to aortic outflow,** thereby preferentially increasing forward output while reducing the amount of regurgitation. Vasodilators also **reduce left ventricular size,** which helps to reestablish mitral competence.

        (4) Anticoagulants. Patients with mitral regurgitation and atrial fibrillation are at some risk for systemic embolism; therefore, anticoagulants usually are indicated.

    b. Surgical treatment. Mitral valve replacement or repair is indicated for chronic severe mitral regurgitation, even if symptoms are mild or absent, if there is evidence of ventricular dysfunction.

        (1) Valve replacement must be performed prior to the onset of significant muscle dysfunction, which limits the success of operative intervention. To help ensure preservation of ventricular function, surgery should occur before the ejection fraction falls below 60% or the end-systolic dimension exceeds 40 mm.

        (2) Valve repair offers several advantages over replacement, including eliminating the introduction of a prosthesis and decreasing the need for anticoagulation therapy. Furthermore, repairing rather than replacing the valve helps preserve left ventricular function because the mitral valve apparatus, which plays an important role in ventricular contraction, is preserved.

E Tricuspid regurgitation

1. Etiology

    a. Infective endocarditis. In drug abusers who inject drugs under septic conditions, infective endocarditis is a common cause of tricuspid regurgitation.

    b. Right ventricular failure. Sustained pressure or volume overload on the right ventricle leads to right ventricular dilation and improper alignment of the papillary muscles, which produces tricuspid regurgitation.

    c. Rheumatic heart disease. In rheumatic heart disease, tricuspid regurgitation may occur secondary to right ventricular pressure overload from left-sided valvular lesions. Tricuspid regurgitation also may occur as a result of primary rheumatic involvement of the tricuspid valve.

2. **Pathophysiology.** During systole, the dysfunctioning tricuspid valve allows blood to flow backward into the right atrium, leading to systemic venous congestion and venous hypertension.

3. **Clinical features**
   a. **Symptoms.** Right-sided failure (i.e., **edema, ascites**) occurs. In severe and acute cases, **hepatic congestion** may be sufficiently extensive to produce **right upper quadrant pain.** Passive hepatic congestion also may lead to hepatocellular damage and **jaundice.**
   b. **Physical signs**
      (1) **Right ventricular lift.** The enlarged right ventricle may be palpated as a systolic lift of the sternum.
      (2) **Murmur.** A holosystolic murmur that increases with inspiration is heard along the left sternal border.
      (3) **Jugular venous pulsation.** A large **v wave** is seen in jugular veins during systole.
      (4) **Pulsatile liver.** Systolic expansion of the liver frequently is present.

4. **Diagnosis**
   a. **Chest radiography** shows right ventricular enlargement as an obliteration of the retrosternal airspace on the lateral view.
   b. **Echocardiography** demonstrates enlargement of the right atrium and right ventricle. Doppler examination is highly effective in demonstrating tricuspid regurgitation.

5. **Therapy.** Left-sided failure frequently is the cause of right-sided failure and tricuspid regurgitation. Effective treatment of left-sided failure reduces right ventricular pressure overload, which may decrease right ventricular size, thereby restoring valvular competence. If tricuspid regurgitation is caused by organic valvular disease, surgical repair or replacement of the tricuspid valve may be necessary.

V CARDIOMYOPATHIES

A Dilated (congestive) cardiomyopathy

1. **Definition.** Dilated cardiomyopathy is defined as a diminution in the contractile function of the left, right, or both ventricles in the absence of pressure overload, volume overload, or coronary artery disease. The loss of cardiac muscle function results in CHF.

2. **Etiology.** The cause of most cases of dilated cardiomyopathy is unknown. Viral infection has been implicated in the pathogenesis of this disease, but proof of cause generally is lacking. The following other conditions have been linked to cardiomyopathy.
   a. **Prolonged ethanol abuse** is the most common reversible cause of cardiomyopathy.
   b. **Doxorubicin therapy.** High doses of doxorubicin, a commonly used chemotherapeutic drug, may result in irreversible dilated cardiomyopathy.
   c. **Exposure to mercury, lead,** or **high-dose catecholamines** may cause myocardial damage and dilated cardiomyopathy.
   d. **Endocrinopathies,** including **thyrotoxicosis, hypothyroidism,** and **acromegaly,** have been reported to cause dilated cardiomyopathy. In thyrotoxicosis and in hypothyroidism, the myopathy usually is reversed when the endocrinopathy is corrected.
   e. **Metabolic disorders** (e.g., **hypophosphatemia, hypocalcemia, thiamin deficiency**) may produce reversible cardiomyopathy.
   f. **Hemoglobinopathies** (e.g., **sickle cell anemia, thalassemia**) are associated with myocardial dysfunction.
   g. **Genetic abnormalities.** In some families, the development of dilated cardiomyopathy is linked to specific genetic abnormalities.
   h. **Prolonged tachycardia** (persisting for weeks or months) may result from uncontrolled atrial arrhythmias, causing a dilated cardiomyopathy that may be reversed within weeks, after heart rate is controlled.

3. **Clinical features, diagnosis,** and **treatment** of dilated cardiomyopathy are similar to left- and right-sided CHF as described in I D–F.
   a. **Symptoms**
   b. **Physical signs**

4. Diagnosis

5. Therapy

B **Hypertrophic cardiomyopathy**

1. **Definition.** Hypertrophic cardiomyopathy is a disorder in which regional hypertrophy of the left ventricle occurs independent of loading conditions. It most commonly involves the interventricular septum but can also involve the apex. When the septum is involved, the hypertrophied septum and the anterior leaflet of the mitral valve may produce dynamic left ventricular outflow obstruction.

2. **Etiology.** Most cases are inherited through an autosomal dominant mode of transmission, but sporadic cases also occur. Specific abnormalities in the genes coding for cardiac myosin and other cardiac proteins have been identified.

3. **Pathophysiology**

   a. **Methods of obstruction** include the following:

      (1) As shown in Figure 2–10, the hypertrophied septum encroaches on the left ventricular outflow tract and comes into close approximation with the anterior leaflet of the mitral valve.

      (2) During systole, a low-pressure zone may develop as blood flow accelerates through the narrowed area between the septum and the anterior leaflet, generating a **Bernoulli effect.** Thus, the anterior leaflet of the mitral valve is drawn into the septum (systolic anterior motion), leading to outflow obstruction.

   b. The **degree of outflow obstruction** varies from patient to patient and from time to time in the same patient.

      (1) Physiologic conditions that enlarge the left ventricle (e.g., increases in preload and afterload) separate the septum and anterior leaflet of the mitral valve and reduce the obstruction.

      (2) Physiologic conditions that make the ventricle smaller or that increase the velocity of blood flow (e.g., dehydration, positive inotropic drugs) increase the degree of obstruction.

   c. The obstruction to outflow may cause secondary cardiac hypertrophy of the nonseptal portions of the ventricle, but septal thickness generally remains greater than that of the free wall of the ventricle.

4. **Clinical features**

   a. **Symptoms**

      (1) **Angina.** Patients with obstructive cardiomyopathy frequently complain of chest pain.

         (a) The pain usually has **atypical features;** that is, the pain may occur at rest and is not always related to exercise.

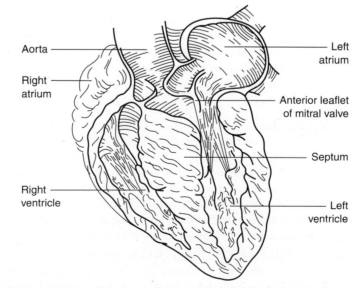

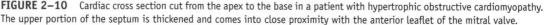

FIGURE 2–10 Cardiac cross section cut from the apex to the base in a patient with hypertrophic obstructive cardiomyopathy. The upper portion of the septum is thickened and comes into close proximity with the anterior leaflet of the mitral valve.

(b) The pathophysiology of angina in hypertrophic obstructive cardiomyopathy is unclear, but coronary blood flow is subnormal, potentially causing ischemia.

(2) Syncope

(a) Syncope usually occurs during or after exercise in patients with obstructive cardiomyopathy as a result of reduced left ventricular size and the consequent increased obstruction to outflow.

  (i) After exercise, **afterload is reduced** because of peripheral vasodilation.

  (ii) **Preload is reduced** because of the decreased activity of the contractions of the leg muscles, which help to return blood to the heart.

  (iii) The **inotropic state remains elevated** because of the increased catecholamine level after exercise.

(b) **Arrhythmias,** which are common in this disorder, also may precipitate syncope or sudden death.

(3) CHF. Dyspnea on exertion, orthopnea, and paroxysmal nocturnal dyspnea occur in patients with obstructive cardiomyopathy. Systolic function usually is normal or supranormal, and the ejection fraction often exceeds 80%.

(a) The symptoms of heart failure usually are not caused by systolic malfunction, but rather occur as a result of increased diastolic stiffness.

(b) The thickened myocardium requires an increased filling pressure for adequate diastolic distention. The increased filling pressure is reflected to the lungs and produces pulmonary congestive symptoms.

(c) In the later stages of the disease, however, systolic dysfunction also may occur, contributing to the symptoms of CHF.

b. Physical signs

(1) Carotid upstroke. In patients with the obstructive form of the disease, the carotid upstrokes have a **spike-and-dome character** (Online Figure 2–11). This configuration indicates early systolic outflow followed by a period of obstruction, during which flow falls. The dome portion of the curve reflects the period near the end of systole when obstruction diminishes and aortic outflow again commences.

(2) Murmur. The murmur is a systolic ejection murmur heard along the left sternal border. Unlike the murmur in aortic stenosis, it does not usually radiate to the neck.

(a) **Increasing the intensity of the murmur:**

  (i) Maneuvers that diminish left ventricular size cause an increase in both the obstruction to outflow and the intensity of the cardiac murmur. Thus, the **Valsalva maneuver,** which diminishes the murmur in valvular aortic stenosis by diminishing flow, increases the murmur in obstructive cardiomyopathy by increasing obstruction.

  (ii) Having the patient stand or inhale amyl nitrite also diminishes left ventricular size and therefore increases the intensity of the murmur.

(b) **Diminishing the intensity of the murmur. Squatting,** which increases myocardial afterload and venous return to the heart, increases cardiac size and therefore diminishes the murmur.

5. Diagnosis

a. Electrocardiography almost always is abnormal. The ECG usually shows evidence of left ventricular hypertrophy, nonspecific ST- and T-wave abnormalities, and left atrial enlargement.

b. Echocardiography establishes the diagnosis in most patients.

(1) In patients with **asymmetric septal hypertrophy without obstruction,** increased septal thickness results in a **ratio of septum to free wall thickness of 1.3:1** or greater.

(2) Findings in the obstructive form of the disease include **systolic anterior motion of the mitral valve, systolic fluttering of the aortic valve leaflets,** and **early closure of the aortic valve,** corresponding to the spike and dome seen in the carotid pulse.

6. Therapy. Unlike aortic stenosis, in which relief of valvular obstruction relieves symptoms and prolongs life, there is no conclusive evidence that surgical relief of obstruction in obstructive cardiomyopathy prolongs life. Therefore, medical therapy is used first in an attempt to improve symptoms.

a. Medical therapy

(1) **β-Blockers** are effective in relieving symptoms in this disease.

  (a) β-Blockade **slows the heart rate,** which increases left ventricular filling and size, diminishing obstruction.

  (b) β-Blockade also reduces the vigor of left ventricular contraction and thus **decreases the velocity of blood flow,** which also reduces the degree of obstruction.

(2) **Calcium channel blocking agents.** These agents are an alternative to β-blockers and have been shown to **diminish the left ventricular outflow gradient. Verapamil** is the calcium channel blocker most widely used in the treatment of this disease. Caution must be exercised in patients with CHF because verapamil may worsen failure and precipitate acute pulmonary edema.

(3) **Digitalis is contraindicated in the hyperdynamic phase** of the disease when obstruction is present and the left ventricular cavity is small, because digitalis increases the vigor of left ventricular contraction and thus increases the outflow obstruction.

b. Surgical therapy

(1) **Myomectomy.** Surgical reduction of the thickness of the left ventricular septum relieves the outflow gradient and symptoms in those patients who have not responded to medical therapy.

(2) **Mitral valve replacement.** Because it is the anterior leaflet of the mitral valve that produces the obstruction, mitral valve replacement is also effective in relieving obstruction.

(3) **Intentional septal infarction.** Transcatheter instillation of ethanol into the septal artery is performed to partially infarct the septum and reduce obstruction.

c. Antiarrhythmic therapy. Most patients with hypertrophic myopathy die suddenly. Patients with a family history of sudden death or a personal history of syncope or ventricular tachycardia are at high risk and should undergo electrophysiologic testing. Many patients receive implantable defibrillators.

C Restrictive cardiomyopathy

1. **Definition.** The restrictive cardiomyopathies are a group of diseases in which the composition of the myocardium has changed so that it becomes stiffer. The **increased stiffness of the myocardium** restricts left ventricular filling, thereby reducing stroke output and increasing left ventricular filling pressure.

2. **Etiology. Infiltrative diseases** of the myocardium, which produce restrictive cardiomyopathy, include **amyloidosis, hemochromatosis, idiopathic eosinophilia, carcinoid syndrome, sarcoidosis,** and **endomyocardial fibroelastosis.**

3. **Pathophysiology.** Systolic function usually is normal in the early stages of the disease, but the altered properties of the myocardium increase diastolic stiffness. Thus, the left ventricular pressure is above normal at any diastolic left ventricular volume. Increased filling pressure produces pulmonary congestion. As the infiltrative process progresses, systolic function also is compromised.

4. **Clinical features**

a. Symptoms of both left-sided and right-sided CHF usually are present; the symptoms of right-sided failure are usually more prominent.

b. Physical signs include those present in left-sided and right-sided CHF.

5. **Diagnosis**

a. Electrocardiography. The ECG frequently shows low QRS voltages and nonspecific ST- and T-wave abnormalities. Conduction abnormalities are common.

b. Radiographs. Signs of pulmonary vascular congestion may coexist with normal heart size because even when left ventricular systolic function fails in the later stages of the disease, the restriction to cardiac filling prevents cardiac dilation.

c. Echocardiography

(1) The echocardiogram may demonstrate thickening of the left and right ventricles. The combination of increased left ventricular thickness on the echocardiogram and decreased left ventricular voltage on the ECG is highly suggestive of restrictive cardiomyopathy.

(2) Doppler examination may reveal evidence of abnormal ventricular diastolic filling or altered compliance.

(3) Left and right ventricular chamber sizes usually are normal, whereas the left and right atria are increased in size.

(4) In amyloidosis, the myocardium may appear brighter than normal.

d. **Cardiac catheterization.** Often it is difficult to distinguish restrictive cardiomyopathy from constrictive pericarditis.

(1) A **dip** and **plateau** in the left and right ventricular filling pressures may be seen in both diseases.

(2) In restrictive cardiomyopathy, **left and right atrial pressures** and **left and right ventricular filling pressures** usually are **not identical,** as they are in constrictive pericarditis.

(3) **Endomyocardial biopsy** during cardiac catheterization may help establish the diagnosis.

6. **Therapy.** Treatment for this group of diseases is limited.

a. In cases with a **reversible etiology** (e.g., hemochromatosis), **direct therapy** such as iron chelation may result in improvement.

b. When the cause of the disease cannot be treated, **symptomatic therapy with diuretics** to reduce the symptoms of congestion is indicated.

VI PERICARDIAL DISEASE

A Acute pericarditis

1. **Etiology**

a. **Myocardial infarction (MI).** Pericarditis may occur in the first 24 hours following transmural MI because the inflamed surface of the infarcted area of myocardium produces **pericardial irritation.** A second type of pericarditis, called **Dressler's syndrome,** also may be seen from 1 week to several months after MI and may occur as the result of an autoimmune reaction to the damaged heart muscle.

b. **Infection. Pericarditis frequently follows upper respiratory tract viral infections** and is seen in many viral infections, including HIV, hepatitis, and many more. Tuberculosis, streptococcal infection, staphylococcal infection, and the sequelae of infective endocarditis also may produce pericarditis.

c. **Collagen vascular disease.** Acute pericarditis may be a clinical manifestation of SLE, rheumatoid arthritis, or, less commonly, scleroderma.

d. **Drugs.** Commonly used drugs that may cause acute pericarditis include **procainamide, hydralazine,** and **isoniazid.**

e. **Malignancy.** Pericarditis may occur secondary to metastatic involvement of the pericardium. **Pulmonary and breast carcinomas** are the most **common primary sites.**

f. **Uremia.** Pericarditis is common in untreated or undertreated severe chronic renal failure.

g. **Postpericardiotomy syndrome.** During open heart surgery, the pericardium is incised. Usually, the pericarditis that arises from this injury is short lived; however, it may be protracted and severe in some patients.

h. **Radiation.** Radiation therapy delivered to the chest for thoracic malignancies may cause pericarditis.

2. **Clinical features**

a. **Symptoms.** The most common symptom in pericarditis is **inspiratory chest pain.**

(1) The pain is located in the left side and often is lessened when the patient sits up and leans forward.

(2) Occasionally the pain may be similar to that of myocardial ischemia and may radiate to the neck and arm.

b. **Physical signs.** The **classic sign** of acute pericarditis is the **pericardial friction rub,** which is a scratchy, leathery sound with three components corresponding to ventricular systole, early diastolic filling, and atrial contraction.

3. **Diagnosis**

a. **Physical examination.** The presence of a **pericardial friction rub** confirms the diagnosis of pericarditis.

    b. **Electrocardiography.** Epicardial inflammation produces a diffuse current of injury with ST-segment elevation throughout the ECG. There is no reciprocal ST-segment depression, as is seen in acute MI. **Depression of the PR segment is unique to pericarditis.**

    c. **Echocardiography.** The echocardiogram frequently demonstrates a pericardial effusion, which helps confirm the diagnosis.

4. Therapy

    a. **Specific therapy** should be directed toward the cause of the pericarditis, if the cause is known.

    b. **Nonsteroidal anti-inflammatory drugs (NSAIDs)** such as **aspirin, indomethacin,** and **ibuprofen** usually are effective in reducing the inflammation and relieving the chest pain.

    c. **Colchicine.** Intractable cases of pericarditis, as may occur with Dressler's syndrome and post-pericardiotomy syndrome, may require glucocorticoid therapy for relief of symptoms. Recently colchicine has replaced steroids at many centers.

B Pericardial effusion

1. Pathophysiology. The inflammation caused by acute pericarditis often produces exudation of fluid into the pericardial space. When fluid accumulates slowly, the pericardium expands to accommodate it, but when fluid accumulates rapidly, it compresses the heart, thus inhibiting cardiac filling. This latter condition is known as **cardiac tamponade** [see VI C].

2. Clinical features

    a. **Symptoms.** The mere presence of a pericardial effusion does not cause symptoms. However, symptoms of acute pericarditis may coexist with a pericardial effusion.

    b. **Physical signs.** As the effusion accumulates, it acts as a cushion around the heart.

       (1) The precordium becomes quiet, palpation of the PMI becomes difficult, and the heart tones become distant and soft.

       (2) Although the accumulation of fluid between the layers of pericardium may diminish a pericardial friction rub, a friction rub still may exist in the presence of a large effusion.

3. Diagnosis

    a. **Electrocardiography.** The ECG demonstrates low voltage; electrical alternans may be seen if a large effusion is present.

    b. **Chest radiography.** Cardiac enlargement occurs as the effusion develops. Typically, the cardiac silhouette has a **"water bottle" appearance.** The presence of an extremely enlarged heart without signs of vascular congestion suggests the diagnosis of pericardial effusion.

    c. **Echocardiography.** An echocardiogram demonstrating an **echo-free space between the two layers of the pericardium** is diagnostic of a pericardial effusion.

    d. **Pericardiocentesis.** The presence of a pericardial effusion may be confirmed by the aspiration of fluid from the pericardial sac. Examination of the fluid helps establish the cause of the effusion.

       (1) The fluid should be sent for a cell count and differential, bacterial and fungal cultures, stains and cultures for *Mycobacterium tuberculosis,* protein content, and lactate dehydrogenase (LDH) and **adenosine deaminase (ADA)** content. ADA has a very high sensitivity for extrapulmonary tuberculosis infection. **QuantiFERON-TB Gold test (QFT-G)** is a whole-blood test that can also be used to aid the diagnosis of tuberculosis infection.

       (2) An additional aliquot of fluid should be centrifuged and examined for tumor cells.

       (3) Bloody effusions are characteristic of certain etiologies (e.g., neoplasia, tuberculosis). However, bloody effusions can also occur if the needle is passed too far and ventricular blood is aspirated by mistake. It is possible to distinguish the two because ventricular blood forms clots, whereas a bloody effusion does not.

    e. **Therapy.** Treatment for a pericardial effusion is the same as that for acute pericarditis but may also involve aspiration.

C Cardiac tamponade

1. Definition and pathophysiology. Cardiac tamponade is a **life-threatening condition** in which a pericardial effusion has developed so rapidly or has become so large that it compresses the heart.

    a. The heart cannot fill adequately, and because the heart can pump out only what it takes in, impaired filling causes a profound reduction in cardiac output.

b. The external pressure produced by the fluid on the four chambers of the heart is dispersed equally. Because external pressure usually rises to a greater level than the normal cardiac filling pressures, intrapericardial pressure, left and right atrial pressures, and left and right ventricular pressures all become equal in diastole.

2. **Clinical features**
    a. **Symptoms.** Most patients with cardiac tamponade complain of **dyspnea, fatigue,** and **orthopnea.**
    b. **Physical signs**
        (1) **Pulsus paradoxus.** The normal fall in systolic blood pressure that occurs during inspiration is exaggerated in tamponade. A decrease of more than 10 mm Hg occurs in 95% of patients with cardiac tamponade. The presence of pulsus paradoxus implies that stroke volume is falling during inspiration, probably as a result of the following mechanisms:
            (a) **Septal shift.** During inspiration, right ventricular filling is augmented by negative intrathoracic pressure, which increases venous return. This causes transient enlargement of the right ventricle and pushes the ventricular septum into the left ventricle, thus reducing the size and output of the left ventricle.
            (b) **Tensing of the pericardium.** Inspiration produces downward traction on the pericardium, further compressing the cardiac structures and reducing left ventricular output.
            (c) **Right ventricular enlargement.** The enhanced right ventricular filling during inspiration also distends the right ventricle, causing it to take up more room in the pericardial space. This further limits left ventricular filling.
            (d) **Negative intrathoracic pressure.** During inspiration, the negative pressure inside the chest subtracts pressure from the extrathoracic vasculature, further reducing blood pressure.
            (e) **Expansion of the pulmonary vascular bed.** The pulmonary vascular bed expands during inspiration, increasing its capacity and thus reducing left atrial filling.
        (2) **Neck vein distention.** The intrapericardial pressure and right atrial pressure are reflected by extreme elevation of the jugular venous pressure. However, Kussmaul's sign (i.e., increased neck vein distention with inspiration) usually is absent in this condition.
        (3) **Narrowed pulse pressure.** Reduction in left ventricular stroke volume leads to a reduction in systolic pressure; the tachycardia that usually occurs as a compensatory mechanism diminishes diastolic runoff and maintains diastolic pressure. Thus, pulse pressure is narrowed; however, less severe cases of cardiac tamponade may coexist with a normal pulse pressure.
        (4) **Shock.** The carotid upstroke is diminished in volume, the systolic blood pressure is reduced, and the periphery is cold and clammy because of the vasoconstriction present in reduced cardiac output states.

3. **Diagnosis.** Elevated neck veins, pulsus paradoxus, and an enlarged cardiac silhouette on chest x-ray in a patient exhibiting symptoms of compromised cardiac output strongly suggest the diagnosis.
    a. **Echocardiography** is an indispensable tool in the evaluation of tamponade. Features consistent with tamponade include the following:
        (1) Presence of a pericardial effusion.
        (2) Collapse of the right atrium and/or right ventricle, which occurs in diastole as the pericardial pressure exceeds the intracavitary pressure.
        (3) Enhanced inspiratory transtricuspid flow and simultaneously reduced transmitral flow. This is the echo equivalent of a pulsus paradoxus.
    b. **Cardiac catheterization,** which could confirm the diastolic equalization of pressures, is less commonly used for diagnosis of tamponade.

4. **Therapy.** The only effective therapy for cardiac tamponade is removal of fluid from the pericardial sac. Thus, **emergency pericardiocentesis** is indicated. The use of **pressor agents** and **volume expansion** is of limited benefit until pericardiocentesis can be performed.

D **Constrictive pericarditis**

1. **Definition.** Constrictive pericarditis is the diffuse thickening of the pericardium in reaction to prior inflammation, which results in reduced distensibility of the cardiac chambers. Cardiac output is limited, and filling pressures are increased to match the external constrictive force placed on the heart by the pericardium.

2. **Etiology.** Most conditions that cause acute pericarditis may lead to chronic constrictive pericarditis.

3. **Clinical features**
   a. **Symptoms.** The clinical picture typically is dominated by **symptoms of right-sided failure** rather than left-sided failure.
      (1) Most patients with constrictive pericarditis complain of **dyspnea on exertion** as a result of limited cardiac output. Although approximately 50% of patients complain of **orthopnea,** paroxysmal nocturnal dyspnea is rare.
      (2) Symptoms related to systemic venous hypertension frequently are reported and include **ascites, edema,** and **jaundice.**
   b. **Physical signs**
      (1) **Jugular venous distention.** The jugular veins are distended, indicating systemic venous hypertension. Neck vein distention increases with inspiration (**Kussmaul's sign**).
      (2) **Heart sounds.** The heart sounds are distant. Early in diastole, a pericardial knock may be heard, which falls in the same cadence as an S_3 but is higher pitched and corresponds to early, abrupt cessation of ventricular filling.
      (3) **Other signs of systemic venous hypertension. Ascites, edema, hepatic tenderness,** and **hepatomegaly** are frequently present. It is not uncommon for constriction to masquerade as end-stage liver disease.

4. **Diagnosis**
   a. **Electrocardiography.** The ECG shows low voltage in the limb leads. **Atrial arrhythmias** are common.
   b. **Chest radiography** reveals **pericardial calcification** in 50% of patients. This finding is seen as a **radiopaque ring around the heart** in the lateral view. The heart usually is normal in size, although cardiomegaly occasionally is noted.
   c. **Echocardiography.** Although pericardial thickening often can be detected, reliable diagnosis of constrictive pericarditis by echocardiography is difficult. However, Doppler interrogation of the hepatic vein can show diastolic flow reversal with expiration and reversion with inspiration, which is a classic finding suggestive of constrictive pericarditis.
   d. **Magnetic resonance imaging (MRI)** gated to the cardiac cycle is an imaging technique capable of measuring pericardial thickness.
   e. **Cardiac catheterization** reveals equal pressures in the four cardiac chambers during diastole; in addition, all pressures usually are elevated.

5. **Therapy.** Surgical removal of the pericardium is curative. However, immediate relief of constrictive symptoms may not occur for up to 6 weeks after **pericardiectomy.**

VII CONGENITAL HEART DISEASE IN THE ADULT

A **Atrial septal defect** (Figure 2–12)

1. **Classification**
   a. An **ostium secundum atrial septal defect** occurs in the **midportion** of the intra-atrial septum and is caused by failure of the septum secundum to form properly.
   b. An **ostium primum atrial septal defect** results from improper septation of the endocardial cushion portion of the septum. It invariably involves the **mitral valve,** which is cleft and often regurgitant.
   c. A **sinus venosus–type atrial septal defect** occurs **high in the atrial septum** and frequently is associated with anomalous drainage of one or more of the pulmonary veins into the right atrium.
   d. **Holt–Oram syndrome** is characterized by the presence of a **secundum defect** together with **bony abnormalities of the forearms and hands.** This syndrome is a **hereditary** disease that is transmitted in an autosomal dominant fashion.

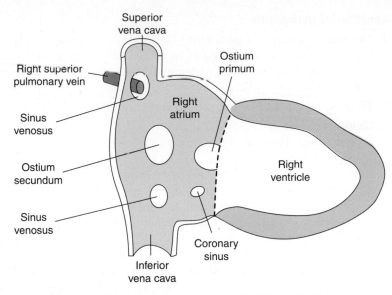

FIGURE 2–12 Atrial septal defects. Shown here are several types of atrial septal defects: sinus venosus defects of the superior vena caval (SVC) and inferior vena caval (IVC) types, ostium secundum and ostium primum defects, and a coronary sinus defect.

2. **Pathophysiology**
   a. Left and right atrial pressures usually are equal in atrial septal defect; thus, no pressure gradient exists between the atria. However, the increased thickness of the left ventricle as compared with the right ventricle makes the left ventricle less compliant and, therefore, harder to fill. Blood flow takes the path of least resistance and thus is shunted from the left atrium to the right atrium. The net effect is to increase the volume work of the right ventricle.
   b. The increased volume pumped through the pulmonary vasculature may lead to architectural changes in the pulmonary vasculature and to the development of irreversible pulmonary hypertension—a serious but rare late complication.

3. **Clinical features**
   a. **Symptoms.** Patients with atrial septal defect may have a **prolonged symptom-free period.** Eventually, symptoms develop and may include **palpitations** as a result of atrial arrhythmias, **fatigue, dyspnea on exertion, orthopnea, frequent respiratory tract infections,** and **symptoms of right ventricular failure.**
   b. **Physical signs**
      (1) **Wide and fixed splitting of the S$_2$ is the classic finding** in atrial septal defect. The increased cardiac flow through the right ventricle delays pulmonic valve closure, widening the normal splitting of the S$_2$. Inspiration produces relatively little change in right-sided flow, so there is little respiratory variation in the splitting of the S$_2$.
      (2) **Murmur.** Under low pressure, blood flow from the left to the right atrium occurs through a wide aperture and produces no turbulence or murmur. However, the increased pulmonary blood flow in atrial septal defect produces a **systolic ejection murmur,** which is **heard in the pulmonic area.** The increased flow also may produce a **diastolic rumble across the tricuspid valve** if the left-to-right shunt ratio is greater than 3:1.
      (3) **Neck vein distention, ascites,** and **edema** are indicative of right ventricular failure.

4. **Diagnosis**
   a. **Electrocardiography.** In ostium secundum defects, incomplete right bundle block and right axis deviation are common findings. Ostium primum defects usually involve the anterior fascicle of the left bundle, producing left anterior hemiblock and left axis deviation.
   b. **Chest radiography**
      (1) Increased pulmonary blood flow produces increased pulmonary vascular markings in the lungs, which is called **shunt vascularity.**
      (2) Right ventricular enlargement may encroach on the retrosternal airspace, reducing it in the lateral view.

        (3) Enlargement of the pulmonary artery segment in the posteroanterior view also may be seen.

   c. Echocardiography

        (1) The echocardiogram shows dilation of the right ventricle, and the atrial septal defect itself may be seen in many cases.

        (2) A saline injection, which carries with it microbubbles of air, shows a **negative-contrast image at the site** of the defect.

        (3) Doppler examination of the interatrial septum demonstrates the abnormal presence of left-to-right blood flow across the septum.

   d. Cardiac catheterization

        (1) During cardiac catheterization, the diagnosis can be confirmed by passage of the catheter across the atrial septal defect.

        (2) Left and right atrial pressures usually are equal.

        (3) Oxygen samples drawn from the superior vena cava and right atrium demonstrate a **step-up in oxygen concentration** in the right atrium as highly oxygenated left atrial blood is shunted into the right atrium. Oxygen saturations can be used to quantitate the magnitude of the left-to-right shunt.

5. Therapy

   a. Surgical correction, which has a low operative mortality rate, is indicated for shunts with a pulmonary-to-systemic flow ratio of greater than 2:1, even in asymptomatic patients. Shunts of this magnitude may lead to the development of pulmonary hypertension, usually become symptomatic, and worsen with age.

   b. Alternatively, several catheter-based devices for defect closure are now approved for use.

B   **Ventricular septal defect**

1. Pathophysiology. In ventricular septal defect, the left ventricle actively propels the blood into the right ventricle, resulting in the taxation of both ventricles and in increased pulmonary blood flow. Pulmonary hypertension is more severe and more frequent in ventricular septal defect than in atrial septal defect.

2. Clinical features. Because most ventricular septal defects lead to symptoms and are corrected in childhood, significant congenital ventricular septal defect rarely is diagnosed for the first time in adulthood.

   a. Symptoms of ventricular septal defect are those of both **left-** and **right-sided CHF.**

   b. Physical signs

        (1) Displacement of the PMI to the left is indicative of left ventricular enlargement.

        (2) Sternal lift is indicative of right ventricular enlargement.

        (3) Murmur. A **harsh, holosystolic murmur** is heard along the left sternal border. The murmur often is accompanied by a **thrill** and radiates to the right of the sternum.

        (4) Aortic regurgitation. Ventricular septal defects may involve the right coronary cusp of the aortic valve, producing insufficient support for this valve leaflet and, hence, aortic regurgitation. Approximately 6% of patients with ventricular septal defect have signs of aortic insufficiency.

3. Diagnosis

   a. Electrocardiography. The ECG typically shows **biventricular hypertrophy.**

   b. Chest radiography. Cardiac enlargement is the rule. If the shunt is greater than 2:1 in magnitude, **shunt vascularity** usually is present.

   c. Echocardiography. The septal defect frequently can be demonstrated during two-dimensional echocardiography. Left atrial and ventricular dilatation with right ventricular hypertrophy may be seen as well. Doppler examination reveals abnormal blood flow from the left ventricle to the right ventricle.

   d. Cardiac catheterization

        (1) A left ventriculogram obtained in the left anterior oblique position demonstrates flow of contrast from the left ventricle across the septum into the right ventricle.

        (2) During cardiac catheterization, an **oxygen step-up** occurs at the level of the right ventricle. Pulmonary hypertension, if present, can be quantified.

4. Therapy. Because patients with ventricular septal defects are prone to pulmonary vascular complications and bacterial endocarditis, ventricular septal defects with a magnitude of 2:1 or greater should be corrected surgically.

C **Patent ductus arteriosus**

1. **Pathophysiology.** In patent ductus arteriosus, blood flows from the aorta into the pulmonary artery after the takeoff of the left subclavian artery. Volume overload is imposed on the left ventricle, which must pump blood into both the systemic and pulmonary circulations and, in time, may lead to left ventricular failure. The increased pulmonary blood flow created by this lesion may lead to the development of pulmonary hypertension, imposing a pressure overload on the right ventricle.

2. **Physical signs**
   a. **Murmur.** Throughout the cardiac cycle, the vascular resistance and pressure in the pulmonary circuit are lower than the resistance and pressure in the aorta. Therefore, blood is shunted from left to right in both systole and diastole, and a **continuous murmur** with systolic and diastolic components is heard.
   b. **Pulses.** The presence of a low-pressure, low-resistance pathway allows for increased aortic runoff in diastole, which produces **bounding, full pulses** similar to those found in aortic insufficiency.

3. **Diagnosis**
   a. **Chest radiography** reveals an enlarged cardiac silhouette with the presence of shunt vascularity. In adults, the patent ductus may become calcified, rendering it visible on the chest radiograph.
   b. **Echocardiography** may reveal the patent ductus. Doppler interrogation detects abnormal flow of blood from the aorta to the pulmonary artery.
   c. **Cardiac catheterization**
      (1) During cardiac catheterization, the catheter usually can be passed from the pulmonary artery into the descending aorta, confirming the presence of a patent ductus arteriosus.
      (2) **Oximetry** can be used to quantify the magnitude of the left-to-right shunt.
      (3) **Aortography** demonstrates the flow of contrast from the aorta through the patent ductus into the pulmonary artery.
   d. **Cardiac multislice CT** or **MRI** may also demonstrate a patent ductus arteriosus.

4. **Therapy.** Catheter-based closure or surgical closure of the patent ductus is indicated in adults with a shunt ratio of greater than 2:1.

D **Coarctation of the aorta**   This defect is a stenosis of the aorta, usually at the site of the ductus arteriosus.

1. **Pathophysiology.** Coarctation of the aorta often leads to hypertension.
   a. If the stenosis is severe, it limits aortic blood flow distal to the constriction. Distal tissues are perfused by an extensive collateral arterial circulation.
   b. Whereas renal blood flow and renal function usually are normal in adults with coarctation of the aorta, the kidneys still are perfused at a subnormal blood pressure.

2. **Clinical features.** If the coarctation does not cause heart failure due to pressure overload in childhood, it may not be detected until it manifests as hypertension in the adult.
   a. **Symptoms.** Patients with coarctation may complain of **headache, claudication,** and **leg fatigue.**
   b. **Physical signs**
      (1) **Blood pressure** determined in the arms usually is elevated, whereas pulses and blood pressure in the legs usually are reduced, representing the gradient across the coarctation.
      (2) **Habitus.** The upper body usually is well developed, whereas the legs occasionally appear underdeveloped.
      (3) **Murmur.** Typically, a **midsystolic** murmur is heard over the back. If the stenosis is severe, a continuous murmur may be heard. Continuous murmurs also may be heard diffusely over the chest cavity as the result of increased flow through collateral vessels.

3. **Diagnosis**
   a. **Electrocardiography.** The ECG shows left ventricular hypertrophy.
   b. **Chest radiography. Cardiac enlargement** usually is seen. Dilation of the aorta proximal and distal to the coarctation with indentation at the site of the coarctation may cause the aorta to assume a **"figure 3" appearance.** Dilation of chest wall arteries forming the collateral pathways produces **rib notching.**
   c. **Cardiac catheterization.** During cardiac catheterization, the gradient across the coarctation can be measured. Aortography also allows visual demonstration of the coarctation.
   d. **Cardiac multislice CT** or **MRI** may also reveal a coarctation of the aorta.

4. **Therapy. Surgical correction** of the coarctation is standard therapy. **Percutaneous balloon aortoplasty** with or without stenting may be a suitable alternative for selected patients.

5. **Complications. Hypertension, infective endocarditis, dissection of the thoracic aorta,** and **rupture of cerebral (berry) aneurysms** are seen frequently. Hypertension may persist even after the coarctation is repaired.

E Ebstein's anomaly of the tricuspid valve

1. **Pathophysiology.** In Ebstein's anomaly, the septal hinge point of the tricuspid valve is abnormally apically displaced within the right ventricle. Thus, a portion of the right ventricle actually lies above the AV groove and is "atrialized," reducing the size of the right ventricle and usually resulting in **tricuspid regurgitation.** A **coexistent atrial septal defect** occurs in approximately 75% of cases.

2. **Clinical features**
   a. **Symptoms.** Depending on the degree of tricuspid regurgitation and whether an atrial septal defect exists, a patient's status may **range from asymptomatic to cyanotic.**
      (1) Dyspnea on exertion, peripheral edema, and other **symptoms of right ventricular failure** frequently are encountered.
      (2) Palpitations also are common in this anomaly, which is associated with **Wolff-Parkinson-White (WPW) syndrome** in approximately 10% of patients. WPW syndrome is characterized by abnormal ventricular conduction as the result of a congenital short circuit of the conducting system. Tachyarrhythmias are common.
   b. **Physical signs**
      (1) **Tricuspid regurgitation.** A **large v wave** in the neck veins and a pulsatile liver reflect tricuspid regurgitation.
      (2) **Heart sounds.** Wide splitting of the S_1 and S_2 is heard. Because an S_3 and an S_4 often also exist, a quadruple or quintuple cadence is a common auscultatory finding.
      (3) **Murmur.** The **holosystolic murmur of tricuspid regurgitation** is heard along the sternal border and may be accompanied by a systolic thrill.

3. **Diagnosis**
   a. **Electrocardiography.** The ECG may show evidence of WPW syndrome (a short PR interval and a slurred QRS upstroke). Other findings include right atrial enlargement and right-bundle-branch block.
   b. **Echocardiography.** The echocardiogram in Ebstein's anomaly shows exaggerated apical displacement of the septal hinge point of the tricuspid valve, which is characteristic. Tricuspid regurgitation is usually present.

4. **Therapy.** Tricuspid valve replacement and closure of the atrial septal defect may be useful in patients who have developed early signs of right ventricular failure.

F Eisenmenger's syndrome

1. **Pathophysiology.** In Eisenmenger's syndrome, which can occur with any intracardiac shunt, the **left-to-right shunt is reversed** to produce a right-to-left shunt. Reversal occurs as a result of pulmonary vascular disease that leads to increased pulmonary vascular resistance. Increased pulmonary vascular resistance leads to decreased right-sided compliance and increased right-sided pressures, which produce right-to-left shunting.

2. **Clinical features**
   a. **Cyanosis** may be constant or noted only during exercise. **Differential cyanosis** may occur in the presence of a patent ductus arteriosus; the preductal tissues (including the upper trunk) are pink, and the postductal tissues are cyanotic.
   b. **Angina.** Patients with Eisenmenger's syndrome may experience exertional chest pain, which occurs even in the presence of normal coronary arteries. Reduced myocardial oxygenation and increased right ventricular wall stress may be factors causing the symptom.
   c. **Heart failure.** Dyspnea on exertion, ascites, and peripheral edema are common.

3. **Diagnosis**
   a. **Electrocardiography.** Right ventricular hypertrophy invariably is present.
   b. **Echocardiography. Saline injection** demonstrates right-to-left shunting of microbubbles in the presence of either an atrial or a ventricular septal defect. **Doppler examination** also demonstrates the abnormal right-to-left blood flow at the site of the shunt.
   c. **Laboratory data.** Due to chronic hypoxemia, patients with Eisenmenger's syndrome are **polycythemic.** Hemoglobin concentrations in excess of 20 g/dL are common.
   d. **Cardiac catheterization.** Right-sided pressures are extremely elevated. Oximetry is used to quantitate the right-to-left shunt. Administration of 100% oxygen via a rebreathing mask does not significantly correct the arterial desaturation.

4. **Therapy.** Surgical therapy generally is not successful.
   a. **Closure of the shunt site,** which acts as an escape valve for the right ventricle, increases right ventricular pressures and causes worsening of right ventricular failure.
   b. **Phlebotomy** may be necessary to avoid hyperviscosity by maintaining the hemoglobin level at less than 20 g/dL.

VIII VENOUS THROMBOSIS

A **Deep venous thrombosis**

1. **Definition.** Deep venous thrombosis occurs when a blood clot forms in the lower extremities or in the pelvic veins. The gravity of deep venous thrombosis stems from the tendency of the thrombi to become pulmonary emboli. This tendency is especially pronounced for clots located above the popliteal fossa.

2. **Predisposing factors**
   a. **Immobilization.** The muscles in the legs act as pumps to maintain venous return from the lower extremities. Inactivity of these muscles leads to **venous stasis,** with subsequent development of **thrombophlebitis.** Stasis is likely to occur during surgery, prolonged bed rest, and prolonged periods in one position.
   b. **Venous incompetence.** Venous valvular incompetence and the presence of varicose veins increase the incidence of thrombophlebitis.
   c. **CHF.** In CHF, cardiac output is reduced, as is venous return from the legs.
   d. **Injury.** Direct mechanical injury to the lower extremities may lead to blood clot formation and the development of thrombophlebitis.
   e. **Hypercoagulable states, malignancy, estrogen use,** and **hyperviscosity syndrome** may produce a hypercoagulable state, increasing the risk of thrombophlebitis.

3. **Clinical features**
   a. **Symptoms.** The patient usually presents with **unilateral leg pain** and **swelling.**
   b. **Physical signs.** In general, the physical examination is unreliable. Tenderness on compression of the calf muscles, increased resistance during dorsiflexion of the foot (**Homans' sign**), and an increase in the circumference of the affected leg by at least 1 cm suggest the presence of deep venous thrombosis.

4. **Diagnosis**
   a. **Noninvasive studies. Impedance plethysmography** and **Doppler ultrasonography** are useful tests for the detection of deep venous thrombosis.
   b. **Invasive studies. Contrast venography** currently is the most effective way to demonstrate the area of blood clot. This technique is associated with complications, including adverse reactions to the contrast agent and postvenography thrombophlebitis.

5. **Therapy. Anticoagulants** prevent additional clot formation and allow the body's autolytic system to lyse effectively and heal deep venous thrombosis. Anticoagulation therapy is usually maintained for 3–6 months.

    a. Anticoagulation with **intravenous heparin** is indicated in the acute treatment of deep venous thrombosis. LMWH appears to be as effective as unfractionated heparin. Although the low–molecular-weight form is more expensive, it does not require laboratory monitoring. In cases of heparin-induced thrombocytopenia, a direct thrombin inhibitor should be substituted for heparin.

    b. After adequate treatment with heparin, **oral anticoagulation with warfarin** is begun.

6. **Prophylaxis.** There is substantial medical evidence that the incidence of deep venous thrombosis for hospitalized patients can be reduced by the following methods.

    a. **Rapid mobilization.** Prolonged bed rest should be avoided when possible. The increasingly rapid mobilization of patients following MI has significantly reduced the incidence of thromboembolic complications following this disease.

    b. **Increasing deep venous flow**

        (1) **Antithromboembolic stockings** and **pneumatic compression devices** compress the superficial veins, thereby increasing deep venous flow and reducing stasis and the incidence of thromboembolism.

        (2) **Foot exercises** and **avoidance of leg crossing** are further methods of preventing deep venous thrombosis.

    c. **"Minidose" heparin.** Intermittent doses of subcutaneous heparin given at 8- hour intervals inhibit factors X and XI in the clotting cascade without producing overt anticoagulation. This treatment significantly reduces the incidence of deep venous thrombosis in both medical and surgical patients on bed rest.

B **Superficial thrombophlebitis** Unlike deep venous thrombosis, in which a thrombus may break off and become a pulmonary embolism, superficial thrombophlebitis has **little potential for embolic complications.** Patients with superficial thrombophlebitis may present with a painful tender cord that can be easily palpated in the lower extremities. In the absence of concomitant deep venous thrombosis, **anticoagulation is not indicated.** Superficial thrombophlebitis is **treated with elevation of the legs,** heat, and **administration of salicylates or other NSAIDs.**

IX CARDIOVASCULAR SYNCOPE

A **Definition** Syncope is a sudden loss of consciousness of brief duration.

B **Pathophysiology** Cardiovascular syncope occurs when the brain's metabolic needs cannot be met by the available blood supply. Adequate perfusion is dependent on an adequate systemic blood pressure: $BP = CO \times SVR$, where BP is blood pressure, CO is cardiac output, and SVR is systemic vascular resistance. Therefore, a fall in cardiac output or a fall in systemic vascular resistance can precipitate a fall in blood pressure, leading to syncope. Because $CO = SV \times HR$, where SV is stroke volume and HR is heart rate, either inadequate stroke volume or inadequate heart rate reduces cardiac output, potentially leading to hypotension and syncope.

C **Etiology**

1. **Reduced cardiac output**

    a. **Bradycardia**

        (1) **Heart block.** A block in the cardiac conduction pathway may prevent the SA nodal electrical signal for ventricular contraction from being transmitted, in turn causing bradycardia. Whether syncope occurs depends on whether an alternative, lower pacemaker (e.g., the AV junction) produces an escape rate that is sufficiently fast to maintain blood pressure.

        (2) **Sick sinus syndrome** occurs when there is a deficit in impulse generation from the SA node, which may lead to bradycardia and syncope.

            (a) Profound sinus bradycardia, sinus arrest, and the tachycardia–bradycardia syndrome are the arrhythmias that constitute the sick sinus syndrome. The tachycardia–bradycardia syndrome is one of atrial instability where supraventricular tachycardia halts abruptly and is followed by severe bradycardia.

      (b) Sick sinus syndrome may result from ischemic heart disease and idiopathic or inflammatory degeneration of the SA node.

   b. Impaired stroke volume. The rhythmic filling and emptying of the left ventricle generates its stroke volume; therefore, conditions that either inhibit left ventricular filling or inhibit left ventricular emptying can severely reduce stroke volume, leading to hypotension and syncope.

    (1) Conditions that limit left ventricular filling

      (a) Obstruction to inflow. Any mechanical block in the cardiovascular system that inhibits filling of the left ventricle impairs its output. Such obstructions include mitral stenosis, left atrial myxoma, right atrial myxoma, pulmonary embolism, and pulmonic stenosis.

      (b) Tachycardia. Both ventricular tachycardia and very rapid supraventricular tachycardia reduce the diastolic filling period of the left ventricle, limiting its filling and reducing its stroke volume. In ventricular tachycardia, the shortened diastolic filling period is compounded by incomplete ventricular relaxation, which further limits filling.

      (c) Impaired systemic venous return. Failure of adequate systemic venous return to the right heart subsequently impairs its output to the left heart, impairing left ventricular stroke volume.

        (i) Typically, impaired venous return occurs when the supine patient assumes the upright posture.

        (ii) Normally, the tendency for gravity-induced venous pooling of blood in the legs is offset by venous vasoconstriction, which helps maintain venous return. However, in the face of dehydration, antihypertensive drugs, or autonomic dysfunction, impaired venous return may produce **orthostatic syncope.** Autonomic dysfunction may be idiopathic, familial, surgically induced, or result from diabetes, alcoholism, or pyridoxine deficiency.

    (2) Conditions that impair left ventricular emptying. The left ventricle may be impaired from emptying either as a result of a severe, sudden depression in myocardial contractile function or as a result of outflow obstruction.

      (a) Decreased myocardial contractility. The sudden and severe degree of contractile depression required to cause syncope is almost invariably caused by global ischemia produced by left main or triple-vessel coronary disease, acute MI, ventricular tachycardia, or ventricular fibrillation.

      (b) Obstruction to outflow. Obstruction of left ventricular outflow that produces syncope is caused by valvular aortic stenosis and hypertrophic cardiomyopathy.

 2. Reduced total peripheral resistance. If cardiac output is maintained but total peripheral resistance falls, blood pressure also falls, potentially causing syncope.

   a. An inappropriate fall in total peripheral resistance is usually operative in the **common fainting spell.** Increased blood flow to the skeletal muscles due to a fall in total peripheral resistance may divert flow from the brain and result in fainting. Venodilation and relative bradycardia may further compound the **"vasovagal faint"** by reducing venous return and cardiac output.

   b. Reduced total peripheral resistance leading to syncope may also occur in drug-induced, familial, or idiopathic autonomic dysfunction.

 D **Diagnosis** A single fainting episode or episode of light-headedness occurs in more than 50% of the population at some point in a lifetime. It would be impossible to explore the cause of the event extensively in every affected patient. A good history and physical examination should be adequate to exclude potentially serious causes of a single episode of syncope. However, recurrent syncope requires a more extensive workup.

 1. History. A thorough patient interview can reveal clues that may point to a specific etiology for the recurrent syncope.

   a. A history of palpitations might indicate an arrhythmia.

   b. The observation that syncope occurred upon assumption of an upright position suggests orthostatic hypotension.

   c. A history of chest pain might indicate an ischemic event or pulmonary embolism.

   d. A change in antihypertensive medication or a recent episode of dehydration are additional clues.

  e. A history of a prior MI and reduced left ventricular function suggests the possibility of a ventricular arrhythmia.

2. Physical examination. Those maneuvers that might reveal a reason for hypotension and possible syncope should be emphasized.

  a. Blood pressure

   (1) The blood pressure should be recorded in both arms in both the supine and the sitting or standing positions.

   (2) On assuming an upright posture, it is normal for a patient's systolic blood pressure to fall slightly while diastolic pressure increases. There is also usually a slight increase in heart rate.

    (a) A frank decline in systolic and diastolic pressure on assuming an upright posture may indicate volume depletion or sympathetic compensation that is inadequate to counteract the change in posture.

    (b) A fall in diastolic pressure of more than 10 mm Hg is significant and may suggest an orthostatic etiology of the syncope.

  b. Heart rate and rhythm. The pulse should be examined for an extended period of time in an effort to detect arrhythmia or bradycardia.

  c. Valvular obstruction. The murmurs and physical findings associated with mitral stenosis, aortic stenosis, pulmonic stenosis, or idiopathic hypertrophic subaortic stenosis should be recognized as indications of potentially correctable mechanisms for syncope.

  d. Thromboembolism. Thrombophlebitis in the lower limbs indicates a source of pulmonary emboli, which can cause syncope. Physical evidence that a pulmonary embolus is present includes wheezing, increased intensity of the pulmonary component of the S_2, and jugular venous distention.

3. Electrocardiography. If second- or third-degree AV block is detected, it demonstrates the likely cause of the syncope. Bundle-branch block, arrhythmias, or both on the standard ECG should raise suspicion that heart block or arrhythmia are syncopal etiologies.

4. Holter monitoring. If the history, physical examination, and ECG point to an arrhythmia as the potential cause of the syncope, Holter monitoring may be performed. It records each heart beat over a 24-hour period, which is then reviewed for arrhythmia. Unfortunately, because most arrhythmias occur sporadically, most Holter monitor examinations are negative even when an arrhythmia is the source of the syncope.

5. Event monitors. These devices are worn or carried for several weeks. They are activated by the patient at the time of symptoms and document the rhythm before and after activation. The recording is then reviewed for arrhythmia.

6. Electrophysiologic testing. If the initial workup demonstrates that heart disease is present but fails to demonstrate a specific cause of syncope, electrophysiologic stimulation may provoke the arrhythmia responsible for the syncope. With an arrhythmic cause established, the proper therapy may then be instituted.

E **Therapy**

1. Therapy for bradyarrhythmias. When a bradyarrhythmia has been established as the cause of the syncope, drug-induced bradycardia should be ruled out as a cause by discontinuing potentially offending drugs. If symptomatic bradycardia persists, a permanent pacemaker is indicated.

2. Therapy for tachyarrhythmias

  a. Drug therapy for both ventricular and supraventricular tachyarrhythmias that have caused an episode of syncope is clearly indicated [see II D 1 b (3)]. In general, such therapy should be guided by electrophysiologic testing.

  b. Antitachycardia pacemakers or **implantable defibrillators** may be used to electrically correct arrhythmias if drug therapy fails.

3. Therapy for autonomic dysfunction. If autonomic dysfunction is the cause of orthostatic hypotension and syncope, little can be done directly to treat the underlying cause. Instead, therapies to protect the patient from possible hypotension should be instituted. These include high salt intake or fludrocortisone to ensure volume expansion, support stockings to prevent venous pooling, or midodrine to increase peripheral vascular resistance. There may be a role for permanent cardiac pacing in a select group of patients for whom other forms of therapy have failed.

4. **Correction of mechanical obstructions to cardiac inflow or outflow.** Any fixed valvular lesion that has caused an episode of syncope should be corrected. If idiopathic hypertrophic subaortic stenosis is determined to be the cause of the syncope, standard therapy with propranolol or verapamil is indicated to reduce the amount of outflow obstruction. If medical therapy fails, myomectomy or alcohol septal ablation may be necessary.

Study Questions

A 52-year-old man presents with fever, chills, and arthralgia. On physical examination: temperature is 102.2°F, pulse is 106 bpm, blood pressure is 100/60 mm Hg, and respiratory rate is 22. S_1 is soft. There is a short II/VI diastolic blowing murmur at the left sternal border. There are no rashes or petechiae. The results of the rest of the examination are unremarkable.

1. What is the most likely diagnosis?
   - (A) Viral syndrome with flow murmur
   - (B) Acute systemic lupus erythematosus with aortic valve involvement
   - (C) Infective endocarditis of the aortic valve with probably mild insufficiency
   - (D) Infective endocarditis of the mitral valve
   - (E) Infective endocarditis of the aortic valve with probably severe insufficiency

2. Which of the following statements is true of the condition of the patient in question 1?
   - (A) The cardiac physical examination is hyperdynamic.
   - (B) S_1 is soft because of aortic valve preclosure.
   - (C) Mitral valve preclosure indicates a poor prognosis without aortic valve replacement.
   - (D) The appearance of a diastolic murmur is usually benign.
   - (E) Hill's sign is a good predictor of severity.

3. The diagnostic test(s) that should be performed next is/are
   - (A) A chest x-ray
   - (B) Blood cultures
   - (C) Cardiac catheterization
   - (D) A radionuclide ventriculogram
   - (E) Exploratory thoracotomy

A 56-year-old man enters the emergency department complaining of dyspnea that began about 3 weeks ago and has progressed so that he now has difficulty walking across a room. He has begun sleeping on three pillows. On physical examination: temperature is 99°F, pulse is 102 bpm, blood pressure is 130/90 mm Hg, and respiratory rate is 24. There is jugular venous distention, and estimated central venous pressure is 10 cm H_2O. Other findings include bibasilar rales and an S_3 gallop.

4. What is the most likely diagnosis in this patient?
   - (A) Pulmonary embolism
   - (B) Congestive heart failure
   - (C) Emphysema
   - (D) Pneumonia
   - (E) Atrial septal defect

5. Which of the following tests is most appropriate to aid in establishing therapy for this patient?
   - (A) A chest x-ray
   - (B) An echocardiogram
   - (C) An electrocardiogram
   - (D) A heart catheterization
   - (E) A radionuclide ventriculogram

6. Which of the following is true about the treatment of the condition of the patient in question 4?
   - (A) The cause of the condition should be treated whenever possible.
   - (B) Systolic versus diastolic dysfunction usually cannot be established.
   - (C) ACE inhibitors improve symptoms but do not prolong life.
   - (D) Diuretics are the court of last resort.
   - (E) β-Blockers are dangerous and should be avoided.

On a routine office visit, a 45-year-old man complains that recently he has noted right-sided chest pain while mowing his lawn with a push lawn mower. The pain develops suddenly, lasts 2–3 minutes, and subsides when he rests. He denies smoking or a history of hypertension, diabetes, or hyperlipidemia. His physical examination is unremarkable. An ECG shows nonspecific T-wave abnormalities.

7. This patient most likely has which of the following?

   A Angina pectoris
   B Hiatal hernia
   C Pleuritis
   D A nonspecific chest pain syndrome
   E There is not enough information to arrive at a diagnosis.

8. What should be the next step in establishing the diagnosis for this patient?

   A Repeat the ECG.
   B Perform a cardiac catheterization.
   C Obtain cardiac enzymes and a troponin level.
   D Perform a stress ECG.
   E Perform a stress echocardiogram.

9. If coronary disease is found in this patient, indications for surgical revascularization would include which of the following?

   A Occasional angina
   B Left main coronary stenosis of 20%
   C Three-vessel coronary artery disease with left ventricular systolic dysfunction
   D Disease of the right and circumflex arteries
   E A severe lesion in one coronary artery

A 56-year-old man with a history of hypertension is seen for the evaluation of chest pain that began an hour ago. The pain was centered in the left side of the chest and radiates to the left arm. It was associated with nausea and vomiting. His physical examination findings are:

   Blood pressure 80/60 mm Hg, pulse 58 bpm, and respiratory rate 16
   Chest: clear
   Heart: no gallops or murmurs
   ECG: acute anterior myocardial infarction and sinus bradycardia

10. What should be the next step in management of this patient?

   A Insertion of a temporary pacemaker
   B Administration of nitrates
   C Fluid resuscitation
   D Insertion of an intra-aortic balloon pump
   E Administration of a β-blocker

11. After the patient in question 10 is stabilized, he should:

   A Be transferred to the critical care unit
   B Undergo immediate percutaneous coronary angioplasty if available
   C Receive warfarin
   D Receive nifedipine
   E Receive intravenous lidocaine

12. On the second hospital day, the patient becomes diaphoretic and hypotensive. A III/VI holosystolic murmur is heard. Which of the following is likely?

   A He has developed pericardial tamponade.
   B There has been acute ventricular septal rupture.
   C He has an acute atrial septal defect.
   D He has developed mitral valve endocarditis.
   E The murmur was old but obscured by the reduced cardiac output from his MI.

13. Ultimately this patient's prognosis will be determined most by which of the following?

[A] The amount of myocardial damage he has sustained.
[B] His LDL cholesterol level
[C] His HDL cholesterol level
[D] The ratio of LDL to HDL cholesterol
[E] Blood pressure control

A 25-year-old woman presents with chest pain that worsens when she inspires. Her physical examination findings are blood pressure of 120/70 mm Hg; pulse 76 bpm; respiratory rate 14; and heart, three-component friction rub.

14. Which of the following statements is true of the friction rub?

[A] It is generated by movement of the parietal and visceral layers of the pericardium.
[B] It is generated by the visceral layers of the pericardium and pleura.
[C] It indicates the absence of an effusion.
[D] It indicates that the cause of the pericarditis is a malignancy.
[E] It often persists through effective therapy.

15. What would be the best first-line therapy for the patient in question 14?

[A] Acetaminophen
[B] Aspirin
[C] Ibuprofen
[D] Prednisone
[E] Colchicine

16. Several days later, the patient develops dyspnea and jugular venous distension. The likely diagnosis now is:

[A] Right-sided heart failure
[B] Myocardial infarction
[C] Pulmonary embolism
[D] Pericardial tamponade
[E] Pneumonia

A 75-year-old man complains of chest pain while climbing stairs. On physical examination, there is a II/VI systolic ejection murmur that radiates to the neck. The carotid upstrokes are delayed and diminished in volume.

17. The most likely diagnosis is:

[A] Hypertrophic cardiomyopathy
[B] Aortic stenosis
[C] Mitral stenosis
[D] Pulmonary stenosis
[E] Vasovagal syncope

18. The best test to confirm the diagnosis is:

[A] An ECG
[B] An exercise stress test
[C] An echocardiogram
[D] A radionuclide ventriculogram
[E] A chest x-ray

19. The recommended therapy is:

[A] Urgent aortic valve replacement
[B] An ACE inhibitor

C Nitroglycerin
D A calcium channel blocker
E A β-blocker

A murmur is detected on the routine examination of a 35-year-old woman. She is entirely asymptomatic and engages in aerobic exercise classes without difficulty. On physical examination, there is II/VI systolic ejection murmur heard best in the left second interspace. S_1 is normal. S_2 is widely split and does not vary with respiration.

20. The likely diagnosis is:
A Pulmonary stenosis
B Aortic stenosis
C Ventricular septal defect
D Atrial septal defect
E A flow (innocent) murmur

21. Which of the following is true about this abnormality?
A This abnormality, when identified, should always be repaired.
B All types of this defect are associated with an increased risk of endocarditis.
C Uncorrected, this defect may lead to pulmonary hypertension and right heart failure.
D Ventricular arrhythmias are frequently associated with this abnormality.
E The murmur is due to turbulent flow across the defect.

A 50-year-old man presents with mild dyspnea on exertion of recent onset. He was told that he had "a murmur" during childhood, but he has not seen a physician in many years. On examination, his pulses are bounding and his blood pressure is 160/60 mm Hg. S_1 is soft and S_2 is normal. There is a soft apical diastolic low-pitched rumble heard at the apex, and there is a diastolic decrescendo murmur heard along the left sternal border extending to S_1. Chest x-ray demonstrates cardiomegaly.

22. The most likely diagnosis is:
A Aortic stenosis
B Aortic insufficiency
C Mitral stenosis
D Mitral insufficiency
E Mixed aortic insufficiency and mitral stenosis

23. An echocardiogram confirms your clinical suspicions. The left ventricular function is normal, but the left ventricle is dilated to 6 cm at end-systole. You should recommend which of the following treatments?
A Careful titration of a β-blocker
B Afterload reduction with an ACE inhibitor
C Mitral valve replacement
D Aortic valve replacement
E Mitral and aortic valve replacement

A 35-year-old white woman enters the emergency department complaining of episodic chest pain that usually lasts for 5–10 minutes. Sometimes it is related to exercise, but on other occasions it occurs at rest. The pain does not radiate. The woman is a nonsmoker and has no history of hypertension. Two other family members have died of heart disease, one at 50 years of age and the other at 56 years of age. On physical examination, the patient is in no acute distress. Her blood pressure is 120/70 mm Hg, and her pulse is 70 bpm. Examination of the precordium finds that the PMI is forceful. There is a II/VI systolic ejection murmur heard along the left sternal border that increases in intensity when the patient stands up. The ECG shows nonspecific ST-segment and T-wave abnormalities.

24. Which of the following is the most likely diagnosis?

    A. Innocent flow murmur
    B. Aortic stenosis
    C. Hypertrophic cardiomyopathy
    D. Mitral stenosis
    E. Pulmonic stenosis

25. Which of the following tools would be best to use when diagnosing this patient?

    A. Chest radiograph
    B. Cardiac catheterization
    C. Thallium scanning
    D. Echocardiography
    E. Myocardial biopsy

26. Which of the following therapies is most appropriate for this patient?

    A. Immediate surgery
    B. A β-blocker
    C. Vasodilators
    D. Digoxin
    E. Furosemide

27. Which of the following is true regarding percutaneous coronary intervention?

    A. There is no benefit over the use of intravenous thrombolytic agents for the treatment of acute myocardial infarction.
    B. In patients with stable anginal symptoms it provides symptom relief and a mortality benefit.
    C. Stents bonded with drugs such as sirolimus or paclitaxel have eliminated the risk of restenosis.
    D. One third of patients who undergo balloon angioplasty alone will develop restenosis within 6 months.
    E. Periprocedural administration of glycoprotein IIb/IIIa antagonists enhances short-term but not long-term patency rates and clinical success.

Answers and Explanations

1. The answer is E [IV C 3 b (2)]. The diastolic murmur is typical of that of aortic insufficiency. The fever chills and arthralgia suggest infection, making infective endocarditis the most likely diagnosis. The soft S_1 suggests mitral valve preclosure, indicating severe disease. This syndrome could be seen in acute lupus, but this is less likely in a man without other evidence of the disease. Increased flow from any cause does not produce aortic insufficiency. A lesion on the mitral valve creates systolic, not diastolic, murmurs.

2. The answer is C [IV C 3 b]. Mitral valve preclosure, caused by high ventricular diastolic filling pressure greater than left atrial pressure, indicates severe disease that is usually fatal without aortic valve replacement. In acute aortic insufficiency such as that seen in endocarditis, left ventricular dilation has not yet occurred, stroke volume is not increased very much, and thus the circulation is not hyperdynamic. Therefore Hill's sign is also absent. In general, diastolic murmurs are not benign and indicate valve pathology.

3. The answer is B [IV C 4]. Blood cultures to confirm a bloodstream infection and echocardiography to identify valve lesions and valve function are the mainstays of diagnosis in infective endocarditis. Although a chest x-ray might be useful, it is never diagnostic of endocarditis. Valve surgery would not be contemplated without the diagnosis of endocarditis being established first. Cardiac catheterization is rarely indicated in endocarditis today because echocardiography provides more information more safely. A radionuclide ventriculogram would give information about cardiac performance but would not confirm the diagnosis.

4. The answer is B [I D 1–2]. The gradual onset of dyspnea, the pulmonary rales, and the S_3 gallop are all typical of congestive heart failure. Although a pulmonary embolus could cause all of the findings in this patient, even a right-sided S_3, sudden onset is the norm in that condition. The other conditions all could cause dyspnea but would not cause gallop rhythm.

5. The answer is B [I E 3]. An echocardiogram will yield data about systolic and diastolic function, chamber size, and valvular abnormalities. All of the other tests are useful, but all except catheterization give less information than the echocardiogram. Cardiac catheterization has a higher risk and is only employed when the information gained outweighs that risk. Thus, in CHF, echocardiography provides the "biggest bang for the buck."

6. The answer is A [I F 1]. Congestive heart failure is a syndrome, and its cause should be sought and treated directly whenever possible. It is usually helpful to establish whether the root cause is systolic or diastolic dysfunction, a distinction made easily with echocardiography. Diuretics form the mainstay of therapy, but adding both ACE inhibitors and β-blockers prolongs life.

7. The answer is E [III A 5 a (1)]. His presentation with exertional pain is typical of angina, but the location, duration, and lack of risk factors are atypical. No diagnosis can be made based on this information.

8. The answer is E [III A 5 a (3) (c)]. A stress echocardiogram will give information about cardiac function and the presence of coronary disease (90% sensitivity). Repeating the ECG is unlikely to give new information. The brevity of the pain makes it very unlikely that myocardial damage has occurred, and thus troponin is likely to be normal. The stress ECG will be of limited use because the resting ECG is already abnormal. Cardiac catheterization could be employed, but because of its invasive nature, it is usually not the first step in arriving at a diagnosis.

9. The answer is C [III A 5 a (4) (e)]. Surgical revascularization has shown a mortality benefit for patients with disease of $>70\%$ of all three epicardial coronary arteries and associated left ventricular dysfunction. In addition, a mortality benefit has been shown for patients with $>50\%$ stenosis of the left main coronary artery, irrespective of ventricular function. Given the risks of surgical revascularization, medical therapy and/or percutaneous intervention should be considered first for patients who are not likely to experience a mortality benefit from bypass surgery.

10. The answer is C [III A 5 b (4)]. The patient is hypotensive, as he has no signs of volume overload or heart failure; thus, fluid resuscitation should be performed first. Although both β-blockers and nitrates are indicated in MI, their use here would only exacerbate the hypotension. A pacemaker might improve blood pressure, but only if AV sequential pacing were used, a sometimes complex procedure. In fact, pacemakers are rarely used for mild sinus bradycardia. Intra-aortic balloon pumping would be used only if other measures failed to restore blood pressure.

11. The answer is B [III A 5 b (4) (b)]. If acute angioplasty is available, it should be performed immediately to restore coronary blood flow without transferring the patient to the coronary care unit (CCU) because every minute counts in preserving myocardium. Dihydropyridine calcium channel blockers such as nifedipine are contraindicated in MI because they increase mortality. Lidocaine is no longer used prophylactically against cardiac arrhythmias because of possible cardiac standstill. Although heparin is an essential part of therapy, warfarin, which takes days to become effective, is not.

12. The answer is B [III A 5 b (6) (f)]. Hemodynamic decompensation and a new cardiac murmur after MI indicate either acute ventricular septal rupture or acute mitral valve dysfunction. Atrial septal defect is not a consequence of MI. There is no indication that the patient has developed endocarditis. If anything, the patient's output has been still further reduced, as indicated by his change in vital signs. There are no signs of tamponade, such as pulsus paradoxus or neck vein distention.

13. The answer is A [III A 5 b (5) (a)]. Prognosis is dependent most on the amount of muscle damage (and therefore the amount the ventricular dysfunction that develops), the patient's age, and the extent of coronary disease. Although improving the status of known coronary risk factors such as hyperlipidemia and hypertension reduces subsequent risk, the effect on prognosis is not as large as are muscle damage, age, and extent of disease.

14. The answer is A [VI A 2 b]. The rub is caused by movement of the inflamed parietal and visceral layers of the pericardium. A rub is indicative of pericarditis from any cause and does not imply malignancy. Rubs can still occur even when an effusion separates the two layers of the pericardium. Rubs usually disappear with effective therapy.

15. The answer is C [VI A 4]. Nonsteroidal anti-inflammatory drugs (NSAIDs) such as ibuprofen form the first line of therapy. High-dose aspirin is effective but is more likely to cause gastrointestinal tract side effects. Although acetaminophen might relieve the pain, it would not treat the inflammation. Prednisone and colchicine are reserved for NSAID failures.

16. The answer is D [VI C 2]. The onset of dyspnea and neck vein distention should immediately trigger concern for tamponade in a patient with known pericarditis. As fluid builds up in the pericardial sac, it compresses the heart, limits its output, and raises the pressure in all four cardiac chambers—hence the neck vein distention. Although MI, right-sided failure, pulmonary embolism, and pneumonia are all possible occurrences, there are no findings to confirm their presence in this otherwise healthy young woman.

17. The answer is B [IV A 3 a–b]. The murmur and delayed carotid upstrokes are typical of the fixed LV outflow obstruction of aortic stenosis. Pulmonary stenosis also can cause chest pain and a systolic ejection murmur but would not cause carotid delay. Hypertrophic cardiomyopathy causes a spike and dome of the carotid upstrokes, that is, a sharp upstroke followed by fall and a flatter secondary rise. The murmur of mitral stenosis is diastolic. Although the syncope could have been attributable to a vasovagal faint, this could only be a diagnosis of exclusion in the face of obvious aortic stenosis.

18. The answer is C [IV A 4 b]. Echocardiography with Doppler interrogation of the valve will show the aortic stenosis, quantify its severity, and assess left ventricular function. The ECG and chest x-ray are nonspecific in this disease. Although useful in asymptomatic patients, stress testing is dangerous in symptomatic aortic stenosis. A radionuclide study would give information about left ventricular function but not about lesion severity.

19. The answer is A [IV A 5 b]. The only accepted therapy for symptomatic aortic stenosis is aortic valve replacement. Nitrates can be used cautiously for angina until the valve is replaced, but only as a temporizing measure. The other agents listed could cause hypotension and should not be used.

20. The answer is D [VII A 3 b]. The widely split S_2 that does not vary with respiration is pathognomonic of atrial septal defect. The murmur is caused by increased flow across the pulmonic valve, which is not stenotic. The murmur of a ventricular septal defect is holosystolic. The murmur of aortic stenosis is associated with a soft single S_2 because the aortic valve neither opens nor closes well.

21. The answer is C [VII A 3 a]. Atrial septal defects may occur in different locations and may be of different sizes. Large, nonrestrictive defects may lead to pulmonary hypertension and eventual right-sided heart failure if left uncorrected. Not all atrial septal defects are associated with an increased incidence of endocarditis. Endocarditis is more common in ostium primum atrial septal defects due the associated abnormality of the anterior mitral valve (cleft mitral valve). Ostium secundum defects, the most common type, are not associated with an increased risk. Atrial arrhythmias commonly occur late in the natural history of the disease, but ventricular arrhythmias are not commonly associated with atrial septal defects. The murmur associated with an atrial septal defect is due to the relative increase in blood flow across the pulmonic valve and is not directly related to shunt flow across the atrial septal defect.

22. The answer is B [IV C 1–2]. The bounding pulses and widened pulse pressure are characteristic of significant aortic insufficiency and represent both the increased stroke volume and the enhanced aortic "run-off" due to the incompetent valve. Because of retrograde diastolic flow across the aortic valve into the left ventricle, the left ventricular diastolic pressure rises rapidly, leading to a nearly or completely closed mitral valve at the time of ventricular systole, accounting for the soft S_1. In mitral stenosis, S_1 is usually loud until very late stages of the disease. The "preclosure" of the mitral valve is also possibly the cause of a relative mitral stenosis/diastolic rumble, termed the "Austin Flint" murmur. Cardiomegaly is present in the volume-overloaded state of severe aortic insufficiency. By comparison, the left ventricle is protected from volume overload with pure mitral stenosis, and it is generally small in size.

23. The answer is D [IV C 5]. Patients with severe aortic valvular insufficiency with left ventricular dilation to this degree should be referred for aortic valve replacement. Medical therapy at this point is more likely to result in worse postoperative left ventricular function and more symptoms of heart failure. The use of β-blockers in patients with significant aortic insufficiency is controversial, as they prolong the diastolic interval and therefore may increase the regurgitant fraction of blood. Afterload reduction in patients with significant aortic regurgitation but without this degree of ventricular dilation would be prudent and can delay left ventricular dilation and compromise of function.

24. The answer is C [V B 4]. The most likely diagnosis is hypertrophic cardiomyopathy, as evidenced by the increased intensity of the systolic ejection murmur when the patient stands. When a patient with hypertrophic cardiomyopathy stands, blood pools in the legs, decreasing left ventricular size and bringing the anterior leaflet of the mitral valve in closer contact with the hypertrophied ventricular septum. This increases the obstruction and makes the murmur louder. Conversely, innocent flow murmurs and the murmurs associated with pulmonic and aortic stenosis decrease when the patient stands because the temporary pooling of central volume in the legs decreases forward cardiac output, thereby decreasing turbulent flow in the valve. The murmur of mitral stenosis is a diastolic murmur, not a systolic murmur.

25. The answer is D [V B 5 b]. The echocardiogram is a highly effective diagnostic tool in hypertrophic cardiomyopathy, provided the patient can be visualized adequately. Asymmetric hypertrophy of the septum compared with the free cardiac wall confirms the diagnosis. If obstruction is present, there will also be systolic anterior motion of the mitral valve. There are no particular features of hypertrophic cardiomyopathy demonstrable on a chest radiograph. Thallium scintigraphy may show the hypertrophied septum, but this is not the optimum form of imaging. Cardiac catheterization can certainly confirm the diagnosis, but this invasive test needs to be performed in only a minority of patients when echocardiography cannot adequately visualize the patient's heart.

26. The answer is B [V B 6 a]. Symptoms of hypertrophic cardiomyopathy may be relieved with propranolol, a β-adrenergic blocking agent. By decreasing heart rate, propranolol allows increased left ventricular filling, thereby increasing separation of the anterior leaflet of the mitral valve and the septum and reducing the amount of obstruction. Unlike valvular aortic stenosis (where death may be imminent after the development of symptoms unless surgery is performed) in hypertrophic cardiomyopathy, there is no evidence that surgery prolongs life. Both digoxin (by increasing the force of that contraction) and furosemide (by decreasing left ventricular size) would worsen the obstruction and likely exacerbate the patient's symptoms.

27. The answer is D [III A 5 a (4) (d) (ii)]. The restenosis rate associated with balloon angioplasty alone is 33% within 6 months. Stents were developed, in part, to decrease the incidence of restenosis. While they have achieved this goal, they have not eliminated the risk totally. The use of glycoprotein IIb/IIIa antagonists has improved both short- and long-term clinical success rates and angiographic patency rates. When percutaneous intervention is readily accessible for patients undergoing treatment for acute myocardial infarction, the angiographic patency rates and clinical outcomes are better with the use of direct PCI. Patients with stable anginal symptoms may have symptomatic benefit from PCI but do not enjoy a mortality benefit related to the procedure.

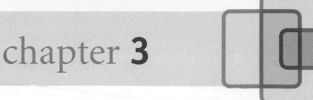

chapter 3

Pulmonary Diseases

LEANN SILHAN • NEVINS TODD

I PULMONARY FUNCTION STUDIES AND PULMONARY PHYSIOLOGY

(Online Figures 3–1 to 3–4; Online Table 3–1)

II APPROACH TO PATIENT WITH PULMONARY DISEASE

A Introduction

1. The approach to pulmonary disease diagnosis consists of the history, physical exam, physiologic testing (pulmonary function tests), radiologic imaging (chest x-ray and computed tomography), and lung pathology.

B History

1. Within the **history of present illness (HPI)** it is important to enquire about **cough** (productive or nonproductive, type of sputum, hemoptysis), **chest pain** (pleuritic or nondescript), **dyspnea** (at rest or only with exertion), and **constitutional symptoms** (fever, malaise, anorexia, weight loss, night sweats).

2. In the **past medical history,** it is important to note history of connective tissue diseases, previous malignancy and history of chemotherapy or radiation, and current and previous medications (including herbal and over-the-counter medications), as many drugs can have pulmonary toxicities.

3. **Family history** should include malignancy, cystic fibrosis, asthma, and infectious disease history.

4. **Social history** is very important in pulmonary medicine and includes the following: smoking history—current or previous smoking, amount (in pack-years: multiply number of years by packs per day); illicit substance abuse; alcohol use (enough to pass out?—risk of aspiration); HIV risk factors (sexual history, intravenous drug use); occupational history (exposure to silica, asbestos, chemicals, farming); hobbies (birds, animals); and recent travel history.

C Physical Exam

1. **Vital signs** may reveal dyspnea (labored breathing) or tachypnea (respiratory rate >25 breaths/minute), tachycardia (heart rate >100 bpm), and fever (temperature >38°C or 100.4°F).

2. **Inspection** should examine for "pursed-lip" breathing and accessory muscle breathing (use of sternocleidomastoid, scalene, and abdominal muscles may have paradoxical breathing: abdomen abnormally goes in with inspiration and out with exhalation). A blue hue to the lips and digits is called cyanosis. Clubbing of the digits is a "spongy" enlargement of the fingertips and is a result of unknown physiology. The chest wall can show a "barrel chest," pectus excavatum, pectus carinatum, or kyphoscoliosis.

3. **Palpation** includes palpation for a deviated trachea (displacement of the trachea to the left or right of midline), crepitus (a crackly feeling of the subcutaneous tissue, like bubble wrap), and tactile fremitus (having the patient say "O" or "99" and feeling increased vibration on the chest wall). There is increased fremitus when there is consolidation of the underlying lung, that is, pneumonia. There is decreased fremitus with pathologies that move the lung away from the chest wall—pleural effusion or pneumothorax.

4. **Percussion** is performed by tapping the opposite-hand flattened finger against the chest wall. Normal is resonant. Hyperresonant is hypertympanic and indicates increased air (pneumothorax or hyperinflation). Dullness or "flat" signifies consolidation of the underlying lung, atelectasis, or a pleural effusion.

5. **Auscultation** with the stethoscope should reveal "vesicular" breath sounds, during which one should hear the inspiration clearly but only the initial portion of expiration. Bronchial breath sounds are abnormal and reveal prominent expiratory breath sounds, sometimes more prominent than inspiratory sounds. This is normal if one listens over the trachea but abnormal in the lung. It implies consolidation of the lung (pneumonia). Decreased breath sounds are heard with pneumothorax, effusion, emphysema, or atelectasis. Stridor is heard over the trachea and is a course wheeze heard in the neck and is due to upper airway narrowing (laryngeal narrowing as in anaphylaxis). Crackles or rales are heard at end-inspiration and reflect closed alveoli opening due to diffuse parenchymal fibrosis or pulmonary edema. Terms that can be applied to crackles are wet, dry, fine, coarse, or Velcro-like. Wheezing is a high-pitched musical sound that is heard mostly during expiration, signifying bronchospasm with asthma or chronic obstructive pulmonary disease. Voice-generated sounds include egophony and pectoriloquy. Egophony is performed with the stethoscope on the chest wall and having the patient say "eeeee." If the "eeeee" sounds convert to "aaaay" sounds, there is positive egophony. Pectoriloquy is also performed with the stethoscope against the chest wall and is positive if the area against the stethoscope accentuates the whispered sound so that it is louder. Both egophony and pectoriloquy signify consolidation of the underlying lung. A pleural friction rub is a scratchy or creaking sound that occurs with inspiration and expiration and signifies an inflamed visceral and parietal pleura rubbing together.

D **Pulmonary function tests** 🖰 Online Section I discusses interpretation of pulmonary function tests (PFT).

E **Radiologic imaging** consists of chest x-ray (CXR) and chest computed tomography (CT). CXR is best performed with a posterior–anterior (PA) and lateral view with the patient upright. An alternative method with the patient partially upright is the anterior–posterior (AP) view, with which the cardiac and mediastinal elements will appear enlarged. CT is much more detailed and can be done with or without intravenous (IV) contrast dye.

F **Pulmonary pathology** Specimens can be obtained via bronchoscopy (most commonly), transthoracic needle biopsy, or video-assisted thoracic surgery (VATS). Tests include sputum or lavage staining, cytology, and tissue biopsy with fine cuts and staining.

III   CHRONIC OBSTRUCTIVE PULMONARY DISEASE (COPD)

A **Introduction**

1. **Definition.** Chronic obstructive pulmonary disease is defined as a disease state characterized by the presence of airflow obstruction that is not fully reversible. The diagnosis is established by PFTs. The airflow obstruction is generally progressive and may be accompanied by increased airway reactivity (Figure 3–5). COPD is a common disorder, usually characterized by progressive obstruction to airflow and a history of inhalation of irritants (e.g., tobacco smoke). COPD also is referred to as **chronic obstructive lung disease (COLD), chronic airway obstruction (CAO),** and, either individually or together, as chronic bronchitis and emphysema.
   a. **Chronic bronchitis** is defined in terms of clinical symptoms, and is characterized by excessive secretion of mucus in the bronchial tree leading to productive cough for at least 3 months in two successive years.
   b. **Emphysema** is a lung condition characterized by permanent, abnormal enlargement of air spaces distal to the terminal bronchiole and accompanied by the destruction of bronchiole and alveolar walls. The diagnosis of emphysema is made **radiographically with chest CT** or pathologically.
   c. Many patients with COPD have, in varying degrees, a combination of these two entities. Therefore, the more general term COPD is appropriate.

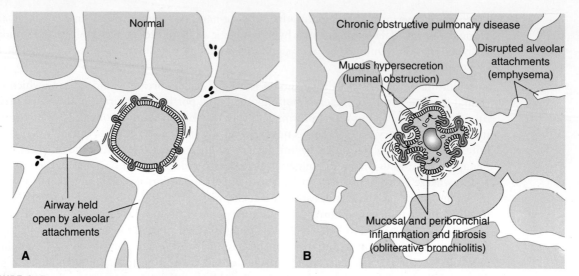

FIGURE 3–5 Examples of normal and COPD small airways. Normal peripheral airways have no evidence of inflammation or goblet cell hypertrophy, and the airways are held open by alveolar attachments. By contrast, in COPD, a loss of alveolar attachments, due to emphysema, contributes to small airway closure. In addition, mucous hypersecretion, and peribronchial inflammation and fibrosis contribute to obliterative bronchiolitis and luminal obstruction.

    2. The **social and economic consequences** of COPD are staggering. Twenty-four million Americans have COPD. Chronic lung disease (a large portion of which is COPD) is the fourth-leading cause of death in the United States. Between 20 and 40 billion dollars are expended annually to treat COPD patients, and more is lost annually because of decreased work productivity.

B | **Etiology** The precise scientific etiology of COPD is unknown; however, the most important environmental etiologic agent is chronic inhalation of tobacco smoke. The Fletcher curve (Figure 3–6) illustrates effects of tobacco smoking on forced expiratory volume in 1 second (FEV_1). Nonsmokers lose approximately 30 mL of FEV_1 per year. Smokers lose twice the amount, 60 mL yearly. If someone stops smoking at a certain age, they will not regain the lung function lost but will slow the rate to that of a nonsmoker. Premature birth, poor lung maturation, lower socioeconomic status, and airways hyperreactivity are believed to be additional important factors.

    1. Tobacco smoke. Smoking in **pack-years** (the number of years a patient has smoked multiplied by the number of packs smoked per day) is directly related to ventilatory dysfunction and pathologic

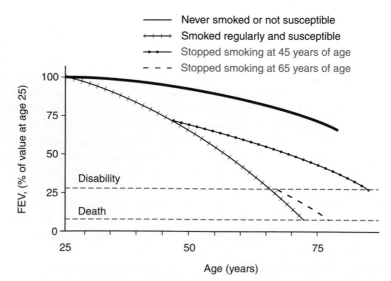

FIGURE 3–6 Age-related rate of decline in lung function in various patient groups. FEV_1, forced expiratory volume in 1 second.

changes in the lung. Smoking stimulates inflammatory cytokines, depresses alveolar macrophages, may reduce the functional integrity of pulmonary surfactant, retards transport of mucus, and enhances the release of lysosomal enzymes believed to be involved in the pathogenesis of COPD [see details in III B 3].

2. **Other environmental factors**
   a. The extent that urban and industrial **air pollution** contributes to the pathogenesis of COPD is not entirely known. Studies comparing patients who live in areas of clean air versus areas of polluted air indicate a higher incidence of COPD in areas of polluted air.
   b. The role of **infections** in the development and progression of COPD is receiving increasing attention. Evidence suggests that upper respiratory **viral infections** in childhood may predispose patients to COPD in adulthood, and viral infections are frequent precipitating factors in symptomatic exacerbations of COPD. **Bacterial infections** also have been reported to be involved in acute exacerbation of chronic bronchitis.

3. Tobacco smoke and other inhalants activate an **inflammatory cascade** that creates an imbalance between **proteinases and antiproteinases.** CD8 T cells and macrophages are activated, and neutrophil chemotactic factors are produced, including interleukin-8 (IL-8) and tumor necrosis factor-α (TNF-α). Neutrophils respond by secreting serine proteinases (neutrophil elastase, shown to cause emphysema in animal models), matrix metalloproteinases, and cysteine proteinases, which result in mucus hypersecretion (chronic bronchitis) and alveolar wall destruction (emphysema). The antiproteinases inhibit these proteinases, but there is a relative deficiency of antiproteinases (ratio of proteinases to antiproteinases is high).

4. α_1-**Protease inhibitor (API) deficiency** (also known as α-1 antitrypsin deficiency) is a well-recognized genetic factor that predisposes patients to emphysema, accounting for approximately 2% of cases. API is a serum protein produced by the liver that **inactivates proteases,** primarily neutrophil elastase.
   a. This deficiency increases the susceptibility of pulmonary tissue to autodigestion by naturally occurring proteases.
   b. The gene for API is on the long arm of chromosome 14. The disease is autosomal recessive. The normal gene is the M allele. Abnormal mutations include the Z, S, or null alleles, and both alleles on chromosome 14 must be abnormal to produce disease (homozygous).
   c. Deficiency of API leads to premature emphysema and cirrhosis of the liver. Cigarette smoking accelerates the process. In its pure form [see also Chapter 6], α_1-antitrypsin deficiency manifests as hepatic cirrhosis, absence of the α_1-globulin peak on serum protein electrophoresis, negligible amounts of serum α_1-antitrypsin, and advanced panlobular emphysema, predominantly in the base of the lungs.
   d. For patients with API deficiency, replacement therapy is available but very expensive.

C **Pathophysiology and pathology**   The pathologic changes of COPD are seen in both the airways and the alveoli.

1. **Chronic bronchitis**
   a. In early disease, the small airways demonstrate mucous plugging, inflammation, narrowing, and obliteration.
   b. In later disease, the chronic bronchitis includes varying degrees of mucous gland hyperplasia, mucosal inflammation and edema, bronchospasm, impacted secretions, and peribronchiolar fibrosis. These elements contribute to airway narrowing and increased airway resistance.
   c. Chronic bronchitis alone does not change the diffusing capacity of the lung for carbon monoxide (D_LCO).

2. **Emphysema**
   a. The destruction of alveolar walls and the supporting structure produces widely dilated airspaces or bullae. The loss of tissue support for the airways is believed to contribute to airway narrowing; the unsupported airways tend to collapse dynamically during expiration, trapping air. In addition, the loss of functioning alveolar capillary units reduces D_LCO or diffusion capacity.
   b. Anatomically, emphysema is classified as **centriacinar (centrilobular), panacinar (panlobular), or distal acinar (paraseptal)** (Figure 3–7).

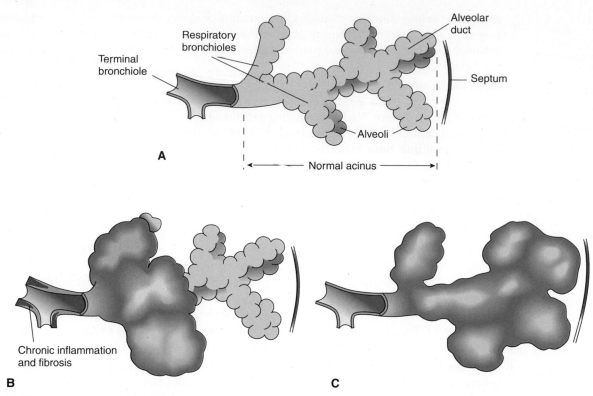

FIGURE 3–7 Emphysema is classified according to the pulmonary lobule that is dilated. **A.** A normal pulmonary lobule. **B.** In centrolobular (centriacinar) emphysema the midportion of the lobule is dilated, including the respiratory bronchiole and alveolar ducts. The terminal alveoli are spared. **C.** In panlobular (panacinar) emphysema the entire pulmonary lobule is dilated.

     (1) Centriacinar (centrilobular) emphysema is the most common type of emphysema encountered in clinical practice and is typically found in smokers. It has a predilection for upper lung zones.

     (2) Panacinar (panlobular) emphysema, in contrast to centriacinar emphysema, has little association with chronic bronchitis and is seen commonly in patients with α_1-antitrypsin deficiency or in those with prior intravenous methylphenidate (Ritalin) abuse. It occurs most commonly in the lung bases.

D **Clinical Features, Diagnosis, and Clinical Course**

1. **Clinical features.** COPD is an insidious, long-term process that presents as follows:
   a. **History of present illness.** Dyspnea is the cardinal symptom in COPD, first with exertion, then with rest as the disease progresses. Cough is present in chronic bronchitis, with or without sputum production. Patients will occasionally experience hemoptysis. COPD symptoms may worsen with a variety of stimuli (pollen, viral infection, smoke, changes in weather), but are much less common than in asthma. When an unrelated health problem places the respiratory system under stress, the presence of COPD becomes evident. Pneumonia, surgery, and trauma are common precipitating events.
   b. **Past medical history** may include other problems related to smoking: cancer, heart disease, peripheral vascular disease.
   c. **Family history** may be nonsignificant, but there are likely genetic factors that influence who develops COPD and who does not. α_1-Protease inhibitor deficiency is inherited in an autosomal recessive fashion.
   d. **Social history** is usually significant for heavy smoking—usually >20 pack-years (e.g., 20 pack-years = 1 pack per day for 20 years or 2 packs per day for 10 years). Occasionally, there may also be occupational exposures.
   e. **Physical exam findings** that may be present include pursed-lip breathing, a barrel-shaped chest, hyperresonance on percussion, wheezing or rhonchi on auscultation, and vital sign abnormalities (in COPD exacerbation). The vital signs may include tachypnea and/or tachycardia.

2. **Clinical syndromes**
   a. **Two classic types of COPD** exist and are given various names. Most patients who carry a diagnosis of COPD have components of emphysema and chronic bronchitis. It is difficult to predict, and it is unclear why some patients develop more of an emphysematous disease and others have more symptoms of chronic bronchitis.
      (1) Patients with a **normal concentration of carbon dioxide in arterial blood ($PaCO_2$)** tend to be thinner, are chronically tachypnic, and are not hypercapnic. Historically, these patients have been referred to as "pink puffers" and tend to have predominant emphysema.
         (a) Pulmonary function testing indicates airway obstruction with a decreased D_LCO, only a mild increase in airway resistance (RAW), and little improvement in airflow after treatment with bronchodilators. Arterial blood gas (ABG) analysis shows mild hypoxemia and normal or low $PaCO_2$.
      (2) Patients with an **elevated $PaCO_2$** are heavier (overweight or obese) and have a chronic respiratory acidosis (hypercapnic). At a relatively young age, they experience chronic cough and expectoration, episodic dyspnea, and weight gain. Wheezing and rhonchi frequently are heard in the chest, and cor pulmonale often develops, accompanied by edema and cyanosis. Historically, these patients have been referred to as "blue bloaters."
         (a) Pulmonary function testing also indicates airway obstruction, increased RAW, improved airflow after treatment with bronchodilators, and relatively preserved lung volumes and D_LCO. ABG analysis often shows moderate-to-severe hypoxemia, and hypercapnia. Patients may develop polycythemia in response to chronic hypoxemia.
         (b) Pathologically, there is minimal emphysema but significant bronchiolitis, bronchitis, mucous gland hyperplasia, and right ventricular hypertrophy.

3. **Diagnosis** COPD may be suspected based on the patient's history, symptoms, and physical signs, but it is diagnosed with PFTs as airway obstruction (with FEV_1/forced vital capacity [FVC] ratio <70%) that is not fully reversible. **Spirometry** will show a flattened volume–time curve and a scooped out flow–volume curve. Lung volumes usually show some degree of hyperinflation (increased total lung capacity [TLC], functional residual capacity [FRC], and residual volume [RV]). There will often be a reduced D_LCO reflective of emphysema.
   a. **Chronic bronchitis** is defined in terms of clinical symptoms of excessive secretion of mucus in the bronchial tree leading to productive cough for at least 3 months in two successive years.
   b. **Emphysema** is a characterized by permanent, abnormal enlargement of air spaces distal to the terminal bronchiole and accompanied by the destruction of bronchiole and alveolar walls. The diagnosis of emphysema is made **radiographically with chest CT** or pathologically.

4. **Clinical course and prognosis**
   a. COPD tends to be a progressive disorder unless there is some form of intervention (i.e., cessation of smoking, removal of other irritants, or medical therapy). Once COPD is advanced, medical treatment will not slow the progression of disease. However, cessation of smoking may alter the decline in pulmonary function in all but far-advanced disease.
   b. The FEV_1 declines by approximately 60 mL/year in typical patients with COPD, as compared with a normal decline of 30 mL/year.
      (1) Survival is statistically related to the degree of ventilatory function that exists when patients are first evaluated. For example, among patients with an initial FEV_1 of less than 0.75 L, the 5-year survival rate is 25%, whereas among those with an initial FEV_1 of 1 L, the 5-year survival rate is approximately 50%.
      (2) **Pulmonary hypertension and right heart failure** may occur in advanced COPD. Increasing number of oxygen-poor areas of the lung causes pulmonary vasoconstriction in an effort to route the blood to oxygen-rich areas. As more vasoconstriction occurs over time, pulmonary hypertension and right heart failure can develop.

E **Therapy (Figure 3–8)**
   1. **Bronchodilation.** Some patients with COPD have a bronchodilator response on PFTs, but obstruction is not usually completely reversible with bronchodilators. However, most patients will have a clinical response and improvement of symptoms.

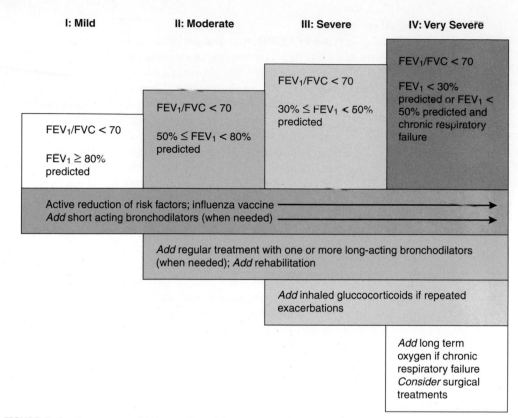

FIGURE 3–8 Management of COPD as adapted from the Global Initiative for Chronic Obstructive Lung Disease guidelines. FEV_1, forced expiratory volume in 1 second; FVC, forced vital capacity.

a. The two major classes of bronchodilators are **β-adrenergic agonists** (albuterol and others) and **anticholinergics** (ipratropium bromide). These agents may be used separately or in combination. The selective β-adrenergic agonists offer advantages over the older agents in terms of a longer duration of bronchodilating action ($β_2$ effect) and reduced cardiac stimulation ($β_1$ effect). Some newer β-agonists have acute as well as long-acting effects. Other therapy may include theophylline (a methylxanthine), but this is used less often in current clinical practice.

2. **Corticosteroid therapy.** The use of corticosteroids in the treatment of the bronchospasm associated with COPD is controversial. However, some patients clearly have a bronchospastic component to their disease and *may* respond to steroid therapy. Delivery of inhaled corticosteroids by a metered-dose inhaler (MDI) is the preferred route of administration. Current guidelines state that inhaled corticosteroids are appropriate for symptomatic COPD patients with an FEV_1 <50% and frequent exacerbations. Systemic steroids (oral prednisone) are used in COPD exacerbations.

3. **Sputum mobilization.** Traditional expectorants and mucolytic agents appear to have little beneficial effect in chronic COPD.

4. **Management of infection.** Patients presenting in exacerbation are most likely to be infected with *Haemophilus influenzae*, *Moraxella catarrhalis*, or *Streptococcus pneumoniae*. Antibiotics (appropriate antibiotics: amoxicillin, azithromycin, or doxycycline) have been shown to be useful if patients have at least two of the following three symptoms: increased dyspnea, increased sputum volume, or increased sputum purulence. In addition, patients with COPD should receive annual vaccination against influenza, as well as a vaccine for pneumococcal infection every 5 years.

5. **Pulmonary rehabilitation programs.** Participation in these programs may improve exercise performance, decrease dyspnea, and improve quality of life. Patients are instructed in exercise programs aimed at increasing exercise tolerance and respiratory muscle stamina. In addition, counseling and nutritional guidance are available.

6. **Surgery**
   a. **In carefully selected patients,** lung volume reduction surgery (LVRS) has been shown to improve lung function, exercise performance, quality of life, and even survival in select patients with emphysema. Upper lobe predominant emphysema on computed tomography (CT) scan appears to be the key prognostic factor in predicting success with LVRS. By decreasing lung volume in the hyperinflated state, LVRS improves respiratory muscle function and chest wall mechanics and increases lung elastic recoil, thereby facilitating enhanced expiratory flow.
   b. Single- and double-lung transplantations have been performed in patients with COPD, and they improve quality of life and exercise tolerance. However, chronic rejection continues to be the major obstacle to long-term success; 5-year mortality still approaches 50%.

7. **Oxygen.** Oxygen administration, in addition to smoking cessation, is the only therapeutic modality other than LVRS that can improve survival. Its value, however, is only demonstrable in those patients with a partial pressure of arterial oxygen (PaO_2) of 55 mm Hg or less on room air, correlating with oxygen saturation of 88% or less.

F **Prevention** Avoidance of smoking is by far the best means of disease prevention. In addition, patients should avoid chronic exposure to other bronchial irritants. Simple spirometric screening of high-risk patients can help detect early disease so that appropriate interventions can be taken to help prevent further deterioration.

IV ASTHMA

A **Introduction**

1. **Definition.** Asthma is an inflammatory disorder of the airways that causes intermittent, recurrent symptoms of coughing, wheezing, dyspnea, and chest tightness. The inflammation is associated with widespread but **variable** airflow obstruction that reverses with treatment or spontaneously.

B **Etiology**

1. Asthma occurs in 3%–8% of the population. It is caused by airway hyperresponsiveness and inflammation. The definitive cause of the inflammatory process leading to asthma has not yet been established. Etiologic or pathologic classification of the disease is difficult; however, asthma traditionally is divided into two forms.
   a. An **allergic form** (also termed extrinsic asthma), responsible for most cases of **asthma in children and many in adults,** is immunologically mediated—it is caused by type I (immediate) hypersensitivity to inhaled antigens.
   b. A **nonallergic form** (also termed intrinsic), which occurs primarily in **adults**, shows no evidence of immediate hypersensitivity to specific antigens.

C **Pathophysiology and Pathology**

1. All patients with asthma have inflammation; the contributors in this inflammatory cascade include CD4 cells, Th2 cytokines, mast cells, and eosinophils.
   a. In the **allergic form of asthma,** the inflammatory cascade is initiated by type I (immunoglobulin E [IgE]–mediated) hypersensitivity reaction to specific antigens, such as pollen, dust mites, animal dander, or viral infections.
      (1) Allergens are presented to CD4 cells (T2 helper cells specifically) that produce IL-4, IL-5, and IL-13 in response. Interleukin-4 induces chemotaxis of eosinophils, induces B cells to produce IgE, and induces maturation of mast cells, which have a large amount of receptors for the Fc end of IgE. Interleukin-5 induces maturation of eosinophils.
      (2) IgE binds to the allergen via the Fab fragment. The Fc fragment of IgE binds to mast cells, cross-linking occurs, and mast cells degranulate. Degranulation of mast cells release vasoactive amines (histamine and serotonin) and lipid mediators (leukotrienes and platelet activating factor). Histamine and serotonin cause edema and mucous hypersecretion. The leukotrienes and platelet activating factor cause smooth muscle contraction (bronchoconstriction) and mucous hypersecretion.

(3) Eosinophils degranulate as well, secreting granule proteins and leukotrienes. The granule proteins include Charcot–Leyden protein, major basic protein, and eosinophilic cationic protein, which produce bronchial edema. The leukotrienes released cause vasoconstriction.

b. In **nonallergic asthma,** there is degranulation of mast cells and eosinophils probably unrelated to IgE mechanisms (degranulation as above). It is usually in response to smoke, perfume, cold air, exercise, or viral infection. There is constriction of airway smooth muscle, mucous hypersecretion, edema, and inflammatory cell infiltration of the airway mucosa and a thickened basement membrane or the underlying epithelium.

D **Clinical Features**

1. History

a. History of Present Illness. Patients with asthma usually present at a young age, although some patients have onset of asthma in middle age. With an asthma exacerbation (attack), patients will experience dyspnea, cough (productive or nonproductive), and chest tightness. They may report audible wheezing. The symptoms are intermittent, may occur at night or in the early morning or may be seasonal. The symptoms occur in response to a variety of stimuli: inhaled allergens (pollen, dust mites, animal dander), viral infection, irritants (tobacco or wood smoke), airborne chemicals (perfumes), exercise, changes in weather, strong emotion (laughing or crying hard), or stress.

b. Past medical history may include other forms of atopy, like eczema, allergic rhinitis, or allergic conjunctivitis.

c. Family history may include a family history of atopy or asthma.

d. Social history can be significant for living conditions: mold, carpet, tobacco, pet exposure.

2. Physical exam. Wheezing on auscultation is the prominent finding, which is a high-pitched "musical" sound, most prominent with expiration, but may be absent in very severe bronchospasm, reflecting severely impaired airflow. There is hyperresonance on percussion. There may be tachypnea or tachycardia, depending on severity of exacerbation. A pulsus paradoxus (inspiratory decrease in systolic blood pressure of more than 10 mm Hg) indicates gross overinflation of the lung and wide swings in pleural pressure. This is present only in severe asthma exacerbations.

3. Chest x-ray is often normal or may show hyperinflation.

4. Sputum may appear purulent because of an increased eosinophil content or an inflammatory response to a viral tracheobronchitis. Sputum smears may reveal **Curschmann's spirals** (i.e., mucus that forms a cast of the small airways) or **Charcot–Leyden crystals** (i.e., breakdown products of the eosinophils).

5. Hematologic studies indicate a modest leukocytosis and eosinophilia in both the allergic and nonallergic forms of the disease.

6. Arterial blood gas. The $PaCO_2$ usually is low (i.e., <36 mm Hg). An increased $PaCO_2$ or normal $PaCO_2$ (40 mm Hg) may indicate severe obstruction and respiratory muscle fatigue. Arterial hypoxemia is common despite the increased ventilation and is due to underventilation of lung segments supplied by narrowed airways (i.e., there is $\dot{V}/\dot{Q}$ **mismatch**).

7. Complication: Status asthmaticus is a complication that may occur with a severe asthmatic attack that does not respond to initial treatment and involves bronchospasm so severe that the patient is at risk for ventilatory failure.

E **Diagnosis**

1. The diagnosis of asthma is made predominantly by history, physical, and pulmonary function testing.

2. History and physical exam. See prior discussion.

3. Pulmonary function testing

a. Pulmonary function tests are typically normal when the patient is not having an exacerbation of asthma. During attacks the FEV_1 and FVC are reduced; the FEV_1/FVC ratio is reduced but usually improves after inhalation of a bronchodilator, reflecting reversibility (the FEV_1 should improve by 12% or more with bronchodilators—albuterol—to be considered reversible). RV, TLC, and lung compliance usually are increased, and the D_LCO frequently is normal or may be increased.

b. After symptomatic recovery, TLC and lung compliance return to normal, but the maximum expiratory flow rate may remain reduced at low lung volumes, and an abnormal distribution of ventilation may persist, reflecting resistant obstruction of small airways.

c. **In the absence of a reduced** FEV_1/FVC ratio but a suspicion for asthma, the methacholine challenge test may be performed to test for increased bronchial hyperresponsiveness and, if abnormal, is consistent with a diagnosis of asthma. It is performed by administering methacholine (a cholinergic agonist) at increasing doses and monitoring for a decline in the FEV_1 (20% decline is abnormal).

F **Therapy** is based on an understanding of the underlying pathophysiologic mechanisms. Effective management of asthma relies on four integral components: objective measures of lung function, pharmacologic therapy, environmental measures to control allergens and irritants, and patient education.

1. **Goals of therapy.** The goals of therapy are as follows:
   a. Maintain near-normal pulmonary function.
   b. Maintain normal activity levels.
   c. Prevent chronic and troublesome symptoms (e.g., cough, nocturnal symptoms).
   d. Prevent recurrent exacerbations.
   e. Have minimal use of short-acting inhaled β_2-agonists.
   f. Avoid adverse effects from asthma medications.

2. **Principles of treatment.** Asthma is a **chronic condition with acute exacerbations.**
   a. **Prevention** of exacerbations is particularly important. Environmental control measures may be employed (carpet removed, no indoor pets, etc.)
   b. **Early intervention** when treating acute exacerbations of asthma is important to reduce the likelihood of developing severe airway narrowing.
   c. **Control of airway inflammation** is a key factor in treating asthma, as suggested by evidence of the presence of airway inflammation in all patients with asthma. Patients should be educated on how to monitor their asthma with a peak flow meter and be given an action plan for what to do when symptoms worsen.

3. **Pharmacologic therapy** can be divided in two categories: quick-relief medication and long-term control medication. Therapy is given in a stepwise approach (Table 3–3).
   a. **Quick-relief medications** include inhaled **short-acting β_2-agonists (SABAs)** and inhaled **anticholinergics.** These are used to treat symptoms when they happen and can be given in inhaler or nebulized form.
   (1) Short-acting β_2-agonists (SABAs) consist of **albuterol** (used most commonly), pirbuterol, and levalbuterol. SABAs induce relaxation of airway smooth muscle causing bronchodilation, inhibit mast cell mediator release, and increase mucociliary clearance.
   (2) **Ipratropium** is the main anticholinergic inhaler that is used as a quick-relief medication. It is not used as commonly in asthma as it is in COPD. Ipratropium works by inhibiting parasympathetic-mediated airway tone, thus leading to relaxation of airway smooth muscle and bronchodilation.
   b. **Long-term control medications**
   (1) **Corticosteroids** have become the mainstay therapy for maintenance of asthma control. Inhaled corticosteroids, including fluticasone, budesonide, and mometasone, are preferred for maintenance therapy over systemic steroids. Systemic steroids should be avoided as long-term therapy due to side effects but are sometimes necessary. Systemic steroids, methylprednisolone, and prednisone are the cornerstones of treatment for acute asthma exacerbations.
   (2) **Long-acting β_2-agonists (LABAs)** include salmeterol and formoterol. The duration of bronchodilation is at least 12 hours after a single dose. They have similar effects to SABAs but last longer and thus work as a preventive medication. They induce relaxation of airway smooth muscle causing bronchodilation, inhibit mast cell mediator release, and increase mucociliary clearance. LABAs should not be used without cotherapy with corticosteroids, as use of LABAs alone in asthma may increase mortality.
   (3) **Leukotriene modifiers** include zafirlukast and montelukast (antagonists of the type 1 cysteinyl leukotriene receptor) and zileuton (a 5-lipoxygenase inhibitor). They inhibit

TABLE 3–3   Asthma Management in Adults According to Classification of Severity

Severity of Asthma	Frequency of Day-time Symptoms	Frequency of Nighttime Symptoms	PEF or FEV$_1$ / PEF Variability	Recommended Management (Includes Short-acting Inhaled β-agonist as Needed)
Mild intermittent	≤2 days/week; asymptomatic and normal PEF between attacks	≤2 nights/ month	≥80% / <20%	None necessary
Mild persistent	>2 times per week but <1 time per day; attacks may affect activity	>2 nights/ month	≥80% / 20%–30%	Low-dose inhaled corticosteroid
Moderate persistent	Daily; attacks affect activity	>1 night/ week	60%–80% / >30%	Low- to medium-dose inhaled corticosteroid plus long-acting β-agonist; *alternative:* medium-dose inhaled steroid plus oral anti-inflammatory*
Severe persistent	Continuous; limited physical activity	Frequent	≤60% / >30%	High-dose inhaled corticosteroid plus long-acting β-agonist, oral anti-inflammatory if needed, and oral glucocorticoid as needed

PEF, peak expiratory flow; FEV$_1$, forced expiratory volume in 1 second.
*Oral anti-inflammatory medications include leukotriene modifiers such as zafirlukast or zileuton, long-acting theophylline.
Adapted from the National Asthma Education and Prevention Program. Available at: http://www.nhlbi.nih.gov/guidelines/asthma/execsumm.pdf.

leukotriene-mediated effects (bronchoconstriction, mucosal edema, and mucous hypersecretion).

(4) **Mast cell stabilizers** include nedocromil and disodium cromoglycate (cromolyn sodium). Through inhibition of cellular activation of mast cells and eosinophils, they modestly reduce inflammation. These tend to be used more in the pediatric population.

(5) **Methylxanthines** (theophylline) are no longer used as widely as they once were due to unfavorable side effects. Theophylline is a phosphodiesterase inhibitor, has a mild bronchodilator effect, and may improve diaphragmatic function.

(6) The **immunomodulator omalizumab** is a monoclonal antibody against IgE that prevents binding of IgE to the high-affinity Fc receptors on mast cells. It should be used only in allergic asthma but has been associated with anaphylaxis and is very expensive.

G **Occupational asthma**   Exposure to various occupational inhalants can cause occupational asthma, often without a demonstrable immunologic mechanism. Affected individuals may or may not be atopic, and the reaction usually occurs several hours after exposure. The history is the most important aspect of diagnosis. The patient will have symptoms of asthma during the work week that improve or resolve on days away from the work place. **Etiologic agents** include simple inorganic chemicals (e.g., platinum salts), simple organic chemicals (e.g., formaldehyde), wood dust, animal dander and excretions, and grain and grain contaminants. Direct confirmation by challenge testing is the most convincing demonstration of the causal relationship. Avoidance of exposure is the most effective treatment. Acute attacks may respond to standard asthma medication.

V   BRONCHIECTASIS, CYSTIC FIBROSIS, AND LUNG ABSCESS

A **Bronchiectasis**

1. **Definition.** Bronchiectasis is a pathologic, irreversible dilation of the bronchi caused by destruction of the bronchial wall, usually resulting from suppurative infection.

2. **Etiology**
   a. The small bronchi of childhood are most susceptible to bronchial infection and to obstruction by impacted secretions, foreign bodies, or compressing lymph nodes. Seventy-five percent of patients can recall experiencing symptoms of bronchiectasis as early as the age of 5 years.
   b. The most common cause of bronchiectasis is bacterial pneumonia, which may be primary or may be a complication of measles, a tumor, or aspiration of gastric contents or particulate matter. Even though bacterial pneumonia is the most common cause, the incidence had decreased drastically due to the advent of antibiotics.
   c. Predisposing conditions include congenital disorders, immune deficiencies [e.g., hypogammaglobulinemia or immunoglobulin A (IgA) deficiency], and cystic fibrosis.

3. **Pathophysiology and pathology:** In bronchiectasis, there are impaired airway clearance mechanisms and host defenses, resulting in an inability to clear secretions, which predisposes patients to chronic infection and inflammation. As the result of frequent infections, most commonly with *Haemophilus influenzae* (35%), *Pseudomonas aeruginosa* (31%), *Moraxella catarrhalis* (20%), *Staphylococcus aureus* (14%), and *Streptococcus pneumoniae* (13%), airways become inspissated with viscous mucus-containing inflammatory mediators and pathogens. The airways slowly become dilated, scarred, and distorted. Histologically, bronchial walls are thickened by edema, inflammation, and neovascularization.

4. **Clinical features.** Symptoms include a chronic cough productive of purulent sputum, recurrent chest colds or pneumonias, occasional hemoptysis, and pleuritic pain. These symptoms cannot be differentiated from those of chronic suppurative bronchitis. Progressive dyspnea, cyanosis, digital clubbing, and cor pulmonale are seen in advanced cases.

5. **Diagnosis**
   a. **Physical examination** reveals rales over the area of involvement on repeated examinations.
   b. **Pulmonary function testing** produces normal results in mild cases, but in moderate or severe cases it may reveal either restrictive or a mixture of restrictive and obstructive ventilatory patterns.
   c. **Chest radiography** shows peribronchial fibrosis in the involved segment. Segmental lung collapse in areas of bronchiectasis is common.
   d. **CT scanning,** particularly **high-resolution computed tomography (HRCT),** is the definitive method for diagnosing bronchiectasis.
   e. **Traction bronchiectasis** in pulmonary fibrosis may appear on CT scan as dilated bronchi but is not caused by suppurative infections.

6. **Therapy.** The proper therapy can markedly improve symptoms.
   a. **Medical treatment** is the mainstay and consists of therapy with antibiotics on a frequent or regular basis (e.g., ampicillin, tetracycline, erythromycin, or as indicated by culture and sensitivity testing), postural drainage, and immunization against influenza and pneumococcal pneumonia.
   b. **Bronchodilator therapy** may be effective in some patients.
   c. **Oxygen therapy** is appropriate if PaO_2 levels are depressed.
   d. **Surgical resection** may be helpful in localized disease.

B **Cystic fibrosis**

1. **Definition.** Cystic fibrosis (CF) is an autosomal recessive disease characterized by dysfunction of the exocrine glands, leading to obstruction in such organs as the lungs, pancreas, and gastrointestinal tract. In 99% of patients with CF, death is caused by respiratory failure, with portal hypertension secondary to biliary cirrhosis accounting for the remainder of deaths.

2. **Incidence**
   a. An estimated 30,000 individuals with CF live in the United States. The disease is most common among whites, occurring in 1 of 2500 births, and 5% of the white population are carriers. Because inheritance is recessive and individuals who are heterozygotic have no disease, a negative family history does not rule out the disease.
   b. Once thought to be unique to children, CF now is recognized as the most common cause of obstructive airway disease among individuals up to age 30 years. The median age of patients with CF has risen from the teens in the 1960s to approximately 37 years in 2006.

3. **Etiology.** The genetic abnormality that is responsible for CF has been identified on the long arm of chromosome 7.

   a. The gene for CF produces a membrane transport protein called **cystic fibrosis transmembrane regulator (CFTR).** More than 200 mutations have been discovered in the CF gene; 70% of patients have a mutation that leads to a deletion of the amino acid phenylalanine at position 508 (ΔF508) in the CFTR protein. This deletion produces an abnormal CFTR protein.

4. **Pathology and pathophysiology.** The abnormality in the CFTR protein results in decreased chloride secretion and increased sodium and water resorption into the epithelial cell, decreasing the hydration of the mucus. This abnormality leads to highly viscous mucus production, causing obstruction of organs served by exocrine glands.

5. **Clinical features.** The manifestations of CF are varied, with pulmonary abnormalities being the overriding clinical concern.

   a. **Pulmonary manifestations**

      (1) The earliest pulmonary manifestation is peripheral airway obstruction resulting from plugged bronchi. Repeated bouts of infection lead to a cycle of obstruction, tissue damage, and infection that ultimately progresses to a loss of pulmonary function.

      (2) The predominant organisms to colonize the lung are the highly resistant mucoid strain of *Pseudomonas aeruginosa* and *Burkholderia cepacia*. Other infections may be due to *Staphylococcus aureus*. Complete eradication of the organisms is virtually impossible.

      (3) Many patients with CF develop sinusitis and nasal polyps, and most have clubbing of the digits.

      (4) Most patients die of respiratory complications due to gradual loss of lung function, the result of chronic inflammation perpetuated by *P. aeruginosa.*

   b. **Nonpulmonary manifestations** also are common and include meconium ileus, malabsorption, fatty infiltration of the liver, focal biliary cirrhosis, glucose intolerance, sterility in males, and a predilection for heat illness due to severe salt depletion. As patients with CF live longer, osteoporosis has become a problem in both males and females. In addition, there appears to be some epidemiologic evidence of an increase in some gastrointestinal cancers.

   c. **Complications** include hypoxia that is only partially responsive to oxygen therapy, cor pulmonale with all the manifestations of right-sided heart failure (e.g., hepatomegaly, peripheral edema), hemoptysis, and possible pneumothorax.

6. **Diagnosis**

   a. **Sweat test (a skin test).** An abnormal sweat test is observed in virtually all cases and, in combination with certain clinical hallmarks, confirms the diagnosis.

      (1) The sodium and chloride concentrations in sweat are elevated dramatically in CF. The **quantitative pilocarpine iontophoresis sweat test** is positive when a sweat chloride concentration is greater than 60 mEq/L.

      (2) A positive sweat test is diagnostic of CF in the presence of at least one of the following three criteria:

         (a) A reliable family history of CF

         (b) Obstructive pulmonary disease

         (c) Pancreatic insufficiency

   b. **Pulmonary function testing** shows limitation of forced expiratory flows and an elevated RV. The $D_L CO$ is usually within normal limits. As the disease progresses, the FEV_1 and ratio of FEV_1 to FVC decline, indicating obstruction.

   c. **Chest radiography** shows striking manifestations that are more pronounced in the upper lobes. Findings include bronchiectasis, hyperinflation, cyst formation, atelectasis, and segmental infiltration.

   d. **CT scanning** demonstrates a characteristic "secular bronchiectasis."

7. **Therapy**

   a. In the **early stages** of the disease, therapy must be individualized according to specific clinical manifestations.

      (1) Salt depletion is a potential problem in warmer climates.

      (2) Nutritional supplementation and pancreatic enzyme replacement often are indicated.

(3) Pulmonary infections may require hospitalization and vigorous treatment with parenteral antibiotics, hydration, humidification, and supplemental oxygen.

b. In the **later stages** of the disease, therapy is aimed at suppressing infection with specific antibiotics, inducing and clearing sputum through chest physiotherapy and postural drainage, and administering supplemental oxygen as required. **Dornase-α,** a drug that hydrolyzes extracellular DNA and makes sputum less viscous, has been approved for use in patients with CF. This drug has been shown to decrease respiratory tract infections and increase pulmonary function. Aerosolized **tobramycin** is an aminoglycoside antibiotic that has demonstrated improved pulmonary function and decreased symptoms when used on a chronic basis. Inhaled **hypertonic saline** increases hydration of airway surface liquid, thereby improving mucociliary clearance.

c. In **end-stage** disease, bilateral lung transplantation (the procedure of choice) can be considered. Results are similar to those obtained with bilateral lung transplantation in other end-stage lung diseases.

d. New therapies aimed at counteracting the pathophysiologic process of CF are being tested. These include gene therapy; manipulation of ion transport and protein trafficking; and administration of anti-inflammatory agents, antibiotics, and antielastases.

C **Lung abscess** [see also Chapter 9 V C 5]

1. Definition. A lung abscess is a localized area of infection within the lung parenchyma that develops from an initial pneumonic stage. The center of the infected area first becomes necrotic and purulent and then becomes well demarcated from the surrounding lung tissue. The wall of the abscess becomes intensely inflamed and lined with fibrous and granulation tissue and abundant blood vessels.

2. Etiology. A solitary lung abscess most commonly results from aspiration of secretions from the oropharynx. Other, less common causes include bronchial obstruction (e.g., from neoplasm), bacterial pneumonia, pulmonary embolism with infarction, transdiaphragmatic spread from intra-abdominal infections, chest trauma, and bacteremic infection.

3. Pathology and pathophysiology. Bacteria and polymorphonuclear white blood cells accumulate in the parenchyma, create tissue destruction, and wall off a cavity or "abscess."

4. Clinical features
a. Initial symptoms are similar to those of acute pneumonia, including fever, cough, and purulent, foul-smelling sputum production.
b. Chronically, lung abscess is associated with constitutional symptoms that include weight loss, low-grade fever, fatigue, and malaise.

5. Diagnosis
a. Physical examination may reveal relatively normal findings, although there is occasionally clubbing of the nail beds. There may be bronchial breath sounds or crackles.
b. Pulmonary function testing usually is not affected by a lung abscess.
c. Chest x-ray and CT scanning make the diagnosis of a lung abscess: irregularly shaped cavity with an air–fluid level inside. The cavity may be thin walled (suggesting a primary suppurative lung abscess) or thick walled (suggesting cavitary carcinoma with or without overriding infection).
d. Bronchoscopy. In general, purulent lung abscesses can be treated with antibiotics alone without drainage or bronchoscopy. If the condition is not responding to treatment or if there is concern for malignancy or foreign body, bronchoscopy may be indicated.

6. Therapy. The treatment of choice is antibiotics, initially with broad-spectrum antibiotic to cover both gram-positive cocci, gram-negative rods, and anaerobic bacteria. Therapy may be narrowed based on culture results. Methicillin-resistant *Staphylococcus aureus* infection requires therapy with vancomycin. The total duration of therapy is 6–8 weeks or until the abscess resolves radiologically.

VI **ACUTE RESPIRATORY FAILURE**

A **Definition** Acute respiratory failure occurs when the respiratory system dysfunction is severe enough to threaten life. There may be hypoxemia (i.e., a PaO_2 of <50 mm Hg) with or without associated hypercapnia (i.e., a $PaCO_2$ of >45 mm Hg).

B **Classification** Acute respiratory failure can be divided into two types.

1. **Hypoxemic respiratory failure without carbon dioxide retention** (i.e., low PaO$_2$ with low or normal PaCO$_2$). This type of respiratory failure is characterized by marked $\dot{V}/\dot{Q}$ abnormalities and intrapulmonary shunting. **Hypoxemic** respiratory failure occurs in such clinical settings as the following:
   a. Acute respiratory distress syndrome (ARDS) [see VI]
   b. Diffuse pneumonia (viral and bacterial)
   c. Aspiration pneumonitis
   d. Fat embolism
   e. Pulmonary edema
   f. Pulmonary embolism

2. **Hypercapnic respiratory failure with carbon dioxide retention**, or **ventilatory failure**, has two basic physiologic abnormalities—$\dot{V}/\dot{Q}$ imbalance and inadequate alveolar ventilation. These patients may have normal or low PaO$_2$ levels. Causes of hypercapnic respiratory failure include the following:
   a. COPD (chronic bronchitis, emphysema) and cystic fibrosis
   b. Acute obstructive lung disease (asthma, severe acute bronchitis)
   c. Disorders of respiratory control (e.g., drug overdose, central nervous system disease, trauma, or cerebrovascular accident)
   d. Neuromuscular abnormalities (e.g., poliomyelitis, myasthenia gravis, Guillain–Barré syndrome)
   e. Chest wall trauma, kyphoscoliosis, upper airway obstruction

C **Pathophysiologic mechanisms of hypoxemia**

1. **$\dot{V}/\dot{Q}$ imbalance** (the alveolar/capillary units have a low ventilation-to-perfusion ratio), the most common pathophysiologic cause of hypoxemia, arises when alveolar ventilation decreases with respect to perfusion in the lung. Hypoxemia resulting from a moderate alteration in the $\dot{V}/\dot{Q}$ can be reversed with relatively small increases in the inspired oxygen concentration. Lobar pneumonia is a good example: There is poor ventilation to that lobe, but it is still perfused.

2. **Intrapulmonary shunting** occurs when ventilation approaches or reaches zero in perfused areas (e.g., due to collapsed or fluid-filled alveoli), so that venous blood is shunted directly to the arterial circulation without first being oxygenated. Hypoxemia due to a shunt frequently cannot be corrected, even with 100% inspired oxygen.

3. **Hypoventilation with resulting hypercapnia** will result in hypoxemia as evidenced by the alveolar gas equation: $P_AO_2 = FiO_2(P_{ATM} - P_{H2O}) - PaCO_2/R$, where P_AO_2 is the alveolar partial oxygen pressure, FiO_2 is the fraction of inspired oxygen, P_{ATM} is the atmospheric pressure, P_{H2O} is the alveolar partial pressure of water vapor, and R is the respiratory quotient (ratio of the volume of CO_2 expired to the volume of O_2 consumed). According to this equation, the P_AO_2 will fall as the PaCO$_2$ rises.

4. An abnormality in the **diffusion of oxygen** across the alveolar–capillary membrane may contribute to hypoxemia during exercise or in conditions of lowered inspired oxygen content (most commonly due to high altitude, e.g., during a commercial airline flight). However, the contribution of this mechanism to respiratory failure is usually not significant.

D **Therapy**

1. **Principles.** Treatment is directed toward the underlying disease as well as toward the ventilatory and hypoxic components. In addition, the acute and chronic aspects of respiratory failure must be considered. Patients with chronic respiratory disease frequently can tolerate a lower PaO$_2$ and a higher PaCO$_2$ than those with acute respiratory failure. In fact, they may depend on their PaO$_2$ level as their CNS drive to breathe, whereas in normal humans, the PaCO$_2$ level drives the CNS respiratory center. In these patients who rely on PaO$_2$ level, care must be taken not to overoxygenate, as this might suppress their drive to breathe. Oxygen saturations in the low 90s are adequate.

2. **Oxygen therapy**
   a. In **hypoxemic respiratory failure,** patients may require high concentrations of inspired oxygen. Oxygen may be delivered by mask or nasal cannula. The use of devices to increase

end-expiratory lung volumes, such as continuous positive airway pressure (CPAP) or, in more severe cases, intubation with mechanical ventilation may be required.

    b. In **hypercapnic respiratory failure,** treatment depends on the cause.

        (1) The basis of therapy is controlled administration of oxygen (i.e., low-flow oxygen treatment), with care taken not to increase the $PaCO_2$. Invasive mechanical ventilation may be needed with severe obstruction causing respiratory failure. **Noninvasive mask ventilation** with bilevel positive airway pressure (BiPAP) or preset volume ventilation has been used with some success, thereby avoiding the need for airway intubation.

        (2) If the cause of hypercapnic respiratory failure is neuromuscular weakness, the underlying cause of respiratory muscle weakness must be treated (e.g., myasthenia gravis flare).

VII   ACUTE RESPIRATORY DISTRESS SYNDROME (ARDS)

A **Definition**

    1. Clinical definition. Acute respiratory distress syndrome is an important form of acute hypoxemic respiratory failure characterized by severe dyspnea, hypoxemia, loss of lung compliance, and pulmonary edema. There is increased extravascular lung fluid (the basic pathophysiologic mechanism underlying this condition).

    2. Physiologic definition

        a. The ratio of **PaO_2 to FiO_2 is ≤ 200,** regardless of the presence or level of positive end-expiratory pressure (PEEP). There is a finding of bilateral **pulmonary opacities** on imaging. There is pulmonary capillary wedge pressure (**PCWP**) of ≤ 18 **mm Hg** or no clinical evidence of elevated left atrial pressure. [See VII D for further details.]

B **Etiology**   ARDS can be initiated by many different events and conditions, including shock, aspiration of fluid, disseminated intravascular coagulation (DIC), bacteremia, trauma, blood transfusion, pancreatitis, smoke inhalation, and heroin overdose. Causes of ARDS can be divided in two categories: direct and indirect.

    1. Direct causes of ARDS include direct injury to the lung: toxin inhalation, acute infectious pneumonia (viral, bacterial, fungal), or aspiration.

    2. Indirect causes of ARDS include sepsis, pancreatitis, transfusion-related acute lung injury (TRALI), and trauma.

C **Pathology and pathophysiology**

    1. An insult to the capillary endothelium or alveolar epithelium precipitates ARDS. This insult results in capillary congestion and interstitial edema, leading to disruption of capillary integrity and the extravasation of fluid, fibrin, red blood cells (RBCs), and white blood cells (WBCs) into the lung interstitium, lymphatics, and, ultimately, the alveoli.

        a. Tumor necrosis factor-α (TNF-α) and interleukin-1 (IL-1), "early response" cytokines, are critical for initiating the inflammatory response.

        b. These cytokines then stimulate IL-8, which perpetuates inflammation and coagulation.

    2. The severe hypoxemia is caused by extreme $\dot{V}/\dot{Q}$ imbalance and the shunting of blood in the fluid-filled areas of the lung.

    3. The edema causes the lungs to stiffen and become less compliant, resulting in difficulty with mechanical ventilation and subsequent high airway pressures.

D **Clinical Features, Diagnosis, and Clinical Course**   Symptoms may develop immediately after the insult but usually are delayed 24–48 hours.

    1. Progressive tachypnea with increased minute ventilation usually is the earliest sign, followed by dyspnea.

    2. Physical findings often are absent or limited to bronchial breath sounds and rales.

    3. Arterial blood gas will show acute respiratory alkalosis and hypoxemia.

    4. Chest radiograph or CT shows patchy, diffuse, bilateral, fluffy opacities that are relatively symmetric and often more in dependent areas of the lungs.

5. The ratio of **PaO$_2$ to FiO$_2$ is ≤200,** regardless of the presence or level of PEEP.

6. On right heart catheterization, there is **PCWP of ≤18 mm Hg** or no clinical evidence of elevated left atrial pressure. In other words, the pulmonary edema is not due to left ventricular heart failure.

7. The **prognosis** of ARDS has improved over the last 20 years. Survival is now 60%–70%. Patients with poor prognostic factors include those older than 65 years and those with sepsis as the underlying cause. Most patients with ARDS require invasive mechanical ventilation for at least several days and with improvement, can be liberated from mechanical ventilation.

E Therapy

1. **Oxygenation.** The ultimate goal of therapy is to provide adequate tissue oxygenation. Overall tissue oxygenation can be estimated from the mixed venous oxygen content (CVO$_2$). In addition, concomitant measurement of cardiac output by thermodilution may aid in the correction of abnormal oxygen transport.

   a. The goal of oxygenation is to maintain PaO$_2$ at approximately 60–80 mm Hg. This results in approximately a 90% oxygen saturation, which ensures that tissue oxygen needs are met as long as cardiac output and hemoglobin levels are normal.

   b. **Mechanical ventilation** is required by most patients with ARDS.

      (1) **PEEP** commonly is used to increase lung volume by recruiting alveoli, reducing intrapulmonary shunt, and improving $\dot{V}/\dot{Q}$ relationships. PEEP may cause barotrauma or a reduced cardiac output. In patients whose cardiac output is compromised, the PaO$_2$ increases, but oxygen delivery to the tissues may decrease. Therefore, it is important to measure mixed venous PaO$_2$ (MVO$_2$) when using PEEP.

      (2) A large multicentered National Institutes of Health (NIH)–supported trial showed that the use of a low-tidal-volume strategy (e.g., 6 mL/kg) decreased mortality compared with one using a larger tidal volume (12 mL/kg).

      (3) Other methods of ventilation, such as **inverse-ratio, pressure release,** and **high-frequency ventilation,** may be useful in certain situations.

      (4) Some studies have demonstrated that placing patients in the prone position or using inhaled nitric oxide may improve oxygenation, but neither treatment has been shown to improve survival.

2. **Other measures.** The underlying disease process must be treated. In addition, patients who require more than 24–48 hours of mechanical ventilation should receive nutritional support, preferably through the gastrointestinal tract. Providing diuretic therapy and limiting fluid administration decrease the development of extravascular lung fluid and improve lung compliance.

3. **Possible new treatments.** Other novel therapies have been investigated for treatment of ARDS. None has shown consistent, unequivocal benefit. They include surfactant replacement, β-agonists, inhaled nitric oxide, corticosteroids (given for 3 days), ibuprofen, ketoconazole (inhibition of thromboxane synthesis), TNF-α antibodies, and IL-1–receptor antagonists.

VIII PULMONARY HYPERTENSION

A Definition

1. Pulmonary hypertension (PH) is a condition characterized by a sustained elevation of mean pulmonary artery pressure to >25 mm Hg at rest or >30 mm Hg with exercise.

2. Pulmonary hypertension is classified by the World Health Organization into five major categories. This was recently revised in 2004.

   a. **Group I** pulmonary hypertension is referred to as **pulmonary arterial hypertension (PAH). PAH requires three findings: (1) PH as defined above, (2) a mean pulmonary capillary wedge pressure <15 mm Hg, and (3) an elevated pulmonary vascular resistance >3 Wood units.** Group I encompasses idiopathic (primary), familial, and venous (or capillary)-related pulmonary hypertension. **Idiopathic PAH** (previously termed primary pulmonary hypertension or PPH) is most common in young females (female:male ratio is 2:1). It is a rare disease, with an incidence 2–15 cases per 1 million persons. Mean age of onset is 36 years. Familial

PAH refers to inheritable disorders. Other causes of PH in this group include collagen vascular disease, congenital systemic-to-pulmonary shunts, portal hypertension, HIV infection, drugs or toxins (e.g., anorexigens), glycogen storage disease, hereditary hemorrhagic telangiectasia, and hemoglobinopathies. Venous or capillary-related PH includes veno-occlusive disease and pulmonary–capillary hemangiomatosis.

   b. Group II is PH from pulmonary venous hypertension as a result of left-sided atrial or ventricular heart disease or left-sided valvular (mitral or aortic) heart disease.

   c. Group III encompasses PH associated with chronic hypoxemia, as in COPD, interstitial lung disease, sleep-disordered breathing, alveolar hypoventilation disorders, or chronic exposure to high altitudes.

   d. Group IV PH is due to chronic thrombotic disease, embolic disease, or both. This can be due to chronic thromboemboli to the proximal or distal pulmonary arteries or to pulmonary embolism from tumor or parasites.

   e. Group V is the miscellaneous classification of PH. It includes sarcoidosis, pulmonary Langerhans'-cell histiocytosis, lymphangiomatosis, and external compression of the pulmonary vessels (from adenopathy, tumor, etc.)

B Etiology

1. The underlying cause of PAH (group I PH) is not well understood. PH due to groups II–V PH have underlying disease that results from a secondary cause. Among environmental factors associated with an increased risk of the development of pulmonary arterial hypertension, three mechanisms are plausible: hypoxia, anorexigens, and central nervous system stimulants.

C Pathology and Pathophysiology

1. The pulmonary circulation is normally a low-resistance, high-compliance vascular system. The pulmonary circulation is the only organ to receive 100% of the cardiac output. Pulmonary blood flow can increase four to five times its baseline during exercise or times of stress, by increasing CO and decreasing pulmonary vascular resistance (PVR).

2. The pathologic changes that occur in PAH are vasoconstriction, smooth muscle and endothelial cell proliferation, in situ thrombosis, and plexiform lesions in end-stage PAH.

3. There is a neurohormonal imbalance in PAH. An increase in **endothelin-1,** angiopoeitin-1, plasminogen activator inhibitor-1, and platelet derived growth factor all act to induce pulmonary vasoconstriction and smooth muscle and endothelial cell proliferation and cause a prothrombotic state. Endothelin-1 is the most powerful vasoconstrictor found endogenously. It is the active peptide in sarafotoxin, the venom of the Israeli burrowing asp, one of the deadliest snakes in the world.

4. **Prostacyclin, nitric oxide,** and **vasoactive intestinal peptide** all act to induce vasodilation, control of cellular proliferation, and decrease of platelet aggregation; these are reduced in PAH.

D Clinical Features, Diagnosis, and Clinical Course

1. Symptoms associated with pulmonary hypertension are vague and nondescript. Most patients have symptoms for approximately 2 years before being diagnosed.

   a. Fatigue appears to be the most common symptom and is present in approximately 60% of patients at diagnosis.

   b. Dyspnea occurs in 60% of patients when they initially present but is encountered by all as the disease progresses.

   c. Syncope and angina, particularly with exertion, are late manifestations of the disease, suggesting the presence of severe pulmonary hypertension causing reduced cardiac output.

2. On **physical exam,** there is a loud second heart sound (P2), jugular venous distension (JVD), hepatomegaly, lower-extremity edema, and ascites, and there may be a murmur of pulmonary and/or tricuspid regurgitation.

3. **Diagnosis** of PH is challenging. The presenting symptoms are often nonspecific, the routine outpatient tests (chest radiography and electrocardiogram) are usually not that helpful, and there are no blood tests for PH. An echocardiogram is the best screening test for PH, but to **make the diagnosis,** a **right heart catheterization** must be performed.

a. **Chest radiography** may show peripheral pulmonary hypovascularity ("pruning"), prominent proximal pulmonary arteries, and right ventricular enlargement into the retrosternal space.

b. The **electrocardiogram** can reflect changes in the heart due to PAH. There may be right axis deviation, right atrial enlargement, right ventricular hypertrophy, and right ventricular strain.

c. With an **echocardiogram**, the right ventricle and pulmonary artery pressures can be estimated, right ventricular and left atrial enlargement are seen, and tricuspid and pulmonary valve regurgitation are seen with color Doppler. However, the right ventricle and pulmonary pressures are only *estimated* and may not be accurate.

d. A **right heart catheterization (Swan–Ganz catheter)** is required to confirm a suspected diagnosis of PH. The catheter is inserted into the right internal jugular vein and advanced into the superior vena cava; the balloon at the tip of the catheter is inflated, and pressures are measured in the right atrium, right ventricle, and the pulmonary artery as the catheter is advanced. After the pulmonary artery pressure is measured, the catheter is advanced even further and "wedged" into one of the pulmonary arteries. This reflects the pressure in the left atrium and left ventricle and is called the pulmonary capillary wedge pressure.

e. Other tests to rule out secondary causes of pulmonary hypertension are recommended. Pulmonary function studies are important to evaluate for the presence of other causes (e.g., lung disease) contributing to the development of pulmonary hypertension (group III: PH associated with hypoxemia). Ventilation–perfusion lung imaging is important to exclude chronic thromboembolic disease. Serologic studies are performed to screen for connective tissue diseases. A positive antinuclear antibody test is common in the setting of PPH; however, higher titers or specific antibody patterns should raise the index of suspicion for underlying collagen vascular disease. Whether or not obstructive sleep apnea (OSA) causes pulmonary hypertension has been debated. In patients with pulmonary hypertension, a sleep study should be done before a diagnosis of PAH is given. An HIV test should be performed in all patients with a diagnosis of PH, as the incidence of PH is much higher in HIV patients.

4. **Prognosis**

a. Historically, the prognosis for patients with PAH has been poor, with an estimated median survival of 2.8 years, as noted in the NIH registry reporting in the 1980s. In the registry data, survival rates at 1, 3, and 5 years were 68%, 48%, and 34%, respectively. However, a more recent report in 2006 showed a 1-year survival of 88%.

E Therapy

1. Conventional medical therapy for pulmonary hypertension has centered on the use of supplemental oxygen (with goal oxygen saturation >90%), diuretics, anticoagulants (warfarin with goal international normalized ratio [INR] between 1.5 and 2.5), and vasodilators.

2. **Diuretics** are frequently used to treat excessive edema that compromises the patient's condition, especially when hepatic congestion and ascites are present. However, diuretics must be used with caution in patients with higher right-sided pressures to avoid significant reductions in cardiac preload that could further reduce cardiac output.

3. Data demonstrating the effectiveness of **anticoagulation** are limited. However, based on the poor prognosis and evidence of in situ thrombosis in patients with pulmonary hypertension, anticoagulation is recommended to achieve an INR of 1.5–2.5 times that of normal controls.

4. Digoxin is recommended by some experts; however, it is somewhat controversial. It is always recommended for use in patients who have pulmonary hypertension with evidence of left ventricular dysfunction. However, its role in patients with isolated right ventricular dysfunction secondary to pulmonary hypertension in the absence of left ventricular dysfunction is unclear.

5. **Calcium channel blockers** have historically played a role in the treatment of PH but are currently used less frequently due to the medications listed in Section 6. The rationale for the use of calcium channel blockers was based on the premise that vasoconstriction is a prominent feature of the disease.

a. During a right heart catheterization, an acute response to a vasodilator (adenosine, nitric oxide, or epoprostenol) is present in approximately 10% of patients with PAH and may portend a better prognosis and indicate which patients might respond to high-dose calcium channel blockers. Calcium channel blockers used include nifedipine (dose range, 30–240 mg/day) and diltiazem (120–900 mg/day).

    b. Caution needs to be exhibited when using these agents because they may precipitously reduce cardiac output.

    c. Side effects include systemic hypotension, edema, and hypoxemia, all of which need to be identified under close administration in a structured setting by experienced clinicians.

6. The U.S. Food and Drug Administration–approved targeted therapies for PAH comprise **prostacyclin derivatives, endothelin receptor antagonists, and phosphodiesterase type-5 inhibitors.**

    a. The **prostacyclin** derivatives include intravenous (IV) epoprostenol, inhaled iloprost, and subcutaneous, intravenous, or inhaled treprostinil. **Epoprostenol** is currently the most effective therapy but has a short half-life and must be administered continuously via an IV infusion. Side effects may limit its use and include flushing, headache, nausea, vomiting, diarrhea, jaw pain, hypotension, and delivery-site complications. **Iloprost** is given via inhalation, but its half-life is short, and so it requires six to nine inhalations per day. **Treprostinil** is a longer-acting prostacyclin analog, is infused subcutaneously or intravenously, and is complicated by site infusion pain that can be severe enough to cause discontinuation. The inhaled form was recently approved and requires 2- to 3-minute inhalational treatment four times per day.

    b. The **endothelin receptor antagonists** include bosentan and ambrisentan, both of which are administered orally. **Bosentan** was the first oral therapy approved for PAH therapy, in 2001, and it has been shown to increase exercise capacity. Monthly liver function tests must be done, as it has been shown to cause liver problems in up to 11% of patients. **Ambrisentan** has similar efficacy to that of bosentan, with far lower risk of liver toxicity, but it causes lower-extremity edema more frequently than does bosentan.

    c. Sildenafil and tadalafil comprise the **phosphodiesterase type-5 inhibitors** that have been approved for the treatment of PAH. They work in the same pathway as exogenous nitric oxide by increasing cyclic GMP and causing vasodilation. **Sildenafil** is well tolerated and administered three times a day, but it cannot be used with other nitrates. Hypotension can be a side effect. **Tadalafil** is similar but is administered once daily.

IX   PULMONARY THROMBOEMBOLISM

A Introduction

1. Definition. In pulmonary thromboembolism, a thrombus arises elsewhere in the body and migrates to the pulmonary vascular tree, where it causes obstruction. Nearly all pulmonary emboli derive from deep venous thrombosis. Rarely (e.g., in sickle cell disease), pulmonary arterial thrombosis occurs in situ as a primary event without an embolic source.

2. Incidence. Acute pulmonary thromboembolism is a major cause of morbidity and mortality in the United States. Approximately 50% of cases of deep venous thrombosis are complicated by pulmonary embolism. Each year, 650,000–900,000 individuals in the United States sustain pulmonary emboli, an estimated 150,000 of whom die as a result. This mortality figure has not changed during the last 25 years.

B Etiology

1. Site of thrombus formation. Stasis in the **iliofemoral venous system** with subsequent **deep venous thrombosis (DVT)** is the most common precursor of pulmonary embolism. Other common sites of thrombus formation include the **prostatic and pelvic veins.** A superficial vein is a vein that is close to the surface of the body and not paired with a nearby artery. Deep veins lie close to a main artery, for example, the femoral vein and femoral artery. Superficial veins can develop a thrombus, inducing a problem called superficial thrombophlebitis. These superficial thrombi do not carry the risk of embolizing to cause a pulmonary embolus. An exception is the saphenous vein, which can be a precursor to a DVT. Except in intravenous drug abusers or those patients with indwelling catheters, pulmonary emboli generally originate in the lower extremities.

2. Predisposing factors. Conditions that increase a patient's risk of venous thrombosis and therefore pulmonary thromboembolism are the components of **Virchow's triad:** stasis of blood (as during a long plane trip), hypercoagulobility, and endothelial injury or dysfunction [see Chapter 4 for further details].

C **Pathology and Pathophysiology**

1. **Embolization.** When a thrombus breaks off from its site of origin, it is carried through the inferior vena cava and right ventricle to the pulmonary arteries, where it lodges. Pulmonary emboli may be single or multiple and vary in size from microscopic particles to large emboli that completely block the major branches of the pulmonary artery. A "saddle embolus" is a thrombus that sits over the main pulmonary artery partially or totally occluding the right and left pulmonary arteries.

2. **Hemodynamic consequences**
   a. **Right ventricular failure** and hemodynamic collapse is the major cause of mortality resulting from a pulmonary embolus.
   b. Obstruction of the pulmonary arteries by the embolus increases resistance to blood flow through the pulmonary circuit and increases right ventricular afterload. When more than 50%–60% of the pulmonary perfusion is impeded, pulmonary hypertension, right ventricular strain, and cardiac failure ensue.
   c. The embolism also may cause the release of humoral substances (e.g., histamine, serotonin, prostaglandins), leading to vasoconstriction throughout the lungs. This vasoconstrictive effect further increases pulmonary vascular resistance and the work of the right ventricle.
   d. Fewer than 10% of cases of pulmonary embolism progress to **pulmonary infarction** because the lung parenchyma has three sources of oxygen—the airways, the bronchial artery circulation, and the pulmonary artery circulation.
   d. Recurrent pulmonary emboli progressively occlude the pulmonary vascular bed and lead to chronic progressive pulmonary hypertension and, ultimately, **cor pulmonale.**

3. **Pulmonary consequences**
   a. The primary pulmonary consequence of an embolism is $\dot{V}/\dot{Q}$ **mismatch,** creating a high ventilation-to-perfusion ratio (see 🅟 Online I H on $\dot{V}/\dot{Q}$ mismatch).
      (1) "Wasted" ventilation or "dead space" occurs in the lung segments where the vascular supply is obstructed and perfusion cannot occur.
      (2) The blood must be shunted to other areas of the lung.
   b. Other pulmonary responses include atelectasis of the ischemic segment of the lung, reflex bronchiolar and vascular constriction, and the loss or malfunction of alveolar surfactant.

D **Clinical Features, Diagnosis, and Clinical Course**

1. **Symptoms.** Patients may complain of dyspnea at rest and chest pain that is often pleuritic. Syncope may occur in a large pulmonary embolism as cardiac output declines. Occasionally there is hemoptysis. Recent unilateral leg swelling may indicate a recent DVT. It is important to ask about risk factors for pulmonary thromboembolism and DVT, including recent travel or being bed bound, trauma, malignancy risk factors, signs like unintentional weight loss, and family history of clots.

2. **Physical examination**
   a. Nearly all patients with pulmonary embolism have tachypnea and tachycardia, and many have a low-grade fever.
   b. In **massive pulmonary embolism,** the severe physiologic consequences are manifested as cyanosis, hypotension, hypoxemia, peripheral venous engorgement, and hepatic congestion; there may be evidence of cor pulmonale. In **submassive pulmonary embolism,** the less profound hemodynamic changes may be subtle, so that hypotension, tachycardia, and hypoxia may not be observed.
   c. There is dullness to percussion and decreased breath sounds over the involved area of the lung. Findings are usually normal over the remaining lung segments. Occasionally, a pleural friction rub or wheezing is heard.
   d. Evidence of deep venous thrombosis is seen in approximately 50% of patients.

3. **Chest radiography.** Results are normal or only mildly abnormal in most patients. A few show plate-like atelectasis, a unilaterally high diaphragm, or a small pleural effusion. Occasional

findings include a bulging pulmonary artery and a large oligemic lung segment called Westermark's sign. A wedge-shaped, pleural-based density is typical of a pulmonary infarction, known as Hampton's hump.

4. **Electrocardiography.** The electrocardiogram (ECG) is usually is not specific but may help differentiate between myocardial infarction and pulmonary embolism.

   a. The most common finding is sinus tachycardia with or without premature atrial and ventricular contractions. The mean P axis commonly shifts to the right when right-sided pulmonary obstruction is severe. The classic ECG is a pronounced S wave in lead I and a Q wave and inverted T wave in lead III (denoted $S_1Q_3T_3$).

   b. Right ventricular strain may produce intermittent right-bundle-branch block, P pulmonale (i.e., "peaked" P waves that are most evident in lead II), and right-axis deviation of the QRS.

5. **Blood gas analysis**

   a. **Hypoxemia** (indicated by a decrease in PaO_2), hyperventilation (indicated by a decrease in $PaCO_2$), and a mild acute respiratory alkalosis (indicated by a slightly elevated pH) are the classic changes seen in patients with pulmonary embolism. However, they are **nonspecific** for pulmonary embolism, and pulmonary embolism may occur without these changes.

   b. A more sensitive indicator of abnormal gas exchange is the alveolar-to-arterial oxygen gradient (A–a DO_2 [⊙ Online I H 3]), which is usually elevated in patients with pulmonary embolism.

6. **Imaging.** The diagnosis of pulmonary thromboembolism is made and confirmed with specific imaging: perfusion/ventilation scanning, spiral chest CT, or pulmonary angiography.

   a. In **perfusion scanning,** the patient's blood is labeled with a radioactive tracer. Poorly perfused areas of the lung appear as relatively inactive areas on the scan. The test is not specific for pulmonary embolism because pneumonia and COPD also can produce scanning abnormalities. In **xenon ventilation scanning,** the patient inhales the radioactive tracer. This procedure is performed in conjunction with perfusion scanning to increase the specificity of the test. Finding well-ventilated but poorly perfused areas suggests pulmonary embolism; finding areas with both perfusion and ventilation defects suggests parenchymal lung disease rather than pulmonary embolism.

   b. **Spiral (helical) chest computed tomography** with intravenous contrast is another technique. It has become the standard to diagnose pulmonary embolism over the last 10 years. This technique involves continuous movement of the patient through the scanner with multiple rapid scans of the thorax during a single breath (Figure 3–9). Several studies have reported greater than 95% sensitivity and specificity to diagnose pulmonary embolism. Spiral CT is most sensitive for thromboembolism involving the main, lobar, and segmental arteries.

   c. **Pulmonary angiography** is the time-honored gold standard test for the diagnosis of pulmonary embolism, although has been used much less commonly in clinical practice over the last 10 years due to the risks, and it is invasive. It is unequivocally diagnostic if emboli are visualized.

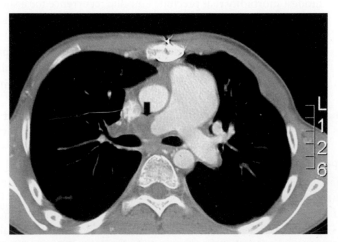

FIGURE 3–9   Spiral CT of the chest with contrast, showing a large clot (*black arrow*) obstructing the right main pulmonary artery.

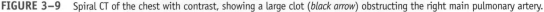

7. When the diagnosis of pulmonary embolism remains in question despite many diagnostic studies, **corroborative evidence** of venous disease in the lower extremities should be sought.

   a. Noninvasive methods include **Doppler ultrasonography,** impedance plethysmography, and leg and thigh scanning with radioiodinated fibrinogen. However, these techniques can produce false-positive results, and they cannot be used to evaluate pelvic veins.

   b. Contrast venography is helpful in diagnosing occlusion of the pelvic, thigh, and leg veins. This invasive technique is not without morbidity. It has been associated with phlebitis, hypersensitivity reactions, and local pain.

   c. D-dimer is a degradation product released during endogenous fibrinolysis. The negative predictive value of D-dimer has been reported to be 97%–98% in several studies. However, the test has a low positive predictive value and low specificity, so it should be used only if the likelihood of thromboembolism is low in order to rule out a DVT or pulmonary embolism. The modified Well's criteria can help determine pretest probability.

E Therapy

1. **Anticoagulants**

   a. Unless contraindicated, the drug of choice for documented or suspected pulmonary embolism is standard unfractionated **heparin** or **low–molecular-weight heparin** (LMWH). Standard unfractionated heparin must be given in doses that maintain the partial thromboplastin time (PTT) at 2–2.5 times normal, given by continuous intravenous administration. LMWH is a type of fractionated natural heparin with a molecular weight of 200–700 daltons (15,000 for standard heparin). It is given subcutaneously. It is an alternative to unfractionated heparin and may enable patients to be discharged earlier or, in some cases, to receive only outpatient therapy. LMWH has a longer half-life than natural heparin, and LMWH also demonstrates efficacy in the prophylaxis and management of venous thrombosis.

   b. After anticoagulation with heparin or LMWH has been achieved for a few days, therapy is changed to **warfarin,** given orally, in doses that maintain the prothrombin time (PT) at 2–2.5 times the normal value or the INR at 2–3. The oral anticoagulant is continued for 3–6 months in the first occurrence of pulmonary thromboembolism or longer if a genetic cause is found.

2. **Oxygen** is given routinely to correct hypoxemia, and **bed rest** ordinarily is prescribed until the dyspnea and pain resolve, after which patients may ambulate while remaining on anticoagulant therapy.

3. **Thrombolytic agents.** Fibrinolytic agents are given when rapid lysis of clots is important.

   a. Because thrombolytic agents increase the risk of hemorrhage, they are reserved for use when occlusion has produced right-sided heart failure and hemodynamic instability.

   b. Thrombolytic agents appear to provide long-term physiologic improvement in the pulmonary vascular bed.

4. **Surgery**

   a. Percutaneous insertion of an "umbrella" filter (Greenfield filter) is a surgical remedy with modest morbidity that preclude embolic recurrence for a short period.

      (1) Collateral venous channels in the pelvis or lower abdomen may develop in patients with chronic vena caval obstruction and may find routes around the obstruction to the pulmonary artery, eventually negating the effectiveness of the procedure.

      (2) Vena caval filters should be reserved for patients in whom embolism recurs despite adequate anticoagulation therapy and for patients in whom anticoagulants are contraindicated (e.g., patients with active bleeding).

   b. Surgical embolectomy remains an alternative treatment for patients who cannot maintain effective cardiac output. Occasionally, embolectomy is life saving, but the overall survival rate is approximately 10%.

5. **Prophylactic "minidose" heparin therapy or LMWH.** Giving small doses of heparin prophylactically has been helpful in preventing pulmonary embolism in certain high-risk patients, with little risk of hemorrhage.

   a. Prophylaxis is particularly applicable for older patients who undergo lower abdominal or pelvic surgery and who are on bed rest postoperatively. It also is helpful for obese patients who are perioperative or who will be bed bound for a time.

b. It also is recommended for patients on prolonged bed rest because of stroke, myocardial infarction, cardiac failure, or cancer or those with a high number of risk factors when admitted to the hospital.

X DISEASES OF THE PLEURA

A Pleural effusion

1. **Definition.** A pleural effusion is an abnormal accumulation of fluid in the pleural space.

2. **Etiology**
   a. In healthy patients, the pleural cavity contains a small volume of lubricating serous fluid, formed primarily by transudation from the parietal pleura and absorbed primarily by the capillaries and lymphatics. The balance between formation and removal of this fluid may be compromised by any disorder that increases the pulmonary or systemic venous pressure, lowers the plasma oncotic pressure, increases capillary permeability, or obstructs the lymphatic circulation.
   b. A pleural effusion may be a transudate or an exudate (Table 3–4).
      (1) Transudates are caused by elevated venous pressure or by decreased plasma oncotic pressure; the primary pathologic process does not directly involve the pleural surface. Transudates are usually noninflammatory pleural effusions that may occur in any condition that causes ascites, obstruction of the venous or lymphatic outflow from the thorax, isolated left- or right-sided congestive heart failure (CHF), or hypoalbuminemia.
      (2) Exudates are caused by increased permeability of the pleural surface (due to inflammation, trauma, or disease) or by obstruction of the lymphatics. Exudates are usually inflammatory, infectious, or malignant pleural effusions that result from abnormal processes adjacent to the pleural surface. The site of inflammation usually is just beneath the visceral pleura within the lung but occasionally is within the mediastinum, diaphragm, or chest wall. Secondary inflammation of larger areas of the pleural surface may result in rapid outpouring of exudate. Removal of the fluid by the normal clearing mechanisms may be considerably retarded by inflammatory obstruction of the lymphatics that drain the thorax.

3. **Clinical Features, Diagnosis, and Clinical Course**
   a. Symptoms result from inflammation of the parietal pleura and compression of the lung.
      (1) Pleuritic pain occurs most commonly with exudative effusions and may be accompanied by a friction rub.
         (a) The pain commonly is a sharp, stabbing sensation that is minimal during quiet respiration but intensifies abruptly during full inflation of the lungs.

TABLE 3–4   Causes of Pleural Effusions

Causes of Exudates
Malignancy (e.g., bronchogenic carcinoma, lymphoma, metastatic tumor)
Inflammatory processes
Infections (e.g., tuberculosis, pneumonia)
Pulmonary embolic disease
Collagen vascular disease (e.g., rheumatoid arthritis)
Subdiaphragmatic process
Asbestosis
Pancreatitis
Hypothyroidism
Trauma

Causes of Transudates
Decreased plasma oncotic pressure
Nephrotic syndrome
Cirrhosis
Increased hydrostatic pressure
Congestive heart failure

(2) **Dyspnea** can occur if the accumulation of pleural fluid compresses the lung and interferes with the movement of the diaphragm.

b. **Physical signs.** Fluid usually accumulates first at the base of the lung, where the earliest physical signs are noted.

(1) Auscultation usually reveals absent or decreased breath sounds. Percussion is dull at the area of the effusion. Fremitus is decreased and pectoriloquy is absent.

(2) The mediastinum may shift away from the side of a large effusion, usually if the volume is greater than 1 L.

c. **Radiographic appearance**

(1) **Chest radiography.** The earliest visible signs of effusion on a plain-film radiograph are blunting of the costophrenic angle and blurring of the posterior diaphragm in the lateral view. A posterior–anterior film may show no abnormality if there is less than 300 mL of pleural fluid. The lateral view may show a small effusion as blunting of the posterior costophrenic angle. A lateral decubitus film may help differentiate free fluid from previous inflammatory adhesions.

(2) **Diagnostic ultrasound** may help localize the effusion more accurately when blind a thoracentesis is difficult or unsuccessful.

d. **Specialized diagnostic procedures**

(1) Unless a cause has been established, the presence of fluid in the pleural cavity is an indication for **thoracentesis.**

(a) The fluid should be removed, the gross appearance noted, and specimens sent to the laboratory for examination.

(b) Routine laboratory procedures include measuring and calculating Light's criteria. This is to determine whether the effusion is a **transudate** or an **exudate. A transudate** (noninflammatory effusion) is defined as follows: pleural fluid/serum total protein ratio of <0.5, pleural fluid/serum lactate dehydrogenase (LDH) ratio of <0.6, and pleural fluid LDH less than two-thirds the upper limit of normal for serum. Transudative pleural effusions occur in congestive heart failure and hepatic hydrothorax or in low-albumin states such as nephritic syndrome.

(c) An **exudate** is defined by Light's criteria as follows: pleural fluid/serum total protein ratio of >0.5, pleural fluid/serum LDH ratio of >0.6, and pleural fluid LDH greater than two-thirds the upper limit of normal for serum. Exudative pleural effusions occur in malignancy, pulmonary embolism, connective tissue diseases, parapneumonic effusion (effusions in the presence of bacterial pneumonia within the lung), subdiaphragmatic inflammatory processes (pancreatitis, hepatic or perinephric abscess), and tuberculosis.

(d) Other tests that should be sent from the pleural fluid include pH, cell count and differential, Gram stain, culture, amylase, glucose, cytology, adenosine deaminase (if tuberculosis suspected), amylase (if pancreatitis or esophageal rupture suspected), and triglycerides (if chylothorax or pseudochylothorax suspected).

(2) **Needle biopsy** of the pleura is performed to determine the cause of an exudate when repeated thoracenteses are nondiagnostic.

(3) When ordinary measures fail to establish a definitive diagnosis, **thoracotomy** or **video-assisted thoracoscopy (VATS)** with exploration of the lung and biopsy of the involved areas of the pleural surface may be essential for accurate diagnosis.

4. **Differential diagnosis.** Laboratory data can help determine the cause of a pleural effusion.

a. It is useful to establish whether the fluid is an exudate or a transudate (see Table 3–4), which is explained earlier.

b. The presence of **gross blood** in the pleural fluid is most common when the effusion is caused by **malignancy,** trauma, or pulmonary infarction.

c. The pleural fluid-to-serum **glucose** ratio is sometimes low when the effusion is caused by tuberculosis or malignancy but usually is very low in effusions that are caused by rheumatoid arthritis.

d. The pleural fluid **amylase** level frequently is elevated when the effusion is attributable to pancreatic disease or rupture of the esophagus and occasionally is elevated moderately in malignant effusions.

    e. The **pH** of pleural fluid usually is 7.3 or greater. Lower values occasionally are seen in tuberculosis and malignant effusions. A pH of less than 7.2 in a parapneumonic effusion suggests an empyema and requires urgent drainage with a chest tube.

5. **Therapy**

    a. Treatment must be directed at the disease causing the effusion. Transudative effusions are usually treated by addressing the underlying cause (e.g., CHF). Appropriate therapy for exudative effusions may call for chest tube placement, antibiotics, antituberculosis therapy, repeated thoracentesis, or chemical pleurodesis to eliminate the pleural space.

    b. Dyspnea may be relieved by thoracentesis, but this procedure carries the risk of pneumothorax (from visceral pleural puncture) or cardiovascular collapse (from removing too much fluid too quickly). An amount of ≤ 1.5 L should be removed at one time to prevent reexpansion pulmonary edema.

B Empyema

1. **Definition and clinical features.** An empyema is an exudative pleural process falling within the broad category of parapneumonic effusions but has become more advanced and complex as there is a true accumulation of pus in the pleural space; it is an occasional complication of both bacterial pneumonia and lung abscess. The fluid usually is thick and has the appearance of frank pus. As previously stated, pleural fluid with a pH of less than 7.2 strongly suggests an empyema.

2. **Therapy.** An empyema almost always requires chest tube drainage as well as antibiotic therapy. Drainage may be straightforward early in the patient's course; however, after several days without adequate drainage, most empyemas become loculated, so that tube drainage becomes more complex and thoracic surgical intervention may become necessary.

C Pneumothorax

1. **Definition.** Pneumothorax is an accumulation of air in the pleural space. If the accumulation is large enough, the underlying lung parenchyma may become collapsed and functionless.

2. **Etiology**

    a. Pneumothorax is a common medical problem, frequently caused by **trauma,** including trauma due to medical procedures. **Primary spontaneous pneumothorax** occurs with the rupture of a bulla, most commonly in an upper lobe. It occurs more frequently in men than in women, and especially in men 20–40 years of age.

    b. Spontaneous pneumothorax also may occur **secondary** to lung involvement in **almost any lung disease** but occurs most commonly in COPD, *Pneumocystis jiroveci* infection, cystic fibrosis, and tuberculosis.

3. **Clinical Features and Diagnosis**

    a. The major **symptoms** of pneumothorax are **chest pain** and **dyspnea.**

    b. **Physical examination** shows hyperresonance and decreased breath sounds over the involved side.

    c. In a "tension pneumothorax" the trachea may be deviated away from the affected side.

    d. **Chest radiographs** obtained during expiration help demonstrate small pneumothoraces because this technique increases the space between the lung and pleural space.

4. **Therapy**

    a. A small spontaneous pneumothorax often resolves by itself and is aided by high-flow oxygen therapy. A more severe pneumothorax calls for reexpansion of the lung through placement of an intercostal chest tube and application of appropriate negative pressure. The treatment is continued for 24–48 hours after the lung is reexpanded, so that the pleural space seals and pleural adhesions prevent recurrence. In select cases, smaller, less-complicated pneumothoraces can be treated with pneumocentesis (e.g., removal of air during a thoracentesis) without placement of a chest tube.

    b. Spontaneous pneumothorax has a tendency to recur, and surgical treatment should be considered after three or more occurrences on a given side. Surgery involves an open thoracotomy or VATS and abrasion of the pleural surfaces (pleurodesis), which produces symphysis of the parietal and visceral pleurae.

5. **Complications.** Although pneumothorax is a relatively benign condition, serious complications can result.
   a. **Bilateral simultaneous pneumothorax** is rare but can cause rapid death and is usually the result of trauma.
   b. Pneumothorax may be accompanied by hemorrhage into the pleural space, which results in **hemopneumothorax.**
   c. **Tension pneumothorax** is a buildup of positive pressure within the pleural space, which rapidly produces severe respiratory and cardiovascular compromise. Patients undergoing positive-pressure mechanical ventilation are particularly at risk.
      (1) Tension pneumothorax presumably results from a ball-valve mechanism at the site of the air leak from the lung, which allows air to enter but not leave the pleural space.
      (2) This leads to progressive collapse of the lung, a contralateral shift of the mediastinal structures, including the trachea, and reduced blood flow to the right side of the heart, impairing cardiovascular function as well as lung function. Prompt decompression of the involved pleural space is indicated.

D **Chylothorax** A chylothorax is another one of the exudative effusions. In the normal adult, the thoracic duct transports up to 4 L of chyle per day. When the thoracic duct is lacerated or obstructed by trauma (cardiovascular surgery) or tumor, lymph may accumulate in the pleural space. This condition, termed chylothorax, is identified by a murky appearance of the pleural fluid, demonstration of fat droplets on staining with Sudan III, and a total neutral fat content of >0.5 g/dL.

E **Primary pleural neoplasia**

1. **Localized fibrous mesothelioma.** This uncommon neoplasm arises from the pleural surface and most commonly is attached to the visceral pleura.
   a. **Symptoms**
      (1) The lesion may cause chest discomfort and dyspnea if it becomes very large. However, most of these neoplasms are discovered before these symptoms develop.
      (2) The syndrome of **hypertrophic pulmonary osteoarthropathy,** which is associated with arthralgia of the hands, ankles, wrists, and knees and with clubbing of the fingers, may occur secondary to pleural-based neoplasms.
   b. **Diagnosis.** Chest radiograph indicates a mass lesion. A pleural effusion occasionally is present.
   c. **Therapy** is surgical resection, which also relieves the symptoms of the hypertrophic pulmonary osteoarthropathy.
   d. **Prognosis.** Most of these neoplasms are benign, and patients have an excellent prognosis. A few of these neoplasms are malignant but have favorable courses.

2. **Diffuse malignant mesothelioma**
   a. **Incidence.** This malignant neoplasm occurs over a wide age range, with the average age at onset being 55 years. The incidence is increased in workers exposed to asbestos; generally, the malignancy develops 20 or more years after exposure.
   b. **Symptoms and diagnosis.** Chest pain and dyspnea are the predominant symptoms. The chest radiograph may show pleural thickening, pleural effusion, or both. The diagnosis is difficult to establish by cytologic examination; pleural biopsy often is necessary.
   c. **Therapy** involves radiation therapy or chemotherapy; results are uniformly very poor.

XI CHEST WALL DISORDERS

A **Etiology** Chest wall disorders may be either mechanical or neuromuscular in origin. They may cause respiratory dysfunction and, in severe cases, respiratory failure.

1. **Mechanical disorders** affecting the chest wall include kyphosis, scoliosis, obesity-associated hypoventilation, thoracoplasty, ankylosing spondylitis, and chest wall trauma.

2. **Neuromuscular diseases** affecting the chest wall are polyneuropathies, motor system diseases, muscular dystrophies, spinal cord injuries, multiple sclerosis, and myasthenia gravis.

B **Kyphoscoliosis,** the most common and best understood chest wall disease, is used in this discussion as a prototype for the pathophysiology, course, and management of all chest wall disorders.

1. **Definition.** Kyphoscoliosis is a common skeletal abnormality characterized by posterior curvature (**kyphosis**) and lateral curvature (**scoliosis**) of the spine. These processes, alone or in combination, decrease the volume and mobility of the lung and chest wall.

2. **Incidence.** Kyphoscoliosis affects 1% of the U.S. population and occurs predominantly in females. The deformity is clinically significant in 2.3% of affected individuals.

3. **Etiology** is not clear in 80% of cases. A major known cause is childhood poliomyelitis. Congenital kyphoscoliosis is uncommon but can potentially result in severe deformity and neurologic abnormalities. Severe osteoporosis may cause multiple thoracic spinal compression fractures, which will result in kyphoscoliosis.

4. **Pathophysiology**
   a. Lung volume is reduced in kyphoscoliosis because the chest wall is distorted. The distortion also causes stiffness of the chest wall, increasing the work of breathing and causing decreased total respiratory system compliance and reduction of FRC. The pressure–volume compliance curve of the lung (as opposed to that of the chest wall) is nearly normal, and forced expiratory flow is preserved relative to lung volume.
   b. Gas exchange is impaired in marked kyphoscoliosis: Alveolar hypoventilation occurs and **$PaCO_2$** rises. The A–a DO_2 is mildly widened because of $\dot{V}/\dot{Q}$ inequality, which results from the compressive effect of atelectasis and inadequate periodic hyperinflation.
   c. Pulmonary hypertension eventually is present at rest as well as during exercise in patients with a moderate chest wall deformity.

5. **Clinical features, diagnosis, and clinical course**
   a. **Symptoms**
      (1) **Exertional dyspnea** is the major respiratory symptom. The onset and severity of dyspnea correlate with the degree of the spinal angulation, as measured on the chest film. Hypoventilation supervenes in those patients whose deformity is severe.
      (2) **Sequelae of prolonged arterial hypoxemia,** including pulmonary hypertension, right ventricular dysfunction, and cor pulmonale, may develop as late manifestations.
   b. **Chest radiograph.** Ribs on the convex portion of the spine are widely spaced and rotated posteriorly. Ribs on the concave aspect are crowded and displaced anteriorly.
   c. **Complications.** Respiratory failure and cor pulmonale, the major complications, result from respiratory infections or injudicious use of sedatives, or both.

6. **Therapy**
   a. Early identification of kyphoscoliosis in adolescence is the key to prevention of symptomatic disease. **Corrective intervention** should be considered when the angulation is greater than 40 degrees. There are two forms of intervention:
      (1) **Mechanical.** A Milwaukee brace can be applied externally during the early stages of the disease.
      (2) **Surgical.** The Harrington procedure, using metal rods and focal spinal fusion, can be performed, after which the patient wears a plaster of Paris jacket cast for several months. Surgery does not improve the maximum breathing capacity but may improve arterial oxygen and oxygen desaturation. At best, surgery appears to preserve whatever pulmonary function is present at the time of intervention.
   b. Periodic hyperinflation with intermittent positive-pressure breathing devices appears to increase **PaO_2** in outpatients. In patients who develop obstructive sleep apnea (OSA) because of cervical spine angulation, continuous positive-pressure breathing (CPAP) during sleep is useful. In those who develop chronic hypercapnic respiratory failure, noninvasive positive-pressure ventilation (NPPV) may be useful.

C **Chest Trauma**

1. **Blunt trauma.** Blunt chest trauma causes injury either by direct application of sudden force to the chest wall and indirect transmission of these forces to the intrathoracic structures or by secondary visceral destruction by chest wall structures.
   a. Injury of extrapulmonary organs often accompanies blunt chest trauma. Disruption of the chest wall may cause rib fractures, hemothorax, pneumothorax, and flail chest. Inertial injury may cause rupture of the bronchial, diaphragmatic, or great blood vessels.

b. **Flail chest** most commonly results from motor vehicle injury or overzealous cardiac resuscitation. The chest wall, or at least one hemithorax, is rendered unstable by multiple fractures of the ribs, sternum, or costochondral joints.

   (1) The injured portion moves **paradoxically,** that is, inward on inspiration as the intrapleural pressure becomes subatmospheric and outward on expiration as the intrapleural pressure increases toward atmospheric.

   (2) Respiratory failure is treated with mechanical ventilation, pain control, and oxygen supplementation.

2. **Penetrating trauma** is characterized by puncture or laceration of the chest wall and intrathoracic fistulae. Vehicular accidents and knife and missile wounds are the usual causes. Exploratory thoracotomies are indicated for persistent hemothorax and sucking chest wounds and to determine the likelihood of mediastinal, diaphragmatic, or cardiac disruption.

XII MEDIASTINAL DISEASES

A **Mediastinal masses**   The mediastinum is divided into three parts: **anterior/superior, middle,** and **posterior.** Mediastinal masses may occur at any age and are characteristic of the mediastinal compartment in which they occur. The lateral chest radiograph and CT of the chest often are the most important initial diagnostic measures.

1. **Masses in the anterior/superior mediastinum**
   a. Masses in this compartment are more likely to be **malignant** than those in other compartments.
   b. **Thymomas** are the most common superior mediastinal masses. **Presentation** frequently involves cough, chest pain, and superior vena caval obstruction. Myasthenia gravis occurs in approximately one third of patients with a thymoma. RBC aplasia and hypogammaglobulinemia are other recognized but rare associations. Surgical excision is recommended.
   c. **Hodgkin's disease** and **non-Hodgkin's lymphomas** may manifest as masses in the anterior or superior mediastinum.
   d. **Intrathoracic thyroid goiters** may occur, particularly in middle-aged women. They usually are asymptomatic but may cause stridor, hoarseness, or dysphagia. Functional goiters can result in hyperthyroidism.
   e. **Dermoid cysts (teratomas)** appear as dense, lobular shadows in the anterior mediastinum, often with calcifications in the walls. Teeth may be recognized within the tumor. Dermoid cysts usually are asymptomatic unless infection or malignant change develops. Other malignant germ cell neoplasms may also occur.

2. **Masses in the middle mediastinum**
   a. **Lymphomas** may also appear in the middle mediastinum.
   b. **Pleuropericardial cysts** occur in the middle mediastinum at the right cardiophrenic angle, characteristically appearing as smooth, sharply demarcated masses of uniform density.
   c. **Bronchogenic cysts** and **duplication cysts of the esophagus** are rare causes of middle mediastinal masses.

3. **Masses in the posterior mediastinum. Neurogenic tumors** are the most common posterior mediastinal tumors and characteristically occur along the paravertebral border. These tumors often are asymptomatic in adults but may cause chest pain with stridor, breathlessness, cough, and tracheal compression. Horner's syndrome and spinal cord compression also may occur.

4. **Aneurysms of the aorta** may occur in any compartment, depending on their location within the aorta.

B **Mediastinitis**

1. **Acute mediastinitis** is a severe, life-threatening illness that most often follows cardiothoracic surgery or rupture of the esophagus. It also may follow vomiting, dental work, endoscopy, or other trauma and is characterized by fever, chest pain, and variable mediastinal enlargement. The disease progresses rapidly and requires emergency medical and surgical treatment.

2. **Chronic mediastinitis and mediastinal fibrosis.** *Histoplasma* spp. or, rarely, other fungi or mycobacteria can produce a chronic granulomatous process in the mediastinum, often with

extensive scar tissue that contracts to cause narrowing of the trachea, bronchi, vena cava, pulmonary arteries, and pulmonary veins.

C **Pneumomediastinum** is the presence of air in the mediastinum. Air is presumed to leak from alveoli and to dissect along bronchi to the hilum, from which it may enter the mediastinum. If pressure builds in the mediastinum, air may expand into the neck tissues, producing subcutaneous emphysema, and there may be chest pain. However, if the mediastinal air is confined, the increasing pressure may interfere with circulation. When this occurs, tracheostomy usually is adequate therapy. Intervention is unnecessary in patients without circulatory problems.

XIII DIFFUSE PARENCHYMAL LUNG DISEASES

A **Definition** Diffuse parenchymal lung disease (DPLD) (a more accurate term than the older term interstitial lung disease) is a broad term for a group of related disorders that are all characterized by inflammation and/or fibrosis of the lung and involve the alveoli and/or interstitium. Regardless of their various causes, DPLDs share certain clinical, radiographic, pathologic, and physiologic characteristics.

B **Etiology**

1. In approximately 50% of cases, diffuse parenchymal disease occurs spontaneously, and many are idiopathic. Table 3–5 list the types of diffuse parenchymal lung diseases.

2. The remaining cases are associated with known or suspected causes. Environmental or occupational exposure to a variety of substances is well known to induce interstitial pulmonary fibrosis (see XIV D on occupational lung diseases); these substances may act as inciting allergens or directly toxic agents. In other cases, DPLD is associated with connective tissue disease, sarcoidosis, vasculitis, or chronic hypersensitivity pneumonitis. Many of these diseases have been associated with cigarette smoking.

TABLE 3–5 Clinical Classification of Diffuse Parenchymal Lung Diseases

Idiopathic Fibrotic Disorders
Idiopathic pulmonary fibrosis
Nonspecific interstitial pneumonia
Cryptogenic organizing pneumonia
Respiratory bronchiolitis–associated interstitial lung disease
Desquamative interstitial pneumonia
Lymphocytic interstitial pneumonia
Acute interstitial pneumonitis

Connective Tissue Diseases
Scleroderma
Polymyositis-dermatomyositis
Systemic lupus erythematosus
Rheumatoid arthritis
Mixed connective tissue disorder

Drug-Induced Diseases
Antibiotics (nitrofurantoin, sulfasalazine)
Antiarrhythmics (amiodarone, propranolol)
Chemotherapeutic agents (mitomycin C, bleomycin, busulfan, methotrexate)
Anticonvulsants (Dilantin)
Therapeutic radiation

Primary (Unclassified) Diseases
Sarcoidosis
Pulmonary Langerhans cell histiocytosis X
Amyloidosis
Pulmonary vasculitis
Lymphangioleiomyomatosis
Tuberous sclerosis

Occupational and Environmental Diseases
Organic (Hypersensitivity Pneumonitis)
Bird feeders lung
Farmer's lung
Grain worker's lung
Humidifier lung

Inorganic
Silicosis
Asbestosis
Hard metal pneumoconiosis
Coal worker's pneumoconiosis

C **Pathology and Pathophysiology**

1. **Inflammation.** Epithelial and/or endothelial injury causes edema; there is infiltration of cells (neutrophils, macrophages, and lymphocytes), tissue necrosis factor-α (TNF-α), and interferon-γ (IFN-γ).

2. **Pulmonary fibrosis.** There is deposition of extracellular matrix by fibroblasts, mediated by Th-2 cytokines and transforming growth factor-β (TGF-β). There is also an increased number of fibroblasts.

3. **Effects on pulmonary function.** Most patients with diffuse parenchymal lung disease will have either a restrictive disease pattern or a mixed restrictive and obstructive pattern on pulmonary function testing. Many will also have a decreased diffusion capacity and will have hypoxemia initially only with exertion and, as the disease progresses, have hypoxemia at rest.

D **Clinical Features, Diagnosis, and Clinical Course**

1. **Symptoms** of interstitial lung disease seen most frequently are dyspnea on exertion and nonproductive cough. Increased fatigability, fever, and weight loss also are common.

2. **Physical findings** include tachypnea, digital clubbing, and late inspiratory crackles. If the disease is severe, cyanosis and evidence of right ventricular failure (elevated jugular venous pressure, hepatomegaly, and lower extremity edema) also may be present.

3. **Laboratory findings** are usually nonspecific. Tests for antinuclear antibodies (ANAs), rheumatoid factor, and immunoglobulin may be positive in specific connective tissue diseases.

4. **Radiographic findings. Chest radiographs** usually show a diffuse reticulonodular pattern throughout both lung fields that is often more pronounced at the lung bases. Chest CT, especially with high resolution, provides more extensive data on the extent of lung involvement and whether fibrosis or alveolitis is the predominant process (Figure 3–10). Other findings include upper or lower lobe opacities, ground glass opacities, mediastinal or hilar lymphadenopathy, and cysts in the parenchyma.

5. **Pulmonary function testing.** As noted earlier, PFTs will show either a restrictive pattern or a combination of restriction and obstruction, with impaired diffusion capacity.

6. **Diagnosis.** The clinical, radiographic, and physiologic findings strongly suggest the diagnosis of diffuse parenchymal lung disease. Definitive diagnosis requires tissue confirmation with a biopsy, either by bronchoscopic biopsy or video-assisted thoracoscopic surgical (VATS) biopsy. The risks of performing the procedure have to be weighed against the benefit of making an accurate diagnosis so that appropriate therapy can be initiated. These procedures, both bronchoscopy and VATS, may carry higher risks in the patient with parenchymal lung disease, especially if the disease

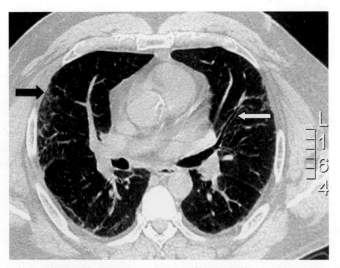

FIGURE 3–10 Chest CT in a patient with idiopathic pulmonary fibrosis (IPF), showing peripheral reticular abnormalities (*black arrow*) and traction bronchiectasis (*white arrow*).

TABLE 3–6 Idiopathic Interstitial Pneumonias

Clinical Diagnosis	Pathology
Idiopathic pulmonary fibrosis	Usual interstitial pneumonia (UIP)
Nonspecific interstitial pneumonia	Nonspecific interstitial pneumonia (NSIP)
Cryptogenic organizing pneumonia	Organizing pneumonia (OP)
Respiratory bronchiolitis–associated interstitial lung disease	Respiratory bronchiolitis (RB)
Desquamative interstitial pneumonia	Desquamative interstitial pneumonia (DIP)
Lymphocytic interstitial pneumonia	Lymphocytic interstitial pneumonia (LIP)
Acute interstitial pneumonitis	Diffuse alveolar damage (DAD)

is advanced. They may be complicated by hypoxemia, cardiopulmonary collapse, and prolonged mechanical ventilation. In the various diffuse parenchymal diseases to be discussed, bronchoscopy is useful when diagnosing sarcoidosis, organizing pneumonia, hypersensitivity pneumonitis, and alveolar proteinosis. Most other diseases will require VATS for accurate diagnosis.

7. **Clinical course.** The clinical course will vary depending upon the underlying disease. The idiopathic interstitial pneumonias (IIPs) are more aggressive, progress rapidly, and generally carry a worse prognosis over a couple of years. However, sarcoidosis and pulmonary vasculitides respond better to therapy and have a better prognosis.

E Therapy

1. Therapy will vary with specific diseases, but the general therapy is corticosteroids and other immunosuppressive agents. **Corticosteroids** have been the mainstay of therapy and are clearly indicated when open-lung biopsy shows an active cellular process without extensive fibrosis. Large doses (e.g., prednisone 1 mg/kg per day) may be used initially; physiologic and radiographic parameters should be monitored closely, and the dose should be tapered after response. If no improvement occurs with steroids alone, **immunosuppressive agents** may be given either alone or in combination with steroids. Azathioprine, cyclophosphamide, and chlorambucil are often used.

    The major diseases within the category of diffuse parenchymal lung diseases will be discussed in the following. It is important not to confuse the clinical disease with the pathologic/histologic diagnosis seen on biopsy. Some clinical diseases are described the same as the histology and some are not (Table 3–6).

F Idiopathic interstitial pneumonia (IIP) is a term used for a group of idiopathic diffuse parenchymal lung diseases that have a specific pathologic/histologic appearance under the microscope. The diagnosis is ultimately made with pathology. There are seven currently recognized distinct types (see Table 3–6).

1. **Interstitial pulmonary fibrosis (IPF)**
    a. **Definition and etiology.** IPF is a chronic, progressive form of lung disease characterized by fibrosis of the supporting framework (interstitium) of the lungs. By definition, the cause is unknown ("idiopathic"). In the British literature, this disease is termed cryptogenic fibrosing alveolitis.
    b. **Pathology and pathophysiology.** Biopsy specimens will show a specific form of pulmonary fibrosis known as **usual interstitial pneumonia (UIP)**. UIP consists of dense areas of interstitial collagen deposition, fibroblastic foci, some areas of cellular inflammation, and areas of honeycomb formation (cysts with mature respiratory epithelium at the alveolar level).
    c. **Clinical features, diagnosis, and clinical course.** Men and women are affected equally and usually diagnosed after the age of 50 years. Symptoms are gradual in onset and include progressive dyspnea, dry cough, and fatigue. On examination, there may be pulmonary crackles on auscultation ("Velcro-like" crackles) and clubbing of the fingers. Chest radiography and chest CT reveal decreased lung volumes and typically prominent reticular interstitial markings in the lung bases; "honeycombing" may be seen in advanced disease and is characterized by multiple cystic spaces within the fibrosed parenchyma, more prominent in the lower lung

fields. There may be traction bronchiectasis. On PFTs, there are the characteristic findings of restriction, along with reduced lung compliance and increased elastic recoil. D_LCO will be decreased, and the degree predicts severity of hypoxemia. The diagnosis is unquestionably made with biopsy via VATS and will show **UIP on histology.** IPF is a fairly aggressive disease, and mean survival after diagnosis is 2–4 years.

   d. Therapy. There are no well-studied therapies that have been found to be extremely beneficial in IPF. A trial of steroids with or without other immunosuppressants should be given and continued if there is a positive clinical effect but tapered and potentially stopped if there is not. Continuous oxygen therapy has shown a survival benefit in COPD patients with a PaO_2 of <55 mm Hg, and IPF patients with hypoxemia probably benefit as well. Patients who are appropriate candidates should be considered for lung transplantation; they have a 1-year survival rate of 90% and a 5-year survival rate of 50%. Bronchodilators are not beneficial. N-acetylcysteine (NAC) has been shown to improve D_LCO and vital capacity and is a safe therapy, but it has not shown survival benefits. Due to the possible benefits and safety profile, NAC is a reasonable therapy to consider.

2. **Idiopathic nonspecific interstitial pneumonia (NSIP)** is a disease entity that has a pathologic appearance distinct from that of UIP. NSIP histologically is characterized by mild-to-moderate cellular interstitial inflammation, varying degrees of interstitial fibrosis, and a general uniformity of these abnormalities throughout the biopsy. In contrast with UIP, NSIP usually does not have honeycomb change, and fibroblastic foci are few. In general the prognosis of patients with idiopathic NSIP generally is better than that of patients with IPF.

3. **Cryptogenic organizing pneumonia (COP)**
   a. Definition and etiology. By definition, there is no known etiology; "cryptogenic" means idiopathic. It was formerly referred to as bronchiolitis obliterans organizing pneumonia (BOOP). It is an inflammatory lung disease with distinctive clinical, radiologic, and pathologic features. Granulation tissue predominates in the alveoli but is also found in the bronchiolar lumen.
   b. Pathology and pathophysiology. Organizing pneumonia (OP) is the pathologic term used to describe the changes in COP. However, pathologic changes of organizing pneumonia may also be seen in pulmonary infections, certain drugs, and connective tissue diseases. By definition, COP has no underlying cause. Histologically, OP shows intra-alveolar buds of granulation tissue consisting of fibroblasts, myofibroblasts, and loose connective tissue. These buds may extend from one alveolus to the next, giving a characteristic "butterfly" pattern. Bronchiolar lesions consist of similar buds. These histologic patterns are distinct from those of UIP and NSIP.
   c. Clinical features, diagnosis, and clinical course. Men and women are affected equally and are usually between 50 and 60 years of age. The onset of symptoms is subacute, and symptoms include fever, nonproductive cough, malaise, anorexia, and weight loss. Hemoptysis, bronchorrhea, chest pain, and night sweats are less common symptoms. Crackles may be heard over affected areas. The radiographic and CT scan are characteristic of COP. They suggest the diagnosis when multiple patchy alveolar opacities with a peripheral and bilateral distribution are present. There may also be air bronchograms. Diagnosis is established by biopsy showing histology of OP. PFTs most commonly show a restrictive ventilatory defect. D_LCO is reduced. Hypoxemia is common to varying degrees. With treatment, most patients with COP do well and in general have a much better prognosis than patients with IPF.
   d. Therapy. Corticosteroids are the current standard treatment of COP. The response to corticosteroids is generally favorable, and patients usually improve subjectively and objectively (PFTS and CT scan). Most patients will require 6–12 months of treatment. A few patients are resistant to corticosteroids and may improve with other immunosuppressives.

4. **Respiratory bronchiolitis–associated interstitial lung disease (RB-ILD)** is an interstitial lung disease that is associated with smoking, and some experts believe that desquamative interstitial pneumonia (DIP; see next paragraph) is within the spectrum of the same disease. The diagnosis of RB-ILD requires the proper clinical setting with recent or current cigarette smoking, clinical manifestations of cough or dyspnea with crackles on auscultation of the lungs, radiographic manifestations of diffuse or patchy ground-glass opacities, fine nodules and air trapping on high-resolution CT scanning, and lung biopsy confirming the diagnosis with histologic findings of respiratory bronchiolitis (RB). Histologically, respiratory bronchiolitis is an inflammatory

process involving the membranous and respiratory bronchioles, with accumulation of tan-brown pigmented macrophages in the respiratory bronchioles and neighboring alveolar ducts and alveoli. Specific treatment does not exist, but smoking cessation, corticosteroid therapy, and/or other immunosuppressive therapies have been tried; data supporting efficacy are lacking.

5. **Desquamative interstitial pneumonia (DIP)** is another IIP associated with smoking and has a better prognosis than IPF. It is differentiated from RB-ILD by pathology. DIP shows alveolar septa infiltrated with plasma cells and occasional eosinophils and numerous macrophages with finely granular brown pigment flecked with tiny black particles in the distal air spaces.

6. **Lymphocytic interstitial pneumonia (LIP)** is an uncommon process characterized by the presence of widespread, monotonous sheets of lymphocytic infiltration in the interstitium of the lung. It is associated with hypogammaglobulinemia, monoclonal or polyclonal gammopathy, Sjögren's syndrome, chronic active hepatitis, HIV infection, and other systemic illnesses. It is usually successfully treated with corticosteroids.

7. **Acute interstitial pneumonitis (AIP)** is also known as Hamman–Rich syndrome.
   a. **Definition and etiology.** It is a rare fulminant form of acute lung injury that presents in a previously healthy individual.
   b. **Pathology and pathophysiology.** The hallmark pathologic findings are those termed diffuse alveolar damage (DAD). Biopsy results will show organizing diffuse alveolar damage due to injury to the alveolar capillary basement membrane. After the endothelial and epithelial injury, there is leakage of serum proteins and red blood cells in the alveolar spaces. The alveolar epithelium becomes necrotic and is sloughed, and the interstitium becomes edematous. Hyaline membranes form within alveolar spaces and create a decrease in ventilation-to-perfusion ratio. The same pathology is seen in acute respiratory distress syndrome (ARDS), but with ARDS, there is an identifiable underlying acute process such as sepsis, infectious pneumonia, or trauma that results in the acute lung injury. With AIP, no identifiable cause can be identified.
   c. **Clinical features, diagnosis, and clinical course.** The most common symptoms of AIP are dyspnea, cough, and fever. The symptoms progress rapidly, usually requiring hospitalization and mechanical ventilation only days to weeks after symptoms begin. Diffuse rales or crackles are heard on auscultation, lower more than upper lung fields. Chest x-ray and CT scanning are similar to ARDS, with patchy, diffuse bilateral, fluffy opacities. The lung biopsy will show organizing diffuse alveolar damage. Mortality is approximately 60%, with mean survival 1.5 months. People who survive usually recover lung function completely and do not have a second episode of AIP.
   d. **Therapy.** Treatment is mainly supportive in an intensive care unit with mechanical ventilation. Therapy with corticosteroids is commonly used, though usefulness has not been established. Lung transplantation has been done successfully on occasion.

G **Connective tissue disease–associated interstitial pneumonia (CTD-IP)** The connective tissue diseases (CTDs) that can involve the pulmonary system include systemic sclerosis (scleroderma), rheumatoid arthritis, systemic lupus erythematosus, Sjögren's syndrome, mixed connective tissue disease, and polymyositis/dermatomyositis.

1. **Definition.** CTDs include various diseases or abnormal states characterized by inflammatory or degenerative changes in connective tissue and are often autoimmune in origin. They are also known as collagen vascular diseases.

2. **Etiology.** The pulmonary complications can include the large airways, the lung parenchyma, the pleura, and/or the pulmonary vasculature as a complication of the autoimmune disease. [See Chapter 11 for the etiology of connective tissue diseases.]

3. **Pathology and pathophysiology.** On lung biopsy, any number of specific pulmonary pathologic patterns of disease (see previous discussion on the idiopathic group for pathologic descriptions and terminology) can be seen: usual interstitial pneumonia (UIP), nonspecific interstitial pneumonia (NSIP), organizing pneumonia (OP), lymphocytic interstitial pneumonia (LIP), or diffuse alveolar damage.

4. **Clinical features, diagnosis, and clinical course.** Symptoms are similar to those of the other chronic forms of DPLD: progressive dyspnea, nonproductive cough, and fatigue. Other symptoms

are specific to the type of connective tissue disease, for example, joint pain and swelling in rheumatoid arthritis. Imaging will reveal fibrosis of the lungs. Diagnosis is made with biopsy, or sometimes it is suspected by CT scanning and biopsy can be avoided. The clinical course and prognosis is generally better than with IPF and the other idiopathic interstitial pneumonias. CTD-related pulmonary diseases are also generally more responsive to treatment.

5. **Therapy.** The underlying connective tissue disease must be treated, and often the pulmonary component of the disease will improve as inflammation decreases. Corticosteroids, immunomodulators, and other immunosuppressants are the mainstay therapies. [See Chapter 11 for specific therapies for the various CTDs.]

H Sarcoidosis

1. **Definition.** Sarcoidosis is a multisystem, noncaseating granulomatous disease that can involve almost any organ in the body but involves the pulmonary system in 90% of cases. Patients with sarcoidosis usually present with mediastinal or hilar lymphadenopathy along with pulmonary infiltration in the parenchyma of the lung, combined with cutaneous or ocular lesions. Less common but important manifestations include peripheral adenopathy, erythema nodosum, arthritis, splenomegaly, hepatomegaly, hypercalcemia, diffuse or localized central nervous system (CNS) involvement, and cardiomyopathy.

2. **Etiology.** The etiology of sarcoidosis is unknown. Theories include infection-induced and immunologic defects. Patients with sarcoidosis show impaired cellular immunity characterized by a complete skin anergy to tuberculin and other common skin antigens. Humoral immunity is normal.

3. **Pathology and pathophysiology**
   a. The fundamental lesion of sarcoidosis is a **noncaseating granuloma.** This cluster of epithelioid cells is similar to the granulomas occurring in other diseases such as fungal disease, mycobacterial disease, and Hodgkin's disease, although these are usually "caseating" granulomas with a central area of necrosis. Granulomatous inflammation is characterized by accumulation of monocytes, macrophages, and activated T lymphocytes, with increased production of key inflammatory mediators—TNF-alpha, INF-gamma, IL-2, and IL-12—characteristic of a Th1-polarized response (T-helper lymphocyte-1 response).
   b. Giant cells frequently are present and contain several types of inclusions. Lymphocytes and rare plasma cells may be present at the periphery of the granuloma; neutrophils and eosinophils are absent.
   c. The inflammation causes stiffness of the lungs, and fibrosis develops over time.

4. **Clinical features, diagnosis, and clinical course**
   a. **Symptoms** vary greatly depending on organ involvement and extent of disease. Fatigue and exertional dyspnea are common. Cough, if present, usually is nonproductive. Hemoptysis is rare. Chest pain occurs infrequently, and pleurisy is uncommon.
   b. **Pulmonary function testing.** Results may be normal but usually show some impairment of gas exchange and some evidence of lung restriction with reduced vital capacity (VC) and $D_L CO$. In many cases, small airway function also is abnormal.
   c. **Chest radiography and CT scan.** Enlarged intrathoracic lymph nodes are seen, termed hilar or mediastinal lymphadenopathy. Parenchymal manifestations vary from a faint interstitial infiltrate, to well-developed diffuse nodular infiltrates, to varying degrees of lung fibrosis, including "honeycombing." The **radiographic staging** of pulmonary involvement in sarcoidosis is as follows:
      (1) **Stage 1:** Bilateral hilar adenopathy and normal lung parenchyma
      (2) **Stage 2:** Bilateral hilar adenopathy and interstitial infiltrate
      (3) **Stage 3:** Interstitial infiltrate only
      (4) **Stage 4:** Fibrosis
   d. **Systemic involvement**
      (1) **Uveitis** is a common presentation and may progress to blindness.
      (2) A variety of infiltrative **skin lesions** occurs in one third of patients and often portends chronic progressive sarcoidosis. An exception is **erythema nodosum,** which may occur early in the disease and is associated with a good prognosis.

(3) **Bone and joint involvement.** Transient polyarthritis is associated with erythema nodosum; a chronic form of arthritis also occurs. Bone involvement may produce cystic destruction and disability.

(4) **Nervous system involvement** may manifest as Bell's palsy and other cranial neuropathies, peripheral neuropathies, and (rarely) granulomatous meningitis.

(5) **Cardiomyopathy** manifests as arrhythmias and conduction disturbances that carry a high risk for sudden death.

(6) **Liver function abnormalities may occur.**

(7) **Disturbances in calcium metabolism** (e.g., hypercalciuria, renal stones, and hypercalcemia) occur in up to 25% of patients.

   e. **Diagnosis.** Sarcoidosis should be suspected in patients with mediastinal or hilar adenopathy and interstitial lung disease (e.g., pulmonary fibrosis). Erythema nodosum, uveitis, skin lesions, hypercalcemia, multisystem disease, and granulomas of any organ should also suggest sarcoidosis. Diagnostic confirmation requires tissue biopsy showing typical granulomas in a patient with consistent clinical presentations; transbronchial biopsy by bronchoscopy is often diagnostic. Because sarcoidosis is a diagnosis of exclusion, all tissue samples should be cultured to rule out infectious causes and should be specially stained for identification of fungal disease.

   f. **Clinical course and prognosis.** The course of sarcoidosis is variable. Approximately one third of patients will have complete resolution of signs and symptoms, one third will have chronic persistent but relatively stable disease, and one third will have progressive deterioration in lung function.

5. **Therapy.** Corticosteroid administration is the principal treatment for sarcoidosis. Occasionally other immunosuppressants are used. However, a decision must be made as to whether a patient's symptoms warrant therapy, as therapy can have adverse side effects. The patients are followed clinically over years, making adjustments to steroid doses, monitoring PFTs, and using other supportive measures. Lung transplantation may be considered in patients with progressive lung disease.

I Occupational lung diseases secondary to organic inhalants

1. **Definition.** Organic dust–caused pulmonary disease is referred to as **hypersensitivity pneumonitis** or **extrinsic allergic alveolitis.** The disease results from inflammation of the alveoli within the lung caused by hypersensitivity to inhaled organic dusts.

2. **Etiology.** The inhalation of organic dusts (e.g., fungal spores, thermophilic actinomycetes, or fragments of animal and vegetable matter) causes a diffuse, granulomatous pulmonary parenchymal reaction. Patients often have antibodies against the offending substances, and the findings suggest a type III hypersensitivity reaction, with tissue damage from the deposition of antigen–antibody complexes.

3. **Pathology and pathophysiology.** The pathology of hypersensitivity pneumonitis consists of loosely, poorly formed granulomas, mononuclear inflammatory cell interstitial infiltrates, and some fibrosis. The granulomas are loosely formed and can usually be distinguished histologically from the very tightly organized noncaseating granulomas of sarcoidosis.

4. **Clinical features, diagnosis, and clinical course.** Several hours after exposure, patients experience malaise, fever, and chills, with chest tightness and persistent dry cough. Radiographs obtained during acute attacks show pulmonary infiltrates. Symptoms abate within a few days but recur with subsequent exposures. Repeated exposures may lead to a fixed restrictive lung disease. Diagnosis is made by history, radiography, and often bronchoscopic lung biopsy.

5. **Therapy** includes avoidance of exposure and corticosteroid treatment for acute attacks.

J Occupational lung diseases secondary to inorganic inhalants

1. **Definition.** Lung disease caused by inhalation of inorganic **dust** is termed **pneumoconiosis.** The major dusts that cause pneumoconiosis are asbestos, silica, coal dust, and hard metals.

2. **Asbestos-related disease.** *Asbestos* is the term applied to several naturally occurring fibrous silicates, whose fibers may be long, curled, and flexible or straight and brittle. Asbestos fibers may cause several distinct types of lesions.

   a. **Asbestosis.** This is a diffuse parenchymal lung disease due to asbestos inhalation. It results in interstitial cellular inflammation and fibrosis. Affected patients complain of breathlessness, and physical signs include digital clubbing and auscultatory bibasilar crackles. The chest film shows small lungs containing hazy infiltrates composed of small, irregular or linear opacities; lower lung zones are more heavily affected. Restrictive ventilatory impairment and a reduced D_LCO are the expected abnormalities on PFTs.

   b. Nonneoplastic pleural disorders. Asbestos exposure may result in several nonneoplastic pleural disorders, including pleural effusion, pleural plaques (which are usually calcified), and diffuse pleural thickening.

   c. Neoplasia. Many years after exposure (latency period of about 20 years), cancer can develop in persons exposed to asbestos at sufficient concentrations.

     (1) Bronchogenic carcinoma (non–small cell and small cell carcinoma) is a recognized consequence of asbestos exposure, especially in individuals who smoke. The risk of bronchogenic carcinoma in patients who smoke and were exposed to asbestos has been estimated to be 100-fold above normal.

     (2) Malignant pleural mesotheliomas [see Chapter 5] are rare tumors. They are almost always caused by prior asbestos exposure but are not associated with smoking.

3. Silica-related disease. Free silica and silicates are abundant components of the earth's crust. To be injurious to the lungs, these particles must exist as respirable aerosols.

   a. Silicosis is a diffuse fibrotic reaction of the lungs to inhalation of free crystalline silica (sand, quartz). Inhaled silica particles are ingested by alveolar macrophages, which soon rupture, releasing cytotoxic enzymes along with the engulfed silica particles. The silica is reingested by other macrophages, and the cycle continues, stimulating a local fibrotic reaction. The final result is the formation of the relatively acellular **fibrous silicotic nodule** that characterizes this disease.

     (1) Simple silicosis. In this stage, the chest radiograph shows numerous small, rounded opacities (isolated nodules) scattered throughout the lungs. Simple silicosis usually is not associated with ventilatory impairment.

     (2) Complicated silicosis. If exposure to silica continues, isolated nodules may coalesce to form larger masses of fibrotic tissue that distort the lungs, and this has been termed progressive massive fibrosis (PMF). PMF often produces a mixture of restrictive and obstructive ventilatory impairment on PFT testing.

   b. Nonfibrotic effects. Silicates such as talc, kaolin, fuller's earth, and bentonite can produce simple or complicated **pneumoconiosis,** without diffuse pulmonary fibrosis.

4. Coal worker's pneumoconiosis (CWP, "black lung")

   a. Although coal dust is less fibrotic than silica, CWP shares with silicosis the radiographic appearance of small, rounded opacities in the simple stage and large, conglomerate masses in the complicated stage. However, simple CWP only occasionally develops into complicated CWP.

   b. Simple CWP has no characteristic functional abnormality. A chronic bronchitis probably accounts for most of the respiratory disability in affected patients. **Complicated CWP** can lead to progressive massive fibrosis (PMF), with restrictive ventilatory impairment.

5. Hard metal lung disease or hard metal pneumoconiosis is a hypersensitivity reaction to hard metal inhalation, including cobalt and powdered tungsten carbide. Cobalt is thought to be the primary offending agent. Cobalt is used to make machine parts that require high heat resistance and to make tools used for drilling, cutting, machining, and grinding. An important aspect of hard metal pneumoconiosis is that it occurs after a fairly short duration of exposure, suggesting that individual susceptibility rather than cumulative exposure plays a major role. Diagnosis is made by identifying a giant cell interstitial pneumonitis (GIP), and an alternative term for this entity is giant cell interstitial pneumonitis. These giant cells on bronchial lavage or biopsy often have a "cannibalistic" appearance, with giant multinucleated cells present.

K Pulmonary Vasculitis

1. Wegener's granulomatosis (or ANCA-associated vasculitis) [see also Chapter 7]

   a. Definition. This disease is the prototype of a group of rare disorders characterized by granulomatous vasculitis and necrosis of the lung and other organs. Individuals of all ages may be affected; males are affected more commonly than females.

(1) Wegener originally described the syndrome as a destructive granulomatous infiltration of the upper respiratory tract and lung parenchyma combined with glomerulonephritis.

(2) Today the disease is recognized as a systemic vasculitis with a predilection for the respiratory tract and kidney. Other commonly involved sites are the skin, joints, and peripheral nerves. Involvement of the eyes, heart, and CNS also can occur.

(3) A variant form affects the respiratory tract, chiefly the lungs, while sparing the kidney.

   b. Etiology of Wegener's granulomatosis is unknown.

   c. Pathology and pathogenesis

     (1) The pathogenic mechanism is thought to be an immunologic injury of vessels, with secondary inflammatory changes.

     (2) The pathologic lesion is a granulomatous angiitis of small vessels with characteristic tissue necrosis surrounded by mononuclear inflammatory cells, forming noncaseating granulomatous vasculitis.

       (a) In the lung, this process commonly results in excavation and destruction of the lung parenchyma, causing hemoptysis and pulmonary insufficiency.

       (b) The renal lesion is a focal glomerulonephritis that can progress to renal failure.

   d. Clinical features, diagnosis, and clinical course

     (1) Symptoms include dyspnea, cough, and fever, but patients sometimes present in acute respiratory failure. Hemoptysis is present in about one third of patients. The **chest x-ray** will show diffuse bilateral alveolar infiltrates. Other testing includes urinalysis and possible kidney biopsy, CT scan of the lung and bronchoalveolar lavage, and testing for **anti–neutrophilic cytoplasmic antibody (ANCA).**

     (2) Diagnosis. Wegener's granulomatosis is identified by the classic clinical triad of upper and lower respiratory involvement and glomerulonephritis, supported by a positive ANCA test and biopsy of the involved tissue. **Cytoplasmic ANCA (c-ANCA)** is more often positive than perinuclear ANCA (p-ANCA).

     (3) Clinical Course. The untreated disease is fatal in most patients within 1 month to several years. Some forms of the disease are associated with longer survival rates, particularly those that do not involve active nephritis.

   e. Therapy. Correct diagnosis is critical because of the remarkable efficacy of **cytotoxic therapy.** Cyclophosphamide alone or with corticosteroids produces rapid reversal of the disease, if introduced early in the course.

2. Microscopic polyangiitis is another pulmonary–renal vasculitis.

   a. Definition. It is a pauci-immune, necrotizing, small-vessel vasculitis without clinical or pathologic evidence of granulomatous inflammation. Glomerulonephritis is universal in these patients, but there is pulmonary involvement in only about 30% of patients.

   b. Etiology is unknown.

   c. Pathology. A focal, segmental necrotizing vasculitis and a mixed inflammatory infiltrate without granulomata are seen.

   d. Clinical features, diagnosis, and clinical course. Symptoms and signs are similar to those of Wegener's granulomatosis, but often joint, skin, central nervous system, and the gastrointestinal system are involved as well. The p-ANCA is positive in about 75% of patients, with the c-ANCA being positive in only 10%–15%. With therapy the prognosis is good.

   e. Therapy with cyclophosphamide and corticosteroids has greatly improved the prognosis, with the 5-year survival being around 12%, down from 50% prior to current therapies.

3. Churg–Strauss syndrome (CSS) is a medium- and small-vessel vasculitis (can affect the arteries, veins, arterioles, and venules). CSS is defined by: (1) a history or current symptoms of **asthma,** (2) peripheral **eosinophilia,** and (3) systemic vasculitis of at least two **extrapulmonary organs** (cardiac, nervous system, skin, or gastrointestinal tract). CCS often presents with a prodrome of allergic rhinitis, nasal polyposis, or asthma. Then peripheral blood and tissue eosinophilia develop. Diagnosis is made via biopsy; the pathologic features include eosinophilic extravascular granulomas and granulomatous or nongranulomatous necrotizing vasculitis. CSS is usually very responsive to therapy, but complications include transient, patchy pulmonary infiltrates, extravascular necrotizing granulomata of the skin, and mononeuritis multiplex. Treatment with corticosteroids and/or other immunosuppressants results in a remission rate of 60%–90% at 5 years.

L **Pulmonary hemorrhage syndromes** include pulmonary vasculitis, Goodpasture's syndrome, connective tissue diseases, and idiopathic causes. With active pulmonary hemorrhage, all will appear as diffuse alveolar hemorrhage on bronchoscopy with bronchoalveolar lavage (BAL) or biopsy. With BAL, specimens show blood with numerous erythrocytes, and the lavage fluid remains hemorrhagic even after sequential sampling. Each vial of recovered saline is as red discolored as the previous one.

1. **Vasculitis.** Pulmonary vasculitic syndromes can cause diffuse alveolar hemorrhage and were discussed previously.

2. **Goodpasture's syndrome** [see also Chapter 7]
   a. **Definition.** Goodpasture's syndrome is a progressive autoimmune disease of the lungs and kidneys that produces **intra-alveolar hemorrhage** and **glomerulonephritis.** The disease is rare, occurs at all ages, and is predominant in males.
   b. **Etiology** is unknown.
   c. **Pathology and pathogenesis**
      (1) Goodpasture's syndrome is caused by an anti–glomerular basement membrane (anti-GBM) antibody, usually immunoglobulin G (IgG), which reacts with glomerular and alveolar basement membranes.
      (2) Linear deposition of the antibody, characteristic of a type II hypersensitivity reaction, occurs along the basement membrane of glomeruli, alveoli, and capillaries.
         (a) The pathologic result in the lung is diffuse capillary leakage and intra-alveolar hemorrhage but little or no inflammation.
         (b) The renal lesion is a proliferative glomerulonephritis that progresses to renal failure.
   d. **Clinical features, diagnosis, and clinical course**
      (1) **Clinical features.** Patients usually present with hemoptysis and dyspnea. However, renal failure without pulmonary complaints can be an initial finding, and a history of respiratory illness often precedes the onset of pulmonary hemorrhage.
      (2) **Diagnosis**
         (a) Bilateral alveolar infiltrates on chest radiograph, hypoxemia, and a restrictive pattern on pulmonary function testing are characteristic.
         (b) The diagnosis is confirmed by demonstration of anti-GBM antibody in the serum or in a biopsy specimen from the kidney or lung.
         (c) **Differential diagnosis** includes Wegener's granulomatosis, systemic lupus erythematosus (SLE), and idiopathic pulmonary hemosiderosis.
            (i) **Wegener's granulomatosis** (see earlier discussion) usually affects both the upper and lower respiratory tract and lacks anti-GBM antibody.
            (ii) **SLE** [see also Chapter 11] is distinguished from Goodpasture's syndrome by the absence of anti-GBM antibody and the findings of free DNA, various ANAs, and depressed serum levels of complement.
            (iii) **Idiopathic pulmonary hemosiderosis** is described later.
      (3) **Clinical course.** Untreated Goodpasture's syndrome is rapidly fatal as a result of renal failure or asphyxia from pulmonary hemorrhage. Treatment can control episodes of pulmonary hemorrhage, but the renal failure will be progressive. Five-year survival is between 60% and 90%, depending on degree of renal failure and underlying conditions.
   e. **Therapy.** Currently, the combination of plasmapheresis to remove circulating anti-GBM antibodies and immunosuppressive therapy with corticosteroids and alkylating agents appears to give the best results. Hemodialysis or kidney transplantation has been used to control end-stage renal disease.

3. **Idiopathic pulmonary siderosis** is characterized by repeated pulmonary hemorrhage but no nephritis. Death caused by massive hemorrhage may occur at any time, but prolonged survival with or without symptoms of pulmonary insufficiency is common. Idiopathic pulmonary hemosiderosis has no known immune mechanisms for pathogenesis, and no successful therapy has evolved.

4. **Connective tissue diseases,** especially SLE, can cause pulmonary hemorrhage.

5. **Other causes of diffuse pulmonary hemorrhage.** Certain drugs, such as intravenous heparin, amiodarone, and propylthiouricil, as well as crack cocaine, infections such as invasive *Aspergillosis* and *Hantavirus*, and coagulopathies are also known causes of alveolar hemorrhage.

M Eosinophilic granuloma (histiocytosis X or Langerhans cell histiocytosis)

1. **Definition.** Histiocytosis X is a generic term for a group of systemic disorders characterized by various degrees of fibrosis with focal infiltrations of tissue by nonmalignant histiocytes and eosinophils. The disease can be localized to one area (e.g., bone or lung) or it can be widely disseminated. **Eosinophilic granuloma** (of bone or lung) is localized; **Letterer–Siwe disease** and **Hand–Schüller–Christian syndrome** are widespread.

2. **Etiology.** An abnormality of the immune system is suspected. The disease is rare, affects men more commonly than women, and affects children and young adults more commonly than individuals in other age groups. Eosinophilic granuloma of the lung is almost always associated with cigarette smoking.

3. **Pathology and pathophysiology.** Proliferating histiocytes show cytoplasmic inclusions, the so-called "X bodies." Pulmonary histiocytosis X produces bilateral, reticulonodular infiltrates, with a predilection for the upper lobes and typical progression to cyst formation, fibrosis, and "honeycombing."

4. **Clinical features, diagnosis, and clinical course**
   a. **Findings** may include cough, chest pain, dyspnea, fever, spontaneous pneumothorax, and a honeycomb appearance on chest radiography. Lytic bone disease may be present. A triad of diabetes insipidus, exophthalmos, and bone lesions is seen occasionally.
   b. **Pulmonary function testing** indicates restriction and impaired gas exchange. In advanced cases, severe obstruction may dominate.
   c. **Definitive diagnosis** requires bronchoscopic or surgical (VATS) biopsy demonstrating "X bodies" on electron microscopy, which appear as pentilaminar cytoplasmic inclusion bodies.
   d. **Clinical course.** The prognosis is variable—some cases result in death, but spontaneous remissions are common.

5. **Therapy.** Smoking cessation is recommended. Corticosteroids are given for pulmonary manifestations, but their efficacy is uncertain. Surgery or radiation therapy is used for localized bone disease.

N Pulmonary alveolar proteinosis (PAP)

1. **Definition.** PAP is a rare disease characterized by massive accumulations of a phospholipid- and protein-rich substance in alveoli. The interstitium usually is not involved, and there is no other organ involvement.

2. **Etiology.** PAP can occur in a primary form or secondarily in the settings of malignancy (e.g., myeloid leukemia), pulmonary infection, or environmental exposure to dusts or chemicals. Rare familial forms have also been recognized, suggesting a genetic component in some cases. It has also been linked to tobacco smoking. The disorder is more common in men than in women and has been described in all ages.

3. **Pathology and pathophysiology.** The substance in the alveoli is closely related to pulmonary surfactant and probably accumulates as a result of impaired clearance. The impaired clearance may be due to deficiency or defect of granulocyte macrophage colony-stimulating factor (GM-CSF) in some cases. Macrophages engorged with the substance also are present, but other inflammatory cells are lacking. The distal air spaces are filled with a granular, eosinophilic material that stains **positively with periodic-acid Schiff (PAS)** reagent.

4. **Clinical features, diagnosis, and clinical course**
   a. **Clinical features.** Dyspnea, nonproductive cough, pulmonary rales, and cyanosis are common. Pulmonary function testing shows a restrictive ventilatory pattern and hypoxia. Chest radiograph shows an alveolar infiltrate, usually in a bilateral perihilar butterfly distribution similar to the pattern seen in pulmonary edema.
   b. **Diagnosis.** Lung biopsy or BAL is necessary to make the diagnosis, which again demonstrates (PAS)–positive material in the alveoli.
   c. **Clinical course**
      (1) Patients are predisposed to lung infection, including nocardiosis and fungal infections, possibly because of a functional impairment of alveolar macrophages.
      (2) The disease may progress to respiratory insufficiency and death, but spontaneous resolution is just as common. Pulmonary fibrosis has been described as a late complication.

5. **Therapy.** Patients with minimal symptoms require no therapy. For dyspnic patients, whole-lung lavage is effective and reverses the physiologic abnormality. Corticosteroids are contraindicated because they increase the risk of infection.

O Lymphangioleiomyomatosis (LAM)

1. **Definition.** LAM is a rare lung disease in which abnormal, muscle-like cells grow out of control in certain organs, especially the lungs, lymph nodes, and kidneys. It main affects premenopausal women. There is a **sporadic** or primary form of LAM and a form that occurs in patients with **tuberous sclerosis**. LAM in tuberous sclerosis is usually less severe. Tuberous sclerosis is rare genetic disease that causes benign tumors to grow in the brain and on other organs such as the kidneys, eyes, lungs, and skin. Symptoms may include seizures, developmental delay, behavioral problems, skin abnormalities, and lung and kidney disease.

2. **Etiology.** The etiology of LAM is unknown; however, the fact that the condition occurs primarily in women who are premenopausal and is exacerbated by high-estrogen states suggests a role of hormones. In tuberous sclerosis, mutations in TSC1 or TSC2 are inherited or occur spontaneously. However, the percentage of LAM in patients with tuberous sclerosis is low.

3. **Pathology and pathophysiology.** Pathology will reveal foci of smooth muscle cell infiltration of lung parenchyma, airways, lymphatics, and blood vessels associated with areas of thin-walled cystic changes. The two actin-positive cell types are that are found in the lesion are small, spindle-shaped cells and cuboidal epithelioid cells. LAM cell proliferation may obstruct bronchioles, leading to airflow obstruction, air trapping, formation of bullae, and pneumothoraces. Obstruction of lymphatics may result in chylothorax and chylous ascites, and obstruction of venules may result in hemosiderosis and hemoptysis.

4. **Clinical features, diagnosis, and clinical course**
   a. **Symptoms** are dyspnea and, less commonly, cough, chest pain, and hemoptysis. There are few signs of disease, but some women have crackles and rhonchi. Many patients present with spontaneous pneumothorax.
   b. **Pulmonary function testing** will reveal obstructive or mixed obstructive and restrictive pattern. **Chest x-ray** will show hyperinflation.
   c. **High-resolution CT scan (HRCT)** will reveal multiple, small, diffusely distributed cysts that are generally pathognomonic for LAM.
   d. **Diagnosis.** If the HRCT is not diagnostic, biopsy with VATS is performed and biopsy will show pathology as described earlier.
   e. **Clinical course.** Prognosis is variable in LAM, but it is usually slowly progressive and leads to respiratory failure and usually death. Median survival is 8–10 years. Women should be advised that progression may be accelerated during pregnancy.

5. **Therapy** includes treatment of pneumothoraces, considering surgical pleurodesis if pneumothorax is recurrent. Treatment of LAM includes antiestrogen therapy, progestin therapy, and lung transplantation.

P Eosinophilic pneumonia syndromes

1. **Definition. Eosinophilic pneumonia (EP)** is a disease in which eosinophils accumulate in the lung and cause disruption of the alveolar spaces.

2. **Etiology.** The EP syndromes are divided into categories based on their etiology, including with an etiology is unknown (idiopathic). Known causes include autoimmune disorders (Churg–Strauss syndrome), certain medications, parasitic infections, and cancer.

3. **Pathology and pathophysiology.** The common characteristic among different causes of EP is eosinophil overreaction or dysfunction in the lung. Biopsy or BAL will show increased eosinophil infiltration.

4. **Clinical features, diagnosis, and clinical course.** Cough, fever, dyspnea, and night sweats are the symptoms associated with EP. Physical exam may reveal a serpiginous or raised rash, evidence of rhinitis/sinusitis, and rales/crackles and wheezing. Diagnosis is made when a complete blood count reveals eosinophilia, a chest x-ray or CT scan identifies abnormalities in the lung, a biopsy identifies increased eosinophils in lung tissue, or increased eosinophils are found in BAL fluid

obtained by a bronchoscopy. EP due to cancer or parasitic infection carries the same prognosis as the underlying disease. EP due to Churg–Strauss or idiopathic causes carry a good prognosis when properly treated.

5. **Therapy.** If EP is due to underlying parasitic infection or cancer, the underlying disease is treated. Other causes of EP are treated with steroids and sometimes other immunosuppressants (mycophenolate mofetil, cyclophosphamide, methotrexate, azathioprine).

6. The following are different causes of EP.
   a. **Drugs** associated with EP include nonsteroidal anti-inflammatory drugs (NSAIDs), phenytoin, nitrofurantoin, ampicillin, cocaine, heroin, and cigarette smoke. Treatment for drug-induced EP is withdrawal of the offending agent, supportive therapy, and often corticosteroids.
   b. **Parasites** can cause EP in three different ways: Parasites can invade the lung, live in the lung as part of their life cycle, or be spread to the lung by the bloodstream. Eosinophils migrate to the lung in order to defend against the parasites, and EP results. Parasites that invade the lung include *Paragonimus* lung flukes and the tapeworms *Echinococcus* and *Taenia solium*. Important parasites that inhabit the lung as part of their normal life cycle include the helminths *Ascaris lumbricoides*, *Strongyloides stercoralis*, and the hookworms *Ancylostoma duodenale* and *Necator americanus*. When EP is caused by worms inhabiting the lung as part of their life cycle, it is called Löffler's syndrome. The final group of parasites cause EP when a large number of eggs are carried into the lungs by the bloodstream. This includes *Trichinella spiralis*, *Strongyloides stercoralis*, the hookworms, and the schistosomes. This form of EP is treated with antiparasitic medications.
   c. **Churg–Strauss syndrome** was discussed earlier with pulmonary vasculitis.
   d. **Idiopathic EP** can be divided into acute eosinophilic pneumonia (AEP) and chronic eosinophilic pneumonia (CEP), depending on the symptoms and duration of symptoms a person is experiencing. Treatment is the same as for Churg–Strauss syndrome.

XIV SLEEP APNEA SYNDROME

A **Definition**   Sleep apnea is a disorder characterized by repetitive periods of **apnea** (i.e., cessation of breathing) occurring during sleep. A period of more than 10 seconds without airflow is considered an apneic episode. Patients with this syndrome can have hundreds of such episodes during the course of one night's sleep. This disorder can be demonstrated in 9% of middle-aged women and 24% of middle-aged men.

B **Etiology**   Sleep apnea may be obstructive, central, or mixed.

1. In **obstructive sleep apnea (OSA),** transient obstruction of the upper airway, usually the oropharynx, prevents inspiratory airflow. The obstruction results from loss of tone in the pharyngeal muscles or the genioglossus muscles (which normally cause the tongue to protrude forward from the posterior pharyngeal wall). Obesity is a major risk factor for OSA.

2. In **central apnea,** there is no drive to breathe during the apneic episode; that is, there is no signal from the respiratory center to initiate inspiration. Rarely, the cause is a neurologic disorder. Why the drive is absent in other individuals is not known.

3. In **mixed apnea,** patients have episodes of both obstructive and central apnea. Polysomnography (sleep study) will delineate the different forms of apnea present in any given patient.

C **Clinical features, diagnosis, and clinical course**

1. **Symptoms.** Usually, sleep partners notice patients' problems. **Loud snoring** is prominent, and patients may thrash about during periods of obstructive apnea. During the daytime, they are **overly somnolent** and may show personality changes or slowed mentation.

2. **Physical signs.** In patients with **central** apnea, monitoring of the chest wall motion reveals no movement; this corresponds to cessation of airflow and oxygen desaturation. In patients with **obstructive apnea,** chest wall and abdominal movement can be detected during fruitless attempts to move air through the obstructed airway.

3. Obesity hypoventilation syndrome (OHS) occasionally may coexist with OSA. The OHS is characterized by extreme obesity and alveolar hypoventilation during wakefulness.

4. **Diagnosis** is made by an overnight polysomnogram or sleep study.

5. **Clinical course.** Sleep apnea is a lifelong, chronic disease and usually requires lifelong therapy. Complications include cardiac arrhythmias, pulmonary hypertension, and cor pulmonale.

D **Therapy**

1. **Central apnea.** Treatment involves respiratory stimulants. A phrenic nerve pacemaker may be implanted to stimulate the diaphragm electrically.

2. **Obstructive apnea.** In those patients requiring intervention, nasal CPAP is the most common treatment. Oral appliances or surgery to debulk the posterior pharynx may be required on occasion. Rarely, in severe cases, tracheostomy to bypass the upper airway may be required. Weight loss is indicated in most patients, but without bariatric surgery, it is rarely successful.

Study Questions

1. A 32-year-old man working on a construction crew falls from the scaffolding and develops multiple long bone fractures. Four hours after presenting to the emergency department, he complains of increased shortness of breath and hypoxemia and has diffuse infiltrates on his chest radiograph, consistent with development of acute respiratory distress syndrome (ARDS). Which of the following findings is almost always present in patients who present with ARDS?

- (A) A small localized mass on chest radiograph
- (B) Reduced lung compliance
- (C) Normal oxygenation with impaired minute ventilation
- (D) Increased arterial PCO_2
- (E) Pulmonary embolism

2. An 18-year-old girl complains of symptoms of an upper respiratory tract infection for 1–2 days, followed by an increase in shortness of breath and greater use of inhaled bronchodilators for treatment of her chronic stable asthma. She presents to the emergency room with increased use of accessory muscles of ventilation, tachypnea, and wheezing. Shortly after the symptoms of her asthmatic attack have resolved, pulmonary function testing is most likely to show which of the following?

- (A) Normal values for peak expiratory flow
- (B) Decreased lung compliance
- (C) Increased residual volume (RV)
- (D) No change in peak expiratory flow after inhalation of bronchodilator
- (E) Elevated FEV_1/FVC ratio

3. A 16-year-old adolescent presents with recurrent respiratory tract infections, poor weight gain, and breathlessness on exertion. Which of the following combinations of findings would provide a definite diagnosis of cystic fibrosis?

- (A) A family history of cystic fibrosis and abnormal pulmonary function
- (B) Abnormal pulmonary function and pancreatic insufficiency
- (C) Pancreatic insufficiency and high electrolyte concentration in sweat
- (D) High electrolyte concentration in sweat and abnormal chest radiograph
- (E) Abnormal chest radiograph and family history of cystic fibrosis

4. A 19-year-old man presents with fatigue, dyspnea, and a mild nonproductive cough. Pulmonary function testing shows a mild decrease in the FVC and FEV_1 with a preserved FEV_1/FVC ratio. D_LCO is mildly decreased. Chest radiograph shows bilateral hilar adenopathy and mild interstitial infiltrates. Which of the following statements is true regarding his most likely diagnosis?

- (A) Open-lung or video-assisted thoracoscopic (VATS) biopsy will be required to confirm the diagnosis.
- (B) Most patients experience a prolonged downhill course, with respiratory failure likely within 5 years.
- (C) Manifestations of the disease are confined to the lungs.
- (D) Corticosteroids are the primary therapy.
- (E) The presence of erythema nodosum at the time of diagnosis portends a poor prognosis.

5. A 36-year-old woman is seen for newly developed lower extremity edema. On further questioning, she admits to progressively worsening exercise tolerance for the past 2–3 years. She has had lightheadedness on occasion, and once had a syncopal episode while rushing for the bus. Her lungs are clear, and heart examination reveals a right ventricular heave and a right-sided fourth heart sound (S_4). She is presumed to have idiopathic pulmonary arterial hypertension (PAH), and further confirmatory testing is ordered. Which of the following statements about PAH in this patient is true?

- (A) If her pulmonary artery pressure and cardiac output respond to vasodilators during cardiac catheterization, then she will likely respond to high-dose calcium channel blockers.
- (B) Echocardiography provides little diagnostic information and should not be performed until late in her work-up, if at all.

[C] Anticoagulant therapy is contraindicated in PAH due to the risk of bleeding with this disease.

[D] If PAH is confirmed, her expected 5-year survival is excellent.

[E] Syncope occurs early in the course of PPH when pulmonary artery pressures are still relatively low.

6. Chronic obstructive pulmonary disease (COPD) is classified as emphysematous or bronchitic, depending on the pathologic changes that occur in the lung. Although these two COPD syndromes rarely exist as pure entities, they may be differentiated on the basis of their clinical presentation. Which of the following clinical features is common to both the emphysematous and bronchitic types of COPD?

[A] Polycythemia

[B] Improved airflow with bronchodilators

[C] Dyspnea

[D] Chronic cough

[E] Hypercapnia

7. A 70-year-old man complains of increased shortness of breath, which has progressed over the previous 2 years. Chest radiographs show bilateral basilar interstitial infiltrates. The patient is noted to have hypoxemia on ambulation. It is considered that the patient may have early manifestations of idiopathic pulmonary fibrosis, or usual interstitial pneumonitis (UIP). Pulmonary function data in this patient would most likely show:

[A] Low lung volumes

[B] A decrease in the ratio of forced expiratory volume in 1 second to forced vital capacity (FEV_1/FVC)

[C] An increased vital capacity (VC)

[D] An increased diffusing capacity (D_LCO)

[E] An increased airways resistance (RAW)

8. A 62-year-old woman with congestive heart failure (CHF) develops pneumonia and a large pleural effusion. Thoracentesis is performed in an effort to establish whether the pleural effusion is due to CHF or pneumonia. Which of the following findings would indicate that the pleural effusion is due to CHF?

[A] A protein content of 6 g/dL with a serum protein level of 8 g/dL

[B] A pH of 7.13

[C] A glucose content of 20 mg/dL

[D] A lactate dehydrogenase (LDH) content of 100 mg/dL (with a serum LDH level of 420 mg/dL)

[E] A pleural fluid to serum protein ratio of 0.7

Answers and Explanations

1. The answer is B [VII]. Acute respiratory distress syndrome (ARDS, "wet lung") begins with a disruption of capillary integrity, which leads to extravasation of fluid, fibrin, and protein into the alveoli. As a result, the lungs become wet and stiff (i.e., noncompliant). This condition is characterized by severe hypoxia caused by extreme ventilation–perfusion ($\dot{V}/\dot{Q}$) imbalance and shunting of blood in the fluid-filled areas of the lung. Clinical features include progressive tachypnea; patchy, diffuse, fluffy infiltrates on chest radiograph; increased minute ventilation; and decreased lung volumes. There usually is an absence of specific physical findings.

2. The answer is C [IV E]. Patients who have had a recent asthmatic attack, even though asymptomatic, still have residual airflow obstruction that may take a couple of months to disappear. During this time, patients still respond to bronchodilators but show abnormal peak expiratory flow, increased lung compliance, and continued maldistribution of ventilation. The FEV_1/FVC ratio is either normal or decreased (due to obstruction) in asthma. It is often increased in restrictive lung diseases.

3. The answer is C [V B 5.]. Although chest radiography and pulmonary function testing show abnormalities, the sweat test is the definitive test for cystic fibrosis. In virtually all cases of cystic fibrosis, sodium and chloride concentrations in sweat are increased significantly, whereas concentrations of these electrolytes are normal elsewhere in the body. To make a diagnosis of cystic fibrosis, this defect must be identified. The diagnosis is confirmed by a positive sweat test combined with any one of the following findings: a family history of cystic fibrosis, obstructive pulmonary disease, or pancreatic insufficiency.

4. The answer is D [XIII C]. The presence of fatigue, dyspnea, and cough combined with restrictive defect on pulmonary function testing and hilar adenopathy and interstitial infiltrates on chest x-ray strongly suggests sarcoidosis. The diagnosis of sarcoidosis frequently requires biopsy, but open-lung biopsy is usually not required, as transbronchial biopsy is typically sufficient. Although the lungs are involved in 90% of cases, almost any system can be involved in sarcoidosis, including cardiac, neurologic, skin, renal, and skeletal systems. In most cases, the disease regresses within 2 years, either with or without corticosteroids, the preferred treatment. In 25% the disease may progress to fibrosis and disabling pulmonary disease. Erythema nodosum signifies a favorable prognosis when present.

5. The answer is A [VIII]. Syncope is a late manifestation of PAH and suggests severely elevated pulmonary artery pressures. The initial response to a vasodilator during right-heart catheterization is associated with a better prognosis and a favorable response to long-term calcium channel blockers. Echocardiography can estimate pulmonary artery pressure and assess right ventricular function and is a useful initial test to confirm the diagnosis of PAH. Anticoagulant therapy has been shown to prolong survival and is prescribed for nearly all patients with PAH. The prognosis for PAH is generally poor, with a 5-year survival rate of approximately 34%.

6. The answer is C [III]. All patients with chronic obstructive pulmonary disease (COPD) experience dyspnea to some degree. The two classic types of COPD—emphysematous and bronchitic—represent extremes of the spectrum and rarely are encountered in their pure form in clinical practice. By definition, individuals with the emphysematous type of COPD present at a relatively older age (>60 years). This form of disease is characterized by progressive exertional dyspnea, weight loss, little or no cough, mild hypoxia, hypocapnia, and only a mild increase in airway resistance (RAW) that shows little improvement with bronchodilation. Persons with the bronchitic type of COPD present at a relatively young age. This form is characterized by episodic dyspnea, fluid retention, chronic cough, severe hypoxemia, hypercapnia, polycythemia, and an increase in RAW that improves with bronchodilation.

7. The answer is A [Online I F 2]. Restrictive disorders are characterized by low lung volumes. D_LCO is usually decreased in pulmonary fibrosis, a type of restrictive disease. A decrease in FEV_1/FVC is the hallmark of obstructive, not restrictive, disease. VC and RAW are decreased in restrictive lung disorders.

8. The answer is D [X A]. With the exception of the LDH findings, all of the pleural fluid findings listed indicate the presence of an exudate. Exudates are caused by inflammation or disease of the pleural surface or by lymphatic obstruction (e.g., due to tuberculosis, lung cancer, or pneumonia). Transudates are caused by elevated systemic or pulmonary venous pressure or by decreased plasma oncotic pressure (e.g., due to CHF or nephrotic syndrome). Therefore, in establishing the etiology of a pleural effusion, it is useful to determine whether the fluid is a transudate or an exudate. This determination often can be made on the basis of a chemical analysis of the pleural fluid. A pleural fluid-to-serum protein ratio of more than 0.5, an LDH content of more than two-thirds the upper limit for serum, or a pleural fluid-to-serum LDH ratio of greater than 0.6 usually indicates the presence of an exudate. Pleural fluid pH values of less than 7.2 and a pleural fluid glucose content of less than 20 mg/dL also are associated with inflammatory effusions (exudates).

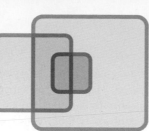

chapter 4

Hematologic Diseases

VICTORIA GIFFI · ANN ZIMRIN

I   **DISORDERS OF DECREASED HEMOGLOBIN (ONLINE FIGURE 4–1)**

A   **Anemia caused by decreased red blood cell production**   Hemoglobin, which represents 95% of the total composition of a red blood cell (RBC), is a mixture of globin and the iron-containing heme compound **protoporphyrin.** Any abnormality in hemoglobin synthesis or iron metabolism results in hemoglobin-deficient cells. As a rule, such deficient cells exhibit **hypochromia** (i.e., diminished hemoglobin concentration) and **microcytosis** (i.e., diminished size). Both conditions may be detected using the RBC indices available by calculation and the Coulter counter along with an examination of a stained blood smear. Disorders causing this type of anemia fall into four major classes.

1. **Microcytic anemias**
   a. **Iron-deficiency anemia** is the most common form of anemia in the United States, where 20% of adult women are reported to be iron deficient.
      (1) **Etiology.** Iron deficiency is most commonly caused by blood loss when the loss of the iron component exceeds the dietary intake of iron. Examples include gastrointestinal blood loss from an ulcer or a tumor and menstrual blood loss. Occasionally, in the neonate and young child, new blood formation and subsequent increased iron use exceed iron intake and result in anemia without concomitant blood loss.
      (2) **Clinical manifestations.** The symptoms of iron-deficiency anemia, like those of all anemias, include fatigue and weakness. Symptoms specific to iron deficiency may include epithelial changes such as brittle nails and atrophic tongue. In addition, the underlying pathology may dominate the symptoms (e.g., peptic ulcer).
      (3) **Diagnosis.** In the appropriate clinical setting (e.g., in a young woman with excessive menstrual blood loss and anemia), a smear showing hypochromia and microcytosis is adequate for the diagnosis (Online Figure 4–2). When more specific tests are needed, a positive diagnosis can be made from low levels of ferritin and a low serum iron level in association with an elevated total iron-binding capacity.
      (4) **Therapy.** Treatment usually involves restoration of the body's iron stores to correct the anemia. As a rule, oral iron in the form of ferrous sulfate suffices; however, for patients who do not tolerate this form, ferrous gluconate and fumarate are available. In difficult cases that are refractory, either physiologically or due to an inability to take oral iron, parenteral iron preparations are given. Reticulocytosis occurs 7 days after appropriate treatment; after 3 weeks, the hemoglobin level increases several grams.
   b. **Anemia of chronic disease.** This mild-to-moderate anemia is associated with inflammatory diseases such as rheumatoid arthritis, serious infections, and carcinoma.
      (1) **Pathophysiology**
         (a) Anemia of chronic disease is characterized by hemoglobin levels of 8–10 g/dL, although lower levels are possible. It is unusual for the hemoglobin level to be less than 7 g/dL.
         (b) Patients with this anemia have plentiful iron but diminished iron utilization by the bone marrow. Therefore, inadequate amounts of iron are available to the bone marrow for RBC formation despite adequate body stores.
         (c) Another important mechanism for this anemia is an impaired marrow response to erythropoietin. Hepcidin, a 25–amino acid peptide, has been found to play a key role

in the condition by regulating the absorption of iron and controlling the efflux of iron from storage sites. Hepcidin levels increase during inflammation, resulting in decreased iron concentration in the blood.

    (2) Diagnosis is based on confirmation of the following findings:

        (a) The anemia associated with chronic inflammation is of moderate degree and reveals slight hypochromia and microcytosis.

        (b) The mean corpuscular volume (MCV) is 80–85 fL, and the mean corpuscular hemoglobin concentration (MCHC) is 30–32 g/dL.

        (c) If stained, the marrow reveals plentiful iron stores. In addition, serum ferritin levels usually are normal or elevated. Serum iron is lowered, as is the total iron-binding capacity, unlike the clinical situation with iron-deficiency anemia.

    (3) Therapy. Hematinics, including iron, are not effective treatment for this disorder.

        (a) Correction of the underlying disease can lead to reversal of the anemia within 1 month.

        (b) Exogenous erythropoietin is effective in certain situations such as perioperatively in rheumatoid patients undergoing joint replacement surgery, in acquired immunodeficiency syndrome (AIDS), and in inflammatory bowel diseases. Because the inflammatory state induces a relative hyposensitivity to erythropoietin, generous doses may be needed.

  c. Sideroblastic anemias

    (1) Pathophysiology. These anemias, caused by disorders in the synthesis of the heme moiety of hemoglobin, are characterized by trapped iron in the mitochondria of nucleated RBCs. Many of the enzymes for protoporphyrin synthesis are located in the nucleated RBC mitochondria. Therefore, derangements in these pathways cause iron accumulation in the perinuclear mitochondria, which gives this anemia its characteristic morphologic finding of **ringed sideroblasts.** The defective heme synthesis causes diminished hemoglobin levels in these cells; as a result, this cell population is hypochromic and microcytic.

    (2) Types. There are two types of sideroblastic anemias.

        (a) Hereditary sideroblastic anemia. This X-linked condition is due to an abnormality in pyridoxine (vitamin B_6) metabolism. It is thought to be a congenital defect in the enzyme **δ-aminolevulinic acid (ALA) synthetase.**

        (b) Acquired sideroblastic anemias are more common than the hereditary type. Lead, alcohol, and the antibacterial drug isoniazid cause sideroblastic anemia by inhibiting enzymes of protoporphyrin synthesis; however, many cases are idiopathic.

    (3) Diagnosis. This anemia may be relatively severe in patients older than 60 years and is characterized by hemoglobin levels of 8–10 g/dL. Coulter counter reveals normocytic or even macrocytic cells, but examination of the blood smear shows a dimorphic population with some very small cells. The bone marrow reveals erythroid hyperplasia, and iron staining demonstrates the ringed sideroblasts. Iron studies show elevated ferritin levels and high serum iron levels with high transferrin saturation. Often, some normal or slightly macrocytic cells are seen intermingling with the hypochromic, microcytic cells, and a blood smear revealing such a condition is diagnostic of this anemia.

    (4) Therapy

        (a) If a drug such as isoniazid, chloramphenicol, or alcohol is involved, the anemia and sideroblastic changes regress with discontinuation of the agent.

        (b) All patients should be given a trial of **pyridoxine** in high doses; however, in all but the hereditary cases, this usually fails. Often, these patients are transfusion dependent. Acute leukemia develops in a portion (10%) of patients with acquired idiopathic disease. In these patients, the sideroblastic anemia is a preleukemic syndrome and is classified as a myelodysplastic syndrome.

        (c) Efficacy using **exogenous erythropoietin** to treat this condition is approximately 20%, and this therapy should be tried in transfusion-dependent patients.

  d. Thalassemias are genetic disorders characterized by diminished synthesis of one of the globin chains. These diseases are due to abnormalities in the genes that are responsible for synthesis of the globin portion of the hemoglobin molecule. Thalassemias are named according to the deficient chain.

(1) Types

(a) α-Thalassemias. These disorders are characterized by deficient α-chain synthesis, usually due to deletion of one or more of the α-globin genes from the genome. There are four such genes and, thus, four α-thalassemias; these range from a silent carrier state to a severe anemia that is fatal in utero. The α-thalassemias are most prevalent in Asian populations.

(b) β-Thalassemias. These disorders are due to the absence or malfunction of the β-globin gene. In the latter case, RNA is present but in reduced amounts or in defective forms. The two β-globin genes in the genome result in two different forms of β-thalassemia. **β-Thalassemia major,** or **Cooley's anemia,** is a severe disease that appears in childhood. Patients with this disease are transfusion dependent. Patients with **β-thalassemia minor,** a mild anemia, are not transfusion dependent and can live full, normal lives. The β-thalassemias are most prevalent in individuals of Mediterranean descent, particularly those from Greece and Italy.

(2) Diagnosis. The thalassemias should be suspected in anemic patients who reveal marked abnormalities on blood smear. Such abnormalities include microcytosis, hypochromia, and poikilocytosis (i.e., the presence of bizarrely shaped RBCs).

(a) α-Thalassemia is most difficult to diagnose when it exists in the carrier state. Patients with the carrier form generally have normal hemoglobin, sometimes with a mild microcytosis. There is no excess of the non–β-hemoglobins because all chains have α components. Therefore, sophisticated studies are required for definitive diagnosis. In neonates, however, the diagnosis can be made from cord blood tests that show an increase in **Bart's hemoglobin.** With the advent of genetic mapping technology, the presence or absence of α-globin genes can be ascertained to make the diagnosis definitively.

(b) The diagnosis of **β-thalassemia** may be confirmed in several ways.

(i) Measurement of minor hemoglobin chains A_2 and F reveals elevations as the erythron attempts to compensate for the diminished synthesis of β chains by making excessive γ and δ chains instead.

(ii) Genetic analysis of hemoglobin mRNA or genetic mapping of the globin genes is now available.

(3) Therapy includes chronic red cell transfusions and folic acid supplementation. The regular use of iron chelation therapy has slowed the development of iron overload in these patients. In selected patients, bone marrow transplantation (BMT) has been curative.

2. Macrocytic anemias are characterized by RBCs that exceed 100 μm. Three major mechanisms are linked to the development of macrocytic anemia.

a. Accelerated erythropoiesis. Reticulocytes and young erythrocytes are larger than normal; therefore, individuals with large numbers of reticulocytes have large numbers of circulating cells of great size. A reticulocyte count confirms the diagnosis.

b. Increased membrane surface area. Patients with excessive plasma lipids absorb these lipids onto RBC surfaces, which creates an enlarged membrane surface area and a macrocytosis in excess of 100 μm. This condition is most common in patients with liver disease and can be diagnosed by a blood smear that reveals the characteristic **target cell** of liver disease (i.e., a round macrocyte with a dark center). Liver disease causes this by diminished hepatic synthesis of lecithin–cholesterol acetyl transferase (LCAT), resulting in excess plasma-free cholesterol, which is absorbed onto RBC membranes.

c. Defective DNA synthesis is the main characteristic of the classic **megaloblastic anemias.** In these conditions, erythroid precursors cannot produce nucleic acid, and so nuclear maturation is arrested. Cytoplasmic maturation proceeds, however, resulting in abnormally large cells. These cells are larger than those seen with accelerated erythropoiesis, and they have an increased membrane surface area. An MCV that exceeds 115 mm^3 is not uncommon.

(1) Etiology. Megaloblastic anemias usually are caused by a deficiency of either vitamin B_{12} or folic acid.

(a) B_{12} deficiency may result from fish tapeworm infestation, strict vegetarian (vegan) diets, or intestinal blind loops with bacterial overgrowth. The most common cause, however, is a lack of the intrinsic factor necessary for vitamin B_{12} absorption into the terminal ileum. Two forms of atrophic gastritis have been described. Type A, pernicious anemia, is a true autoimmune gastritis involving the fundus and body of the stomach and has the gastric parietal cell H^-/K^+-ATPase as the molecular target of the autoimmune process. Type B is nonautoimmune, involves the entire stomach, and is associated with *Helicobacter pylori* infection.

- (b) **Folic acid deficiency** is caused by dietary deficiency due to inadequate intake, inadequate absorption, or both. This condition is most commonly encountered in alcoholics.
- (c) **Drug-induced disorders of DNA synthesis.** Certain drugs used to treat cancer (e.g., methotrexate), bacterial infections (e.g., trimethoprim), and parasitic infections (e.g., pyrimethamine), as well as phenytoin, interfere with folic acid metabolism and cause megaloblastic anemia and bone marrow changes. These diagnoses can be made easily from patient history.

(2) **Clinical manifestations.** Patients with megaloblastic anemia have varying degrees of anemia associated with large RBCs. Because nucleic acid metabolism is necessary for all cellular elements in bone marrow, white blood cells (WBCs) and platelets are diminished. The ineffective erythropoiesis and intramedullary hemolysis associated with this disorder often result in serum **lactate dehydrogenase (LDH)** levels that exceed 500 units/dL and an elevated bilirubin. Both RBCs and WBCs in bone marrow reveal the classic megaloblastic sign of immature, open nuclei in association with mature cytoplasmic components. Blood smear shows characteristic oval macrocytes and hypersegmented polymorphonuclear leukocytes (PMNLs) (Online Figure 4–3).

(3) **Differential diagnosis**
- (a) Serum levels of folate and vitamin B_{12} as well as RBC folic acid levels should be measured to determine whether the deficiency is in folic acid or vitamin B_{12}.
- (b) Vitamin B_{12} has a neurologic function; therefore, when a macrocytic anemia is associated with neurologic symptoms, particularly posterior column signs and symptoms, vitamin B_{12} deficiency should be suspected. The hallmarks of pernicious anemia are macrocytic anemia, neurologic symptoms and signs, and **atrophic glossitis.**
- (c) The **Schilling test** for the presence of intrinsic factor and intestinal function can be performed to differentiate the cause of vitamin B_{12} deficiency. However, clinicians have become less enthusiastic about this test because of its complexity and occasional inaccuracy. Most practitioners prefer to use more refined biochemical testing of the purine synthetic pathways. Currently, measurement of the methylmalonic acid level has replaced the Schilling test as the diagnostic procedure of choice. However, the Schilling test remains useful for study of the physiology of vitamin B_{12}. Serum antiparietal cell antibodies are a relatively specific test finding for the autoimmune type A variant (>90%).

(4) **Therapy.** Specific therapy is determined by the vitamin that is missing. Folic acid alone should never be given in an undiagnosed case of macrocytic anemia; while folic acid can reverse hematologic signs, it will exacerbate neurologic degeneration.
- (a) Patients with pernicious anemia due to vitamin B_{12} deficiency generally require life-long treatment with parenteral vitamin B_{12}. If reversible causes are found (e.g., intestinal bacterial overgrowth), appropriate measures may reverse the deficiency and obviate the need for permanent vitamin B_{12} therapy.
- (b) Folic acid deficiency is treated with oral preparations of folic acid.

3. **Normochromic, normocytic anemias** represent a vast array of conditions characterized by normal cell size and hemoglobin concentration. These anemias are not related by common pathogenic mechanisms; **classification is by the degree of marrow response to the anemia.**
   a. **Anemia associated with impaired marrow response.** The following anemias are characterized by normal or low reticulocyte counts.
   (1) **Hypoplastic,** or **aplastic, anemia** is an intrinsic marrow disease characterized by an absence of stem cells. All myeloid (derived from the bone marrow) cell lines are involved, with a resultant **pancytopenia.** Severe cases of this disease are associated with a high mortality rate. Levels of serum erythropoietin are usually elevated proportionately to the degree of anemia. Treatment that suppresses the immune system, such as antithymocyte globulin (ATG), can result in an improvement in blood counts. In young patients, BMT techniques are curative in cases in which an appropriate marrow donor is available.

(2) Disorders characterized by infiltration of bone marrow (myelophthisic anemias) include myeloma, carcinoma or, more rarely, granulomatous infections such as tuberculosis. Disruption of bone marrow architecture is common; a blood smear that reveals immature WBCs and nucleated RBCs (called leukoerythroblastosis) is a clue to the presence of these conditions. A bone marrow aspirate and biopsy confirm the diagnosis in such cases.

(3) Anemia due to diminished erythropoietin secretion is the anemia of **chronic renal failure.** Erythropoietin is a protein–lipid molecule required by the marrow for adequate RBC formation. With severe kidney disease, the erythropoietin secreted by the kidneys is lost, and anemia ensues. The degree of anemia roughly correlates with the degree of renal failure.

  (a) Proper attention to iron and folic acid stores is important in this group of patients because deficiencies in these nutrients secondarily complicate the anemia of renal failure.

  (b) Erythropoietin has been effective in raising the hemoglobin to normal or near-normal levels in these patients, although it has not been consistently shown to significantly increase patient quality of life. Recent studies have raised concerns about this therapy because of the possibly increased risk of stroke, myocardial infarction, congestive heart failure, and hemodialysis vascular access thrombosis.

(4) Other anemias associated with hypoproliferation of bone marrow include those associated with hypothyroidism, hypopituitarism, and liver disease.

b. Anemia associated with appropriately increased RBC production, such as anemia following hemorrhage. An increased reticulocyte count is the normal marrow response in patients who bleed either overtly (e.g., with surgery) or covertly (e.g., into the gastrointestinal tract) and have adequate iron stores. This condition can be confused with hemolysis; however, an appropriate clinical setting (e.g., a postoperative patient with a large resolving hematoma) and lack of hemolysis markers will lead to the correct diagnosis.

B **Anemia caused by increased RBC destruction** **Hemolytic anemias** represent conditions in which RBC survival is shortened. In most cases, the marrow is intrinsically normal; therefore, adequate new RBCs can be made, and the patients have elevated reticulocyte counts. Diagnostic of these anemias are signs of increased RBC destruction (e.g., increased unconjugated bilirubin, elevated serum LDH, reduced haptoglobin) combined with signs of accelerated marrow activity (e.g., elevated reticulocyte counts and erythroid hyperplasia in the marrow). The diagnosis of hemolysis should be made first and the specific cause of the hemolysis sought later. Hemolytic anemia exists in many forms, which are grouped as follows.

1. Hemolytic anemia due to factors extrinsic to the RBC

a. Autoantibodies can attach to the RBC and cause its destruction by the reticuloendothelial system. A classic example is **Coombs-positive hemolytic anemia** due to either warm [immunoglobulin G (IgG)] or cold (IgM) antibodies. This anemia may be idiopathic or may arise as a complication of collagen disease or lymphoma. In severe cases, steroids and splenectomy may be required to control the anemia.

b. Exogenous agents such as malarial organisms render the RBC vulnerable to hemolysis.

c. Abnormalities in the circulation can cause premature destruction of RBCs. The following are examples of such abnormalities, and disorders associated with each condition are also cited.

  (1) Lipid abnormalities (spur-cell anemia in advanced liver disease)

  (2) Fibrin deposition in the microvasculature with shearing of RBCs (disseminated intravascular coagulation [DIC] syndrome)

  (3) RBC damage due to trauma from prosthetic heart valves

2. Hemolytic anemia due to factors intrinsic to the RBC. These disorders involve congenital abnormalities that render the RBC more likely to hemolyze.

a. Membrane disorders include **hereditary spherocytosis,** in which a defect in the membrane sodium–potassium–ATPase pump causes RBC swelling. This results in the characteristic finding on blood smear of small, round, hyperchromic RBCs without the usual central pallor (i.e., spherocytes). These cells are osmotically fragile and are destroyed in the spleen. Splenectomy usually controls the anemia, although the RBC defect remains.

b. **Hemoglobin disorders—hemoglobinopathies.** These diseases, of which more than 250 are known, are caused by point mutations in the DNA code related to variation in a single amino acid in the globin chains. The most commonly encountered hemoglobinopathies involve amino acid changes near the surface of the globular hemoglobin molecule, which predispose the hemoglobin to polymerization. Such polymerization results in the hemoglobin becoming rigid, with subsequent membrane and cell shape changes. These affected RBCs become liable to hemolysis.

(1) **Hemoglobin S (Hb S).** The most common hemoglobinopathy is Hb S, which causes **sickle cell anemia** (Online Figure 4–4). This disorder occurs in 1% of African Americans. The disease manifestations result from three major pathophysiologic processes (Table 4–1). The polymerized hemoglobin severely deforms RBCs and results in **marked, chronic hemolysis.** This manifests as severe, chronic anemia (with hemoglobin of 5–10 g/dL); predisposition to aplastic crises associated with parvovirus and other infections; elevated bilirubin levels with almost universal gallstone disease; and frequent, chronic ulceration of the legs in the ankle area. Splenic autoinfarction and diminished synthesis of opsonizing immunoglobulins results in frequent infections, especially with encapsulated microorganisms (e.g., pneumococci, *Haemophilus*, *Salmonella* species). **Acute episodes of pain ("painful crises")** are the principal symptom and cause of morbidity in patients with sickle cell disease. Painful crises have been thought to be the result of microvascular occlusion with infarction resulting from local hyperviscosity associated with the rigid, deformed and abnormally adhesive sickle cells. More recently, leukocyte adhesion, inflammatory mediators, and endothelial activation have been proposed as contributing factors.

(2) Other common hemoglobinopathies that cause less severe sickle syndromes include hemoglobin C (Hb C), hemoglobin O (Hb O), and combinations such as hemoglobin SC (Hb SC).

(3) **Diagnosis** is confirmed by hemoglobin electrophoresis, which demonstrates the characteristic changes in mobility caused by specific amino acid changes.

(4) **Therapy,** which is still not satisfactory, continues to evolve. **Supportive medical care** remains the cornerstone of effective therapy and includes transfusions when indicated (e.g., during hypoplastic crises), attention to hydration, and analgesics for the pain of microvascular occlusion.

(5) Newer directions in therapy have moved toward manipulation of the relative hemoglobin concentrations within the cell to diminish the propensity to polymerize. Hemoglobin F (Hb F) has been found to have an inhibitory effect on sickling, and the cytotoxic agent hydroxyurea, which often causes an increase in Hb F, has been investigated in patients with severe sickle cell anemia. A randomized study and multiple observational studies have shown that the use of hydroxyurea results in fewer painful crises and hospital admissions. See more information online.

(6) Specific **complications** are responsible for much of the mortality in sickle cell disease. An important example is the development of **acute chest syndrome.** In this situation, which usually complicates what appears to be a routine painful crisis, the patient develops a

TABLE 4–1 Clinical Manifestations of Sickle Cell Anemia		
Related to Chronic Hemolytic Anemia	**Related to Abnormal Adhesions, Sickling, and Vaso-occlusion**	**Related to Increased Susceptibility to Infection**
Normocytic anemia	Painful crises	Pneumococcal sepsis
Elevated bilirubin and lactate dehydrogenase	Cerebrovascular accident	*Salmonella* sepsis
Gallstone disease	Acute and chronic cardiopulmonary disease (e.g., acute chest syndromes, cor pulmonale)	Osteomyelitis
	Priapism	
	Splenic autoinfarction	
	Skeletal changes (e.g., aseptic necrosis of the hip)	

fever, frequently manifests an unusually brisk leukocytosis, and then develops profound hypoxia. A chest radiograph demonstrates diffuse chest infiltrates, and the clinical syndrome evolves into an adult respiratory distress syndrome (ARDS)–like situation. This complication carries a high mortality if not quickly recognized and treated. The syndrome usually responds very well to exchange transfusions to lower Hb S levels to 30%. Other currently accepted indications for RBC exchange transfusion include stroke and central nervous system (CNS) vascular lesions.

    c. **Disorders of the cytoplasm and enzymes** occur as congenital hemolytic anemias. An RBC lacks a nucleus when it leaves the marrow; therefore, an RBC must survive its 120-day life span with its given complement of enzymes. A cell deficient in necessary enzymes is unable to maintain itself and thus dies prematurely.

        (1) **Glucose-6-phosphate dehydrogenase (G6PD) deficiency** is an extremely common X-linked disorder; more than 150 subtypes are found in more than 100 million individuals worldwide. The red blood cells of affected individuals have decreased reducing capacity and thus are vulnerable to oxidant stress, which occurs with infections and with certain drugs (e.g., sulfa drugs, quinine). Such oxidant stress results in denatured hemoglobin or Heinz bodies, leading to hemolysis of affected RBCs. It is believed that G6PD protects individuals from falciparum malaria; G6PD deficiency is most common in malaria-endemic areas.

        (2) **Diagnosis** is suspected by demonstrating Heinz bodies during an acute hemolytic anemia episode and confirmed by measuring abnormally low levels of enzyme in the steady state. Enzyme levels should not be measured during a hemolytic episode, when they may temporarily become more normal as a result of destruction of old, extremely deficient cells and their replacement by relatively G6PD-rich reticulocytes.

        (3) Other examples of enzyme deficiencies include **pyruvate kinase (PK) deficiency,** which is most common in northern European populations.

II   DISORDERS OF INCREASED HEMOGLOBIN

Increases in hematocrit are caused by either **increased RBC mass** or **decreased plasma volume.** The following discussion deals exclusively with disorders associated with abnormal elevation of hematocrit (i.e., hematocrit ≥55%).

   A **Terminology**   The term **polycythemia** often is used to describe an increase in the number of RBCs, with no reference to fluctuations in leukocytes and platelets. However, this condition is more accurately termed **erythrocytosis.** [There is a condition called **polycythemia vera** in which leukocytes and platelets also increase in number. See II C 2 b (2) (a) for a discussion of this disorder.] Increased hematocrits occur in two ways.

    1. **Relative erythrocytosis** refers to an elevation of hematocrit due to diminished plasma volume; RBC mass remains normal.

    2. **Absolute erythrocytosis** refers to an elevation of hematocrit due to a true increase in RBC mass.

   B **Pathophysiology**   Blood viscosity is directly proportional to hematocrit; therefore, an excessively elevated hematocrit can diminish tissue blood flow, decrease tissue oxygen delivery, and increase cardiac work. In extreme cases, this can result in hyperviscosity syndromes.

   C **Classification**

    1. **Relative erythrocytosis** exists in two forms.

      a. **Stress erythrocytosis,** or **Gaisböck's syndrome,** occurs predominantly in middle-aged men. This disorder is usually asymptomatic. It is important to differentiate patients with stress erythrocytosis from those with early and subtle manifestations of the much more serious condition polycythemia vera. Patients with stress erythrocytosis require no treatment.

      b. **Erythrocytosis occurs secondary to known causes of contracted plasma volume** (e.g., excessive diuresis; nasogastric drainage; severe gastroenteritis, especially in infants; burns). These conditions are apparent clinically; therapy includes fluid and plasma replacement and treatment of the underlying condition.

2. Absolute erythrocytosis is classified according to the mechanism responsible for increased RBC mass.

   a. Hypoxia

   (1) **Etiology.** Causes include severe lung disease, severe heart failure, cyanotic heart disease with right-to-left cardiopulmonary shunts, and abnormal hemoglobins with increased oxygen affinity.

   (2) **Pathophysiology.** The RBC mass rises secondary to tissue hypoxia, which causes an increase in erythropoietin release from the kidneys and subsequent hematocrit elevation.

   (3) **Diagnosis** may be apparent clinically, but blood gas analysis showing arterial oxygen saturation less than 92%, a moderately elevated serum erythropoietin level, and possibly P_{50} analysis (i.e., studies of the oxygen-releasing characteristics of hemoglobin) may be required to confirm the diagnosis.

   (4) **Therapy** is directed at maintaining a hemoglobin that minimizes the patient's symptoms of dyspnea. Phlebotomy to maintain a hematocrit of 55% or less will sometimes attain that goal.

   b. Neoplasia

   (1) **Neoplastic erythropoietin sources** cause the RBC mass to increase.

   (a) **Etiology.** Causes include hypernephroma and renal cysts; such renal pathology accounts for more than 90% of this type of erythrocytosis. Other tumors include cerebellar hemangioblastoma, hepatoma, and uterine fibroids.

   (b) **Diagnosis** requires radiologic demonstration of tumor and the demonstration of inappropriately elevated serum erythropoietin levels.

   (c) **Therapy.** Removal of the tumor corrects the hematocrit.

   (2) **Autonomous bone marrow**

   (a) In the condition **polycythemia vera (PV),** the bone marrow becomes autonomous and synthesizes cells independent of erythropoietin levels. Polycythemia vera represents a true neoplasm of the marrow stem cells. This disorder has been found to be associated with a mutation in the JAK-2 protein in a majority of cases.

   (i) **Diagnosis.** Prior to testing for the JAK-2 mutation, diagnosis was confirmed using major and minor criteria defined by the Polycythemia Vera Study Group. The World Health Organization (WHO) has proposed an amendment of these criteria using separate major and minor criteria that incorporate the JAK-2 mutation. A positive JAK-2 mutation in the setting of erythrocytosis with a low erythropoietin level is diagnostic of PV.

   (ii) **Therapy** involves removal of RBCs, suppression of marrow function, or both. **Phlebotomy** removes RBCs and should be performed to lower hematocrit to below 45%. Marrow suppression is needed for patients at high risk of thrombosis or for progressive splenomegaly. Interferon-α has been shown to be an effective agent to control myeloproliferation and splenomegaly. Chemotherapy with the antimetabolite hydroxyurea is used to control many cases of polycythemia vera. Few if any leukemogenic or second malignancy–inducing effects have been encountered with this agent. Specific JAK-2 inhibitors are being studied in clinical trials.

   (iii) **Complications.** The major causes of morbidity and mortality are thromboembolic and cardiovascular events, which account for almost 50% of deaths. Other complications include bleeding, myelofibrosis, and leukemic transformation.

   (b) **Myelofibrosis,** a chronic myeloproliferative disorder, is pathophysiologically related. It is characterized by splenomegaly, immature granulocytes and erythrocytes in the blood, distorted teardrop-shaped RBC forms, and marrow fibrosis. The disease is a **monoclonal stem cell disease** of primitive hematopoietic stem cells. JAK-2 mutation is found in approximately 50% of cases. The **fibrosis** is a secondary event.

   (i) **Anemia** and signs and symptoms of **massive splenomegaly** are the hallmarks of the disease.

   (ii) Most **therapy is supportive.** In selected cases of true hypersplenism and symptoms from massive splenomegaly, splenectomy is beneficial. JAK-2 inhibitor therapy is being explored in clinical trials.

III   DISORDERS OF PLATELETS

Platelets play a role in the primary arrest of bleeding. Platelet abnormalities are classified according to disorders of number and function.

A   Thrombocytopenia   (i.e., decreased numbers of platelets) is the **most common cause of abnormal bleeding.**

1. **General considerations**
   a. Platelets are derived from megakaryocytes—large multinucleated cells that reside in the bone marrow. Mature megakaryocytes produce elongated cytoplasmic processes that separate from the cell body, become disc shaped, and enter into the circulation as platelets.
   b. With a platelet count of less than $50,000/mm^3$, there is a potential increased risk of bleeding with trauma and surgical procedures. Most individuals experience an increased tendency to bruise with platelet counts of between 30,000 and $10,000/mm^3$. Formation of spontaneous petechiae with bleeding may occur with platelet counts less than $10,000/mm^3$, with serious spontaneous bleeding (e.g., CNS) occurring with platelet counts of less than $5000/mm^3$.

2. **Mechanisms** of thrombocytopenia include impaired platelet production, abnormal platelet pooling in the spleen, and increased peripheral destruction. Various examples, marrow findings, and therapies are summarized in Table 4–2.
   a. **Impaired platelet production**
      (1) **Etiology**
          (a) Megakaryocytes may be selectively suppressed by certain agents (e.g., thiazide diuretics, ethanol).

TABLE 4–2   Mechanisms of Thrombocytopenia

Mechanisms	Marrow Findings	Clinical Conditions	Therapy
Impaired production of platelets	Megakaryocytes reduced or absent	Induced chemically or physically (e.g., chemotherapy, radiation)	Removal of offending agents; supportive
		Aplastic anemia, paroxysmal nocturnal hemoglobinuria, leukemia	Marrow transplantation
		Infection (e.g., viral hepatitis, cytomegalovirus, tuberculosis)	Treatment of infection
Ineffective production of platelets	Abnormal and/or dysplastic megakaryocytes	Megaloblastic disorder (vitamin B$_{12}$ deficiency, folate deficiency)	Vitamin B$_{12}$ or folate supplementation
		Myelodysplasias and myeloproliferative disorders	Treatment of underlying disorder
Enhanced destruction of platelets (immune mediated)	Increased megakaryocytes	Idiopathic thrombocytopenic purpura	See V C 1 b (3)
		Posttransfusion purpura	Plasmapheresis
		Drug induced (e.g., rifampin, methicillin, sulfonamides, phenytoin, quinine, quinidine, heparin)	Removal of offending agent
		Lymphomas	Treatment of underlying disorder
			Steroids
		Immune complex disorder (e.g., systemic lupus erythematosus)	
Enhanced destruction of platelets (not immune related)	Increased megakaryocytes	Thrombotic thrombocytopenic purpura	Plasmapheresis
		Hemolytic uremic syndrome	Plasmapheresis
		Disseminated intravascular coagulation	Treatment of underlying disorders
		Dilution and cardiopulmonary bypass	Supportive
		Splenomegaly	Usually not required; splenectomy may be necessary occasionally

    (b) Impaired platelet production is associated with the megaloblastic hematopoiesis seen in vitamin B_{12} and folate deficiencies, as well as in cases of myelodysplastic and preleukemic syndromes.

    (c) A rare cause is amegakaryocytic thrombocytopenia caused by congenital deficiency of megakaryocyte colony-forming units.

(2) **Diagnosis** is confirmed by a bone marrow smear that reveals too few megakaryocytes or pathology consistent with one of the aforementioned diagnoses.

(3) **Therapy** involves removal of the offending agent, if possible, or treatment of the underlying disease. Patients have essentially normal platelet half-lives and should be transfused with exogenous platelets if they are thrombocytopenic and bleeding. Thrombocytopenia associated with vitamin B_{12} or folate deficiency is rapidly corrected by therapy with the deficient vitamin.

(4) **Associated conditions.** Impaired platelet production is also associated with aplastic anemia, myelophthisic processes (replacement of marrow by tumor or fibrosis), overwhelming infections that suppress the bone marrow, and certain rare congenital syndromes (e.g., thrombocytopenia with absent radii).

b. **Abnormal platelet pooling** results when platelets are sequestered from the circulation. **Splenic platelet sequestration** is the most common cause of abnormal platelet pooling.

(1) **Pathophysiology.** Normally, the spleen holds one third of the circulating platelet pool. As splenomegaly occurs, higher numbers of platelets are sequestered and, thus, are unavailable for hemostasis. In very large spleens, as much as 90% of the platelet pool may be sequestered; however, platelets in the peripheral circulation do have normal survival times.

(2) **Diagnosis** of hypersplenism is suggested by a moderate thrombocytopenia (platelet counts of $<30,000/mm^3$ are unusual), a bone marrow aspirate that reveals adequate marrow megakaryocytes, and evidence of significant splenic enlargement.

(3) **Clinical features** in such cases are dominated by the underlying illness causing the splenomegaly (e.g., cirrhosis with portal hypertension).

(4) **Therapy** usually is not required, although splenectomy may correct the problem. Transfused platelets are sequestered in the same ratio and thus are less effective than in hypoactive marrow states.

c. **Increased peripheral destruction** of platelets is the **most common form of thrombocytopenia.** Conditions involving increased platelet destruction are characterized by shortened platelet survival and increased number of marrow megakaryocytes. Causes include immune-mediated thrombocytopenia, drug-induced thrombocytopenia (including heparin-induced thrombocytopenia; [see Section V]), disseminated intravascular coagulation [see Section IV], and thrombotic thrombocytopenic purpura [see Section V]. **Idiopathic (or immune) thrombocytopenic purpura (ITP)** is seen in all age groups, although the clinical manifestations and course vary across the age spectrum.

(1) **Clinical features.** The **acute variant** of ITP occurs in children between the ages of 2 and 6 years and often occurs after a nonspecific viral illness. The **chronic variant** occurs in young adults, more commonly in young women. All ITP patients show varying degrees of thrombocytopenia, which in some acute cases is severe (i.e., associated with platelet counts of $<1000/mm^3$), and all show increased megakaryocytes. Other blood findings and cell lines are normal. Patients can have mucocutaneous bleeding with petechiae, purpura, mucosal bullae, and excessive bleeding after trauma. ITP can be associated with autoimmune diseases such as systemic lupus erythematosus or other collagen diseases.

(2) **Diagnosis** requires exclusion of other possible causes of thrombocytopenia, including other illnesses or drugs.

    (a) In patients who are younger than 60 years of age with otherwise normal blood counts, bone marrow examination is not required. The clinical diagnosis of ITP can be made as long as splenectomy is not contemplated (in which case a confirmatory marrow examination is performed).

    (b) In patients older than 60 years, a bone marrow examination should be performed because of the increasing incidence of myelodysplasia or other bone marrow abnormalities in such patients.

(c) New epidemiologic studies have shown a high incidence of human immunodeficiency virus (HIV) and hepatitis C as causes of thrombocytopenia, and many authorities suggest testing for them in ITP patients. If appropriate on clinical grounds, lupus testing also should be performed. These conditions can manifest as apparently isolated thrombocytopenia.

(3) Clinical course. The acute childhood variant often resolves within 4–8 weeks; the adult form is generally chronic and demonstrates relapses and remissions.

(4) Therapy for the acute childhood form usually involves protection from trauma and, in some cases, a short course of steroids. Treatment of adult ITP is more complex and protracted.

   (a) High doses of corticosteroids often produce complete remission and remain the core therapy for chronic ITP.

   (b) Steroids induce responses in approximately two thirds of cases and in a minority (5%–30% in various studies) result in sustained remissions requiring no further treatment.

   (c) Splenectomy may be necessary in resistant cases and in two thirds of patients is associated with a response. The need for splenectomy has diminished in recent years.

   (d) Refractory patients, who have a fall in platelet count after corticosteroids are tapered, are often treated with rituximab, a monoclonal antibody directed against the CD20 antigen on lymphocytes.

   (e) An effective therapy that can temporarily elevate platelet counts in an acute crisis is **infusion with intravenous IgG.** The infused IgG competes for and saturates reticuloendothelial binding sites, making fewer of them available for platelet binding and destruction. This maneuver has also gained popularity as a preoperative therapy in ITP patients who require surgery. **Hyperimmune anti-Rh(D) globulin** (e.g., such as that given to women after giving birth to Rh-positive infants) has been found to act in a like manner as an urgent therapy in ITP and can be used in similar settings (i.e., prior to surgery or when thrombocytopenia is extreme) with excellent results. These maneuvers have become the initial therapy in most cases of acute and severe ITP.

   (f) In the event of clinically significant bleeding, platelet transfusions can be given. However, this is not always effective in raising the platelet count because of short platelet survival.

   (g) For patients who relapse after rituximab therapy, the thrombopoietin receptor agonists eltrombopag and romiplostim have been effective at producing sustained increases in platelet counts with minimal toxicity.

(5) Prognosis. The overall prognosis is good; only 2%–3% of ITP patients die from the condition after 5 years.

B **Thrombocytopathia** involves platelets that are adequate in number but unable to function properly in hemostasis and in the primary arrest of bleeding.

1. **Description.** Thrombocytopathia is characterized by the following:
   a. Platelet-type mucocutaneous bleeding
   b. Normal platelet counts
   c. Demonstrated abnormalities in platelet function testing (e.g., aggregometry)

2. **Etiology**
   a. **Drug-related platelet dysfunction** is the most common cause of abnormal platelet function.
      (1) Aspirin permanently acetylates platelet membranes, impairing the platelet prostaglandin synthesis [e.g., impairing synthesis of thromboxane A_2 (TXA_2)] required for proper platelet function. Such impaired platelets may prolong bleeding times and cause bruising and increase hemorrhage with trauma. The aspirin-induced platelet lesion permanently alters circulating platelets and lasts until the platelets are replaced by new, unaffected ones, usually 3–7 days after discontinuation of the aspirin.
      (2) Clopidogrel (Plavix) is a powerful antiplatelet agent that selectively inhibits platelet receptor binding of adenosine diphosphate (ADP) and subsequent activation of the IIb/IIIa complex. Like aspirin, the effect is irreversible and lasts for the remainder of the exposed platelet's life span.

(3) Other anti-inflammatory drugs (e.g., indomethacin) cause similar dysfunction but differ from aspirin in that their effects are not permanent and disappear when the agent is withdrawn.

b. Platelet dysfunction is seen in patients with end-stage renal disease. In bleeding uremic patients, dialysis may evoke a response. Administration of cryoprecipitate or desmopressin (dDAVP) may also improve the coagulopathy.

c. Congenital forms of platelet dysfunction

C **Thrombocytosis** is the existence of too many platelets in the blood. The platelet count can be high secondary to another process or can be the result of a primary hematologic disorder.

1. **Secondary thrombocytosis**
   a. **Reactive thrombocytosis** is a rise in the platelet count above normal in the setting of a metabolically active process such as infection, trauma, major surgery, or chronic inflammatory state. In order to be considered reactive, the platelet count should normalize with resolution of the event.
   b. **Spurious thrombocytosis** refers to a measured platelet count that is high when the actual platelet count is normal. Causes of spurious thrombocytosis include mixed cryoglobulinemia (precipitates may be counted as platelets) and cell fragments such as in severe hemolysis.

2. **Primary thrombocytosis**
   a. **Essential thrombocythemia (ET)** is a **myeloproliferative** disorder in which abnormally high numbers of platelets are produced from precursor megakaryocytes in the bone marrow. JAK-2 mutations are found in approximately 50% of patients with this disorder.
   b. **Thrombocytosis** can also occur autonomously from the bone marrow in **myelodysplastic** syndromes [see Section VII]. Among the myelodysplastic syndromes, thrombocytosis is particularly associated with deletion of the long arm of chromosome 5 ("5q– syndrome").

IV DISORDERS OF IMPAIRED COAGULATION AND INCREASED RISK OF BLEEDING

A **General considerations**   Hemostasis requires an intact coagulation system of vascular and tissue components, platelets, and coagulation proteins. Deficiency or disease of any of these components may cause either spontaneous or trauma-related hemorrhage.

1. **History.** A careful history provides clues to the pathogenesis of bleeding. Immediate, mucocutaneous bleeding suggests vascular or platelet disease; delayed deep tissue bleeding and hemarthrosis suggest coagulation protein deficiency. Genetic transmissions of bleeding disorders (e.g., the X-linked hemophilias) also are elicited by history, as is ingestion of drugs (e.g., aspirin).

2. **Physical findings** aid in differentiation of bleeding syndromes. Mucocutaneous petechiae and purpura suggest platelet disorders; hematomas and hemarthrosis suggest coagulopathy.

3. **Laboratory testing** is vital in the evaluation of bleeding disorders. Single tests rarely provide conclusive results, so various batteries of tests have been developed. The coagulation cascade is shown in Figure 4–5, and the diagnosis of common bleeding disorders based on commonly used tests is shown in Table 4–3.

B **Disorders of blood vessels and vascular tissues**   The following bleeding disorders result from pathology in the vessel area itself, with secondary leakage of blood. Most of these disorders have as their hallmark a visible and usually palpable skin lesion. Testing performed on patients with these bleeding disorders reveals normal coagulation.

1. **Autoimmune (allergic) purpura (Henoch–Schönlein purpura)** occurs most commonly in children and young adults. The syndrome is associated with various infections, chemical exposure, and malignancies. The lesions are symmetric and palpable and are usually found on the distal extremities. There is no standard therapy.

2. **Purpura associated with infections** may be due to embolic occlusion of the microvasculature (e.g., endocarditis) or to endothelial injury by the infectious agent (e.g., *Rickettsia*). Biopsy and culture of the material may be helpful.

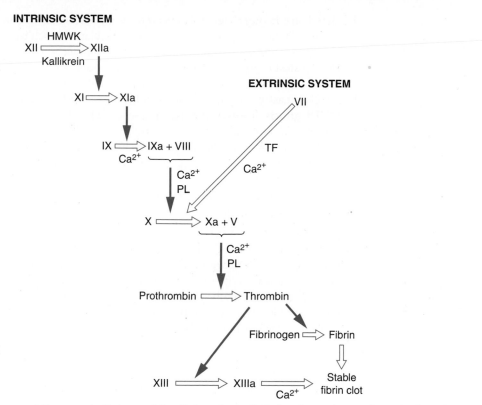

INTRINSIC SYSTEM

EXTRINSIC SYSTEM

FIGURE 4–5 The coagulation cascade. Each coagulation factor, when activated, activates the next factor in the series. (Factors are numbered in order of their discovery, not in order of activation.) In the intrinsic system, factor XII is initially activated by an unknown mechanism and subsequently by kallikrein during the contact phase. Alternatively, factor VII and tissue factor can initiate the extrinsic system. Intrinsic and extrinsic pathways each end with activation of factor X, setting off a final, common pathway that ends with formation of the fibrin clot. Open arrows indicate conversion of a substrate or a reactant to a product. HMWK, high–molecular-weight kininogen; PL, phospholipid; TF, tissue factor.

3. **Structural malformations of vessels and vascular tissues** are associated with the following conditions.

   a. **Scurvy** is caused by vitamin C deficiency; collagen synthesis is impaired as a result of this deficiency. Vessel walls with poor collagen support are pliable and easily ruptured. Physical findings include perifollicular petechiae, gingival bleeding, and subperiosteal hemorrhages. Therapy with 1 g/day of vitamin C rapidly corrects all bleeding.

TABLE 4–3   Presumptive Diagnosis of Common Bleeding Disorders by Primary Screening Tests

Platelet Count	Bleeding Time	PTT	PT	Presumptive Diagnosis	Common Etiologies
Decreased	Prolonged	Normal	Normal	Thrombocytopenia	ITP; drugs
Normal	Prolonged	Prolonged	Normal	von Willebrand's disease	
Normal	Prolonged	Normal	Normal	Thrombocytopathy	Drugs; uremia
Normal	Normal	Prolonged	Normal	Coagulopathy of intrinsic pathway	Hemophilia A or hemophilia B; factor VIII and lupus-type inhibitors
Normal	Normal	Prolonged	Prolonged	Coagulopathy of common or multiple pathways	Liver disease; vitamin K deficiency; DIC; heparin
Normal	Normal	Normal	Prolonged	Coagulopathy of extrinsic pathway	Factor VII deficiency
Normal	Normal	Normal	Normal	Hereditary telangiectasia; allergic purpura	

DIC, disseminated intravascular coagulation; ITP, idiopathic thrombocytopenic purpura; PT, prothrombin time; PTT, partial thromboplastin time.

Adapted with permission from Lee GR, et al. *Wintrobe's Clinical Hematology*. 9th ed. Philadelphia: Lea and Febiger; 1993:1315.

    b. Hereditary hemorrhagic telangiectasia is an autosomal dominant disorder associated with abnormally thin vessel walls and impaired vascular contractility. Such vessels are markedly friable, liable to burst with trauma, and unable to contract appropriately for primary hemostasis.

        (1) Physical findings include small, nodular violaceous lesions on the lips, face, ears, tongue, and gastrointestinal mucosa; these lesions blanch on pressure. Bleeding is common, especially gastrointestinal bleeding and epistaxis, with resultant iron-deficiency anemia.

        (2) Diagnosis involves the association of three factors: recurrent hemorrhage, multiple telangiectases, and familial occurrence.

        (3) Advances in supportive measures such as local measures (nasal emollients), erythropoietin, epsilon amino caproic acid, and safer parenteral iron forms has improved quality of life and prognosis in these patients.

    c. Diminished collagen synthesis due to **steroid therapy** results in a syndrome of vascular fragility and skin bleeding.

  4. Miscellaneous vascular conditions

    a. Paraproteinemias, including cryoglobulinemias and amyloidosis, are associated with skin bleeding. Diagnosis requires demonstration of the paraprotein.

    b. Senile purpura occurs in elderly individuals as a result of degeneration and loss of dermal collagen, elastin, and subcutaneous fat. This disorder, which is thought to be caused by shearing injury to blood vessels from the hypermobility of the skin on the thinned underlying tissue, is characterized by benign purpura of the arms.

C **Hereditary coagulopathies** Disorders of the coagulation system may be classified as hereditary or acquired. The hereditary forms usually result from deficiency of a single coagulation protein. A careful family history will usually elicit information concerning other family members with manifestations of a hemorrhagic tendency.

  1. Hemophilia A is the most common hereditary coagulopathy, accounting for 68%–80% of such conditions.

    a. Pathophysiology. Genetically, hemophilia A is transmitted as a classic X-linked recessive trait; the disorder is carried by females and manifested in males. Factor VIIIc, the procoagulant portion of the factor VIII complex, is deficient or dysfunctional in hemophilia A. The remainder of the factor VIII complex, including von Willebrand factor (vWF), remains present in normal amounts. The genetic locus for hemophilia has been elucidated and studied. The milder forms (Table 4–4) are characterized by single amino acid changes that result in synthesis of abnormal factor VIIIc, antigenically recognizable but functionally defective. Such patients do not make antibodies to factor VIIIc in response to concentrate therapy. Severe forms are characterized by gene deletion, which results in absent antigenically recognizable factor VIII protein material. Exogenous factor VIII given as treatment is seen as foreign protein and is problematic. Anti-VIII antibodies form in 20%–25% of these cases.

TABLE 4–4　Clinical and Laboratory Findings in Hemophilia A and Hemophilia B

Severity	Level of Factor VIII or IX (U/dL)	Partial Thromboplastin Time	Clinical Picture
Severe	0–2	Very prolonged	Hemarthrosis and spontaneous bleeding are severe and frequent; crippling is common
Moderate	2–5	Prolonged	Hemarthrosis and spontaneous bleeding are infrequent; disability is uncommon; severe bleeding occurs from injuries and surgery
Mild	5–25	Variable	Hemarthrosis and spontaneous bleeding are very unusual; unsuspected and severe bleeding occur from injuries and surgery
Subclinical	25–49	Usually normal	Bleeding after major trauma or surgery is possible; diagnosis is often missed

Adapted with permission from Lee GR, et al. *Wintrobe's Clinical Hematology,* 9th ed. Philadelphia: Lea and Febiger, 1993:1428.

    b. **Clinical features** vary with the degree of deficiency and are summarized in Table 4–4. The nature of hemorrhage is deep tissue bleeding with deep hematomas, hemarthrosis, and significant bleeding after stress such as trauma and surgery. Repeated hemarthrosis results in severe disabling arthropathy, which is the clinical hallmark of severe hemophilia A.

    c. **Diagnosis.** The constellation of spontaneous or unexpected hemorrhage, especially hemarthrosis, in a male patient with an appropriate family history is suggestive. Laboratory tests reveal a prolonged **partial thromboplastin time (PTT),** but the PTT may be normal if the factor VIII level is only mildly decreased; other coagulation tests are normal. The diagnosis is confirmed by factor assay demonstrating low levels of VIII. Detection of the abnormal gene itself is now clinically available.

    d. **Therapy** is with factor VIII transfusion in the form of either cryoprecipitate or factor VIII concentrates. The formation of VIII antibodies is a difficult complication in patients with severe hemophilia. Activated factor VII (NovoSeven) can be useful for acute bleeding episodes in patients with inhibitors to factor VIII.

2. **Von Willebrand's disease** (vWD) is a heterogeneous disorder that also involves the factor VIII molecule, but indirectly.

    a. **Pathophysiology.** Von Willebrand factor (vWF) is deficient in amount or is abnormal in function in vWD. VWF is involved in two pathways of hemostasis: vWF is necessary for platelet adhesion and functions as a carrier protein for factor VIII in the blood. Deficiencies in both roles result in a spectrum of bleeding and laboratory abnormalities. VWD is separated into types 1, 2 (with subtypes) and 3, depending on vWF's quantitative and qualitative level of function.

    b. **Clinical features** include immediate, mucocutaneous bleeding due to vWF's role in platelet adhesion and delayed, deep-tissue, posttrauma (i.e., coagulation-type) bleeding due to its role as a carrier for factor VIII. As with hemophilia A, the clinical picture for vWD varies with the degree of deficiency and dysfunction.

    c. **Diagnosis** is suggested by abnormal bleeding, usually mucocutaneous, in an individual with an appropriate family history. Bleeding time and PTT can be abnormal in vWF but are insensitive tests for diagnosis. More sensitive tests include vWF antigen (vWF:Ag) levels, measurement of vWF function, ristocetin cofactor (vWF:RCo) activity, and ristocetin-induced platelet aggregation. The last two tests demonstrate abnormal platelet aggregation in the setting of vWD.

    d. **Therapy** requires the replacement and coordination of both vWF and factor VIII. Factor VIII:vWF concentrates have been developed, but the required repletion varies, depending on the clinical presentation (extent or frequency of bleeding) and situation (surgery, postpartum).

3. **Other hereditary coagulation disorders** are uncommon. Diagnosis requires factor analysis to demonstrate the specific deficiency.

    a. **Hemophilia B (factor IX deficiency)** is identical to hemophilia A in its genetic features and clinical manifestations. Therapy differs in that either plasma or a purified prothrombin complex (which contains concentrated factors II, VII, IX, and X) is used as a source for factor IX.

    b. **Factor XI deficiency** is an autosomal recessive coagulopathy with milder clinical manifestations than those of the hemophilias. PTT is prolonged due to low factor XI levels. Plasma serves as adequate replacement therapy.

    c. **Factor XII, prekallikrein,** and **high–molecular-weight kininogen deficiencies** are unique in that they cause significant prolongation of PTT yet no predisposition to hemorrhage. Diagnosis is suggested by abnormal PTT with no history of bleeding, even with trauma. Factor analysis is necessary to demonstrate the deficient factor.

    d. **Deficiencies of all other factors** have been described but are rare.

D The **acquired coagulation disorders** are more complex than the hereditary forms. The acquired coagulopathies usually involve multiple and mixed factor deficiencies and often are complications of other diseases. Coagulation testing shows abnormalities in multiple pathways; often the bleeding severity correlates poorly with coagulation abnormalities seen in laboratory testing.

1. **Vitamin K–dependent factor deficiency**

    a. **Etiology**

      (1) **Malabsorption** of vitamin K can occur with biliary obstruction as well as with intestinal disease (e.g., sprue). Again, coagulopathy merely complicates the obvious clinical picture.

      (2) Particularly in intensive care units, **nutritional deficiency** occurs in patients with poor oral intake of vitamin K and in those in whom antibiotics have removed the gastrointestinal flora that serve as an alternate source of vitamin K.

      (3) Drugs can interfere with vitamin K metabolism—most specifically, the vitamin K antagonist **warfarin,** which is used to treat thrombotic diseases.

   b. Pathophysiology. The liver synthesizes factors II, VII, IX, and X. The final posttranslational step in their synthesis renders these proteins functional and requires γ-carboxylation of a minimum of 10 terminal glutamic acid residues, with vitamin K as a cofactor. Interference in this mechanism causes functional deficiency of these clotting proteins, particularly impairing Ca^{2+} binding of the proteins at the clot site.

   c. Diagnosis. Because many clotting factors are deficient, laboratory testing shows **prolonged prothrombin time (PT)** and, to a lesser extent, prolonged PTT. Specific measurements demonstrate the deficiency of factors II, VII, IX, and X.

   d. Therapy for vitamin K–related coagulopathy varies with its cause.

      (1) In cases of malabsorption and nutritional deficiency, supplemental (often parenteral) vitamin K corrects the coagulopathy.

      (2) In cases of excess warfarin, withdrawal of the offending drug with supplemental vitamin K is efficacious.

      (3) In patients with normal gastrointestinal tract function, oral administration is more effective (speed and extent of recovery) than subcutaneous administration. Small doses in the 1- to 3-mg range should be used in patients for whom warfarin therapy may be restarted.

2. Disseminated intravascular coagulation (DIC)

   a. Etiology. DIC is a common acquired coagulopathy that occurs secondary to other disease processes such as the following:

      (1) Activation of the intrinsic coagulation pathway by endothelial damage (e.g., in gram-negative sepsis, meningococcemia, and viremia)

      (2) Activation of the extrinsic pathway by abnormal entry of tissue thromboplastins into the circulation (e.g., in obstetric complications, carcinomatosis, and massive trauma)

   b. Pathophysiology. DIC is initiated by stimuli in the systemic circulation that activate the coagulation mechanism and cause the abnormal formation of excessive systemic thrombin. The thrombin, in turn, causes extensive activation of coagulation in the microcirculation, which consumes many coagulation moieties and activates the fibrinolytic system secondarily.

   c. Clinical features vary, depending on the balance between intravascular coagulation and fibrinolysis and factor depletion.

      (1) In florid acute cases (e.g., amniotic fluid embolism), the coagulopathy is dominant, and the major symptoms are bleeding and shock.

      (2) In more chronic cases (e.g., carcinomatosis), thrombosis may predominate.

      (3) Many cases of DIC involve abnormal coagulation parameters but no clinical manifestations of bleeding or clotting.

   d. Diagnosis. Laboratory tests reveal a complicated picture. Many coagulation factors are consumed in the diffuse clotting process; these factor deficiencies prolong both PTT and PT. Platelet consumption results in thrombocytopenia. Fibrinogen deficiency arises from thrombin-mediated clotting, as well as from plasmin-mediated fibrinolysis. The secondary fibrinolysis is demonstrated by the presence of high titers of fibrin degradation products (FDPs), which are measured by D-dimer assays. Fibrinogen levels may be low or deceptively normal; since inflammatory conditions often elevate fibrinogen, the DIC process can lower the fibrinogen into the normal range.

   e. Therapy is directed at addressing the underlying "trigger." Replacement of fibrinogen (with cryoprecipitate) is generally reserved for fibrinogen levels less than 100 mg/dL. Replacement of other deficiencies with plasma is reserved for acute, clinically significant bleeding. Heparin is used only for patients with thrombotic complications (e.g., skin infarction, acral gangrene, recognizable vessel thromboses). Many patients require no specific coagulation therapy and are treated only for their underlying condition.

3. **Liver disease** results in a complex coagulopathy involving many aspects of clotting.

    a. Liver disease results in impaired synthesis of vitamin K–dependent clotting proteins, fibrinogen, antithrombin III, plasminogen, and other protein moieties.

    b. Impaired clearance of FDPs and activated coagulation factors may result in a condition similar to DIC.

    c. Portal hypertension may result in splenomegaly and excessive platelet pooling with thrombocytopenia.

    d. The accumulation of FDPs causes impaired platelet function (thrombocytopathia).

    e. **Therapy.** Sustaining coagulation function and controlling hemorrhage in patients with advanced liver disease is one of the most difficult situations in coagulation medicine. The number of deficient proteins and the short half-lives of some (e.g., factor VII, 4–6 hours) render most concentrates ineffective. Fresh-frozen plasma (FFP) has been used traditionally, but, because of volume complications and short half-life, the results are poor. Genetically engineered activated factor VII can be used for acute bleeding, but its use is limited by its short half-life.

4. **Pathologic inhibitors of coagulation.** Specific inhibitors of coagulation are antibodies with specificity for single coagulation proteins. The most common inhibitor is an antibody to factor VIII, which arises in 20% of patients with hemophilia who have received factor therapy. An acquired variety can also be seen, most often in patients older than 65 years. Other conditions associated with acquired factor VIII inhibitors include autoimmune diseases, underlying cancer, infections, some medications, and the postpartum state.

    a. Clinically, such antibodies cause profound bleeding dyscrasias of severity similar to that of congenital deficiency.

    b. Diagnosis is made by demonstrating a specific factor deficiency that is not corrected by administration of normal plasma (abnormal mixing study).

    c. Therapy is difficult because the antibody also inactivates exogenously administered factors. Steroids, rituximab, and immunosuppressive agents have been used with limited success. In the acute setting, activated factor VII preparations have been used with some success. For patients with low-titer inhibitors, large doses of factor VIII can also be effective.

5. **Other acquired coagulation disorders.** Coagulopathy has been associated with amyloidosis (factor X deficiency), nephrotic syndrome (due to renal wasting of coagulation proteins, especially factor IX), extracorporeal circulation (thought to activate the coagulation system partially and cause low-grade DIC), and massive transfusions (the patient hemorrhages normal blood, but it is replaced with blood bank–derived blood that is poor in coagulation factors and platelets).

V DISORDERS OF HYPERCOAGULABILITY AND INCREASED RISK OF THROMBOSIS

A Anatomic abnormalities of vessels and blood flow Disorders that predispose the patient to thrombosis related to anatomic abnormalities of vessels and blood flow, not to intrinsic abnormalities in the blood itself, include the following.

1. **Stasis** can occur in conditions such as postoperative states, orthopedic injury, and neurologic diseases. Pathogenetic factors include venodilation and localized areas of reduced clearance of activated procoagulant factors.

2. **Turbulence** (e.g., associated with aneurysms) can damage vascular endothelium and expose blood to the interior of the vessel wall, facilitating endothelial–platelet–coagulation protein interaction.

3. **Trauma** to blood vessels can damage and disrupt vessel walls. Tumors can directly invade blood vessels or indirectly render the endothelium procoagulant. The vasculitic syndromes are another example.

B Intrinsic blood disorders Disorders causing abnormalities of platelets can also predispose to thrombosis:

1. **Myeloproliferative diseases** such as polycythemia vera and essential (hemorrhagic) thrombocythemia, especially when the platelet count exceeds $10^6/mm^3$

2. **Paroxysmal nocturnal hemoglobinuria (PNH),** associated with enhanced platelet reactivity and unusual thromboses involving abdominal hepatic veins

C Specific hereditary disorders of enhanced thrombosis associated with abnormalities of plasma proteins

1. **Abnormal fibrinogens** (dysfibrinogens) that are too sensitive to thrombin or that clot too tightly and do not allow for physiologic lysis by plasmin and **abnormal plasminogens** that are unable to dissolve clots physiologically are rare.

2. **Deficiencies of coagulation inhibitors**
   a. **Antithrombin (also called antithrombin III) deficiency** can be quantitative or qualitative. The defect has variable phenotypic penetrance but can cause recurrent venous thrombosis in young patients.
   b. **Protein C deficiency.** Protein C is a vitamin K–dependent factor synthesized by the liver that inhibits factors VIIIa and Va. The homozygotic condition causes purpura fulminans in neonates. The heterozygotic condition results in enhanced venous thrombosis and a possible predisposition to skin necrosis when a patient is placed on warfarin without concomitant heparin.
   c. **Activated protein C resistance [factor V (Leiden)]** is a genetic defect in factor V that renders it refractory to the inhibitory activity of protein C. This condition is now known to be the most common congenital hypercoagulable state. Some studies report a 20% incidence in hypercoagulable state workups. Data now demonstrate that this lesion alone is frequently not sufficient to cause thrombosis. The heterozygous condition acts as a comorbid risk factor with other events such as childbirth, long bone fracture, oral contraceptive use, and surgery to cause thrombosis. This "multiple-hit" pathophysiology appears to be common in most hypercoagulable situations.
   d. **Protein S deficiency.** Protein S is a cofactor that facilitates factors VIIIa and Va inhibition by protein C. Its deficiency results in a thrombotic diathesis syndrome similar to protein C deficiency.
   e. **Mutations in the prothrombin protein** (G20210A) and elevated homocysteine also increase thrombosis.

D Specific acquired disorders of enhanced thrombosis associated with abnormalities of plasma proteins

1. **Pregnancy and oral contraceptive agents** are associated with statistically increased incidence of stroke, acute myocardial infarction (MI), and venous thrombosis. Pregnancy and oral contraceptives cause elevation in most procoagulant proteins and diminution of most fibrinolytic and inhibitor proteins, thus altering the hemostatic balance in favor of clotting.
   a. **Therapy.** Patients who have an increased tendency to develop thrombosis are at increased risk during pregnancy and especially in the postpartum period. For pregnant patients who need anticoagulation, heparin therapy is used. Warfarin must be avoided because it crosses the placenta and is teratogenic. Low–molecular-weight heparins are quite effective and are more convenient to use. The anticoagulation period must extend through to the peripartum period because the month after delivery may be the period of highest risk.

2. **Nephrotic syndrome** is associated with urine wasting of antithrombin III and, more important, hypoalbuminemia, which may result in enhanced platelet aggregation.

3. **Lupus inhibitor (antiphospholipid antibody) syndrome.** The presence of the so-called lupus inhibitor is associated with increased thrombosis, especially in patients with systemic lupus erythematosus (SLE). Most cases, however, are not associated with SLE or other underlying conditions. Lupus inhibitor is becoming one of the more common diagnosable conditions related to hypercoagulability, with an incidence of thrombotic complications ranging from 9% to 28% in affected patients.
   a. **Pathophysiology.** The lupus inhibitor or antiphospholipid antibodies or both interact with the coagulation pathway at the X–V–Ca complex.
   b. **Clinical manifestations.** Despite prolonged laboratory clotting times, thrombosis (both arterial and venous), placental dysfunction, and recurrent miscarriage are the major symptoms and signs of this disorder. Abnormal bleeding does not occur, except in patients for whom an

antibody against prothrombin results in increased clearance of prothrombin and thus a prothrombin deficiency.

    c. **Diagnosis.** Laboratory findings include prolongation of the PTT that does not reverse when the patient's plasma is mixed with normal plasma. Further diagnostic testing includes a confirmation that the inhibitor is phospholipid dependent, detection of anticardiolipin antibodies (IgG or IgM), or anti–β2-glycoprotein-1 antibodies (IgG or IgM). This testing needs to be repeated 12 weeks later to confirm the diagnosis since these antibodies can be transient.

    d. **Therapy. Aggressive anticoagulation** initially with heparin and followed by warfarin is indicated in cases of lupus inhibitor syndrome accompanied by clinical thrombosis. Warfarin anticoagulation to an international normalized ratio (INR) of 2–3 has recently been shown to be adequate.

4. **Heparin-induced thrombocytopenia (HIT) syndrome** is associated with thrombosis of venous and arterial sites in patients using heparin. This syndrome has become more commonly recognized.

    (1) **Incidence** is 1%–5% of patients on heparin therapy. Most data suggest that this is more common in settings such as coronary artery bypass grafting (CABG) and other situations involving intense vascular manipulation.

    (2) **Pathogenesis** involves heparin-dependent antiplatelet IgG antibody. The platelet undergoes an "activating event" (as with vascular surgery), which results in expression of PF4 on its membrane. The heparin binds to the PF4, creating a neoantigen to which an IgG heparin-dependent antibody is made. The antibody activates platelets and causes release of platelet microparticles into the circulation, resulting in both platelet hyperreactivity and plasma hypercoagulability.

    (3) **Diagnosis** is made by means of an enzyme-linked immunosorbent assay. Since this test has a relatively high false-positive rate, confirmation can be obtained if necessary with a serotonin release assay. For patients in whom HIT is strongly suspected on clinical grounds, treatment should be given regardless of the test results. Thrombocytopenia usually precedes thrombosis, so platelet counts should be monitored in heparin patients and heparin discontinued if the platelet count significantly declines.

    (4) **Therapy** involves the use of direct thrombin inhibitors such as lepirudin and argatroban. Lepirudin, a recombinant hirudin, is excreted by the kidney; extreme caution is required in the setting of elevated creatinine and renal failure. Argatroban, a small peptide that inhibits the thrombin catalytic site, is excreted solely by hepatic metabolism; caution is required in the setting of liver dysfunction and elevated bilirubin. As with hirudin, there is no antidote. These agents have markedly improved the management and prognosis of HIT.

5. **Thrombotic thrombocytopenic purpura (TTP)**

    a. TTP is characterized by a deficiency or inhibition of the vWF-clearing protease ADAMTS 13, leading to the accumulation of large vWF multimers in circulation. These multimers lead to abnormal platelet aggregation and deposition within vascular beds. Although all organ systems may be involved, the classic pentad of TTP consists of thrombocytopenia, anemia, mental status changes (symptoms may vary from confusion to seizure), renal failure, and fever. All five abnormalities are rarely seen, but microangiopathic hemolytic anemia with schistocytes on peripheral smear and thrombocytopenia are key to making the diagnosis (Online Figure 4-9).

    b. **Treatment.** Plasmapheresis therapy adds the missing enzyme and also removes factor VIII:Ag macroaggregates. Pheresis has resulted in a reversal in mortality from ≥80% before pheresis to <20% now. Plasma infusion is less effective than plasmapheresis but can be used as a means of replacing the enzyme until plasmapheresis can be initiated, often with improvement in the patient's symptoms and/or the platelet count. Laboratory measurements of platelets and LDH are used to assess response to treatment. In refractory cases, rituximab may be used; it is a monoclonal antibody to the B cell surface marker CD20, so it reduces production of the antibodies against ADAMTS-13.

    c. **TTP syndrome** occurs idiopathically but is also seen as a complication of advanced AIDS, drugs (e.g., antirejection drugs, cyclosporine), or infections.

6. **Malignancy associated with chronic DIC (Trousseau's syndrome)** causes a pronounced hypercoagulability. The mechanism for enhanced thrombosis is chronic DIC initiated by tumor cells releasing thromboplastic substances, activating factor XII, or both.

   a. Migratory thrombophlebitis of superficial veins is uniformly associated with chronic DIC in classic Trousseau's syndrome. Common neoplasms are adenocarcinomas of lung, pancreas, stomach, and prostate. This condition requires heparin therapy for control.

   b. Marantic endocarditis is another DIC variant; it results in fibrin vegetation in the heart and recurrent embolization.

   c. Routine deep venous thrombosis and pulmonary embolism are also statistically associated with malignancy. In one large study, 7% of patients with idiopathic disease developed neoplasia at 2 years, compared with 2.5% in age-matched controls.

E **Diagnostic and therapeutic approach to hypercoagulability**

1. **Diagnostic approach**

   a. Clinical settings in which investigation for a hypercoagulable state is indicated include the following:

      (1) Family history of documented thromboembolic events

      (2) Age younger than 40 years at onset of thromboembolic events

      (3) Recurrent thromboembolic events

      (4) Unusual sites of thrombosis (e.g., mesenteric or cerebral veins)

      (5) Resistance to standard therapy for thrombosis

   b. Table 4–5 summarizes several causes of hypercoagulability.

2. **Treatment depends on the underlying cause.**

   a. In myeloproliferative disorders, treatment of the underlying disease with hydroxyurea and anagrelide is effective.

   b. Vessel abnormalities can be surgically repaired if found at angiography.

   c. Most congenital protein deficiency states, including those of protein C, are managed with lifelong warfarin therapy once a thrombotic event has occurred. No treatment is given to asymptomatic carriers because many of these individuals never develop a thrombosis. Such individuals should be given aggressive prophylaxis, however, when in high-risk situations such as after a fracture or surgery.

   d. Lupus-inhibitor patients who have manifested thrombosis are managed with warfarin.

   e. Hypercoagulability associated with cancer usually requires long-term subcutaneous heparin therapy because warfarin does not control the thrombotic diathesis in these cases. When

---

TABLE 4–5   Hypercoagulable Syndromes

Inherited Forms

Relatively Common	*Rare*
Factor V (Leiden) and protein C resistance	Abnormal fibrinogens
Antithrombin III deficiency	Plasminogen deficiency
• Quantitative	• Qualitative
• Qualitative	• Quantitative
Protein C deficiency	Decreased release of plasminogen activator
Protein S deficiency	Increased levels of histidine-rich glycoprotein
Prothrombin variant (G20210A)	
Hyperhomocysteinemia	

Acquired Forms

Pregnancy (especially postpartum period)
Oral contraceptive and estrogen use
Lupus anticoagulants and anticardiolipin antibodies
Malignancy (chronic disseminated intravascular coagulation)
Myeloproliferative diseases (polycythemia vera, essential
  thrombocytopenia) and paroxysmal nocturnal hemoglobinuria
Nephrotic syndrome
Heparin-induced thrombocytopenia syndrome

TABLE 4–6 Management of Hypercoagulable States According to Venous Thromboembolism (VTE) Risk Stratification

Moderate Risk
- Carriers of inherited thrombophilias who have never experienced a thrombotic event
- Patients with an acquired thrombophilia who have not experienced a thrombotic event (e.g., antiphospholipid antibodies, malignancy)
- Patients with one thrombotic event associated with a provocative reversible comorbid stimulus (e.g., leg casting, hormonal therapy)

Aggressive VTE prophylaxis when exposed to high-risk situations (e.g., pregnancy, prolonged immobility)

High Risk
- Two or more documented VTE events
- One VTE event of life-threatening nature (e.g., massive pulmonary embolism)
- One documented VTE event plus
  - Presence of multiple inherited defect
  - Presence specifically of antithrombin III deficiency, protein C/S deficiency
  - Presence of antiphospholipid antibody syndrome or active malignancy
  - Idiopathic VTE event (?)

Indefinite anticoagulation using an accepted regimen

effective therapy for the tumor is available, as it is for prostate cancer, it often resolves the coagulopathy for as long as the tumor is controlled.

    f. Table 4–6 summarizes therapeutic principles for the common hypercoagulable states.

VI   BENIGN DISORDERS OF WHITE BLOOD CELLS

The white blood cells (WBCs) include lymphocytes, monocytes, basophils, eosinophils, and neutrophils (PMNLs). Disorders of WBCs can be considered in terms of level of maturity, number, and function. This section examines disorders involving the five types of mature WBCs.

A **Lymphocytes** exist in bone marrow as well as in the lymphoid tissue of the body. Lymphocyte functions include delayed hypersensitivity, which is performed by T lymphocytes (**T cells**), and antibody production, which is performed by B lymphocytes (**B cells**) and plasma cells.

    1. Lymphopenia refers to a diminished number of lymphocytes.

        a. Lymphopenia without significant immune deficiency is seen in many illnesses that cause elevated serum cortisol levels, such as acute infections and inflammatory states. Chemotherapy, radiotherapy, and Hodgkin's disease also are associated with lymphopenia. In none of these conditions is antibody production severely affected.

        b. Congenital lymphopenia with immune deficiency is associated with specific immune deficiency syndromes.

            (1) Varieties

                (a) B cell deficiency

                    (i) Bruton's agammaglobulinemia

                    (ii) Other B cell–deficiency states include common variable hypogammaglobulinemia and IgA deficiency.

                (b) T cell deficiency. Thymic hypoplasia (DiGeorge syndrome).

                (c) Deficiency of both B and T cells

            (2) Diagnosis. For all of the conditions discussed, diagnosis requires the clinical setting of repeated infections combined with the following findings:

                (a) Lymphocyte counts of B and T cells, including surface subset markers

                (b) Measurement of specific immunoglobulin levels

                (c) Demonstration of the absence of specific B cell areas (i.e., germinal centers and plasma cells) or T cell areas (i.e., thymus and lymph node medullary cords)

            (3) Therapy. BMT has been curative in many of these conditions.

        c. Acquired immunodeficiency syndrome (AIDS). For a discussion of AIDS, see Chapter 9 VIII C 3.

2. **Lymphocytosis** is defined as an excessive number of lymphocytes (i.e., $>5000/mm^3$). The differential diagnosis of absolute lymphocytosis is limited.

   a. **Infection.** Certain infections cause lymphocytosis. In children, both pertussis and acute infectious lymphocytosis may cause counts that exceed $50,000/mm^3$. In adults, lesser elevations are seen with hepatitis and infectious mononucleosis.

   b. **Hematopoietic disorders** associated with lymphocytosis include acute lymphocytic leukemia (ALL), chronic lymphocytic leukemia (CLL), and certain lymphomas. For a discussion of these diseases, see Section VII.

3. **Monocytosis and monocytopenia.** Monocytes are **phagocytic cells** that are an important component of the cellular immune system and that secrete many cytokines, including tumor necrosis factor (TNF), all of the interferons (IFNs), granulocyte–macrophage colony-stimulating factor (GM-CSF), and granulocyte colony-stimulating factor (G-CSF).

   a. Monocytopenia in combination with decreases in other cell lines occurs with aplastic anemia, hairy cell leukemia, and steroid use. Familial monocytopenia has also been described.

   b. **Benign monocytosis** can occur in many infectious diseases (e.g., tuberculosis, subacute bacterial endocarditis [SBE], cytomegalovirus infection [CMV]), and inflammatory diseases (e.g., rheumatoid arthritis, sarcoid). The finding is nonspecific.

   c. Monocytosis can accompany essentially all of the hematologic and lymphatic malignancies.

B **Basophils, eosinophils, and neutrophils**   Disorders in these cells also are classified according to fluctuations in cell numbers and to functional deficiency.

1. **Basophils.** An abnormally increased number of basophils is called **basophilia.** This uncommon condition usually is associated with the myeloproliferative syndromes, particularly chronic myelogenous leukemia (CML).

2. **Eosinophils.** An abnormally increased number of eosinophils is called **eosinophilia.** This condition is more common than basophilia and occurs most commonly secondary to other disease processes, including the following:

   a. Neoplasia, including lymphoma, myeloid leukemias (CML, AML, MDS), and nonhematologic malignancies

   b. Addison's disease

   c. Allergic and atopic diseases, including asthma, allergic rhinitis, atopic dermatitis, and drug hypersensitivity reactions

   d. Connective tissue disease (collagen vascular disorders, Sjögren's syndrome, serum sickness)

   e. Gastrointestinal diseases (inflammatory bowel disease, eosinophilic gastroenteritis)

   f. Parasitic infestation

   g. Primary hypereosinophilic symptoms are uncommon. These syndromes are characterized by very high (15,000 or higher) levels of sustained eosinophilia, invasive toxic effects to the heart and lungs, and chromosomal clonal aberrations typical of malignancy.

3. **Neutrophils**

   a. **Neutrophilia** is an excessively increased number of neutrophils in the blood. Causes of neutrophilia include the following:

      (1) Most cases of neutrophilia result from conditions such as infection, tumor, stress, collagen disorders, and steroids; the underlying disease may not be apparent clinically.

      (2) In unusual cases, more than 50,000 neutrophils/mm^3 appear in the blood. These so-called **leukemoid reactions** can be differentiated from the leukemias by the absence of the circulating blast forms, the presence of a normal erythrocyte count, an elevated leukocyte alkaline phosphatase (LAP) value, and the absence of the JAK-2 and BCR–ABL mutations characteristic of the myeloproliferative disorders.

      (3) Neutrophilia also results from **neoplastic marrow diseases** such as polycythemia vera and CML. For a discussion of CML, see Section VII.

   b. **Neutropenia** is an absolute decrease in the number of circulating neutrophils. Neutropenia occurs rarely as an early manifestation of intrinsic marrow disease (e.g., acute leukemia) but more commonly secondary to exogenous stimuli.

      (1) **Infections.** Certain viral infections (e.g., hepatitis, influenza) and bacterial infections (e.g., typhoid fever) cause neutropenia.

(2) Drugs (e.g., phenothiazines, fluoxetine, antithyroid medications) are associated with neutropenia and, in severe instances, can cause agranulocytosis. Agranulocytosis is characterized by the following:

    (a) Profoundly lowered neutrophil counts (i.e., <500/mm^3)

    (b) Severe prostration, high fever, and often a necrotic pharyngitis

    (c) Bone marrow showing **maturation arrest** (i.e., large numbers of immature WBC forms in an otherwise normal marrow)

    (d) High mortality rates unless treated early and aggressively with supportive measures and potent bactericidal antibiotics. Use of genetically engineered G-CSF and other marrow growth factors has been encouraging. G-CSF has been shown to reduce febrile days and hospital days.

(3) The **collagen vascular diseases** (e.g., SLE, rheumatoid arthritis) can cause neutropenia via immune destruction of WBCs.

(4) Familial forms of neutropenia include familial benign chronic neutropenia, cyclic neutropenia, and chronic idiopathic neutropenia. These disorders have good prognoses, although they are associated with an increase in minor infections (e.g., boils) when the neutrophil count is less than 500/mm^3. They respond well to G-CSF.

(5) Chemotherapeutic agents used in the therapy of malignant disease are the most common cause of neutropenia. Chemotherapy-induced neutropenia can be markedly ameliorated by the judicious use of G-CSF.

c. Functional disorders of neutrophils involve a compromised ability to fight infection. These conditions are rare; affected individuals have recurrent infections.

    (1) Chédiak–Higashi syndrome

    (2) Chronic granulomatous disease (CGD)

VII MALIGNANT DISORDERS OF WHITE BLOOD CELLS: LEUKEMIAS, MYELODYSPLASIA, LYMPHOMAS, MYELOMA

A Acute leukemias The acute leukemias are disorders in the maturation of hematopoietic tissue that are characterized by the presence of immature leukocytes in the marrow and peripheral blood. The immature cells are arrested in the earliest phases of differentiation and are referred to as **blasts.**

1. Classification and epidemiology. It is important both prognostically and therapeutically to distinguish the lymphocytic from the nonlymphocytic (myelogenous) leukemias. Classification of cells involves special histochemical stains (e.g., peroxidase in myelogenous leukemia), marker enzymes (e.g., terminal transferase in ALL), and specific cell-surface antigenic markers; use of these methods in combination allows classification that approaches 95% accuracy. Cytogenetic analysis, marker chromosome defects, and chromosomal banding techniques have even further refined the classification of acute leukemias. In addition, such chromosomal groupings appear to identify subgroups within specific leukemia types that have different responses to therapy and different prognoses. Currently, acute leukemias are classified into two major types: acute lymphocytic leukemia (ALL) and acute myelogenous leukemia (AML) [Online Table 4–7].

a. ALL is common in children: 85% of cases of ALL occur in children, and 90% of leukemia that occurs in children is ALL. Conversely, ALL is not a common leukemia in adults. Techniques such as membrane surface markers and antibody detection of surface antigens have enabled investigators to characterize ALL subsets.

(1) The most common ALL variant (75% of cases) is of B cell lineage of null variety (i.e., there is absent rosette formation). This variant also expresses the common ALL antigen (CALLA) on the cell surface.

(2) T cell ALL and other less common varieties constitute the remainder of cases.

(3) Most ALL varieties express terminal deoxynucleotidyl transferase (TdT), and staining for this enzyme is useful in differentiating ALL from myelogenous leukemias.

(4) Differentiating subtypes has prognostic significance in that, for example, T cell varieties of ALL are more resistant to therapy and have far worse prognoses than common variety B cell ALL.

    b. AML, or **acute nonlymphocytic leukemia (ANLL),** is common in adults, and the incidence increases with age. Specific environmental risks include moderate-to-high doses of ionizing radiation, chemicals such as benzene and petroleum products, and prior exposure to cytotoxic chemotherapy agents such as alkylating drugs (e.g., cyclophosphamide, chlorambucil). The AML cell of origin probably arises at different levels of hematopoiesis in different patients, which accounts for the clinically well-defined subtypes of AML. In most cases, the AML clone arises from a multipotent precursor capable of differentiating into granulocyte, erythrocyte, macrophage, or megakaryocyte colony-forming units (CFUs). Therefore, in most patients, lymphoid and erythroid lineages are not involved in the leukemic process (Online Figure 4–7).

2. **Clinical features** of acute leukemia reflect the effects of marrow infiltration by nonmaturing, functionless blast cells, including subsequent bone marrow failure.

    a. Physical findings include fatigue and pallor (due to anemia); fever and infection (due to neutropenia); and petechiae, purpura, and epistaxis (due to thrombocytopenia). Infiltrative symptoms may include splenomegaly, gingival hypertrophy, and bone pain.

    b. Laboratory findings include almost universal pancytopenia and circulating blast forms. Increased cell turnover results in elevated uric acid levels. In promyelocytic leukemia (M3), DIC is usually present with hypofibrinogenemia and elevated fibrin split products.

3. **Diagnosis.** The diagnosis of acute leukemia is confirmed by the finding of blast infiltration of the bone marrow. Special histochemical stains (e.g., peroxidase, Sudan black), enzyme markers (e.g., TdT), surface antigenic markers, and chromosome cytogenetic studies are performed to identify the specific subtype of leukemia involved.

4. **Therapy.** Initial therapy consists of chemotherapeutic ablation of the leukemic cell line. In AML, it is necessary to ablate the normal marrow as well. Because normal marrow has a shorter generation time than leukemic blasts, recovery with normal marrow tissue is possible. This initial marrow ablation is termed **induction therapy** and is followed by several cycles of consolidation therapy.

    a. ALL induction therapy. ALL blasts are initially more selectively sensitive to chemotherapy than AML blasts. It often is possible to destroy ALL blasts with some sparing of normal marrow. Thus, induction therapy for ALL is associated with lower morbidity and mortality rates than it is for AML. ALL induction is generally followed by less intensive maintenance therapy. [See more information online.]

    b. AML induction therapy

    c. Radiotherapy

    d. BMT

    e. Supportive therapy is extremely important and serves as a prototype for supportive therapy in other forms of neoplasia. The following principles apply to the use of chemotherapy regimens, as well as to bone marrow ablation and transplantation.

        (1) Transfusion with packed red cells is necessary to avoid severe anemia. Leukodepleted and radiated blood is used to avoid allosensitization in the event of later BMT.

        (2) Prophylactic transfusion of platelet concentrates avoids serious spontaneous bleeding when the platelet count declines below 10,000/mm^3, and platelet transfusion is used to maintain platelet counts above 10,000/mm^3. This practice has lowered the incidence of fatal hemorrhage in acute leukemia from 80% to less than 20%.

        (3) Control of infection is a major determinant of survival for patients being treated for acute leukemia.

            (a) Infections are treated early and aggressively. Neutropenic patients (those with neutrophils <500/mm^3) are susceptible to all organisms, especially gram-negative rods and fungi (e.g., *Candida*, *Aspergillus*).

                (i) Initial temperature elevations require thorough clinical evaluation, appropriate cultures, and immediate and empiric treatment with broad-spectrum bactericidal antibiotic combinations of cephalosporins, aminoglycosides, vancomycin, and semisynthetic penicillins (e.g., imipenem).

                (ii) Secondary temperature elevations that occur after treatment with potent broad-spectrum antibiotics may require the empiric use of antifungal agents (e.g., amphotericin B). Prevention of fungal infections with prophylactic triazoles (e.g., fluconazole) has proved effective and has contributed to diminished morbidity and mortality from fungal infections. [See more information online.]

      (b) Strict hand-washing and skin-care techniques, the use of long-term central catheters to avoid peripheral indwelling lines, and the practice of good hygiene decrease the likelihood of infection.

5. Prognosis

    a. The prognosis for **children** with **ALL is very good;** more than 95% obtain complete remission. Approximately 70%–80% of patients are disease free at 5 years and are likely cured. If relapse occurs, second complete remissions are possible in most cases. Patients in second remissions are candidates for BMT, with 35%–65% probability of long-term survival. In **adults,** the prognosis for **ALL is poor;** 5-year survival is estimated to be 40%, and possibly lower for patients older than 60 years. Unlike in children, if relapse occurs in adults, a second complete remission is unlikely to be achieved.

    b. The prognosis of **AML** depends on the subtype, which is generally determined by cytogenetic analysis. For patients with acute promyelocytic leukemia, the combination of all *trans*-retinoic acid and chemotherapy has resulted in complete remission rates of 90% with cure rates of approximately 75%. For other subtypes, however, the remission and cure rates are lower. Overall, approximately 75% of patients obtain complete remissions after induction chemotherapy. Intensive postremission therapy has decreased the risk of relapse from leukemia, with disease-free survival rates at 4 years of 44% in patients less than 60 years of age. Older patients have a less favorable prognosis.

      Bone marrow transplantation (BMT), both allogeneic and autologous, is the treatment of choice for younger patients after obtaining a first complete remission in subtypes with poor prognosis. Current results indicate that 50% of young patients with AML who undergo allogeneic BMT experience prolonged disease-free intervals and may be cured.

B **Chronic leukemias** are disorders of clonal overproduction of mature white blood cells. Like the acute leukemias, these mature WBCs can come from the lymphocytic or the myelogenous cell lines.

    1. Chronic lymphocytic leukemia (CLL). An adult who is older than 50 years and who manifests a mature lymphocytosis most likely has CLL. The cells associated with CLL are mature lymphocytes that accumulate in the body.

      a. Diagnosis. A peripheral blood smear showing a mature lymphocytosis is highly suggestive. Corroborative findings include marrow infiltration by mature lymphocytes, an enlarged spleen, and lymphadenopathy. Lymphocyte markers can also be determined. The technique of flow cytometry is diagnostic (Online Figure 4–6).

      b. Staging

        (1) **CLL** is staged using the Rai or Binet system, which use the presence of cytopenias, lymphadenopathy, and splenomegaly to measure tumor burden. More recently, other factors have been shown to have prognostic significance, especially cytogenetic analysis. Other factors of interest include β2-microglobulin levels, the mutational status of the heavy-chain gene, and expression of CD38 and ZAP-70.

        (2) With the Rai system, stage 0 is characterized by peripheral lymphocytes only, stage I by lymphocytosis and lymphadenopathy, stage II by splenomegaly, stage III by anemia, and stage IV by thrombocytopenia.

      c. Therapy

        (1) **Early-stage CLL.** As a rule, patients with stage 0 disease should be monitored without therapy.

        (2) Patients with stage I and II are sometimes monitored without therapy, but treatment would be considered if there is evidence of massive disease or rapidly increasing lymphocyte count.

        (3) Patients with stage III and IV disease are generally treated with monoclonal antibodies (rituximab, alemtuzumab), chemotherapeutic agents (fludarabine, chlorambucil), or combination regimens.

    2. Chronic myelogenous leukemia (CML). CML is suspected in patients with high WBC counts and splenomegaly. Peripheral blood smears reveal a spectrum of cell forms in the myeloid line ranging from mature polymorphonuclear neutrophils to immature blasts. CML develops as a result of a transformation of a primitive hematopoietic precursor cell caused by a chromosomal translocation that juxtaposes the ABL gene on chromosome 9 and the BCR gene on chromosome 22. The fusion protein of the BCR–ABL gene in CML is detectable, as is the abnormal genetic material itself. The fusion protein results in a functional, mutant tyrosine kinase that results in a lack of control of basic cellular processes such as proliferation rate, adherence, and physiologic death (apoptosis). Affected stem cells manifest a proliferative advantage over normal stem cells, reduced adherence to marrow stroma, and decreased apoptosis.

a. **Diagnosis.** CML is now diagnosed using polymerase chain reaction (PCR) or fluorescent in situ hybridization (FISH) to demonstrate the presence of this abnormal genetic material. These techniques can reveal the abnormal chromosomal fusion even when the marrow appears normal using morphology and routine cytogenetics.

b. **Clinical course.** Patients often progress through three distinct phases of the disease: (1) a chronic phase, characterized by minimal to moderate constitutional symptoms, (2) an accelerated phase marked by worsening symptoms and increased myeloblasts, white cells, and spleen size, and (3) a blast crisis that is clinically similar to acute leukemia.

c. **Treatment and prognosis**

(1) The first treatment option, in all nonpregnant patients, is the tyrosine kinase inhibitor imatinib mesylate (Gleevec), which inhibits the function of the BCR–ABL fusion protein. It induces a compete hematologic response in 98% of patients and major cytogenetic reversal in approximately 90% of cases. It is given orally and is quite well tolerated. Drug resistance can develop over time, generally as a result of additional mutations involving the BCR–ABL protein. This is managed by increasing the dose of imatinib or switching to a different tyrosine kinase inhibitor such as desatinib or nilotinib.

(2) **α-Interferon (α-IFN)** is the preferred treatment for pregnant patients. It is administered three times weekly and induces remission in 70% of patients. It can sometimes convert the patient's marrow to Philadelphia chromosome–negative status and may be curative in some patients. Responses are most likely to occur in patients treated early in their disease course.

(3) **Hydroxyurea** can be used to rapidly lower counts and can be used in conjunction with tyrosine kinase inhibitors at the initiation of therapy.

(4) **Marrow transplantation** is an option for patients younger than 60 years and results in cure for 80% of patients with a matched sibling donor (🔊 Online IV D 4).

C **Myelodysplastic syndrome (MDS)** The myelodysplasias are clonal disorders characterized clinically and morphologically by defective and ineffective hematopoiesis. They are the result of pathology in the hematopoietic stem cells and are thus characterized by cytopenias of varying degree in red cell, white cell, and megakaryocytic lines and abnormal morphology (dysplasia) of the myeloid precursors in the bone marrow. These disorders can occur de novo or as a result of exposure to toxic substances, such as chemotherapy, benzene, or radiation therapy. They are thought to arise as a result of clonal chromosomal abnormalities causing impaired cellular maturation and function of the myeloid cells. Some of the more commonly seen mutations include loss of chromosome 5 (13%) and chromosome 7 (5%), trisomy 8 (5%), and deletions of parts of chromosomes 17 and 20. 🔊 The French–American–British (FAB) classification system uses morphologic criteria to sort the myelodysplastic syndromes into five groups (🔊 Online Table 4–8). The World Health Organization (WHO) adds cytogenetic information and immunophenotyping, producing a more complex system that allows more accurate prediction of prognosis.

1. **Clinical features** of the myelodysplasias relate to bone marrow failure.

a. MDS is seen almost exclusively in patients older than 50 years, and the incidence rises with age. History and physical findings include progressive fatigue, dyspnea on exertion, pallor, frequent infections, and bleeding or bruising.

b. Laboratory findings include cytopenias, with anemia being the most frequent presenting feature (90%).

2. **Diagnosis.** The diagnosis is suspected in an elderly patient with cytopenias and normal iron, B_{12}, and folate levels. Peripheral smear demonstrates a variety of abnormalities that are suggestive (teardrop forms, Pelger–Huet hypogranulated hypolobular WBC forms, and abnormal platelet forms) (🔊 Online Figure 4–8). Examination of bone marrow shows morphologic abnormalities

including megaloblastoid erythroid precursors, asynchronous maturation of cytoplasm and nucleus, ringed sideroblast forms, micromegakaryocytes, and excess blast forms. Cryptogenic analysis reveals chromosomal abnormalities in approximately 40% of patients. Other disorders with similar presentations, such as HIV infection, copper deficiency, and paroxysmal nocturnal hemoglobinuria (PNH), should be excluded.

3. **Therapy**
   a. Supportive therapy is the most widely offered strategy. The use of erythropoietin (EPO) and G-CSF to ameliorate anemia and severe neutropenia is supported by evidence-based trials. Because EPO is effective only in the minority of cases, transfusions are used for symptomatic anemia. Aggressive and judicious use of antibiotics and platelet transfusion techniques are similar to those used in AML situations.
   b. Novel agents are continuously being evaluated in this difficult patient population. They include lenalidomide, an immunomodulatory agent, and azacitidine, an antimetabolite that impairs DNA methylation.
   c. In patients of appropriate age group, allogeneic stem cell transplantation has been successfully used and is the only curative therapy available.

4. **Prognosis** is variable. From 10% to 40% of patients will progress to AML, and others will die of complications of their cytopenias. Median survivals range from 6 months to 6 years, depending on a complex set of variables, including number and severity of cytopenias, presence or absence of cytogenetic abnormalities, and percentage of myeloblasts in the bone marrow. An International Prognostic Scoring System has been developed that uses these factors to predict median survival.

D Lymphomas

1. **Hodgkin's Lymphoma**
   a. **Incidence.** In the United States, more than 8000 new cases of Hodgkin's disease are reported each year. In industrialized countries, the disease is most common in young adults and has a slight male predominance. In developing countries, the disease occurs most commonly in childhood.
   b. **Etiology**
      (1) Molecular studies have demonstrated the presence of **Epstein–Barr virus (EBV)** within the Reed–Sternberg cells (the malignant cell in Hodgkin's lymphoma) in approximately 50% of cases in Western countries and in a much higher percentage of cases in developing countries. Other viruses have been suspected of playing a role in EBV-negative cases, but there is no evidence supporting this.
      (2) An increased incidence of Hodgkin's lymphoma in family members supports a genetic predisposition in a minority of cases.
   c. **Screening.** There are currently no screening guidelines for early detection in asymptomatic people.
   d. **Pathology.** Hodgkin's lymphoma is divided into classic Hodgkin's lymphoma (95% of cases) and nodular lymphocyte-predominant Hodgkin's lymphoma (5% of cases). There are four major histologic variants of classic Hodgkin's disease: nodular sclerosis, mixed cellularity, lymphocyte rich, and lymphocyte depleted. The most common histologic type is nodular sclerosis. The malignant cell, a binucleate giant cell called the Reed–Sternberg cell, has been shown to be derived from B lymphocytes. It comprises less than 1% of the cellular mass in most patients; the remainder of the cells are reactive.
   e. **Clinical features.** Hodgkin's disease patients, especially young patients, usually have **asymptomatic swelling of a lymph node.** Some patients may present with such **systemic symptoms** as **fever, weight loss,** and **drenching sweats,** known as "B" symptoms.
   f. **Diagnosis.** Excisional biopsy of a lymph node is diagnostic (see d.). Further workup includes the following:
      (1) Complete blood count (CBC), chemistry panel, erythrocyte sedimentation rate
      (2) Thorough history and physical examination
      (3) Computed tomography (CT) scans of the chest, abdomen, and pelvis or, more commonly, a positron emission tomography (PET) CT scan
      (4) Percutaneous bilateral bone marrow biopsies

g. Prognosis. Outcome varies mainly with the stage of disease and, to a lesser extent, with histology.

    (1) Patients with stage I or stage II disease have a 5-year disease-free survival rate exceeding 80%.

    (2) Patients with stage III and stage IV disease have long-term survival rates approaching 70%.

    (3) Prognostic models using clinical features and laboratory results allow the physician to predict which patients are likely to respond to therapy.

h. Staging. Hodgkin's disease tends to spread in an orderly fashion from node group to node group. This contiguous nature is in marked contrast to non-Hodgkin's lymphomas, which are more likely to spread hematogenously. The modified **Ann Arbor classification** is used for **staging Hodgkin's disease** (for full staging information, see the most recent edition of the *AJCC Cancer Staging Handbook*).

i. Therapy. Treatment for Hodgkin's lymphoma continues to evolve. However, certain principles have been established and should be firmly adhered to because **even advanced disease is curable.** Individual variations in treatment should be avoided unless there is a strong clinical indication.

    (1) Early stage (stages I, II) disease is treated with **chemotherapy** plus involved-field **radiation therapy.** The chemotherapy most commonly used is a combination of doxorubicin (Adriamycin), bleomycin, vinblastine, and dacarbazine (ABVD).

    (2) Advanced stage (stages III, IV) disease is treated with combination chemotherapy. Regimens that are used include ABVD, BEACOPP, and Stanford V.

    (3) Patients who relapse after attaining a complete remission can be cured with autologous bone marrow transplantation.

2. Non-Hodgkin's Lymphoma

a. Incidence. More than 65,000 patients are diagnosed with non-Hodgkin's lymphoma (NHL) in the United States each year. Non-Hodgkin's lymphomas (especially the aggressive subtypes) are more common in patients with acquired immunodeficiency syndromes and in patients receiving immunosuppressive drugs.

b. Etiology

    (1) Cytogenetic abnormalities such as chromosomal translocations are commonly observed in lymphoma cells. Specific translocations are associated with certain NHL subtypes, such as the (11;14) translocation with mantle cell lymphoma or the (8;14) translocation with Burkitt lymphoma, which can be quite useful diagnostically.

    (2) Infectious agents can play an etiologic role in lymphoma in several distinct ways.

        (a) Infections can act primarily as a stimulus for lymphoid proliferation, which can indirectly lead to mutagenesis, such as *H. pylori* infection in the stomach.

        (b) Infection can lead to generalized immune suppression, decreasing the body's immune surveillance and allowing proliferation of a malignant clone, as is seen in HIV infections.

        (c) The primate T cell leukemia/lymphoma viruses appear to play a more direct role in the development of adult T cell leukemia/lymphoma. Evidence suggests that a viral transactivator protein increases the transcription of cellular proteins that ultimately lead to the malignant phenotype.

c. Pathology. Most non-Hodgkin's lymphomas arise from B cells, although lymphomas can also arise from T cells and, more rarely, NK cells. A number of histologic classification schemes are in use; the one most widely used in the clinical literature is the WHO classification system. The WHO classification for lymphoid neoplasms is found in the *AJCC Cancer Staging Handbook* and delineates a large number of lymphoma subtypes. Broadly speaking, the non-Hodgkin's lymphomas fall into two groups.

    (1) Indolent lymphomas. Pathologic subtypes in this group include follicular lymphoma, small lymphocytic lymphoma, and marginal zone lymphoma. Follicular lymphoma is the most common of these and accounts for approximately 40% of all NHL cases in the United States.

    (2) Aggressive lymphomas include diffuse large B cell lymphoma, comprising 30% of all NHL cases, Burkitt lymphoma, primary CNS lymphoma, anaplastic large cell lymphoma, and others.

d. Clinical features. Patients with non-Hodgkin's lymphoma can be asymptomatic, can present for evaluation of a mass, or can have symptoms caused by obstruction or interference with normal organ function by the lymphoma. Twenty percent of patients have **fever, night sweats, or weight loss,** known as "B" symptoms. Patients with indolent lymphomas may have **waxing and waning adenopathy** for several months before diagnosis, although **persistent nodal enlargement** is more common.

e. **Diagnosis**

(1) A complete **history** and **physical examination,** with particular emphasis on all lymph node–bearing areas, including Waldeyer's ring, as well as liver and spleen size.

(2) **Hematologic studies,** including a CBC, differential, platelet count, liver and kidney function studies, LDH, and uric acid level. Serum protein electrophoresis rules out hypogammaglobulinemia or a monoclonal gammopathy.

(3) **Bone marrow biopsies** and **aspirates.**

(4) An adequate surgical lymph node **biopsy** examined by an experienced pathologist.

(5) **Radiologic studies,** including chest radiography, CT of the chest, abdomen, and pelvis or, more commonly, a PET CT scan.

f. **Prognosis.** Many patients who achieve a complete response, particularly those with diffuse large cell lymphoma, remain disease free for an extended period and will be cured. Aggressive combination chemotherapy regimens containing doxorubicin have high complete response rates ranging from 40% to 80%. Prognostic factors (known as the International Prognostic Indicators or IPI score) for large cell lymphoma include patient age, stage, LDH level, performance status, and the presence of more than one site of extranodal disease. The performance status used in the IPI score was devised by the Eastern Cooperative Oncology Group (ECOG) and ranges from 0 (fully functional) to 5 (deceased).

g. **Staging.** The Ann Arbor staging system used to classify Hodgkin's disease is also used to stage non-Hodgkin's lymphomas (see the *AJCC Cancer Staging Handbook*).

h. **Therapy.** Treatment usually requires a multidisciplinary approach. Radiation therapy and chemotherapy after surgical biopsy are the most common treatment modalities.

(1) **Chemotherapy**

(a) **Low-grade indolent lymphomas** may not require treatment for many years. When therapy is indicated, there are a number of options available, including single-agent or multiagent chemotherapy, often combined with the anti-CD20 antibody rituximab. Radiolabeled monoclonal antibodies ibritumomab tiuxetan (Zevalin) and tositumomab (Bexxar) are now approved for salvage therapy in patients who have failed rituximab and conventional chemotherapy. Other monoclonal antibodies are being studied.

(b) **Aggressive lymphomas** require treatment with multiagent chemotherapy.

(i) The most common regimen involves cyclophosphamide–doxorubicin–vincristine (Oncovin)–prednisone (CHOP) plus rituximab.

(ii) For patients with the most aggressive disease, such as Burkitt's or lymphoblastic lymphoma, protocols similar to those used in the treatment of acute lymphoblastic leukemia (ALL) are used.

(iii) **Colony-stimulating factors** hasten granulocyte recovery and may permit higher doses and better cure rates.

(iv) Prophylactic intrathecal chemotherapy may also be given for high-grade lymphomas.

(v) **Salvage combination chemotherapy** can produce second complete or partial remissions but is rarely curative unless the patient undergoes a stem cell transplant.

(2) **Radiation therapy.** Non-Hodgkin's lymphomas are highly radiosensitive.

(a) **Localized indolent lymphomas.** Long-term patient follow-up after involved or extended field radiation therapy for localized stage I and stage II low-grade lymphoma reveals a 10-year relapse-free survival rate of greater than 50%, especially in younger patients.

(b) Electron beam therapy has been used in the management of cutaneous lymphomas such as the early stages of mycosis fungoides.

(c) Radiation therapy is used **palliatively** in disseminated disease or to "consolidate" a complete response to chemotherapy in areas of bulky disease.

E Multiple Myeloma

1. **Incidence.** Myeloma is a neoplasm of the plasma cells, which are derived from B lymphocytes. It is an uncommon neoplasm, accounting for approximately 1% of adult cancers in the United States. The incidence of myeloma increases with advancing age and is twice as common in blacks. Approximately 20,000 new cases of multiple myeloma are diagnosed each year in the United States.

2. **Etiology**
   a. Although no specific underlying causes have been proven, genetic factors, as well as exposure to petroleum, asbestos, metals, and radiation, may increase the risk of developing myeloma.
   b. Benign monoclonal gammopathies can progress to multiple myeloma, although most do not.
   c. Myeloma cells are characterized by genetic instability, and karyotype analysis often reveals multiple abnormalities, which can provide prognostic information.

3. **Screening.** There are currently no screening guidelines for early detection in asymptomatic people.

4. **Pathology.** Multiple myeloma is a type of mature B cell lymphoid neoplasm characterized by accumulation of malignant plasma cells in the bone marrow compartment.

5. **Clinical features**
   a. **Weakness, fatigue, infection,** and **bleeding** due to marrow failure.
   b. **Osteolytic lesions** resulting from myeloma-induced bone resorption with subsequent pain and bone fractures.
   c. **Recurrent infections** due to acquired hypogammaglobulinemia and leukopenia.
   d. **Renal abnormalities** due to myeloma infiltration of the kidney, hypercalcemia, toxic effects of light chains on tubules, amyloid deposition, and hyperuricemia.
   e. **Hypercalcemia** due to myeloma-stimulated osteoclast activity causing lethargy, polyuria, polydipsia, constipation, nausea, and vomiting.
   f. **Hyperviscosity** due to a high concentration of the M protein, which can cause impaired circulation resulting in visual impairment, headache, and mental status changes.
   g. **Compression of the spinal cord** caused by growth of a plasmacytoma (plasma cell tumor) or collapse of a weakened vertebral body can cause weakness or paralysis of the lower extremities, as well as bowel or bladder dysfunction. If this diagnosis is suspected, it should be considered a medical emergency and investigated promptly.

6. **Laboratory features**
   a. The **major feature** of myeloma is the demonstration of an abnormal monoclonal protein (**M protein**) in the **blood, urine,** or **both.** This M protein usually consists of either one or a combination of heavy chains (IgG and IgA) and light chains (κ and λ).
      (1) M proteins consisting of the whole immunoglobulin molecules IgG and IgA account for 50% and 25% of the cases, respectively.
      (2) M proteins consisting of only light chains account for 25% of cases. These can be measured as serum free light chains and can also be seen excreted in the urine as "Bence Jones" protein.
      (3) Infiltration of the marrow by large numbers of plasma cells, which are usually morphologically abnormal
      (4) Decrease in normal immunoglobulin levels
      (5) Lytic bone lesions on bone survey
      (6) Anemia
      (7) Elevated creatinine
      (8) Hypercalcemia

7. **Prognosis** is variable but can be predicted based on the stage of the disease, cytogenetic analysis, and laboratory data, such as β2-microglobulin and albumin. Mean survival for patients requiring therapy is 3 years.

8. **Staging.** The International Prognostic Index, proposed in 2005, is a simple and widely used staging system. The Durie–Salmon staging system is also commonly employed.

9. **Therapy**
   a. Patients with stage I or **smoldering myeloma** (normal renal function, no bone lesions) should be examined at 3- to 4-month intervals for evidence of disease progression but do not need therapy.

b. Therapy should be given to patients with symptoms of progressive disease, such as bone pain, hypercalcemia, renal dysfunction, and bone marrow suppression. For patients less than 70 years of age with no major comorbidities, autologous stem cell transplant (ASCT) should be considered as a treatment option. These patients are first treated with "induction" chemotherapy to provide relief of their symptoms and decrease the tumor burden.

(1) **Chemotherapy** used prior to ASCT includes combinations of bortezomib, dexamethasone, and thalidomide or lenalidomide.

(2) For older patients or patients with other health problems these same regimens are quite effective. If ASCT is not being considered, melphalan can also be used as part of a combination chemotherapy regimen.

(3) **Autologous stem cell transplantation** has been shown to improve survival in randomized studies and is commonly offered to patients younger than 70 years with no other major health problems.

(4) **Supportive therapy** is extremely important in the management of myeloma and includes the following:

(a) **Bisphosphonate therapy** for all patients with bone disease

(b) **Radiation therapy** for local bone disease

(c) **Hydration** and proper **management of hypercalcemia**

(d) **Orthopedic support** and care

(e) **Plasmapheresis** for hyperviscosity syndrome

(f) **Prophylaxis** against thrombosis for those patients receiving thalidomide or lenalidomide

Study Questions

1. An 83-year-old woman received a hip replacement in her left leg 2 months previously. At that time, a mild anemia of 10 g/dL was noted, and she had been started on iron therapy by her primary care physician. She has mild hypertension. There was remote gastric surgery for presently unknown reasons 40 years ago. She denies symptoms of weakness or fatigue or shortness of breath with exertion. However, her ambulation has been somewhat limited by her hip surgery. Her appetite is "good," but her family reports that her oral intake has been poor for some time. She denies all other symptoms.

Physical examination reveals a thin-appearing woman in no distress. There is pallor of her conjunctival and oral mucous membranes. The tongue is papillated except for the lateral edges, which are smooth. Heart examination reveals regular rhythm 96 bpm with a grade II systolic murmur along the left sternal border. Abdomen is soft without masses or hepatosplenomegaly. A well-healed midline laparotomy incision is present. Neurologic examination results were normal. Stool was Hemoccult negative.

Complete blood count revealed WBC of 5800/mm^3 and platelets 190,000/mm^3. However, hemoglobin is 8.2 g/dL (hematocrit 25%) with a mean corpuscular volume (MCV) of 111 mm^3. Reticulocytes were 25,000/mm^3 (1.4%). An outpatient iron panel obtained after her hip surgery admission showed serum iron 80, transferrin 360, and ferritin 50 µg/dL. Which of the following is the most appropriate management for this patient?

- A Increase the iron dose and add vitamin C to her regimen.
- B Obtain vitamin B_{12} and folic acid levels and initiate therapy with both, pending results.
- C Initiate a course of parenteral iron therapy.
- D Obtain a bone marrow aspirate and initiate erythropoietin therapy for myelodysplasias.

2. A 61-year-old woman is admitted for urgent cardiac catheterization. The patient had experienced ischemic cardiac pain at an outside hospital and was treated in standard fashion including IV heparin, but she continued to decompensate. She was transferred for cardiac catheterization, which demonstrated triple-vessel coronary artery disease. She received full-dose intravenous heparin as well as nitrates for 3 days then was taken to the operating room for CABG. The patient had nonremarkable preoperative blood counts. On the third postoperative day, she was found to have right lower-extremity venous thrombosis and was restarted on IV heparin with rapid attainment of therapeutic PTT. The next day, the right foot became cool, cyanotic, and painful. Doppler study demonstrated extensive deep venous thrombosis (DVT) in the right proximal venous system and arterial occlusion in the right iliac artery. Blood studies showed hemoglobin 12 g/dL, WBC 21,000/mm^3, and platelets 33,000/mm^3. Blood smear was unremarkable save for decreased platelets. Which of the following is the most likely diagnosis for these events?

- A Inadequate heparin dose with recurrent thrombosis
- B Thrombotic thrombocytopenic purpura (TTP)
- C Heparin-induced thrombocytopenia syndrome (HIT)
- D Cardiac embolism
- E Homocystinemia

3. A 20-year-old African American man is admitted for management of sickle cell anemia. He started to experience pain in his joints and lower back, consistent with his usual sickle cell pain pattern, about 48 hours before admission. He has Percocet at home for such episodes but has not received much relief from it. He does well with his sickle cell anemia, requiring hospital admission about two or three times per year for pain management. He holds a full-time job in retail and is engaged to be married. His CBC in the receiving ward showed hemoglobin 7.9 g/dL and WBC 24,000/mm^3, which compare to known baseline levels of 7.8 g/dL and 14,000/mm^3, respectively. Chest film was scheduled for first thing in the morning.

You examine him on morning rounds and find him to be in mild respiratory distress. He has developed moderate pleuritic pain. Vital signs are temperature 38.6°C, blood pressure 110/70 mm Hg, pulse 110 bpm, and respirations 24 breaths/minute. He has mild scleral icterus. Chest examination shows a few rales in both bases without signs of consolidation.

Morning laboratory findings demonstrate a hemoglobin of 7.2 g/dL with a reticulocyte count of 230,000/mm³ and a WBC of 33,000/mm³ with a left shift. Bilirubin is 4 mg/dL, but other liver functions are normal. The chest film shows small, bilateral infiltrates in the bases. An O_2 saturation on room air is 90%. What is the most appropriate definitive management for this patient?

[A] Arrange for an exchange transfusion.

[B] Perform an ultrasound and CT scan of the abdomen to exclude ascending cholangitis.

[C] Initiate heparin for acute pulmonary embolism.

[D] Initiate antibiotics with specific pneumococcus and salmonella coverage.

[E] Initiate hydroxyurea 1000 mg/day.

4. A 19-year-old man experiences moderate trauma while playing in an intramural football game. That evening he experiences worsening pain and swelling in the left thigh. On evaluation, he manifests marked swelling in the left thigh, hemoglobin of 9 g/dL, and PTT of 56 seconds. Magnetic resonance imaging shows a large hematoma. The most likely diagnosis is which of the following?

[A] Uremia

[B] Hemophilia A

[C] Therapy with aspirin

[D] Factor XII deficiency

[E] Idiopathic thrombocytopenic purpura (ITP)

5. A 29-year-old woman presents with new purpura and petechiae on both lower legs. She has also experienced menorrhagia in her last two menstrual cycles. On examination, in addition to the afore-mentioned purpura and petechiae, several petechiae are noted on her tongue and hard palate. Blood count reveals hemoglobin 12 g/dL, WBC 8000/mm³, and platelets 9000/mm³. Which of the following is an expected part of her diagnostic evaluation or management?

[A] Bone marrow megakaryocytes are generally decreased.

[B] Platelet-associated immunoglobulin G (IgG) is diagnostic.

[C] Splenomegaly and other cytopenias are usually present.

[D] The platelet life span is prolonged.

[E] Intravenous immunoglobulin is an effective therapy.

6. A 64-year-old man that you have been following for hypertension and diabetes presents for a routine follow-up. He has no complaints aside from occasional exertional dyspnea. On examination you notice that his conjunctivae and nail beds are pale. His CBC is significant for hemoglobin of 9 g/dL with an MCV of 74 fL; his peripheral blood smear is shown 🔾 online. His chemistries, including liver function tests and bilirubin, are normal. In addition to iron studies, which of the following is the next best step to evaluate this patient's anemia?

[A] Serum B_{12} and folate levels

[B] Bone marrow examination

[C] Colonoscopy

[D] LDH and haptoglobin

[E] Bone scan

7. A 28-year-old white woman is in the 30th week of gestation and notes persistent swelling and dis-comfort in the right calf. She was previously healthy without prior major medical problems. She used barrier contraception before her pregnancy. There is no family history of venous thromboembolism (VTE). A Doppler study confirms DVT of the right lower extremity. Which of the following is most likely in this patient?

[A] Antithrombin III deficiency

[B] Protein C deficiency

[C] Factor V (Leiden) deficiency

[D] Hemophilia A

[E] Trousseau's syndrome

8. A 59-year-old asymptomatic white male with chronic renal insufficiency, hypertension, and diabetes is seen in follow-up after a heart catheterization. He has no complaints and feels well. On physical exam you notice bilateral nontender posterior cervical and axillary lymphadenopathy and splenomegaly. The rest of his examination is normal. A CBC reveals a hemoglobin of 12.8 g/dL, a platelet count of 190,000/mm³ and a WBC count of 41,000/mm³. His peripheral blood smear is shown 🌑 online (low power on left; high power on right). What is the most likely diagnosis?

- [A] Chronic myelogenous leukemia
- [B] Chronic lymphocytic leukemia
- [C] Acute myelogenous leukemia
- [D] Myelodysplastic syndrome
- [E] Leukemoid reaction

9. A 62-year-old man has had an elevated hematocrit for at least 3 years. His past medical history and review of systems are negative, except for mild, well-controlled hypertension. His latest complete blood count reveals the following: hemoglobin 18 mg/dL; hematocrit 56%; and WBC count 17,500/mm³ with platelets 800,000/mm³. On further investigation, which of the following findings is the most typical and expected?

- [A] Ringed sideroblasts on bone marrow examination
- [B] Arterial blood oxygen saturation less than 88%
- [C] Presence of a Philadelphia chromosome on cytogenetic testing
- [D] Very low to absent erythropoietin titer
- [E] Many Pelger–Huet cells on peripheral blood smear

The response options for Items 10–13 are the same. Select one answer for each item in the set.

QUESTIONS 10–13

- [A] Protein C deficiency
- [B] Paroxysmal nocturnal hemoglobinuria (PNH)
- [C] Lupus inhibitor syndrome
- [D] Trousseau's syndrome

Match each of the following clinical vignettes with the most likely diagnosis.

10. A 30-year-old woman with a history of rash and arthritis has deep vein thrombosis; in addition, she has had a problem with recurrent abortions.

11. A 45-year-old man who has been followed by his physician for 4 years for chronic iron-deficiency anemia with unknown source of blood loss has portal vein thrombosis.

12. A 60-year-old man had deep vein thrombosis of his left leg last month and is being appropriately managed with warfarin. He has symptoms of new clot formation in the right leg, as well as a clot in his left forearm.

13. A 67-year-old woman with mitral stenosis is started on warfarin by her cardiologist. On the third day, painful red areas appear on her thigh and breast.

14. An 18-year-old man presents with swollen lymph nodes in his neck for 2 weeks. He has been treated with antibiotics for 10 days, but the lymph nodes continue to grow. He has had a 10-pound weight loss in the last 2 months and is experiencing drenching night sweats. He reports fatigue and inability to play basketball like he used to. He has not been sexually active in the last 1 year. The next best course of action is:

- [A] Change of antibiotics
- [B] CT scan of the chest
- [C] Reference to a surgeon for lymph node biopsy
- [D] Check of his HIV status
- [E] Assurance that he has a self-limiting viral illness

15. Eventually he is diagnosed with nodular sclerosing Hodgkin's lymphoma. His bone marrow biopsy is negative, and he is found to have disease in both sides of the diaphragm (stage III). Treatment of choice in the United States is:

- A Chemotherapy with the ABVD regimen
- B Radiation to all the affected lymph nodes
- C Surgical resection of all the affected lymph nodes
- D Treatment with rituximab
- E High-dose chemotherapy with stem cell support

16. The most serious long-term side effect of this treatment is:

- A Congestive heart failure
- B Peripheral neuropathy
- C Myelodysplastic syndrome/acute myelogenous leukemia
- D Early myocardial infarction
- E Early onset cataract

17. A 55-year-old African American man is seen in the emergency room with a 2-day history of hematuria, back pain, double vision, and altered mental status. He is an engineer with an office-based occupation with no exposure to chemicals or radiation. Family history is positive for an uncle with "bone cancer." He smokes half a pack of cigarettes a day but does not drink alcohol. Laboratory evaluation in the emergency department shows an elevated total protein of 22 mg/dL, elevated gamma globulins, a serum creatinine of 2.5 mg/dL, and hemoglobin of 9 g/L. Blood smear shows rouleaux formation. You suspect:

- A Acute renal failure of unknown etiology
- B Hyperviscosity syndrome secondary to multiple myeloma
- C A genitourinary malignancy
- D Drug toxicity
- E Intravascular hemolysis

18. Best management option at this point is:

- A Plasmapheresis
- B Transfusion of red blood cells
- C Hemodialysis
- D Broad-spectrum antibiotics
- E Supportive care

Answers and Explanations

1. The answer is B [I A 2]. The patient's findings suggest the presence of at least one of the common nutritional anemias—iron deficiency, folate deficiency, or B_{12} deficiency. Her diet seems poor. In addition, there is a history of and evidence for some type of a gastric surgery—either total or partial resection in the past. The most common anemia after gastric resection is iron deficiency that results from removal of acid-secreting cells, which are needed to reduce iron to its ferrous form, the absorbable form of iron. In addition, loss of absorptive surface and the presence of stomal erosions and bleeding also contribute to this pathophysiology. However, this patient's serum ferritin does fall within the normal range, which strongly suggests that the lack of iron is not what is interfering with blood formation in this patient at this time. Furthermore, the patient is displaying macrocytic indices with an MCV of 111 mm^3, which again almost assuredly means that iron-deficient erythropoiesis characterized by deficient hemoglobin synthesis and microcytosis are not the driving force of the anemia in this situation. Thus, answer A, increasing iron dose and adding ascorbic acid to facilitate absorption, although based on sound physiologic principles in this instance, might not be expected to reverse this anemia. Answer C is another iron maneuver that can sometimes be required in true malabsorptive situations. The newer parenteral forms are less allergenic than traditional preparations and have made this therapy safer. However, this still requires a time-consuming infusion, and all avenues of oral iron therapy should be employed before resorting to this. In this case, data do not point to iron deficiency as the primary lesion here.

Myelodysplasia has become the most common cause for anemia in the geriatric population and is an important consideration in this setting. Typically, patients with MDS manifest a slight macrocytosis but only rarely to the degree seen here. MDS can be classified by studying bone marrow findings, and in approximately 25% of cases the anemia responds to pharmacologic doses of EPO. However, before the diagnosis of MDS can be made, reversible causes of macrocytic anemia such as B_{12} and folic deficiency *must* be excluded, so answer D is not appropriate for this patient.

The appropriate management for this patient is answer B—obtaining B_{12} and folic acid levels and initiating therapy pending results. Her significant macrocytosis and subtle physical findings of tongue atrophy suggest B_{12} deficiency, including true type A autoimmune gastritis involving the fundus and body of the stomach, which is the classic Addisonian pernicious anemia. This patient had some form of gastric surgery and a history of peptic ulcer disease (PUD). Thus, she may have B_{12} deficiency associated with total gastric resection, which, although less common than iron deficiency, affects patients who had had that operation about a decade later, or type B *H. pylori*–associated atrophic gastritis (which affects fundus, body, and antrum) related to her PUD. A variety of excellent biochemical tests can determine whether there is B_{12} deficiency (serum B_{12} level by radioimmune assay, methylmalonic acid levels) and whether there is true autoimmune pernicious anemia and its causes (the presence of circulating intrinsic factor autoantibodies). Because there is a possibility of folate deficiency, a folic acid level should be obtained. Because ongoing B_{12} deficiency–related neurologic morbidity can progress and become irreversible, therapy can and should be initiated with parenteral B_{12} while waiting for the biochemical confirmation. Thus, answer B is the most appropriate course of management here.

2. The answer is C [V D 4]. This explosive situation is typical of the HIT with thrombosis syndrome. Heparin is a widely used anticoagulant across many indications. In approximately 3% of cases, patients develop a clinically and biologically active antibody to a heparin–PF4 neoantigen on the platelet, which in the further presence of heparin causes platelet activation, aggregation, thrombocytopenia, and release of tissue factor. If the heparin is still continued, paradoxical thrombosis associated with massive platelet aggregates ("white clot") may ensue. The time course is usually with 5–10 days of heparin exposure, although in patients with prior exposure to heparin, HIT may occur much faster. There is a hierarchy of incidence risk, with full-dose intravenous use causing more HIT than subcutaneous and other less intense regimens. However, all forms and routes can elicit the reaction. In studies, LMWH forms less commonly incite HIT. However, LMWH will cross-react and trigger HIT in sensitized patients. When HIT proceeds into thrombosis, both arterial and venous thrombosis can occur and can be limb and life threatening in up to 50% of cases. When HIT is suspected, all heparins by all routes (including dialysis) must be discontinued. Alternative anticoagulants (hirudin, Argatroban) are now available for patients who require ongoing anticoagulation. HIT is frequently a clinical diagnosis initially—the development of thrombocytopenia without other obvious cause in a patient on heparin. There are confirmatory laboratory tests, such as the enzyme-linked immunosorbent assay HIT antibody assay.

Thrombosis can propagate or recur in heparinized patients (answer A). However, the development of a significant new thrombocytopenia in association with the clots would not be expected and is more typical of HIT. TTP (answer B) does manifest the combination of thrombosis and thrombocytopenia. However, the thrombotic aspects of TTP are in the microcirculation rather than in large arteries or veins, and a cardinal finding is microangiopathic hemolysis with red blood cell fragmentation and schistocytes, which were absent here. Cardiac embolism (answer D) would not be expected to involve the venous system. Homocystinemia (answer E) is a hypercoagulable syndrome that indeed can involve both arterial and venous circulations with premature and recurrent thrombotic events. This patient's presentation should elicit a homocysteine measurement. However, thrombocytopenia would not be expected as part of homocystinemia.

3. The answer is A [I B 2 b (1)]. This patient is manifesting clear findings consistent with acute chest syndrome (ACS), the leading cause of death and second-most-common cause for hospitalization in patients with sickle cell anemia. Typical findings demonstrated here include fever, shortness of breath, tachypnea, striking leukocytosis, chest infiltrates, and hypoxemia. Initiating events can be infectious or noninfectious (e.g., bone marrow embolism from vaso-occlusive events), but once established, the pathophysiology seems similar to that of acute respiratory distress syndrome (ARDS). The syndrome can result in respiratory failure with requirement for ventilation and mortality in as many as 9% of cases. ACS is one of the accepted criteria for exchange transfusion of red cells, and that is the most appropriate choice here. The procedure is usually easily performed in the intensive care unit setting and has excellent results, with an 81% recovery even after mechanical ventilation, which is far superior to that of other patients with ARDS. Simple transfusion may be adequate in mild cases, but exchange is preferred in rapidly deteriorating cases as seen here. Other accepted indications for exchange transfusion in sickle cell patients include neurologic complications such as stroke, priapism, and the less common hepatic sequestration crisis, which causes exquisitely tender and massive hepatomegaly and extreme elevations of bilirubin.

The patient has had cholecystectomy, which is usual for an adult sickle cell patient. These patients have lifelong hemolysis and universally form bilirubin gallstones. The prior cholecystectomy, absence of abdominal symptoms, normal liver function studies, and only minimally elevated bilirubin are strong negatives for the diagnosis of ascending cholangitis. The bilirubin elevation is quite consistent with the hemolytic anemia present. Thus, answer B would not be the initial diagnostic or therapeutic pathway of choice.

Although newer studies have indicated that ACS can be caused frequently by bone marrow fat emboli from infarcted marrow, which occurs during an initial painful crisis, the pathophysiology of ACS is quite different from that of traditional thromboembolism. The emboli are small fat emboli, not clots, and initiate ARDS via cytokine and surfactant mechanisms. In the absence of DVT, which was not suspected epidemiologically or clinically here, heparin (choice C) would not be the preferred therapy.

Patients with homozygous sickle cell anemia have been shown to be predisposed to serious infections from encapsulated organisms, particularly *Pneumococcus* and *Salmonella* species. These patients have increased incidence and severity from such infections, which should be in the differential of a febrile sickle cell patient. However, this patient also displays the entire spectrum of ACS findings and so is past the point of using antibiotics alone for therapy. He requires aggressive pulmonary measures (oxygen, bronchodilators, etc.) and a transfusion maneuver in addition to any antibiotics. Furthermore, recent studies have expanded the universe of infectious agents seen with ACS and suggest the addition of a macrolide in such cases. Answer D is inadequate on many counts as therapy in this situation.

Hydroxyurea has been used *chronically* in selected homozygous sickle cell anemia patients. Earlier theories suggested that its ability to raise hemoglobin F (Hb F) levels and reduce sickling were the basis for its use. More recent data suggest that its role is much more complex and involves lowering WBCs (an independent mortality predictor in sickle cell patients) and modulating cytokine levels in patients, which may be as important as or more so than Hb F levels. Nonetheless, hydroxyurea requires weeks to have effect and thus is not an appropriate acute therapy.

4. The answer is B [IV C 1]. Hemophilia A involves coagulation factor VIII; platelet function is not affected in this disease. This results in a coagulation-type bleeding syndrome with delayed, deep tissue–type bleeding. Although the exact mechanism is unclear, uremia is believed to cause platelet dysfunction by toxins that alter the factor VIII antigen polymers required for normal platelet function. Aspirin causes thrombocytopathia by inhibiting synthesis of thromboxane A_2, a strong inducer of platelet aggregation. Factor XII deficiency results in prolongation of the PTT but is not associated with abnormal bleeding.

5. The answer is E [III A 2 c]. Except when thrombocytopenia has caused chronic bleeding with iron-deficiency anemia, isolated thrombocytopenia is the rule in ITP. Splenomegaly and other cytopenias are not part of ITP, and their presence should bring the diagnosis into doubt. ITP is the prototypical thrombocytopenia due to increased peripheral destruction. Platelet life span is markedly shortened, and, in response, the bone marrow megakaryocytes are increased. Platelet-associated antibodies can usually be found on platelets and in plasma, although their significance remains controversial. Long-term therapy involves intravenous immunoglobulin, particularly in the acute setting, corticosteroids, and splenectomy. Immunosuppression or treatment with drugs that stimulate platelet production (thrombopoietin analogs) can be used in refractory cases.

6. The answer is C [I A 1 a]. This patient has a microcytic anemia, most commonly caused by occult blood loss. Further evaluation with serum iron, ferritin, and total iron-binding capacity can confirm the diagnosis. Once the diagnosis of iron-deficiency anemia is made, it is imperative to find the underlying etiology of blood loss. In this setting, evaluation for a gastrointestinal malignancy such as colon cancer is the appropriate next step in management. Colonoscopy is the test of choice. Vitamin B_{12} and folate deficiencies present as megaloblastic anemia with macrocytosis (MCV of 100 fL or greater). LDH and haptoglobin testing are used when a hemolytic anemia is suspected. These anemias are not as common, are usually normocytic to slightly macrocytic, and are associated with an elevated reticulocyte count. Hemolytic anemias do not have the characteristic findings of this patient's peripheral blood smear.

7. The answer is C [V C 2 c; Table 4–6]. One of the newer developments in hypercoagulability has been the finding of a situation in which the defect for the coagulation inhibitor agonist protein C is located in the receptor molecule rather than in the amount of function of protein C itself. The defective factor V molecule, which is named for the place it was discovered—Leiden, Belgium—is the abnormal protein that is insensitive to the physiologic inhibition by protein C.

Most experts agree that this factor V defect may be the most common diagnosable inborn defect associated with a hypercoagulable state; some studies found an incidence as high as 20% in hypercoagulability workups. A common setting for VTE associated with factor V Leiden is a comorbid risk factor such as pregnancy or use of oral contraceptives. Protein C and antithrombin III deficiencies are traditional defects in the inhibitors themselves, either due to qualitative defects in the inhibitor or quantitative deficiency of the molecules. They have been found to have a higher VTE potential than factor V Leiden and are less commonly associated with a second risk factor. Trousseau's syndrome is another known hypercoagulable state, but it is acquired rather than genetic. The condition is the result of a form of disseminated intravascular coagulation (DIC) caused by carcinoma, especially mucin-producing adenocarcinoma. Hemophilia, although hereditary and caused by a variety of molecular lesions, is associated with profound bleeding rather than clotting.

8. The answer is B [VII B 1]. CLL is the most common leukemia affecting older adults. In the majority of cases patients are asymptomatic but may present with fatigue and weakness. Typical physical exam findings include lymphadenopathy and splenomegaly. A peripheral blood smear showing mature small lymphocytes constituting the majority of white blood cells suggests the diagnosis, which can be confirmed by flow cytometry. In AML, leukemic cells are immature myeloid blasts. Peripheral blood smears in CML reveal a spectrum of cell forms ranging from immature blasts to mature polymorphonuclear neutrophils. The myelodysplastic syndromes are characterized by defective hematopoiesis, which leads to cytopenias, anemia being the most common. Leukemoid reactions are characterized by myeloid cells, not lymphocytes.

9. The answer is D [II A 1; II C 1, 2]. The very elevated hemoglobin and hematocrit, which strongly correlate with true elevations in red blood cell (RBC) mass rather than plasma contraction, are consistent with polycythemia. Polycythemia then is broken down into autonomous or primary polycythemia vera, a stem cell disease, in which the marrow is autonomously creating too many cells, versus reactive or secondary forms, in which the marrow is responding to increased erythropoietin from some alteration of normal physiology. The elevations of the other cell lines suggest polycythemia vera because this stem cell disease involves all marrow cell lines. Ringed sideroblasts and Pelger–Huet cells are seen in myelodysplasia, which is another condition resulting from abnormal marrow clonal stem cells. However, in this condition, cytopenias rather than increases in counts are expected. On occasion, CML, another marrow stem cell clonal proliferative disease, may manifest with elevated counts—specifically the WBC count and, to a lesser extent, platelets. In CML, a hemoglobin and hematocrit elevated to this degree would be unusual and are much more typical of polycythemia vera.

High hemoglobin and hematocrit from secondary causes such as tissue hypoxia (as with certain cardiac and pulmonary diseases) result from physiologic increases in erythropoietin seen in these states. With renal and other tumors, one can also see an elevated hematocrit due to increased erythropoietin secretion. The low oxygen saturation could cause a secondary elevated hemoglobin but not the elevations in the other cell lines manifested by this patient.

10–13. The answers are: 10—C [V D 3]; **11—B** [V B 2]; **12—D** [V D 6]; **13—A** [V C 2 b]. The lupus inhibitor is found in one third of patients with SLE. In these patients, the association with thrombosis risk is 10%–15%. In patients without SLE who display a similar inhibitor-type antibody, there is less risk of thrombosis, but the risk is still far in excess of normal.

PNH is a difficult diagnosis to make, and the disorder can masquerade as chronic iron deficiency (due to urine losses), chronic hemolysis, or both. PNH is associated with increased thrombotic risk and has a tendency to involve intra-abdominal veins.

Recurrent thrombosis associated with adequate warfarin anticoagulation, especially when migratory and involving superficial veins, suggests the presence of chronic DIC with an occult adenocarcinoma (Trousseau's syndrome). Warfarin can, in the early phases of administration, lower the vitamin K–dependent, short–half-life protein inhibitor protein C more rapidly and create an imbalance with coagulation factors II, VII, IX, and X, thus affecting the hemostatic balance toward clotting. Characteristically, it occurs soon after the initiation of warfarin without concomitant administration of heparin.

14. The answer is C [VII D 1 f]. Any lymph node that does not respond to the usual treatment, such as two courses of different antibiotics, should raise the suspicion of the treating physicians. For easily accessible lymph nodes, the preferred method of investigation is a full excisional biopsy. The examination of an intact lymph node allows pathologists to examine the lymph node architecture and arrive at a definitive diagnosis. Although a CT scan might eventually be needed, it should not be the first choice. In addition, the HIV status of a patient with high-risk behavior needs to be determined, but there is no indication from the case presentation that this patient falls into this category, and it should not be the first choice.

15. The answer is A [VII D 1 i (2)]. This combination chemotherapy is the treatment of choice in most parts of the United States. Other multiagent chemotherapy regimens are also acceptable. Ongoing clinical trials are comparing effective regimens to determine whether there are superior alternatives to the ABVD regimen. There is no indication that the removal of all involved lymph nodes is surgically feasible or therapeutic. Disseminated Hodgkin's lymphoma is a systemic disease and should be treated as such. In addition, radiation therapy is reserved for cases in which there is either bulky disease or a focal area of the body is involved. Delivery of radiation to multiple sites is generally not feasible because of the toxicity of this approach. Choice D, treatment with rituximab, is for non-Hodgkin's lymphomas.

16. The answer is C [VII A 1 b]. Cytotoxic chemotherapy could lead to various chromosomal abnormalities that could result in acute leukemia or myelodysplastic syndrome. The risk of secondary myeloid malignancies approaches 2% with the ABVD regimen, and increased incidence of non-Hodgkin's lymphoma is noted as well. A number of chemotherapeutic agents that alkylate DNA are thought to be involved in this process. In general, high-dose therapy with any of these agents is associated with the development of AML/MDS. Congestive heart failure as a result of exposure to doxorubicin (Adriamycin) is known to occur. However, usually this toxicity is seen with doses exceeding 480 mg/m2. The risk of myocardial infarction at a young age should not be an issue if radiation to the chest and thorax is not needed. Peripheral neuropathy is also a manageable toxicity seen with vinca alkaloids such as vincristine.

17. The answer is B [VII E 5 f]. This case requires a close examination of the laboratory results and of the patient presentation in an attempt to arrive at a unifying diagnosis to explain all of the observed abnormalities. The elevated total protein and the presence of rouleaux formation on the blood smear are classic signs of paraproteinemia. The history of change in mental status and double vision in a patient with elevated total protein should raise concerns for hyperviscosity syndrome. Once the presence of anemia and renal insufficiency has been established, the diagnosis of multiple myeloma should strongly be considered. A genitourinary malignancy usually does not lead to an elevated total protein or changes in the blood smear as discussed in this case.

18. The answer is A [VII E 9 b (4) (e)]. Plasmapheresis offers the only option for reducing the amount of protein in the circulation to alleviate some of the symptoms. Blood transfusions could be detrimental until the hyperviscosity has been improved, because blood transfusions will raise blood viscosity. The other two options would not address the issue with high protein content in the circulation.

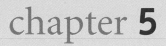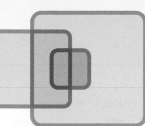

chapter 5

Oncologic Diseases

KRISTI MOORE • THOMAS MACHARIA • KATHERINE TKACZUK

I U.S. CANCER STATISTICS AND SCREENING GUIDELINES

(Figure 5–1; for cancer screening guidelines refer to Chapter 1)

A Bias in Cancer Screening Tests A bias occurs when screen-detected cases appear to have a longer survival than cases detected by symptoms.

1. **Lead-time bias** is an apparent increase in survival due to the longer interval after a diagnosis is made based on a screening test, compared with a diagnosis after onset of symptoms. In truth, the disease retains the same overall survival.

2. **Overdiagnosis bias** occurs when a disease that would have otherwise never been symptomatic in a patient's lifetime is detected at screening, hence giving an apparent prolonged survival. In truth, the disease either does not progress or progresses so slowly that the patient would have died of other causes before clinically apparent disease.

3. **Length bias** refers to the phenomenon in which a large proportion of patients have relatively slowly progressive and asymptomatic cancers that remain detectable only through screening. In truth, the appearance of longer survival is ascribed to the indolent nature of the cancers rather than the screening strategy.

II CANCER PREVENTION

A Classifications

1. **Primary prevention** prevents malignancy in healthy individuals.

2. **Secondary prevention** addresses precancerous lesions to reduce the risk of malignant transformation.

3. **Tertiary prevention** reduces the chance of disease relapse, reduces the risk of developing a second primary tumor, and utilizes measures to limit morbidity and mortality due to superimposed conditions or due to toxic treatments in patients with known malignancy.

B Prevention Strategies

1. Address **modifiable risk factors** [See Chapter 1].

2. Reduce the impact of **infectious diseases**
   a. **Infectious disease prevention**
      (1) **Human papilloma virus (HPV) vaccination** is recommended for girls aged 11–18 years to reduce cervical cancer caused by this virus [see X B 2 b].
      (2) **Hepatitis B vaccination** has been shown to reduce the incidence of hepatocellular carcinoma by preventing chronic hepatitis B infection [see VIII E 2].
   b. **Infectious disease therapy**
      (1) Chronic ***Helicobacter pylori*** infection increases the risk of gastric cancer. In patients with early gastric cancer, the American College of Gastroenterology recommends diagnosis and treatment of *H. pylori*. Although there is no consensus on treatment of patients who are at high risk without a known malignancy, trials suggest that this population also derives benefit from therapy [see VIII C 2 a].
      (2) Therapy for **hepatitis B and C** decreases the risk of hepatocellular carcinoma in individuals with chronic infection; those who have a virologic or biochemical response to therapy have a greater benefit [see VIII E 2].

Estimated New Cases*

Males **Females**

Males				Females		
Prostate	192,280	25%		Breast	192,370	27%
Lung & bronchus	116,090	15%		Lung & bronchus	103,350	14%
Colon & rectum	75,590	10%		Colon & rectum	71,380	10%
Urinary bladder	52,810	7%		Uterine corpus	42,160	6%
Melanoma of the skin	39,080	5%		Non-Hodgkin lymphoma	29,990	4%
Non-Hodgkin lymphoma	35,990	5%		Melanoma of the skin	29,640	4%
Kidney & renal pelvis	35,430	5%		Thyroid	27,200	4%
Leukemia	25,630	3%		Kidney & renal pelvis	22,330	3%
Oral cavity & pharynx	25,240	3%		Ovary	21,550	3%
Pancreas	21,050	3%		Pancreas	21,420	3%
All Sites	**766,130**	**100%**		**All Sites**	**713,220**	**100%**

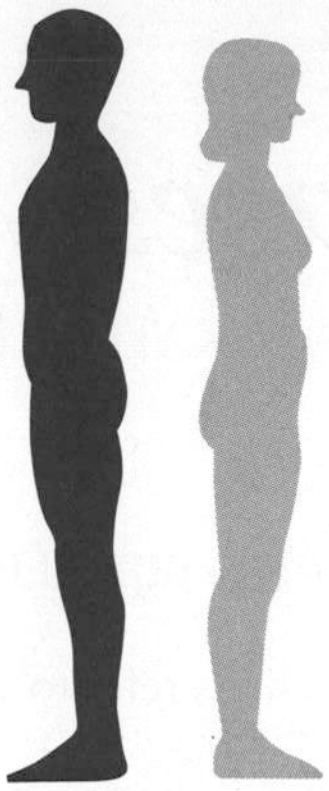

Estimated Deaths

Males **Females**

Males				Females		
Lung & bronchus	88,900	30%		Lung & bronchus	70,490	26%
Prostate	27,360	9%		Breast	40,170	15%
Colon & rectum	25,240	9%		Colon & rectum	24,680	9%
Pancreas	18,030	6%		Pancreas	17,210	6%
Leukemia	12,590	4%		Ovary	14,600	5%
Liver & intrahepatic bile duct	12,090	4%		Non-Hodgkin lymphoma	9,670	4%
Esophagus	11,490	4%		Leukemia	9,280	3%
Urinary bladder	10,180	3%		Uterine Corpus	7,780	3%
Non-Hodgkin lymphoma	9,830	3%		Liver & intrahepatic bile duct	6,070	2%
Kidney & renal pelvis	8,160	3%		Brain & other nervous system	5,590	2%
All Sites	**292,540**	**100%**		**All Sites**	**269,800**	**100%**

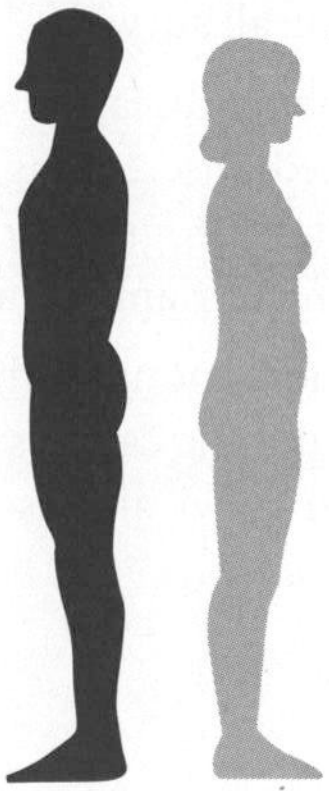

*Excludes basal and squamous cell skin cancers and in situ carcinoma except urinary bladder. Estimates are rounded to the nearest 10.

FIGURE 5–1   Ten leading cancer types for estimated new cancer cases and deaths, by gender, United States, 2009. Reprinted with permission from Jemal A, Siegel R, Ward E, et al. Cancer statistics, 2009. CA Cancer J Clin. 2009; 59:225–49.

(3) **HIV** therapy with highly active antiretroviral therapy (HAART) decreases the incidence of AIDS-related lymphomas [see Chapter 4].

3. **Chemoprevention**
   a. **Breast cancer**
      (1) **Tamoxifen,** a selective estrogen reuptake inhibitor (SERM), is approved for the primary prevention of breast cancer in premenopausal and postmenopausal women who are at high risk as defined by the Gail model [see IX C 4]. It is also used to prevent recurrence in women with estrogen and/or progesterone receptor–positive breast cancer.
      (2) **Raloxifene** is a second-generation SERM with a lower risk of endometrial cancer. It is approved for the prevention of breast cancer in high-risk postmenopausal women aged 60 years or older.
      (3) **Aromatase inhibitors** (AIs) are approved for adjuvant therapy of early-stage estrogen and/or progesterone receptor–positive breast cancer in postmenopausal women to prevent recurrent disease.
   b. **Colon cancer**
      (1) **Aspirin** use is associated with decreased risk of certain colon cancers; however, at this time there is not enough data to recommend routine prophylaxis with aspirin in individuals of average risk.

      (2) Celecoxib is recommended in patients with familial adenomatous polyposis syndrome (FAP) to decrease the incidence of colonic polyps and lower the risk of invasive colon cancer [see VIII A 2 a].

   c. Prostate cancer

      (1) 5-Alpha reductase inhibitors (e.g., finasteride) decrease the overall prostate cancer incidence in men at high risk, although there is a slight increase in high-grade cancers in those receiving treatment.

   d. Skin cancer

      (1) Retinoids are used prophylactically in patients at moderate to high risk of skin cancer. Isotretinoin, an oral vitamin A derivative, has also been shown to reduce the incidence of skin cancers in patients with xeroderma pigmentosum who are predisposed to these cancers.

      (2) Topical diclofenac is approved for the treatment of actinic keratoses, which are considered premalignant skin lesions.

   e. Ovarian cancer

      (1) Oral contraceptives (OCPs) have decreased the incidence of ovarian cancer since their introduction in the 1950s. Women who have used OCPs have sustained protection even several years after discontinuation. The mechanism is not well understood but may be related to direct suppression of ovarian activity.

  4. Surgical therapy

   a. Breast cancer

      (1) Mastectomy should be considered for women with *BRCA1* or *BRCA2* gene mutations [see IX B 1 b (2)]. Women without a history of cancer should be offered bilateral prophylactic mastectomies, and women with known breast cancer should consider contralateral mastectomy to reduce the risk of a cancer in the contralateral breast.

      (2) Bilateral salpingo-oophorectomy reduces the risk of breast cancer in women with *BRCA1* or *BRCA2* mutations, likely by decreasing hormone levels.

   b. Ovarian cancer

      (1) Bilateral salpingo-oophorectomy should be offered to women with known *BRCA1* or *BRCA2* mutations at the time of hysterectomy, after the completion of childbearing, or by age 40–50 years [see IX B 1 b (2)].

   c. Gastrointestinal cancer

      (1) Resection of precancerous lesions (e.g., colonic polyps, Barrett's esophagus) is performed via colonoscopy and/or esophagogastroduodenoscopy.

      (2) Total or subtotal **proctocolectomy** is recommended for patients with FAP or related disorders as these patients have nearly a 100% lifetime risk of colon cancer.

   d. Skin cancer

      (1) Resection of precancerous lesions (e.g., actinic keratosis, dysplastic nevi) reduces the risk of malignant transformation.

III   TUMOR GROWTH

Uncontrolled growth and a loss of responsiveness to growth-inhibitory signals distinguish malignant cells from normal cells. More rapidly growing tumors may be poorly differentiated, but they may be more sensitive to certain kinds of therapy.

A **Patterns of tumor growth**   Cancer growth follows two general patterns:

  1. Direct invasion of the tissue in which the cancer arose.

  2. Metastasis (dissemination) to distant organs via the bloodstream, lymphatic system, or by intracavitary extension.

   a. Different types of **tumors vary in metastatic potential.** For example, primary brain cancers tend to remain localized and rarely spread to distant foci. Other carcinomas, such as small cell lung cancer (SCLC), are already widely disseminated in the majority of patients at the time of diagnosis.

   b. Each cancer also exhibits a distinct **pattern of spread** dictated by the biology of the tumor cell–host interaction. For example, common sites of metastases in colon cancer include the liver, lungs, and peritoneal cavity, and common sites in SCLC include the lungs, liver, bones, and neuraxis.

B **Tumor growth rate and prognosis**   Growth rate and patterns of spread are important determinants of prognosis in the absence of treatment and in the response to therapeutic modalities such as surgery, chemotherapy, or radiation therapy.

1. **Rapidly growing neoplasms** such as acute leukemias, SCLC, and lymphomas are generally highly responsive to chemotherapy and radiation therapy and, therefore, are frequently curable. However, there are numerous exceptions.

2. **Slow-growing tumors** such as low-grade sarcomas are less responsive to systemic treatment modalities. Surgical resection and radiation therapy are more effective treatment options for such neoplasms.

3. Growth rates can be estimated using **flow cytometry** to determine the percentage of tumor nuclei in the S phase of the cell cycle or by determination of Ki-67 levels by immunohistochemical staining.

C **Genetic changes and cancer**   Cancers are genetic diseases characterized by mutations or changes in the expression of genes that regulate vital cell processes.

1. **Oncogenes** (cancer-promoting genes) interfere with the regulatory controls of the cell. Most oncogenes are derived from **proto-oncogenes**—normal genes that ordinarily regulate cell growth processes. Each oncogene induces only a subset of changes associated with the development of a malignancy; therefore, a series of genetic changes is typically required.

   a. Oncogenes modify the affected cell, resulting in the acquisition of malignant characteristics such as changes in shape, autocrine growth factor secretion, loss of contact inhibition, and anchorage independence. Oncogenes may function in a number of ways:

      (1) They may cause the tumor cell to secrete mitogenic growth factors that then stimulate growth of the same cell, leading to autostimulation of cell growth, or **autocrine growth.**

      (2) They may **affect growth factor–induced signal transduction.** Typically, cell surface receptors engaged by their respective ligands transmit signals through a series of defined intracellular pathways that culminate in the regulation of DNA synthesis or transcription. Mutations or altered gene expression in any of these pathways may disturb such regulated signaling, leading to a loss of regulated cell growth or function. The protein products of some oncogenes, such as *ras*, mutate so that they constitutively promote cell growth in the absence of growth factor interactions with their receptors.

   b. **Activation of proto-oncogenes**

      (1) **Point mutations** are single-base changes in a gene. A single mutation in codon 12 of the *ras* gene causes activation of *ras,* the most commonly activated oncogene in solid malignancies.

      (2) **Gene fusion.** In chronic myelogenous leukemia, the *abl* proto-oncogene is fused with a fully unrelated gene, *BCR*. The protein encoded by the *BCR–abl* hybrid has a novel structure and function.

      (3) **Amplification.** Differences in the expression of encoded proteins can cause proto-oncogenes to become oncogenic. For example, in childhood neuroblastoma, the amount of the N-*myc* gene is increased from a diploid number to many dozens per cell. N-*myc* gene amplification is associated with a poor prognosis.

2. **Tumor suppressor genes** function in normal cells to regulate cellular proliferation. The inactivation these genes can promote tumorigenesis.

   a. Inactive alleles of tumor suppressor genes may be acquired in two ways:

      (1) Somatic mutation

      (2) Incorporation in the germ line to create a congenital predisposition to cancer (e.g., as in retinoblastoma)

   b. Inactivation of tumor suppressor genes is associated with neuroblastoma, SCLC, kidney cancer, colon carcinoma, Wilms' tumor, bladder cancer, osteoblastoma, and liver cancer, among other malignancies.

   c. Specific mutations in *BRCA1*, a heritable somatic gene prevalent in Ashkenazi Jews, in affected women increase the risk of early-onset breast cancer. The *BRCA1* gene normally affects estrogen receptor function.

IV   CANCER STAGING

For full staging information, see the seventh edition of the American Joint Committee on Cancer's *AJCC Cancer Staging Handbook* (New York: Springer, 2010).

Conventional tumor–node–metastasis (TNM) staging systems define a series of categories or stages, each of which defines a prognostic stage of a tumor.

V   TREATMENT MODALITIES

A   General principles

1. Most cancer treatment programs are multimodality and may be either **curative** or **palliative** in intent. **Curative** treatments aim to permanently eradicate the tumor, and **palliative** treatments seek to slow tumor growth and control cancer-related symptoms. Therapy is multidisciplinary and must be customized to meet the specific needs of individual patients.

2. **Clinical trials,** which are essential to progress in cancer therapy, are integrated into the routine care of many cancer patients.
   a. **Phase I trials** are small trials evaluating the pharmacokinetics, pharmacodynamics, and safety of a new drug or combination of drugs.
   b. **Phase II trials** are more focused and seek to evaluate the efficacy and safety of a single drug or combination of drugs in a particular tumor type.
   c. **Phase III trials** are larger randomized controlled trials to compare the new treatment to the current standard of care.

B   Radiation therapy   Nearly 60% of all cancer patients require radiation therapy at some point during the course of their disease.

1. **Definition.** Radiation therapy is the use of ionizing radiation for therapeutic purposes. Ionizing radiation is a form of energy emitted via subatomic particles or electromagnetic waves that can displace electrons from atoms or molecules, thereby producing ions (charged atoms or molecules).

2. **Mechanism of action.** Ionization of atoms in DNA causes DNA damage. Noncancerous cells have the ability to repair much of this damage or regenerate new cells. Cancer cells are thought to have impaired repair mechanisms, and cell death occurs after exposure to ionizing radiation.

3. **Uses of radiation therapy**
   a. **Curative,** if there is a survival benefit (e.g., Hodgkin's lymphoma, prostate, breast, gynecologic, and head and neck malignancies)
   b. **Palliative,** when a cure is not possible (e.g., brain metastases, compression of the vena cava or airway)

4. **Timing of radiation therapy**
   a. **In combination with chemotherapy**
   b. **Adjuvant.** Radiation therapy administered **in addition to** the main treatment, whether surgery, chemotherapy, or hormonal therapy.
   c. **Neoadjuvant.** Radiation therapy administered **before** the main treatment.

5. **Sources of Radiation**
   a. **X-rays.** A form of electromagnetic radiation (EMR) emitted by atomic electrons. They are produced by specialized machines called linear accelerators.
   b. **Gamma rays.** EMR emitted by the nuclei of certain radioisotopes (e.g., cobalt, radium), produced when electrons collide with positrons.
   c. **Particle beams.** Ionizing protons or carbon ions directed at the tumor, where the radiation dose peaks, then drops abruptly (known as the Bragg peak), hence minimizing effects on the adjacent nonmalignant tissues.
   d. **Radioisotopes.** Specific radioactive isotopes (e.g., iodine-125, iodine-131, strontium-89, phosphorus-32, or cobalt-60) administered orally, intravenously, or implanted near the tumor.

6. **Types of radiation therapy**
   a. **Systemic (unsealed source).** Radiopharmaceuticals are administered orally or intravenously to treat a malignancy (e.g., strontium-90 for treatment of bony metastases, iodine-131 for treatment of thyroid cancer, and yttrium-90 for treatment of neuroendocrine malignancy).
   b. **External beam (teletherapy).** The source of radiation is external to the body, and the beam is created by a collimator. The intensity of the radiation diminishes the further away the source is located. Variations of external beam radiation include the following;

(1) **Conventional two-dimensional external beam radiation** is applied to an area defined by width and height.

(2) **Three-dimensional (3D) conformal radiation therapy** is a more precise fitting of each beam to the profile of the target by use of height, width, and depth.

(3) **Intensity-modulated radiation therapy** is an advance of 3D conformal radiation therapy in which radiation beams of different intensities are directed to small areas of the field at the same time while avoiding adjacent structures.

(4) In **stereotactic radiation therapy** the tumor field is specifically defined in 3D space by the use of computer-aided image processing, and radiation is precisely directed at the tumor from multiple angles. Stereotactic radiation can also be applied using several smaller doses over time (**fractionated**). Examples include the following:

(a) **Gamma Knife radiosurgery.** Used for intracranial tumors; the patient's skull is immobilized with a 3D reference frame screwed on during the procedure, and the radiation is emitted through cobalt-60 sources arranged around the patient's skull with the beams converging at the tumor from several points.

(b) **CyberKnife robotic radiosurgery.** Used for tumors anywhere in the body. The linear accelerator is housed in a computer-controlled robotic arm that swivels to direct radiation precisely at the tumor from any angle. The body part is not immobilized since the system uses sophisticated image guidance software to accurately locate the tumor and adjust for the patient's movements during the procedure (e.g., breathing movements).

c. **Internal radiation therapy (brachytherapy).** Sealed sources are placed at the target, either adjacent to or inside the tumor.

7. **Side effects.** Radiation therapy is associated with local and systemic side effects, especially in patients who are receiving high-dose radiation.

a. **Time course**

(1) **Acute effects,** principally inflammation, occur within days or weeks of treatment.

(2) **Chronic effects** such as fibrosis, scarring, and memory or cognitive defects may not be apparent until months or years after therapy.

b. The **severity** of adverse reactions is a function of the treatment site, the size of the radiation port, the amount of radiation energy, and dosage variables (e.g., total dose, radiation dose per fraction, and dose rate).

c. **Systemic effects** include malaise, fatigue, anorexia, and depressed blood counts. These generalized symptoms are especially common in patients treated concurrently with radiation and chemotherapy.

d. **Skin reactions** occur after high-dose therapy directed to sites on or near the skin surface (e.g., chest wall after mastectomy, vulva) and are less common after high-energy photon beam therapy. **Acute reactions** consist of erythema and moist or dry desquamation with pruritus. Retreatment or the use of overlapping fields may result in severe and persistent skin reactions. Management of radiation-induced skin reactions includes the following:

(1) Keeping the affected area as clean and dry as possible

(2) Topical application of corticosteroids, vitamin A and D ointment, moisturizers, baby oil, or cornstarch

(3) Avoiding irritating clothing and direct exposure to the sun

e. **Oral cavity** and **pharyngeal** reactions such as mucositis, xerostomia, pain, and dental caries occur after high-dose radiation to the head or neck.

(1) Strict attention to dental hygiene, topical anesthetics, artificial saliva preparations, and nutritional counseling may be helpful.

(2) Severe cases may require insertion of a gastric feeding tube or percutaneous gastrostomy to maintain adequate oral intake.

f. **Gastrointestinal reactions** occur with cumulative radiation doses exceeding 4000–5500 cGy.

(1) **Esophagitis** usually subsides in 7–10 days but predisposes patients to superimposed *Candida* infections. Treatment measures include use of antacids, a bland diet, and topical anesthetics.

(2) **Radiation gastritis** or **enteritis** may manifest as nausea, vomiting, diarrhea, abdominal pain, anorexia, or bleeding. Management includes antiemetics; antidiarrheals; a bland, low-fat, low-residue, high-gluten diet; and dietary supplements.

(3) Rectal inflammation (proctitis) may result in bleeding or pain. A low-residue diet, stool softeners, or steroid enemas may give relief.

g. **Radiation pneumonitis,** characterized by cough, dyspnea, and chest pain, usually occurs 2–3 months after radiation exposure to a significant lung volume. Corticosteroids may be effective for symptom management.

h. **Central nervous system (CNS) symptoms** may occur during therapy or may not appear until weeks or months after treatment cessation.

(1) Acute symptoms accompanying intracranial irradiation include headache and signs of increased intracranial pressure (ICP); gastrointestinal symptoms (e.g., nausea and vomiting) may also occur. Dexamethasone usually provides rapid relief.

(2) Delayed symptoms, including short-term memory loss, visual disturbances, and white matter abnormalities (e.g., calcifications, ventricular dilation), are particularly common in patients undergoing prophylactic cranial irradiation for small cell lung cancer.

(3) A **somnolence syndrome** characterized by hypersomnia and fatigue has been observed weeks or months after intracranial irradiation, especially in patients receiving concurrent intrathecal chemotherapy.

i. **Bone marrow suppression** may follow large-field radiation treatments in Hodgkin's lymphoma or pelvic malignancies, especially if patients are receiving concurrent chemotherapy. Leukopenia or thrombocytopenia may require suspension of therapy; however, anemia is rare.

j. In Hodgkin's disease, mediastinal irradiation is associated with long-term toxicities such as hypothyroidism and coronary artery disease. Late effects of radiation to the neck and mediastinum include an increased risk of breast and thyroid cancers.

k. Side effects can be minimized by the following procedures:

(1) Accurately targeting the tumor area by using sophisticated radiologic imaging (e.g., computed tomography [CT], magnetic resonance imaging [MRI]) and by the use of newer techniques such as stereotactic body radiation therapy or stereotactic radiation surgery.

(2) Directing radiation to avoid organs with low tolerance to radiation (e.g., spinal cord) using 3D conformal radiation therapy, intensity modulated radiation therapy, or proton beam radiation therapy.

(3) Blocking or protecting normal tissue from radiation (e.g., by the use of amifostine [Ethyol] to protect against radiation-induced mucositis).

(4) Reducing the treatment field over the course of therapy and dividing the total dose over several days (fractionation), which allows nontumor cells time to regenerate. It may also allow tumor cells that are in a relatively radioresistant phase (e.g., late G1 and S phase) to move into a more susceptible phase.

C **Chemotherapy and Other Pharmacologic Therapies of Cancer**

1. **Uses.** Chemotherapy should only be used when patients benefit from the treatment. If cure is the objective, complete responses are generally required, and considerable host toxicity is acceptable. However, if palliation is the goal, acceptable toxicity must be coupled with an absence of disease progression.

2. **Indications** for chemotherapy

a. To **cure** certain disseminated malignancies (e.g., acute leukemia, lymphoma, small cell lung cancer).

b. To **palliate** symptoms of disseminated malignancy when the control of symptoms is desired, but only if the perceived benefits outweigh the risks.

c. **Adjuvant chemotherapy** involves treating patients with no evidence of clinically detectable disease after surgical resection but who are at high risk for future relapse. In early-stage breast, colon, and lung cancers, it has been shown to lower the risk of disease relapse and improve survival.

d. **Neoadjuvant chemotherapy** is an approach of initial chemotherapy prior to the final surgical excision of the tumor. This may be offered in conjunction with radiotherapy and is usually recommended when the tumor is not surgically resectable initially, if surgical resection would cause significant mutilation, or if organ preservation is the goal. An example of this approach is treatment of rectal cancer with neoadjuvant chemotherapy and radiotherapy prior to rectal sphincter-sparing surgery to avoid permanent colostomy. An excellent response to neoadjuvant chemotherapy (complete pathologic response) has been associated with improved outcomes in many solid tumor malignancies.

3. **Contraindications** to chemotherapy
   a. When the expertise of the facilities is inadequate to administer, monitor, and manage the side effects of chemotherapy.
   b. When the patient is unable to understand the risks and benefits of chemotherapy and/or unable or unwilling to comply with the proper follow-up after treatment.
   c. When the patient is unlikely to derive benefit from the treatment even if tumor shrinkage is achieved (e.g., a severely debilitated patient with multiple other comorbid conditions and limited life expectancy).
   d. When the patient is asymptomatic from a slow-growing and incurable tumor, in which case the treatment can be postponed until disease-related symptoms occur and need to be palliated.

4. **Monitoring the response to therapy**
   a. **Measurable disease** is defined as the presence of at least one measurable lesion. **Measurable lesions** are defined as lesions that can be accurately measured in at least one dimension with greatest diameter ≥20 mm using conventional techniques or ≥10 mm with CT scan.
   b. **Nonmeasurable lesions** include small lesions (greatest diameter <20 mm with conventional techniques or <10 mm with CT scan) and disease that is **truly nonmeasurable** (e.g., leptomeningeal disease, ascites, pleural or pericardial effusion, inflammatory breast disease, lymphangitis cutis or pulmonis, cystic lesions, and also abdominal masses or organomegaly).
   c. All target lesions are evaluated by **imaging or physical examination** during therapy (on average every two or three treatment cycles or every 6–8 weeks) using standardized **Response Evaluation Criteria in Solid Tumors (RECIST)** to determine whether therapy is effective (Table 5–1).

5. **Combination therapy** utilizes two or more active agents in the treatment of potentially curable or highly chemotherapy-responsive cancers (e.g., acute leukemia and testicular cancer). In chemotherapy-sensitive cancers, combination therapy is usually far more effective than single-agent therapy.
   a. Combinations are selected based on evidence of therapeutic synergy or additivity with acceptable host toxicity. When possible, highly active agents with nonoverlapping toxicity profiles are chosen.
   b. Combinations of marginally active chemotherapeutic agents tend to be relatively inactive and more toxic than the use of single agents with comparable efficacy profiles.
   c. Combination chemotherapy may prevent or delay the development of drug resistance that commonly develops when malignant cells are exposed to a single agent over a given period.

6. **Drug resistance.** This phenomenon may be either **innate** or **acquired.** Certain malignancies (e.g., pancreatic and hepatocellular carcinomas) exhibit innate drug resistance and rarely respond to conventional chemotherapy. Other cancers (e.g., SCLC, ovarian and breast cancers) initially respond well to chemotherapy before the emergence of drug resistance that leads to disease progression. Several mechanisms of drug resistance have been identified;

TABLE 5–1 Response Evaluation Criteria in Solid Tumors (RECIST 1.1) of Target and Nontarget Lesions	
Complete response (CR)	No clinically detectable cancer is found after the completion of therapy, all pathologic lymph nodes must resolve (defined as <10 mm on short axis of CT imaging), and tumor markers must normalize if elevated prior to treatment
Partial response (PR)	The measurable tumor shrinks by ≥30% after treatment, no new areas of tumor develop, and no other area of tumor increases in size
Progressive disease (PD)	The measurable tumor mass increases in size by ≥20% and by at least 5 mm, new lesions appear, or the patient dies as a result of tumor progression
Stable disease (SD)	Persistent lesions, maintenance of tumor marker levels above normal limits, or neither sufficient shrinkage to qualify for PR nor sufficient increase to qualify for PD

Information adapted from Eisenhauer EA, Therasse P, Bogaerts J, et al. New response evaluation criteria in solid tumours: revised RECIST guideline (version 1.1). *Eur J Cancer* 2009;45:228–247.

TABLE 5–2   Classes of Common Chemotherapeutic Agents Used in Oncologic Disease

Alkylating Agents	**Topoisomerase Inhibitors**
Nitrogen Mustards	*Topoisomerase I*
Mechlorethamine	Irinotecan
Cyclophosphamide	Topotecan
Ifosfamide	
Melphalan	*Topoisomerase II*
Chlorambucil	Etoposide
	Antibiotics
Platinum Analogs	Anthracyclines
Cisplatin	Daunorubicin
Carboplatin	Doxorubicin
Oxaliplatin	Epirubicin
	Idarubicin
Nitrosoureas	
Carmustine (BCNU)	*Other*
Lomustine (CCNU)	Mitoxantrone
Streptozocin	Mitomycin-C
	Bleomycin
Alkyl Sulfates	Actinomycin-D
Busulfan	
	Antimetabolites
Ethyleneimines and Methylmelamines	5-Fluorouracil (5-FU)
Thiotepa	Methotrexate
Hexamethylmelamine/altretamine	6-Mercaptopurine (6-MP)
Triazenes	Fludarabine
Temozolomide	Cytarabine (Ara-C)
	Capecitabine
Mitotic Spindle Agents	Gemcitabine
Vinca Alkaloids	Floxuridine (FUDR)
Vincristine	Pemetrexed
Vinblastine	Pentostatin
Vinorelbine	
	Miscellaneous Agents
Taxanes	Procarbazine
Paclitaxel	Hydroxyurea
Docetaxel	Retinoids
	ʟ-Asparaginase
Estramustine	Bortezomib
Epothilones	
Ixabepilone	

a. Inhibition of drug accumulation or active drug efflux.

b. Overexpression of the drug target.

c. Accelerated repair of chemotherapy-induced cellular damage.

d. Inhibition of cell death (apoptosis) pathways.

7. Types of therapeutic agents in cancer

   a. **Chemotherapy** The most often used chemotherapeutic drugs and their mechanisms of action, therapeutic uses, and toxicities are discussed in the following sections (Table 5–2).

     (1) **Alkylating agents**

      (a) **Mechanism of action**

      (b) **Drug resistance**

      (c) **Therapeutic uses and toxicities** (Online Tables 5–3 through 5–8)

     (2) **Mitotic spindle agents**

      (a) **Mechanism of action**

      (b) **Therapeutic uses and toxicities** (Online Table 5–9)

        (3) Antibiotics

        (a) Mechanism of action

        (b) Therapeutic uses and toxicities (Online Table 5–10)

        (4) Antimetabolites

        (a) Mechanism of action

        (b) Therapeutic uses and toxicities (Online Table 5–11)

        (5) Topoisomerase inhibitors

        (a) Mechanism of action

        (b) Therapeutic uses and toxicities (Online Table 5–12)

        (6) Miscellaneous agents. Procarbazine, hydroxyurea, L-asparaginase, bortezomib, and the retinoids are in this category.

        (a) Therapeutic uses and toxicities (Online Table 5–13)

    b. Hormonal agents

        (1) Androgens

        (a) Mechanism of action

        (b) Therapeutic uses

        (c) Toxicities

        (2) Antiandrogens

        (a) Mechanism of action

        (b) Therapeutic uses

        (c) Toxicities

        (3) Estrogens

        (a) Mechanism of action

        (b) Therapeutic uses

        (c) Toxicities

        (4) Antiestrogens

        (a) Mechanism of action

        (b) Therapeutic uses and toxicities (Online Table 5–14)

        (5) Aromatase inhibitors

        (a) Mechanism of action

        (b) Therapeutic uses

        (c) Toxicities

        (6) Luteinizing hormone–releasing hormone agonists

        (a) Mechanism of action

        (b) Therapeutic uses

        (c) Toxicities

        (7) Progestins

        (a) Mechanism of action

        (b) Therapeutic uses and toxicities

        (c) Toxicities

        (8) Adrenocorticosteroids

        (a) Mechanism of action

        (b) Therapeutic uses

        (c) Toxicities

(9) Adrenal Inhibitors

(a) Mechanism of action

(b) Therapeutic uses

(c) Toxicities

c. **Monoclonal antibodies** against specific tumor antigens have the advantage of selectivity and specificity with a relative lack of toxicity. Targets for monoclonal antibodies include antigens that are **selectively expressed** by malignant cells or that exert important **functional effects** on malignant cell growth or viability.

   (1) **Diagnostic uses.** Monoclonal antibodies targeting cancer antigens facilitate histopathologic diagnosis. They have particular value in staging leukemias and lymphomas and in identifying the origin of poorly differentiated tumors.

   (2) **Therapeutic uses.** Table 5–15 notes the U.S. Food and Drug Administration (FDA)–approved antibodies, their targets, and therapeutic indications.

   (3) **Other uses**

   (a) Antibodies may be used ex vivo to purge autologous bone marrow of residual tumor cells before reinfusion after high-dose cytotoxic chemotherapy.

   (b) Antibodies also have potential utility as vehicles for the delivery of radioisotopes and chemotherapeutic agents.

   (i) **Radiolabeled monoclonal antibodies** are capable of delivering lethal radiation doses directly to tumor cells (see Table 5–15).

   (ii) **Immunotoxins** are monoclonal antibodies containing a bacterial (e.g., *Pseudomonas* exotoxin) or plant (e.g., ricin A chain) toxin (see Table 5–15).

   (c) **Anti-idiotypic antibodies** induce the production of host antibodies that recognize tumor-associated cell-surface antigens. These agents are being investigated as possible **tumor vaccines.**

d. **Cancer vaccines** may result from new understanding of tumor immunology and the components and regulation of the human antitumor immune response.

TABLE 5–15 Monoclonal Antibodies

Drug	Molecular Target	Therapeutic Uses
Trastuzumab (Herceptin)	Extracellular domain of HER2/*neu* oncogene-derived protein	Early-stage and metastatic breast cancer in tumors that overexpress HER2/*neu*
Rituximab (Rituxan)	CD20 antigen on the surface of mature B cells	Non-Hodgkin's lymphoma
Bevacizumab (Avastin)	Vascular endothelial growth factor	Advanced colorectal and nonsquamous non–small cell lung cancers
Alemtuzumab (Campath-1H)	CD52 antigen on the surface of B and T lymphocytes, NK cells, monocytes, and macrophages	T cell prolymphocytic leukemia and relapsed or refractory B cell chronic lymphocytic leukemia
Cetuximab (Erbitux)	EGFR	EGFR-expressing metastatic colon cancer, squamous cell carcinoma of head and neck
Panitumumab (Vectibix)	EGFR receptors on normal and tumor cells	EGFR-expressing colorectal cancer
Radiolabeled Monoclonal Antibodies		
Ibritumomab tiuxetan with ^{90}Yttrium (Zevalin)	CD20 antigen on normal and malignant B cells	Low-grade refractory non-Hodgkin's lymphoma
Tositumomab with ^{131}Iodine (Bexxar)	CD20 antigen on normal and malignant B cells	Low-grade refractory non-Hodgkin's lymphoma
Immunotoxins		
Gemtuzumab ozogamicin with calicheamicin (Mylotarg)	CD33 antigen on myeloid cells	Chemotherapy-refractory, CD33-positive acute myelogenous leukemia for patients ≥60 years old who are not candidates for chemotherapy

EGFR, epidermal growth factor receptor.

TABLE 5–16 Tyrosine Kinase Inhibitors

Drug	Therapeutic Uses
Imatinib (Gleevec)	First-line therapy for newly diagnosed chronic myelogenous leukemia; gastrointestinal stromal tumors, myelodysplastic/myeloproliferative diseases, systemic mastocytosis, hypereosinophilic syndrome, dermatofibrosarcoma protuberans
Sunitinib (Sutent)	Advanced renal cell carcinoma; gastrointestinal stromal tumors; trials underway to evaluate the use in advanced thyroid cancer
Erlotinib (Tarceva)	Metastatic non–small cell lung cancer, pancreatic cancer
Dasatinib (Sprycel)	Chronic, accelerated, or blast-phase chronic myelogenous leukemia with resistance or intolerance to prior therapy
Gefitinib (Iressa)	Non–small cell lung cancer after failure of both platinum- and taxane-based chemotherapies
Lapatinib (Tykerb)	Metastatic breast carcinoma that overexpresses HER2/*neu* in patients who have received prior therapy with trastuzumab, anthracycline, and taxanes
Nilotinib (Tasigna)	Chronic, accelerated, or blast-phase chronic myelogenous leukemia with resistance or prior intolerance to imatinib
Sorafenib (Nexavar)	Metastatic renal cell carcinoma and unresectable hepatocellular carcinoma

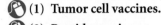 **(1) Tumor cell vaccines.**

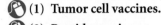 **(2) Peptide vaccines.**

    (3) Anti-idiotype approach.

  e. Tyrosine kinase inhibitors (TKIs) are a novel class of oral anticancer agents that target intracellular tyrosine kinase signal transduction receptors, which play important roles in clonogenicity, tumorigenicity, apoptosis, tumor growth and progression, pathologic angiogenesis, and tumor metastasis in various solid and hematologic malignancies. FDA-approved TKIs and their therapeutic uses are summarized in Table 5–16.

  f. Biologic response modifiers are agents that alter the growth characteristics or antigenicity of a tumor, resulting in a therapeutic enhancement of host response. The mechanism of action may be immunologic or nonimmunologic.

    (1) BCG. An attenuated strain of *Mycobacterium bovis*, BCG has demonstrated activity when administered locally in direct contact with tumor cells.

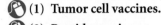 **(a) Therapeutic indications.**

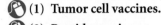 **(b) Toxicity.**

    (2) The interleukins affect totipotent **stem cells,** or immature hematopoietic precursors. In addition, these cytokines have widespread physiologic effects on lymphocytes and other organs.

 (a) Interleukin-2 (IL-2), a lymphokine secreted by activated T lymphocytes, modifies the proliferation and function of T and B cells and is essential for the growth of T cells and peripheral blood lymphocytes.

 (i) Therapeutic indications.

 (ii) Side effects.

    (3) Colony-stimulating factors act to regulate the proliferation, differentiation, maturation, and function of blood cells.

    (a) Erythropoiesis-stimulating agents (ESAs) are synthetic derivatives of endogenous erythropoietin, a hormone made by the kidney that regulates red blood cell production. ESAs administered subcutaneously or via the intravenous route result in a marked increase in reticulocytes and increases in the hemoglobin and hematocrit.

      (i) Therapeutic indications. ESAs must be prescribed under a risk management program to ensure the safe use of these drugs. ESAs are only recommended for patients with severe anemia due to concurrent chemotherapy in whom a complete cure is not anticipated. The lowest effective dose to prevent transfusion should be used.

      (ii) Side effects. ESAs can increase the risk of tumor progression and may reduce survival in cancer patients. Studies also show that ESAs can increase the risk of heart attack, heart failure, stroke, or blood clots in patients using these drugs for other conditions.

        (b) Granulocyte-macrophage colony-stimulating factor (GM-CSF) primarily stimulates the production of neutrophils, eosinophils, granulocytes, and monocytes, whereas **granulocyte-colony stimulating factor (G-CSF)** stimulates neutrophils and granulocytes.

            (i) Therapeutic indications.

            (ii) Side effects.

    (4) Interferons (IFNs) are glycoproteins that possess antiviral and antiproliferative activities. They enhance T cell and macrophage activity, stimulate the expression of tumor-specific cell surface antigens, alter oncogene expression, and promote cell differentiation.

        (a) Therapeutic indications.

        (b) Toxic reactions.

VI. HEAD AND NECK CARCINOMAS

A. Incidence Head and neck carcinomas account for 3% of the cancers reported each year in the United States. These tumors occur nearly three times more frequently in men than in women. Patients are typically between 50 and 60 years of age. The most frequently affected sites are the oral cavity (40%), larynx (25%), oropharynx and hypopharynx (15%), and salivary gland (10%).

B. Risk factors

1. **Tobacco use,** including cigarette smoking and chewing tobacco use, is the main risk factor.

2. **Heavy alcohol consumption** works in synergy with cigarette smoking to increase the incidence of head and neck cancer 10- to 40-fold.

3. **Nickel exposure** increases the risk of nasal cavity and paranasal sinus cancers.

4. **Syphilis** is associated with an increased incidence of cancer of the tongue.

5. **Prolonged sun exposure** increases the incidence of lip cancer.

6. The **Epstein–Barr virus** and certain **food dyes** have been linked to nasopharyngeal cancers in Asians.

7. **Human papilloma virus** infection, particularly HPV-16, increases the risk of cancer of the oropharynx.

C. Screening There are currently no screening guidelines for early detection in asymptomatic people. The U.S. Preventative Task Force does recommend counseling for cessation of tobacco use and limitation of alcohol intake.

D. Pathology Most (95%) of head and neck cancers are squamous cell carcinomas, which vary from well-differentiated varieties to invasive, poorly differentiated, or undifferentiated tumors. Nodal involvement is a factor of the primary tumor site, size, and degree of differentiation. Thyroid carcinoma, lymphoma, and skin cancers also occur in the head and neck region and are discussed in separate sections.

1. **Tumors of the salivary gland** are most commonly of the mixed type, although adenoid cystic carcinomas are not uncommon.

2. **Nasopharyngeal cancers** may be squamous cell cancers, lymphoepitheliomas, or lymphomas.

E. Clinical features Common symptoms include dysphagia, persistent hoarseness, head or neck pain, ear pain, and swelling. Affected patients with large lesions may present with nonhealing ulcerations or white patches (leukoplakia). Some patients present with adenopathy in the absence of an obvious primary source.

F. Diagnosis

1. **Detection**
   a. **Tissue diagnosis** relies on biopsy of the nonnecrotic portion of the tumor, tumor edge, and adjacent normal mucosa. Open biopsy of the neck lymph nodes should be avoided if squamous cell cancer is suspected.

    b. Radiologic studies may include the following:

       (1) Radiographs of the mandible, sinus, or nasopharynx.

       (2) CT, positron emission tomography (PET), PET/CT, and/or MRI scans to evaluate the nasopharynx, thymus, oral cavity, and oral pharynx and to check nodal involvement. PET/CT is also useful in assessing the extent of involvement and evaluating tumor viability after radiation therapy.

       (3) Barium swallow (in patients with evidence of tumor encroachment on the cervical esophagus).

2. Pretreatment evaluation

    a. A thorough **dental evaluation** is necessary before radiation therapy to help prevent and manage osteoradionecrosis, hyposalivation, and rapid tooth decay that often complicate radiation therapy.

    b. If a mutilating surgical procedure is anticipated, a **prosthodontist** should be consulted to plan reconstructive cosmetic surgery.

    c. Many patients with head and neck cancer are malnourished because of their inability to swallow and chew. They should undergo a complete **nutritional assessment,** and attempts should be made to bring the patient into positive nitrogen balance to reduce the complications of treatment.

G Staging   For full staging information, see the most recent edition of the *AJCC Cancer Staging Handbook.*

H Prognosis   The most important determinant of prognosis is stage at diagnosis. The 5-year survival rates for stage I exceeds 80% but is less than 40% in stages III and IV disease. The presence of a palpable lymph node in the neck decreases the survival rate by 50% compared to the same T stage without node involvement. Advanced primary tumor, pathologic evidence of neck lymph node spread, and gross or microscopic extracapsular spread predict metastatic disease and hence a poorer prognosis. The lifetime risk of developing a new cancer is 20%–40%.

I Therapy   Multimodality therapy and a multidisciplinary approach are key to optimizing outcomes. Operability depends on anatomic extent of tumor, functional consequences of resection, presence of metastases, and comorbid conditions that affect suitability for surgical procedures. Small lesions can be treated with curative surgery and radiation therapy. Patients with advanced, unresectable disease can benefit from radiation therapy or combined-modality approaches.

1. Surgery

    a. Surgical resection should not be undertaken in metastatic disease except in some slow-growing salivary gland tumors and well-differentiated thyroid neoplasms or when complete resection is not possible.

    b. Primary tumors should be excised with negative margins, which may require skin flaps.

    c. Patients with neck lymph node involvement require **radical neck dissection** (i.e., dissection of the superficial and deep cervical fascia and close lymph nodes; sternocleidomastoid muscles; internal, external, and jugular veins; spinal accessory nerve; and submandibular glands).

    d. Patients with cancers of the oral cavity, oral pharynx, or supraglottic larynx and no evidence of nodal involvement are treated with a **functional neck dissection** for better functional and cosmetic results. In tumors of the larynx, attempts can be made to further preserve the larynx by use of neoadjuvant chemotherapy and radiotherapy.

    e. Surgery is associated with **morbidity,** including cosmetic deformities, speech impediments, aspiration pneumonia, shoulder droop, and pain.

2. Radiation therapy. Adjuvant radiation therapy is indicated for stage III–IV cancers, perineural involvement, and vascular tumor embolism. For nonresectable tumors, positive margins, or extracapsular extension, chemoradiation therapy is required. Most patients are treated with radiation over a 5- to 6-week interval. Side effects include dry mouth, loss of taste, mouth ulcers, osteoradionecrosis of the mandible (which can be prevented by appropriate pretreatment dental extractions, antibiotics, and fluoride administration), laryngeal edema, and, rarely, hypothyroidism. Intensity-modulated radiation therapy decreases radiation injury to nearby tissues.

3. **Chemotherapy** for locally unresectable or metastatic disease may include cisplatin, 5-fluorouracil (5-FU), methotrexate, and taxanes.
   a. Newer drugs such as irinotecan, pemetrexed, epidermal growth factor receptor antagonists, and p53 gene therapy are being tested in clinical trials and show promise.
   b. Combination chemotherapy with cisplatin and 5-FU has a reported response rate as high as 90% in patients with unresectable disease.

VII — LUNG CANCER

A **Incidence/Epidemiology**   The frequency of lung cancer is increasing rapidly. Originally a disease that primarily afflicted men older than age 60 years, lung cancer has become the second-most-common cause of cancer in women. The annual incidence of lung cancer in the United States is 219,440 new cases per year, and it is the leading cause of cancer death in both men and women.

B **Etiology/Risk Factors**

1. **Cigarette smoking.** "Passive smoking" is also associated with a small but significant increase in the incidence of lung cancer.

2. **Industrial carcinogens.** Exposure to beryllium, radon, hydrocarbons, mustard gas, nickel, radiation, and asbestos has been linked to lung cancer. Cigarette smoking exacerbates the risk associated with such exposure. Smoking and asbestos exposure increase the risk 53-fold.

3. **Air pollutants** (e.g., diesel exhaust, tar, arsenic, chromium, cadmium, nickel).

4. **Existing lung damage.** Adenocarcinomas of the lung may develop in areas scarred by **tuberculosis** or other lung conditions associated with **fibrosis.** These tumors are called **scar carcinomas.**

5. Patients with **lymphoma** or **malignancies of the head, neck,** and **esophagus** have an increased incidence of lung cancer.

C **Screening**   Routine screening by the use of chest radiography, sputum cytology, or low-dose computerized tomography in asymptomatic persons at risk for lung cancer is not recommended at this time. The American Cancer Society recommends that persons with a history of heavy smoking who seek screening should first discuss the risks and benefits with their physicians and that such testing only be performed in experienced centers with multidisciplinary specialty groups for diagnosis and follow-up. Of course, the best prevention is smoking cessation.

D **Pathology**   Lung cancer is divided into two major histologic subtypes: non–small cell lung cancer (NSCLC), which represents 85% of lung carcinomas, and small cell lung cancer (SCLC), which is much less common and represents the remaining 15% of newly diagnosed lung cancer cases.

1. **Non–small cell lung cancer**
   a. **Squamous cell carcinomas** (20%–25% of NSCLC) were once the most common type of NSCLC, but they have become less common than adenocarcinomas. Squamous cell tumors more commonly arise centrally near the hilum, where they present as endobronchial disease.
   b. **Adenocarcinoma** (50%–60% of NSCLC) is the most frequently diagnosed form of NSCLC in both men and women. The lesions are often peripheral, occurring in more distal airways. More than half of patients with adenocarcinoma who have apparently localized disease as a peripheral nodule have regional nodal metastases. **Bronchoalveolar cell cancer (BAC),** a variant of adenocarcinoma, is characterized by a spreading pattern within the bronchioles without apparent invasion. BAC is frequently misdiagnosed initially as pneumonia due to its multicentric and infiltrative pattern on chest radiographs. BAC is more common in young female nonsmokers and is thought to be more sensitive to tyrosine kinase inhibitor therapy (e.g., erlotinib).
   c. **Large cell and other unspecified lung cancers** account for 5%–10% of all lung cancers. These tumors are usually peripheral lesions. Large cell lung cancers and adenocarcinomas have similar natural histories with a tendency to spread rapidly and widely hematogenously, commonly involving the liver, lung, and bone.

2. **Small cell lung carcinoma** (15% of all lung cancers) comprises several histologic subtypes (polygonal cell, lymphocytic, spindle cell, oat cell), which all have similar natural histories. The

tumor is thought to arise from neural crest neuroendocrine or amine precursor uptake and decarboxylation cells and progresses rapidly without treatment. The average survival time in the absence of treatment is only 2–4 months.

3. **Uncommon tumors of the lung** include bronchial carcinoids, cystic adenoid carcinomas, carcionosarcomas, and mesotheliomas.

E Clinical features

1. **Local symptoms** of intrathoracic disease include cough, hemoptysis, obstructive pneumonia (due to endobronchial tumors), chest pain, pleural effusion, hoarseness (from recurrent laryngeal nerve compression), wheezing, stridor, and superior vena cava syndrome (due to obstruction of the vessel by a mediastinal tumor). Patients with bronchoalveolar cell cancer may have a severe cough productive of clear sputum.

2. **Systemic manifestations** include the following:
   a. Anorexia and weight loss
   b. Bone pain from distant metastases
   c. Hepatomegaly, tenderness, and fever caused by liver involvement
   d. CNS signs or seizures from brain metastases or carcinomatous meningitis
   e. Hypercalcemia from bone metastases or other humoral substances

3. Patients with lung cancer may present with symptoms of ectopic hormone production or other **paraneoplastic syndromes** [see XVIII].
   a. **Ectopic adrenocorticotropic hormone (ACTH) secretion** causes hypokalemia and muscle wasting.
   b. **Syndrome of inappropriate antidiuretic hormone secretion (SIADH)** results in hyponatremia.
   c. **Eaton–Lambert syndrome** results in myasthenia-like symptoms.
   d. **Ectopic production of parathyroid hormone–related peptide** results in hypercalcemia.

F Diagnosis

1. **Sputum cytology** or **bronchoscopy** confirms the diagnosis in patients with endobronchial disease. Bronchoscopy also assesses proximal endobronchial tumor extension and the status of the contralateral lung. It should be performed in all patients with centrally located tumors and in selected patients with peripheral tumors, especially if they are potential surgical candidates.

2. **Transthoracic needle biopsy,** guided by CT, is often necessary for the diagnosis of peripheral lesions. The false-negative rate is 15%.

3. **Transbronchial needle aspiration** of mediastinal nodes may obviate the need for more-invasive procedures.

4. **Thoracotomy** or **mediastinoscopy** is required in approximately 5%–10% of patients. These invasive procedures are especially useful in the diagnosis of SCLC, which grows centrally in the mediastinum rather than endobronchially. Mediastinoscopy or mediastinotomy also can be used to assess the resectability of mediastinal and hilar nodes.

5. **Video-assisted transthorascopic surgery (VATS)** is less invasive than thoracotomy and involves three or four incisions (1–2 cm) in the chest wall to view the diaphragm, lung parenchyma, and mediastinal structures. Visible lesions may be removed by biopsy.

6. **Lymph node biopsy** is used to evaluate suspicious supraclavicular or neck lymph nodes.

7. **CT scans** of the chest, abdomen, brain, and adrenal glands are performed for staging to establish the **extent of distant metastatic disease** and can provide information about mediastinal node involvement and chest wall invasion.

8. **Radionuclide bone scans** may be used to rule out metastatic skeletal disease.

9. **MRI** of the chest is most useful for evaluating spread to cardiovascular organs (e.g., heart, aorta, superior vena cava).

10. **PET scan** is now widely used in the initial staging of patients with lung cancer. It provides additional information regarding metastatic involvement and can therefore affect the staging of disease. PET or PET/CT also plays a role in posttreatment assessment of response to therapy and follow-up phases of patient care.

G **Staging** For full staging information, see the most recent edition of the *AJCC Cancer Staging Handbook.*

1. NSCLC.

2. SCLC.

H **Prognosis**

1. **NSCLC**
   a. **Tumor stage** based on the American Joint Committee on Cancer (AJCC) TNM staging system is an independent prognostic factor. Five-year survival ranges range from 40% to 50% in stage I disease and from 15% to 30% in stage II disease. Patients who have distant metastatic disease have a median survival of approximately 12 months.
   b. **Performance status (PS).** Patients who feel well and have few disease-related symptoms (PS 0 or 1) survive longer than ill patients.
   c. Involuntary **weight loss** of ≥5% is an independent negative prognostic factor.
   d. Molecular prognostic factors such as mutated p53 tumor suppressor gene or oncogene overexpression (*c-myc, K-ras, erb-B2*) are associated with poor prognosis.

2. **SCLC**
   a. Patients with **limited SCLC** (disease confined to one hemithorax) have approximately 25% 5-year survival rates and a median survival of 23 months with appropriate therapy. Prophylactic cranial irradiation (PCI) results in approximately a 5% improvement in survival in limited-stage disease with minimal cognitive dysfunction if total dose of 3000 cGy in 200-cGy/day fractions is used.
   b. **Extensive SCLC** is not curable, and the median survival in patients with PS of 0–1 is less than 1 year, and the 2-year survival rate is approximately 20%. Despite initial responsiveness to chemotherapy, only 15%–20% of patients achieve complete response.

I **Therapy**

1. **NSCLC**
   a. **Pretreatment considerations**
      (1) A tumor is resectable if all of the tumor can be completely excised with pathologically negative margins.
      (2) Mediastinoscopy or mediastinotomy should be used only if positive findings will prevent a curative thoracotomy.
   b. **Therapeutic modalities**
      (1) **Surgery** is the primary treatment modality for patients with stage I and stage II disease. Stage III patients with more extensive mediastinal nodal involvement and/or involvement of mediastinal structures are often resectable but invariably relapse, with a 5-year mortality rate of 90%–95%. Combination chemotherapy and radiation therapy is now frequently employed in the management of these patients.
         (a) **Operable tumors.** If the cardiopulmonary status of the patient is compatible with surgery, surgical options include lobectomy or pneumonectomy, depending on the extent of disease.
         (b) **Resectable tumors.** The surgeon should aim to remove the tumor completely with adequate margins of resection while conserving as much normal lung tissue as possible.
         (c) **Advanced local cancer.** Selected patients may undergo surgical resection with or without chest irradiation.
            (i) Patients with small tumors in the ipsilateral mediastinal nodes or large primary tumors without mediastinal node involvement have 5-year survival rates as high as 35% with a combination of surgery and radiation therapy.
            (ii) Tumors of the superior sulcus (**Pancoast's tumor**) are typically treated with combination chemotherapy and radiation therapy, which results in median survival rates of 37 months and 5-year survival rates of 42%.
      (2) **Radiation therapy**
         (a) Routine use of adjuvant radiation therapy in completely resected stage I, II, and III NSCLC tumors cannot be recommended at this time.

    (b) Patients who cannot tolerate surgery because of insufficient cardiopulmonary reserve should receive chest irradiation. Survival rates at 5 years range from 5% to 20%.

    (c) **Definitive radiation therapy** is often used in patients with **unresectable but localized cancers,** with less than 5% long-term survival. **Palliative radiation therapy** can relieve the symptoms of pain, hemoptysis, superior vena cava syndrome, or pneumonitis that are associated with obstructive lesions or metastatic disease.

    (3) Chemotherapy

        (a) An international study (International Adjuvant Lung Trial [IALT]) of more than 1800 patients with NSCLC who were treated with platinum-based combination chemotherapy after complete resection of their primary tumors showed that adjuvant chemotherapy resulted in a 5% absolute improvement in long-term overall survival. Two additional trials (National Cancer Institute of Canada Clinical Trials Group JBR.10 and Adjuvant Navelbine International Trialist's Association [ANITA]) also showed nearly a 10% reduction in mortality. Several studies have shown that neoadjuvant chemotherapy improves survival in stage III patients. In one study, researchers found that administration of two courses of cisplatin and vinblastine before radiation therapy in stage III unresectable patients was superior to that of radiation alone. The survival rates were 55% (vs. 40%) at 1 year, 26% (vs. 13%) at 2 years, and 23% (vs. 11%) at 3 years. Studies have also shown that concurrent chemoradiation therapy is superior to sequential treatment.

        (b) **Combination chemotherapy** has a response rate of approximately 10%–30% in patients with metastatic NSCLC. Response rates double in ambulatory patients who have not lost weight. The most commonly used drugs include carboplatin, paclitaxel, cisplatin, etoposide, gemcitabine, irinotecan, vinorelbine, and docetaxel, in some combination.

    (4) Nonchemotherapy agents may be beneficial in a small group of patients. **Erlotinib,** an epidermal growth factor receptor blocker, is FDA approved for second- and third-line therapy of NSCLC and achieves a 5%–10% radiographic response rate. Women with adenocarcinoma, younger patients, and nonsmokers are more likely to respond. The major toxicities include skin rash, diarrhea, and, rarely, pneumonitis.

2. SCLC

  a. Pretreatment considerations. With **limited disease,** the highest long-term survival rates (10%–25%) are obtained with **concurrent radiation therapy** and cisplatin-based **chemotherapy.** Hyperfractionated radiation therapy combined with chemotherapy may improve treatment outcome.

  b. Therapeutic modalities

    (1) Chemotherapy is the mainstay of treatment. For **extensive disease, combination chemotherapy** with etoposide plus carboplatin or cisplatin is standard therapy. Other active drugs include ifosfamide, vincristine, paclitaxel, and topotecan. Irinotecan in combination with cisplatin has shown significant promise in a recent phase II trial.

    (2) Radiation therapy. Prophylactic cranial irradiation should be considered in responsive patients with limited disease. Radiation therapy has only palliative benefit in patients whose conditions have failed to respond to chemotherapy or who have brain metastases.

    J **Mesothelioma**   This neoplasm arises from the mesothelial lining of the pleural and peritoneal cavities. It has a very poor prognosis, with a median survival of 6–18 months, and so far there are no effective treatments. A very select group of patients are surgically treated, but the overall survival is poor. Smoking and asbestos exposure increase the risk of development of mesothelioma by 90-fold. Several chemotherapeutic agents have been evaluated for the treatment of this condition, including doxorubicin, gemcitabine, cisplatin, and carboplatin. Most recently, multitargeted antifolate pemetrexed (Alimta) has received much attention as a possible new and effective agent in the treatment of mesothelioma. The combination of this agent with a platinum agent is superior to the use of platinum alone.

VIII   GASTROINTESTINAL CANCERS

  A **Carcinoma of the colon, rectum, and anus**

    1. Incidence. Cancers of the colon and rectum occur in 152,260 individuals annually in the United States and account for 50,630 deaths each year.

2. **Etiology/risk factors.** Up to 70% of patients diagnosed with colon cancer have no identifiable risk factors. However, genetic and epidemiologic studies have linked colon and rectal cancer to the following factors:

   a. **Inherited predisposition.** Familial syndromes such as familial adenomatous polyposis (FAP)—an autosomal dominant disorder caused by mutations in the adenomatous polyposis coli (APC) gene on chromosome 5—may lead to an increased risk of colon cancer. In FAP, cancers commonly develop in adolescence and young adulthood, and the incidence of colorectal neoplasms is nearly 100% by age 50 years. Hereditary nonpolyposis colon cancer (HNPCC or Lynch syndrome) is associated with a lower but significant risk of cancer of the colon and rectum. Mutations in tumor suppressor genes such as *MCC, DCC, BRCA1*, and p53 also confer higher risks for colorectal neoplasms.

   b. **Somatic mutations** that accompany the progression from epithelial hyperplasia through polyp formation and eventual cancer development form a continuum. These changes indicate an association among inherited predispositions (e.g., mutated p53) and acquired mutations in either tumor suppressor genes such as *DCC* or in oncogenes such as *ras*.

   c. **Dietary influence.** The higher incidence of colorectal cancer in industrialized societies has led to hypotheses that high-fat, low-fiber diets deficient in calcium, selenium, folate, vitamins D and E, and other trace elements predispose to the development of colorectal neoplasms.

   d. **Inflammatory bowel disease,** particularly ulcerative colitis with pancolitis, is associated with a higher incidence of colorectal neoplasms.

3. **Screening**

   a. Adults with signs or symptoms consistent with colorectal neoplasm should undergo testing to exclude the presence of a mass.

   b. All average-risk adults aged 50 years or older should undergo one or more of the following: annual fecal occult blood test (FOBT) or fecal immunochemical test (FIT), flexible sigmoidoscopy every 5 years, double-contrast barium enema (DCBE) every 5 years, CT colonography every 5 years, or colonoscopy every 10 years. All positive tests should be followed up with a colonoscopy.

   c. High-risk patients, including those with a personal or family history of colorectal cancer or adenomatous polyps, a history of FAP or HNPCC, or a history of inflammatory bowel disease, should be screened earlier and more frequently.

4. **Pathology**

   a. The large majority of colorectal neoplasms are **adenocarcinomas,** and most are well or moderately differentiated. Poorly differentiated neoplasms are associated with poor prognosis.

   b. **Squamous cell carcinomas** can arise in the anus. Such neoplasms differ from adenocarcinomas in terms of biology and therapy.

5. **Clinical features**

   a. **Local symptoms** include a change in bowel habits that may involve constipation, diarrhea, a change in stool caliber, crampy abdominal pain, and rectal bleeding. Signs of obstruction, perforation, or early satiety may occur. Patients with locally advanced rectal carcinoma may present with symptoms of tenesmus or perineal pain.

   b. **Systemic manifestations** are more often seen in metastatic disease and may include anorexia, fatigue, weight loss, hepatomegaly, abdominal pain, or fever.

6. **Diagnosis**

   a. **Colonoscopy** is the preferred diagnostic test for colorectal cancer since it can be used to visualize the tumor and allows for biopsy and/or removal of polyps or suspicious lesions. **Barium enema** and **flexible sigmoidoscopy** may also be useful, but the diagnostic yield with this combined procedure is less than that of colonoscopy alone. **CT colonography** may be used for patients in which colonoscopy is not possible to achieve a radiologic diagnosis (e.g., in the event of an obstructing tumor or tortuous colon).

   b. **Biopsy** of suspicious lesions is required to establish a diagnosis.

   c. **Tumor markers** such as **carcinoembryonic antigen (CEA)** or **carbohydrate antigen (CA) 19-9** have a poor sensitivity and specificity and are not useful in the diagnosis or screening of colorectal cancer.

   d. Radiologic studies are used to evaluate the extent of local disease and to screen for metastatic disease.

    (1) CT scans of the pelvis, contrast-enhanced MRI, and/or **endorectal ultrasound** may be appropriate for rectal neoplasms.

    (2) CT scans of the chest and abdomen can screen for the presence of intra-abdominal (e.g., mesenteric or retroperitoneal lymph node enlargement), hepatic, or pulmonary metastases.

    (3) Contrast-enhanced MRI has improved sensitivity for the evaluation of suspected hepatic metastases.

    (4) PET scan and **PET/CT** are used to localize the site of recurrence in patients with rising levels of tumor markers or to determine the extent of hepatic metastases in patients being evaluated for hepatic resection surgery.

7. Staging. For full staging information, see the most recent edition of the *AJCC Cancer Staging Handbook.*

8. Prognosis. Five-year survival rate for stage 0–I is >90%; for stage II is 75%–85%; for stage III is 45%–65%; and for stage IV is <10%. Cure rates for lymph node–negative T_1–T_3 lesions are 75%–90% and decrease to 35%–45% when regional lymph nodes are involved. The cure rates decrease with increasing numbers of involved regional lymph nodes and increasing tumor size.

    a. Colorectal cancer. Key prognostic factors include the **extent of tumor invasion, lymph node involvement,** and **the presence or absence of distant metastases.** Genetic mutations, including p53 gene mutation and loss of the long arm of chromosome 18, result in an adverse prognosis.

    b. Anal cancer. Long-term survival rates in patients with **localized squamous cell carcinoma of the anus** are approximately 80% after combined chemotherapy and radiation therapy. However, metastatic disease is not curable, despite the initial responsiveness to chemotherapy.

9. Therapy

    a. Colorectal cancer

        (1) Surgery

            (a) Colon cancer. Treatment of cancers above the peritoneal reflection usually involves **partial colectomy,** unless the extent of metastatic disease necessitates systemic chemotherapy. Principles of surgical oncology, including establishing wide surgical margins, should be followed to optimize outcomes. In experienced hands, a laparoscopic procedure is acceptable.

            (b) Rectal cancer. Treatment involves abdominoperineal resection or, if the lesion is higher in the rectum, a low anterior resection that preserves sphincter function and does not require colostomy. Another approach for low rectal tumors includes initial chemotherapy and radiation followed by a segmental rectum resection and the formation of a coloanal anastomosis.

        (2) Radiation therapy

            (a) Colon cancer. Prospective randomized trials have not established the value of adjunctive radiation for enhancement of surgical cures. Nevertheless, adjunctive radiation, frequently in combination with chemotherapy, is commonly offered to patients with T_4 lesions in the ascending or descending colon or to patients with positive operative margins.

            (b) Rectal cancer. Adjunctive radiation, in conjunction with chemotherapy, enhances cure rates in patients with transmural or lymph node–positive rectal neoplasms.

        (3) Chemotherapy

            (a) Adjuvant therapy for colon cancer. Surgery cures only 30%–60% of patients with lymph node–positive (e.g., any T, N_1 or N_2, M_0) colon cancer. The addition of adjuvant chemotherapy with **5-FU** and **leucovorin** has been shown to reduce the incidence of recurrence by up to 41%.

                (i) The role of adjuvant chemotherapy in the management of patients with lymph node–negative stage II lesions (e.g., $T_3N_0M_0$) remains controversial. The American Society of Clinical Oncology panel concluded that the routine use of adjuvant chemotherapy for patients with stage II disease could not be routinely recommended based on the review of 37 randomized studies that found no statistically significant survival benefit.

(ii) Combination regimens such as **FOLFOX4 (oxaliplatin, 5-FU, and leucovorin)** are now the standard therapy for patients with stage III colon cancer. **Irinotecan** and **capecitabine** are other emerging adjuvants.

(b) **Adjuvant therapy for rectal cancer.** The combined administration of **radiation therapy** and **5-FU** improves cure rates. Typically, combined-modality therapy is administered postoperatively, followed by an additional 4 months of chemotherapy alone. Excellent results are also obtained when the chemoradiation precedes surgery.

(c) In some cases, chemotherapy is given **following the resection of metastases.** Rarely, individuals present with metastases that are solitary or restricted to a solitary organ and are amenable to either resection or an ablative procedure such as cryosurgery. In patients who undergo hepatic lobectomies to resect metastases, the combined use of a systemic 5-FU–based compound and intrahepatic chemotherapy is associated with a survival benefit compared with surgery alone.

(d) **Disseminated metastatic disease** is common, and chemotherapy is offered with palliative intent. **5-FU** and **LV** in combination with **oxaliplatin (FOLFOX)** is the standard first-line therapy for metastatic colorectal cancer. A newer agent, **irinotecan,** has a similar degree of efficacy and is commonly used in combination with **5-FU/LV (FOLFIRI)** as second-line therapy. A new oral formulation of 5-FU, **capecitabine,** has improved drug administration and offers continuous drug exposure to maximize antitumor properties.

(e) The angiogenesis inhibitor **bevacizumab** (Avastin) improves both the response rate and overall survival in patients with newly diagnosed metastatic colon cancer when used in conjunction with contemporary chemotherapy regimens and is FDA approved for patients with metastatic colorectal cancer.

(f) **Cetuximab,** a chimerized IgG1 antibody to the epidermal growth factor (EGFR), is approved by the FDA for the treatment of EGFR-positive colorectal cancer that is refractory to or intolerant of irinotecan chemotherapy.

(g) **Capecitabine** alone, or **irinotecan in combination with 5-FU and leucovorin,** improves response rates and survival. In metastatic disease that is refractory to chemotherapy with 5-FU plus leucovorin, irinotecan treatment improves response rates, time to progression, survival, and quality of life in comparison with either therapy alone. **Oxaliplatin** is another approved option.

(h) Other agents that are infrequently used include single-agent administration of **mitomycin-C or nitrosoureas.**

b. **Anal cancer. Combined-modality chemotherapy and radiation therapy** for localized cancers usually involve **5-FU and mitomycin-C.** The majority of patients with localized cancers are cured, and function of the anal sphincter is preserved.

B Carcinoma of the pancreas

1. **Incidence.** Cancers of the pancreas occur in approximately 42,470 individuals annually in the United States and account for more than 35,240 annual deaths.

2. **Etiology.** A small portion of pancreatic cancers are familial and are linked to mutations in common tumor suppressor genes such as p16 and p53. Carriers of the *BRCA-2* mutation also have a higher risk of developing the disease. Other risk factors include the following:
   a. **Cigarette smoking**
   b. **Dietary carcinogens**
   c. **Environmental carcinogens**
   d. **Age** greater than 60 years old
   e. **Male gender**
   f. **African American ethnicity**
   g. **Chronic pancreatitis** (minor increase in risk)

3. **Screening.** There are no good screening tests for pancreatic cancer. CA 19-9 is elevated in 70%–90% of patients with pancreatic cancer; however, it is not useful as a screening test due to low specificity.

4. **Pathology.** Most pancreatic neoplasms are adenocarcinomas, and most are poorly or moderately differentiated.
   a. **Adenocarcinomas** can arise in the head, body, or tail of the pancreas.

    b. Neuroendocrine tumors such as carcinoid tumors or islet cell tumors are less common but are frequently associated with early hepatic metastases. In contrast to exocrine tumors, these malignancies may have relatively indolent natural histories. These tumors may produce hormones that induce **carcinoid syndrome,** which is characterized by flushing, hypotension, diarrhea, and valvular heart disease.

5. Clinical features

    a. Local symptoms may include painless jaundice, epigastric fullness, or symptoms of gastric outlet obstruction. When adjacent nerves are involved, patients may complain of abdominal pain radiating to the back.

    b. Systemic manifestations are common and may include the following:

        (1) Anorexia, weight loss

        (2) Hepatomegaly, pain, or fever attributable to liver involvement

        (3) Hematologic disorders manifested by either recurrent superficial thrombophlebitis (Trousseau's syndrome), deep thrombophlebitis, or disseminated intravascular coagulation (DIC)

        (4) Glucose intolerance

6. Diagnosis. Pancreatic cancer is notoriously difficult to diagnose, and patients frequently present with unresectable disease. Frequently used diagnostic modalities include the following:

    a. A dedicated **pancreatic CT scan** may identify a suspicious mass lesion.

    b. Biopsy of suspicious lesions is required to establish a diagnosis. This may be accomplished by endoscopic retrograde cholangiopancreatography (ERCP), percutaneous fine-needle aspiration (FNA), or exploratory laparoscopy or laparotomy.

    c. Endoscopic ultrasound (EUS) is frequently used to determine the extent of tumor invasion and can be performed concurrently with ERCP.

    d. Additional studies may be necessary to evaluate the extent of local disease and to screen for metastatic disease.

        (1) Patients who are potential candidates for curative-attempt surgery often undergo **CT scans of the chest and abdomen,** along with **angiography** or **MRI imaging** to assess patency and integrity of key vascular structures such as the superior mesenteric artery.

        (2) Bone scans and brain imaging are not indicated in patients with no symptoms of brain or bone metastases.

7. Staging. For full staging information, see the most recent edition of the *AJCC Cancer Staging Handbook*.

8. Prognosis

    a. Surgically resectable cancer. Only 15%–20% of patients with pancreatic cancer are candidates for surgical cure. Patients who undergo surgery followed by adjuvant chemoradiation may have long-term survival rates as high as 40%.

    b. Locally advanced, unresectable cancer. These patients cannot be cured, but the use of concurrent chemotherapy with radiation therapy increases average survival to approximately 1 year.

    c. Metastatic cancer. The survival of untreated patients averages about 3 months. This increases to almost 6 months when gemcitabine chemotherapy is used. Long-term survival is exceedingly rare.

9. Therapy

    a. Localized disease

        (1) Surgery. Surgery is the treatment of choice for patients with localized pancreatic cancer. With an experienced surgeon, a pancreaticoduodenectomy or Whipple procedure may be performed with acceptable operative morbidity and mortality. However, only 20%–30% of patients who undergo this operation or total pancreatectomies are cured of pancreatic cancer.

        (2) Adjuvant chemotherapy and radiation therapy. Postoperative radiation therapy administered in conjunction with **5-FU** or **gemcitabine chemotherapy** has been shown to improve cure rates.

    b. Metastatic disease

        (1) The approach to metastatic disease is purely palliative. Narcotic analgesics or celiac plexus blocks may palliate pain. Either operative bypass or biliary stenting is used to palliate obstructive jaundice. Expandable duodenal stents are also being employed to reduce duodenal and gastric outlet obstruction.

(2) Chemotherapy using the antimetabolite **gemcitabine** improves quality of life and survival. 5-FU has less palliative benefit but can be used as an alternative agent.

    c. Neuroendocrine tumors. Many patients with neuroendocrine tumors have hepatic metastases at the time of diagnosis. However, due to the indolent nature of carcinoid tumors, patients may be followed for years before needing therapeutic intervention. Chemotherapy with **5-FU** and **streptozocin** can provide palliation. **Locoregional approaches** to liver metastases such as chemoembolization or intrahepatic arterial chemotherapy may be appropriate in selected patients. Metastatic **islet cell tumors** are responsive to chemotherapy with **streptozocin** and **doxorubicin.** Patients with **carcinoid syndrome** may benefit from treatment with **somatostatin analogs** (e.g., octreotide).

C Carcinoma of the stomach

1. **Incidence.** Cancers of the stomach occur in approximately 21,100 individuals, with more than 10,600 deaths annually in the United States. The incidence of gastric adenocarcinomas has decreased in the last 50 years; however, the causes of this change are not known. The incidence of cancer of the cardia and gastroesophageal junction, however, has been rising rapidly.

2. **Etiology.** Although the etiology of stomach cancers remains largely unknown, the following have been implicated in the development of gastric cancer:
   a. **Precursor conditions,** including chronic atrophic gastritis, intestinal metaplasia, pernicious anemia, partial gastrectomy for benign disease, *Helicobacter pylori* infection, and gastric adenomatous polyps.
   b. **Family history.** Patients with hereditary nonpolyposis colorectal cancer (Lynch syndrome) are at increased risk.
   c. **Tobacco use**
   d. **Diet and vitamin deficiencies.** Diets that are high in salt and nitrosamines, such as fermented and smoked foods, are considered risk factors for gastric cancer. Deficiencies in vitamins A, C, and E, selenium, β-carotene, and fiber are also risk factors for cancer.

3. **Screening.** Currently, there are no recommendations for screening in asymptomatic individuals.

4. **Pathology.** The vast majority of stomach neoplasms are adenocarcinomas. Most are poorly or moderately differentiated.
   a. **Adenocarcinomas** may originate in any part of the stomach.
   b. **Lymphomas** may arise in the stomach.

5. **Clinical features**
   a. **Local symptoms** may include abdominal pain, early satiety, gastrointestinal bleeding, nausea, vomiting, dyspepsia, dysphagia, odynophagia, or symptoms of gastric outlet obstruction.
   b. **Systemic manifestations** are common and may include the following:
      (1) Anorexia, weight loss, fatigue
      (2) Nausea
      (3) Pain due to bone metastases
      (4) Hepatomegaly, abdominal pain, or fever due to liver involvement
      (5) Hematologic disorders including deep thrombophlebitis, recurrent superficial thrombophlebitis (Trousseau's syndrome), or DIC

6. **Diagnosis**
   a. An **upper gastrointestinal series** or **upper gastrointestinal endoscopy** establishes the presence of a mass. Occasionally, gastric cancer manifests as **linitis plastica,** without an obvious epithelial lesion, but with a submucosal tumor infiltrating the organ.
   b. **Biopsy** should be performed in all gastric ulcers, even those that appear to be benign (if deemed safe). Ulcers should be followed carefully to ensure that complete healing occurs. Typically, endoscopic biopsy diagnoses the presence of a gastric cancer.
   c. Commonly used **staging procedures** include the following:
      (1) Endoscopic ultrasound is used to determine the depth of invasion
      (2) CT scanning may identify perigastric or celiac lymph node involvement. In addition, it can identify the presence of pulmonary, mediastinal, liver, retroperitoneal lymph node, or pelvic metastases.

    (3) Laparoscopy may be used preoperatively to evaluate the omentum, a common site of metastasis that is poorly visualized on CT scans.

    (4) Bone scans and brain imaging are not indicated in patients with no symptoms of brain or bone metastases.

7. Staging. For full staging information, see the most recent edition of the *AJCC Cancer Staging Handbook.*

8. Prognosis. Pathologic staging remains the most important determinant of prognosis. Other negative prognostic factors include older age, weight loss >10%, diffuse versus intestinal histology, and proximal location of the tumor.

    a. Surgically resectable cancer. Cures result in the majority of patients who undergo surgery for early (e.g., $T_1N_0M_0$) lesions, but surgical cure rates decline rapidly with advancing disease stage.

    b. Metastatic cancer. The average survival of untreated patients is approximately 6 months, and treatment with combination chemotherapy increases this time by only several months.

9. Therapy

    a. Surgery. Surgery is the treatment of choice for patients with localized gastric cancer. The **probability of surgical cure is directly related to the stage of the cancer.** Patients with transmural, lymph node–involved cancers have low surgical cure rates of only 15%–20%.

        (1) Gastric cancer is typically diagnosed at relatively advanced stages in the United States, and relatively few patients are cured. More extensive surgery, pioneered in Japan, has not been shown to improve outcomes in patients with locally advanced cancers.

        (2) Adjuvant chemotherapy and radiotherapy. Postoperative radiation therapy has not been shown to improve surgical outcomes in patients who have undergone surgery with curative intent. However, adjuvant therapy with radiation therapy plus 5-FU chemotherapy improves survival. Newer agents including epirubicin are also used in combination chemotherapy with 5-FU.

    b. Palliative approach to metastatic disease. Narcotic analgesics or celiac plexus blocks may reduce pain, and either operative bypass or the placement of biliary stents or catheters may palliate obstructive jaundice. Chemotherapeutic agents such as 5-FU, doxorubicin, mitomycin-C, etoposide, methotrexate, paclitaxel, docetaxel, or cisplatin have modest single-agent activity and may provide palliation of symptoms, but they have no meaningful impact on survival. Combination therapy may improve quality of life and survival, but the overall impact is minimal.

    c. Eradication of *Helicobacter pylori* infection is recommended by the American College of Gastroenterology for all patients with a diagnosis of early gastric cancer.

D Carcinoma of the esophagus

1. Incidence. Cancers of the esophagus occur in approximately 16,500 individuals, with 14,500 deaths annually in the United States. Striking increases in the incidence of esophageal adenocarcinomas have been noted in the United States since the early part of the twentieth century for unclear reasons.

2. Etiology. The etiology of esophageal cancers remains largely unknown. Most **adenocarcinomas** arise in areas of intestinal metaplasia found in the distal esophagus known as **Barrett's esophagus,** but relatively few individuals with Barrett's esophagus develop esophageal malignancies. Gastroesophageal reflux disease (GERD) may contribute to the formation of Barrett's esophagus. **Alcohol abuse** and **tobacco use** predispose to squamous cell carcinomas.

3. Screening

    a. Patients with frequent and chronic **GERD** symptoms (e.g., symptoms occurring several times weekly over 5 or more years) should be screened with an initial endoscopy and biopsy. If no dysplasia is found, screening is no longer indicated.

    b. Endoscopy with multiple biopsies should be performed in all patients with visible areas of **Barrett's esophagus**.

        (1) If no dysplasia is found, repeat endoscopy in 1 year. If biopsies remain negative, screening is lengthened to every 3 years.

        (2) For low-grade dysplasia, endoscopy every 6 months for 12 months and then yearly is recommended.

(3) For high-grade dysplasia, definitive treatment is indicated. Esophagectomy is the gold standard; endoscopic resection and photodynamic therapy are alternatives for nonsurgical candidates or if the patient declines surgery. In this case, surveillance endoscopy should be performed every 3 months.

4. **Pathology.** The vast majority of esophageal adenocarcinomas are poorly or moderately differentiated. **Adenocarcinomas** typically arise in or near the gastroesophageal junction in an area of Barrett's esophagus.

5. **Clinical features**
   a. **Local symptoms** include dyspepsia, dysphagia or odynophagia, epigastric or retrosternal pain, and occasionally gastrointestinal bleeding.
   b. **Systemic manifestations** are common and include anorexia, weight loss, fatigue, bone pain, hepatomegaly, abdominal pain, and fever.

6. **Diagnosis**
   a. Barium swallow or upper gastrointestinal endoscopy establishes the presence of a mass lesion.
   b. **Endoscopic biopsy** diagnoses the presence of an esophageal cancer.
   c. Commonly used **staging studies** include the following:
      (1) **CT scan** may identify mediastinal or celiac lymph node involvement and can identify the presence of pulmonary, liver, retroperitoneal lymph node, or pelvic metastases.
      (2) **EUS** may define the extent of tumor invasion in the esophagus and the presence of periesophageal lymph node enlargement. EUS may also identify liver metastases and provide endoscopic guidance for needle biopsies.
      (3) **PET scans** can determine the presence of occult metastases.
      (4) **Laparoscopy** is controversial, but it can be used preoperatively to determine the presence of peritoneal metastases, which are poorly visualized on CT scans. This is rarely necessary due to the advanced PET and CT techniques available today.
      (5) **Bone scans and brain imaging are not indicated** in patients with no symptoms of brain or bone metastases.

7. **Staging.** For full staging information, see the most recent edition of the *AJCC Cancer Staging Handbook*.

8. **Prognosis.** Esophageal cancer is highly curable in its earliest stages; however, the majority of patients present with locally advanced or metastatic disease and many require neoadjuvant chemoradiation therapy to achieve resectability.
   a. **Surgically resectable cancer.** Most patients who undergo surgery for early (e.g., $T_1N_0M_0$) lesions are cured, but surgical cure rates decrease rapidly as the stage of cancer increases.
   b. **Metastatic cancer.** The survival of untreated patients averages about 6 months, and chemotherapy increases average survival by several months in responsive patients.

9. **Therapy**
   a. **Localized cancer**
      (1) **Surgery.** Surgery, either alone or with neoadjuvant chemoradiation therapy, is the most commonly used curative treatment modality in esophageal disease. The probability of surgical cure relates directly to cancer staging. A minority of patients with transmural or lymph node–involved cancers are cured by esophagectomy. A curative approach is not usually taken for supraclavicular or celiac lymph node metastases. Patients with carcinoma in situ and very early stage cancers who are not candidates for esophagectomy may benefit from endoscopic mucosal ablation and photodynamic therapy.
      (2) **Preoperative radiation therapy and chemotherapy** using 5-FU and cisplatin improves surgical outcomes in patients who undergo surgery with curative intent. When used alone, neither chemotherapy nor radiation therapy improves surgical outcome.
   b. **Metastatic disease.** Treatment is palliative.
      (1) **Radiation therapy in conjunction with chemotherapy** may palliate local symptoms caused by esophageal obstruction.
      (2) **Esophageal stents and feeding tubes** may improve the patient's ability to maintain enteral nutrition.

(3) **Single-agent or combination chemotherapy** with 5-FU, etoposide, irinotecan, paclitaxel, docetaxel, or cisplatin may display moderate activity and provide palliation of symptoms but without meaningful impact on survival.

E Carcinoma of the hepatobiliary system

1. **Incidence.** Hepatobiliary cancers occur in approximately 32,400 individuals annually in the United States, with more than 21,500 deaths each year.

2. **Etiology. Hepatocellular carcinoma (HCC)** is associated with diseases that cause chronic liver injury such as **chronic active hepatitis** caused by **hepatitis B virus (HBV), hepatitis C virus (HCV), alcoholic cirrhosis, hemochromatosis,** dietary iron overload, and Wilson's disease. Biliary tract neoplasms such as **cholangiocarcinoma** and **gallbladder cancer** have increased incidence in individuals with **inflammatory bowel disease.**

3. **Screening.** The American Association for the Study of Liver Diseases recommends surveillance for HCC in individuals at increased risk with biannual **serum alpha fetoprotein (AFP)** measurement and **liver ultrasound.** Patients recommended for screening include those with chronic hepatitis B or C infection, alcoholic cirrhosis, genetic liver disease, including hemochromatosis, primary biliary cirrhosis, or autoimmune hepatitis, and all patients who are on the liver transplant list.

4. **Pathology.** Most hepatobiliary neoplasms are adenocarcinomas.

5. **Clinical features**
   a. **Local symptoms of hepatocellular carcinoma** include **pain** resulting from distention of the liver capsule, palpable mass in the right upper quadrant, or abdominal distention. **Obstructive jaundice** is a characteristic presentation for **cholangiocarcinoma.** Jaundice may be a manifestation of **gallbladder cancer.**
   b. **Systemic manifestations** are common and may include the following:
      (1) Signs and symptoms of liver failure such as edema, ascites, pruritus, and portal hypertension
      (2) Anorexia, weight loss, nausea, and vomiting
      (3) Fatigue and anemia
      (4) Pain due to bone metastases or peritoneal metastases
      (5) Dyspnea or cough due to pulmonary metastases

6. **Diagnosis. Hepatocellular carcinoma** may be initially suspected in at-risk individuals by a rise in the **AFP serum tumor marker** or by the presence of mass on a screening liver **ultrasound.** Occasionally **gallbladder carcinoma** is discovered incidentally at the time of cholecystectomy.
   a. **CT scans** and **MRI** may identify a mass or masses in the liver. Typically, the diagnosis of hepatocellular carcinoma is established by a CT-guided or ultrasound-guided fine-needle aspiration biopsy.
   b. **CT scan** or **ERCP** may detect a mass, obstruction of biliary flow, or a filling defect in a major biliary radicle. Fine-needle aspiration biopsy or ERCP-guided biopsy can establish a diagnosis of **cholangiocarcinoma.**
   c. Commonly used **staging studies** include the following:
      (1) **CT scans** may identify mediastinal or celiac lymph node involvement. They can identify the presence of pulmonary, liver, retroperitoneal lymph node, or pelvic metastases.
      (2) **PET** scans can detect occult metastases and may be used to determine a patient's eligibility for liver transplantation.
      (3) **Bone scans and brain imaging are not indicated** in patients with no symptoms of bone or brain metastases.

7. **Staging.** For full staging information, see the most recent edition of the *AJCC Cancer Staging Handbook.*

8. **Prognosis**
   a. **Surgically resectable cancer.** Surgical cure rates decrease rapidly with increasing disease stage.
   b. **Metastatic cancer.** The average survival of untreated patients is approximately 6 months.

9. **Therapy**
   a. **Localized cancer**

(1) **Surgery**
   (a) In **localized hepatobiliary neoplasms,** surgery alone may provide a cure. Some patients with technically unresectable but liver-confined neoplasms may be candidates for **liver transplantation.** Radiation therapy and standard systemic chemotherapy have no defined roles in the management of hepatocellular carcinoma, although chemotherapy is occasionally used to reduce tumor size and facilitate curative-attempt surgery.
   (b) In **biliary tract neoplasms,** adjunctive 5-FU–based chemotherapy plus external beam or high–dose-rate intraluminal radiation is commonly used.

(2) **Other locoregional approaches.** Patients with small (<4 cm), unresectable lesions may benefit from **radiofrequency ablation (RFA)** or the instillation of **intralesional ethanol.** For larger lesions not amenable to resection, **transarterial chemoembolization (TACE),** which involves the injection of a suspension of chemotherapeutic agents directly into the vessel supplying the neoplastic lesion, offers a modest survival advantage. **Cryoablation** is used for unresectable lesions that are not candidates for RFA due to concerns about excessive thermal damage. **Stereotactic radiotherapy** and **selective internal irradiation** are other promising methods used for HCC that are still undergoing trials.

(3) **Metastatic disease.** Standard chemotherapeutic agents are ineffective in patients with advanced HCC, and the administration of chemotherapy is complicated by comorbidities associated with liver failure. No one chemotherapeutic agent or regimen has emerged as a standard of care in biliary neoplasms, but several agents are used with palliative intent. In addition, bile duct **stenting** can palliate obstructive jaundice.

IX BREAST CANCER

A **Incidence** Although the incidence of breast carcinoma increased over the last several decades, there has been a recent decrease of approximately 7%, probably due to lower rates of hormone replacement therapy (HRT) use in postmenopausal women. It is the most common cancer diagnosed in women and second only to lung cancer as cause of death from cancer in the United States. The incidence of invasive breast cancer in the United States in 2009 was 194,280 cases. As many as one in eight women will develop breast cancer during their lifetime.

B **Risk factors**

1. **Family history.** At least two hereditary patterns are characteristic of breast cancer; however, the majority of breast cancers are sporadic.
   a. **Familial aggregation** is associated with a modest increase in risk, especially among first-degree relatives, and is relatively common.
   b. **True genetic pattern.** Linkage to a specific gene with high penetrance accounts for fewer than 5% of all cases of breast cancer. Cancer tends to occur at a younger age and is more likely to be bilateral. Multiple family members over three or more generations are affected.
      (1) **p53** is a tumor suppressor gene that appears in carriers and patients in Li–Fraumeni families. The gene is located on chromosome 17.
      (2) Mutations in the ***BRCA1* and *BRCA2* genes,** located on chromosome 17q21 and chromosome 13q12, respectively, are seen in some patients with a family history of breast and ovarian cancer and confer increased risk. Both genes are autosomal dominant with incomplete penetration. Patients who have *BRCA1* have a 50%–87% estimated cumulative risk of developing breast cancer and a 15%–45% risk of developing ovarian cancer by the age of 70 years. *BRCA1* tumors frequently lack the expression of estrogen receptors (ERs), progesterone receptors (PRs), and HER2/*neu* receptors ("triple negative" or "basal" breast cancer phenotype).

2. **Early menarche,** before 12 years of age.

3. **Late menopause,** after 55 years of age.

4. **Nulliparity or a late first pregnancy,** after age 30 years.

5. **Prior history of invasive or noninvasive breast cancers.**

6. **Age;** approximately 75% of cases are diagnosed in postmenopausal women.

7. **Hormone replacement therapy (HRT)** is associated with a modest increase in the risk of breast cancer.

8. **Prolonged use of oral contraceptives** before the first pregnancy.

9. **Dietary factors,** e.g., high-fat diet (unproven), alcohol consumption.

10. **Early exposure to ionizing radiation.**

11. **Mammographically dense breast tissue.**

12. **Atypical ductal or lobular hyperplasia.**

C Screening

1. **Breast self-examination.** According to the American Cancer Society (ACS), all women should know how their breasts normally look and feel and should report any change to their health care provider. Brease self examination is an option for all women starting in their 20s. Such examinations are best performed monthly, 5–7 days after the menstrual period when breast swelling and fibrocystic changes are less likely to interfere with the detection of a lump or mass. Women should undergo **clinical breast examination** every 3 years between the ages of 20 and 39 years and annually after age 40 years.

2. **Mammography.** All women should have a baseline mammogram at age 40 years. Depending on the presence of known risk factors, patients should undergo mammography either yearly or every other year between age 40 and 50 years and yearly after age 50 years. Women with risk factors for breast carcinoma should have a yearly mammogram at an earlier age.

3. **High-risk women.** Although there are not sufficient data to recommend a specific surveillance strategy for high-risk women, the ACS guidelines recommend earlier initiation of screening, screening at shorter intervals, and screening with additional modalities such as ultrasound or MRI. Female family members at high risk for breast cancer, especially with *BRCA1* and *BRCA2* mutations, are advised to undergo mammographic screening from the age of 25 years or at an age 5 years prior to that of the index case.

4. **The Gail model.** This model has been incorporated into the Breast Cancer Risk Assessment Tool of the National Cancer Institute and estimates the risk of breast cancer in a woman with certain risk factors, including age, age at menarche, age at first live birth, number of first-degree relatives with breast cancer, number of previous breast biopsies, history of lobular or ductal carcinoma in situ or atypical hyperplasia on previous biopsy, and race. The tool computes risks of breast cancer based on these factors for the purpose of medical counseling of individuals at average risk. It may not accurately estimate risk for women less than 35 years old, individuals with history of irradiation for Hodgkin's lymphoma, and nonwhite females.

D Pathology Breast cancers are adenocarcinomas.

1. **Classification.** Most breast cancers are irregular, firm masses detected by clinical breast examination and ultrasound or areas of mammographically detected densities frequently associated with microcalcifications.

   a. **Infiltrating ductal carcinomas** (70%) are characterized by nests and cords of tumor cells surrounded by a dense collagenous stroma.

   b. **Infiltrating lobular carcinomas** (10%–15%) are characterized by abnormal single cell radial pattern of growth called "Indian filling" on light microscopy, causing them often to be clinically nonpalpable and mammographically silent. Invasive lobular carcinomas are more likely to be bilateral compared to infiltrating ductal carcinomas.

   c. Special subtypes with a favorable prognosis include **papillary, tubular, mucinous,** and **pure medullary carcinomas** (<10% of breast cancers).

   d. **Inflammatory carcinomas** (<1%) invade the dermal lymphatics and cause skin redness, induration, warmth, and an erysipeloid margin resembling mastitis.

   e. **Cytosarcoma phyllodes** (1%)—a rare, predominantly benign type of breast tumor (10% are malignant)—can recur locally or metastasize. Surgical excision with large margins improves local control.

   f. **Paget's disease** of the breast is a unilateral eczematous change of the nipple that is frequently associated with noninvasive breast carcinoma.

2. **Hormone receptor and HER2/*neu* status.**
   a. Breast cancer can be classified according to the presence or absence of **estrogen receptors (ERs) and progesterone receptors (PRs).** These cellular proteins are found by immunohistochemical staining (IHC) of tumor tissue, and nearly 60% of breast cancers are ER and/or PR positive. **ER-positive** tumors are more common in postmenopausal patients; premenopausal women are more likely to have **ER-negative** tumors. Presence of ER and/or PR ($>1\%$ by IHC) is associated with a higher response to hormonal/endocrine therapy and a better prognosis.
   b. Approximately 20%–30% of breast cancer patients also have **HER2/*neu*** oncogene gene amplification and overexpression, which is associated with higher propensity for metastases. HER2/*neu* overexpression is associated with higher chance of response to trastuzumab therapy but poorer prognosis overall.

E Clinical features

1. **Local symptoms** include a breast lump, skin thickening or dimpling, alteration of the shape of the breast, erythema, peau d'orange, dimpling of the skin, nipple inversion or crusting (Paget's disease of the nipple), and unilateral nipple discharge. However, the majority of patients diagnosed in the United States do not have any clinical signs or symptoms of breast cancer and are diagnosed by routine screening mammography.

2. Patients may also present with signs and symptoms of **metastatic disease** to local nodal areas (axillary, infraclavicular, supraclavicular, internal mammary, mediastinal, and cervical lymph nodes) or common sites of distant metastases including bone, lung, and liver.

F Diagnosis

1. **Pretreatment evaluation**
   a. In addition to a **medical history, physical examination, chest radiograph,** and **routine laboratory tests,** all women with newly diagnosed breast cancer should have a bilateral diagnostic **mammogram to detect multicentricity** or **bilateral involvement.** Breast MRI with gadolinium contrast can be considered to further rule out multicentric or contralateral disease. In addition, ultrasound of the tumor mass and ipsilateral axilla should be performed before final surgical recommendations are made to rule out axillary involvement.
   b. **Radiologic (staging) tests** may include a bone scan and CT or PET/CT scans as dictated by clinical presentation. If metastatic disease is detected, then, if technically feasible, an effort should be made to pathologically confirm the presence of metastatic disease by tissue biopsy.
   c. **Excisional surgical biopsy** for the pathologic diagnosis of breast cancer is indicated only for patients if a **core needle biopsy** is not possible.
   d. Patients with metastatic disease may have elevation in CA 15-3, CA 27-29, or CEA **tumor markers.** The value of these markers to monitor disease status remains controversial.

G Staging   For full staging information, see the most recent edition of the *AJCC Cancer Staging Handbook.*

H Prognosis   Approximately 50% of patients with operable breast cancer develop recurrent or metastatic disease. Prognostic factors include the following:

1. **Tumor size.** Tumors larger than 5 cm are associated with a decreased survival rate and an increased risk of recurrence. The 20-year disease-free survival rate for women with lymph node–negative breast cancers treated with mastectomy alone is 75%–80% for T_{1c} (1–2 cm) tumors and 92% for $T_{1a\text{-}b}$ (<1 cm) tumors.

2. **Axillary lymph node status** is the strongest prognostic factor. Seventy percent of patients with negative nodes are disease-free at 10 years. Disease-free survival declines to 40% of patients with no more than 3 positive nodes and 15–25% for patients with 4 or more positive nodes.

3. **Distant metastases.** Many patients survive for prolonged periods of time with metastatic disease, and prognosis depends on the number and location of metastases, response to therapy, and rate of progression of disease. The median survival is approximately 24 months.

4. **Tumor grade.** Breast tumors are graded morphologically by assessing for tubule formation, nuclear pleomorphism, and number of mitoses. Each factor is graded on a 3-point scale, for a maximum of 9 points for a poorly differentiated (grade 3) tumor, which has higher recurrence rates.

5. **Hormone receptor status.** Of primary breast cancers, 60%–70% express ERs and 40%–50% express PRs. Patients with hormone receptor–positive tumors have lower rates of local and distant recurrence initially and prolonged survival rates compared with those with receptor-negative tumors. However, these patients appear to have higher rates of "late" recurrence after 5 or more years from the time of the initial diagnosis and treatment.

6. **S-phase fraction and DNA index.** The S-phase fraction (i.e., the percentage of tumor cells in the S phase of the cell cycle) is proportional to the tumor growth rate. Patients with aneuploid tumors or high S-phase fractions, as determined by flow cytometry, generally have a poorer prognosis compared to those with slow-growing diploid tumors.

7. **Overexpression.** Expression of the HER2/*neu* oncogene is associated with a poorer prognosis. All breast cancers should be tested for the presence of HER2/*neu* expression by IHC, and only tumors that are +3 positive are considered truly positive and should be considered for trastuzumab therapy.

8. **Other factors associated with a poor prognosis** include the presence of lymphatic, vascular, or perineural infiltration; cathepsin-D; mutated p53; epidermal growth factor receptor; and tumor growth factor-β (TGF-β).

I Therapy   The primary goal of local therapy is to provide optimal control of the disease in the breast and regional tissues while providing the best possible cosmetic result. Systemic therapy should be given to patients at high risk for developing metastatic disease to eradicate micrometastases. Patients should be seen by a medical oncologist, radiation oncologist, and breast surgeon to determine the best course of initial treatment, which may include surgery, radiation therapy, adjuvant chemotherapy, adjuvant endocrine therapy, trastuzumab, or a combination of these.

1. **Surgery**
   a. The optimal surgical **approach** is determined by disease stage, tumor size, tumor location, breast size and configuration, number and location of tumors in the breast, available surgical and radiotherapeutic techniques, and patient preference concerning breast conservation.
   b. **Procedures.** In the past, most patients underwent modified radical mastectomy; however, multiple clinical trials have shown that breast conservation procedures such as lumpectomy plus whole-breast irradiation allow adequate control of the tumor and improve cosmetic outcomes. Breast-conserving therapy is considered the standard of care when technically feasible if this approach does not negatively impact systemic control. Contraindications for breast conservation therapies are summarized in Table 5–17.
   (1) **Modified radical mastectomy** involves removal of the breast and axillary contents with preservation of the pectoral muscles. Patients may undergo breast reconstruction during surgery or at a later time.
   (2) **Partial mastectomy, quadrantectomy,** or **lumpectomy** involves excision of the tumor and an adjacent rim of normal tissue.
      (a) **Sentinel node biopsy (SNB)** is a useful means for limiting axillary lymph node dissection. It is a minimally invasive procedure in which dye is injected around the tumor bed and the identified sentinel lymph node(s) are excised.

TABLE 5–17   Contraindications for Breast Conservation Therapy

Large tumor in a small breast (increases likelihood of poor cosmetic results)
Subareolar primary tumors or inflammatory breast cancer
More than one tumor in the breast (multicentricity)
Contraindications to radiation therapy
Advanced disease (i.e., beyond stage II)
Large areas of intraductal disease or microcalcifications
Tumors with an extensive intraductal component (i.e., >25% of the primary tumor is in situ and there is at least one focus of breast cancer that is in situ in normal breast tissue and is separate from the breast primary)

      (b) Axillary dissection is performed for adequate staging and local control only if the SNB is positive.

2. **Radiation therapy**
   a. **Patients treated with lumpectomy and SNB or full axillary dissection** should receive whole-breast radiation therapy with a boost to the tumor bed. Patients with more than three positive lymph nodes or extranodal extension of the tumor should also receive radiation to the lymphatic bed.
   b. **After mastectomy,** postoperative radiation should be considered if there are any of the following risk factors for local recurrence:
      (1) Primary tumor >4 cm
      (2) More than three positive axillary nodes
      (3) Tumor involving the surgical margin, invasion of pectoral fascia or muscle, or extranodal extension into the axillary fat
   c. In **patients at high risk for metastases,** radiation therapy is delayed until the completion of adjuvant chemotherapy. The risk of ipsilateral arm lymphedema is increased by postoperative axillary radiation.

3. **Adjuvant chemotherapy** delays or prevents recurrence and improves survival in patients with positive axillary nodes as well as in some patients with negative axillary nodes. Premenopausal patients with positive axillary nodes are most likely to benefit from adjuvant combination chemotherapy. A course of 6 months of adjuvant combination chemotherapy reduces the annual risk of breast cancer death by about 38% for women aged <50 years and by approximately 20% for women aged 50–69 years. Addition of trastuzumab to chemotherapy results in 52% reduction in the risk of recurrence and a 33% reduction in the risk of death for patients with HER2/*neu*-amplified early-stage breast cancer.
   a. **Drug regimens.** Maximally tolerated doses should be used unless significant toxicity develops.
      (1) The most commonly used adjuvant therapy regimens contain combinations of doxorubicin, cyclophosphamide, methotrexate, and 5-FU. Taxanes are important components of adjuvant therapy in patients with node-positive disease. The anti-HER2/*neu* monoclonal antibody trastuzumab (Herceptin) is FDA approved for adjuvant therapy in patients with HER2/*neu*-positive cancers.
      (2) Patients at higher risk for developing recurrent or metastatic disease are typically offered doxorubicin- or taxane-containing regimens.
   b. **Combination chemotherapy** is commonly used in the high-risk adjuvant setting (patients with stage II–III disease and some patients with stage I disease), and a course of 4–6 months of treatment (four to eight cycles of combination chemotherapy every 2–3 weeks) is usually sufficient to obtain maximum benefit. Patients at higher risk for developing recurrent or metastatic disease are typically offered doxorubicin and taxane-containing regimens (six to eight cycles). The two short (four cycle) regimens frequently used as adjuvant therapy include AC (doxorubicin and cyclophosphamide) or TC (docetaxel and cyclophosphamide). The more extended regimens are reserved for patients with lymph node–positive breast cancer and include TAC (docetaxel, doxorubicin, and cyclophosphamide) for six cycles or AC for four cycles every 2 weeks (dose-dense) followed by paclitaxel for four cycles every 2 weeks. Four to eight cycles of therapy (depending on the regimen) over 3–6 months are as effective as longer treatment periods.
   c. **Trastuzumab and combination chemotherapy.** Patients who have HER2/*neu*-positive cancers also should receive 52 weeks of trastuzumab therapy in conjunction with chemotherapy. Trastuzumab is never combined with anthracyclines due to increased risk of cardiotoxicity.
   d. **Metastatic breast cancer.** The use of sequential single-agent therapy is as effective as combination chemotherapy regimens, which are more likely to be toxic. Response rates are generally higher with combination chemotherapy, although this does not lead to significant improvements in overall survival. High-dose chemotherapy with autologous stem cell rescue does not improve treatment outcomes in women with early-stage or metastatic breast cancer and is not recommended. Several chemotherapy agents, including paclitaxel, docetaxel, ixabepilone, vinorelbine, gemcitabine, and capecitabine, are considered effective for the treatment of advanced breast cancer as single agents or in combination and may be used to palliate

patients with metastatic disease. Trastuzumab and lapatinib (Tykerb), a TKI inhibitor, are used successfully in combination with various chemotherapy agents for treatment of HER2/*neu*-positive metastatic breast cancer.

    4. Endocrine therapy

        a. Adjuvant endocrine/hormonal therapy. Both premenopausal and postmenopausal patients with positive hormone receptors (ERs and/or PRs) are offered endocrine therapy after completion of chemotherapy.

            (1) The selective estrogen receptor modulator (SERM) tamoxifen and aromatase inhibitors (AIs) such as anastrozole, letrozole, and exemestane are the preferred agents. AIs are FDA approved for postmenopausal women only and can be used up front for 5 years or sequentially after 2–5 years of tamoxifen therapy for a total of 5–10 years of adjuvant hormonal therapy. Tamoxifen and AIs delay recurrence and improve survival.

            (2) **Surgical oophorectomy** and **ovarian suppression** with luteinizing hormone–releasing hormone (LHRH) agonists are effective therapies for premenopausal patients with ER-positive tumors. Data from clinical trials indicate that the benefit is similar to that of chemotherapy with cyclophosphamide, methotrexate, and 5-FU. Two clinical trials are evaluating the benefit of LHRH plus aromatase inhibitors compared to LHRH plus tamoxifen and tamoxifen alone in premenopausal, ER-positive early-stage breast cancer (Suppression of Ovarian Function Trial [SOFT] and Tamoxifen and Exemestane Trial [TEXT]).

            (3) Patients with ER-negative tumors exhibit little or no response to hormonal therapy; therefore, it is not indicated in either the adjuvant or metastatic setting.

        b. Hormonal therapy for metastatic breast cancer

            (1) Hormonal therapy is appropriate for patients with subcutaneous metastases, lymph node involvement, pleural effusions, bone metastases, and nonlymphangitic lung metastases. Most patients with liver metastases, lymphangitic disease of the lung, pericardial metastases, or other potentially life-threatening metastases are treated initially with chemotherapy to obtain a rapid response, but such treatment decisions must be customized.

            (2) Patients with ER-positive primary tumors exhibit response rates of at least 30% to hormone therapy. If the tumor contains high expression of both ERs and PRs, response rates are higher.

            (3) Postmenopausal patients whose hormone receptor status is unknown may respond to hormone therapy, but a tissue biopsy should be attempted to restain the tissue for ER, PR, and HER2/*neu* receptors.

            (4) Patients with a previous response to hormonal therapy may respond to substitution of the original agent for a second agent.

            (5) Hormonal therapy options include tamoxifen, toremifene, fulvestrant (Faslodex), anastrozole (Arimidex), Letrozole (Femara), exemestane (Aromasin), megestrol (Megace), fluoxymesterone (Halotestin), and LHRH antagonists.

        c. The results of studies of **ovarian ablation by radiation, oophorectomy,** or **chemical ablation** in premenopausal patients have been mixed. Certain subgroups may gain long-term benefits.

    5. Other types of breast cancer and treatment recommendations

        a. Intraductal breast cancer (ductal carcinoma in situ [DCIS]). Because the tumor is noninvasive (i.e., confined to the ducts), careful pathologic review is necessary to confirm the diagnosis. The risk of lymph node involvement or distant metastases is minimal, and the prognosis is generally excellent with local therapy alone (surgery and/or radiation therapy to the breast).

            (1) Patients may be treated by total mastectomy with or without lymph node biopsy or by lumpectomy followed by radiation to the whole breast. Negative margins of resection of at least 1 mm are required.

            (2) Axillary lymph node dissection is controversial; most experts believe it is unnecessary.

            (3) Tamoxifen is widely used in the postoperative setting to prevent recurrence and to prevent second primaries in the ipsilateral and contralateral breast.

        b. Lobular CIS. Patients with this noninvasive lesion are at higher risk for development of invasive cancer in both breasts. Treatment options include rigorous observation and follow-up and tamoxifen prophylaxis therapy. Rarely bilateral mastectomy is performed for prophylaxis.

   c. Stage I and stage II disease. Most patients have the option of either breast conservation with lumpectomy or modified radical mastectomy with sentinel node biopsy (SNB). Axillary lymph node dissection is reserved for patients with positive SNB. Postoperative radiation therapy is also recommended for all patients who had a lumpectomy and is administered after completion of adjuvant chemotherapy but can be given concurrently with hormonal therapy and trastuzumab. Adjuvant therapy (chemotherapy, hormonal therapy, and trastuzumab) should be offered to high-risk stage I patients and all stage II patients; the choice of therapy is based on the ER, PR, and HER2/*neu* tumor status.

   d. Stage III disease

     (1) Patients with operable tumors are generally treated with modified radical mastectomy and postoperative radiation therapy. These patients also receive adjuvant chemotherapy and trastuzumab where indicated followed by hormonal therapy when the tumor is ER and/or PR positive.

     (2) Patients with inoperable stage III disease have poor survival rates.

       (a) A combined-modality approach is required, using systemic neoadjuvant chemotherapy with trastuzumab for HER2/*neu*-positive cancers in addition to surgery and radiation and hormonal therapy for ER/PR-positive cancers.

       (b) In most cases, aggressive combination chemotherapy is initiated after biopsy to reduce tumor bulk, facilitate local treatment, and treat distant micrometastases.

X   GYNECOLOGIC MALIGNANCIES

A **Ovarian cancer**

   1. Incidence. Ovarian cancer develops in approximately 1 in 71 women, with the highest incidence rates in industrialized nations. In 2009, there were 21,550 new cases of ovarian cancer diagnosed, with 14,600 deaths in the United States.

   2. Risk factors for ovarian cancer include the following:

    a. Nulliparity

    b. Family history of ovarian cancer

    c. History of endocrine disorders

    d. Age

    e. Early menarche before age 12 years or late menopause after age 50 years

    f. Use of postmenopausal estrogen therapy

    g. Genetic risk factors, including hereditary breast and ovarian cancer syndromes associated with *BRCA1* and *BRCA2* [see IX B 1 b (2)] and hereditary nonpolyposis colorectal cancer syndrome (Lynch syndrome).

   3. Screening. Ovarian cancer is rarely diagnosed before the disease has reached an advanced stage (stage III or IV).

    a. Screening is recommended in women with known high-risk genetic syndromes such as *BRCA1* and *BRCA2* mutations and Lynch syndrome and for women with a strong family history of ovarian cancer. Pelvic examination, pelvic ultrasound, and CA-125 are utilized for screening.

    b. Early detection. Women with average risk for ovarian cancer should obtain routine gynecologic examinations. No existing diagnostic modality exhibits sufficient sensitivity and specificity to permit the reliable early detection of surgically curable ovarian cancers in average-risk women.

   4. Pathology. The majority of ovarian cancers are epithelial in origin and include serous, mucinous, endometrioid, transitional, and clear cell types. Clear cell has the worse prognosis. Less common are the germ cell and stromal tumors.

   5. Clinical features

    a. Local symptoms include abdominal discomfort, low back pain, bloating, and abdominal distention.

    b. Systemic manifestations include the following:

     (1) Virilization from germ cell tumors

     (2) Precocious puberty in premenarchal women, **amenorrhea** in women of reproductive age, and **vaginal bleeding** in postmenopausal women can be caused by granulosa cell tumors.

6. **Diagnosis**
   a. **Initial evaluation**
      (1) **Pelvic ultrasound** detects small lesions in the ovary, even those that cannot be palpated during bimanual examination.
      (2) **Tumor marker CA-125** levels and an annual **pelvic ultrasound** are recommended in patients with a family history of ovarian cancer. However, elevations of CA-125 are not specific and may be elevated in patients without ovarian cancer.
   b. **Pretreatment evaluation**
      (1) All patients with ovarian cancer should undergo abdominal and pelvic CT scanning and/or MRI and a pelvic ultrasound. Chest radiography, cystoscopy, flexible sigmoidoscopy, and barium enema may be considered, depending on the presentation of the disease.
      (2) An elevated CA-125 is found in 80%–85% of patients with metastatic disease. If a germ cell tumor is suspected, the tumor markers lactate dehydrogenase (LDH), alpha-fetoprotein (AFP), and human chorionic gonadotropin (β-hCG) should be drawn.
      (3) A careful laparotomy establishes the stage and extent of the disease and may permit the reduction of tumor masses.
         (a) The entire abdominal contents should be explored, and any suspicious lesions should be removed and examined by biopsy.
         (b) In addition to checking the primary tumor for rupture or adherence, the surgeon should note the amount and type of ascites (if present). Samples of fluid should be collected for cytologic analysis by peritoneal washing.
         (c) The renal hilar para-aortic nodes should be biopsied.
         (d) The diaphragmatic surfaces should be carefully explored.

7. **Staging.** For full staging information, see the most recent edition of the *AJCC Cancer Staging Handbook.*

8. **Prognosis**
   a. The **stage of disease** is the most important prognostic factor.
      (1) Patients with distant metastases are rarely cured, even after combination chemotherapy.
      (2) Disease limited to the ovary may be cured with surgery alone.
      (3) Patients with minimal disease have a good prognosis with debulking surgery followed by combination chemotherapy, especially if the residual tumor masses measure less than 2 cm in diameter.
   b. **Histologic grade** has greater prognostic significance than type. Borderline tumors, which display nuclear characteristics of malignancy but lack stromal invasion, behave in an indolent fashion but are not responsive to chemotherapy.

9. **Therapy**
   a. **Surgery**
      (1) **Procedures**
         (a) **Transabdominal hysterectomy and bilateral salpingo-oophorectomy** (TAH/BSO) with resection of gross residual disease is indicated.
         (b) Since ovarian cancer is frequently associated with omental and peritoneal seeding, the entire abdominal and pelvic cavities should be explored, a **partial omentectomy** performed, and the paracolic gutters inspected.
      (2) **Adjuvant therapy and follow-up**
         (a) Patients with stage IA or stage IB disease with well-differentiated or moderately differentiated tumors require no additional therapy after surgery. Patients with stage III and IV disease should receive adjuvant therapy, which usually consists of **carboplatin and paclitaxel** for six cycles postoperatively. Advanced ovarian cancer is not curable by surgery alone. However, **reduction** of bulky cancer is associated with an improved response to either radiation or chemotherapy if the largest residual mass is reduced to <2 cm in diameter. Less extensive reductions are not beneficial, even if large amounts of the tumor are removed.
         (b) **Second-look surgery.** Surgical reexploration after the conclusion of chemotherapy can detect remission, assess response, and allow further cytoreductive surgery in an attempt to prolong survival. However, this is rarely recommended.

b. Chemotherapy. Systemic chemotherapy results in high response rates in patients with ovarian cancer and increases the likelihood of a cure in patients with resectable disease.

   (1) **Drug regimens.** Contemporary combination regimens commonly use **paclitaxel** in conjunction with **carboplatin** or **cisplatin.**

   (a) Renal-adjusted carboplatin is equivalent in efficacy to cisplatin and is associated with less emesis, peripheral neuropathy, and ototoxicity, although it has an increased rate of bone marrow toxicity compared with cisplatin. Because carboplatin can be administered easily in the outpatient setting, it is generally preferred over cisplatin to treat ovarian cancer.

   (b) Taxanes are associated with approximately 30% response rates in patients who have failed to respond to other therapies. Taxane–platinum combinations induce complete clinical remission in more than 60% of women with previously untreated stage III ovarian cancer.

   (2) **Treatment of residual disease after induction chemotherapy**

   (a) **Intraperitoneal chemotherapy** is based on the slow peritoneal clearance of many chemotherapeutic agents relative to total body clearance. Some studies demonstrate that intraperitoneal chemotherapy is advantageous compared with systemic chemotherapy in the treatment of ovarian cancer. Typical agents include paclitaxel and cisplatin administered in large volumes (1–2 L) through semipermanent catheters.

   (b) **Salvage chemotherapy** options in platinum-resistant disease include docetaxel, etoposide, gemcitabine, and topotecan.

   (c) **Radiation therapy.** In advanced disease, localized radiation therapy is an option for palliation of symptoms.

B **Cervical cancer**

1. **Incidence.** Cervical carcinoma, once one of the most common causes of death from cancer, has been decreasing in incidence over the last 30 years, likely due to the use of the Papanicolaou (Pap) smear for cervical cancer screening. Cervical cancer affects 11,270 women annually, with more than 4070 deaths per year. Invasive cancer is most frequently seen in patients between 45 and 55 years of age from lower socioeconomic groups.

2. **Etiology**

   a. **Risk factors** for cervical cancer include the following:

   (1) Early initial sexual activity or multiple sexual partners
   (2) Early age at first pregnancy and multiple pregnancies
   (3) History of venereal infection
   (4) Oral contraceptive use

   b. Cervical cancer has been associated with **human papillomavirus (HPV) infection,** particularly types 16 and 18, which account for 60%–75% of invasive squamous cell cervical cancers and 70% of adenocarcinomas of the cervix. The oncogenes *c-myc* and *ras* have also been implicated.

3. **Screening.** The **Pap smear** is useful for detecting early lesions and has a sensitivity of 90%–95%.

   a. Women should be screened every 2 years beginning at age 21 years, then every 3 years after the age of 30 years if they have had three consecutive negative results. Women with risk factors, including HIV, immunosuppression, history of diethylstilbestrol (DES) exposure in utero, or history of cervical intraepithelial neoplasia (CIN) or cervical cancer, should be tested more frequently. Screening should end at age 70 years if a woman has had no abnormal cytology tests within the previous 10 years or earlier if she has had a complete hysterectomy.

   b. Hemorrhage, inflammatory reactions (e.g., a fungating mass), or invasive cancer may result in false-negative smears.

4. **Pathology**

   a. **Squamous metaplasia,** the precursor of **cervical intraepithelial neoplasia (CIN),** is subdivided into three grades according to severity.

   (1) Grade I (mild-to-moderate dysplasia)
   (2) Grade II (moderate-to-severe dysplasia)
   (3) Grade III (severe dysplasia and CIS)

b. CIS exhibits cytologic evidence of neoplasia without invasion of the basement membrane. This stage can persist as long as 3–10 years before progressing to invasive cervical carcinoma.

5. Clinical features
  a. Local symptoms include abnormal vaginal bleeding or vaginal discharge.
  b. Systemic features include the following:
   (1) Fatigue and anemia secondary to chronic bleeding
   (2) Pain in the lumbosacral or gluteal area suggesting hydronephrosis or involvement of the iliac or periaortic lymph nodes
   (3) Urinary or rectal symptoms
   (4) Leg pain or **edema** resulting from lymphatic or venous blockage

6. Diagnosis
  a. Early detection. Women with abnormal Pap smears or women with visible cervical lesions should undergo **cervical biopsy.** If there are no visible lesions, colposcopy (using a binocular microscope and light source) reduces the need for cervical conization.
  b. Pretreatment evaluation should include basic lab work, chest radiography, CT scans of the abdomen and pelvis, and a barium enema in patients with symptoms involving the colon or rectum.
   (1) Because of the possibility of upper extension of the tumor, **curettage** of the endocervical canal and endometrium is recommended during the initial evaluation.
   (2) Cystoscopy and **rectosigmoidoscopy** are performed in selected patients with advanced disease.

7. Staging. For full staging information, see the most recent edition of the *AJCC Cancer Staging Handbook.* Clinical staging is often inaccurate, with more than 30% of patients having more extensive disease by laparotomy than is suggested by clinical staging procedures.

8. Prognosis. The 5-year survival rates for stage I, II, III, and IV cervical cancers are 75%–95%, 65%–70%, 35%–40%, and 10%–20%, respectively.
  a. Tumor volume and grade are important prognostic factors. Histologic subtype has little significance, except for some unusual variants.
  b. Lymph node metastases are associated with a poor prognosis.
  c. Other poor prognostic factors include **high tumor grade, depth of invasion,** and **lymphovascular space invasion.**

9. Therapy. Cervical cancer is treated with combinations of **surgery, radiation therapy, and/or cisplatin-based chemotherapy.**
  a. Total abdominal hysterectomy is the usual treatment for CIS, stage I microinvasive cancer (i.e., an invasion of <3 mm in depth), and high-grade CIN in women who have completed childbearing. In women who wish to bear children, management with **cervical conization** and careful follow-up may be appropriate. The risk of central recurrence and lymph node metastasis is increased when the tumor exceeds 3–5 mm in depth; in these cases, hysterectomy and pelvic lymphadenectomy are indicated.
  b. Radical hysterectomy, pelvic lymphadenectomy, and **radiation therapy** have similar results in stage IB and stage IIA cancers. Because of the 15%–25% incidence of lymph node metastases, treatment consists of radical hysterectomy and bilateral pelvic lymphadenectomy.
   (1) Postsurgical complications include bladder and urethral dysfunction or fistulas.
   (2) Radiation therapy (brachytherapy or external beam radiation) is indicated after surgery for microscopic parametrial extension, lesions greater than 4 cm, nodal metastases, lymphatic or vascular invasion, positive margins, and grade III lesions.
  c. Radiation therapy or **surgery** is appropriate for patients with invasion beyond the cervix but without distant metastatic involvement. If there is parametrial spread (i.e., the tumor extends through the pelvic wall or into the vagina), radiation therapy may be preferred.

C Endometrial cancer

1. Incidence. Endometrial carcinoma accounts for 6% of all malignant tumors in women and is the most common gynecologic malignancy. Approximately 42,160 new cases are diagnosed annually, resulting in more than 7780 deaths.

2. **Risk factors**
   a. **Obesity, diabetes, hypertension, polycystic ovarian disease, late onset of menopause, increasing age, and Lynch syndrome** are risks.
   b. **Unopposed estrogen therapy** also poses an increased risk. Progesterone decreases the risk associated with the use of postmenopausal estrogens. Use of combination oral contraceptives appears to decrease risk.
   c. Other risk factors include tamoxifen use, chronic anovulation, and irregular menses.

3. **Screening.** There are currently no screening guidelines for early detection in asymptomatic women without a history of genetic predisposition.

4. **Pathology.** Most endometrial cancers (75%–80%) are **adenocarcinomas.** Other types include papillary serous and clear cell carcinoma, both of which are highly aggressive tumors. Squamous cell endometrial carcinoma is rare.

5. **Clinical features**
   a. **Local symptoms** include **abnormal vaginal bleeding,** which is seen in approximately 90% of cases. In premenopausal women symptoms may include prolonged or heavy menses and intermenstrual spotting.
   b. **Systemic manifestations** include bowel obstruction, jaundice, ascites, and pelvic pain.

6. **Diagnosis**
   a. Most women with endometrial cancer have abnormal uterine bleeding.
   b. Less than 20% of cases of endometrial cancer are identified by Pap smear. Other diagnostic procedures include transvaginal ultrasound, endometrial biopsy, hysteroscopy with dilatation and curettage (D&C), and endometrial brush techniques.
   c. **Pretreatment evaluation** includes routine laboratory testing, urinalysis, chest radiograph, and, occasionally, hysteroscopy or hysterography.
      (1) **CT** and **cystoscopy** should be performed if there is evidence of bladder dysfunction.
      (2) Patients with lower gastrointestinal symptoms should undergo **proctosigmoidoscopy** and **barium enema.**

7. **Staging.** For full staging information, see the most recent edition of the *AJCC Cancer Staging Handbook.* More than 75% of women have stage I disease at the time of diagnosis.

8. **Prognosis**
   a. **Stage at diagnosis** is the most important prognostic factor. Five-year survival rates are 85%–90% for stage I, 74%–83% for stage II, 50%–66% for stage III, and 20%–25% for stage IV disease.
   b. Other important prognostic factors include the patient's **age, extent of cervical and myometrial invasion or vascular invasion, lymph node involvement** (especially pelvic or para-aortic nodes), and **histologic grade. Clear cell or papillary serous tumors** have a worse prognosis. Of lesser importance are uterine size and positive peritoneal cytology.

9. **Therapy.** Treatment measures include **surgery, radiation therapy, hormone therapy,** and, occasionally, **chemotherapy.**
   a. **Early-stage disease**
      (1) Low risk (stage IA, IB, IC, grade 1): total abdominal hysterectomy and bilateral salpingo-oophorectomy (TAH/BSO) only.
      (2) Intermediate risk (stage II, grade 1): TAH/BSO with para-aortic and selective pelvic lymph node dissection. Adjuvant radiation therapy may be offered for tumors with deep myometrial invasion, high-grade histology, cervical involvement, and vascular space invasion.
      (3) High risk (stage IB or IC high grade, any stage II or III): TAH/BSO and periaortic lymph node sampling and postoperative radiation.
      (4) For stage IIB or higher disease, adjuvant chemotherapy may be recommended. Doxorubicin, cisplatin, carboplatin, and paclitaxel are the most commonly used agents.
   b. **Metastatic disease**
      (1) Synthetic progestational agents are the most commonly used hormone therapy agents, with response rates of approximately 15%–20%. The probability of response depends on the histologic grade of the tumor and the presence of progesterone receptors. Well-differentiated tumors have the highest response rates.

(2) SERMs including **tamoxifen** have a 20%–30% response rate in patients who do not respond to standard progesterone therapy. Low-grade tumors that are PR positive respond best to tamoxifen.

(3) Chemotherapy response rates range from 10% to 50% using doxorubicin, cisplatin, and/ or paclitaxel.

c. Specific treatment recommendations. Adenomatous endometrial hyperplasia can be treated with hysterectomy or hormone therapy, depending on the patient's desire to bear children.

(1) Continuous combination estrogen and progesterone contraceptive agents or high-dose progestins are used in hormone therapy. Ovulation can be induced with clomiphene, if necessary.

(2) Patients maintained on hormone therapy should be carefully monitored and undergo routine endometrial sampling.

XI TESTICULAR CANCER

A **Incidence** Testicular cancer is the most common malignancy in men aged 15–35 years, with an average age at diagnosis of 32 years. In 2009, 8400 cases and 380 deaths were seen in the United States, accounting for 1% of all male cancers.

B **Risk factors** include **hypospadias,** a **cryptorchid testicle, abnormal testicular development, Klinefelter's syndrome,** and a **prior history** of testicular cancer. **Familial testicular germ cell tumors** have an autosomal recessive inheritance, with 4- to 10-fold increased risk in first-degree relatives. There may be an association between testicular germ cell tumors and **organochlorine compounds.**

C **Screening** Because of the low prevalence of testicular cancer and the limited accuracy of screening tests, routine screening in asymptomatic men is not recommended. The ACS, however, does recommend annual testicular exams.

D **Pathology** Testicular tumors are classified as **germ cell** and sex-cord or **gonadal stromal tumors.** Germ cell tumors, which comprise 95% of all testicular tumors, are further classified as **seminomatous** or **nonseminomatous** tumors.

1. Seminomas are further classified as **classical, anaplastic,** or **spermatocystic.**

2. Nonseminomatous tumors include embryonal carcinoma, teratoma, yolk sac carcinoma (also known as endodermal sinus tumor), and choriocarcinoma

E **Clinical features**

1. More than 90% of patients have a **painless, solid testicular swelling,** which may be found incidentally. Occasionally, patients with painful testicular masses are erroneously diagnosed as having epididymitis or orchitis.

2. Para-aortic lymph node involvement can manifest as **ureteral obstruction,** back pain, or new-onset varicocele.

3. Patients also may have **abdominal complaints** from abdominal masses or pulmonary symptoms from multiple nodules.

4. Gynecomastia and **hyperthyroidism** may occur in patients with elevated β-hCG levels. Gynecomastia may occur as a consequence of testicular failure and low testosterone levels after successful chemotherapy.

F **Diagnosis**

1. Radiologic evaluation

a. Scrotal ultrasound may show suspicious intratesticular echogenic foci and can define invasion of the spermatic cord, epididymis, and scrotum.

b. Chest radiograph and/or **CT scans** of the chest, abdomen, and pelvis, as well as the brain (in patients with neurologic symptoms).

c. **Bone scan** (if there is skeletal pain).

d. Excretory urography and venacavogram are rarely used.

2. **Inguinal exploratory surgery,** including high ligation of the spermatic cord with orchiectomy, is necessary for patients with suspicious scrotal masses without a confirmed diagnosis. Open biopsy and scrotal exploration are contraindicated because of the possibility of tumor spread. In addition, vascular control must be achieved before manipulation of the tumor.

3. **Elevated blood levels of AFP** or **β-hCG** are diagnostic of nonseminomatous germ cell tumors. Levels are often normal in seminomas.

G **Staging** For full staging information, see the most recent edition of the *AJCC Cancer Staging Handbook.*

H **Prognosis** is subdivided into good, intermediate, and poor.

1. **Prognosis** for nonseminomas and seminomas is determined by the presence of metastases and the level of AFP, β-hCG, and LDH.

2. **Survival rates.** Five-year survival rates for **nonseminomas** for good, intermediate, and poor prognosis are 92%, 80%, and 48%, respectively. The 5-year survival rates for **seminomas** for good and intermediate prognosis are 86% and 72%, respectively. No poor prognosis category exists for seminomas.

I **Therapy**

1. **Nonseminomatous tumors.** In the absence of advanced metastases requiring immediate chemotherapy, most patients undergo orchiectomy for definitive treatment. Approximately 30% of patients with clinical stage I nonseminomatous germ cell tumors have occult retroperitoneal lymph node metastases. The risk is higher (approximately 50%) if the primary tumor is predominantly embryonal carcinoma and shows vascular invasion.

   a. **Clinical stage I disease** (limited to the testis).

   (1) Unilateral **retroperitoneal lymph node dissection** is used if lymph nodes are negative, allowing the preservation of ejaculatory function. Otherwise, a bilateral procedure is performed. Rigorous follow-up with CT imaging and marker studies may be appropriate.

   (2) Primary chemotherapy with bleomycin, etoposide, and cisplatin effectively prevents relapse and "overtreats" 50% of patients.

   (3) The treatment chosen depends on several factors, including patient age, reliability, feasibility of close follow-up, risk of relapse (as estimated from primary tumor histologic features and CT scan), need to maintain fertility, and patient preference.

      (a) In TN_1-, TN_2-, or M_0-staged patients with nonseminomatous cancer, those with seminomas and elevated AFP levels, or seminomas with persistent β-hCG elevation after orchiectomy, a bilateral retroperitoneal lymph node dissection is performed.

      (b) Observation is an option for clinical N_0 patients.

   b. **Stage II disease** involves surgery or chemotherapy.

   (1) Patients with tumors less than 3 cm in diameter may be treated with node dissection for curative intent.

   (2) Patients with retroperitoneal tumors more than 5 cm in diameter should receive chemotherapy.

   (3) Adjuvant chemotherapy after complete resection is optional. Patients who have proven extranodal extension, any node more than 2 cm in diameter, or at least six positive nodes have a relapse rate after node dissection of greater than 50%. With adjuvant chemotherapy, however, the relapse rate approaches zero.

2. **Seminomatous tumors**

   a. **Stage I seminomas** are usually treated with retroperitoneal and pelvic radiation therapy after surgery. In the United States, radiation therapy remains the standard approach, but there is emerging evidence that surveillance may be a viable alternative. With this approach, approximately 15% of patients relapse, but salvage therapy using chemotherapy or radiation therapy is effective in almost all cases. After treatment, patients should be reevaluated every month for the first year and every 2 months for a second year.

b. **Stage II seminomas.** All patients with stage II seminoma have retroperitoneal node metastases.
  (1) **Radiation therapy** is the treatment of choice for patients with N_1 and N_2 disease. Because of bone marrow toxicity from mediastinal radiation therapy, prophylactic radiation to the mediastinum is no longer indicated.
  (2) Patients with N_3 retroperitoneal adenopathy have a high relapse rate after radiation therapy; these patients should receive **chemotherapy** instead. Bleomycin, etoposide, and cisplatin may be used.
c. **Stage III or IV seminomas (and nonseminomatous germ cell tumors)** are generally treated with **cisplatin** in combination with **etoposide** and **bleomycin** (BEP) at 3-week intervals for three or four cycles. Four cycles of etoposide plus cisplatin have been shown to be equivalent to three cycles of bleomycin plus etoposide plus cisplatin.
  (1) Other chemotherapeutic options for patients with recurrent disease include ifosfamide, paclitaxel, and vinblastine.
  (2) Surgical removal of residual masses after chemotherapy is usually recommended. Such masses contain viable cancer in 10%–15% of cases, fibrosis or necrosis in 40%–45%, and teratomas in 40%. Radiologic studies cannot distinguish among these possibilities. Patients with viable residual tumors should receive two additional cycles of chemotherapy. Surgery also may be considered as a "salvage" therapy for patients who are refractory to cisplatin-based chemotherapy in resectable disease confined to one anatomic site.
  (3) High-dose chemotherapy with carboplatin, etoposide, and cyclophosphamide may be combined with an autologous bone marrow transplant or peripheral blood stem cell support in selected patients with chemotherapy-sensitive relapses.

XII CANCERS OF THE KIDNEY, BLADDER, AND PROSTATE

A Renal cell cancer (hypernephroma)

1. **Incidence.** Cancer of the kidney accounts for 3%–4% of all cancers, with 57,760 new cases diagnosed each year. The ratio of affected men to women is approximately 1.5:1, with an average age of 55–60 years at presentation.

2. **Risk factors. Cigarette smoking** and **obesity** are the strongest risk factors. Patients with **von Hippel–Lindau disease** or **acquired polycystic kidney disease** have a higher incidence of renal carcinoma. **Familial** types of renal cell carcinoma have been associated with abnormalities of chromosome 3 and the p53 gene. Other risk factors include hypertension, high consumption of fried or sautéed meats, chronic hepatitis C infection, chronic dialysis therapy, and exposure to asbestos or petroleum products. **Renal medullary carcinoma** is associated with **sickle cell trait.**

3. **Screening.** There are currently no screening guidelines for early detection in asymptomatic persons.

4. **Pathology**
   a. Most renal tumors are clear cell adenocarcinomas; together with chromophobe and papillary cell carcinomas, these account for 85%–90% of renal cell cancers. Other types include granular cell tumors, mixed tumors, and aggressive carcinosarcomas (adenocarcinomas with sarcomatous degeneration). Rarely, tumors arise in renal cysts, especially in chronic dialysis patients.
   b. Renal cancers are usually **extremely vascular, readily metastasizing** to the lung, bone, liver, brain, and other sites. Dissemination also may occur when tumor emboli enter the renal vein and inferior vena cava or by nodal spread in the para-aortic, paracaval, hilar, and mediastinal areas.

5. **Clinical features**
   a. Hematuria (40%–70% of patients)
   b. Abdominal mass with flank pain (20%–40% of patients)
   c. Weight loss (30% of patients)
   d. Fever, malaise, night sweats, or anemia (15%–30% of patients)
   e. Paraneoplastic syndromes, including hypercalcemia, polycythemia, hyponatremia, or hypertension

6. **Diagnosis.** Diagnostic procedures including hematologic studies, renal ultrasound, chest radiographs, abdominal CT, and radionuclide bone scans are used to detect the presence of metastases. **CT scans** are adequate for initial diagnosis and staging. **MRI** is superior for visualizing tumor or thrombus in the renal vein and vena cava.

7. **Staging.** For full staging information, see the most recent edition of the *AJCC Cancer Staging Handbook*.

8. **Prognosis.** Radical nephrectomy yields a 5-year survival rate in 75% of patients with localized tumors. Patients with high-grade stage III lesions and invasion of major vascular structures have a survival rate of only 30%–40%.

9. **Therapy**
   a. **Surgery**
      (1) **Radical nephrectomy** with lymph node dissection is the treatment of choice for stage I, stage II, and stage III renal cell carcinomas. Nephrectomy should also be considered for patients with disseminated disease to relieve hematuria, flank pain, or paraneoplastic syndromes.
      (2) In certain cases, **selective renal arterial embolization** permits surgical resection or halts life-threatening hematuria.
      (3) Patients with few metastatic lesions, indolent tumor growth, and no evidence of progressive metastasis may be candidates for aggressive **surgical resection of metastases.**
   b. **Radiation therapy** has only limited value because most tumors are relatively radioresistant. However, radiation therapy offers the best palliative options for painful bone metastases or nerve root compressions.
   c. **Chemotherapy** is also relatively ineffective, with transient tumor regression occurring in fewer than 5% of patients. Sunitinib (Sutent) and sorafenib (Nexavar) are oral agents directed against the intracellular tyrosine kinases that have demonstrated promising efficacy and are now FDA approved for therapy of advanced renal cell cancer. A related kinase inhibitor, temsirolimus, is also FDA approved for advanced disease.
   d. **Biologic response modifiers**
      (1) **IFN-α** yields response rates of 13%–20% in patients with soft tissue or lung metastases. It can be combined with bevacizumab, an angiogenesis inhibitor approved by the FDA in 2009.
      (2) High-dose **IL-2** therapy yields partial or complete tumor regression in approximately 15% of cases. However, the treatment is extremely toxic and requires a high level of supportive care and admission to the intensive care unit. Although most responses are limited in duration, complete responses tend to be durable.

B **Urothelial (transitional cell) carcinomas** (bladder, ureter, and renal pelvis)

1. **Incidence.** These tumors account for approximately 3% of the cancer deaths in the United States. The annual incidence is approximately 73,250 cases, with 15,120 deaths. From 80% to 85% of patients present with superficial tumors without muscle-wall invasion at diagnosis. Bladder carcinomas are three times more common in men and usually occur in patients who are 50–70 years of age.

2. **Risk factors**
   a. **Tobacco** use.
   b. **Occupational carcinogens** in the rubber, dye, printing, and chemical industries (aromatic amines, polycyclic hydrocarbons, and solvents).
   c. **Schistosomiasis** of the bladder has been strongly correlated with squamous cell carcinoma.
   d. Other etiologic agents include **cyclophosphamide, phenacetin** (banned in the United States in the 1970s), **renal stones, chronic bladder infection,** and possibly **aristholochic acid.**
   e. **Molecular alterations** in the **p53** and **Rb** tumor suppressor genes are involved in 20%–40% of tumors. The prognosis worsens when one or more of these genes are mutated.
   f. **Saccharin** has been shown to cause bladder tumors in animals, but its role in humans is unproven.

3. **Screening.** There are currently no screening guidelines for early detection in asymptomatic people.

4. **Pathology.** Bladder tumors are generally of transitional cell origin, with the exception of the schistosome-related variant, which is of squamous cell origin.

5. **Clinical features.** Eighty-five percent of patients present with **hematuria,** and 25% present with **bladder irritability** or **infection.** Constitutional symptoms such as weight loss and abdominal or bone pain may be present in advanced disease.

6. **Diagnosis**
   a. **Cystoscopy,** with bimanual palpation and subsequent biopsy, is the definitive diagnostic procedure. This technique is nearly 100% accurate.
   b. **Radiologic procedures** include pelvic and abdominal CT scans, chest radiography, bone scan, and retrograde pyelography for renal pelvic or ureteral tumors.
   c. **Urine cytology with flow cytometry** is an option for high-risk patients.

7. **Staging.** For full staging information, see the most recent edition of the *AJCC Cancer Staging Handbook.*

8. **Prognosis**
   a. Major prognostic factors are the **tumor stage** at time of diagnosis and **degree of tumor differentiation.** Other adverse prognostic factors include older age, expression of p53, aneuploidy, tumor multifocality, and presence of a palpable mass. Although women have a lower incidence of urothelial carcinoma of the bladder, they more often present at advanced stages and have a relatively worse survival than men.
   b. Five-year survival rates for patients with superficial, muscle-invasive, and metastatic bladder cancer are 95%, 50%, and 6%, respectively.

9. **Therapy**
   a. **Surgery**
      (1) **Superficial lesions** (stages T_a, T_1, and sometimes T_{2a}) are treated with **endoscopic resection** and **fulguration,** followed by cystoscopy every 3 months. Recurrent or multiple lesions are treated with intravesicular instillation of thiotepa, mitomycin, or BCG.
         (a) The recurrence rate after transurethral resection (TUR) is 50%–70%. The recurrence rate is higher if the size of the tumor is greater than 3 cm, if it is multifocal and associated with CIS, or if it is a high-grade T_1 lesion.
         (b) Even with BCG prophylaxis after TUR, most patients develop recurrences, and some progress to muscle-invasive disease.
      (2) **Recurrent cancer, diffuse transitional cell CIS,** or **stages T_2 and T_3 invasive cancers** are treated with **radical cystectomy.**
      (3) Tumors of the renal pelvis or ureter are treated by **removal of the affected kidney or ureter.**
   b. **Combination chemotherapy**
      (1) In randomized studies, combination chemotherapy with **gemcitabine and cisplatin** has been shown to be as effective as and better tolerated than methotrexate-vinblastine-doxorubicin-cisplatin (MVAC) in patients with advanced disease. However, these studies were not powered to detect a survival benefit with this regimen.
      (2) Newer combination regimens include gemcitabine plus paclitaxel, cisplatin plus paclitaxel, and paclitaxel plus carboplatin.

C **Prostate carcinoma**

1. **Incidence.** Cancer of the prostate accounts for 13% of all new cancers in the United States each year, with more than 192,300 cases diagnosed. Incidence rates are higher among blacks and increase with age. In the United States, the risk of death is approximately 9%.

2. **Risk factors** include **age, family history,** and **race.** Geographic location has also been implicated, with rates of prostate cancer lowest in Asia and higher in Scandinavia and the United States.

3. **Screening.** Currently there is insufficient evidence regarding the value of testing for early prostate cancer in the average-risk man. However, the ACS recommends that prostate-specific antigen (PSA) testing and digital rectal exam (DRE) should be offered annually beginning at age 50 years to men of average risk whose life expectancy is at least 10 years, at the age of 40 years for African American men, and for those with a family history of prostate cancer.

4. **Pathology.** Nearly all prostate cancers are adenocarcinomas.
   a. Prostate adenocarcinomas are classified as **well differentiated, moderately well differentiated, or poorly differentiated** according to the **Gleason prognostic classification system,** which assigns a grade between 0 and 5 to the primary and secondary differentiation patterns.
   b. Most prostatic tumors originate in the peripheral zone; only 25% originate in the central zone.
   c. More than 90% of distant metastases involve bone, but soft tissue metastases also can occur in the lymph nodes, lung, and liver.

5. **Clinical features.** The majority of prostate cancers are nonpalpable at the time of diagnosis and are identified by elevated PSA levels. Symptoms, if present, may include a palpable nodule, dysuria, urinary retention, hematuria, and urinary dribbling, frequency, or urgency. Systemic manifestations of metastatic disease include bone pain, weight loss, and, rarely, spinal cord compression.

6. **Diagnosis**
   a. **Digital rectal examination** remains the diagnostic gold standard for prostate carcinoma, even though only 10% of the prostatic tumors found as nodules on rectal examination are sufficiently localized for cure.
   b. Ten percent of **pathologic specimens** removed for treatment of obstructive prostatic hypertrophy show malignancy. Other cases of prostate cancer are found in advanced stages; often these cancers are **revealed in investigations for metastatic bone disease.**
   c. **Prostate-specific antigen** is an established diagnostic marker, but false positive values may occur. If the PSA is >10 ng/mL, then 66% of the prostate biopsies indicate prostate cancer. If the PSA is between 4 and 10 ng/mL, then 22% of the biopsies will be positive. The percentage of free PSA (e.g., unbound to plasma α_1-antichymotrypsin) may increase diagnostic specificity, but this occurs at the cost of overall sensitivity.
   d. **Transrectal ultrasonography (TRUS)** is most useful for evaluation of prostate size and for the precise biopsy of lesions that are not palpable. However, as a sole diagnostic tool, it is insensitive and nonspecific.
   e. Rectal, perineal, or urethral **needle biopsy** confirms the diagnosis.
   f. **Laboratory studies** are used to assess renal function.
   g. **Radiologic studies,** including bone scans, radiographs, and pelvic or abdominal CT, confirm the presence of metastatic disease.

7. **Staging.** For full staging information, see the most recent edition of the *AJCC Cancer Staging Handbook*. Staging techniques are used along with the histologic grade (Gleason score) and the PSA level to determine the probability that carcinoma limited to the prostate is curable by surgery or radiation. Clinical staging alone is not accurate.
   a. Stage T_{1a} and T_{1b} tumors
   b. Stage T_2 tumors
   c. Stage T_3 tumors
   d. Stage T_4 tumors

8. **Therapy and prognosis** are determined by the clinical stage of disease, PSA level, and histologic (Gleason) grade at diagnosis. Comorbidities and life expectancies also factor into treatment decisions.
   a. **Early disease** is treated with radical prostatectomy, external beam radiation, or brachytherapy. In selected cases, no treatment (e.g., expectant management) is appropriate.
      (1) **Prostatectomy** is performed in patients with at least a 10-year life expectancy. Patients with cancers of stage T_{1b}, T_{2a}, and T_{2b} and younger patients with T_{1a} disease are candidates for surgical cure. Up to 16% of patients with clinical T_{1a} disease progress.
      (2) **Nerve-sparing radical prostatectomy** is appropriate for patients with small lesions. This approach preserves sexual function in some men but has a 5%–15% rate of postsurgical urinary incontinence and depends on the expertise and training of the surgeon.
      (3) **Radiation therapy** is used for older patients, patients with other medical disorders, patients with large prostatic lesions precluding surgery, and men who wish a better chance to retain normal sexual activity. With modern techniques, including conformal radiation therapy, 70–75 Gy provides good local control with acceptable morbidity. External beam radiation is useful in palliating metastatic bone disease. Strontium-89 or samarium-153

may be useful when administered intravenously to palliate pain in patients with widespread bone disease. Intensity-modulated radiation therapy (IMRT) can be used to deliver high radiation dose with improved normal tissue tolerance. Diarrhea, rectal bleeding, and proctitis are sometimes associated with this form of treatment.

b. Stage IV tumors cannot be cured, but prolonged survival (>5 years) may be possible in subgroups of patients with low-grade tumors. The early use of androgen suppression also may improve survival.

(1) Endocrine therapy is generally the initial mode of treatment.

(a) Orchiectomy is the preferred therapy in patients with cardiovascular or thrombotic risk. Postsurgical administration of exogenous estrogens such as diethylstilbestrol (DES) further suppresses testosterone levels.

(b) Pharmacological approaches include the LHRH analog **leuprolide** (Zoladex), either alone or in combination with an antiandrogen (e.g., **flutamide**). **Aminoglutethimide or ketoconazole plus a corticosteroid** is an option for patients who fail to respond to primary hormone treatment. These hormonal manipulations induce remission in 50%–80% of patients, although cures are rare. Typically, prostate and soft tissue lesions regress, acid phosphatase and PSA levels decline, and bone pain decreases, with an average duration of the initial hormone response of 9–18 months.

(2) Chemotherapy has improved and is destined to be used in earlier stages of disease. The most frequently used agents are estramustine with vinblastine, paclitaxel, docetaxel, or etoposide. Mitoxantrone plus a corticosteroid has established palliative value beyond that of corticosteroids alone, and the FDA has approved the use of this combination in hormone-refractory prostate cancer. Doxorubicin and cyclophosphamide also may produce palliation. Treatment options may be limited for metastatic hormone-refractory prostate cancer because of advanced age and additional comorbidities.

XIII CENTRAL NERVOUS SYSTEM CANCERS

A Incidence The incidence of primary malignant brain and central nervous system tumors (excluding lymphomas, leukemias, pineal, and pituitary tumors) in the United States is 6.4 per 100,000 with a slightly higher rate in men. They comprise 1.4% of all primary malignant cancers.

B Histologic classification for central nervous system tumors is based on the cell type that originates the abnormal growth.

C Clinical Presentation

1. **Symptoms due to generalized cerebral disturbance** include cognitive decline, seizures, malaise, and personality changes.

2. **Symptoms due to raised intracranial pressure** include headache, nausea, vomiting, and sixth nerve palsy. Uncal herniation may lead to third nerve palsy, stupor, coma, bilateral upper motor neuron deficits, decerebrate posturing, apnea, and death, while cerebellar tonsillar herniation may cause apnea, asystole, hypotension, and death. Compression of the cerebral peduncle leads to contralateral upper motor neuron deficits. Parinaud's syndrome, or paralysis of upward gaze, may occur with tumors of the pineal region.

3. **Focal neurologic deficits** depend on the site affected. For example, seizures may occur in cortical involvement. Frontal lobe involvement may result in disinhibition, aphasia, and cognitive decline. Sensory disturbance, apraxia, and acalculia may occur in parietal lobe involvement. Depersonalization and auditory hallucinations may occur in temporal lobe lesions. Cerebellar lesions may cause ataxia, and occipital lobe lesions may lead to visual disturbances.

D Diagnosis

1. **Imaging.** Noncontrast **CT scan** is diagnostic for meningioma and can detect hydrocephalus and a midline shift. CT may miss structural tumors, especially those of the posterior fossa, and nonenhancing tumors (e.g., low-grade gliomas); **MRI** with gadolinium contrast is the test of choice. **PET** scans can supplement MRI (e.g., hypometabolism on PET suggests low-grade behavior).

2. **Cerebral arteriography** is important in distinguishing between a pituitary adenoma and an aneurysm in tumors of the sellar region.

3. **Open surgical biopsy** is performed when possible; otherwise, a stereotactic biopsy is an option for tumors that are nonresectable.

4. Lumbar puncture may be dangerous due to risk of herniation.

E **Staging** For full staging information, see the most recent edition of the *AJCC Cancer Staging Handbook*.

F **Treatment** Treatment is variable and depends on the type of tumor.
1. **Surgery**
   a. **Total resection** is attempted for most tumors whenever feasible, except for primary cerebral lymphomas. Total resection may be impossible if the tumor involves critical regions or large areas of the brain.
   b. **Ventricular shunting** may relieve increased intracranial pressure.
   c. **Carmustine (BCNU)-impregnated wafers** implanted at the time of surgery have modest survival benefits in patients with recurrent glioma.

2. **Radiation therapy** is administered for a majority of brain tumors, with the exception of ependymomas, which are not radiosensitive.
   a. **Whole-brain irradiation** is recommended for carcinomatous meningitis and multiple lesions.
   b. **Stereotactic radiation therapy and radiation surgery,** including Gamma Knife and CyberKnife, are used for focal lesions ≤3cm size

3. **Chemotherapy** has limited survival benefits in most primary CNS malignancies. **Temozolomide** in addition to radiation therapy is recommended for high-grade gliomas, and methotrexate is used for cerebral lymphoma. Other agents used as salvage therapy include etoposide, carboplatin, irinotecan, and procarbazine–lomustine–vincristine (PCV), but this therapy does not significantly improve survival.

G **Prognosis** depends on several factors, including the following.
1. **Histological type.** High-grade tumors such as glioblastoma multiforme have poorer prognosis than more differentiated neoplasms such as gliomas.

2. If the **location** of a tumor or its **extent** limits surgical resectability, the prognosis is poor. For example, brainstem gliomas are usually unresectable, and the complete excision of astrocytomas or craniopharyngiomas is usually not possible. On the other hand, many pituitary adenomas, oligodendrogliomas, and meningiomas are often completely resectable, with associated improved survival. Carcinomatous meningitis has a very poor prognosis.

3. **Performance status and age of patient.** The 5-year survival for patients aged <19 years is 66%, compared to only 4.7% for those >75 years old. There is also a slight trend toward higher survival in **women.**

4. Use of **combination radiation therapy and chemotherapy** may also improve survival in several types of tumors, such as astrocytomas and lymphomas. **Temozolomide** improves survival in selected patients with astrocytomas.

5. **Status of the patient's immune system.** Survival in primary cerebral lymphoma in patients with HIV correlates with the absolute CD4 count.

XIV ENDOCRINE SYSTEM CANCERS

A **Thyroid cancer**
1. **Incidence** of thyroid cancer in the United States is 37,200 cases, with 1630 deaths. Papillary carcinoma is typically diagnosed in patients aged 30–50 years, while follicular carcinoma occurs in patients aged 40–60 years.

2. **Risk factors** include **female sex** and a history of **childhood radiation exposure.** Familial syndromes, including **multiple endocrine neoplasia (MEN) types 2a and 2b,** increase the risk of developing medullary thyroid carcinoma. A **low-iodine diet** is a risk factor for follicular thyroid carcinoma.

3. **Screening.** Routine screening is not indicated in healthy patients of average risk. In patients with higher risk, thyroid ultrasound is recommended.

4. **Pathology**
   a. **Papillary carcinoma** is the most common subtype of thyroid cancer, occurring in nearly 80% of cases.
   b. **Follicular carcinoma** (10%–15%) is difficult to distinguish from follicular adenoma, a benign condition, by fine needle aspiration alone. Pathologic determination of capsular or vascular invasion is required.
   c. **Medullary carcinoma (MTC)** (5%–10%) begins in the parafollicular cells (C cells), which are responsible for **calcitonin** production.
   d. **Anaplastic carcinomas** (1%–2%) are highly aggressive tumors typically found in patients older than 50 years and have a nearly 100% mortality rate.

5. **Clinical Features**
   a. **Local symptoms** may include a painless thyroid nodule, hoarseness from recurrent laryngeal nerve involvement, or dysphagia from esophageal compression. Many patients are asymptomatic at the time of diagnosis.
   b. **Systemic manifestations** may arise from a functional thyroid nodule and may include palpitations, heat intolerance, and/or weight loss.

6. **Diagnosis.** Thyroid cancer is diagnosed by the detection of a **palpable thyroid nodule** on physical examination or as an **incidental finding** on a CT scan performed for other indications. **FNA** with histologic evaluation is required for all suspicious thyroid nodules. **Radioactive iodine scan** may distinguish between functioning ("hot") and nonfunctioning ("cold") thyroid nodules. All cold nodules should be surgically excised and sent for pathologic examination. Preoperative evaluation with **ultrasound** can identify lymphatic involvement, and **PET scans** can help determine the presence of distant metastasis.

7. **Staging.** For full staging information, see the most recent edition of the *AJCC Cancer Staging Handbook*.

8. **Prognosis.** Negative prognostic factors for **papillary carcinoma** include age >45 years, a large or bilateral tumor, presence of vascular or soft tissue invasion or distant metastasis at the time of presentation, and a high percentage of vascular endothelial growth factor tumor receptors. Capsular extension, vascular invasion, and high-grade histology are risk factors for decreased survival in **follicular carcinoma.**

9. **Therapy**
   a. **Papillary and follicular carcinomas** are initially treated with total or subtotal **thyroidectomy** followed by adjuvant **radioactive iodine (RAI)** therapy. **Thyroxine** should be given to prevent hypothyroidism and to suppress thyroid-stimulating hormone. Combination doxorubicin-based **chemotherapy** and **radiation therapy** may prolong survival. Sorafenib has also shown some promise in ongoing trials for the treatment of thyroid cancer.
   b. Patients with **medullary thyroid cancer** should receive total thyroidectomy with cervical lymph node dissection. Adjuvant radiation therapy has been shown to improve disease-free survival; chemotherapy with doxorubicin provides minimal improvements in survival rates. Octreotide may be used to palliate symptoms.
   c. Most **anaplastic thyroid carcinomas** are unresectable at the time of diagnosis, and treatment is **palliative.** Chemotherapy with paclitaxel has a 50% initial response rate, but response is not durable. External-beam radiation may provide palliation of symptoms.

B **Parathyroid carcinoma** is rare, although incidence increased over the last decade. Patients may present with profound **hypercalcemia,** a neck mass, and bone or renal disease. **Surgery** is the mainstay of treatment, and there is little role for adjuvant chemotherapy or radiation therapy. Additional treatment involves control of hypercalcemia with hydration, bisphosphonates, and, more recently, **cinacalcet,** an FDA-approved calcimimetic used to treat secondary hyperparathyroidism.

C **Adrenal**

1. **Adrenocortical carcinoma (ACC)** is a rare, aggressive tumor that occurs in children <5 years of age and in adults in the fourth and fifth decades. Most cases are sporadic, although there is a

higher incidence in familial cancer syndromes such as MEN1 and Li–Fraumeni syndrome. Other risk factors include smoking and oral contraceptive use. Nearly 60% of ACCs are functional and produce virilization and/or Cushing's syndrome. They may also present with symptoms due to local mass effect in larger tumors, or they may be found incidentally on routine imaging (e.g., "incidentaloma"). Prognosis is poor, with a 5-year survival of approximately 30%. Treatment is primarily surgical, although local recurrence is common if the tumor capsule is violated. Options for adjuvant therapy include mitotane with etoposide, doxorubicin, and cisplatin or with streptozocin. Adjuvant radiation therapy is controversial but is currently recommended for stage III disease or for patients with incomplete resection.

2. **Pheochromocytomas** are catecholamine-secreting tumors of the adrenal chromaffin cells, and 10% are malignant. Surgery is indicated for all pheochromocytomas, and intensive medical management with sequential perioperative alpha- and beta-blockade is necessary. Adjuvant combination chemotherapy or local radiation may be used in malignant disease. Metastases can occur decades after initial diagnosis, so long-term follow-up is necessary.

XV SKIN CANCER [See Chapter 13]

XVI SARCOMAS

A **Incidence** Approximately 9500 sarcomas are diagnosed in the United States each year, constituting 1% of adult malignancies.

B **Risk factors**

1. Exposure to **radiation.**

2. Exposure to **chemicals** (e.g., wood preservatives, herbicides, vinyl chloride, asbestos).

3. Certain **medications** (e.g., tamoxifen increases risk of uterine sarcoma).

4. **Genetic abnormalities,** including Li–Fraumeni and Gardner syndromes, von Recklinghausen's disease, and the retinoblastoma (Rb) gene increase risk.

5. **Preexisting bone disease.** Osteosarcomas occur in 0.2% of patients with Paget's disease.

C **Screening** There are currently no screening guidelines for early detection in asymptomatic persons.

D **Pathology** Soft tissue sarcomas are classified according to the presumptive tissue of origin. Examples include perivascular, fibrohistiocytic, fibroblastic, myofibroblastic, and extraskeletal cartilaginous or osseous tumors.

E **Clinical features**

1. **Soft tissue sarcomas** often manifest as a **mass, swelling,** or **pain** in the trunk or extremities.

2. Patients with **retroperitoneal tumors** generally experience **weight loss** or **deep-seated pain.**

3. **Abnormal bleeding** is the most common presenting feature of **gynecologic** and **gastrointestinal sarcomas.**

4. Most patients with osteosarcomas present with **pain** and/or a **mass.**

F **Diagnosis**

1. **Biopsy** should be performed in any rapidly growing mass or a mass larger than 5 cm, especially if it is firm, deep, or fixed. These lesions generally require an excisional biopsy or a large incisional biopsy; needle biopsy is inadequate. The biopsy site must be selected carefully to allow for the possibility of limb-sparing surgery.

2. **Imaging procedures. MRI** is preferred for evaluation of soft tissue sarcoma and may be used to evaluate liver or bone involvement. **CT** and **bone scan** are also useful for bony evaluation.

G **Staging** For full staging information, see the most recent edition of the *AJCC Cancer Staging Handbook.*

H **Prognosis**

1. **Histologic grade** is determined by the mitotic rate, nuclear grade, extent of necrosis, nuclear morphology, and cellularity.

2. **Tumor size** is an independent prognostic factor. Small (<5 cm), completely excised, low-grade lesions rarely recur locally and have a low metastatic rate.

3. **Other factors** associated with an increased risk of local recurrence include age older than 53 years, presentation with recurrent disease, high-grade, painful mass, limb-sparing surgery, and inadequate surgical margins.

I **Therapy**

1. **Surgery** is the mainstay of therapy.
   a. **Definitive resection** may consist of extensive surgical excision, including a 2- to 4-cm pathologically documented margin of normal tissue, or conservative resection with documented tumor-free margins, supplemented with radiation therapy. Reexcision should be considered after biopsy if microscopically involved margins are demonstrated.
   b. **Limb-sparing surgery** is considered in most extremity sarcomas. This results in a 90% local control rate and an overall disease-free survival rate of 60%. This is similar to that seen with amputation or radical resection. **Neoadjuvant intra-arterial chemotherapy** and **radiation therapy** may facilitate limb-sparing surgery in borderline resectable tumors.
   c. If seeding of the surgical field occurs during the procedure, a wide excision should be performed, followed by 6600-cGy radiation therapy.
   d. Surgery may be curative in patients with few pulmonary metastases.

2. **Radiation therapy** may be used when the tumor margins are less than 2–4 cm or if tumor seeding has occurred.

3. **Chemotherapy**
   a. **Adjuvant chemotherapy** has no clear benefit except in young patients with osteosarcoma, rhabdomyosarcoma, or Ewing's sarcoma. Doxorubicin-based combination regimens have been shown to improve disease-free and overall survival rates in adults with extremity sarcomas.
   b. **Advanced sarcomas.** Previously treated patients may respond to doxorubicin (15%–35%), dacarbazine (17%), or ifosfamide (20%–40%). Studies suggest that combination chemotherapy, particularly with doxorubicin and ifosfamide, may yield improved results. The combination of gemcitabine plus docetaxel is highly active in patients with leiomyosarcomas.

4. **Targeted molecular therapy** with the tyrosine kinase inhibitor imatinib is used for gastrointestinal stromal tumors and dermatofibroma protuberans. Gefitinib is undergoing trials for treatment of advanced synovial sarcomas, while bevacizumab is being evaluated for the treatment of Kaposi's sarcoma.

XVII CANCER OF UNKNOWN PRIMARY SITE

A **Incidence**   Patients with cancer of unknown primary site (CUPS) have metastatic carcinoma in the absence of a known primary site. Approximately 5% of patients with newly diagnosed cancer have CUPS. Even at autopsy, the primary site remains obscure in 15%–25% of these patients.

B **Screening**   Because the primary site is unknown, there are no identifiable risk factors or screening recommendations.

C **Pathology**

1. **Histologic subtypes**
   a. **Adenocarcinoma** is most common, occurring in nearly 70% of patients.
   b. **Poorly differentiated carcinomas** make up 15%–20% of CUPS.
   c. **Squamous cell carcinomas** are present in 5% of patients.
   d. Other types include lymphomas, germ cell tumors, melanomas, neuroendocrine tumors, and sarcomas.
      (1) **Lymphoma** can sometimes be distinguished from undifferentiated carcinoma by special immunohistochemical stains for leukocyte markers such as leukocyte common antigen.

(2) **Metastatic small cell endocrine tumors** can be identified by staining for S-100 or neuron-specific enolase.

(3) **Germ cell tumors** may stain positive for AFP or β-hCG.

2. Light microscopy, electron microscopy, and immunohistochemical techniques may be useful in identifying the histologic subtype or tissue origin.

   a. Visualization of the cellular architecture by **light microscopy** may identify the histologic subtype of origin. However, since CUPS is often anaplastic, differentiation by light microscopy is not always possible.

   b. **Immunohistochemical markers** are important pathologic tools. For example, a positive keratin stain implies an epithelial origin.

   c. **Electron microscopy** detects **intercellular bridging,** characteristic of squamous cell carcinomas; **neurosecretory granules,** characteristic of neuroendocrine tumors; **melanosomes,** characteristic of melanoma; and **intracellular structures** such as myofibrils, characteristic of sarcomas.

D **Clinical features** Most patients present with symptoms due to metastatic disease. Nonspecific symptoms are common, including anorexia, weight loss, and fatigue.

E **Diagnosis** Due to advances in molecular diagnostics, many cases of CUPS can achieve a specific diagnosis based on immunohistochemical evaluation of biopsy specimens. In addition, because lung, pancreatic, and colon cancers are the most likely primary sources of undifferentiated adenocarcinoma, routine diagnostic procedures include a chest radiograph, fecal occult blood test (accompanied by colonoscopy in positive cases), and/or abdominal CT. PET scans may also be used to identify the primary site of disease in 20%–30% of cases.

1. Women should undergo **mammography, pelvic examination,** and **pelvic ultrasound.**

2. **PSA levels** and a testicular examination should be performed in men.

3. Patients with suspected germ cell carcinomas should also receive β-hCG and AFP determinations. The use of other tumor markers (e.g., CEA, CA 19-9) is not recommended due to low specificity.

4. Patients with clavicular lymphadenopathy should be evaluated with a CT scan of the head and neck, direct laryngoscopy, and nasopharyngoscopy to evaluate for head and neck squamous cell carcinomas.

F **Prognosis** Median survival is only 5–6 months after diagnosis, although the range is broad; 5%–11% of patients may be alive after 5 years.

G **Therapy**

1. **Empiric combination chemotherapy** with gemcitabine, platinum compounds, taxanes, and/or irinotecan is an option for adenocarcinomas of unknown primary site. Antiangiogenesis agents such as bevacizumab are also being investigated in the treatment of CUPS.

2. Women with suspected adenocarcinoma in an axillary node should be considered to have stage II breast cancer and be treated accordingly.

3. Patients with **squamous cell carcinoma metastatic to the neck** from an unknown primary site without distant metastases should be treated with neck dissection and radiation therapy to the neck.

4. Individuals—particularly men—with midline-dominant CUPS lesions (e.g., para-aortic or mediastinal lymphadenopathy) and pulmonary nodules should be treated for poor-prognosis nonseminomatous germ cell tumors.

5. Young men with **anaplastic tumors of the mediastinum or retroperitoneum** may respond to treatment modalities used for germ cell tumors of the testes, especially if AFP or β-hCG levels are elevated.

XVIII PARANEOPLASTIC SYNDROMES

A **Endocrine syndromes** resulting from ectopic polypeptide hormone production are the most common and best understood of the paraneoplastic processes. Many tumors produce more than one biologically active hormone, leading to multiple endocrine paraneoplastic syndromes.

1. **Criteria** for establishing ectopic hormone secretion by tumor cells include the following:
   a. **Increased hormone levels** on laboratory analysis. Note that some patients with elevated hormone levels do not have clinical symptoms.
   b. **Decreased hormone levels after removal or treatment of the tumor**
   c. **Persistent hormone elevation after removal of the normal gland** that usually secretes the hormone
   d. An **arteriovenous gradient for hormone levels** across the tumor vascular bed

2. **Types**
   a. **Ectopic growth hormone secretion** has been detected in patients with **lung and gastric carcinomas.** The elevated hormone levels may lead to hypertrophic pulmonary osteoarthropathy. Organomegaly may occur with slow-growing carcinoid tumors.
   b. **Ectopic ACTH secretion** was the first paraneoplastic endocrine syndrome described in the literature.
      (1) The most common **tumors associated with ectopic ACTH production** are **SCLC** and **atypical carcinoids.** High cortisol levels have also been described in patients with adenocarcinoma and large cell carcinoma of the lung, other carcinoid tumors, thymoma, neural crest tumors, medullary thyroid carcinoma, and bronchial adenomas.
      (2) **Clinical features.** Most patients have **hypokalemia** and **metabolic alkalosis.**
         (a) Patients rarely live long enough for frank Cushing's syndrome to develop. However, diabetes, hypertension, edema, muscle wasting, central obesity, moon facies, and striae may develop in those with extremely high cortisol levels.
         (b) Alterations in mental status, fatigue, and anorexia caused by opiate-like peptide fragments are rare symptoms.
      (3) **Diagnosis** is confirmed by a plasma ACTH level of >200 pg/mL, a plasma cortisol level of >40 mg/dL without diurnal variation, or a positive dexamethasone suppression test.
   c. **SIADH** can occur due to ectopic hormone production by a malignancy or may result from the use of certain medications or chemotherapy.
      (1) **Small cell lung cancer** is most the common malignancy associated with ectopic ADH secretion. SIADH is also associated with head and neck cancer, primary or metastatic CNS cancer, hematologic malignancies, and, rarely, breast, prostate, pancreatic, or other gastrointestinal malignancies. In addition, chemotherapy agents such as vincristine, vinblastine, cyclophosphamide, high-dose melphalan, thiotepa, and cisplatin may initiate SIADH, or the syndrome may develop as a side effect of general anesthesia or the use of antidepressants, antipsychotics, narcotics, carbamazepine, or chlorpropamide in cancer patients.
      (2) **Clinical features.** Patients present with **hypo-osmolar hyponatremia** and **inappropriately concentrated urine.**
         (a) Patients with mild hyponatremia may present with fatigue, nausea, anorexia, and headache.
         (b) Confusion, lethargy, hallucinations, seizures, coma, and death may result from serum sodium levels less than 115 mEq/L.
      (3) **Diagnosis.** Other causes of hyponatremia, including volume depletion, gastrointestinal electrolyte losses, diuretic use, abnormal fluid retention, cortisol deficiency, and hypothyroidism, must first be ruled out. SIADH is suggested by a low plasma osmolality (<280 mmol/kg) and a urine sodium excretion of >20 mEq/L without diuretic use in the setting of serum hyponatremia.
      (4) The initial **treatment** is **fluid restriction** (<500 mL/day) for patients without life-threatening symptoms. Patients who do not respond to conservative measures may be treated with demeclocycline, which inhibits renal response to ADH. If seizures or coma are present, therapy consists of infusion of 3% hypertonic saline with or without intravenous furosemide in the intensive care setting. Complete resolution of the disorder is frequently not possible unless the underlying malignancy is completely eradicated.
   d. **Ectopic secretion of parathyroid hormone–related protein (PTHrP)** is termed **humoral hypercalcemia of malignancy** and accounts for greater than 80% of cases of hypercalcemia in cancer. Tumors associated with this are head and neck squamous cell carcinomas, lung, breast, and gynecologic malignancies, renal carcinoma, lymphoma, and multiple myeloma.

(1) Secretion of PTHrP increases calcium resorption from bone and reduces calciuresis. PTHrP may also have paracrine effects to induce osteoclastic differentiation resulting in increased osteolysis.

(2) See XIX C for information on diagnosis, treatment, and prognosis.

B **Hematologic syndromes**

1. **Paraneoplastic syndromes of cellular blood components**

   a. **Erythrocytosis** occurs in renal cancer and hepatoma.

   b. **Pure red cell aplasia.** Severe anemia due to a complete lack of RBC production is uncommon. However, 50% of patients with pure red cell aplasia have **thymoma.** Many patients may also have other immunologic abnormalities, such as hypogammaglobulinemia, paraproteinemia, positive antinuclear antibodies, or autoimmune hemolytic anemia.

      (1) **Etiology.** The cause may relate to effects of suppressor T cells on red blood cell (RBC) production, leading to a severe reticulocytopenic anemia.

      (2) **Therapy.** In thymoma, surgery and radiation are not uniformly successful in reversing the anemia. **Corticosteroids, splenectomy,** or cyclophosphamide **immunosuppressive therapy** may be useful.

   c. **Autoimmune hemolytic anemia,** or **cold agglutinin disease,** is usually caused by an immunoglobulin produced by lymphoma or chronic lymphocytic leukemia cells.

      (1) **RBC indices** may be high or low, depending on the reticulocyte response. For example, if the reticulocyte count is high, the indices are normal or high. If immune hemolysis is present, multiple **spherocytes** are present.

      (2) **Therapy** with **prednisone** is often effective; **splenectomy** is occasionally useful. In most cases, however, therapy is not effective for long periods unless the underlying cancer is effectively treated.

   d. **Microangiopathic hemolytic anemia** occurs with mucin-producing adenocarcinomas, especially gastric cancer. There is no effective **treatment** except treating the underlying tumor.

   e. **Granulocytosis** may occur even in the absence of bone marrow involvement, and other causes of inflammation or infection must be excluded. The most common malignancies associated with granulocytosis include gastric, lung, and pancreatic carcinoma; melanoma; CNS tumors; Hodgkin's disease; and large cell lymphomas.

   f. **Thrombocytosis** occurs in as many as one third of all cancer patients. If essential thrombocythemia is present, hydroxyurea should be given to keep the platelet count below 500,000/mm^3.

   g. **Thrombocytopenia** is often due to secondary effects of chemotherapy, bone marrow involvement, or radiation therapy but is also seen in severe microangiopathic hemolytic anemia and DIC. A syndrome resembling autoimmune thrombocytopenia has been described in some leukemias and lymphomas and in certain solid tumors. This form of idiopathic thrombocytopenic purpura (ITP) is treated with corticosteroids, splenectomy, or immunosuppressive drugs.

2. **Paraneoplastic syndromes of the coagulation system**

   a. **DIC** occurs most frequently with mucin-producing adenocarcinomas such as pancreatic, gastric, lung, prostate, and colon cancers. Both acute and chronic DIC are associated with thrombophlebitis, arterial emboli, endocarditis, circulating inhibitors of coagulation, and abnormal circulating proteins that may precipitate hemorrhagic complications.

      (1) **Acute DIC** is often observed in acute promyelocytic leukemia as the result of the release of a procoagulant contained in the abnormal granules of the leukemia promyelocyte.

         (a) **Clinical features.** Early signs include elevation of the prothrombin time (PT) and fibrin split products and decreased fibrinogen. An increase in the partial thromboplastin time (PTT) occurs in more severe cases.

         (b) **Treatment** includes **aggressive transfusion support** to maintain a platelet count of 35,000–50,000/mm^3, **intravenous vitamin K,** and **clotting factor replacement** with fresh-frozen plasma or cryoprecipitate if the fibrinogen level is <75 mg/dL. **Heparin** is controversial but can be administered cautiously to refractory patients.

TABLE 5–18   Central Nervous System Paraneoplastic Syndromes and Associated Malignancies

Syndrome	Associated Malignancy
Limbic encephalitis	Small cell lung cancer
Subacute cerebellar degeneration	Ovarian cancer, small cell lung cancer
Subacute motor neuropathy	Lymphoma
Subacute sensory neuropathy	Small cell lung cancer
Sensorimotor polyneuropathy	Small cell lung carcinoma, Hodgkin's lymphoma
Eaton-Lambert myasthenia	Lung cancer, ovarian cancer
Polymyositis or dermatomyositis	Varied; breast, lung, gastrointestinal, and ovarian carcinomas are most common

      (2) Chronic DIC is most common in patients with adenocarcinomas.

         (a) Clinical features include mild prolongations of the PT, normal to slightly elevated fibrinogen levels, and elevation of the fibrin split products. Patients often have thrombophlebitis or pulmonary emboli.

         (b) Heparin is the treatment of choice; **thrombolytic therapy** may also be considered if there are no contraindications.

    b. Syndromes associated with paraproteins

      (1) Coagulopathy. Abnormal hemostasis and coagulation may develop in patients with plasma cell dysplasias (e.g., multiple myeloma) as a result of the effects of paraproteins on normal clotting factors and platelet receptor function. Paraproteins can also inhibit fibrin monomer aggregation and act as inhibitors of factor VIII. If patients have intractable bleeding, plasmapheresis may be required in combination with chemotherapy.

      (2) Hyperviscosity. In multiple myeloma and macroglobulinemia, patients with a serum viscosity greater than 4 (relative to water) may have signs of decreased blood flow, including headaches, dizziness, epistaxis, seizures, hearing loss, altered mental status, and cardiac disease. Treatment consists of prompt plasmapheresis to remove the excessive paraprotein and avoid dehydration, as well as treatment of the underlying plasma cell dyscrasia.

C **CNS syndromes** are rare. The most common are listed in Table 5–18.

XIX   ONCOLOGIC EMERGENCIES

A **Spinal cord compression (SCC)**

  1. Etiology. Most cases of SCC are due to metastatic breast, lung, or prostate cancer; lymphoma; multiple myeloma; or renal or gastrointestinal tumors.

  2. Clinical features include back or radicular pain with or without neurologic symptoms such as muscle weakness; changes in bowel or bladder function; sensory loss; or autonomic dysfunction. These symptoms should prompt a thorough physical and neurologic examination.

  3. Diagnosis. MRI with gadolinium contrast is the gold standard for diagnosing SCC because of its high sensitivity and specificity.

  4. Therapy. The goals of therapy for SCC include pain control, recovery of normal neurologic function, local tumor control, and avoidance of complications. All patients who are symptomatic and have an abnormal neurologic examination should receive corticosteroids immediately. In addition, surgery and radiation oncology consultations should be pursued immediately upon clinical suspicion of SCC in a patient with malignancy.

B **Superior vena cava syndrome (SVCS)**

  1. Etiology. SVCS is primarily caused by direct extrinsic compression of the superior vena cava (SVC) by bronchogenic carcinomas or non-Hodgkin's lymphoma of the anterior mediastinum. Other causes include metastatic mediastinal disease, central line thrombosis, fibrosing mediastinitis, or a retrosternal goiter.

  2. Clinical features of SVCS may be acute or chronic. Many patients will exhibit neck or chest wall superficial venous distension; facial, periorbital, or upper extremity edema; facial plethora; and/or cyanosis. Other symptoms include dyspnea, orthopnea, cough, and hoarseness.

3. **Diagnosis.** Although the diagnosis of SVCS can be made on physical examination alone, noninvasive imaging such as CT with contrast, MRI, and Doppler ultrasonography examination of the jugular or subclavian veins can be used to facilitate the diagnosis.

4. **Therapy.** If there is evidence of respiratory compromise or CNS involvement, emergent radiation therapy and airway stabilization are indicated. Nonemergent treatment consists of symptom relief and treatment of the underlying cause of SVCS. If at all possible, it is important to obtain a tissue diagnosis prior to treatment.

C **Hypercalcemia** Up to 20%–30% of patients with cancer develop hypercalcemia, making this the most common metabolic disorder associated with malignancy and the second most common cause of hypercalcemia as a whole.

1. **Etiology**
   a. A large proportion of patients with hypercalcemia of malignancy have **metastases to the bone,** which increases osteolytic activity. This is most commonly associated with breast cancer and multiple myeloma.
   b. The most common etiology of hypercalcemia in patients with nonmetastatic tumors is systemic secretion of **PTHrP** [see XVIII A 2 d].
   c. A rare cause of hypercalcemia is excessive production of active **vitamin D (1,25-dihydroxycholecalciferol),** seen in some lymphomas, which promotes the increase of osteoclastic bone resorption and increased calcium absorption from the gut.

2. **Clinical features.** Hypercalcemia may be found either in a patient with known malignancy or as the initial presentation of an undiagnosed cancer. Fatigue, mental status changes, dehydration (which can be severe), constipation, urolithiasis, cardiac arrhythmia, and generalized pain may occur.

3. The **diagnosis** is made upon finding hypercalcemia (>10.5 mg/dL and often >14 mg/dL) in a patient with an associated cancer. The serum intact parathyroid hormone (iPTH) is low or undetectable, serum PTHrP levels may be elevated, and both 1,25-dihydroxycholecalciferol and inorganic phosphate levels are low or normal. In a minority of lymphomas, the vitamin D level is elevated.

4. **Therapy**
   a. **Intravenous normal saline** repletes volume and increases the renal excretion of calcium.
   b. **Intravenous bisphosphonates** (e.g., zolendronate, pamidronate) prevent bone resorption by inhibiting osteoclasts.
   c. **Loop diuretics** inhibit renal calcium resorption in the ascending loop of Henle and induce a natriuresis, both of which cause calciuresis. Loop diuretics should only be administered after adequate volume expansion.
   d. **Calcitonin** increases distal tubular calciuresis and reduces bone resorption by decreasing osteoclast activity. It is given if a more rapid reduction in calcium levels is desired but becomes less effective after about 48 hours due to tachyphylaxis.
   e. **Glucocorticoids** are used in hypercalcemia associated with lymphoma or multiple myeloma to reduce gastrointestinal calcium absorption.
   f. **Specific treatment of the malignancy** is very important.

5. **Prognosis** depends on the associated malignancy, but survival is generally poor. Half of these patients die within 30 days of diagnosis of hypercalcemia.

D **Tumor lysis syndrome (TLS)**

1. **Etiology.** Cell death, with subsequent release of intracellular contents, commonly occurs after chemotherapy or in tumors with rapid cell turnover such as leukemias. This often results in life-threatening lactic acidosis, hyperkalemia, hyperphosphatemia, hyperuricemia, and hypocalcemia.

2. **Clinical features.** Many of the symptoms of TLS are associated with electrolyte abnormalities. For instance, patients can develop cardiac arrhythmias from severe hyperkalemia or hypocalcemia. Hyperphosphatemia and hyperuricemia of TLS may result in acute renal failure.

3. **Diagnosis.** Laboratory diagnosis of tumor lysis syndrome is based on having two or more electrolyte abnormalities, including elevated **uric acid** ($\geq$8 mg/dL), **potassium** ($\geq$6 mmol/L), or **phosphorus levels** ($\geq$4.5 mg/dL) and/or a low **calcium level** ($\leq$7 mg/dL).

4. **Therapy.** Corrective measures should be directed toward the metabolic derangements. Often these patients require close monitoring either in a telemetry or intensive care unit. The treatment of hyperuremic acute renal failure following chemotherapy consists of loop diuretics, intravenous fluids, and possibly recombinant urate oxidase (rasburicase). Patients at high risk for TLS should receive prehydration, allopurinol, and metabolic monitoring for 24–48 hours prior to the initiation of chemotherapy.

E **Fever and Neutropenia**

1. **Etiology.** Neutropenia may occur in cancer patients due to the direct myelosuppressive effects of chemotherapy, or it may be due to bone marrow infiltration. Neutropenia of brief duration (<7 days) is most likely associated with bacterial infections, with gram-positive bacteria representing approximately 66% of isolates and gram-negative bacteria account for 33%. In patients who remain profoundly neutropenic for ≥10 days, fungal infections, particularly *Candida* and *Aspergillus* species, must be considered.

2. **Clinical features.** By definition, neutropenic fever occurs in patients with an absolute neutrophil count (ANC) of ≤500 cells/mm^3 (or an ANC of ≤1000 cells/mm^3 with an anticipated continued decline) who present with a single oral temperature of ≥38.3°C (101°F) or fever of ≥38.0°C (100.4°F) persisting for more than 1 hour. Apart from fever and chills, the majority of patients do not have any localizing symptoms, but, if present, the most common symptom is pain at the site of infection. This paucity of clinical signs and symptoms is likely due to a lack of an inflammatory reaction.

3. **Diagnosis.** A thorough **physical examination,** including a detailed evaluation of the ocular fundus, oropharynx, teeth, lungs, perineum, anus, and skin, including vascular catheter sites, should be performed, remembering that the classic signs of infection may not be present. Digital rectal and pelvic exams are deferred to limit mucosal trauma and to reduce the risk of bacteremia. Bacterial and fungal **blood cultures** should be drawn from a peripheral vein, and urine and stool cultures are indicated if there are signs or symptoms of infection at these sites or if a urinary catheter is in place. Lumbar puncture is not routinely recommended but can be considered if the patient has altered mental status and meningeal signs. CSF fluid should always be sent for cytology as well as cultures. Biopsy and culture of skin lesions may also be indicated. A two-view **chest radiograph** is recommended as part of the initial evaluation. Other imaging studies such as CT scan, MRI, or nuclear imaging studies should be performed if any abnormality is found or if the patient continues to have unresolved or worsening symptoms.

4. **Therapy.** Since fever is often the only presenting symptom, empiric broad-spectrum antibiotics are begun immediately after cultures are obtained. Antibiotic resistance should always be considered in patients who are not improving on therapy.

   a. Low-risk patients may be treated as outpatients with close monitoring using oral ciprofloxacin or levofloxacin and amoxicillin–clavulanate.

   b. Most patients are treated in the hospital setting with intravenous antibiotics including a broad-spectrum carbapenem (e.g., imipenem–cilastatin or meropenem), a fourth-generation cephalosporin (e.g., cefepime), or an extended-spectrum penicillin and beta-lactamase inhibitor (e.g., ticarcillin–clavulanate or piperacillin–tazobactam). Vancomycin is added if a central venous catheter infection is suspected or if the patient was previously infected by or colonized with a resistant gram-positive organism. An aminoglycoside may also be added.

   c. Consideration should be given to catheter removal for severe infections or if bacteremia does not resolve within 72 hours.

   d. Infectious disease and medical oncology consultations should be considered early in the management of the febrile neutropenic patient.

Study Questions

1. A 55-year-old, postmenopausal woman presents for a yearly visit. A 1-cm nodule is palpated in the upper, outer quadrant of her right breast. Her most recent mammogram 6 months ago was negative. Her family history is significant for her mother and a sister both diagnosed with breast cancer in their early to mid-50s. She has hypertension and hypercholesterolemia. What is the most appropriate next step in her management?

- A Repeat mammogram and ultrasound now.
- B Repeat mammogram in 6 months.
- C Repeat clinical examination in 1 month and refer for mammography if there is an increase in the size of the nodule.
- D Begin tamoxifen.
- E Refer her to a surgeon.

2. The yearly mammogram of a 65-year-old postmenopausal woman shows an irregular area of micro-calcification that has grown in size compared with her mammogram from 2 years ago. She missed her mammogram last year. Physical examination is unrevealing without lymphadenopathy or nodularity in the breasts. You refer her to a surgeon, and a 2-cm invasive ductal carcinoma is removed from her left breast. Sentinel node biopsy shows two positive lymph nodes, and axillary dissection reveals five additional positive nodes. The tumor expresses the estrogen receptor (ER+). Which of the following interventions would increase her chance of cure?

- A Chemotherapy followed by hormonal therapy
- B Radiation therapy
- C Total mastectomy
- D Hormonal therapy alone
- E High-dose chemotherapy with stem cell support

3. A 65-year-old man who is being treated with neoadjuvant combination chemotherapy for stage IIIb non–small cell lung cancer presents to the emergency room with a 3-hour history of subjective fevers. His last chemotherapy treatment was 5 days ago. On examination, his oral temperature is 100.6°F, pulse is 115 bpm, and blood pressure is 92/54 mm Hg. He has a tunneled central venous catheter in the right internal jugular vein; there is erythema and mild tenderness to palpation at the insertion site. Cardiac, pulmonary, and abdominal examinations are normal. Laboratory data reveal a white blood cell count of 4.1 cells/mm^3 (82% lymphocytes, 12% neutrophils, 6% eosinophils), hemoglobin of 7.1 g/dL, and creatinine of 1.7 mg/dL. What is the most appropriate next step in this patient's management after cultures are drawn?

- A Begin intravenous cefepime and admit the patient.
- B Begin intravenous cefepime and vancomycin and admit the patient.
- C Begin oral ciprofloxacin and discharge the patient to home.
- D Begin oral penicillin and discharge the patient to home.
- E Begin intravenous amphotericin B and admit the patient.

4. A 61-year-old man with a history of gastroesophageal reflux disease and Barrett's esophagus is undergoing a screening endoscopy. The biopsy results show high-grade dysplasia. What is the recommended treatment approach?

- A Refer the patient to a surgeon for esophagectomy.
- B Repeat surveillance endoscopy in 6 months.
- C Repeat surveillance endoscopy in 1 year.
- D No further endoscopy is indicated unless the patient becomes symptomatic.
- E Initiate chemotherapy.

5. A 59-year-old postmenopausal woman returns for a regularly scheduled follow-up visit. She was diagnosed with irritable bowel syndrome 6 months ago after complaints of mild lower abdominal discomfort.

Today, she reports no improvement in her symptoms. She is otherwise well and has not lost weight. A 5.5-cm left adnexal cyst is discovered on abdominal ultrasound. The patient has a sister who died of breast cancer at 55 years of age and another sister who was treated for ovarian cancer at 50 years of age. The best management for this patient is:

- A. Initiate a trial of combination oral contraceptive pills with repeat pelvic and transvaginal ultrasound in 6 weeks to determine if the mass is still present.
- B. Provide reassurance and book a follow-up visit in 3 months.
- C. Check a CA-125 level.
- D. Undertake immediate exploratory laparotomy.
- E. Undertake colonoscopy now.

6. A 65-year-old man is evaluated for a 2 cm by 2 cm anterior cervical lymph node that is mobile and nontender and has been present for 4 months. He had successful treatment for glottic carcinoma 7 years previously, and subsequent examinations had suggested no recurrence. He has no hoarseness, dysphagia, epistaxis, fever, or oral discomfort. He stopped smoking 4 years ago but continues to drink four to five shots of bourbon daily. A careful oral examination does not yield any obvious lesions. What is the best next step in this patient's management?

- A. Direct examination of the nasal, nasopharyngeal and oropharyngeal passages including the larynx. If negative, provide reassurance and follow up in 6 months.
- B. Empiric antibiotic therapy with reevaluation in 2 weeks. If the lymph node has not resolved, then an excisional biopsy should be performed.
- C. Immediate fine needle aspirate and biopsy. If the results are not diagnostic, then an excisional biopsy should be performed.
- D. An incisional biopsy should be obtained, and if results are indeterminate, proceed to an excisional biopsy.
- E. Perform a random glottic biopsy since his glottic carcinoma could have recurred.

7. A 42-year-old woman presents to clinic for a routine visit. Her father and brother were diagnosed with colon cancer at ages 49 and 43, respectively. She denies abdominal pain, weight loss, melena, hematochezia, or changes in stool caliber. The best option for colorectal cancer screening in this patient is:

- A. Colonoscopy beginning at age 50 years
- B. CEA and CA 19-9 testing now
- C. Screening for *Helicobacter pylori* infection and treatment, if positive
- D. Barium enema with CEA and CA 19-9 testing beginning at age 50 years
- E. Colonoscopy now

8. A 75-year-old woman with metastatic breast cancer to the skeleton presents to the emergency department because she fell at home while getting up from her chair. Her family states that she has been lethargic and nauseated and notes that she has complained of dizziness and increasing thirst. She is found to be orthostatic on examination. Laboratory studies reveal the following: blood urea nitrogen 42 mg/dL, total serum calcium 12.2 mg/dL, serum creatinine 1.4 mg/dL, and serum albumin 2.8 g/dL. What is the most appropriate initial treatment?

- A. Slow rehydration with half-normal saline
- B. Intravenous administration of a bisphosphonate
- C. Vigorous rehydration with normal saline
- D. Intravenous administration of furosemide along with saline rehydration
- E. Intravenous administration of corticosteroids

9. A 50-year-old executive undergoes his first screening colonoscopy. He has been constipated for 1 year, relieved by laxatives. There has been no blood in his stools. A fungating mass is seen in the sigmoid colon, and subsequent surgery shows a lesion that has penetrated through the muscularis propria. Three regional lymph nodes are positive for adenocarcinoma. His best chance for cure would occur with which form of therapy?

- A. No further therapy needed
- B. Adjuvant chemotherapy

[C] Radiation treatment
[D] Concurrent chemotherapy and radiation therapy
[E] Immunotherapy

10. A 26-year-old woman underwent a Pap smear, which revealed a low-grade squamous intraepithelial lesion. There was no inflammation found. She was also found to be HIV negative, and a Pap smear 2 years ago was negative. The most appropriate next step in her treatment is:

[A] Colposcopy and biopsy
[B] Cervical conization
[C] Cryotherapy or laser therapy
[D] Return in 4–6 months for repeat Pap smear
[E] Hysterectomy

11. A 45-year-old premenopausal woman who completed adjuvant chemotherapy treatment for a stage II, ER/PR-positive breast cancer is presenting for a discussion regarding initiation of hormonal treatment with tamoxifen. The optimal duration of treatment with this agent is:

[A] 10 years
[B] 5 years
[C] 2 years
[D] Lifetime
[E] Intermittent treatment for 5 years

12. A 67-year-old man with a significant smoking history has had a persistent right upper lobe infiltrate. A CT scan shows a 3-cm solitary lesion with irregular borders, and a fine-needle aspiration shows adenocarcinoma. Appropriate staging workup at this point includes:

[A] Bone marrow biopsy
[B] Posteroanterior and lateral chest radiograms
[C] Lymphangiogram
[D] CT scans of the chest, abdomen, and pelvis and a PET scan
[E] Video-assisted thoracic surgery (VATS)

13. A 48-year-old female smoker with a history of Hodgkin's disease treated with chest radiation at age 29 years has developed a squamous cell lung carcinoma. Staging workup shows only a 2.5-cm solitary lesion in the left upper lobe. Her forced expiratory volume in 1 second (FEV_1) and forced vital capacity (FVC) are 75% of the predicted values. The best treatment option to increase her chance for cure is:

[A] Radiation
[B] Chemotherapy with carboplatin and Taxol
[C] Lobectomy
[D] Concurrent chemotherapy and radiation
[E] Radiation followed by surgery

14. A 60-year-old man with newly diagnosed prostate cancer comes to see you. He underwent transrectal ultrasonography with a needle biopsy showing adenocarcinoma. Except for elevated PSA, he is currently asymptomatic. The first test to order in staging for his prostate cancer is:

[A] Full-body plain film x-rays
[B] Bone scan
[C] CT of head
[D] CEA level
[E] Repeat PSA now

Answers and Explanations

1. The answer is A [IX C]. A palpable mass on examination warrants immediate evaluation. Even though she had undergone mammography 6 months ago, most clinicians would repeat this study. In addition, an ultrasound might reveal whether this is a cyst or a solid mass. Repeating the mammogram in 6 months is not a good option as this will delay treatment if the abnormal finding is in fact a malignancy. The same is true for answer C. One would not begin therapy without a firm diagnosis; therefore, answers D and E are incorrect.

2. The answer is A [IX I]. This patient is at high risk of recurrence by virtue of having disease in her lymph nodes. Radiation therapy or surgical excision of the breast cancer usually provides local control and adequate protection against recurrence of disease in the tumor bed. However, micrometastatic disease can only be addressed through the administration of systemic therapy such as cytotoxic chemotherapy. In patients with hormonally sensitive tumors (e.g., estrogen-receptor positive), hormonal therapy has been shown to be very effective in the prevention of disease recurrence after chemotherapy. Randomized clinical trials have shown that lumpectomy and radiation therapy is equal to a total mastectomy in terms of overall survival. For tumors that can be completely removed with adequate margins (>10 mm), lumpectomy offers better cosmetic and psychological results, is less invasive, and allows for faster recovery time.

3. The answer is B [XIX E]. This patient is neutropenic, with an absolute neutrophil count (ANC) of 492/mm^3 [ANC = white blood cells × (% neutrophils + % bands)]. He is experiencing fever with clinical signs of infection, and this should be treated as a medical emergency. Hospital admission and intravenous antibiotics are the most appropriate therapy. A broad-spectrum agent such as cefepime is appropriate initial therapy. In addition, this patient should receive intravenous vancomycin to treat a suspected central venous catheter infection based on symptoms of pain and erythema at the insertion site. Select patients may be managed as outpatients with oral ciprofloxacin, but this patient is too ill based on his tachycardia and hypotension, making choice C incorrect. Oral penicillin is never an option in the treatment of febrile neutropenia. Fungal infections are usually only seen after prolonged neutropenic episodes. Since this patient's last chemotherapy dose was within 5 days, it is unlikely that he has been neutropenic for longer than 10 days, and he is at low risk for fungal infection at this time. Antifungal coverage alone is inappropriate regardless. Therefore, choice E is incorrect.

4. The answer is A [VIII D 3]. Barrett's esophagus with high-grade dysplasia requires definitive treatment, and referral for esophagectomy is recommended. For patients who are medically unstable or for those who refuse surgery, endoscopic resection or photodynamic therapy are viable alternatives. Surveillance alone is inappropriate, making B and C incorrect. (Surveillance endoscopy at 6 months and 1 year are recommended for patients with Barrett's esophagus with low-grade dysplasia and no dysplasia, respectively.) Chemotherapy is not indicated unless carcinoma in found; therefore E is not correct.

5. The answer is D [X A]. The risk of ovarian cancer is significantly increased in women with a strong family history of breast and ovarian cancer syndromes associated with *BRCA1* and *BRCA2* mutations and/or hereditary nonpolyposis colorectal cancer syndromes. In postmenopausal women, an adnexal mass that is more than twice the size of the contralateral ovary or is larger than 5 cm should immediately be ruled out for ovarian cancer. This patient's symptoms of persistent abdominal pain, bloating, and a change in bowel habits occur commonly in patients with ovarian cancer, and these nonspecific symptoms may lead to a delay in diagnosis. Although a colonoscopy may be indicated in the future, it is imperative to evaluate the large ovarian cyst first, especially since the patient has such a strong family history of ovarian and breast cancer. Oral contraceptives are not indicated in this patient; since the patient is postmenopausal, this is not a physiologic or functional cyst associated with ovulation. Therefore, choice A is incorrect. CA-125 levels have a low specificity and may be elevated in postmenopausal women without ovarian cancer, and so C is not correct.

6. The answer is C [VI F]. Tobacco and alcohol abuse and a prior history of head and neck cancer are the strongest risk factors for head and neck cancer. Given the prolonged course of symptoms, reassurance or a trial of antibiotics is not the best choice. If possible, an open biopsy of the neck lymph nodes should be avoided if squamous cell cancer is suspected since it interferes with subsequent management. Therefore, a fine needle aspiration biopsy is the most appropriate initial procedure. If this is nondiagnostic, a careful excisional biopsy with frozen section analysis should be arranged. A random biopsy of the glottis would be unlikely to be diagnostic since there are no obvious masses in this area, making choice E incorrect.

7. The answer is E [VIII A 3]. Screening for colon cancer in average-risk patients should begin at age 50 years; however, this patient has two first-degree relatives with colorectal cancer, making her high risk for developing the disease. Patients with a family history of early colon cancer should begin receiving screening at age 40 years or 10 years before the age at which cancer was diagnosed in the family member, whichever is first. CEA and CA 19-9 levels may be elevated in patients with colorectal neoplasms, but this is not specific and is not used for screening. *H. pylori* is a risk factor for gastric cancer, but there is no evidence of increased risk of colorectal cancers.

8. The answer is C [XIX C 4]. The patient has hypercalcemia, the most common metabolic complication of malignancy. She is profoundly dehydrated, as seen by her orthostasis and subsequent fall at home. The patient should be adequately rehydrated initially with normal saline prior to administration of furosemide. A bisphosphonate would not be appropriate in the acute setting because of the patient's volume depletion. For the same reason, while corticosteroids can be considered an adjunctive therapy in a patient with a potentially hormone-responsive tumor, the main priority in this severely dehydrated patient should be volume repletion.

9. The answer is B [VIII A 9 a (3)]. Of the options presented, only adjuvant chemotherapy would increase the likelihood of cure for a patient who has had resection of stage III (e.g., lymph node positive, T_{any}, $N_{1 \text{ or } 2}$, M_0) adenocarcinoma of the colon. Once cancer has been found in the lymph nodes, the patient has a high rate of systemic dissemination.

10. The answer is A [X B 6 a]. The correct answer is colposcopy with biopsy. Cervical cancer mortality is so preventable because it is easily revealed by Pap smear, but this is only a screening test. If the Pap smear returns with low- or high-grade squamous intraepithelial lesion, a punch biopsy is required for diagnosis of CIN or invasive carcinoma. If the biopsy shows CIN I (slight dysplasia), this may resolve and does not require treatment. CIN I is managed with follow-up and a repeat Pap smear in 4–6 months. CIN II and III (moderate and severe dysplasia) are treated with ablative therapy using either laser or cryotherapy. If the punch biopsy returns showing invasive carcinoma, staging is performed, and the patient is treated with hysterectomy and/or radiation therapy. If the biopsy is inconclusive, then cervical conization is indicated.

11. The answer is B [IX I 4 a]. The optimal duration of treatment with tamoxifen is 5 years. Large randomized clinical trials have proven that shorter treatment duration is not as protective, and longer duration (10 years) is associated with more side effects such as thromboembolism.

12. The answer is D [VII F]. The goal in the initial staging of a patient with lung cancer is to rule out the presence of gross disease in all areas where lung cancer can potentially metastasize, including liver, adrenal glands, mediastinal lymph nodes, and contralateral chest. Routine chest films are not sufficiently sensitive to detect smaller lymph nodes in the hilar region. Neither bone marrow biopsies nor lymphangiograms are indicated for staging of lung cancer. In fact, lymphangiograms are no longer routinely performed. PET scans are increasingly used in the initial staging of patients with lung cancer because of their sensitivity in detecting minimal disease. Accurate staging information has a major impact on the choice of therapy for this disease. A patient who, based on initial CT scans, is considered to be a candidate for potentially curative surgery might be found to have metastatic disease by PET scan and therefore be a candidate for palliative chemotherapy. VATS is a useful surgical modality to obtain a tissue biopsy for diagnosis or as a method of surgical excision. However, this patient already has a diagnosis, and staging must be completed before consideration of treatment options.

13. The answer is C [VII I 1 b (1)]. Treatment of choice for stage I lung cancer is surgical resection. This can be accomplished by a lobectomy or a wedge resection of the involved lung segment. Surgical resection for stage I or II non–small cell lung cancer is potentially curative, with 5-year survival of close to 70%. Neither chemotherapy alone nor concurrent chemoradiation therapy is appropriate for a young, otherwise healthy patient with early-stage lung cancer.

14. The answer is B [XII C 6]. The correct answer is to do a bone scan. This is the first staging test done in the workup of prostate cancer. If abnormalities are found on the bone scan, you then proceed to do plain film x-rays of the areas to exclude other possible causes. Then you would perform surgical staging with removal and examination of the surrounding nodes (often done with prostatectomy).

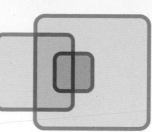

chapter **6**

Gastrointestinal Diseases

ARUL THOMAS · DARRYN POTOSKY · BRUCE GREENWALD

I **DISEASES OF THE ESOPHAGUS**

The esophagus is basically an organ of transport, with no significant absorptive or secretory function.

A **Features common to clinical disorders**

1. **Dysphagia,** or difficulty in swallowing, is a symptom often described as a **sticking sensation.**
   a. **Dysphagia for solids** indicates an esophageal obstruction as a result of:
      (1) Carcinoma
      (2) Benign esophageal stricture
      (3) An esophageal web or ring
   b. **Dysphagia for solids and liquids generally** indicates an esophageal abnormality as a result of motor dysfunction, such as:
      (1) Achalasia
      (2) Scleroderma
      (3) **Nutcracker esophagus or** diffuse esophageal spasm (DES) (🔊 see online)
   c. **Transfer dysphagia** indicates a difficulty in initiating swallowing and is often associated with:
      (1) A neuromuscular disorder of the pharynx or proximal esophagus (e.g., after a cerebrovascular accident)
      (2) Proximal muscle weakness of the pharynx or esophagus (e.g., polymyositis)
      (3) Other neuromuscular disorders (myasthenia gravis, myotonia dystrophica, or Parkinson's disease)
      (4) **Hypothyroidism**

2. **Odynophagia,** or pain on swallowing, may be due to:
   a. **Motor disorders** of the esophagus, especially achalasia and DES
   b. **Mucosal disruption** caused by:
      (1) Severe peptic esophagitis
      (2) Severe infections of the esophagus (candidal esophagitis, herpetic esophagitis, cytomegalovirus [CMV])
      (3) Drug-induced esophagitis (see I B 4 g)
      (4) Radiation esophagitis
      (5) Ingestion of lye or other caustic agents

3. **Heartburn** is a substernal burning sensation that radiates toward the mouth and may be initiated by bending forward.

B **Specific disorders**

1. **Gastroesophageal reflux disease (GERD)** is caused by the recurrent reflux of gastric contents into the distal esophagus.
   a. **Etiology and pathogenesis**
      (1) **Lower esophageal sphincter (LES) dysfunction.** Normally, the LES blocks reflux of gastric contents into the esophagus. GERD is thought to stem from defects in the LES mechanism, including:
         (a) Inappropriate transient relaxation of the LES
         (b) Anatomic disruption of the LES due to hiatal or paraesophageal hernia

215

(c) Decreased resting LES tone

(d) Transient increase in abdominal pressure

(2) **Secondary causes** of GERD should always be suspected and corrected if possible. The following conditions appear to decrease LES tone:

(a) **Pregnancy.** Especially during the last trimester, heartburn may be severe and probably is caused by inhibitory effects on the LES by progesterone.

(b) **Drugs.** Medications that decrease LES tone due to smooth muscle relaxation include:

(i) Anticholinergic agents

(ii) β_2- Adrenergic agonists and theophylline

(iii) Calcium channel–blocking agents and nitrates

(c) **Scleroderma.** Decreased motility in the esophageal body plus weakened LES causes severe GERD.

b. **Clinical features**

(1) **Heartburn** or **acid regurgitation** is a specific symptom of gastroesophageal reflux.

(2) **Dysphagia** in the GERD patient generally is for solids and may indicate a developing stricture.

(3) **Substernal chest pain** may be indistinguishable from the pain of myocardial ischemia or infarction and can radiate to the neck or jaw.

(4) **Anemia** may occur if recurrent esophageal bleeding is present due to severe esophagitis.

(5) **Extraesophageal manifestations** include hoarseness, recurrent laryngitis, globus sensation (feeling of something caught in the throat), reflux-induced asthma, cough, dental enamel erosion, earache, and hiccups.

c. **Diagnosis**

(1) **GERD is generally diagnosed by the appropriate clinical history. Diagnostic tests for uncomplicated GERD are rarely needed.**

(2) **Endoscopy with biopsy.** This procedure is indicated in the patient with dysphagia or anemia and is helpful in evaluating for Barrett's esophagus [see I B 1 e (5)]. Erosive changes are seen in only a minority of patients who undergo endoscopy.

(3) **Barium swallow/videoesophagram and upper gastrointestinal series.** This is the least sensitive test and is rarely performed. Generally, it is positive only in severe gastroesophageal reflux with a very weakened LES or in the presence of esophageal ulceration.

(4) **The following tests are generally not performed except in cases where the diagnosis is unclear or in evaluation for antireflux surgery [see I B 1 d (1) (d)].**

(a) **Twenty-four–hour esophageal pH and impedance monitoring.** These tests measure the number of episodes and length of time for esophageal reflux episodes, including acid reflux (pH monitoring) and non–acid reflux (impedance monitoring).

(b) **Esophageal manometry.** This procedure evaluates esophageal motility and LES pressure. Pressures consistently measured at less than one third of the lower limit of normal usually are associated with significant reflux.

d. **Therapy**

(1) **Increasing the reflux barrier** may be accomplished by:

(a) Lifestyle modification, including elevating the head of the bed 4–6 inches, avoiding eating within 3 hours of bedtime, avoiding fatty or large-volume meals, and reducing caffeine and alcohol intake

(b) Administration of alginic acid and antacid combinations

(c) Administration of drugs that increase LES tone (e.g., metoclopramide, bethanechol, domperidone)

(d) Antireflux surgery, especially Nissen fundoplication

(2) **Decreasing gastric acid effects** may be accomplished by:

(a) Administration of antacids, which produce rapid onset of relief but of short duration

(b) Administration of histamine$_2$ (H$_2$)-receptor antagonists (e.g., cimetidine, famotidine, ranitidine, and nizatidine), which have a relatively short time to onset and longer duration of action than antacids

(c) Administration of proton pump inhibitors such as dexlansoprazole, esomeprazole, lansoprazole, omeprazole, pantoprazole, and rabeprazole. These are the most potent inhibitors of gastric acid secretion but slowest time to onset of effect.

(3) Maintaining LES pressure. The following agents decrease LES pressure and should be avoided:

(a) Medications: anticholinergics, β-adrenergics, calcium channel blockers, and nitrates

(b) Foods: chocolate, fats, and peppermint

(c) Other: nicotine and caffeine

e. Complications

(1) Benign esophageal stricture occurs in a small portion of all GERD patients, specifically those with reflux esophagitis cases, and is best diagnosed by endoscopy, although barium esophagram may also be used.

(2) Esophageal ulceration may be accompanied by dysphagia or bleeding. It may be asymptomatic but can be associated with pain.

(3) Reflux-induced laryngeal disease is a common cause of recurrent hoarseness in adults.

(4) Pulmonary aspiration is a serious sequela of GERD. Patients older than 30 years of age who develop recurrent pneumonia or new symptoms of asthma should be evaluated for esophageal reflux.

(5) Barrett's esophagus refers to a condition in which metaplastic columnar epithelium replaces the normal squamous epithelium of the esophagus. Patients with Barrett's esophagus have a lifetime risk of 5%–6% for developing esophageal adenocarcinoma. Periodic endoscopy with biopsy is recommended. Cancer development is generally preceded by the development of dysplasia, which is detected by biopsy. Low-grade dysplasia is generally not treated. High-grade dysplasia carries a 5%–6% annual risk for developing esophageal adenocarcinoma. Treatment options include endoscopic resection, endoscopic ablation (with radiofrequency ablation, spray cryotherapy, or photodynamic therapy), and surgical esophagectomy.

2. Obstructive esophageal conditions

a. Carcinoma

(1) Epidemiology. In the United States, the incidences of esophageal adenocarcinoma and esophageal squamous cell carcinoma are equal. Carcinoma occurs predominantly in men and with varying incidence throughout the world. The population of the United States is considered at low risk, with more than 16,000 cases estimated in 2009; most advanced cases are fatal.

(2) Etiology. Certain factors appear to increase the risk of esophageal cancer.

(a) Tobacco smoking increases the risk of squamous cell carcinoma twofold to fourfold.

(b) Alcohol consumption has been shown to increase the risk of squamous cell carcinoma up to 12 times in France. Alcohol and tobacco appear to have an additive effect.

(c) Geographic factors. Incidence levels were found to be 400 times greater in certain regions in China and Iran and may be attributable to a diet that includes increased amounts of pickled food, nitrosamines, and molds as well as decreased amounts of selenium, fresh fruits, and vegetables. See other factors online.

(d) Barrett's esophagus [see I B 1 e (5)]. This is the strongest risk factor for adenocarcinoma.

(e) Obesity. Epidemiologic studies show an increased risk of adenocarcinoma in the obese. See other factors online.

(3) Clinical features

(a) Progressive dysphagia for solids indicates the presence of an ongoing obstructive lesion. Usually, when the esophageal lumen narrows to 1.2 cm or less, **persistent dysphagia** for solid food is observed.

(b) Pain usually signifies extension of the tumor beyond the wall of the esophagus.

(c) Dysphagia for liquids, cough, hoarseness, and **weight loss** generally are symptoms of advanced esophageal carcinoma, with cough suggesting the presence of a tracheoesophageal fistula.

(4) Diagnosis

(a) Endoscopy with biopsy and cytologic study, if performed together, establishes a diagnosis in approximately 90% of cases and is the diagnostic procedure of choice.

(b) Endoscopic ultrasound (EUS) is useful for staging esophageal carcinomas.

(c) **Computed tomography (CT)** and **positron emission tomography (PET)** should be used to evaluate for the presence and extent of nodal and visceral metastases and invasion into adjacent organs.

(d) **Bronchoscopy** is indicated in proximal tumors to assess for airway invasion.

(5) **Therapy** (see Chapter 5 VII I)

b. **Benign esophageal stricture** may be a sequela of prolonged reflux esophagitis. Heartburn may lessen as solid-food dysphagia worsens with progression of the stricture. Diagnosis is established by endoscopy or barium esophagram. Treatment includes control of acid reflux and dilation of the stricture endoscopically with tapered dilators (bougies) or with balloon dilation catheters.

c. **Esophageal webs** seen in the **upper one third** of the esophagus may be caused by a failure of complete embryologic recanalization. Webs in this area also may be associated with iron-deficiency anemia in the **Plummer–Vinson (Paterson–Kelly) syndrome.** Effective treatment of this syndrome includes administering iron for the anemia and esophageal dilation to fracture the webs.

d. **Esophageal rings** most commonly occur at the **squamocolumnar junction** and are called **Schatzki's rings.** Dysphagia for solids often is intermittent in this condition, especially if the narrowest point of the esophagus measures between 1.2 and 2 cm. Esophageal dilation often is effective therapy.

3. **Esophageal motor disorders**

a. **Oropharyngeal dysphagia (transfer dysphagia)** is a descriptive term applied to disorders of the neuromuscular apparatus of the distal pharynx and upper esophagus. Symptoms include difficulty in initiating swallowing, nasal regurgitation, and cough with pulmonary aspiration.

b. **Achalasia**

(1) **Epidemiology.** Achalasia occurs in approximately 1 in 100,000 individuals in the United States and equally in both sexes. The most common age of onset is between 20 and 40 years.

(2) **Pathology.** Histologic findings include a loss of inhibitory neurons at the lower esophageal sphincter and loss of myenteric ganglion cells in the esophageal body. The cause of these changes is unknown.

(3) **Clinical features**

(a) Dysphagia for solids and liquids in 95%–100% of patients

(b) Weight loss in 90% of patients

(c) Chest pain, which is severe in 60% of patients

(d) Nocturnal cough in 30% of patients, indicating possible overflow aspiration of unemptied esophageal contents and, in such cases, the need for immediate treatment

(e) Recurrent bronchitis or pneumonia in approximately 7%–8% of patients

(4) **Diagnosis.** Diagnosis involves excluding malignancy (i.e., carcinoma or lymphoma) at the esophagogastric junction, which may mimic achalasia ("pseudoachalasia"). Pseudoachalasia may be characterized by greater weight loss, shorter duration of symptoms, and less esophageal dilatation in an older person.

(a) **Radiography** may reveal a flaccid, dilated, fluid-filled esophagus with a **beak-like tapering** over the LES region. CT scan of the chest and abdomen or endoscopic ultrasound of the esophagogastric junction may be needed to rule out pseudoachalasia.

(b) **Manometry** is the most sensitive diagnostic method and should reveal:

(i) Absence of normal peristalsis in the entire esophagus

(ii) Elevated LES pressure

(iii) Incomplete relaxation of the LES, resulting in a persistent obstructing barrier after swallowing

(5) **Therapy**

(a) **Drugs** such as nitrates and calcium channel–blocking agents are effective in less than 50% of patients.

(b) **Pneumatic dilation** performed at endoscopy is effective in 70%–90% of patients, has a mortality rate of approximately 0.2%, and has a perforation rate of roughly 2%–3%.

(c) **Endoscopic injection of botulinum toxin** into the LES results in decreased LES pressure and decreased dysphagia in 70%–80% of patients. Repeated injections may be necessary, and long-term efficacy is noted in less than 50% of patients.

        (d) Surgical therapy. The favored procedure is **Heller myotomy,** which has a 65%–90% success rate and a 3%–4% surgical complication rate. For operations that do not incorporate an antireflux procedure, the rate of postoperative reflux may increase to 25%–30% after several years. Laparoscopic techniques are favored.

  c. Other motility disorders of the esophagus. These include nutcracker esophagus, diffuse esophageal spasm (DES), and nonspecific esophageal motility disorder (see ⊙ online).

  d. Systemic sclerosis (scleroderma) is a systemic collagen vascular disease involving the skin in 98% of cases. The esophagus is found to be abnormal in 75% of autopsies and in 80% of cases studied manometrically.

    (1) Pathology. The early esophageal effects are thought to be neural because no anatomic abnormality of the smooth muscle can be identified at a time when marked weakness of the esophagus is noted. A late defect may include a disuse type of atrophy of the circular smooth muscle elements of the esophagus; the longitudinal muscular layers remain intact.

    (2) Clinical features

      (a) Dysphagia for solids and liquids

      (b) Severe heartburn in 50% of patients

      (c) Esophageal stricture in 25% of long-term survivors

    (3) Diagnosis

      (a) Radiography. Supine esophagography may indicate poor esophageal emptying because of an absence of peristalsis.

      (b) Manometry. This procedure, which is the most reliable diagnostic technique, reveals:

        (i) Decreased LES pressure

        (ii) Very weak, low-amplitude peristaltic contractions in the distal smooth muscle portion (lower two thirds) of the esophagus

    (4) Therapy. The esophageal disorder is treated with antireflux measures [see I B 1 d].

4. Other esophageal disorders

  a. Diverticula

    (1) Zenker's diverticulum is a mucosal herniation (not a true diverticulum) above the cricopharyngeal region. Obstructive symptoms may occur if there is incomplete emptying of this diverticulum. Large diverticula are treated surgically.

    (2) Traction diverticula occur in the mid and distal regions and are thought to be secondary to an adjacent inflammatory process such as tuberculosis.

    (3) Epiphrenic diverticula occur in the distal esophagus, above the LES, and often are asymptomatic.

  b. Infections. Several infectious agents are of particular interest.

    (1) Candidal esophagitis usually occurs in diabetic patients, immunocompromised hosts (e.g., patients infected with human immunodeficiency virus [HIV] or patients undergoing cancer chemotherapy or steroid treatment), and in those with poor esophageal emptying (e.g., patients with achalasia or severe stricture). Odynophagia is a major symptom, and diagnosis is made by endoscopy and cytologic studies. Treatment is with nystatin, fluconazole, or, in resistant cases, low doses of amphotericin B.

    (2) Herpes simplex virus (HSV) may cause esophagitis in immunocompromised hosts and less commonly in nonimmunocompromised hosts. The esophagitis is characterized by relatively small, isolated ulcers. Biopsy of the ulcerating edges may show characteristic multinucleated cells with nuclear inclusions. Treatment is with acyclovir or valacyclovir.

    (3) CMV infection of the esophagus is typically seen in immunocompromised patients and may produce very large ulcerations of the esophagus. Intranuclear inclusion bodies are observed on biopsy. Treatment is with ganciclovir or valganciclovir.

    (4) HIV esophagitis may result in a diffuse inflammatory esophagitis. The diagnosis is one of exclusion once other infectious etiologies have been evaluated. Treatment of isolated acquired immunodeficiency syndrome (AIDS) esophagitis is with steroids.

  c. Eosinophilic esophagitis. Eosinophilic inflammation and submucosal fibrosis can occur in all ages. About half of patients have a history of food allergy or peripheral eosinophilia.

       (1) Pathology. The chemokine eotaxin-3 mediates inflammatory damage. Mucosal biopsies show increased eosinophils per high-power field. Microabscesses can also form.

       (2) Clinical symptoms. Symptoms are often seen in young children and males. Children can present with failure to thrive and refusal to swallow. Other symptoms described in children are regurgitation, heartburn, dysphagia, and vomiting. Adults can present with intermittent dysphagia and frank food impaction.

       (3) Diagnosis. A small-caliber esophagus, small areas of narrowing, and esophageal rings may be seen on barium studies. Longitudinal fissures, concentric rings, proximal strictures, and white specks can be seen on endoscopy. Other conditions to consider are reflux esophagitis, eosinophilic gastroenteritis (see online), and esophageal rings and strictures.

       (4) Treatment. Swallowed fluticasone for 12 weeks, in addition to the identification and elimination of offending foods, is the treatment. Esophageal dislodging of impacted food and luminal dilation can be performed cautiously. Esophageal perforation can occur at a higher rate during endoscopy.

    d. Caustic esophageal injury. Ingestion of caustic agents (i.e., strong alkali or acid) can cause serious esophageal burns. Ingestion of lye or detergents such as chlorine bleach is a common suicidal gesture in adults and a common accident in children. Radiographs and CT scans are done initially to exclude perforation. Emergency endoscopy should be performed to assess the extent of damage. Broad-spectrum antibiotics are recommended initially in management of esophageal burns. Steroids may also be prescribed. Long-term sequelae in survivors may include esophageal stricture and esophageal carcinoma.

    e. Esophageal tears. These conditions are seen most commonly after vomiting (75% of cases), straining, or coughing.

       (1) A mucosal tear (**Mallory–Weiss syndrome**) produces significant hematemesis after an initial nonbloody vomitus. Surgery is required in less than 10% of these cases.

       (2) A rupture of the esophagus (**Boerhaave's syndrome**) usually occurs above the esophagogastric junction. Mediastinal air suggests the diagnosis, and immediate surgical intervention is necessary if the patient is to survive.

    f. Paraesophageal hernia. Unlike the much more common hiatal hernia, a paraesophageal hernia may lead to gastric vascular compromise. The esophagogastric junction traverses the diaphragm in the appropriate location. The body of the stomach travels above the diaphragm, and gastric volvulus with incarceration may occur. Surgery may be necessary to alleviate symptoms of pain, upper gastrointestinal bleeding, and ischemia.

    g. Pill-induced esophagitis. This condition is often caused by medications such as **oral bisphosphonates (particularly alendronate),** aspirin and other nonsteroidal anti-inflammatory drugs (NSAIDs), potassium chloride tablets, iron preparations, quinidine, tetracyclines, and other antibiotics. These medications are often temporarily lodged in the esophagus because of either inadequate liquid with swallowing or a relative narrowing of the esophagus. Diagnosis is largely clinical, although upper endoscopy is most sensitive in patients with difficult presentations. Severe erosions and strictures may develop in a minority of cases. Treatment is symptomatic.

II   DISEASES OF THE STOMACH

A **Gastritis**

  1. Acute gastritis is an inflammation of the gastric mucosa, which may be diffuse or localized and usually is self-limited.

    a. Etiology

      (1) Drugs that can damage the mucosal barrier and lead to backdiffusion of acid and pepsin include:

        (a) Aspirin and NSAIDs

        (b) Alcohol, which may produce an additive effect with aspirin

      (2) Accidental ingestion of caustic substances such as strong alkali (e.g., lye), strong acid (e.g., sulfuric or hydrochloric acid), or fixatives [e.g., formaldehyde, trinitrophenol (picric acid)] can be fatal. Patients who survive the ingestion of such corrosives sustain injuries that leave considerable scars and subsequent antral narrowing.

      (3) Stress related to severe illness, especially multiorgan failure, burns, and central nervous system (CNS) injuries, can causes acute gastritis. Ischemia and gastric acid, even at normal levels, may be involved.

      (4) Infections

        (a) *Helicobacter pylori* infectious gastritis (see III C 2)

        (b) Infections with CMV, herpesvirus, *Mycobacterium avium* complex (MAC), *Candida*, *Treponema pallidum*, and *Mycobacterium tuberculosis* have been associated with gastritis, especially in immunocompromised patients.

  b. Clinical features (present in 70% of patients)

    (1) Epigastric burning and **pain, nausea,** and **vomiting**

    (2) Gastrointestinal bleeding, which may be severe and associated with hematemesis and shock

  c. Diagnosis. In most cases, diagnosis is made on the basis of endoscopic visualization with or without biopsy. Congestion, friability, superficial ulceration, and petechiae frequently are seen in the gastric mucosa.

  d. Therapy. Treatment begins with removal of offending agents. Antacids, antiviral and antifungal agents, H_2-receptor antagonists, proton pump inhibitors, and surface-acting agents (e.g., sucralfate) are useful as well. Patients with acute hemorrhagic gastritis usually respond to fluid or blood replacement combined with intravenous proton pump inhibitors (or H_2-receptor antagonists if proton pump inhibitors are contraindicated). Surgery rarely is necessary for these patients and is associated with high morbidity and mortality rates.

2. Chronic gastritis is characterized by a superficial lymphocyte infiltrate in the lamina propria.

  a. Etiology. Chronic gastritis can be caused by:

    (1) Prolonged use of alcohol, aspirin, and other irritating drugs

    (2) Radiation or thermal injury

    (3) Immunologic factors

    (4) Infections (e.g., *H. pylori*). **H. pylori** infectious gastritis is caused by a gram-negative, spiral-shaped bacterium that survives in the acidic milieu of the stomach by producing urease, which liberates ammonia. Chronic gastritis involving *H. pylori* has been associated with 80%–90% of duodenal ulcer patients (see III C 2) and with 60%–70% of gastric ulcer patients.

  b. Types

    (1) Chronic type A gastritis involves the fundus and body of the stomach; the antrum is spared. This type of gastritis is associated with parietal cell antibodies, high serum gastrin levels, and pernicious anemia.

    (2) Chronic type B gastritis involves the antrum of the stomach; the body and fundus are relatively spared. Gastrin cell antibodies have been detected in some patients with this gastritis. More commonly, reflux of duodenal or biliary secretions or *H. pylori* infections are linked causatively to type B gastritis.

  c. Clinical features. Clinical evidence may be limited in patients with chronic gastritis. Type A gastritis is associated with little to no gastric acid production (hypochlorhydria or achlorhydria), whereas type B gastritis is associated with normal or low acid levels. Hypothyroidism, diabetes mellitus, and vitiligo occur more frequently with type A than with type B gastritis.

  d. Clinical course. Data suggest that these lesions may remain unchanged for several years. Gastric atrophy develops in approximately 50% of patients with superficial gastritis over 10–20 years. There is an increased association with gastric polyps, gastric ulcer, and gastric cancer in both types of chronic gastritis, with type B being associated with a higher incidence of gastric cancer than type A.

  e. Therapy. Treatment usually is unnecessary; however, conditions associated with gastritis (e.g., pernicious anemia, *H. pylori* infections, hypothyroidism, and diabetes) should be treated accordingly.

3. Special types of gastritis

B **Gastric neoplasms** (see Chapter 5 VIII C). The most common types of gastric neoplasms are **gastric adenocarcinoma** and **gastric lymphoma.** An important type of gastric lymphoma is mucosa-associated lymphoid tissue (**MALT**) lymphoma.

1. **MALT lymphoma** most commonly occurs in the stomach but has been observed in the orbit, intestine, lung, and other organs. Almost 95% of MALT lymphomas are associated with ***H. pylori* infection.** Endoscopic biopsy can be attempted in many cases, with some patients requiring surgical biopsy. Endoscopic ultrasound can help define the extent of gastric involvement. Histologically, MALT lymphoma is a well-differentiated, superficial process. It is typically localized. Eradication of *H. pylori* can achieve remission, but long-term remission is uncertain. Radiation and surgery can also treat local disease, and single-agent chemotherapy can be used for more extensive disease.

2. **Other gastric tumors**

C Disorders of gastric emptying

1. **Gastroparesis** is a disorder of gastric emptying that is not caused by an obstruction. The diagnosis should be made by a nuclear solid-phase gastric emptying study after mechanical obstruction has been ruled out by an upper gastrointestinal series and endoscopy. Gastroparesis most frequently is caused by type 1 (insulin-dependent) diabetes mellitus of longer than 10 years duration. Other associated conditions include systemic sclerosis, postvagotomy states, and therapy with anticholinergic agents or narcotics. In diabetes, loss of gastric phase III activity is noted on electrical recordings, with other signs of diabetic visceral neuropathy often being seen as well. Treatment with prokinetic agents such as metoclopramide, domperidone, or erythromycin has been effective. Electrical gastric pacing may be helpful in resistant cases.

2. **Pyloric stenosis**

3. **Gastric bezoars**

4. **Gastric diverticula**

5. **Gastric volvulus**

III   PEPTIC ULCER DISEASE

A Introduction   Peptic ulcer disease refers to a group of disorders of the gastrointestinal tract involving discrete tissue destruction caused by acid and pepsin. Peptic ulcers occur most commonly in the stomach or proximal duodenum, less commonly in the distal esophagus, and rarely in the small intestine. (Peptic ulcers in the distal small intestine usually are associated with a Meckel's diverticulum that contains gastric mucosa.) In general, the clinical features and treatment of peptic ulcer disease are similar regardless of location, although peptic esophagitis caused by reflux of gastric contents has some unique features (see I B 1).

B Incidence   Peptic ulcer disease occurs more commonly in men than in women. Duodenal ulcers are three times more common than gastric ulcers and occur approximately 10 years earlier; the peak incidence for duodenal ulcers is at approximately 40 years of age, as opposed to 50 years of age for gastric ulcers. Duodenal ulcers have a 1-year relapse rate of approximately 80% (much lower if associated with *H. pylori* that has been eradicated). Patients with gastric ulcers have a 33% chance of developing subsequent duodenal ulcers.

C Pathogenesis   Acid and pepsin are necessary for development of ulcers. However, several factors, especially *H. pylori* infection, are thought to contribute to the pathogenesis.

1. **Social factors**
   a. **Tobacco smoking** increases the risk of peptic ulcer disease. Smoking also raises the morbidity and mortality rates and lowers the healing rate for peptic ulcers.
   b. **Drugs** such as NSAIDs are implicated in ulcer disease, with an antiprostaglandin effect suggested as an underlying factor. Ulcers develop in approximately 30% of arthritis patients who take high doses of aspirin. Steroids also are thought to break the mucosal barrier and may increase the risk of peptic ulcer disease, especially with concordant aspirin or NSAID use.
   c. **Alcohol** compromises the mucosal barrier and increases gastric acid secretion.

2. *Helicobacter pylori*
   a. **Microbiology.** *H. pylori* has been identified in the gastric antrum in up to 90% of patients with duodenal ulcer disease or antral type B gastritis, and the association for patients with gastric ulcer disease is 60%–70%.

b. **Pathophysiology.** *H. pylori* is found on gastric epithelium and does not penetrate the cell. If it is a primary offender, it may act as a "barrier breaker," allowing acid backdiffusion and peptic ulcer disease to develop. *H. pylori* elaborates ammonia, which damages cell surfaces, and liberates a number of other inflammatory cell-recruiting factors and adhesion molecules.

c. ***H. pylori* detection.** *H. pylori* liberates urease, and a biopsy of the gastric antrum may change a pH color monitor. *H. pylori* may also be recognized histologically on gastric biopsies, although special stains may assist in identification. A urea breath test using carbon-13 (^{13}C)– or ^{14}C-labeled urea measures exhaled labeled carbon dioxide. Antibodies to *H. pylori* detected by enzyme-linked immunosorbent assay (ELISA) indicate active or prior infection. A stool test for *H. pylori* is also available. Stool or breath testing may be falsely negative if performed while the patient is taking a proton pump inhibitor, which can suppress *H. pylori* growth.

d. **Treatment. Antibiotics** are used to treat *H. pylori* infection. Regimens typically involve combinations of antibiotics, a proton pump inhibitor, and sometimes a bismuth-containing product. Treatment is for approximately 2 weeks, with a 70%–90% response rate, depending on the regimen selected (see III F 3).

e. **Outcome.** Studies have shown a decreased relapse rate in peptic ulcers in cases where *H.* pylori is successfully eradicated.

3. **Associated diseases.** Some patients with **multiple endocrine neoplasia type I (MEN I)** present with gastrin-secreting tumors.

D Clinical features

1. **Pain** is the predominant symptom, although it may be absent in 25% of gastric ulcer patients. The pain characteristically is described as an epigastric burning sensation and may be accompanied by bloating or nausea. Eating may exacerbate the pain in gastric ulcer patients, whereas in duodenal ulcer patients, the pain usually is diminished by eating, only to recur 2–3 hours later. Pain may awaken patients from sleep, especially those with duodenal ulcers.

2. **Upper gastrointestinal hemorrhage** may be the presenting sign of peptic ulcer disease, and anemia from chronic blood loss may be seen.

3. **Less common symptoms**
   a. **Repeated vomiting,** which may indicate gastric outlet obstruction
   b. **Weight loss,** which is somewhat more common with gastric ulcer

E Diagnosis
Because patients may complain only of vague symptoms, a high index of suspicion is needed.

1. **Endoscopy** is the primary diagnostic maneuver to identify or confirm a radiographic diagnosis. Because 5% of gastric ulcers that occur in the United States are malignant, endoscopic biopsies at the margin of the ulcer and simultaneous cytologic brushings are obtained, with subsequent endoscopy in 6–8 weeks to document healing.

2. **Radiography** is a useful screening tool; however, an upper gastrointestinal series may miss up to 30% of gastric ulcers, and scarring of the duodenal bulb from chronic or recurrent ulcer disease may make radiographic interpretation difficult. Double-contrast techniques may improve diagnostic accuracy. **Duodenal ulcers always are benign; however, gastric ulcers may be benign or malignant.**

3. ***H. pylori* detection** (see III C 4 c).

F Therapy
Treatment is virtually the same for esophageal, gastric, and duodenal ulcers.

1. **Intensive antacids,** while they have been shown to promote the healing of gastric and duodenal ulcers, are generally of historical significance only.

2. **H$_2$-receptor antagonists (cimetidine, ranitidine, famotidine,** and **nizatidine) and proton pump inhibitors (dexlansoprazole, esomeprazole, lansoprazole, omeprazole, pantoprazole, and rabeprazole)** are the mainstay of treatment because of patient convenience, sustained acid reduction, and increased healing rates with diminished relapse rates—**particularly in combination with antibiotics if *H. pylori* is present.**

3. **Antibiotics** are used to treat *H. pylori* infection (see III C 4 d). The most common therapy is amoxicillin, clarithromycin, and a proton pump inhibitor for 7–14 days. Alternative treatment

plans utilize metronidazole, tetracycline, and a bismuth preparation. Regimen compliance and drug resistance are important factors for successful treatment.

4. **Dietary factors** may be of some importance. There is no proof that bland diets promote healing in peptic ulcer disease. In fact, milk may be harmful because it increases acid secretion, probably by calcium- and protein-stimulated gastrin release. Caffeine and alcohol stimulate gastric acid secretion and therefore should be restricted in acute cases. Decaffeinated coffee also may stimulate acid release. Ulcer patients who smoke should be urged to stop smoking, as relapse rates are higher in smokers.

5. **Other therapeutic agents and approaches**

G **Complications**

1. **Hemorrhage** occurs in 20% of patients and is the most serious complication, having a 10% mortality rate. Significant bleeding is often due to a visible vessel in the ulcer crater, which can be treated with endoscopic injection, coagulation, or clipping. If blood requirements exceed 3 units in 24 hours for longer than 48–72 hours or if in-hospital rebleeding occurs, surgical intervention may be indicated, especially if endoscopic treatment failures.

2. **Perforation** occurs in approximately 5%–10% of all peptic ulcers and is far more common with duodenal ulcers than with gastric ulcers. Of ulcers that perforate, 10% bleed simultaneously. Symptoms and signs are those of peritonitis, which include intense pain, a rigid abdomen, decreased bowel sounds, and direct or rebound tenderness. This catastrophic complication is confirmed in approximately 75%–85% of cases by an erect abdominal radiograph showing free air under the diaphragm. Most cases require immediate surgical intervention, but selected patients have been treated successfully with nasogastric suction and antibiotics.

3. **Gastric outlet obstruction** occurs when luminal narrowing develops from ulcer formation in the pyloric area, with edema or scarring. Early satiety, epigastric fullness, nausea, and vomiting of undigested food (frequently ingested hours earlier) suggest the diagnosis. Weight loss is common. Treatment consists of gastric decompression via a nasogastric tube, treatment of active peptic ulcer disease as described previously, and possibly endoscopic balloon dilation of the obstruction. Approximately 25%–40% of patients require surgery due to recurrent obstruction.

4. **Penetration** into an adjacent organ usually is a complication of posterior duodenal ulcers, with penetration into the pancreas. Pain usually is sudden in onset and radiates to the back. Serum amylase and lipase levels frequently are elevated. Treatment is surgical.

H **Postsurgical complications**

I **Zollinger–Ellison syndrome** refers to a non–β islet cell tumor that produces gastrin and is associated with gastric acid hypersecretion and peptic ulcer disease. The tumors are biologically malignant in 60% of cases and most commonly involve the pancreas. Other tumor sites include the stomach, duodenum, spleen, and lymph nodes. Tumor size varies from 2 mm to 20 cm. Approximately 10% of patients with Zollinger–Ellison syndrome have a resectable lesion.

1. **Clinical features**
2. **Diagnosis**
3. **Therapy**

J **Other disorders of the stomach**

1. **Portal hypertensive gastropathy** is the term given to diffuse submucosal dilation of gastric vessels in the setting of portal hypertension. It accounts for upper gastrointestinal bleeding in approximately 10% of patients with portal hypertension. A mosaic-like pattern to the mucosa with or without diffuse, irregular areas of red spots produces a characteristic appearance at endoscopy. Treatment is aimed at reducing the underlying portal hypertension and endoscopic treatment of active focal lesions.

2. **Dieulafoy's lesion** is a difficult-to-diagnose vascular lesion generally seen in the proximal stomach. This may be a cause of significant recurrent upper gastrointestinal bleeding. Men older than 50 years of age are most commonly affected. The lesion appears as an exposed, large-caliber

submucosal penetrating arteriole, with no or minimal mucosal ulceration. Endoscopic therapy with injection, cautery, clipping, or banding is effective in stopping the bleeding, but angiography or surgery may be necessary because of the difficulty of identifying the small vascular defect during endoscopy.

IV DISEASES OF THE SMALL INTESTINE

A **Intestinal obstruction** is a term used to denote failure of passage of intestinal contents and may be due to mechanical obstruction or adynamic ileus.

1. **Mechanical obstruction**
   a. **Etiology**
      (1) **Extrinsic causes:** Adhesions from prior surgery, incarcerated hernia, metastatic tumors, volvulus, endometriosis, and NSAID-induced strictures (often multiple)
      (2) **Intramural causes:** Hematomas from trauma, strictures, and intramural tumors
      (3) **Intraluminal causes:** Epithelial tumors (especially colonic), intussusception, and foreign bodies
   b. **Clinical features**
      (1) Crampy pain that waxes and wanes in intensity
      (2) High-pitched bowel sounds with rushes and tinkles
      (3) Constipation and obstipation
      (4) Vomiting, which is more prominent in proximal intestinal obstruction
      (5) Distention, which is more prominent in distal intestinal obstruction
      (6) Intestinal ischemia, leading first to edema, then to petechial hemorrhages, and finally to necrosis and gangrene (this is secondary to increased intraluminal pressure occurring after 6–12 hours of obstruction, when absorption ceases and secretion commences)
   c. **Diagnosis** usually is made with plain and upright abdominal radiographs. Characteristic air–fluid levels exist above the area of obstruction, and no air is seen in the rectum. A barium enema may be useful in diagnosing colonic obstruction. Reflux of barium into the small bowel also may be helpful in the diagnosis of low small bowel obstruction.
   d. **Therapy**
      (1) Replacement of fluid and electrolytes
      (2) Intestinal decompression with nasogastric suction or small bowel intubation
      (3) Surgery, which is required for complete small bowel obstruction and those with partial small bowel obstruction who do not improve with conservative measures

2. **Adynamic,** or **paralytic, ileus** is a nonobstructive lack of propulsion through the intestinal tract.
   a. **Etiology.** Adynamic ileus commonly is linked to the following conditions:
      (1) Recent abdominal surgery, which results in transient ileus usually lasting 2–3 days
      (2) Electrolyte imbalance, especially hypokalemia
      (3) Chemical or bacterial peritonitis
      (4) Severe intra-abdominal inflammation such as pancreatitis and cholecystitis
      (5) Systemic illness such as pneumonia
   b. **Clinical features.** Physical examination shows a distended abdomen and diminished bowel sounds.
   c. **Diagnosis.** Radiographs show diffuse intestinal gas and air in the rectum, and CT scan contrast studies show movement of contrast into the colon.
   d. **Therapy**
      (1) Bowel rest and placement of a nasogastric tube
      (2) Correction of underlying causes
      (3) Intravenous neostigmine (with careful cardiac monitoring) may be used in resistant cases.

B **Intestinal pseudo-obstruction** is a rare but important entity characterized by apparently recurrent episodes of mechanical obstruction but with no demonstrable source of obstruction.

1. **Classification**
2. **Diagnosis**

 C Small bowel diverticula

D **Diarrhea** is defined as an increase in stool frequency and volume. The stool usually is liquid, and 24-hour output exceeds 250 g. Patients may experience lower abdominal crampy pain and fecal urgency.

1. **Classification.** Pathophysiologic criteria are used to classify diarrhea as one of three distinct types.

   a. **Secretory diarrhea**

      (1) **Pathophysiology.** Secretory diarrhea occurs when the secretion of fluid and electrolytes is increased or when the normal absorptive capacity of the bowel is decreased.

         (a) Agents that activate the adenyl cyclase–cyclic adenosine 3′,5′-monophosphate (cAMP) system include cholera toxin, heat-labile *Escherichia coli* toxin, *Salmonella* enterotoxin, and vasoactive intestinal peptide (VIP).

         (b) Agents that probably do not activate the adenyl cyclase–cAMP system include heat-stable *E. coli* toxin, a variety of other bacterial enterotoxins (e.g., those produced by *Clostridium perfringens*, *Pseudomonas aeruginosa*, and *Klebsiella pneumoniae*), castor oil, and phenolphthalein.

         (c) Chronic secretory diarrhea is seen in the pancreatic cholera syndrome with VIP secretion, medullary carcinoma of the thyroid gland with calcitonin secretion, carcinoid syndrome with serotonin secretion, and villous adenoma of the rectum.

      (2) **Diagnosis.** Persistent diarrhea in the absence of food intake or the presence of a stool osmotic gap [stool osmolarity – 2(stool Na^+ + stool K^+)] less than 50.

      (3) **Therapy.** Fluid and electrolyte support should be given while the cause of the diarrhea is being determined. In general, diarrhea secondary to bacterial enterotoxin is self-limited. Any contributing exogenous agent must be withdrawn.

   b. **Osmotic diarrhea** is caused by the presence of nonabsorbable substances in the intestine, with the secondary accumulation of fluid and electrolytes. Such nonabsorbable substances include lactose in a patient with lactase deficiency, laxatives (e.g., magnesium citrate and sodium phosphate), and foodstuffs in a patient with malabsorption. The diagnosis is suggested by the absence of diarrhea after a 48- to 72-hour fast (with concurrent intravenous fluid replacement). There is a stool osmotic gap [stool osmolarity – 2(stool Na^+ + stool K^+)] of greater than 50.

   c. **Abnormal intestinal motility** causes or contributes to the diarrhea seen in diabetes, irritable bowel syndrome, postvagotomy states, carcinoid syndrome, and hyperthyroidism. Mechanisms of abnormal intestinal motility include the following:

      (1) If small bowel peristalsis is too rapid, an abnormally large amount of fluid and partially digested food may be delivered to the colon.

      (2) Extremely slow peristalsis may allow bacterial overgrowth to occur and bile salt deconjugation to cause secondary malabsorption.

      (3) Rapid colonic motility may not allow adequate time for the colon to absorb fluid delivered to the cecum. (Normally, 90% of the fluid is absorbed.)

2. **Diagnosis**

   a. **Tests** performed on stool samples include the following:

      (1) **Culture and sensitivity testing** to detect a pathogenic bacterial strain. A positive stool culture is found for 40% of patients who have white blood cells (WBCs) in the stool and fever.

      (2) **Microscopic examination** to identify ova and parasites (samples should be sent on 3 separate days to increase yield)

      (3) **Fecal** occult blood testing

      (4) **Sudan staining** to detect fat droplets

      (5) **Fecal leukocytes** or stool lactoferrin may be positive in patients with invasive bacterial colitis (such as *Salmonella*, *Shigella*, *Campylobacter*, *Clostridium difficile*, and invasive *E. coli*) and other inflammatory colitides. Toxigenic *E. coli*, viruses, Norwalk agent, and *Giardia lamblia* are not invasive. Irritable bowel syndrome, malabsorption syndrome, and laxative abuse do not cause pus in the stool. *Staphylococcus aureus*, *C. perfringens*, and *Entamoeba histolytica* also may be present with fecal leukocytes.

      (6) Testing for the presence of **C. difficile toxin** in stool.

(7) Fecal fat (see IV E 3 a). A qualitative exam of a spot stool specimen in malabsorption will show increased number and size of fat droplets, and a quantitative exam (usually a 2- to 3-day collection) will show increased proportion of fat (normally <5%–7%). These exams must be done while the patient maintains dietary fat intake, typically 80–100 g/day.

b. Sigmoidoscopy or colonoscopy also is performed, especially to exclude or confirm a diagnosis of inflammatory bowel disease.

3. Specific causes of persistent diarrhea

a. Irritable bowel syndrome (IBS) is an intestinal disorder characterized by chronic abdominal pain and altered bowel habits in the absence of any organic cause. It is the most commonly diagnosed gastrointestinal condition and comprises 25%–50% of all referrals to gastroenterologists. Although IBS can affect any individual, it is more common in young patients and women, with an estimated 2:1 female predominance in North America.

(1) Pathophysiology. The exact pathophysiology of IBS remains uncertain. Many believe there is interplay between abnormal gastrointestinal motility (altered basal contractions, prolonged motor activity after meals, abnormal response to stress) in the small bowel and colon, abnormal and hypersensitive visceral nerve perception in the gut, and psychological factors. Researchers are also exploring the possibility of the development of IBS following a bout of infectious enteritis, particularly with *Campylobacter*, *Salmonella*, and *Shigella*. Although investigations are ongoing, no physiologic or psychological abnormality has been found to be specific to IBS.

(2) Clinical features. The primary complaints in patients with IBS are chronic abdominal pain and altered bowel habits. Abdominal pain is typically intermittent, variable in intensity, and crampy in nature. The pain is not usually progressive in nature, associated with weight loss or anorexia, or found to prevent patients from sleeping. The pain may improve with defecation. Bowel habits with IBS are widely variable. Complaints range from diarrhea or constipation predominant, to alternating diarrhea and constipation, to normal stools alternating with diarrhea and constipation. Patients often complain of extreme urgency prior to a bowel movement followed by a sense of incomplete evacuation. Lastly, there is also a sense of bloating and increased abdominal gas in patients with IBS.

(3) Diagnosis includes careful history, clinical suspicion, and diagnostic testing to rule out organic disease. Guidelines recommend fecal occult blood testing and complete blood count (CBC), the results of which are usually normal. Stool osmolality, serum chemistries and albumin, ova and parasite examination, thyroid function tests, sedimentation rate, and testing for celiac disease should be performed if symptoms are consistent with diarrhea-predominant disease. Colonoscopy should be used in patients older than 50 years to exclude neoplasm or microscopic colitis and may be used in younger patients to exclude inflammatory bowel disease in the appropriate setting.

(4) Therapy. Treatment includes stool-bulking agents, antispasmodics, and patient reassurance. Constipation is often treated with fiber supplements, and the chloride channel activator lubiprostone may be used for severe cases. Pain is treated with antispasmodic agents or tricyclic antidepressants. Diarrhea is treated with loperamide. Psychological therapies, including cognitive-based therapy, have been effective in studies, and selective serotonin reuptake inhibitors (SSRIs), commonly used to treat coexisting anxiety and depression, may be used.

b. Lactase deficiency usually is not complete (i.e., patients have some enzyme activity), and presenting symptoms occur after puberty. It affects 60%–80% of African Americans and occurs to a lesser extent in Asian and Mediterranean populations. Symptoms of lactase deficiency include abdominal bloating, cramping, and watery diarrhea after milk ingestion. Lactose breath tests measure increased H^+ excretion from bacterial digestion of lactose in the bowel. A relative lactase deficiency may occur after an acute episode of viral enteritis or in association with celiac disease, Whipple's disease, or cystic fibrosis.

c. Incontinence is a disturbing symptom that patients may find difficult to discuss with a physician. It is often not true diarrhea but is associated with inflammatory diseases of the anal canal (e.g., acute gonococcal proctitis, Crohn's disease, and ulcerative colitis) or with systemic neuromuscular diseases (e.g., diabetes mellitus and scleroderma). Incontinence also may be a complication of anal surgery (e.g., fistulectomy and hemorrhoidectomy).

       d. Laxative abuse, which may be associated with psychiatric problems and a desire to lose weight, should be considered in difficult cases. The type of laxative ingested determines the clinical features. Magnesium sulfate, nonabsorbable sugars (e.g., lactulose), and sodium phosphate result in osmotic diarrhea. Dihydroxy bile salts, castor oil, and dioctyl sodium sulfosuccinate (docusate sodium) cause secretory diarrhea. Surreptitious laxative use is difficult to document.

       e. Systemic mastocytosis

   4. Infectious causes of diarrhea are listed in Table 6–1. Some organisms, such as *C. difficile* and *E. histolytica*, primarily attach to the colon.

       a. *E. coli* is the most common cause of **traveler's diarrhea,** which is the often severe diarrhea that occurs within 2 weeks of a visit to a tropical area. Traveler's diarrhea usually is self-limited.

          (1) A toxigenic, heat-labile *E. coli* can activate cAMP or cyclic guanosine 3′,5′-monophosphate (cGMP) to cause a secretory diarrhea. Species of *Shigella*, *Salmonella*, and *Campylobacter* as well as *E. histolytica* and *G. lamblia* are other known causes of traveler's diarrhea.

          (2) Quinolone antibiotics, rifaximin, azithromycin, and bismuth subsalicylate have been shown to be effective in treatment and prevention.

       b. *Giardia lamblia,* a flagellate protozoan, is the most common cause of **water-borne infectious diarrhea** in the United States. Treatment with metronidazole usually is successful.

       c. Viruses commonly cause **acute self-limited diarrhea.** Although many different viruses may cause gastroenteritis, causes of viral gastroenteritis that can be identified with certainty are the **noroviruses** and **rotavirus.**

       d. *Salmonella* **infection,** or salmonellosis, may be highly variable in its presentation. Gastroenteritis, the most common form of salmonellosis, is an acute self-limited diarrheal syndrome. Enteric fever is a severe illness primarily caused by *Salmonella typhi* or *Salmonella paratyphi* but also is seen with infection by other types of *Salmonella*. *Salmonella* septicemia may be seen in patients with osteomyelitis, mycotic aneurysms, or abscesses with no evidence or history of gastrointestinal disease.

       e. *Shigella* infection, or shigellosis, is characterized by acute diarrhea with fever and crampy abdominal pain. If left untreated, the disease progresses to a chronic bloody diarrhea without fever but with weight loss and debilitation, which may last for weeks.

       f. *Campylobacter* infection is the most common cause of bacterial diarrhea in the United States. It presents often as a febrile prodrome followed by diarrhea that can be bloody. Diagnosis is made by positive stool culture but requires special media and handling. Treatment is generally supportive, but erythromycin or azithromycin can be used for those at risk of complications. Resistance to fluoroquinolones is increasing.

       g. *Cryptosporidium* infection, or cryptosporidiosis, is a protozoal infection seen commonly in immunocompromised patients.

       h. *Isospora belli* infection occurs similarly to cryptosporidiosis.

       i. *E. histolytica* causes bloody dysentery with fever.

       j. Hemorrhagic *E. coli* **serotype O157:H7** produces Shiga toxin and causes bloody diarrhea. A life-threatening complication is the **hemolytic–uremic syndrome.**

   5. Nonbacterial food poisoning

E **Malabsorption** of food or nutrients results from a defect at any step of the digestive process or in any of the organs that participate in normal digestion. The clinical features vary widely because malabsorption may involve a single nutrient or multiple nutrients.

   1. Etiology

       a. Maldigestion refers to a defect either in intraluminal hydrolysis of triglycerides or in micelle formation, which results from the following conditions:

          (1) Pancreatic insufficiency caused by chronic pancreatitis, pancreatic carcinoma, or cystic fibrosis

          (2) Deficiency of conjugated bile salts because of cholestatic or obstructive liver disease (e.g., cholangiocarcinoma)

          (3) Bile salt deconjugation attributable to bacterial overgrowth in blind loops (e.g., after Billroth II gastrectomy see online) or in jejunal diverticula, or in association with enterocolonic fistulae or motility disorders (e.g., scleroderma, pseudo-obstruction)

TABLE 8-1   Food Poisoning Syndromes

Organism	Incubation Period	Symptoms	Sources of Contamination	Pathogenic Mechanisms	Comments
Bacteria					
Staphylococcus aureus	2–8 hours	SP, SV, D	Meat and dairy products	Toxin	Sudden onset; intense vomiting; no therapy needed in most cases
Bacillus cereus	2–8 hours	SP, SV, SD	Reheated fried rice	Tissue invasion	Early vomiting, later diarrhea; recovery within 24 hours
Clostridium perfringens	8–14 hours	V, SD	Reheated meat	Toxin	Profuse diarrhea
Vibrio parahaemolyticus	6 hours– 4 days	V, SD, F	Saltwater seafood	Toxin; tissue invasion	Outbreaks usually associated with ingestion of oysters, clams, and crabs
Salmonella species	8–48 hours	V, SD, F, P, H, systemic disease	Food	Mild tissue invasion; possible toxin	Diarrhea with low-grade fever; carrier state possible; should not be treated
Pathogenic *Escherichia coli*	1–3 days	SD	Food and water	Toxin; tissue invasion	Traveler's diarrhea; prophylaxis or therapy with quinolone, azithromycin, or rifaximin
Hemorrhagic *E. coli*, serotype 0157:H7	1–7 days	SP, SD, B	Raw beef; unprocessed milk; water	Toxin; tissue invasion	Severe pain and bloody diarrhea; may be associated with hemolytic–uremic syndrome or TTP; high mortality rate; therapy is supportive; antibiotics not generally recommended
Vibrio cholerae	1–3 days	V, SD	Poor hygiene	Toxin	Life-threatening diarrhea; therapy is intravenous replacement of fluid and electrolytes; epidemic occurrence
Shigella species (mild cases)	1–3 days	SD, F, B	Fecal–oral spread; flies	Toxin; tissue invasion	Therapy with ciprofloxacin if stool culture is positive or severe infection; generally self-limited
Clostridium botulinum	1–4 days	V, H, RE	Canned foods	Toxin	Severe CNS symptoms; ventilatory support needed; high mortality rate
Campylobacter jejuni	2–8 days	SD, B	Fecal–oral spread; pets	Tissue invasion	Most common cause of bacterial diarrhea in the United States; antibiotics for severe cases only
Clostridium difficile	?	SD, F, B	Fecal–oral spread	Toxin	Postantibiotic diarrhea; therapy with vancomycin or metronidazole
Yersinia enterocolitica	24–48 hours	SP, SD, B	Fecal–oral spread; pets	Tissue invasion; possible toxin	May be seen with polyarthritis in children; usually self-limited; aminoglycosides if severe
Protozoa					
Giardia lamblia	usually 1–2 weeks; range 1–45 days	Variable; SD, P, bloating and flatulence	Water	Noninvasive mechanism of pathogenesis not completely understood	Most common cause of waterborne infectious diarrhea in the United States; therapy with metronidazole usually is successful

(continued)

TABLE 6-1   Food Poisoning Syndromes (Continued)

Organism	Incubation Period	Symptoms	Sources of Contamination	Pathogenic Mechanisms	Comments
Cryptosporidium	7–10 days	SD, P	Fecally contaminated food or water; swimming pools	Interferes with intestinal absorption and secretion	Commonly affects immunocompromised patients; rarely occurs in normal individuals; no effective therapy is available
Isospora belli	7–10 days	F, D, H, M–S, D	Fecally contaminated food and water	Mucosal alteration in small and large bowel	Therapy is trimethoprim-sulfamethoxazole; rare in United States; unlike other protozoal infections, eosinophilia may be present
Entamoeba histolytica	Usually 2–4 weeks range: few days to several months	B, F, S, D, P variable	Fecally contaminated food and water	Penetration through mucosal layer	Therapy is metronidazole or iodoquinol
Viruses					
Rotavirus	2 days	V, D, F, P	Food, water, person to person	Tissue invasion toxin	Self-limited; supportive treatment; live oral vaccine available
Norovirus	24–28 hours	F, D, V, H	Food	Noninvasive	Self-limited; supportive treatment

B, blood in stool; CNS, central nervous system; D, diarrhea; F, fever; H, headache; M, mild; P, abdominal pain; S, severe; RE, respiratory embarrassment; TTP, thrombotic thrombocytopenic purpura; V, vomiting.

(4) **Inadequate mixing of gastric contents with bile salts and pancreatic enzymes** as a result of previous gastric surgery, especially Billroth II gastrectomy (🖱 see online)

b. **Intrinsic small bowel disease**

(1) **Celiac disease** causes flattening of the villi and inflammatory cell infiltration in the lamina propria (see IV E 4 c).

(2) **Collagenous sprue** refers to the deposition of a collagenous substance in the lamina propria in a patient who otherwise has the clinical and histologic features of celiac disease. Treatment is gluten-free diet and steroids.

(3) **Whipple's disease,** a systemic disease linked to *Tropheryma whippelii* infection, causes mucosal damage and lymphatic obstruction (see IV E 4 d).

(4) **Amyloidosis** (either primary or secondary) may affect the small intestine in 70% of cases by amyloid infiltration of the submucosa. Altered motility that allows bacterial overgrowth also may contribute to malabsorption. Occult gastrointestinal bleeding may be observed in approximately 25% of cases. Diagnosis is made by biopsy (usually of a rectal valve or stomach) with special stains (e.g., Congo red). Treatment primarily is supportive. A trial of antibiotics for bacterial overgrowth may be given.

(5) **Crohn's disease** may cause malabsorption by mucosal damage, by multiple strictures with bacterial overgrowth, or as a result of the need for multiple bowel resections (see IV G).

c. **Inadequate absorptive surface** (short bowel syndrome) results from extensive small bowel resection, usually for Crohn's disease or vascular compromise of the small intestine.

(1) Resection of up to 50% of the small intestine is well tolerated if the remaining bowel is normal, especially if ileum is preserved. Survival is possible after more extensive resection but requires careful management. If the proximal small bowel is resected, calcium, folic acid, and iron may not be absorbed; tetany may result. If the ileum is removed, bile acid and vitamin B_{12} absorption is impaired greatly. Hepatic dysfunction, oxalate kidney stones, and increased gastric acid secretion are common complications of extensive bowel resection. D-Lactic acidosis is a rare but life-threatening complication.

(2) Initial therapy includes intravenous fluid and electrolyte administration or parenteral hyperalimentation. Oral feedings should include medium-chain triglyceride (MCT oil), fat-soluble vitamins, and iron. Intramuscular vitamin B_{12} injections and antidiarrheal agents (to slow the transit time) may be needed. Cholestyramine resin may bind nonabsorbed bile salts and lessen the diarrhea; however, this drug also depletes the total body bile salt pool and usually is not used if more than 100 cm of distal ileum has been resected.

d. Lymphatic obstruction

(1) **Intestinal lymphangiectasia** may be primary (congenital) or secondary to intestinal tuberculosis, Whipple's disease, trauma, neoplasia, or retroperitoneal fibrosis. In advanced disease, dilated lymphatic channels rupture and leak into the intestinal lumen, causing lymphopenia, low serum protein levels, and massive peripheral edema. Small bowel biopsy reveals the characteristic dilated lymphatics. Treatment is with low-fat diet and MCT supplementation.

(2) **Intestinal lymphoma** may mimic Crohn's disease or adult celiac disease both clinically and radiographically. Clues to the differential diagnosis include persistent fevers and a short duration of symptoms. Enlarged lymph nodes or hepatosplenomegaly may be found on physical examination, and CT may show enlarged retroperitoneal nodes. Diagnosis is made usually only after surgical biopsy. Therapy includes local resection and radiation therapy. Chemotherapy is used for disseminated disease.

e. Multiple defects contribute to malabsorption in the following settings.

(1) **After gastrectomy.** Malabsorption can result after Billroth II gastrectomy, (🅟 see online) when poor mixing of gastric contents with pancreatic enzymes and stasis in the afferent loop with bacterial overgrowth are present. Therapy includes surgical correction of the afferent loop and broad-spectrum antibiotics.

(2) **Radiation enteritis.** This condition interferes with the blood supply to the intestine. Bacterial overgrowth also may occur secondary to the radiation-induced intestinal stricture. Lymphatic obstruction due to edema or fibrosis also may be a part of the syndrome.

(3) **Diabetes mellitus.** Altered gut motility from diabetic neuropathy, bacterial overgrowth, and exocrine pancreatic insufficiency all have been implicated as mechanisms.

🅟 **f. Other causes of malabsorption**

2. **Clinical features** are variable. Patients may present with some or all of the following clinical manifestations.

   a. Passage of abnormal stools, which are greasy, soft, bulky, and foul smelling and may float in the toilet because of their increased gas content; a film of grease or oil droplets may be seen on the surface of the water.

   b. Weight loss, which may be severe and involve marked muscle wasting

   c. Edema and ascites secondary to hypoalbuminemia

   d. Anemia secondary to altered absorption of iron, vitamin B_{12}, folate, or a combination of these

   e. Bone pain or fractures from vitamin D deficiency

   f. Paresthesias or tetany from calcium deficiency

   g. Bleeding from vitamin K deficiency

3. **Diagnosis** is based on clinical evidence, with confirmation by laboratory tests.

   a. **Stool fat analysis.** This test may be qualitative or quantitative. A positive Sudan stain indicates excretion of greater than 15 g fat per day in the stool. A 72-hour fecal fat collection can be used (while the patient maintains an intake of 80–100 g of fat/day) to quantify the amount of fat absorption. Normally, an individual absorbs 93%–95% of all dietary fat ingested. Pancreatic disease often is associated with fecal fat excretion in excess of 20–30 g/day on a diet of 100 g/day of fat.

   b. **D-Xylose absorption testing.** Because D-xylose, a five-carbon sugar, does not require enzymatic degradation or micelle formation for absorption, it can be used to measure intestinal mucosal integrity. After a 25-g oral dose, a 5-hour urine collection should contain at least 4–5 g of D-xylose. Alternatively, a 2-hour serum sample may be used.

   c. **Testing for unabsorbed carbohydrate.** Lowered stool pH occurs when unabsorbed carbohydrates reach the colon and bacterial fermentation occurs. This is particularly common in lactase deficiency but also may be seen in celiac disease and short bowel syndrome.

    d. Pancreatic function testing. Testing involves measuring the bicarbonate and total fluid output from the duodenum after secretin stimulation. Measuring fecal elastase can also be helpful for evaluation of pancreatic exocrine function. It is sensitive, specific, and independent of pancreatic enzyme replacement therapy.

    e. Measurement of serum carotene levels. Because vitamin A is fat soluble and the serum carotene level is a reflection of vitamin A metabolism, a low serum carotene level with normal vitamin A intake may be a useful screening test for fat malabsorption.

    f. Bacterial overgrowth testing

    g. Small bowel radiography. This procedure can be useful for identifying structural abnormalities. Thick folds may be seen in Whipple's disease, lymphoma, amyloidosis, radiation enteritis, Zollinger–Ellison syndrome, and eosinophilic enteritis, and a pseudo-Whipple's appearance is observed in patients with AIDS enteropathy.

    h. Schilling test. This technique is rarely used to diagnose vitamin B_{12} malabsorption.

    i. Small bowel biopsy. This procedure is essential for the diagnosis of many cases of malabsorption. In properly prepared specimens, normal villous crypt ratios are 3:1 or 4:1. Flattening of the villi with inflammatory cell infiltration is characteristic of celiac disease, but flattened villi alone may be seen in infectious enteritis, giardiasis, lymphoma, and bacterial overgrowth.

  4. Characteristics and management of specific causes of malabsorption

    a. Pancreatic insufficiency may be caused by chronic pancreatitis, pancreatic carcinoma, or cystic fibrosis. Treatment is pancreatic enzyme replacement. Most agents are enteric coated to minimize inactivation by gastric acid.

    b. Bacterial overgrowth may be attributable to altered motility (e.g., in diabetes, amyloidosis, and intestinal pseudo-obstruction), small bowel diverticula, strictures (e.g., in lymphoma and Crohn's disease), or blind loops after Billroth II gastrectomy (see online). Surgical correction of the anatomic problems may be considered, but treatment with antibiotics frequently is successful. Many antibiotics have been used successfully, including ampicillin, amoxicillin clavulanate, tetracycline, ciprofloxacin, or co-trimoxazole. The nonabsorbable antibiotic rifaximin has also been used with success. Some patients require continuous therapy, and in these cases, antibiotics should be rotated.

    c. Celiac disease (nontropical sprue)

      (1) Abnormal sensitivity to gluten, a protein component of wheat, causes damage to the intestinal mucosa of these patients. The importance of genetic factors is demonstrated by abnormal small bowel biopsies in 10%–15% of first-degree relatives of patients. The incidence may be as high as 1 in 120 to 1 in 150 of the U.S. population. Celiac patients have proximal intestinal involvement with a relative sparing of the distal ileum.

      (2) Clinical features include diarrhea, steatorrhea, weight loss, and abdominal bloating. Symptoms may begin in childhood and then lessen, only to reappear in the third to sixth decades of life. Only 30%–40% of adult patients present with the classic symptoms of diarrhea, abdominal bloating, weight loss, and steatorrhea. Most of the patients have insidious presentations, including infertility, abnormal liver function tests, osteoporosis, anemia, autoimmune diseases such as type 1 diabetes mellitus, rheumatoid arthritis, or systemic lupus erythematosus. Iron-deficiency anemia unassociated with gastrointestinal blood loss may be seen because iron is preferentially absorbed in the more severely involved proximal small intestine. Unexplained CNS symptoms such as depression, neurologic deficit, or even seizures may be more common in celiac patients.

      (3) Diagnosis requires small bowel biopsy, which shows villous atrophy, crypt hypertrophy, and cuboidal change in the epithelial cells. Inflammatory cell infiltration in the lamina propria at endoscopy may show "scalloped folds" in the proximal duodenum. **Tissue transglutaminase antibody** (TTG-immunoglobulin A [IgA]) is currently the diagnostic antibody of choice with the highest sensitivity and specificity for celiac disease. All antibodies may decrease or disappear with treatment. Because approximately 5%–7% of patients with celiac disease may be IgA deficient, a total IgA level may be necessary if relying on IgA celiac antibodies for diagnostic purposes. Antiendomysial antibodies are less sensitive but more specific.

      (4) Therapy is based on withdrawal of gluten from the diet by eliminating wheat, rye, barley, and oats. Clinical response to gluten withdrawal often is dramatic and may be seen in a few days. Histologic recovery demonstrated on repeat small bowel biopsy may be delayed for months and, in up to 50% of patients, may never be demonstrated. In severely ill patients, steroids may be of short-term benefit.

  (5) Complications
    (a) Lymphoma or carcinoma
    (b) Intestinal ulcers or strictures
    (c) Dermatitis herpetiformis
    (d) Collagenous sprue
    (e) Increased incidence of autoimmune diseases
    (f) Refractory sprue
  d. **Whipple's disease** is a systemic disorder most commonly occurring in middle-aged men.
    (1) **Etiology and pathogenesis.** Numerous small gram-positive cocci are seen in macrophages in individual organs, and the organism *Tropheryma whippelii* has been isolated as the infectious agent. Malabsorption is caused by mucosal damage and lymphatic obstruction.
    (2) **Clinical features** depend on organ involvement. In the intestine, periodic acid–Schiff (PAS)–positive macrophages (i.e., macrophages that contain bacilli) are found in the lamina propria. The mesenteric lymph nodes, heart, spleen, lungs, and CNS also may be involved. Fever occurs in one third to one half of patients. Arthralgia and arthritis are present in 60% of patients and may precede the gastrointestinal symptoms.
    (3) **Diagnosis** is made by intestinal biopsy with a PAS stain. A small bowel radiograph may show thickened folds. In rare cases, the disease is focal and the biopsy specimen is normal.
    (4) **Therapy** with penicillin, ampicillin, or tetracycline is required for at least 4–6 months and may be continued intermittently (i.e., every other day) thereafter. The relapse rate is approximately 10%.

F **Protein-losing enteropathy (PLE)**

G **Crohn's disease (regional enteritis)** is a chronic granulomatous disease that may occur anywhere in the gastrointestinal tract from the mouth to the anus. The ileum most often is involved, with ileocolitis in more than 50% of patients. The first peak of incidence occurs between the ages of 12 and 30 years; a secondary peak occurs at age 50 years.

1. **Etiology**
   a. **Genetic factors** appear to play a role, with an increased incidence of disease noted in monozygotic twins and siblings. Approximately 17% of patients with Crohn's disease have first-degree relatives with the disease. Men are affected more often than women, and the disease is more common among Jews. Compared with the general population, Jewish men have six times the risk of Crohn's disease. The condition can be associated with Turner's syndrome, hypogammaglobulinemia, and selective IgA deficiency.
   b. An **immunologic mechanism** is the most prominent theory. The mucosal immune system becomes reactive to luminal contents. Abnormal numbers, subsets, and functions of T cells have been identified in cases of Crohn's disease. Hyperresponsive immune function, rather than abnormal function, is characteristic. Activated T cells spark a cascade of inflammatory mediators. Luminal bacteria or gut infection may initiate or propagate this response.

2. **Pathologic features**
   a. Marked thickening of the involved intestinal wall with transmural inflammation
   b. Enlarged and matted mesenteric lymph nodes
   c. Focal granulomas in 50% of specimens
   d. Deep serpiginous or linear ulcerations leading to cobblestoning and fistula formation
   e. Stricture formation secondary to scarring
   f. Alternating areas of normal and involved mucosa

3. **Clinical features** are characterized by periodic exacerbations and remissions.
   a. **Pain** often is colicky, especially in the lower abdomen, and may be increased after meals because of the obstructive nature of the pathologic process.
   b. **Systemic symptoms** are common and include fever, weight loss, malaise, and anorexia.
   c. **Diarrhea** is the usual presenting symptom.
   d. **Intestinal obstruction** is the presenting symptom in approximately 25% of cases.

    e. Extraintestinal manifestations are numerous.

        (1) Anemia as well as growth or sexual retardation probably is attributable to inadequate caloric intake.

        (2) Hepatobiliary disorders include fatty liver, pericholangitis, nonspecific hepatitis, cirrhosis, and **sclerosing cholangitis.** There is an increased risk of gallstones. Liver enzyme or liver biopsy abnormalities occur in 50%–70% of patients with Crohn's disease.

        (3) Renal disorders include right ureteral obstruction secondary to contiguous bowel involvement and nephrolithiasis. An increase in calcium oxalate stones is caused by increased oxalate absorption, and an increase in uric acid stones is ascribed to increased cell turnover and concentrated acidic urine.

        (4) Peripheral arthritis occurs in 10%–12% of patients and ankylosing spondylitis in 2%–10%.

        (5) Skin problems include **erythema nodosum** and, rarely, pyoderma gangrenosum.

        (6) Episcleritis or uveitis may occur in 3%–10% of patients.

    f. Fistulas to the skin or other organs occur in approximately 20% of patients. Perianal fistulas or abscesses are especially common in Crohn's colitis. Perianal skin tags are characteristic of colonic Crohn's disease.

4. Diagnosis is based on clinical signs and symptoms combined with characteristic radiographic findings, including deep (collar button) ulcerations, long strictured segments (string sign), and skip areas. Colonoscopy may be helpful when there is colonic involvement, and biopsies may show **granulomas.** Laboratory studies are not specific but may show multifactorial anemia, leukocytosis, an increased sedimentation rate, and evidence of malabsorption or protein loss. Serologic perinuclear antineutrophil cytoplasmic antibodies (**pANCAs**) and anti–*Saccharomyces cerevisiae* (**ASCAs**) antibodies can help diagnose Crohn's disease and identify phenotypes. ASCA antibodies are positive in 60%–70% of Crohn's disease patients, and pANCA positivity is found in 60%–70% of ulcerative colitis patients. Sensitivity and specificity of these antibodies depends on the prevalence of inflammatory bowel disease in a given population. The differential diagnosis for Crohn's disease includes lymphoma, tuberculosis, radiation enteritis, *Yersinia* infection (especially in acute enteritis), and glycogen storage disease type 1B (in children).

5. Therapy is aimed at treating the underlying inflammation and managing complications. No cure exists.

    a. Supportive measures include short-term, broad-spectrum antibiotics; antidiarrheal agents; bowel rest with intravenous fluid support (i.e., nothing by mouth); enteral nutrition with tube feedings; total parenteral nutrition; and vitamin supplementation.

    b. Medical treatment

        (1) 5-Aminosalicylic acid preparations may be used alone or in combination with corticosteroids to treat acute disease. This may be more effective in Crohn's colitis. Ethyl cellulose–coated oral 5-aminosalicylic acid preparations may be useful in small bowel disease.

        (2) Vitamin B$_{12}$ injections are indicated when ileal disease causes malabsorption of this vitamin.

        (3) Oral calcium, vitamin D, or **both** may be helpful in patients with calcium oxalate stones by binding oxalate in the bowel and decreasing urinary oxalate.

        (4) Metronidazole, quinolone antibiotics, or **both** may be effective in treatment of perineal and perianal fistulas and colonic disease.

        (5) Corticosteroids are effective in acute disease but have no role in maintenance of remission. Budesonide, a corticosteroid that is inactivated by first-pass metabolism through the liver, minimizes systemic side effects and is effective for ileal and right colon disease.

        (6) 6-Mercaptopurine, azathioprine, and **methotrexate** also have been used and are effective in prolonging and inducing remission.

        (7) Biologic agents are antibodies administered to target certain cytokines and inflammatory mediators. Patients treated with such agents should be considered immunosuppressed in regard to infectious complications.

            (a) Tumor necrosis factor (TNF) inhibitors include **infliximab, adalimumab, and certolizumab.** Infliximab is a chimeric mouse–human antibody that destroys macrophages and T cells that make TNF while also directly blocking TNF in the serum. Response rates approach 60%–70% for conventional treatment-refractory Crohn's patients, as well as for the treatment of perianal and enterocutaneous fistulas. Adalimumab blocks the interaction between TNF and cell surface receptors, with less immunogenicity in patients.

   (b) Natalizumab is a humanized monoclonal antibody to alpha-4 integrin. This antibody blocks leukocyte adhesion and migration into inflamed tissue. Data have shown improvements in Crohn's disease severity, except in fistulizing disease.

   c. Surgery may be necessary for recurrent intestinal obstruction, enterocutaneous or intra-abdominal fistulas, and perforation, as well as for growth retardation that does not respond to increased caloric intake. The recurrence rate after initial resection may be as high as 80% within 15 years, especially with initial small bowel involvement.

H Small bowel tumors

   1. **Malignant tumors** of the small intestine are rare and include **adenocarcinoma, carcinoid tumors, lymphoma, and leiomyosarcoma.** Capsule endoscopy and push enteroscopy are techniques used to evaluate the small bowel. (For gastrointestinal stromal tumors [GISTs] see Online II B.)

   a. **Etiology and pathogenesis**

   b. **Pathology**

   c. **Clinical features**

   d. **Therapy and prognosis**

   2. **Benign tumors** of the small intestine include **adenomas, lipomas,** and **leiomyomas,** which may be associated with obstruction or bleeding but usually are asymptomatic.

I Acute appendicitis is a common and curable cause of an acute abdomen. Appendicitis develops at any age and in both sexes but most often occurs in males between 10 and 30 years of age.

   1. **Pathogenesis.** It is believed that the primary event is an obstruction of the appendiceal lumen by a fecalith, inflammation, foreign body, or neoplasm. After obstruction of the lumen, increased intraluminal pressure and infection may cause appendiceal necrosis and perforation.

   2. **Clinical features.** Appendicitis is characterized by pain in the right lower quadrant, which initially is vague but becomes localized to McBurney's point, peritoneal signs, fever, and leukocytosis in the range of $10,000–20,000/mm^3$. Rectal tenderness is common in pelvic appendicitis, and retrocecal appendicitis causes psoas muscle pain on hip extension. Patients at the extremes of age, greatly obese patients, and patients taking corticosteroids may have nonspecific complaints and a relatively benign physical examination. A high index of clinical suspicion must be maintained in these cases.

   3. **Diagnosis**
      a. **Differential diagnoses.** Possible diagnoses include acute gastroenteritis, mesenteric adenitis, Meckel's diverticulum, and Crohn's disease. In young women, ovarian torsion, ruptured ovarian cyst, and pelvic inflammatory disease (PID) should be considered. In elderly patients, diverticulitis, cholecystitis, incarcerated hernia, cecal carcinoma, and mesenteric thrombosis should be ruled out.
      b. **Diagnostic modalities.** In difficult-to-diagnose cases, a **CT scan** shows a mass-like effect in the right lower quadrant. On **ultrasound,** a classic "bull's-eye" appearance of the right lower quadrant is believed to be relatively diagnostic of appendicitis.

   4. **Therapy.** Surgery should be performed as early as possible to prevent perforation.

V   DISEASES OF THE COLON

A Constipation

   1. **Simple constipation** is the result of delayed transit of intestinal contents. The highly refined, low-fiber diets of industrialized nations probably contribute to this problem. Although the epidemiologic definition of constipation is less than three stools per week, individual differences exist. Treatment of simple constipation is directed toward increasing intestinal bulk by increasing dietary fiber content with fruits, vegetables, and bulking agents such as psyllium hydrophilic

colloids, which trap water and electrolytes within the bowel lumen. Long-term use of potent laxatives should be avoided because they may result in destruction of colonic intramural nerve plexuses and cathartic colon.

2. **Constipation** may occur with a variety of diseases, including ulcerative proctitis, rectal fissures or abscesses, and rectal strictures, as well as the varied causes of diffusely decreased intestinal activity discussed in IV A and B. Irritable bowel syndrome, which may present as either constipation or diarrhea, is discussed in IV D 3 a.

3. **Colonic inertia** is a motility disorder of the colon characterized by poor propulsion and ineffective mixing. When radiopaque markers are ingested, they often remain in the colon for beyond 7 days. These markers are distributed throughout the colon, indicating poor total colonic motility. **Outlet obstruction** usually occurs when a problem with internal or external sphincteric relaxation develops. In this setting, markers accumulate in the rectum before defecation.

B **Colonic diverticula** are outpouchings of the mucosa only and, therefore, are not true diverticula. In the United States, colonic diverticula occur in approximately 50% of individuals older than 60 years of age.

1. **Pathogenesis.** In industrialized nations, colonic diverticula have been linked to low-fiber diets. Diets low in fiber and bulk are thought to cause an increased intraluminal pressure, particularly in the narrow sigmoid colon. Eventually, the increased intraluminal pressure causes a mucosal herniation at the site of a perforating arteriole carrying blood from the serosal surface to the mucosa.

2. **Clinical features.** Symptoms often are absent in uncomplicated colonic diverticula; however, patients may complain of crampy abdominal pain in the left lower quadrant, with alternating diarrhea and constipation. Often, there is relief of these symptoms after a bowel movement.

3. **Therapy.** Treatment is aimed at increasing stool bulk with high-fiber foods and hydrophilic colloids, thereby decreasing intraluminal pressure. This results in symptomatic improvement, probably by regulating bowel frequency.

4. **Complications**
   a. **Diverticulitis** occurs in approximately 10%–25% of patients with diverticulosis. Generally, there is a microperforation (rarely, a free perforation) with a peridiverticular abscess. Symptoms include left lower quadrant abdominal pain, fever, and constipation. Treatment with antibiotics, intravenous fluids, and bowel rest is effective in most cases. Metronidazole, ciprofloxacin, or ampicillin sodium/sulbactam sodium is used most commonly. Severely ill or toxic patients may require additional antibiotics for adequate coverage of *Pseudomonas* and anaerobes. If an abscess occurs, a fistula to the bladder or vagina may develop.
   b. **Bleeding** occurs in up to 15% of cases and usually is brisk, painless, and not associated with straining. In most cases, bleeding stops spontaneously with only supportive therapy. Arteriography or rapid-sequence nuclear scanning using technetium sulfur colloid or technetium-labeled erythrocytes may localize the bleeding portion of the colon and allow segmental surgical resection, if necessary.

C **Hirschsprung's disease**

D **Ulcerative colitis** is a chronic inflammatory disease of the colonic mucosa and submucosa. Ulcerative colitis and Crohn's disease share some features and, despite their dissimilarities, often are placed together under the generic heading of inflammatory bowel disease. The major peak of incidence occurs between the ages of 15 and 30 years, with a lesser peak between the ages of 50 and 65 years, with males and females affected equally.

1. **Etiology and pathogenesis** are similar to those of Crohn's disease (see IV G). Family members have an increased risk of inflammatory bowel disease; up to 20% of patients have a family member with inflammatory bowel disease. The incidence is increased twofold to fourfold in those of Jewish descent. Whereas smoking increases the risk of Crohn's disease, it decreases the risk of ulcerative colitis to approximately half that of the general population. There is an increased risk of ulcerative colitis in patients who have recently discontinued smoking. For patients with ulcerative colitis patients who are HLA-B27 positive, there is a strong association with arthritis, and especially with ankylosing spondylitis.

2. **Pathology.** The hallmarks of ulcerative colitis are the microabscesses of the crypts of Lieberkühn, which are seen in approximately 70% of cases. The inflammatory response generally is limited to the mucosa. Macroscopic ulcerations are noted with confluence of the inflammatory response. Pseudopolyps occur when normal mucosa is isolated by severe ulcerations, but there are no skip areas. The rectum and distal colon are involved most commonly. Pancolitis is seen in 25% of cases. Ulcerative colitis with rectal sparing is extremely uncommon.

3. **Clinical features** are mild when the disease is limited to the rectum (ulcerative proctitis). Moderate-to-severe symptoms may occur with extensive disease, particularly pancolitis, and include bloody diarrhea, weight loss, fever, abdominal pain, and nocturnal passage of a small volume of blood and mucus. Fulminant disease occurs in 15% of cases. Extraintestinal manifestations are similar to those of Crohn's disease and are evident in 10%–15% of patients. Extraintestinal signs and symptoms include nonsymmetric large-joint arthritis, sacroiliitis (especially in HLA-B27–positive patients), erythema nodosum, pyoderma gangrenosum, sclerosing cholangitis, and uveitis.

4. **Diagnosis** is based on clinical presentation along with the exclusion of infectious, parasitic, and neoplastic etiologic factors. Serologic analysis for p-ANCA may aid in differentiation between ulcerative colitis and Crohn's disease (see IV G), although overlap exists. These antibodies occur in up to 70% of patients with ulcerative colitis.

   a. **Stool examination** reveals mucus, blood, and white blood cells without parasites or bacterial pathogens. It is important to rule out the usual causes of dysentery, including *Salmonella*, *Shigella*, *Campylobacter*, pathogenic *E. coli* (especially *E. coli* O157:H7), amebiasis, and *C. difficile* infection.

   b. **Colonoscopy or proctosigmoidoscopy** reveals friability, edema, and hyperemia of the mucosa. Ulcerations and a mucopurulent exudate may be present. Islands of normal tissue may have the appearance of pseudopolyps. Numerous biopsy samples should be obtained.

   c. **Barium enema** should not be performed in severely ill or toxic patients. If the symptoms are subacute, a barium radiograph after minimal preparation may show a lack of haustral markings, fine serrations (compatible with small ulcerations), large ulcerations, and pseudopolyps.

5. **Therapy** varies with the severity and extent of disease.

   a. In acute flares, **bowel rest with intravenous fluids** may be useful for short periods. Total parenteral nutrition allows prolonged bowel rest with repletion of vitamins, minerals, electrolytes, and calories in the form of carbohydrate, protein, and fat but is rarely used except in severe disease.

   b. **5-Aminosalicylic acid and sulfasalazine** have been shown to induce remission and decrease relapse rates in ulcerative colitis patients. Side effects include headache, nausea, rash, and agranulocytosis. 5-Aminosalicylic acid enemas are effective in left-sided colitis.

   c. **Corticosteroids,** which are administered by enema (especially in distal disease such as ulcerative proctitis) or systemically, may be effective in inducing remission. Prednisone is given orally in doses of 20–60 mg/day.

   d. **Immunomodulating agents** such as 6-mercaptopurine, azathioprine, and cyclosporine have been tried in the hopes of avoiding or delaying emergent surgery or as a steroid-sparing agent in steroid-resistant patients.

   e. **Biologic agents.** In clinical trials, up to 52% of refractory patients responded to infliximab, with up to 37% maintaining remission at 30 weeks.

   f. **Surgery** requires the removal of the entire colon with the creation of an ileostomy or creation of an ileal pouch and ileoanal anastomosis. Surgery is generally reserved for the following conditions:

      (1) Toxic megacolon that is unresponsive to 24–72 hours of intensive conservative medical measures

      (2) Perforation

      (3) Massive hemorrhage that is unresponsive to conservative treatment (rare)

      (4) Carcinoma

      (5) Suspected carcinoma in colonic strictures

      (6) Growth failure in adolescents that is unresponsive to conservative treatment

      (7) Dysplasia noted on biopsy at the time of sigmoidoscopy or colonoscopy

      (8) Cure, as the ileoanal anastomotic procedure that strips the colonic mucosa and avoids the need for a permanent ileostomy has become widespread.

6. **Complications.** The systemic complications noted for Crohn's disease (see IV G 3 e) often occur in ulcerative colitis. Additional complications occur with ulcerative colitis that usually are not seen in Crohn's disease.

   a. **Toxic megacolon** refers to an acute dilation of the colon (usually the transverse portion) to a diameter in excess of 6 cm. This complication of ulcerative colitis probably is attributable to severe inflammation, which affects large segments of the colonic musculature as well as neural control of the colon. Anticholinergic and antidiarrheal medications also may contribute. Patients usually are severely ill, with high fever, abdominal pain, and a marked leukocytosis. Treatment is intensive medical therapy for 48–72 hours. Patients who do not respond should undergo an emergency total colectomy.

   b. **Carcinoma** of the colon is associated with longstanding disease of great extent (usually pancolitis). The risk of cancer increases 0.5%–1% per year after 8–10 years of pancolitis disease. The malignancies often are multicentric and aggressive. Strictured areas of the colon present a particularly difficult problem because of the difficulty in differentiating intensive inflammatory disease from ischemic narrowing or carcinoma. Regular colonoscopic examinations with biopsy samples obtained every 10–20 cm should be performed in patients with longstanding disease, typically after 8–10 years in pancolitis and after 15 years in left-sided disease. If high-grade dysplasia is noted, a prophylactic total colectomy is recommended.

7. **Prognosis.** Mortality rates are approximately 20% in toxic megacolon, with higher rates noted in patients older than 60 years. Approximately 10% of patients do not experience a recurrent attack after the initial onset of disease. Continuous symptoms occur in 10% of patients. Approximately 70%–80% of patients have recurrent remissions and relapses, and approximately 20% of patients eventually require total colectomy.

E **Angiodysplasia/angioectasia** refers to small vascular abnormalities that usually are seen in the ascending colon or cecum in patients older than 60 years of age. Involvement of the small bowel or stomach also occurs. Associations with aortic stenosis and chronic renal insufficiency have been reported.

1. **Pathogenesis.** Angiodysplasia is believed to result from obstruction of intestinal capillaries and venules as these vessels pass through the muscularis propria.

2. **Clinical features.** Most patients are asymptomatic, but the abnormal vessels are a common cause of painless lower gastrointestinal bleeding in older individuals.

3. **Diagnosis.** Angiographic or colonoscopic demonstration of intraluminal extravasation of blood during the acute episode may be used to make the diagnosis.

4. **Therapy.** Bleeding usually can be managed conservatively with colonoscopic treatment using thermal methods or endoscopic clipping, but colon resection occasionally is needed for recurrent or massive bleeding.

F **Endometriosis** involves the colon in approximately 10% of cases. Symptoms include pain or rectal bleeding during menses. A barium enema often reveals extrinsic compression of the rectosigmoid or descending colon. Treatment is hormonal. Rarely, surgery is necessary to alleviate obstruction, pain, or recurrent bleeding.

G **Tumors of the colon**

1. **Benign tumors.** There are several histologic types of benign colonic polyps. **Adenomatous polyps** are considered to be precursors of adenocarcinoma, and the risk increases when the polyps are larger than 2 cm, villous rather than tubular, and sessile (flat-based) rather than pedunculated. Approximately 5%–10% of individuals older than age 40 years have colonic polyps, but most of these polyps are small **hyperplastic** lesions that carry no malignant potential. Other benign tumors include leiomyomas, lipomas, and fibromas.

   a. **Clinical features.** Small polyps are asymptomatic. In large polyps (>1 cm), rectal bleeding may occur and may be microscopic or macroscopic. Large polyps may cause symptoms of an incomplete intestinal obstruction with occasional crampy abdominal pain.

   b. **Diagnosis.** Imaging is by colonoscopy or radiographic study. Barium enema or CT scan is possible.

c. **Therapy**
(1) Therapy for pedunculated lesions is colonoscopic removal with snare electrocautery. Sessile lesions may require surgical excision.
(2) Because carcinoma occurring in an adenomatous polyp may be focal, careful histologic sectioning of the entire polyp, not just a biopsy, is necessary to exclude carcinoma. If malignancy invades the stalk of a polyp, a segmental resection of the colon is indicated to rule out lymphatic spread.
(3) Synchronous polyps occur in 20% of cases, and metachronous lesions occur in approximately 30% of cases. Therefore, full colon evaluation, generally by colonoscopy, must be performed. Follow-up colonoscopy is indicated, and the interval between studies depends on completeness of polyp resection, size and number of polyps removed, and whether polyps are found on subsequent examinations.
(4) First-degree relatives of a patient with colonic polyps or carcinoma are at increased risk of development of a similar lesion. The daily use of aspirin or other NSAIDs may be associated with decreased polyp formation.

2. **Hereditary polyposis syndromes**
a. **Familial adenomatous polyposis (FAP)**
b. **Peutz–Jeghers syndrome**
c. **Turcot's syndrome**
d. **Juvenile polyposis**
e. **Cronkhite–Canada syndrome**
f. **Cowden's disease**

3. **Adenocarcinoma of the colon.** This type of cancer has been steadily increasing in frequency in the United States and ranks second to lung cancer in men and third to breast cancer and lung cancer in women (overall second in men and women) as the major life-threatening malignancy.
   a. **Epidemiology.** The incidence of colorectal carcinomas is increased in developed countries, especially those with a diet high in red meat and low in fiber. In the United States, the incidence is decreased in Seventh-Day Adventists, who practice strict vegetarianism, which also suggests an association with diet. The incidence of colorectal carcinomas is higher in asbestos workers, machinists, and factory woodworkers than in the general population. Increased calcium and folic acid intake in men and women, as well as postmenopausal hormone therapy in women, may be protective. Daily use of aspirin or other NSAIDs also may decrease the risk of developing colon cancer.
   b. **Etiology**
      (1) **Dietary factors.** Diet has been the focus of most etiologic studies. The increased amounts of red meat and animal fat in the diet in the United States promote the growth of bacterial strains that produce carcinogens in the colonic lumen. Bile salts also may contribute to this process. Vitamins A, C, and E in certain foods may inactivate the carcinogens, and broccoli, turnips, and cauliflower induce benzpyrene hydroxylase, which also may inactivate ingested carcinogens.
      (2) **Genetic factors.** The role of genetic factors is demonstrated by FAP and by the fact that first-degree relatives of patients with carcinoma or polyps have a threefold to fivefold increased risk of colorectal carcinoma. FAP accounts for approximately 1% of colorectal cancer (Online IV B). Hereditary nonpolyposis colorectal cancer (HNPCC) family syndromes account for 10% of all colorectal cancer and are autosomal dominant syndromes characterized by an abnormality in mismatch repair genes. One should consider a genetic cause of colorectal cancer if the patient is younger than age 50 years or has a first-degree relative with a colon cancer syndrome.
         (a) **HNPCC type I** is an autosomal dominant inherited form of colon cancer. HNPCC often develops before patients reach 45 years of age and frequently involves the ascending colon.
         (b) **HNPCC type II** is associated with carcinoma of the endometrium, ovary, ureter, renal pelvis, stomach, pancreas, and biliary tree and otherwise is similar to HNPCC type I.

(3) **Other risk factors**
    (a) Ulcerative colitis, especially pancolitis and disease of greater than 10 years' duration
    (b) History of colon cancer or adenoma
    (c) Family history of colon cancer or adenomatous polyp
    (d) History of female genital or breast cancer
    (e) History of juvenile polyps
    (f) Immunodeficiency diseases
    (g) *Streptococcus bovis* **bacteremia**
    (h) Tobacco use

c. **Clinical features.** Signs and symptoms vary, depending on the location and size of the tumor. Tumors in the left colon, especially those in the distal 25 cm, may manifest as obstruction. Right colon tumors frequently present as iron-deficiency anemia and fatigue. Other common symptoms include a change in bowel habit, a decrease in stool size, obvious blood in the stool, and crampy abdominal pain. Metastatic disease usually involves the liver; however, the bone, lung, and brain also may be affected.

d. **Screening guidelines** are based on age and risk of colorectal cancer. These guidelines are listed in Table 6–2.

e. **Diagnosis**
    (1) Diagnosis is made by colonoscopy or air contrast barium enema demonstration of polyps or tumors followed by endoscopic visualization with biopsy and cytologic study. The air contrast barium enema is far more sensitive than the single-contrast examination. Despite these techniques, it can be difficult to differentiate the tumor from diverticulitis, benign stricture, and Crohn's disease. Computed tomography colonoscopy can detect polyps between 6 and 10 mm with high sensitivity and specificity per multicenter trials. There is debate over what an acceptable cutoff size is for follow-up colonoscopy. This modality is not

---

TABLE 6–2   **Colorectal Cancer Screening Recommendations**

Risk for Colorectal Cancer	Recommendations
Average-risk patients (choose one)	Colonoscopy every 10 years after age 50 years
	Fecal occult blood testing or fecal immunochemical test yearly after age 50 years
	Flexible sigmoidoscopy up to 40 cm or the splenic flexure every 5 years
	Double-contrast barium enema every 5 years
Increased-risk patients	
FAP	Genetic testing/counseling
	Flexible sigmoidoscopy beginning age 10–12 years (consider total colectomy if genetic test is positive)
HNPCC	Genetic testing/counseling
	Colonoscopy every 1–2 years after age 20 years, or 10 years earlier than the youngest age of colon cancer diagnosis in the immediate family
Ulcerative colitis	Colonoscopy every 1–2 years after 8 years of disease in patients with pancolitis or colonoscopy every 1–2 years after 15 years in patients with left-sided colitis
First-degree relatives with colon cancer	Same screening as average-risk patients, except begin at age 40 years or 10 years earlier than the first-degree relative's age at diagnosis
Personal history of colon cancer	Complete colonoscopy prior to, during, or within 6 months of resection if no metastatic disease found
	At 1 year and 3 years after surgery; after 3 years, follow-up interval determined by presence or absence of new adenomas
Adenomatous polyps	1 or 2 small (<1 cm) tubular adenomas: colonoscopy at 5–10 years
	3–10 adenomas, 1 or more adenomas >1 cm, adenoma with villous features or high-grade dysplasia: colonoscopy at 3 years
	>10 adenomas: colonoscopy <3 years, consider screening for familial syndrome

FAP, familial adenomatous polyposis; HNPCC, hereditary nonpolyposis colorectal cancer syndrome.
From Levin B, Lieberman DA, McFarland B, et al. Screening and surveillance for the early detection of colorectal cancer and adenomatous polyps, 2008: a joint guideline from the American Cancer Society, the US Multi-Society Task Force on Colorectal Cancer, and the American College of Radiology. *CA Cancer J Clin* 2008;58(3):130–160.

a first-line screening test for high-risk patients (including those with positive fecal occult blood in stool). It could potentially lead to better adherence to colorectal screening.

  (2) Carcinoembryonic antigen (CEA) determinations, although not useful for screening purposes, may be used for periodic follow-up in patients with a history of carcinoma of the colon, with an increasing titer being indicative of recurrent or metastatic disease.

 f. Therapy (see Chapter 5 VIII A 9 a)

 g. Prognosis. The overall 10-year survival rate is 45% and has not changed significantly over the last several years. Staging uses the TNM classification.

  (1) Stage I disease. Cancer confined to the mucosa is often detected by screening. Stage I also includes cancers that penetrate into the muscularis propria, and 5-year survival rate is reported as 93%.

  (2) Stage II disease. Cancer that penetrates through the serosa without lymph node involvement is associated with a 78% 5-year survival rate.

  (3) Stage III disease. Cancer that has spread to regional lymph nodes is associated with a 64% 5-year survival rate. Better prognosis is seen in those with fewer than five lymph nodes involved by cancer.

  (4) Stage IV disease. Cancer that has metastasized to distant organs is associated with a survival rate of less than 25%.

H **Microscopic colitis** refers to two separate entities: **collagenous colitis** and **lymphocytic colitis.** Both are recently described and typically present with chronic watery diarrhea, especially seen in middle-aged women. Laboratory data are usually normal, although 50% of patients may have an increase in erythrocyte sedimentation rate. Hypoalbuminemia and mild steatorrhea have been reported. Colonoscopic examination findings are normal, but biopsy indicates an increase in mononuclear cells in both and a thick layer of subepithelial collagen deposition greater than 10 μm in thickness in collagenous colitis. Treatment is with antidiarrheal agents, 5-aminosalicylates, or steroids, including budesonide. Immunomodulators such as azathioprine have been used in steroid-resistant or steroid-dependent cases.

I **Pseudomembranous colitis** is an acute, potentially severe disease of the colon characterized by exudative plaques that cover the intestinal mucosa. Hospital outbreaks are common. Severe pseudomembranous colitis is rare (<5% of cases) but is associated with mortality of up to 65%.

 1. Pathogenesis. The disease is caused by an enterotoxin produced by *C. difficile,* an anaerobic bacterium. It is thought that antibiotic therapy may "select out" the *C. difficile* organism, allowing proliferation and toxin production. Symptoms begin 3 days to 4 weeks after initiating antibiotic therapy. Virtually all antibiotics have been associated with this disease, but clindamycin, fluoroquinolones, and the cephalosporins are the most common offenders.

 2. Clinical features. Signs and symptoms include watery diarrhea, crampy abdominal pain, lower abdominal tenderness, and fever. Leukocytosis is common. Dehydration and electrolyte disturbances may develop in severely ill patients. Toxic megacolon and colonic perforation are rare but serious complications that may require surgical intervention. Approximately 20% of patients relapse after primary treatment.

 3. Diagnosis. Demonstration of *C. difficile* toxin in the stool is the most common method of diagnosis. Endoscopic visualization of the characteristic yellow-white plaques in an erythematous and edematous mucosa suggests the diagnosis. Biopsy of the plaques shows a mucinous, fibrinous, polymorphonuclear exudate. Most patients have disease throughout the colon; however, the disease may be confined to the right colon, and in such cases sigmoidoscopic findings are negative.

 4. Therapy. The first step in treatment is to discontinue unnecessary antibiotics, which results in improvement in most patients. **Metronidazole** is first-line therapy, and **oral vancomycin** should be used in severe cases. Relapse is treated with a second course of therapy. Multiple relapses can be treated with tapering or pulsed doses of vancomycin or probiotics, including *Lactobacillus* or *Saccharomyces boulardii* or cholestyramine. Early data suggest rifaximin to be effective. Severe relapse cases have been treated with fecal transplantation or intravenous immunoglobulins.

J Anal carcinoma

K **Volvulus of the colon** generally involves either the sigmoid colon (slightly more common) or the cecal region. Sigmoid volvulus usually occurs in individuals older than 60 years of age who live in nursing homes, have CNS disease, or take antimotility drugs. Men are more susceptible, especially those with chronic constipation. Cecal volvulus is associated with previous surgery. Acute cases require emergency colonoscopy or barium enema. Surgical resection may be necessary in 70%–90% of cases.

L **Cytomegalovirus (CMV) colitis** is often seen in patients with AIDS, severe diabetes, renal failure, or inflammatory bowel disease. Bloody diarrhea may occur because of a deeply ulcerated colon. Intranuclear inclusion bodies may be noted on biopsy. The ulcers of CMV colitis may lead to perforation. Ganciclovir has been used for treatment.

M Diversion colitis

VI DISEASES OF THE RECTUM AND ANUS

A **Ulcerative proctitis** is a localized form of ulcerative colitis, which has a better prognosis and a greatly decreased risk of malignancy.

1. **Clinical features.** Symptoms typically include rectal urgency, pain, and bleeding, as well as tenesmus. Some patients may complain of constipation. Only rarely do fever, weight loss, and the systemic complications of ulcerative colitis occur.

2. **Diagnosis.** Other causes of proctitis, especially infection (see later discussion), should be ruled out. The absence of inflammation above the rectum should be verified by sigmoidoscopy.

3. **Therapy.** Corticosteroid or 5-aminosalicylic acid suppositories are often effective. More proximal rectal disease can also be treated with corticosteroid or 5-aminosalicylic acid enemas and oral sulfasalazine or 5-aminosalicylic acid preparations.

4. **Outcome.** In approximately 15%–20% of cases, ulcerative proctitis progresses to diffuse ulcerative colitis.

B Infectious proctitis

1. **Sexually transmitted diseases** that cause infectious proctitis include syphilis, gonorrhea, lymphogranuloma venereum, and herpes simplex. These diseases are especially common in men who have sex with men or patients who may have multiple simultaneous infections (see Chapter 9 VI D).

2. **Amebiasis** (i.e., infection with *E. histolytica*) may present as a diffuse colitis or extraintestinal disease (e.g., meningitis, liver abscess), or it may be confined to the rectosigmoid colon, especially in men who have sex with men. Symptoms range from mild diarrhea to bloody dysentery. Diagnosis is made by demonstrating the organism in the stool or in biopsy specimens with characteristic flask-shaped ulcers. Treatment is metronidazole or iodoquinone.

C **Solitary rectal ulcer** is a syndrome consisting of a superficial ulceration of unknown cause combined with passage of mucus or blood and dull rectal pain. The ulcers usually are 2 cm in diameter on the anterior rectal mucosal wall and located 7–10 cm from the anal verge. They are multiple in 25% of patients. A weakness in the rectal sling musculature may be a contributing cause. Diagnosis is made by excluding other causes of rectal ulcers, including infections, inflammatory bowel disease, and carcinoma. Treatment is supportive, with aggressive treatment of constipation.

D **Hemorrhoids** are dilated internal or external veins of the hemorrhoidal plexus located in the lower rectum. In the United States, 60%–70% of the population experiences symptoms of hemorrhoids at some time. Signs and symptoms include perianal pruritus, rectal bleeding (especially small amounts on the toilet tissue or bright droplets into the toilet bowl), anal pain, and a palpable mass in the anal region. The diagnosis is made by anoscopy or sigmoidoscopy. Treatment goals include reducing constipation with stool softeners and fiber supplements, supportive care with heat and anti-inflammatories, and definitive treatment. Internal hemorrhoids may be treated with rubber band ligation, sclerotherapy, coagulation with a number of different devices, or surgical hemorrhoidectomy, depending on their severity.

E **Anal fissures, abscesses, and fistulas** are tears, infections, and hollow channels from the rectum to the perianal skin, respectively. Locally applied heat, sitz baths, and antibiotics may be effective. However, surgical drainage or excision of an abscess or a fistulous tract may be necessary.

F **Pruritus** of the perianal skin has many causes, including infection (bacterial, fungal, or parasitic), localized anorectal disease (e.g., fistulas, fissures), dermatologic diseases (e.g., psoriasis, eczema), poor hygiene, diarrhea, and systemic diseases such as diabetes mellitus. The underlying condition should be treated. In addition, local care with careful cleaning following defecation and nightly application of hydrocortisone cream may be helpful in controlling symptoms.

G **Squamous cell carcinoma** of the anus is a rare malignancy that manifests as bleeding, pain, a mass, and change in bowel habits. Treatment may involve surgery, chemotherapy, and external beam radiation. The 5-year survival rate is high if recognized early.

VII DISEASES OF THE PANCREAS

A **Acute pancreatitis**

1. **Etiology**
   a. **Common causes.** Approximately 80% of cases of acute pancreatitis that occur in the United States are attributable to either alcohol abuse or gallstones.
      (1) In alcoholic pancreatitis, proteinaceous plugs develop in the pancreatic ducts and calcify in the body of the pancreas, leading to stasis and atrophy of distal segments. Alcoholic pancreatitis is most common in men who have ingested large amounts of alcohol over at least 10 years.
      (2) In gallstone pancreatitis, the passage of a common duct stone (multiple small stones, or even microlithiasis) may initiate reflux of biliary or intestinal contents into the pancreatic gland.
   b. Less common causes of acute pancreatitis
      (1) Postoperative pancreatitis, which may be severe and is especially common after hepato-biliary tract surgery
      (2) Abdominal trauma
      (3) Hypertriglyceridemia: serum values of greater than 1000 mg/dL, seen in types I, II, and V familial hyperlipidemia
      (4) Drugs such as azathioprine, 6-mercaptopurine, estrogens, thiazides, furosemide, sulfonamides, tetracyclines, corticosteroids, valproic acid, pentamidine, 2–3 dideoxyinosine, and 5-aminosalicylic acid
      (5) Hypercalcemia
      (6) Uremia
      (7) Peptic ulcer disease, with penetration into the pancreas
      (8) Cystic fibrosis (in rare cases)
      (9) Endoscopic retrograde cholangiopancreatography (ERCP)
      (10) Infections, including:
           (a) Viral: mumps, coxsackievirus, CMV
           (b) Bacterial: *Mycoplasma*, *Legionella*
           (c) Fungal: *Aspergillus*
           (d) Parasitic: *Toxoplasma*, *Cryptosporidium*, *Ascaris*
      (11) Vascular insufficiency: vasculitis, shock, embolism
      (12) Pancreatic cancer, causing ductal obstruction, including ampullary and duodenal lesions
      (13) Hereditary pancreatitis, which may be inherited in an autosomal dominant pattern and carries an increased risk for development of pancreatic carcinoma
      (14) Pancreas divisum, in which the main portion of the pancreas drains into the smaller accessory duct
      (15) The bite of the scorpion *Tityus trinitatis*, which causes increased pancreatic enzyme secretion.
      (16) Idiopathic causes

2. **Clinical features**
   a. **Abdominal pain,** which often is a steady or severe in the periumbilical or epigastric region and may radiate to the back

    b. Nausea and vomiting, which occur in 70% of cases

    c. Abdominal tenderness, usually without guarding or rebound

    d. Diminished or absent bowel sounds

    e. Epigastric fullness or mass, which usually is found late in the course of the disease

    f. Retroperitoneal bleeding, causing a hematoma at the umbilicus (**Cullen's sign**) or flank (**Turner's sign**), seen in hemorrhagic pancreatitis

3. **Diagnosis** usually is based on characteristic clinical presentations, especially in patients with a history of previous pancreatitis.

    a. Elevated serum amylase levels almost always exist during an acute attack but also may be caused by perforated ulcer, intestinal infarction, obstruction, or ruptured ectopic pregnancy.

    b. Elevated serum lipase levels also are found in acute attacks. This is more specific than elevated amylase levels.

    c. Abdominal radiographs may show a localized ileus (sentinel loop) in the small bowel region adjacent to the pancreas. CT scanning is very helpful for diagnosis and staging of disease. The severity of the pancreatitis and the presence or absence of necrotic tissue can be delineated by CT scan.

4. **Therapy** is supportive and includes aggressive administration of intravenous fluids along with analgesics and bowel rest. Nasogastric suction should be used if severe vomiting is present. In protracted illness, enteral tube feeding or intravenous hyperalimentation may be used. If an impacted gallstone causes pancreatitis, then the combination ERCP, sphincterotomy, and stone removal is the treatment of choice.

5. **Complications** account for the 10% mortality rate associated with acute pancreatitis.

    a. Hemorrhagic pancreatitis is considered an extension of edematous pancreatitis caused by chemical mediators (e.g., elastase), which leads to retroperitoneal hemorrhage and widespread tissue necrosis. Hemorrhagic pancreatitis is more common after trauma, postoperative pancreatitis, and the initial attack of acute pancreatitis and may require peritoneal lavage or surgical intervention for placement of drains. Blood may be present in the peritoneal cavity. The diagnosis is suggested by a declining hematocrit in a severely ill patient.

    b. Acute respiratory distress syndrome (ARDS) is caused by increased alveolar capillary permeability and may cause severe hypoxia requiring mechanical ventilation.

    c. Pancreatic abscess is suggested when high fever, elevated serum amylase levels, and leukocytosis persist beyond 7–10 days. Gas shadows in the region of the pancreas may be visualized by an abdominal flat plate or by CT. Treatment includes surgical drainage and antibiotics.

    d. Pancreatic pseudocyst refers to a collection of fluid and debris within the pancreas or in a space lined by the pancreas and other adjacent structures. Diagnosis is made by imaging (CT or ultrasonography) and/or by an elevated amylase in the cyst aspirate in a patient with a known history of pancreatitis. Approximately 50% of pseudocysts (usually smaller ones) resolve spontaneously. Large pseudocysts persisting beyond 6–10 weeks require drainage to avoid potentially serious complications such as hemorrhage, rupture, and impingement on other abdominal organs causing obstruction (e.g., stomach).

    e. Pancreatic ascites may occur because of a leaking pseudocyst with pancreatic ductal disruption. The diagnosis is suggested by very high serum amylase levels in peritoneal fluid. Conservative therapy with total parenteral nutrition and repeated paracentesis may lead to resolution. Often, ERCP with pancreatic duct stenting or pancreatic resection may be necessary.

B **Chronic pancreatitis** results in permanent structural damage of pancreatic tissue.

1. **Etiology.** Most of the causes of acute pancreatitis in the United States also can result in chronic pancreatitis. A notable exception is gallstones, which cause only recurrent acute attacks of pancreatitis. Alcohol abuse accounts for 90% of cases of chronic pancreatitis in adults. Cystic fibrosis is the most common cause of chronic disease in children.

2. **Clinical features**

    a. Pain, the usual presenting symptom, typically occurs in the epigastrium after eating and radiates to the back.

    b. Malabsorption occurs in association with **steatorrhea** and **weight loss.**

    c. Jaundice occurs because of edema and fibrosis in the pancreatic head, resulting in obstruction of the pancreatic portion of the common bile duct.

    d. Diabetes is common; however, ketoacidosis, nephropathy, and diabetic vascular disease rarely occur.

3. Diagnosis. The development of continuous pain and signs of pancreatic insufficiency in a patient with known recurrent pancreatitis is suggestive, especially when attributable to alcohol ingestion. Specific tests include:

    a. Abdominal radiographs, which show pancreatic calcification in 30%–40% of cases

    b. Secretin-stimulation testing with duodenal intubation and aspiration, finding a low bicarbonate concentration in the pancreatic secretion and low enzyme output

    c. ERCP or magnetic resonance cholangiopancreatography (MRCP), which show diffuse pancreatic ductal dilation with an irregular, beaded ("chain of lakes") appearance

4. Therapy. Treatment is aimed at controlling the manifestations of the disease because the underlying damage to the gland is permanent. In addition, agents that may promote further damage (e.g., alcohol) should be withdrawn.

    a. Control of pain may require narcotic analgesics, but care must be taken to avoid addiction. With abstinence from alcohol over time, some patients experience a lessening of pain.

    b. Replacement of pancreatic enzymes may be indicated for the treatment of steatorrhea or for the relief of pain. Typically, non–enteric -coated preparations are used for this purpose. H_2-receptor antagonists may increase the effectiveness of oral enzyme preparations.

    c. Insulin may be needed in patients who develop diabetes.

    d. Medium-chain triglycerides, which are more easily absorbed than longer-chain fatty acids, can be given.

    e. Endoscopic therapy—dilation of pancreatic duct strictures and removal of pancreatic duct stones—has been used in select cases.

    f. Surgery is a last resort and is generally used for severe pain or recurrent, severe attacks. Subtotal (80%) pancreatectomy and the Puestow procedure (i.e., anastomosis of the pancreatic duct lengthwise to a loop of the jejunum) are used most commonly.

C **Neoplastic cystic lesions** of the pancreas include serous and mucinous cystadenomas and adenocarcinomas. These lesions are true cysts of the pancreas, with multiple small cysts (serous) or large cysts (mucinous). These are not seen to communicate with the pancreatic duct on ERCP. They do not contain amylase, and the serum amylase level is usually normal (as discussed, the serum amylase level is elevated in approximately 60%–75% of cases of pseudocysts). Cyst assessment by endoscopic ultrasound with fluid aspiration (for CEA, amylase, and cytology with mucin stain) can assist in delineating the type of cyst present. Treatment of mucinous cystadenomas is surgical removal—often with complete cure.

D **Adenocarcinoma** of the pancreas accounts for more than 90% of pancreatic malignancies.

1. Epidemiology. The adenocarcinoma is ductal in approximately 95% of patients. This tumor, which increased in incidence during the twentieth century, is the fourth-leading cause of cancer-related death in the Unites States among both men and women. Men are affected more commonly than women, and the average age at presentation is 55–65 years. Seventy percent of adenocarcinomas of the pancreas occur in the head of the pancreas, with 30% occurring in the body or tail.

2. Etiology. The risk of pancreatic carcinoma is increased in patients with hereditary pancreatitis, obese individuals, smokers, patients with chronic pancreatitis, and diabetes mellitus.

3. Clinical features

    a. Common symptoms. Approximately 75% of patients have pain that has been present for 3–4 months by the time of diagnosis. The pain typically is postprandial epigastric or periumbilical discomfort, which radiates to the back and is relieved by sitting up or bending both knees. Jaundice is present in approximately 65% of patients, and weight loss occurs in 60% of patients. Diarrhea and steatorrhea may be present. The gallbladder may be palpable (Courvoisier's sign) in some patients. A palpable epigastric mass may be found on physical examination.

    b. Less common symptoms include unexplained thrombophlebitis (Trousseau's sign), depression, new-onset diabetes mellitus, or acute pancreatitis.

4. **Diagnosis.** A high index of suspicion often is required in patients with constant epigastric or periumbilical distress.

   a. **Laboratory tests** are usually nonspecific. High serum amylase levels are found in 25% of patients. CA 19-9, a tumor marker, has been associated with carcinoma of the pancreas. Although not useful as a screening test, it has an approximate 80% sensitivity and 90% specificity for carcinoma of the pancreas and may be a marker for recurrent diseases or metastasis after primary resection.

   b. **Spiral CT, magnetic resonance imaging (MRI),** or **ultrasonography** of the pancreas demonstrates a mass in 75%–80% of patients. Image-guided needle biopsy can provide a histologic diagnosis.

   c. **ERCP** is abnormal in approximately 85%–90% of patients and generally shows a discrete stricture in the main pancreatic duct with proximal dilatation. The **double duct sign,** or simultaneous dilation of the common bile duct and pancreatic duct from a mass in the head of the pancreas, may also be seen. Cytology of the ducts can be performed, allowing a tissue diagnosis to be made.

   d. **EUS** visualizes most tumors and can provide important staging information, including displacement or encasement of the adjacent vasculature and local lymph node involvement. EUS-guided fine needle aspiration provides a histologic diagnosis.

5. **Therapy and prognosis** (see Chapter 5 VIII B 8, 9)

E **Islet cell tumors** account for 5% of pancreatic carcinomas. They may be multicentric and tend to grow more slowly than tumors of ductular origin. Islet cell tumors frequently are associated with endocrine adenomas in the pituitary and parathyroid glands (e.g., in MEN I syndrome).

VIII DISEASES OF THE BILIARY TRACT

A **Gallstones** are extremely common, occurring in 15%–20% of the population of the United States.

1. **Types**

   a. **Cholesterol gallstones.** Most gallstones that occur in Western populations are composed primarily of cholesterol, which is thought to precipitate from supersaturated bile, especially at night when bile is concentrated in the gallbladder. For women, the risk of cholesterol gallstones increases with age, use of oral contraceptives (at least during the first 5 years of use), and pregnancy. Rapid weight loss, family history of diabetes mellitus, ileal disease (Crohn's disease), ileal resection resulting in a decreased bile salt pool, the use of agents such as clofibrate, ceftriaxone, or octreotide, and total parenteral nutrition all may increase the risk of cholesterol gallstones.

   b. **Pigmented gallstones.** Composed primarily of calcium bilirubinate, pigmented gallstones are found in patients with chronic hemolysis (e.g., sickle cell disease), as well as in Asian populations. In Asia, biliary infection with β-glucuronidase–producing organisms leads to increased amounts of poorly soluble deconjugated bilirubin in bile.

2. **Therapy.** One third to one half of patients with gallstones are asymptomatic and should be treated expectantly. Surgical removal of asymptomatic gallstones is considered in those at high risk for complications, including, Native Americans, children, and patients with morbid obesity or heart or lung transplants.

B **Acute cholecystitis**

1. **Etiology.** In 90%–95% of cases, acute cholecystitis is caused by obstruction of the cystic duct by an impacted gallstone, which leads to edema of the gallbladder wall with submucosal hemorrhage and mucosal ulceration. Acalculous cholecystitis typically occurs in the setting of hospitalization for severe illness, including trauma or sepsis.

2. **Clinical features**

   a. An attack of acute cholecystitis starts with crampy pain in the epigastrium or right upper quadrant, which may radiate to the back near the right scapular tip (biliary colic). The pain is thought to be generated by ductal obstruction and often is postprandial.

   b. An elevated temperature or WBC count, fever, nausea, vomiting, and ileus also may be present.

  c. Cessation of inspiration precipitated by deep palpation of the right upper quadrant is known as **Murphy's sign.**

  d. Jaundice occurs in 20% of patients and is attributable to common duct stones or edema of the common bile duct.

3. Diagnosis. The characteristic clinical picture, especially in a patient known to have gallstones, suggests the diagnosis.

  a. Most gallstones consist of cholesterol and are radiolucent; 10%–15% of gallstones contain enough calcium to appear radiopaque.

  b. Although gallbladder ultrasonography can show the presence of stones (i.e., the fluid-filled gallbladder appears lucent, whereas the stones within it are sono-opaque and cast shadows), this test cannot be used solely to demonstrate cystic duct obstruction. It may demonstrate gallbladder wall thickening, edema and pericholecystic fluid, and an ultrasonographic Murphy's sign.

  c. Failure to visualize the gallbladder during radionuclide scanning (hepatobiliary scan) strongly suggests cystic duct obstruction.

4. Therapy

  a. Supportive treatment should be provided initially, with intravenous fluid replacement, analgesia, and nasogastric suction if intractable vomiting or ileus is present. Antibiotics may also be used. Later, the gallbladder may be removed surgically.

  b. Laparoscopic cholecystectomy is the treatment of choice and often allows gallbladder removal on a "same-day surgery" basis.

  c. Other less commonly used therapies include the following.

  (1) Dissolution is rarely used to dissolve cholesterol stones in patients who are not surgical candidates. **Ursodeoxycholic acid** or **chenodeoxycholic acid** may be used. If several small stones are present and floating, a 50%–70% chance of dissolving the stones may be expected over a period of 12–24 months.

  (2) Lithotripsy may be tried if the gallbladder is functional, the stone mass is less than 3 cm, and the patient has no acute symptoms (approximately 20%–25% of patients).

  (3) Drainage of the gallbladder through a percutaneous cholecystostomy tube may be indicated in high-risk patients who are critically ill.

5. Complications. Surgical intervention generally is required.

  a. Empyema refers to a pus-filled gallbladder. Patients may be toxic and are at high risk for perforation.

  b. Perforation

  (1) Localized perforation occurs several days to 1 week after the onset of acute cholecystitis and leads to a pericholecystic abscess.

  (2) Free perforation into the abdominal cavity, which has a 25% mortality rate, occurs early in the clinical course, probably because inflammation in the early stages is insufficient to wall off the abscess.

  (3) Perforation into an adjacent organ may involve the duodenum, jejunum, colon, or stomach. If a large stone is passed into the lumen, intestinal obstruction (gallstone ileus) may result.

  c. Emphysematous cholecystitis is caused by gas-forming bacteria (often clostridia, *E. coli*, or streptococci) in the gallbladder lumen and wall. Men are affected more commonly than women, and 20%–30% of patients have diabetes mellitus. Early surgical intervention is indicated to prevent perforation.

  d. Postcholecystectomy syndrome refers to abdominal pain that persists after cholecystectomy. The usual cause is an initially mistaken diagnosis, with pain persisting from the underlying process (e.g., pancreatic disease or irritable bowel syndrome). Some patients may have common duct stones.

C **Chronic cholecystitis** is a clinical term used to describe a condition of recurrent subacute symptoms caused by gallstones. Patients with chronic cholecystitis show wide variability in the thickening and fibrosis of the gallbladder wall and in the inflammatory infiltrate. The diagnosis is based on symptoms and low gallbladder ejection factor measured by a quantitative nuclear hepatobiliary scan using cholecystokinin. After other sources of chronic abdominal pain (e.g., peptic ulcer disease, pancreatitis, and irritable bowel syndrome) are ruled out, a cholecystectomy may be performed to relieve symptoms.

D **Choledocholithiasis**

1. **Pathophysiology.** Choledocholithiasis usually occurs when a gallstone is passed into the common duct from the gallbladder or when a gallstone that was missed during operative cholangiography or common duct exploration is retained. Occasionally, a stone forms de novo in the common duct, especially when there is stasis from ductal obstruction.

2. **Clinical features.** Symptoms frequently are intermittent and include colicky pain in the right upper quadrant. Fever, chills, and jaundice accompanied by elevated serum levels of alkaline phosphatase and the transaminases indicate the development of cholangitis. Sepsis may result from ascending cholangitis, which is a closed-space infection. This is an emergency and requires antibiotics and urgent decompression of the bile duct.

3. **Therapy.** Antibiotics are given as needed to control infection, but definitive treatment consists of endoscopic sphincterotomy and stone extraction via ERCP, percutaneous drainage, or surgical removal of the stone.

E **Biliary dyskinesia** (sphincter of Oddi dysfunction) is a clinical syndrome of right upper quadrant symptoms similar to chronic calculous cholecystitis.

1. **Pathophysiology.** An abnormality of biliary motor function is proposed, and manometric findings may indicate elevated basal sphincter of Oddi pressure (usually 40 mm Hg greater than intraduodenal pressure), a paradoxical contraction of the sphincter of Oddi after cholecystokinin injection, or both.

2. **Therapy.** Patients may respond to smooth muscle relaxants (e.g., nitrates, calcium channel–blocking agents) or to endoscopic or surgical sphincterotomy of the sphincter of Oddi.

F **Biliary stricture**

1. **Pathophysiology.** Biliary stricture is a narrowing of the common bile duct generally caused by surgical injury or scarring subsequent to exploration of the common bile duct. Chronic pancreatitis, pancreatic cancer, or bile duct malignancies can also result in biliary strictures. Rarely, trauma or choledocholithiasis may be a cause.

2. **Clinical features.** Patients usually have intermittent obstructive jaundice with or without pain. Cholangiography demonstrates the presence of a narrowing of the duct with proximal dilation.

3. **Therapy.** First-line treatment often is dilation via ERCP or percutaneous transhepatic access with biliary stent placement. If this fails, surgical anastomosis of the bile duct to the intestine may be required.

G **Primary sclerosing cholangitis (PSC),** a rare disease that causes progressive narrowing of the bile ducts, generally is diagnosed in the third or fourth decade of life and is three times more common in men than in women.

1. **Clinical features.** Approximately 70% of patients have inflammatory bowel disease (usually ulcerative colitis), but the biliary and intestinal diseases have independent clinical courses. The usual presenting symptom is pruritus. There is an increased risk of cholangiocarcinoma, gallbladder abnormalities, and colon cancer (if coexistent inflammatory bowel disease) in these patients.

2. **Diagnosis.** Early diagnosis is possible in asymptomatic patients who show marked elevation of serum alkaline phosphatase levels on routine biochemical screening. MRCP, ERCP, or percutaneous cholangiography should establish the diagnosis.

3. **Therapy**
   a. **Medical treatment.** Corticosteroids, ursodeoxycholic acid, methotrexate, long-term antibiotics, or varying combinations of these medications have been used with poor success. There is currently no specific medical therapy recommended for the treatment of PSC.
   b. **Surgical treatment.** Endoscopic or percutaneous dilation of strictures is possible in some cases. Liver transplantation is the treatment of choice with advanced disease.

H **Recurrent pyogenic cholangitis**

I **Cystic malformation of the bile ducts**

J **Tumors of the gallbladder**

1. **Adenocarcinoma** of the gallbladder is commonly a disease of **older women.** The tumor affects three times as many women as it does men, and the average age at diagnosis is 65–75 years. Although most patients have associated gallstones, cancer develops in less than 1% of all patients with stones. Symptoms generally mimic those of acute or chronic cholecystitis. On physical examination, a mass may be palpable in the right upper quadrant, and obstructive jaundice may be seen secondary to local spread of the tumor to the common bile duct. A calcified gallbladder may be seen on abdominal radiographs. An operation consisting of cholecystectomy, lymph node dissection, and removal of a small portion of the adjacent liver is indicated if no obvious metastatic disease is found, but prognosis generally is poor.

2. **Benign tumors** of the gallbladder include abnormalities of the mucosal lining (e.g., adenomatous hyperplasia, cholesterolosis, and cholesterol polyps), cystic changes in the glands, and papillary adenomas. These lesions usually are asymptomatic. In some patients with no other demonstrable causes for abdominal pain, however, cholecystectomy has provided relief of symptoms.

K **Tumors of the bile duct** Adenocarcinoma of the bile duct (cholangiocarcinoma) is typically a disease of **older men** and is not associated with gallstones.

1. **Etiology.** An increased risk is observed in patients with primary sclerosing cholangitis and in patients exposed to benzene or toluene derivatives. Parasitic infection of the biliary system, especially with *Clonorchis,* has been linked to the high rate of cholangiocarcinoma in Asian populations.

2. **Pathology.** Most tumors are of the sclerosing or papillary type. An extensive desmoplastic reaction may make diagnosis difficult. Two thirds of the tumors are located in the common bile duct or at the bifurcation of the common hepatic duct (**Klatskin tumors).**

3. **Clinical features.** Jaundice, with or without pain, is present in most patients, and weight loss also is common. Pruritus may be severe. Common duct tumors causing obstruction distal to the cystic duct result in a palpable gallbladder that is not tender.

4. **Laboratory data.** Serum alkaline phosphatase levels are markedly increased, as are total and direct bilirubin levels. Serum transaminase levels show smaller increases and generally are less than 200 mg/dL.

5. **Diagnosis.** Dilation of the intrahepatic ducts is shown by ultrasonography, CT, or MRI. ERCP or percutaneous cholangiography findings can suggest the diagnosis and also provide tissue sampling. The differential diagnosis includes pancreatic carcinoma, choledocholithiasis, biliary stricture, and sclerosing cholangitis.

6. **Therapy** (see Chapter 5 VIII E 9)

IX DISEASES OF THE LIVER

A **Spectrum of liver disease**

1. **Viral hepatitis,** one of the most common health problems in the world, is caused by any one of several viruses (Table 6–3).
   a. **Etiology**
      (1) **Hepatitis A virus** (HAV) is an RNA virus transmitted primarily by the fecal–oral route. Acute infection is anicteric in 50% of cases. HAV does not lead to chronic disease or to a carrier state.
      (2) **Hepatitis B virus** (HBV) is a DNA virus transmitted parenterally or perinatally (through birth). Individuals at high risk include intravenous drug abusers, men who have sex with men, and individuals exposed to blood and blood products. Chronic HBV disease or a persistent carrier state develops in 1%–20% of patients worldwide, depending on the mode of transmission and age at infection. Certain populations of patients with HBV are at high risk for hepatocellular carcinoma (HCC).
      (3) **Hepatitis C virus** (HCV) is an RNA virus that **formerly accounted for** 90% of posttransfusion hepatitis. The modes of transmission (parenteral, sexual, and, perhaps, perinatal) are similar to those of HBV. Chronic hepatitis develops in up to 85% of patients. Cirrhosis

TABLE 6–3   Viral Hepatitis

	Hepatitis A	Hepatitis B	Hepatitis C	Hepatitis D	Hepatitis E
Type of virus	RNA	DNA	RNA	RNA (hepatitis B required for replication)	RNA
Incidence of positive antibody in the United States (%)	40	10	2–3	Low	Very low
Incidence after blood transfusion (%)	0 to extremely rare	10–20	60–90	?	0 to extremely rare
Incubation period	2–6 weeks	1–6 months	2–24 weeks	1–6 months	2–8 weeks
Infectivity stage	Last 3 weeks of inoculation to 1–2 weeks after jaundice occurs	During hepatitis B surface antigen positivity	?	?	?
Complications	Fulminant hepatitis (rare)	Fulminant hepatitis (rare but more common than with hepatitis A); chronic active hepatitis	Fulminant hepatitis (rare but more common than with hepatitis A); chronic active hepatitis	Present in 20%–50% of cases of fulminant hepatitis and/or chronic active hepatitis	Fulminant hepatitis in pregnant women with 10%–20% mortality
Mechanism of spread	Fecal–oral	Parenteral	Parenteral	Parenteral	Fecal–oral
Prevention	Pooled immune serum globulin; vaccination	Hepatitis B immune globulin; vaccination	Pooled immune serum globulin	?	Good hygiene
Carrier state	Rare, if ever	1%–20% worldwide	Yes (50% of patients)	?	?

may develop in 20% of patients, with an increased risk of HCC. Genotype I accounts for most hepatitis C infections in the United States and does not respond as readily to antiviral therapy as other genotypes.

(4) **Delta hepatitis [hepatitis D virus (HDV)]** is caused by a small, defective RNA virus (delta agent) that is infectious only in the presence of HBV infection because it relies on HBV proteins for replication. It therefore can complicate acute HBV infection but is seen more commonly as a "superinfection" with an increase in abnormal liver function tests in a patient with chronic HBV. HDV generally has a chronic, severe clinical course.

(5) **Hepatitis E virus** is a small RNA virus that has been described in cases of acute hepatitis in the Middle East, Asia, Central America, and Africa. It has a short incubation period and is spread by fecally contaminated water in endemic areas. Sporadic cases have been reported and are believed to be from zoonotic transmission. Fulminant liver failure rarely develops but occurs more commonly in pregnancy. The clinical course is otherwise similar to that of HAV with no risk of chronic hepatitis.

(6) **Other viruses** that can cause acute hepatitis include Epstein–Barr virus, CMV, HSV, and those causing yellow fever and rubella.

b. **Pathology.** The lesions of acute viral hepatitis are similar regardless of etiology and include mononuclear cell infiltration, cellular ballooning and necrosis, and condensed cytoplasm with pyknotic nuclei (acidophilic bodies).

c. **Clinical features**
   (1) Malaise, anorexia, and fatigue
   (2) Arthritis and urticaria, which are especially common in HBV, are ascribed to circulating immune complexes. Polyarteritis nodosa or glomerulonephritis may be seen in HBV or HCV patients.
   (3) Influenza-like syndrome is especially common in HAV.
   (4) Jaundice (with dark urine or light stools) is seen in 50% of cases.
   (5) Hepatic enlargement and tenderness
   (6) Splenomegaly occurs in 20% of patients.
   (7) HCV only: Concomitant porphyria cutanea tarda, **lichen planus,** mixed cryoglobulinemia, **thyroiditis,** or membranoproliferative glomerulonephritis. Immune complex disease is relatively common in HCV patients.

d. **Diagnosis.** Acute viral hepatitis is diagnosed based on clinical features as well as elevated levels of the transaminases (i.e., aspartate aminotransferase [AST], alanine aminotransaminase [ALT]), serum bilirubin, and serum alkaline phosphatase. The increase in bilirubin exceeds the increase in alkaline phosphatase.
   (1) In HAV, the IgM antibody is elevated early in the course, followed by an elevation of the IgG antibody in 2–3 months.
   (2) In HBV, a positive surface antigen usually is diagnostic. However, because this is an early finding, it may be necessary to follow the increase of IgM anticore (HB$_c$Ab) and later of antisurface antibodies (HB$_s$Ab) to document acute infection (Figure 6–1). Patients with acute infection will also have detectable HBV DNA in the serum.
   (3) HCV can be diagnosed by antibodies to hepatitis C or the presence of HCV RNA in the serum.
   (4) HDV may be diagnosed by an elevated delta antibody titer, often with the disappearance of B surface antigen from the serum. A persistently high or slowly falling hepatitis delta antibody is seen in chronic states. HDV RNA can also be detected in the serum by polymerase chain reaction (PCR).

e. **Therapy.** Treatment for acute or active disease is supportive and includes hydration with intravenous fluids, correction of electrolyte abnormalities, provision of nutritional support if

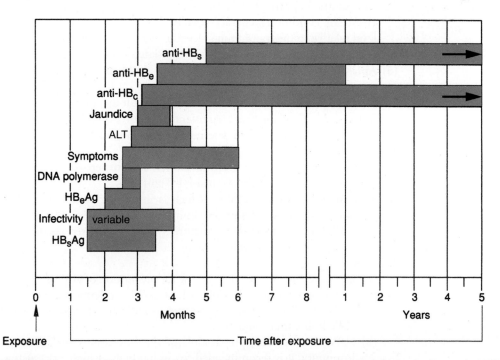

FIGURE 6–1 Typical clinical course of acute HBV infection. Recombinant and pooled-plasma vaccines against HBV do not transmit active HB$_s$Ag and do not contain HB$_e$Ag or hepatitis core antigen. Consequently, the serologic profile of a vaccinated individual consists of anti-HB$_s$ only. SGPT, ALT, alanine aminotransferase; anti-HB$_c$, hepatitis B core antibody; anti-HB$_e$, hepatitis B e antibody.

severe nausea and vomiting are present, and early recognition of complications (bleeding, encephalopathy, infections). Vitamin K should be given if the prothrombin time (PT) is elevated and there is concern or evidence of bleeding. For chronic cases of HBV, interferon or various nucleoside analogs are effective in clearing active viral replication. For chronic HCV, pegylated interferon (PEG-IFN) in combination with ribavirin results in sustained viral clearing rates of between 30% and 70%, depending on the viral load, patient demographics and characteristics, and genotype of the virus (genotype I responds less favorably).

f. **Clinical course and complications.** Nearly all cases of acute viral hepatitis are benign, with most patients showing normal results on liver function testing by 8–10 weeks. However, complications may occur.

(1) **Fulminant hepatitis,** a rare complication of HAV, HCV, and HEV, occurs in 1%–2% of patients with HBV. It is an especially common complication of delta agent superinfection in patients with chronic hepatitis B antigenemia. Patients usually have progressive jaundice, hepatic encephalopathy, and ascites. Hepatorenal syndrome is common. Elevated PT is an early sign. The initially elevated serum transaminase levels later decline, and liver size decreases as a result of necrosis of the liver parenchyma. The mortality rate varies with age and approaches 90%–100%, especially in patients older than 60 years of age.

(2) **Chronic hepatitis** is a complication of HBV and HCV in which serum transaminase levels are elevated for more than 6 months. Fifteen percent of patients with chronic HCV may have hepatitis C antibody but no actively replicating virus; they are individuals who have recovered from acute and chronic HCV infection.

Pathologically, inflammation, necrosis, and fibrosis bridging portal areas or between portal areas and central veins occurs. The disease may progress to cirrhosis over time. On physical examination, patients may have splenomegaly, spider angiomata, caput medusae, and other signs of chronic liver disease. Liver biopsy is not always necessary for diagnosis.

(3) **A chronic carrier state** for hepatitis B surface antigen exists in 0.2% of the population of the United States. A carrier state also exists for HCV because blood donated by apparently normal individuals may transmit this disease when transfused. Carriers of HBV or HCV may have an increased risk of hepatocelluar cancer.

(4) **Cholestatic hepatitis** may occur, particularly with hepatitis E and rarely with HAV and HCV. This condition is characterized by disproportionately elevated alkaline phosphatase level relative to the transaminase level. The clinical course is typical of acute viral hepatitis, but the presentation must be differentiated from that of biliary tract obstruction.

(5) **Aplastic anemia** is seen rarely after acute viral hepatitis. The mortality rate is high, and no treatment has proved effective.

g. **Therapy of acute disease.** PEG-IFN alone can result in a high rate of clearance of hepatitis C virus after acute infection (e.g., parenteral exposure, blood transfusion). It is reasonable to wait 12 weeks after exposure to determine if spontaneous clearance occurred.

h. **Prevention**

(1) **Immune serum globulin** is effective when administered after exposure to HAV and also may be partially protective against HBV and HCV.

(2) **Hepatitis B immune globulin,** which is immunoglobulin that contains high titers of antibody to HBV, conveys passive immunity and is recommended after confirmed exposure to HBV (e.g., from skin puncture by a contaminated needle) and perinatally when there is risk for vertical transmission.

(3) **Vaccines**

(a) **HAV vaccine.** An effective vaccine for prevention of HAV is available. It is particularly recommended for individuals who travel to endemic areas or who have other forms of chronic liver disease. The vaccine also may be effective for secondary prevention in HAV household contacts.

(b) **HBV vaccine.** This preparation of the hepatitis B surface antigen conveys active immunity. It is recommended for individuals at high risk, such as dialysis patients, medical personnel with frequent exposure to blood products, and individuals who are hepatitis B antibody–negative and who have had confirmed exposure to HBV. Infants are routinely vaccinated.

TABLE 6–4 Agents of Drug-Induced Liver Disease

Drugs Causing Direct Toxicity	Drugs Causing Altered Metabolism	Drugs Causing Immune-Mediated Reactions			
		Viral Hepatitis-like	Granulomatous Hepatitis	Inflammatory Cholestasis	Chronic Active Hepatitis
Acetaminophen	Androgens	Halothane	Allopurinol	Chlorpromazine	Acetaminophen
Amiodarone	Corticosteroids (?)	Isoniazid	Hydralazine	Chlorpropamide	Aspirin
Aspirin	Estrogens	Oxacillin	Phenylbutazone	Erythromycin	Isoniazid
Alcohol	Ethanol	Phenytoin	Phenytoin	Estolate	Methyldopa
Carbon	Intravenous	Sulfonamides	Quinidine	Propylthiouracil	Nitrofurantoin
tetrachloride	tetracycline	Valproic acid	Sulfa drugs	Thiazides	Oxyphenisatin
Heavy metals					
Methotrexate					
Mushroom toxins					
(phalloidin					
and phallin)					
Niacin					
Phosphorus					

2. **Drug-induced liver disease** may follow exposure to virtually any drug and manifests as a variety of clinical syndromes and histologic findings (Table 6–4). Any drug may induce liver disease that overlaps two or more categories of disease mechanisms.

   a. **Direct toxicity** by a chemical (e.g., carbon tetrachloride) or a metabolite (e.g., acetaminophen) usually represents a dose-related injury. Niacin may cause a dose-related toxicity at greater than 3 g/day in crystalline form or 1–2 g/day in sustained-release form. Acetaminophen overdose can be treated with *N*-acetylcysteine, which binds to the toxic metabolite and provides cysteine for glutathione synthesis. Smaller doses of acetaminophen (3–4 g) ingested with alcohol may induce hepatic necrosis, marked by high levels of hepatic AST (3000–24,000 IU). Such cases have a high mortality rate.

   b. **Indirect toxicity** may result from interference with the metabolism of bilirubin (e.g., by estrogens and androgens) or with protein synthesis (e.g., by intravenous tetracycline, which causes microvesicular fat accumulation in hepatocytes).

   c. **Immunologic drug reactions** can cause a variety of syndromes, including cholestatic jaundice (a syndrome that mimics acute viral hepatitis), a condition with a histologic picture indistinguishable from that of chronic active hepatitis, and granulomatous hepatitis. Skin rashes, eosinophilia, and fever may be present. In some cases, it has been postulated that a drug or metabolite binds to the liver cell membrane and acts as a **hapten.**

   d. **Commonly used drugs** such as isoniazid, phenytoin, and general anesthetics can cause specific patterns of drug-induced liver injury. (See 🄟 online.)

   e. **Treatment** of drug-induced liver disease involves identification and discontinuation of the offending agent. Depending on the degree of liver injury, it can take months for the transaminases and bilirubin to normalize. Symptomatic treatment for jaundice and pruritis may be needed.

3. **Alcoholic liver disease** refers to the group of liver disorders caused by acute and chronic alcoholism. Acute effects include alcoholic fatty liver and alcoholic hepatitis. Chronic alcoholism is a major cause of cirrhosis of the liver. In the United States, alcoholic liver disease represents the fourth-most-common cause of death of adults 35–55 years of age. It appears that alcohol consumption of less than 80 g/day in men and 40 g/day in (nonpregnant) women generally is not associated with alcoholic liver disease.

   a. **Alcoholic fatty liver** occurs because alcohol alters normal lipid metabolism. Most patients have hepatomegaly but otherwise are asymptomatic unless they have other systemic problems related to alcohol use (e.g., pancreatitis and delirium tremens). Laboratory abnormalities include increases in γ-glutamyl transpeptidase (GGT), serum transaminases, and alkaline phosphatase. Histologic examination shows large-droplet fatty change in the liver. The prognosis is excellent for patients who completely abstain from alcohol consumption.

b. Alcoholic hepatitis is an acute syndrome that generally occurs in the setting of heavy alcohol consumption. Many patients are reported to have ingested more than 100 g of alcohol daily for more than 1 year. (Approximately 100 g of alcohol are contained in 8 ounces of 100-proof whiskey, in 30 ounces of wine, and in eight 12-ounce cans of beer.) The role of decreased vitamin and protein intake is controversial.

    (1) Clinical features include fever, jaundice, hepatomegaly, and liver tenderness. Ascites, encephalopathy, and variceal bleeding may be present.

    (2) Laboratory data include leukocytosis, increased AST (usually <350 IU/mm^3), elevated serum bilirubin, decreased serum albumin, and a modest increase in serum alkaline phosphatase. Occasionally, a cholestatic phase is present with marked elevations in the alkaline phosphatase and direct bilirubin. The ALT is almost always lower than the AST because of decreased pyridoxine intake and conversion to pyridoxal phosphate. Alcohol-induced thrombocytopenia is present in 10% of patients.

    (3) Diagnosis is based on clinical history. Liver biopsy will show large-droplet fatty liver, polymorphonuclear infiltration, alcoholic hyaline (Mallory bodies), hepatocyte necrosis, and, occasionally, sclerosis of central veins.

    (4) Therapy is supportive and includes a daily diet of 2500–3000 kcal with supplemental B vitamins (especially thiamine) and folate. Absolute abstinence from alcohol is crucial. Corticosteroids and pentoxifylline have a controversial therapeutic role but may be useful in severe cases.

4. Nonalcoholic fatty liver disease (NAFLD) and nonalcoholic steatohepatitis (NASH) describe patients who lack a history of significant alcohol consumption but have liver biopsy findings indistinguishable from those of alcoholic hepatitis. Most cases occur between the ages of 40 and 60 years, and the disease is more common in women. Although the etiology of NASH is unknown, it is frequently associated with obesity, type 2 diabetes mellitus, and hyperlipidemia, also known as the metabolic syndrome. NASH has also been described in association with total parenteral nutrition, abdominal surgery, and medications such as amiodarone and tamoxifen.

    (1) Clinical course. NASH is generally considered to be a clinically stable disorder with a markedly better prognosis than alcoholic hepatitis. In most patients, there is little change in liver function tests throughout the course of the disease; however, in some patients, histologic progression occurs, and patients may progress to end-stage liver disease. Unfortunately, no clinical or laboratory features can predict progression; one must rely on liver biopsy.

    (2) Diagnosis and laboratory data. Most patients with NASH are asymptomatic, although fatigue, malaise, and vague right upper abdominal discomfort may be present. The most common presentation is elevated liver function tests. Hepatomegaly is also a frequent finding. Serum AST and ALT levels are elevated in almost 90% of patients, with an AST/ALT ratio usually less than 1. Alkaline phosphatase is less frequently elevated, and hyperbilirubinemia is uncommon. Liver biopsy is the only way to confirm or exclude the diagnosis.

    (3) Therapy. Currently there is no proven effective treatment for NASH. Modification of risk factors, including weight loss, lipid control, and improved diabetic management, is recommended. Weight reduction should be gradual since rapid weight loss has been associated with worsening of liver disease. Studies evaluating the hypoglycemic agents metformin, pioglitazone, and rosiglitazone as potential therapy have shown mixed results, and these agents are not currently recommended for routine care. A recent study suggests that vitamin E may be effective.

5. Autoimmune hepatitis is a chronic hepatitis of unknown etiology characterized by liver injury with the presence of circulating autoantibodies and high serum globulin concentrations. One clue to diagnosis is the presence of other diseases with autoimmune features. This disease can also be seen as a result of drug-induced or viral injury.

a. Clinical features can range from asymptomatic elevated transaminases to debilitating malaise and fatigue to fulminant hepatic failure. Physical exam may be normal until advanced disease develops.

b. Diagnosis is based on liver biopsy that shows piecemeal necrosis and bridging fibrosis. The serum transaminases are persistently elevated to levels that often are 10 times the normal levels. Positive antinuclear antibody (ANA) is present in two thirds of patients, and anti–smooth muscle antibody (ASMA) is found in greater than 80%.

   c. **Therapy** with high-dose corticosteroids, azathioprine, or both is beneficial in the immune-mediated type of chronic hepatitis but usually not in the drug- and virus-associated diseases. Treatment of autoimmune chronic active hepatitis is continued until the serum transaminase levels return to normal. Often treatment is continued lifelong with a steroid-sparing immunomodulator such as azathioprine, as relapse is common.

6. **Primary biliary cirrhosis** is a disease of unknown etiology. The usual patient age at diagnosis is 40–60 years, and 95% of patients are women.

   a. **Pathogenesis** is thought to be immunologic, involving inflammatory destruction of small intrahepatic biliary ducts. Early histologic changes include lymphocytic infiltration and periductal granuloma formation. Later in the disease process, the portal areas may show an absence of ducts.

   b. **Clinical features**

     (1) There is a lack of symptoms early in the course of this disease. However, an early diagnosis often is suspected on the basis of a marked increase in the alkaline phosphatase level noted on routine biochemical screening.

     (2) The first symptom usually is **pruritus,** which may be devastatingly severe, especially at night.

     (3) **Jaundice** occurs in later stages of the disease, as do **osteopenia** (in 25% of patients) and **xanthomas** (in approximately 10% of patients).

     (4) Primary biliary cirrhosis is associated with Sjögren's syndrome (in 75% of patients), the presence of antithyroid antibody (in 25% of patients), rheumatoid arthritis (in 5% of patients), and limited systemic sclerosis (in 3% of patients).

   c. **Diagnosis** is made by the constellation of increased serum cholesterol, markedly increased alkaline phosphatase (four to six times normal), increased direct bilirubin, and the presence of antimitochondrial antibodies, which is found in more than 90% of patients. The liver biopsy shows characteristic changes. Extrahepatic biliary obstruction must be ruled out.

   d. **Therapy** is supportive and includes administration of antipruritic agents and supplementation of vitamins and calcium, as well as bisphosphonates for prevention of osteoporosis. The pruritus may respond to cholestyramine, which binds bile salts in the intestine. The most promising medical treatment is ursodeoxycholic acid, which may improve hepatic structure and function if initiated before advanced stages of the disease. Intravenous naloxone therapy may be useful for severe pruritus. Surgical therapy is liver transplantation, with has excellent 5-year survival rates for this condition.

7. **Secondary biliary cirrhosis** usually occurs after several years of biliary tract obstruction.

   a. **Etiology** includes common bile duct stones, common duct strictures, cholangiocarcinoma, ampullary carcinoma, sclerosing cholangitis, and chronic pancreatitis with compression of the common duct as it traverses the pancreatic head.

   b. **Clinical features** are similar to those of primary biliary cirrhosis but may be superseded by manifestations of the underlying disease. In addition, patients may develop cholangitis with shaking chills, fever, leukocytosis, and jaundice. Antimitochondrial antibodies usually are not present.

   c. **Therapy** is aimed at relieving the obstruction and includes surgery, external drainage, and placement of an indwelling stent.

8. **Primary sclerosing cholangitis** (see VIII G)

9. α_1-**Antitrypsin deficiency** is a genetic defect of the glycoprotein that normally inhibits proteolytic enzymes such as trypsin, chymotrypsin, and elastase. (See online for more information.)

10. **Hemochromatosis** is an autosomal recessive disorder in which mutations in the HFE gene cause increased intestinal iron absorption. This leads to iron deposition in the liver, heart, pancreas, and other organs. Men are more commonly affected than women (at a ratio of 8:1). In the United States, approximately 8%–9% of the population are heterozygotes, and 1 in every 220 are homozygotes, making hemochromatosis one of the most common genetic liver diseases.

   a. **Clinical features**

   b. **Laboratory findings**

(🖱) c. **Therapy**

(🖱) d. **Prognosis**

11. **Infiltrative disease of the liver**

    a. **Granulomatous hepatitis**

        (1) **Etiology.** Granulomatous hepatitis most often is secondary to systemic infections (e.g., tuberculosis), sarcoidosis, fungal infections, syphilis, and viral infections (e.g., infectious mononucleosis, CMV infection, and varicella). Q fever, parasitic diseases, MAI (especially in HIV-infected patients), Hodgkin's disease, and beryllium toxicity also may cause granulomatous hepatitis. Granulomatous hepatitis may be a manifestation of drug reactions involving sulfa drugs, hydralazine, or allopurinol. Occasionally, no cause can be found.

        (2) **Clinical features.** Symptoms include weakness, fatigue, markedly increased erythrocyte sedimentation rate, and fever.

        (3) **Diagnosis.** Liver biopsy is used to make the diagnosis.

        (4) **Therapy.** Treatment of the secondary form includes withdrawal of the offending agent and treatment of the underlying lesion. The idiopathic form may respond to corticosteroid therapy.

    b. **Sarcoidosis.** Approximately 70% of patients with sarcoidosis have granulomas in the liver. Patients usually do not have symptoms referable to the liver but may have increased serum alkaline phosphatase levels. Forty percent of patients have hepatomegaly. A liver biopsy showing noncaseating granulomas may aid in the diagnosis. Treatment is with corticosteroids and immunomodulators (azathioprine)

    c. **Amyloidosis** involves the liver in 50% of cases. Patients have hepatomegaly on physical examination but usually are asymptomatic. Results of liver function testing often are normal but may indicate a marked elevation of serum alkaline phosphatase.

12. **Wilson's disease** is an autosomal recessive disease characterized by excessive copper deposition, which, if untreated, may lead to fulminant hepatic failure. Copper may also be deposited in the brain, kidney, and cornea; copper depositions in the cornea cause Kayser–Fleischer rings. (🖱 See online for more information.)

13. **Vascular problems that mimic cirrhosis**

  (🖱) a. **Budd–Chiari syndrome,** or **hepatic vein thrombosis,** is associated with hypercoagulable states, pregnancy, tumors, abdominal trauma, and use of oral contraceptives.

  (🖱) b. **Splenic vein thrombosis** is due to abdominal trauma, pancreatitis, and tumor.

  (🖱) c. **Veno-occlusive disease**

(🖱) 14. **Cardiac cirrhosis**

(🖱) 15. **Nodular regenerative hyperplasia**

B **Cirrhosis of the liver** represents a late stage of progressive hepatic fibrosis characterized by distortion of the hepatic architecture and the formation of regenerative nodules. Regardless of the cause, it is generally considered to be irreversible in its advanced stages, at which point the only curative option is liver transplantation. Patients with cirrhosis are susceptible to a variety of complications, and their life expectancy is markedly reduced compared to that of the general population.

1. **Causes of cirrhosis (see IX A 1–15)**

2. **Complications of cirrhosis**

    a. **Ascites**

        (1) **Pathogenesis.** Increased backpressure into capillaries, as well as decreased oncotic pressure as the result of decreased albumin synthesis, allows accumulation of a transudative fluid in the peritoneal cavity. In addition, increased activity of the renin–angiotensin–aldosterone system contributes to sodium and water retention.

        (2) **Diagnosis.** If fluid accumulation is large, diagnosis may be obvious on physical examination. Ultrasonography is effective for detecting small amounts of fluid. Paracentesis, which may require guidance through ultrasonography, yields a straw-colored fluid with less than 2.5 g/dL total protein, WBC count of less than 300/mm^3 (usually mononuclear),

normal glucose level, and low serum amylase level. A serum albumin–ascites gradient (SAAG) greater than 1.1 g/dL is indicative of portal hypertension.

(3) Therapy. Treatment is based on sodium restriction and diuretic therapy. Aldosterone antagonists (e.g., spironolactone) and loop diuretics (e.g., furosemide) are used. If there is concern for hypotension or fluid shifts, albumin can be given periprocedurally. Some studies suggest that 10 g of albumin for each 1 L of ascitic fluid removed is effective. Placement of a transjugular intrahepatic portosystemic shunt (TIPS) to connect the hepatic and portal veins can reduce portal hypertension and relieve ascites.

(4) Complications. Respiratory compromise and rupture of an umbilical hernia may occur in cases of massive ascites. Infection of the fluid (e.g., due to spontaneous bacterial peritonitis) can be fatal unless treated appropriately.

b. Varices occur as a result of the development of collateral vessels that bypass the obstructed liver. Varices are common in the esophagus and somewhat less common in the stomach, duodenum, and hemorrhoidal plexus. **Portal hypertensive gastropathy** involves dilation of venous and capillary vessels in the mucosa and submucosa with minimal inflammatory infiltrate. Affected patients may suffer bleeding from the mucosal lining of the stomach itself. In most patients, portal decompression results in a decrease of portal hypertensive gastropathy and cessation of bleeding.

(1) Diagnosis of esophagogastric varices may be suggested by imaging studies but is best made by endoscopy. Endoscopy is essential in the acutely bleeding patient because the mortality rate is high (40%–50% for each episode of bleeding), and early treatment can be life saving.

(2) Short-term therapy with octreotide by continuous intravenous infusion is effective in 60%–70% of patients. Balloon tamponade with a Sengstaken–Blakemore tube controls refractory bleeding in 80% of patients but is associated with a risk of aspiration and esophageal rupture. This is typically used as a bridge to endoscopy or TIPS. Endoscopic band ligation or sclerotherapy is effective in approximately 80%–90% of acute cases. Use of TIPS can stop variceal bleeding that is not responsive to endoscopic therapy.

(3) Long-term therapy to reduce the chance of rebleeding includes repeat endoscopic band ligation to obliterate all varices, nonselective β-adrenergic blockers (e.g., propranolol and nadolol) to reduce portal pressure, or TIPS. Surgical shunting is high risk in these patients and only performed in specialized centers.

c. Portosystemic encephalopathy is a reversible neurologic syndrome characterized by mood changes, confusion, drowsiness, disorientation, and coma.

(1) Etiology. The primary cause of hepatic encephalopathy is unclear. Elevated ammonia levels may be found in the blood but do not clearly correlate with disease. It is essential to rule out secondary causes of hepatic encephalopathy, which include:

(a) Azotemia, due to increased nitrogen load

(b) Increased production of ammonia or increased protein load due to constipation, increased dietary protein, or gastrointestinal bleed

(c) Infection, which leads to increased tissue metabolism and increased protein load

(d) Sedatives, whose direct depressant effect on the brain is compounded by decreased hepatic catabolism of the drugs

(e) Electrolyte abnormalities, including hypokalemia and alkalosis, which lead to impaired renal excretion of ammonia and to increased transfer of ammonia across the blood–brain barrier

(2) Therapy. Treatment includes reversal of any of the secondary causes. In addition, the following measures may be effective.

(a) Lactulose effectively decreases colonic pH and traps ammonium ion (NH_4^+) in the gastrointestinal tract. It also is an effective cathartic.

(b) Antibiotics such as metronidazole, rifaximin, and neomycin may decrease intestinal flora that convert gastrointestinal proteins into ammonia. Long-term therapy with some antibiotics can result in significant nonreversible side effects.

(c) Dietary protein should be limited to less than 40 g/day if other measures are ineffective.

(d) Predisposing factors (e.g., hypokalemia, constipation, and alkalosis) should be corrected.

    d. Hepatorenal syndrome is a progressive renal failure that occurs in patients with severe liver disease. It represents the end stage of a sequence of reductions in renal perfusion induced by severe hepatic injury.

        (1) Etiology. Although the exact mechanism of hepatorenal syndrome is not known, several factors are implicated, including the following:

            (a) Splanchnic arterial vasodilation triggered by portal hypertension.

            (b) Intense renal vasoconstriction

            (c) Decreased glomerular filtration rate (GFR)

            (d) Decreased renal blood flow

        (2) Diagnostic criteria

            (a) Chronic or acute hepatic disease with advanced hepatic failure and portal hypertension

            (b) Plasma creatinine >1.5 mg/dL

            (c) Absence of any other cause for renal disease (shock, infection, obstruction, nephrotoxins)

            (d) Urine red blood cells <50 cells/per high-power field, urine protein <500 mg/day

            (e) Lack of improvement in renal function after volume expansion with albumin and withdrawal of diuretics

        (3) Treatment is focused on lowering renal vascular tone, improving hepatic function, or ultimately liver transplantation. Current options include the following:

            (a) Midodrine and octreotide: Increase mean arterial pressure and decrease splanchnic vasodilation

            (b) Norepinephrine: Increases mean arterial pressure

            (c) Vasopressin analogs (terlipressin—not approved in the United States): reduces splanchnic vasodilation

            (d) TIPS: may provide short-term benefit in selected patients through portal decompression and increased plasma volume

            (e) Hemodialysis as a bridge to transplantation

        (4) Prognosis is poor when hepatorenal syndrome develops. Outcomes are strongly dependent on the reversal of hepatic failure, either through medical therapy or liver transplantation. Rate of recovery of kidney function after liver transplantation is unknown; however, a substantial proportion of patients do improve.

    e. Coagulation defects usually are attributable to decreased hepatic synthesis of clotting factors. In addition, splenomegaly may contribute to thrombocytopenia.

    f. Hepatopulmonary syndrome is a hypoxic state caused by intrapulmonary vascular shunting (effectively, a right-to-left shunt). Exercise or standing-induced hypoxia is noted, and clubbing may occur in severe cases. This syndrome is probably present in 30% of patients with cirrhosis and may be severe in 10% of patients. Treatment is with oxygen and eventual liver transplantation.

3. Therapy. The goals of treating patients with cirrhosis include slowing or reversing the progression of liver disease, preventing superimposed insults to the liver, preventing and treating complications, and determining the appropriateness and optimal timing for liver transplantation. As liver transplantation is the definitive treatment for decompensated cirrhosis, eligible patients should be referred as early as possible. Eligibility is determined by severity of disease, complications, and potential for survival after transplantation, which is numerically classified by the model end-stage liver disease (MELD) score.

C **Other conditions affecting the liver**

1. Liver abscess

    a. Pyogenic liver abscess is usually due to biliary tract disease, including acute cholecystitis and cholangitis. Other infections (e.g., appendicitis and diverticulitis), as well as intrinsic hepatic lesions, also are important causes. In 10% of cases, the causative factor cannot be determined. Approximately 70% of abscesses contain mixed flora; the most commonly found organisms are anaerobes, *E. coli*, *Klebsiella* species, *Staphylococcus aureus*, and streptococci.

        (1) Clinical features. Fever, chills, right upper quadrant pain, anorexia, and nausea may be present. Pleuritic pain occasionally occurs, and weight loss is common. Tender hepatomegaly is present in 50% of cases. The alkaline phosphatase level is elevated in approximately 80% of patients, jaundice is present in approximately 33%, and blood cultures are positive in 40%.

    (2) Diagnosis. The clinical presentation suggests the diagnosis, which can be confirmed by CT- or ultrasonography guided aspiration.

    (3) Therapy. Antibiotics, with or without external drainage, frequently are successful. Treatment usually is continued for 4–6 weeks. Occasionally, surgical drainage is required.

  b. Amebic liver abscess. Of the six *Entamoeba* species found in the human colon, *E. histolytica* is the only true pathogen. In the United States, men who have sex with men and institutionalized individuals are at greatest risk for amebic liver abscess. This disease also is common where diarrheal disease due to *E. histolytica* is endemic.

    (1) Clinical features

    (2) Laboratory data

    (3) Diagnosis

    (4) Therapy

    (5) Complications

  c. Hepatosplenic candidiasis is an entity consisting of hepatic and splenic granulomas containing *Candida albicans* hyphae in immunocompromised hosts. Most patients have a hematologic malignancy and have recently recovered from a period of neutropenia.

    (1) Clinical features

    (2) Diagnosis

    (3) Therapy

2. Hepatic cysts

  a. Solitary cysts, generally found in the right lobe of the liver, usually are asymptomatic but may cause pain and fever secondary to bleeding, infection, or rupture.

  b. Polycystic liver disease is the presence of multiple cysts that range from several millimeters to greater than 10–15 cm in diameter. Like solitary cysts, most cysts in polycystic liver disease are asymptomatic except in cases involving hemorrhage, infection, or rupture. Renal cysts are found in 50% of patients; cysts also may be found in the pancreas, spleen, and lungs. Results of liver function testing usually are normal, although mild elevation of serum alkaline phosphatase levels may be seen. Surgical aspiration or decompression occasionally is necessary.

  c. Echinococcal (hydatid) cysts are most common in individuals who live in Greece, France, Italy, the Middle East, South America, and Iceland. This disease may be found elsewhere in the descendants of individuals from these regions.

    (1) Etiology

    (2) Clinical features

    (3) Diagnosis

    (4) Therapy

    (5) Complications

  d. Peliosis hepatis is a rare condition involving multiple blood-filled hepatic cysts associated with hepatic tumors, cholestatic jaundice or drugs. (See online for more information.)

3. Liver diseases of pregnancy

  a. Cholestasis usually is seen in the last trimester of pregnancy and is benign. Patients may complain of severe pruritus and jaundice, and all symptoms disappear rapidly after delivery. (See online for more information.)

  b. Acute fatty liver is a severe disease usually occurring in a primigravida in the last trimester of pregnancy. Fulminant liver failure may develop. Treatment includes rapid delivery of the fetus. (See online for more information.)

  c. HELLP syndrome (hemolysis, elevated liver enzymes, low platelet count) is usually seen in the third trimester of pregnancy. This condition is associated with preeclampsia/eclampsia in approximately 50% of patients. Abdominal pain and vomiting may be severe. Treatment is delivery of the fetus.

    d. Hepatic rupture rarely occurs after necrosis of the liver in eclamptic patients in their last trimester. Patients with hepatic rupture are generally older and multiparous.

D **Inherited disorders of bilirubin metabolism**

1. Gilbert's syndrome

2. Crigler–Najjar syndrome exists in two forms: type I and type II.

3. Rotor's syndrome

4. Dubin–Johnson syndrome

5. Alagille's syndrome

E **Tumors of the liver**

  1. Benign tumors

    a. Hepatic adenomas usually occur in women of childbearing age and are more common in those with a history of oral contraceptive use.

      (1) Clinical features

      (2) Diagnosis

      (3) Therapy

    b. Focal nodular hyperplasia also occurs primarily in women. The theory that this lesion is associated with oral contraceptive use is controversial. Most are discovered incidentally. The lesion is composed of central connective tissue with radiating septa, which divide the mass into nodules. CT and angiography demonstrate a hypervascular mass. There is no potential for malignant transformation, and hemorrhage, rupture, and necrosis are rare. Management is conservative.

    c. Hemangiomas are the most common benign tumors of the liver and are found at autopsy in 5%–7% of patients. Women are affected more commonly than men.

      (1) Clinical features

      (2) Diagnosis

      (3) Therapy

  2. Malignant tumors (see Chapter 5 VIII E)

X DISEASES OF THE PERITONEUM, MESENTERY, AND ABDOMINAL VASCULATURE

A **Diseases of the peritoneum**

  1. Ascites refers to the accumulation of fluid in the peritoneal cavity.

    a. Pathogenesis. The following mechanisms lead to ascites formation:

      (1) Increased hydrostatic pressure, which may be due to cirrhosis, hepatic vein occlusion (Budd–Chiari syndrome), inferior vena cava obstruction, constrictive pericarditis, and congestive heart failure (CHF).

      (2) Decreased colloid osmotic pressure, which may result from end-stage liver disease with poor protein synthesis, nephrotic syndrome with protein loss, malnutrition, and protein-losing enteropathy (PLE).

      (3) Increased permeability of peritoneal capillaries, which may result from tuberculous peritonitis, bacterial peritonitis, or malignant disease of the peritoneum.

      (4) Leakage of fluid into the peritoneal cavity, leading to bile ascites, pancreatic ascites (usually secondary to a leaking pseudocyst), chylous ascites (secondary to lymphatic duct disruption due to lymphoma or trauma), or urine ascites.

      (5) Miscellaneous causes may include myxedema, ovarian disease (Meigs' syndrome), or chronic hemodialysis.

    b. Diagnosis. The presence of ascites usually is apparent on physical examination by abdominal distention, a fluid wave, or shifting dullness. Abdominal ultrasonography can reliably detect small amounts of fluid. Paracentesis can be performed with or without ultrasound guidance, allowing analysis of the ascitic fluid.

        (1) From measurement of the albumin concentration in the ascitic fluid and the serum albumin concentration, a SAAG can be determined.

           (a) If the SAAG is greater than 1.1 g/dL, the patient has portal hypertension (accuracy of approximately 97%). This may be due to cirrhotic or noncirrhotic causes.

           (b) If the SAAG is less than 1.1 g/dL, the patient may have peritoneal carcinomatosis, infection (e.g., peritonitis or tuberculosis), nephrotic syndrome, or pancreatic or biliary ascites.

        (2) The amylase concentration is elevated in pancreatic ascites.

        (3) The triglyceride concentration is elevated in chylous ascites.

        (4) Cytologic findings are frequently positive in malignancy.

        (5) An absolute polymorphonuclear leukocyte (PMN) count greater than 250/mm^3 is diagnostic of infection. When mononuclear cells predominate, tuberculosis or fungal infection should be considered.

        (6) A red blood cell count greater than 50,000/mm^3 denotes hemorrhagic ascites, which usually is due to malignancy, tuberculosis, or trauma. Hemorrhagic pancreatitis, a ruptured aortic aneurysm, and a ruptured hepatic adenoma may cause frank bleeding into the peritoneal cavity.

        (7) Bacterial infection is documented by culture, as Gram stains of ascitic fluid have low sensitivity.

    c. Therapy. Treatment depends on the underlying cause. High-SAAG (>1.1) ascites may be treated with sodium restriction and careful use of diuretics. Paracentesis may provide relief of acute respiratory distress secondary to tense ascites. Intravenous albumin can be used to replace volume and prevent renal insufficiency associated with large-volume paracentesis. TIPS also has been shown to be useful in treating refractory or diuretic intolerant ascites.

2. Bacterial peritonitis

    a. Pathogenesis

        (1) **Primary** or **spontaneous bacterial peritonitis (SBP)** usually develops in the setting of preexisting ascites.

        (2) **Secondary** or **acute bacterial peritonitis** usually results from a perforated viscus, a ruptured appendix, an intestinal infarction, or ulcerative colitis.

    b. Clinical features

        (1) Abdominal pain, with or without guarding and rebound

        (2) Fever

        (3) Leukocytosis

        (4) Paralytic ileus

        (5) It is common for there to be no symptoms.

    c. Diagnosis

        (1) **Paracentesis** aids in determining the etiology of ascites (SAAG) and the presence or absence of infection (PMN count greater than 250/mm^3). Inoculation of an anaerobic culture tube with freshly drawn ascitic fluid (i.e., at the patient's bedside) and inoculation of blood culture bottles are often useful. If the initial ascitic fluid total protein content is less than 1 mg/dL, patients have an increased risk for spontaneous bacterial peritonitis.

        (2) **Radiographic examination** indicates free air under the diaphragm in the presence of a perforated viscus, may show a nonspecific ileus, or may show centralization of bowel, consistent with ascites.

    d. Therapy

        (1) Antimicrobial therapy for spontaneous bacterial peritonitis includes a third-generation cephalosporin to cover gram-negative organisms, pneumococcus, other streptococci, and anaerobic organisms.

        (2) Administration of intravenous albumin should be used in all cases of SBP to prevent acute kidney injury.

        (3) Surgical intervention is necessary in cases of secondary bacterial peritonitis.

3. Other causes of peritonitis

    a. Bile peritonitis

    b. Starch peritonitis

    c. **Gonococcal peritonitis (Fitz-Hugh–Curtis syndrome)** usually is seen in young women and is caused by an ascending infection originating in the pelvis. Chlamydia has been reported to cause an identical syndrome.

      (1) **Clinical features**

      (2) **Diagnosis**

      (3) **Therapy**

4. **Subphrenic abscess** refers to a collection of pus located inferior to the diaphragm and above the liver, spleen, or stomach.

5. **Tumors of the peritoneum**

    a. **Metastatic lesions** are the most common peritoneal tumors. The primary lesion usually is adenocarcinoma of the gastrointestinal tract, pancreas, or ovary. However, sarcomas, lymphomas, leukemias, and carcinoid tumors all may involve the peritoneum.

      (1) **Diagnosis.** Paracentesis with low SAAG ascites (<1.1), a moderately increased lymphocyte count, and positive cytologic findings are diagnostic. Needle biopsy of the peritoneum also may be used.

      (2) **Therapy.** Treatment is directed at the underlying malignancy. A peritoneal drain can be used for palliation of severe recurrent disease.

    b. **Mesothelioma** is seen most commonly in men older than 50 years of age and is associated with asbestos exposure.

      (1) **Clinical features** include abdominal distention, abdominal pain, nausea, vomiting, and weight loss.

      (2) **Diagnosis** requires demonstration of malignant cells through paracentesis with cytologic testing, needle biopsy, or laparotomy with biopsy.

      (3) **Therapy** includes radiation therapy, chemotherapy, or both, but patient response usually is poor.

    c. **Pseudomyxoma peritonei** is a rare condition characterized by the presence of thick gelatinous material in the peritoneal cavity that can lead to intestinal obstruction and death.

B Diseases of the mesentery

1. **Mesenteric panniculitis (mesenteric Weber–Christian disease)** is a rare condition usually seen in older men that causes inflammation and fibrosis of the mesentery.

2. **Mesenteric cysts** are congenital anomalies of the mesenteric lymphatic system that occur as slowly enlarging, painless, round, smooth, mobile masses. Treatment is drainage or excision. Mesenteric cysts are benign but rarely may cause symptoms because of rupture, bleeding, or torsion.

3. **Mesenteric adenitis** is an inflammatory condition of the mesenteric lymph nodes generally seen in children and young adults and mimics acute appendicitis.

C Diseases of the abdominal vasculature

1. **Abdominal aortic aneurysm** usually manifests as an asymptomatic pulsatile mass, but some patients have abdominal pain, back pain, and leg ischemia. The cause usually is atherosclerosis. Leakage of blood into surrounding tissues with associated abdominal, back, or flank pain may precede overt rupture by several weeks. Rupture into the duodenum—presenting as massive gastrointestinal hemorrhage—or into the abdomen may be catastrophic. Treatment is surgical, with repair of the aneurysm with a synthetic graft. Postoperative aortoenteric fistulas with erosion of the graft into the duodenum (usually in the setting of an infected graft) may be seen several years after aneurysmectomy and may result in fatal bleeding if not recognized early.

2. **Acute mesenteric ischemia** is a classic syndrome of decreased blood supply, usually involving the superior mesenteric artery. Patients have advanced arteriosclerotic cardiovascular disease, often with a history of CHF, acute myocardial infarction (MI), cerebrovascular disease, or peripheral vascular disease. Embolic disease (which affects 25% of patients) often is associated with unstable cardiac rhythms. Thrombosis and nonocclusive mesenteric ischemia are the leading

causes of acute mesenteric ischemic syndromes, each accounting for 25% of cases. Mesenteric venous infarction and inferior mesenteric arterial disease account for the rest of the cases.

    a. Clinical features. Sudden severe periumbilical pain is the most common symptom. Nausea and vomiting are common. A benign but hypoperistaltic abdomen is observed. Anteroposterior (flat plate) radiograph of the abdomen often shows normal findings but may show separation of bowel loops or "thumbprinting" (submucosal hemorrhage and edema).

    b. Diagnosis. An increased WBC count (often >20,000/mm^3) supports the diagnosis, although no laboratory studies are specific. Confirmation is by abdominal imaging or angiography. Doppler ultrasonography also may show decreased flow through the superior mesenteric arterial or celiac tree.

    c. Therapy. Treatment is surgical removal of the embolus or thrombus, although occasionally antithrombotic agents, balloon angioplasty of narrowed vessels, or bypass surgery is used. Resection of nonviable bowel is also performed.

3. Chronic mesenteric ischemia usually is seen only when there is significant occlusion of two of the three major splanchnic arteries. The syndrome usually is seen in older patients with a history of cardiovascular disease.

    a. Clinical features include intermittent crampy abdominal pain occurring 15–30 minutes after eating and lasting several hours. Because of the association of pain with eating, patients characteristically become fearful of eating and decrease their intake to the point of substantial weight loss. Physical examination frequently discloses evidence of peripheral vascular disease, but there are no specific findings indicating intestinal ischemia. The presence or absence of an abdominal bruit is not helpful.

    b. Diagnosis is difficult and must be based on strong clinical suspicion combined with angiographic demonstration of significant narrowing (>50%) of two of the three major splanchnic arteries.

    c. Therapy is surgical vascular reconstruction. Vasodilators have not been shown to be effective.

4. Ischemic colitis is due to a decrease in the arterial blood supply to the colon. Although any portion of the colon may be affected, the most common site is the left colon and, in particular, the so-called "watershed area" at the splenic flexure. This area is vulnerable because it is the site where the superior mesenteric arterial supply ends and the inferior mesenteric arterial supply begins. The rectum usually is spared because it has a generous dual blood supply.

    a. Clinical features include bloody diarrhea, lower abdominal pain, and occasional vomiting. Infarction rarely occurs. The older adult who has a history of heart disease or abdominal aortic aneurysm surgery (with ligation of the inferior mesenteric artery) is particularly susceptible.

    b. Diagnosis is suggested by negative findings for other causes of bloody diarrhea in the elderly population (i.e., polyp, carcinoma, diverticulosis, and angiodysplasia). The WBC count may be elevated to approximately 20,000/mm^3. A flat-plate radiograph of the abdomen may show thumbprinting. Abdominal CT scan may show segmental thickening of the bowel wall. Pneumatosis and gas in the mesenteric veins may be seen in more advanced stages. Sigmoidoscopy or colonoscopy show mucosal inflammation, edema, and ulceration with an abrupt transition to normal mucosa.

    c. Therapy is supportive, with bowel rest, intravenous fluids, blood replacement, and empiric antibiotics in severe cases.

    d. Prognosis generally is good. Late strictures may develop, which can require balloon dilation or surgery.

5. Vasculitis. Involvement of the mesenteric vessels by polyarteritis nodosa, lupus erythematosus, or rheumatoid vasculitis mimics arterial embolization (causing bowel infarction) or chronic mesenteric ischemia. The diagnosis is suggested by the systemic features of the disease. Surgery is required for acute infarction. Otherwise, medical treatment with corticosteroids, immunosuppressive agents, or both frequently is effective.

6. Splenic infarction is characterized by severe abdominal pain in patients who have primary hematologic disease (sickle cell disease, myeloproliferative disease, lymphoma), a hypercoagulable state, or embolic diseases. An abscess may develop with hemorrhage or rupture. Diagnosis is suggested by CT or spleen scan with ^{99}Tc. Treatment is surgical.

Study Questions

1. A 30-year-old man has had difficulty swallowing both solids and liquids over the last 6 months. What is the most likely diagnosis?

- A Esophageal carcinoma
- B Achalasia
- C Schatzki's rings
- D Benign esophageal stricture
- E Barrett's esophagus

2. A 52-year-old man with a history of heartburn was diagnosed with carcinoma of the esophagus. What is the most likely cell type of this tumor?

- A Squamous cell
- B Small cell
- C Transitional cell
- D Adenocarcinoma
- E Primary esophageal melanoma

3. An 84-year-old woman was found to have an esophageal web (Plummer–Vinson syndrome). Which one of the following statements is correct?

- A It is caused by folate deficiency.
- B It is located in the distal esophagus.
- C It causes gastroesophageal reflux.
- D Treatment includes esophageal dilation.
- E It results in elevated iron stores in the blood.

4. A 54-year-old obese woman has chronic gastroesophageal reflux. Which of the following drugs are known to exacerbate her GERD?

- A Glyburide
- B Metoclopramide
- C Theophylline
- D Acetaminophen
- E Omeprazole

5. A 32-year-old man with HIV has pain on swallowing. Which of the following is the most likely cause?

- A Scleroderma
- B Esophageal varices
- C Herpes simplex virus (HSV) infection
- D Achalasia
- E Schatzki's rings

6. A 23-year-old woman reports a 2- to 3-year history of postprandial lower abdominal discomfort and bloating with no specific food predilection. Physical examination and laboratory studies are normal. Celiac antibodies were negative. Which of the following statements concerning the most likely diagnosis is correct?

- A Lactase deficiency is the preferred term.
- B An underlying nervous system abnormality is likely with visceral hypersensitivity.
- C An underlying immunologic defect is likely.
- D The syndrome may be a premalignant state.
- E Incontinence is a common clinical feature.

7. A 29-year-old internal medicine resident who had received recombinant hepatitis B vaccine most likely had which of the following immunologic markers?

- [A] Hepatitis B surface antigen (HB_sAg)
- [B] Hepatitis B core antibody (anti-HB_c)
- [C] Hepatitis B e antibody (anti-HB_e)
- [D] Hepatitis B surface antibody (anti-HB_s)
- [E] Anti-HB_c and anti-HB_s

8. A 51-year-old man with recurrent peptic ulcer disease had a fasting gastrin level of 1000. A presumptive diagnosis of Zollinger–Ellison syndrome was made. Which of the following organs is the most common site of origin of the tumor associated with this syndrome?

- [A] Stomach
- [B] Duodenum
- [C] Lymph nodes
- [D] Spleen
- [E] Pancreas

9. A 79-year-old male smoker with a history of coronary artery disease and peripheral vascular disease developed bloody diarrhea. No infectious pathogens were identified. Which part of the colon is most vulnerable to ischemic insult?

- [A] Splenic flexure
- [B] Cecum
- [C] Rectum
- [D] Sigmoid colon
- [E] Hepatic flexure

10. An otherwise healthy 28-year-old man has a 4-month history of epigastric discomfort and heartburn. Symptoms are usually exacerbated postprandially, especially after eating spicy foods. The patient denies dysphagia, weight loss, or decreased appetite. He does not take any medications. Physical examination is normal. Routine lab work is normal. Which of the following is most appropriate at this time?

- [A] Barium swallow
- [B] Upper endoscopy
- [C] 24-hour ambulatory esophageal pH monitoring
- [D] Trial of acid-suppressive therapy
- [E] Esophageal manometry

11. A 42-year-old intravenous drug abuser was found to have both hepatitis B and hepatitis C with chronic elevations of hepatic transaminases (AST, ALT). Which of the following epidemiologic statements is most appropriate?

- [A] Chronic hepatitis will develop in approximately 30%–50% of such patients.
- [B] There is a high 1-year mortality rate after active infection.
- [C] Vaccine protection is available to protect against both diseases.
- [D] The coexistence of HBV and HCV is rare in intravenous drug abusers.
- [E] There is an increased risk for hepatoma.

12. A 32-year-old man recently returned from a ski vacation in New England. Nonbloody diarrhea developed toward the latter stages of his trip. Stool samples tested for fecal leukocytes were negative. Which of the following is the most likely diagnosis?

- [A] *Shigella* infection
- [B] *Escherichia coli* serotype O157:H7 infection
- [C] Ulcerative colitis
- [D] *Giardia lamblia* infection
- [E] Colonic ischemia

13. A 22-year-old woman with changes in her bowel habits was found to have multiple discrete polyps. On family history, two first-degree relatives were noted to have colon cancer. In which of the following conditions are multiple polypoid lesions highly associated with malignancy?

- [A] Ulcerative colitis
- [B] Crohn's disease
- [C] Gardner's syndrome
- [D] Peutz–Jeghers syndrome
- [E] Juvenile polyposis

14. A 32-year-old woman was found to have severe iron-deficiency anemia. An upper endoscopy, colonoscopy, and capsule endoscopy were all normal. Family history revealed osteoporosis in her 39-year-old brother, which is currently being investigated. Her only gastrointestinal symptoms were those of occasional postprandial abdominal bloating with episodes of diarrhea, previously diagnosed as irritable bowel syndrome. Her mother has a known diagnosis of rheumatoid arthritis. All laboratory studies are normal. Which of the following is the most likely diagnosis?

- [A] Ulcerative colitis
- [B] Crohn's disease
- [C] Lactose intolerance
- [D] Irritable bowel syndrome
- [E] Celiac disease

15. Which of the following findings is likely to be found in this patient?

- [A] Prominent villi on small intestine biopsy
- [B] 3 g of D-xylose in a 5-hour urine collection
- [C] High carotene level with normal vitamin A intake
- [D] 4 g of fat on a 72-hour fecal fat collection
- [E] Negative Sudan stain

16. A 22-year-old college student was found to have right lower quadrant pain, fever, leukocytosis, and localization to McBurney's point. On rectal examination, he had right lower quadrant tenderness. The most likely diagnosis is:

- [A] Diverticulitis
- [B] Ulcerative colitis
- [C] Appendicitis
- [D] Tubo-ovarian abscess
- [E] Cholecystitis

17. A 52-year-old man comes in for routine examination. He feels well, takes no medications, and has no family history of colorectal cancer. Physical examination and complete blood count are normal. He returns three fecal occult stool test cards, with one window testing positive for occult blood. What is the appropriate next step in management?

- [A] Repeat fecal occult blood testing in 3 months
- [B] Double-contrast barium enema
- [C] Flexible sigmoidoscopy
- [D] Digital rectal examination
- [E] Colonoscopy

18. A 48-year-old woman was referred to a gastrointestinal clinic for recurrent nausea with occasional episodes of diarrhea alternating with constipation. A solid-phase gastric emptying study indicated markedly delayed gastric emptying. The most likely explanation for gastroparesis in this setting is:

- [A] Cholinergic drug therapy
- [B] Duodenal ulcer
- [C] Diabetes mellitus
- [D] Scleroderma
- [E] Gastric varices

19. A fourth-year medical student rotating on a radiology elective was presented an x-ray of the abdomen, which showed multiple air–fluid levels with dilated loops of small bowel, paucity of air in the colon, and no air in the rectum. The radiology attending asked the student which of the following clinical features would most likely be found in this patient.

[A] Hypoactive bowel sounds
[B] Pain out of proportion to physical examination
[C] Crampy abdominal pain that waxes and wanes
[D] Diarrhea
[E] A flat, rigid abdomen

20. A 50-year-old man undergoing screening colonoscopy with no associated symptoms was found to have a single small colonic polyp. Inquiring about his risk of cancer, which of the following circumstances indicates the greatest risk for cancer in an individual polyp?

[A] When they are of tubular histology
[B] When they are associated with active bleeding
[C] When they are larger than 2 cm in diameter
[D] When they are pedunculated
[E] When patients are younger than 50 years of age

21. A 56-year-old patient with advanced alcoholic cirrhosis and known ascites is found to have abdominal pain, fever to 102°F, and a peripheral white blood cell count of 17,000 with a shift to the left. Which of the following statements regarding the primary diagnosis is correct?

[A] It is more likely when ascitic fluid total protein exceeds 1 mg/dL.
[B] It develops in the setting of preexisting ascites.
[C] The ascitic polymorphonuclear count is less than 100 cells/mm^3.
[D] It is often associated with aspergillosis.
[E] It is associated with a perforated viscus.

22. A 76-year-old man with a history of an acute myocardial infarction and peripheral vascular disease is seen in the emergency department for very severe abdominal pain, out of proportion to clinical findings. On physical examination, his abdomen is soft, with hypoactive bowel sounds. Which of the following is associated with the most likely diagnosis?

[A] A normal white blood cell (WBC) count
[B] Involvement of the inferior mesenteric artery
[C] Constipation
[D] A definitive clinical presentation
[E] Lack of a significant medical history

23. A 32-year-old woman with Raynaud's phenomenon has had heartburn and regurgitation for 2 years. What is the most likely mechanism for these symptoms in this case?

[A] Presence of *Helicobacter pylori* in the gastric mucosa
[B] Decreased lower esophageal sphincter (LES) pressure
[C] Increased gastric acid secretion
[D] Decreased peristalsis in the upper one third of the esophagus
[E] Esophageal muscular spasm

24. A 52-year-old man developed dysphagia for solids. An upper gastrointestinal series showed a mass lesion in the distal esophagus. Endoscopy confirmed the presence of adenocarcinoma of the esophagus. Which of the following is the most important predisposing factor in his disease?

[A] Achalasia
[B] Palmoplantar keratosis (tylosis)
[C] Barrett's esophagus
[D] Celiac sprue
[E] Alcohol intake

25. A 38-year-old man from Taiwan recently moved to this country and was found to have hepatitis B (HBV) on blood studies. Which of the following laboratory tests most reliably distinguish a chronic healthy carrier state from chronic active hepatitis B disease?

(A) Serum hepatitis B surface antigen (HB$_s$Ag)
(B) Serum hepatitis B core antibody (anti-HB$_c$)
(C) Serum anti–smooth muscle antibody
(D) Liver biopsy
(E) Serum α-fetoprotein (AFP)

26. A 35-year-old man with acquired immunodeficiency syndrome (AIDS) with a CD4 count of 150 cells/mm^3 has had jaundice and fever for 1 month. Liver function tests indicate the following:

Total bilirubin: 3.2 mg/dL
Direct bilirubin: 2.7 mg/dL
Alkaline phosphatase: Elevated (three times normal)
AST and ALT: Normal

Liver ultrasound shows hepatomegaly with normal caliber bile ducts, and liver biopsy indicates granulomatous liver disease. Which of the following is the most likely diagnosis?

(A) Polycystic liver disease
(B) Hepatitis C virus (HCV)
(C) *Mycobacterium avium-intracellulare* (MAI)
(D) Sclerosing cholangitis
(E) Hepatitis B virus (HBV)

27. Results of hepatitis serology are as follows:

Positive hepatitis A IgG antibody
Negative hepatitis A IgM antibody
Positive hepatitis B surface antibody (anti-HB$_s$)
Negative hepatitis B core antibody (anti-HB$_c$)
Negative hepatitis C antibody
Which of the following is the most likely diagnosis?

(A) Acute hepatitis A virus (HAV)
(B) Acute hepatitis B virus (HBV)
(C) Immunity against hepatitis C virus (HCV)
(D) Previous vaccination against hepatitis B virus (HBV)
(E) Past exposure to hepatitis B virus (HBV)

28. A 35-year-old man with a history of intravenous drug abuse was found to have chronic fatigue and markedly elevated transaminases. Polyarteritis nodosum was subsequently diagnosed by vascular biopsy. The most likely diagnosis is:
(A) Hepatitis B
(B) Hepatitis C
(C) Hepatitis A
(D) Hepatitis E

29. Which of the following is indicative of active viral replication in this patient?
(A) Hepatitis B DNA level
(B) Hepatitis C DNA level
(C) Hepatitis C RNA level
(D) Hepatitis B RNA level
(E) Hepatitis C antibody

30. The best means to protect his first-degree relatives in the absence of any prior evidence of hepatitis would be:

- A Vaccination
- B Pooled immune globulin (gamma globulin)
- C Avoidance of household contact
- D Avoidance of shellfish ingestion
- E Hepatitis immunoglobulin

Answers and Explanations

1. The answer is B [I A 1 b (1)]. Esophageal motor disorders such as achalasia are characterized by dysphagia for both solids and liquids. Obstructive esophageal conditions such as carcinoma, stricture, and Schatzki's rings cause dysphagia for solids but allow free passage of liquids. The dysphagia associated with Schatzki's rings is intermittent; in carcinoma and stricture, however, the dysphagia is constant. Barrett's esophagus is the replacement of normal squamous epithelium with columnar epithelium; there is no dysphagia unless an ulceration or stricture complicates this condition.

2. The answer is D [I B 2 a (1)]. Adenocarcinoma of the esophagus has been the second fastest rising cancer in the United States, second only to malignant melanoma. In this patient, a history of reflux places him at risk for adenocarcinoma. Primary small cell carcinoma is rare in the esophagus. Transitional cell carcinoma and melanoma are not primary malignancies of the esophagus.

3. The answer is D [I B 2 c]. Esophageal webs are seen in the upper one third of the esophagus and may be caused by failure of complete embryologic recannulation or by mucosal proliferation secondary to iron deficiency—the Plummer–Vinson (Paterson–Kelly) syndrome. Because of the associated iron deficiency, treatment includes iron supplementation, in addition to fracturing the webs with an esophageal dilator.

4. The answer is C [I B 1 a (2) (b) (ii)]. Theophylline, a bronchodilator for treating asthma and chronic bronchitis, is a smooth muscle–relaxing agent that exacerbates GERD. Other smooth muscle–relaxing agents that can exacerbate gastroesophageal reflux disease include diltiazem, isosorbide dinitrate, and atropine. Glyburide, an oral hypoglycemic agent, has no effect on the LES. Metoclopramide is a prokinetic agent that has constricting effects on the LES and improves gastric emptying. Acetaminophen has no direct irritating effects on gastrointestinal mucosa. Omeprazole, a proton pump inhibitor, is helpful in the management of resistant gastroesophageal reflux disease.

5. The answer is C [I A 2, I B 4 b (2)]. Odynophagia, or pain on swallowing, may be caused by motor disorders of the esophagus (e.g., diffuse esophageal spasm) or mucosal disruption (e.g., as a result of infection or drug-induced esophagitis). The most important infectious agents are *Candida,* HSV, CMV, and HIV, infections that are commonly seen in immunocompromised hosts. Severe gastroesophageal reflux with ulcerative esophagitis and radiation esophagitis can lead to severe odynophagia as well. Drugs that may cause mucosal disruption include potassium chloride tablets, tetracycline preparations, clindamycin, quinidine, ascorbic acid, and iron sulfate. Scleroderma is a motor disorder that affects the smooth muscle portion of the esophagus, causing weak, simultaneous, ineffective peristalsis. Dysphagia and heartburn are the typical symptoms. Esophageal varices caused by portal hypertension are generally found incidentally at the time of upper endoscopy or when acute upper gastrointestinal bleeding is present. Schatzki's rings are benign esophageal strictures primarily seen in the distal esophagus, in which dysphagia is the only symptom present.

6. The answer is B [IV D 3 a]. Irritable bowel syndrome, a common cause of alternating diarrhea and constipation, is a functional disorder of motility that probably involves abnormal nervous system perception. Lactase deficiency is a separate entity that may contribute to irritable bowel syndrome but also may be totally unrelated. There is no evidence of an immunologic defect, and the syndrome is not considered a premalignant state. Incontinence is a symptom of altered anorectal physiology that is seen with inflammatory diseases of the anal canal and with systemic neuromuscular disorders such as diabetes or scleroderma. Although incontinence occasionally occurs with explosive diarrhea, incontinence is not a common feature of irritable bowel syndrome and should suggest a systemic disorder.

7. The answer is D [IX A 1 d; Figure 6–1]. The vaccine against HBV, in either the recombinant or the pooled plasma form, does not contain hepatitis B e or hepatitis B core antigen (HB_eAg or HB_cAg, respectively). Therefore, the antibody produced is simply that against hepatitis surface antigen (HB_sAg). Because no active HB_sAg is transmitted, tests for hepatitis B surface antigenemia are negative.

8. The answer is E [III I]. The Zollinger–Ellison syndrome is a non–β islet cell tumor that produces gastrin and is associated with gastric acid hypersecretion and peptic ulcer disease. Tumors are biologically malignant in 60% of cases, and the most common site involved is the pancreas. Tumor size ranges from 2 mm to 20 cm.

9. The answer is A [X C 4]. Ischemic colitis is caused by a lack of arterial blood supply to the colon. Although any portion of the colon may be affected, the most common site is the left colon, particularly the so-called "watershed" area at the splenic flexure.

10. The answer is D [I B 1 d (2)]. This patient has the classic findings and symptoms of uncomplicated gastroesophageal reflux disease. A response to acid-suppressive therapy is the best way to confirm the diagnosis since additional testing is not indicated if the patient's symptoms resolve with therapy. Further workup would be indicated with the patient had any specific warning signs (dysphagia, weight loss, odynophagia) or did not respond to acid-suppressive therapy.

11. The answer is E [IX A 1]. Patients who are chronic carriers of HBV and those with chronic active HBV and HCV infection are at increased risk for developing hepatoma. HBV is parenterally transmitted, putting intravenous drug abusers, men who have sex with men, and those exposed to blood or blood products at risk. There is a 10% risk of chronic disease or becoming a chronic carrier. HCV is transmitted through parenteral, sexual, and perhaps perinatal methods and accounts for 90% of cases of posttransfusion hepatitis. Approximately 30%–50% of patients develop chronic hepatitis. Fulminant HBV is associated with a high mortality rate, whereas fulminant HCV rarely occurs. Vaccination provides adequate protection against HBV; however, currently there is no HCV vaccine.

12. The answer is D [IV D 4 b, e, j; V D; X C 4; Table 6–1]. *Giardia lamblia* is the most common cause of waterborne infectious diarrhea in the United States. The organism preferentially resides in the upper small intestine, and infected patients may be asymptomatic, have mild diarrhea, or develop a prolonged illness characterized by malabsorption, diarrhea, bloating, and crampy abdominal pain. Organisms such as *Shigella* and *E. coli* serotype O157:H7 are invasive pathogens that can cause fever, crampy abdominal pain, and bloody diarrhea. Ulcerative colitis is an inflammatory bowel disease characterized by bloody diarrhea. Colonic ischemia is characterized by the acute onset of crampy abdominal pain and bloody diarrhea caused by a low-flow state to the colon.

13. The answer is C [V G 2, 🔍 Online IV B 1 (a)]. Gardner's syndrome, characterized by familial adenomatous polyposis associated with osteomas or soft-tissue tumors, has an extremely high risk for the development of colorectal cancer. Peutz–Jeghers syndrome is characterized by mucocutaneous pigmentation of the buccal mucosa and hamartomatous polyps in the stomach, small bowel, and colon. These polyps carry a very low risk for malignant transformation. Both ulcerative colitis and Crohn's disease do carry an increased risk of colon cancer, but these disorders are not associated with adenomatous colonic polyps. If multiple colonic polyps are seen in ulcerative colitis, they are generally pseudopolyps and are not neoplastic. Juvenile polyposis commonly leads to gastrointestinal bleeding from polyps of the colon, small bowel, and stomach, and the risk of malignancy is slightly increased later in life.

14. The answer is E [IV E 4 c]. Celiac (nontropical) sprue is a disease characterized by abnormal sensitivity to gluten, a protein component of wheat. Celiac patients have proximal intestinal involvement with relative sparing of the distal ileum. Iron is absorbed in the duodenum, and therefore iron-deficiency anemia is common in this setting. Crohn's disease and ulcerative colitis are active inflammatory diseases that would be associated with changes on intestinal visualization. Lactose intolerance would not be associated with iron-deficiency anemia. A coexisting autoimmune disease in her mother (rheumatoid arthritis) and osteoporosis in a young male are clues that she most likely has associated family members with either celiac disease or other autoimmune disorders.

15. The answer is B [IV E 3 a, b; 🔍 Online IV E 1)]. After a 25-g oral dose of D-xylose, a 5-hour urine collection should contain at least 5 g of D-xylose. The finding of less than 4–5 g of D-xylose in the stool is indicative of the malabsorption syndromes seen with celiac disease. Flat villi with inflammatory cell infiltration on small bowel biopsy are characterized by celiac disease. The serum carotene level is a reflection of vitamin A metabolism. Because vitamin A is a fat-soluble vitamin, a low serum carotene level with normal vitamin A intake may be useful in screening for fat malabsorption. A positive Sudan stain is indicative of an underlying malabsorptive process. However, the gold standard test for fat malabsorption is a 72-hour stool collection for fecal fat. The coefficient of fat absorption in the small intestine is 7%. As a result, a patient consuming a 100-g fat diet should have no more than 7 g fat in the stool each day; more than 7 g fat would be consistent with a malabsorption syndrome.

16. The answer is C [IV I]. Acute appendicitis most often occurs in males between the ages of 10 and 30 years. Clinical features include right lower quadrant (McBurney's point) pain, fever, and leukocytosis. Differential diagnoses include acute gastroenteritis, mesenteric adenitis, Meckel's diverticulum, Crohn's disease, ovarian torsion, ruptured ovarian cyst, pelvic inflammatory disease (PID), and, in elderly patients, diverticulitis, cholecystitis, incarcerated hernia, and mesenteric thrombosis.

17. The answer is E [V G 3]. Colonoscopy is the most appropriate test for patients with a positive fecal occult blood test. Annual fecal occult blood testing, followed by colonoscopy if the test is positive, reduces colorectal cancer mortality by as much as 33%. Colonoscopy can detect subtle mucosal abnormalities such as telangiectasias, areas of inflammation or ulceration, and neoplasms. In addition, most polyps and some early-stage cancers can be removed during the procedure.

18. The answer is D [II C 1]. Gastroparesis is a disorder of gastric emptying and is not associated with mechanical obstruction. It is most frequently associated with a greater than 10-year history of type 1 (insulin-dependent) diabetes mellitus. Other conditions associated with gastroparesis include systemic sclerosis, postvagotomy states, and the use of anticholinergic agents. Prokinetic agents (e.g., metoclopramide, domperidone, erythromycin, and cisapride) have been used to treat gastroparesis. Gastric varices have no effect on gastric emptying.

19. The answer is C [IV A 1]. The patient has a mechanical intestinal obstruction, as the description of the air–fluid levels indicates a mechanical intestinal obstruction. Mechanical intestinal obstruction may be the result of extrinsic, intramural, or intraluminal causes. Symptoms include crampy abdominal pain that waxes and wanes, obstipation or constipation, nausea and vomiting, and abdominal distention. Physical examination of the abdomen reveals high-pitched bowel sounds and rushes and tinkles, as well as marked abdominal distention and tympany on percussion. Pain out of proportion to the physical examination is most suggestive of acute mesenteric ischemia.

20. The answer is C [V G 1]. Adenomatous polyps that represent an increased risk for adenocarcinoma are greater than 2 cm in diameter, villous rather than tubular, and sessile rather than pedunculated. There is no association with increased risk related to bleeding or patient age.

21. The answer is B [X A 2]. The clinical features of spontaneous bacterial peritonitis, which develops in a setting of preexisting ascites, include abdominal pain, fever, leukocytosis, and paralytic ileus. The initial ascitic fluid total protein count is usually less than 1 mm^3/dL. The absolute polymorphonuclear count in the ascitic fluid is generally greater than 250 cells/dL. Bacterial peritonitis associated with a perforated viscus is secondary bacterial peritonitis.

22. The answer is D [X C 2]. This patient has acute mesenteric ischemia, which is a classic syndrome characterized by decreased blood supply; usually the superior mesenteric artery is involved. In general, patients have comorbid conditions such as atherosclerotic cardiovascular disease, CHF, acute MI, cerebrovascular disease, or peripheral vascular disease. The clinical presentation is the basis of the diagnosis. Symptoms include sudden, severe periumbilical pain with a benign physical examination (symptoms are out of proportion to the physical examination). Abdominal radiographs may show separation of bowel loops or "thumbprinting." The leukocyte count is generally greater than 20,000 cells/mm^3, and metabolic acidosis is present.

23. The answer is B [I B 3 d]. This patient has scleroderma with associated Raynaud's phenomenon. The most likely mechanism for gastroesophageal reflux in patients with scleroderma is decreased LES pressure. Presence of *H. pylori* in gastric mucosa is not a predisposing factor for gastroesophageal reflux.

Although increased gastric acid secretion may cause and aggravate gastroesophageal reflux, it is not the mechanism in this case. Decreased esophageal peristalsis can be observed in patients with scleroderma but occurs in the lower one third of esophagus. Esophageal muscle spasm is not associated with gastroesophageal reflux.

24. The answer is C [I B 2 a (2) d, I B 1 e (5)]. Barrett's esophagus is the major predisposing factor in patients with adenocarcinoma of the esophagus. Smoking, alcohol ingestion, geographic factors, achalasia, and tylosis are important predisposing factors for squamous cell carcinoma of the esophagus. Achalasia and celiac sprue are associated with squamous cell carcinoma of the esophagus.

25. The answer is D [IX A 1 f (2)]. The characteristic histologic findings in patients with chronic hepatitis are inflammation of portal triad with piecemeal necrosis. Chronic healthy carriers of HBV have normal liver histology. HB_sAg and anti-HB_c are detected in healthy carriers and patients with chronic hepatitis. Anti–smooth muscle antibody and α-fetoprotein (AFP) are not markers for HBV.

26. The answer is C [IX A 11 a]. In immunocompromised patients, MAI can cause fever. The presence of granuloma in an HIV patient with a low CD4 count should raise the suspicion for a mycobacterial infection. Polycystic liver disease generally does not cause increased liver tests. HBV and HCV cause necroinflammatory parenchymal liver disease, and patients present with elevated AST and ALT. Although sclerosing cholangitis may occur in patients with AIDS, granuloma is not the usual histologic finding in these individuals.

27. The answer is D [IX A 1 d]. The presence of anti-HB_s in the absence of anti-HB_c indicates previous vaccination against HBV. Patients with acute HAV have hepatitis A IgM antibody, and those with acute HBV are positive for HB_sAg.

28. The answer is A [IX A]. Hepatitis B.

29. The answer is A [IX A]. Hepatitis B DNA level.

30. The answer is A [IX A]. Vaccination. Polyarteritis nodosa or glomerulonephritis may develop in patients with HBV. Intravenous drug abusers, men who have sex with men, and individuals exposed to blood and blood products from patients with HBV are at high risk. Hepatocellular carcinoma, cirrhosis, and chronic hepatitis may develop in patients with HBV, HCV, and HDV. HDV is a small, defective RNA virus (delta agent). Cryoglobulinemia occurs in patients with HCV only and not those with other forms of hepatitis. Fulminant hepatitis develops in HAV, HBV, and HCV. With hepatitis E virus infection, the mortality rate in pregnant women may be 10%–20%. Vaccines for the prevention of both HAV and HBV infections are available and are far more effective in preventing transmission than recommendations to avoid contact or exposure to hepatitis patients. Hepatitis B immune globulin (HBIG) has been shown to decrease the perinatal transmission of hepatitis B but is not effective as a long-term measure to prevent hepatitis B in potential contacts.

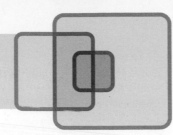

chapter **7**

Renal Diseases, Fluid and Electrolyte Disorders, and Hypertension

NEDA FRAYHA · DONNA HANES

PART I ● **RENAL DISEASES**

I CLINICAL ASSESSMENT OF RENAL FUNCTION

A Urinalysis

B Renal function testing

C Radiography

D Renal biopsy

II ACUTE KIDNEY INJURY

This sudden, rapid, but potentially reversible deterioration in renal function is sufficient to cause nitrogenous waste accumulation in body fluids. Previously referred to as acute renal failure, acute kidney injury (AKI) is especially common in the inpatient setting and carries a 20%–70% mortality rate.

A **Etiology** Causes may be prerenal, postrenal, or parenchymal (Table 7–1).

B **Clinical features**

1. **Azotemia.** Rising blood urea nitrogen (BUN) and serum creatinine levels are the most readily available laboratory signs of a decrease in glomerular filtration rate (GFR). These biochemical changes may be independent of clinical symptoms. Confounding variables that influence BUN and creatinine must be considered before renal failure is confirmed.

   a. **BUN** level is affected by rates of urea production, a function of the amount of dietary protein or protein breakdown (e.g., catabolic drugs or tissue injury), and by resorption of gastrointestinal or soft-tissue hemorrhage.

   b. **Creatinine** level is affected by endogenous creatinine production (increased by breakdown of muscle tissue), by renal creatinine secretion (which is blocked by such drugs as cimetidine and trimethoprim), and by noncreatinine chromogens (usually drugs) that cause measurement errors.

2. **Derangement of urine volume**

   a. **Anuria** (urine output of <100 mL/day). Usually an ominous sign, anuria often indicates either complete arterial occlusion or severe renal injury. However, urine volume per se confers very little diagnostic specificity.

   b. **Oliguria** (urine output <500 mL/day). Such output is insufficient to excrete the daily osmolar load. Although most patients with acute kidney injury are oliguric, 25%–50% of such patients are not and produce more than 800 mL of urine daily.

TABLE 7–1 Causes of Acute Kidney Injury

Classification	Pathophysiology	Example
Prerenal	Severe extracellular volume depletion	Gastrointestinal bleeding
	Decreased renal perfusion	Congestive heart failure
	Renal arterial obstruction	Renal embolus
Postrenal*	Intratubular obstruction	Acute urate nephropathy
	Intrarenal pelvic obstruction	Staghorn calculus
	Ureteropelvic obstruction	Kidney stone
	Ureteral obstruction	Stone, clot, compression by extrarenal lymph nodes
	Bladder-outlet obstruction	Prostatic hypertrophy
Renal parenchymal	Acute tubular necrosis	Sepsis
	Nephrotoxicity	Aminoglycoside antibiotics, radiocontrast dyes
	Intrinsic renal diseases	
	Glomerulonephritis	Poststreptococcal glomerulonephritis
	Tubulointerstitial nephritis	Drug induced
	Vasculitis	ANCA-associated vasculitis

*Must be bilateral, except in patients with only one kidney.

    c. Polyuria. Patients may have acutely rising BUN and serum creatinine levels yet produce more than 3 L of urine daily. This condition may represent a less severe form of acute kidney injury, with preservation of small amounts of glomerular filtration in the presence of tubular damage. Patients with partial urinary tract obstruction frequently present with polyuria.

C Diagnosis

  1. Patient history. Acute kidney injury usually results from several, often synergistic, renal injuries. A history should include information concerning:

    a. Recent surgical and radiographic procedures

    b. Past and present use of medications (e.g., aminoglycosides or nonsteroidal anti-inflammatory drugs [NSAIDs])

    c. Allergies

    d. Underlying chronic renal disease

    e. Family history of renal disease

    f. History of voiding difficulties (suggestive of obstructive uropathy) or symptoms of bladder dysfunction (e.g., hesitancy, urgency)

  2. Physical examination. The physical examination should be organized to parallel the differential diagnosis.

    a. Prerenal failure is suggested by clinical signs of:

      (1) Intravascular volume depletion (e.g., orthostatic changes in blood pressure and pulse, poor skin turgor)

      (2) Congestive heart failure (CHF)

    b. Acute allergic interstitial nephritis is suggested by eosinophilia, eosinophiluria, fever, and maculopapular rash.

    c. Lower urinary tract obstruction is suggested by a suprapubic or flank mass.

  3. Urinalysis

    a. Sediment. Microscopic examination of urinary sediment provides information for the differential diagnosis.

      (1) The presence of few formed elements or only **hyaline casts** is suggestive of prerenal or postrenal failure.

      (2) An abundance of **erythrocytes** is uncommon in the absence of calculi, trauma, infection, or tumor.

      (3) An abundance of **leukocytes** may signify infection, immune-mediated inflammation, or an allergic reaction somewhere in the urinary tract.

      (4) Eosinophiluria occurs in up to 95% of patients with acute allergic interstitial nephritis. Hansel's stain often is helpful to distinguish eosinophils from neutrophils in urine.

      (5) Brownish pigmented cellular casts and many renal tubular epithelial cells are observed in 75% of patients with acute tubular necrosis (ATN). Pigmented casts without erythrocytes in the sediment from urine with a positive dipstick for occult blood indicate either hemoglobinuria or myoglobinuria.

      (6) Red blood cell (RBC) casts are virtually pathognomonic for acute glomerulonephritis (Online Figure 7–1).

  b. Culture. Urine culture should be performed in all patients.

  c. Urine and blood chemistries. Several biochemical indices aid in evaluation. Mainly, these tests distinguish acute oliguria due to prerenal azotemia from that due to parenchymal renal disease (ATN) on the basis that renal tubular function is preserved in the former condition and severely disturbed in the latter.

      (1) The **fractional excretion of sodium** is the ratio of the urine-to-plasma sodium ratio to the urine-to-plasma creatinine ratio expressed as a percentage $[(U_{Na}/P_{Na})/(U_{Cr}/P_{Cr}) \times 100]$. Values less than 1% in oliguric patients suggest prerenal failure, and values greater than 1% suggest ATN.

      (2) Abnormal blood chemistries occasionally aid in the diagnosis of renal failure. A BUN-to-serum creatinine ratio greater than 20 is common in prerenal azotemia.

4. Radiography

  a. Ultrasonography is the method of choice for identifying the presence of two kidneys, for evaluating kidney size and shape, and for detecting **hydronephrosis** or **hydroureter.** Renal calculi, abdominal aneurysms, and renal vein thrombosis sometimes are detected by ultrasonography.

  b. Isotopic flow scans are marginally useful for evaluating the degree of renal perfusion and the presence of obstructive uropathy. Particularly useful is the radiopharmaceutical agent **diethylenetriamine pentaacetic acid (DTPA),** which is excreted only when there is free flow. Scanning using **hippurate** is useful in assessing whether tubular function is intact. Isotopic scans are most helpful in evaluating the function of the renal allograft.

  c. Computed tomography (CT) scans are especially useful in evaluating the nature of **cystic masses** (i.e., benign or malignant).

  d. Retrograde pyelography is performed by injecting contrast material into the ureteral orifice during cystoscopic examination. Specific indications include certain cases of suspected obstructive uropathy in which intervention to relieve the obstruction is contemplated.

5. Biopsy is relevant in only a select group of candidates because the histologic severity and clinical course of acute kidney injury usually do not correlate well. It is reserved for patients in whom the cause of nephrotic syndrome is sought or in whom an acute inflammatory lesion such as vasculitis is suspected and requires cytotoxic therapy for treatment. (Patients who follow a classic laboratory and clinical course of ATN usually do not benefit from renal biopsy.)

6. Cystoscopy is indicated in all cases of urethral obstruction and in some cases of ureteral obstruction.

D **Clinical course**

1. Stages. Acute kidney injury due to ATN typically occurs in three stages: **azotemic, diuretic,** and **recovery.** The initial, azotemic stage can be either oliguric or nonoliguric (Figure 7–2).

2. Morbidity and mortality. The occurrence of oliguria negatively affects morbidity and mortality rates.

  a. Gastrointestinal bleeding, septicemia, metabolic acidemia, and neurologic abnormalities are more common in patients with oliguria.

  b. The risk of mortality is more than two times greater in patients with oliguria, although other factors such as concomitant respiratory or cardiac failure also increase mortality dramatically.

3. Prognosis. Both the severity of the underlying disease and the clinical setting in which acute renal failure occurs affect outcome. For example, the mortality rate among patients with ATN is 60% when ATN is a result of surgery or trauma, 30% when it occurs as a complication of medical illness, and 10%–15% when pregnancy is involved. Ischemia-associated ATN has nearly twice the mortality risk as nephrotoxic ATN. In patients with no complicating factors who survive an episode of acute kidney injury, the chance of complete recovery of kidney function is 90%.

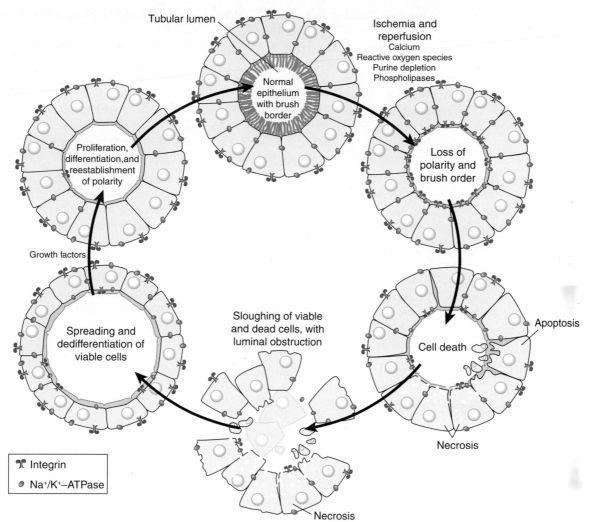

FIGURE 7–2 Stages of acute tubular necrosis.

E **Therapy**

1. **Preliminary measures**
   a. **Exclusion of reversible causes.** Obstruction should be relieved, nephrotoxic drugs should be withdrawn, infection should be treated, and electrolyte derangements should be corrected.
   b. **Correction of prerenal factors.** Intravascular volume and cardiac performance should be optimized.
   c. **Maintenance of urine output.** Although the prognostic importance of oliguria is debated, management of patients without oliguria is clearly easier than management of patients with oliguria. Hemodynamic parameters and intravascular volume should be optimized. Loop diuretics are rarely useful to convert the oliguric form of ATN to the nonoliguric form.

2. **Conservative measures**
   a. **Management of fluids, electrolytes, and anemia.** Patients with acute kidney injury are catabolic and usually lose 0.3 kg of body weight daily. Weight gain or stability usually indicates salt and water retention.
   (1) Total oral and intravenous water administration should equal daily **sensible losses** (via urine, stool, and nasogastric or surgical tube drainage) plus estimated **insensible** (i.e., respiratory and dermal) losses, which usually equal 600–800 mL/day.
   (2) Combined dietary and intravenous sodium and potassium intake should not exceed the measured 24-hour urinary losses of these electrolytes.
   (3) Sodium bicarbonate should be administered if acidemia becomes severe (i.e., if serum bicarbonate concentration drops below 16 mEq/L).

      (4) Oral phosphate-binding antacids (e.g., **calcium acetate**) should be given if the serum phosphate concentration exceeds 6.0 mg/dL.

      (5) Magnesium-containing drugs (e.g., magnesium citrate, magnesium hydroxide–containing antacids) should be withheld.

      (6) Erythropoietin and iron supplements should be administered to maintain hemoglobin levels between 10 and 12 mg/dL if they should fall below this threshold.

  b. Dietary management. Adequate caloric intake is essential for patients with renal failure. Generally, a diet that provides 40–60 g of protein and 35–50 kcal/kg lean body weight is sufficient. However, in some patients, severe catabolism occurs, and protein supplementation to achieve 1.25 g of protein/kg body weight is required to maintain nitrogen balance.

3. Drug usage. Patients who develop renal failure abruptly show only a 1-mg/dL/day increase in serum creatinine because endogenous creatinine production remains constant. Therefore, it is impossible to calculate appropriate drug doses based on serum creatinine level until a new steady state is achieved. Measurement of serum drug levels often is necessary for safe drug use.

4. Dialysis. This procedure is indicated in the management of progressive renal failure that leads to severe uremia, intractable acidemia, hyperkalemia, or volume overload. Clinical research has demonstrated that the use of artificial **biocompatible membranes** improves the mortality of patients with acute kidney injury who require dialysis. In addition to hemodialysis and peritoneal dialysis, **chronic venovenous hemofiltration (CVVH or CVVHD)** is a highly effective form of renal replacement therapy. This modality utilizes highly permeable membranes, which allow the dialysis or filtration processes to occur at very low hydrostatic pressures and flows.

F **Complications** of acute kidney injury are summarized in 🔗 Online Table 7–2.

III   CHRONIC KIDNEY DISEASE

Chronic kidney disease is defined as a substantial and irreversible reduction in renal function that develops over a period of months or years. The stages of chronic kidney disease are outlined in Table 7–3.

A **Etiology**

1. Prerenal causes include severe, longstanding renal artery stenosis and bilateral renal arterial embolism.

2. Renal causes include diabetes mellitus, hypertension, chronic glomerulonephritis, chronic tubulointerstitial nephritis, systemic lupus erythematosus (SLE), amyloidosis, cystic diseases, neoplasia, and human immunodeficiency virus (HIV).

3. Postrenal causes derive from longstanding urinary obstruction.

B **Clinical features**   Presenting manifestations are highly variable. The following constellation of signs and symptoms is referred to as **uremia.**

1. Neurologic signs of lethargy, somnolence, confusion, and neuromuscular irritability develop either gradually or abruptly. Asterixis is a typical finding.

2. Cardiovascular signs of hypertension, CHF, and pericarditis also may be precipitous.

TABLE 7–3   **Stages of Chronic Kidney Disease**

Stage	Description	Estimated GFR	Treatment
1	Kidney damage with normal or increased GFR	>90	Diagnose and treat cause, slow progression, and evaluate risk of cardiovascular disease
2	Kidney damage with mild decrease in GFR	60–89	Estimate progression
3	Kidney damage with moderate decrease in GFR	30–59	Evaluate and treat complications
4	Kidney damage with severe decrease in GFR	15–29	Prepare for renal replacement therapy
5	Kidney failure	<15	Initiate renal replacement therapy

GFR, glomerular filtration rate.

3. **Gastrointestinal signs,** particularly anorexia, nausea, vomiting, and a metallic taste, are very common.

4. **Metabolic signs** can either be nonspecific (e.g., fatigue, pruritus, sleep disturbances) or be referable to a specific defect (e.g., bone pain from secondary hyperparathyroidism).

C Diagnosis The important aim of the diagnostic approach is to establish the chronicity of the renal disease as well as the potential etiologies.

D Therapy

1. **Dietary restrictions** are vital to the proper care of patients to reduce symptoms and, possibly, retard the progression of renal failure. Dietary protein is restricted to 0.6 g/kg lean body weight in early chronic kidney disease, and dietary sodium is restricted to 4 g/day unless residual urine output obligates greater daily losses. (In these cases, urine sodium excretion should be measured and replaced, but not exceeded, in the diet.) Dietary intake of potassium, magnesium, and phosphorus is restricted, and a fluid intake limit is established based on daily losses. It should be noted that most patients with chronic renal failure who do not yet require dialysis do not need severe fluid restriction.

2. **Renal replacement therapy** is necessary for maintenance care of end-stage renal disease.
   a. **Indications** include clinical uremia, severe azotemia (i.e., GFR <15 mL/minute), intractable hyperkalemia or acidemia, and intravascular volume overload.
   b. **Modalities** include hemodialysis, peritoneal dialysis, and renal allograft transplantation.

E Complications Various disorders arise in the course of chronic renal failure and during long-term renal replacement therapy.

IV MEDICAL COMPLICATIONS OF RENAL REPLACEMENT THERAPY

A Introduction

B Hemodialysis

C Peritoneal dialysis

D Renal allograft transplantation

V PROTEINURIA

A Definition Normal adults excrete less than 150 mg of protein in a 24-hour period; **low–molecular-weight proteins** are the major component. Urinary protein excretion exceeding 300 mg/24 hours is termed **proteinuria**. Albumin normally is excreted in the urine at a rate of less than 25 mg/day. Higher rates suggest an abnormality in glomerular barrier function, which normally keeps the albumin molecule from crossing the glomerular basement membrane (GBM). **Macroalbuminuria** refers to an excretion rate of albumin greater than 300 mg/day, a condition detectable with routine screening methods. **Microalbuminuria** refers to a urine albumin excretion rate that exceeds 20 µg/minute but is less than 200 µg/minute (i.e., 30–300 mg/24 hours). Low–molecular-weight proteins are excreted at an increased rate if proximal reabsorptive function is impaired (as in **tubular proteinuria**).

B Etiology

1. **Orthostatic proteinuria** refers to an increase in urinary protein that is detectable only when the patient has been standing. The 24-hour urinary protein output tends to remain constant at about 0.5–2.5 g/24 hours, renal function remains normal, and the prognosis is excellent.

2. **Tubulointerstitial nephritis** involves the excretion of tubular proteins such as **Tamm–Horsfall protein and β₂-microglobulin** in addition to albumin. Tubulointerstitial nephritis is typically seen in patients with drug-induced disease, chronic inflammatory disease (e.g., sarcoidosis), or analgesic nephropathy.

3. **Glomerulonephritis** typically produces albuminuria (>2 g/24 hours). Nephrotic syndrome (hypoalbuminemia, edema, and hyperlipidemia) occurs when protein excretion exceeds 3 g/24 hours.

C **Diagnosis**

1. **Urinalysis**
   a. The most common screening test for proteinuria is the urine dipstick and sulfosalicylic acid precipitation (albumin, paraproteins, immunoglobulins, and amyloid). If positive, characterization of protein (i.e., albumin vs. immunoglobulin) can be performed with urine protein electrophoresis.
   b. Quantification of protein is easily accomplished using a spot urine protein-to-creatinine ratio. A ratio of greater than 0.3 is indicative of significant proteinuria.
   c. Lipiduria is suggested by oval fat bodies on microscopic study.

2. **Urine and blood chemistries** in patients with macroalbuminuria should include quantitative protein measurement and urine protein electrophoresis. Elevated blood lipids and hypoalbuminemia support a diagnosis of nephrotic syndrome.

3. **Biopsy** is indicated in the evaluation of patients with significant proteinuria and nephrotic syndrome when no obvious cause is identified by noninvasive means. Pathologic study should include electron microscopy, immunofluorescence, and the use of special stains (e.g., Congo red for amyloid).

D **Therapy**

1. **Orthostatic proteinuria.** Treatment is not required.
2. **Tubulointerstitial proteinuria.** The underlying disorder must be identified and treated.
3. **Glomerulonephritic proteinuria.** The importance of reducing proteinuria cannot be overemphasized. It not only indicates underlying glomerular disease, but it can perpetuate it. Several therapies have proved useful in reducing proteinuria and retarding progression of renal disease. These include angiotensin-converting-enzyme (ACE) inhibitors, angiotensin-receptor binders (ARBs), lipid-lowering agents, aggressive blood pressure control, smoking cessation, and dietary protein restriction. In addition, diuretics may be useful for symptom relief.

E **Complications** The consequences of hyperlipidemia (atherosclerosis and coronary artery disease), vitamin D deficiency (bone disease), urinary loss of certain proteins impeding spontaneous coagulation (thrombosis), and marked salt retention (massive edema, or anasarca) may result. It has been suggested that patients with nephrotic syndrome are more susceptible to bacterial infections, particularly spontaneous bacterial peritonitis secondary to *Pneumococcus* in children.

VI HEMATURIA

A **Definition** Normal adults excrete 500,000–2,000,000 erythrocytes per 24 hours, which amounts to less than three erythrocytes per high-power field (HPF) of resuspended urinary sediment.

B **Etiology** Causes of hematuria are summarized in Table 7–5.

TABLE 7–5 Causes of Hematuria

Etiology	Clinical Features
Diffuse glomerulonephritis (e.g., systemic lupus erythematosus, vasculitis)	Gross or microscopic hematuria, abnormal proteinuria, red blood cell casts, dysmorphic red cells by phase-contrast microscopy
Focal glomerulonephritis (e.g., immunoglobulin A nephritis, thin basement membrane disease)	Gross or microscopic hematuria without proteinuria, dysmorphic red cells by phase-contrast microscopy
Vascular disease	Gross or microscopic hematuria without proteinuria, isomorphic red cells by phase-contrast microscopy
Tumors (e.g., hypernephroma, bladder cancer)	Isomorphic red cells by phase-contrast microscopy
Trauma	
Kidney stones	
Systemic coagulopathies	

C **Diagnosis**

1. **Urinalysis**
   a. Dipstick testing cannot differentiate hematuria from pigmenturia (i.e., hemoglobinuria or myoglobinuria). A positive **orthotolidine test** in the absence of microscopically detected erythrocytes practically confirms the diagnosis of pigmenturia.
   b. Urine culture should be performed routinely.

2. **Radiography**
   a. Intravenous urography can demonstrate renal masses, cysts, vascular malformations, papillary necrosis, ureteral stricture or obstruction by calculus, bladder tumor, and ureteral deviation. CT scanning is the preferred modality for assessment of renal masses or cysts for malignant characteristics.
   b. Special studies (e.g., angiography, nuclear scanning) occasionally are of value in delineating mass lesions.

3. **Biopsy** occasionally may assist in diagnosing immunoglobulin (Ig) A nephropathy or in characterizing the lesion of a primary glomerular disease.

4. **Cystoscopy** is indicated in the evaluation of hematuria when physical examination, urinalysis, and other imaging studies fail to reveal the cause.

D **Therapy**

1. The underlying disorder must be identified and treated.

2. Urine volume should be maintained to prevent clots and obstruction in the lower urinary tract.

E **Complications**

1. **Iron-deficiency anemia** rarely may complicate chronic, significant hematuria.

2. **Lower urinary tract clots** can induce obstruction.

VII NEPHROLITHIASIS

A **Definition** **Renal calculi** or **stones** arise due to papillary calcification or precipitation in urine of organized crystalline bodies of calcium salts, uric acid, cystine, or struvite. The etiologies of nephrolithiasis are given in Table 7–6.

B **Clinical features** **Signs and symptoms may vary considerably.**

1. **Occult passage** of small, asymptomatic stones may occur.

2. **Hematuria** accompanies stone movement within the urinary tract 85% of the time and may be microscopic or gross. Hematuria may occur with or without pain.

3. **Frequency** and **dysuria** are common complaints of patients with stones lodged in the intravesical segment of the distal ureter and may be mistaken for the symptoms of **cystitis.** Dysuria also occurs during the passage of **sludge.**

TABLE 7–6 **Etiology of Nephrolithiasis**

Stone Type	Etiology or Associated Condition
Calcium phosphate	Hyperparathyroidism, distal renal tubular acidosis, idiopathic hypercalciuria, and medullary sponge kidney
Calcium oxalate	Idiopathic hypercalciuria, excess diet oxalate, vitamin C abuse, small bowel diseases, primary hyperoxaluria, and hypercalcemia; 50% of patients have no identifiable abnormality
Uric acid	Persistently concentrated and acid urine, hyperuricosuria, hyperuricemia (in gout), and excess dietary purine
Cystine	Cystinuria
Struvite (triple phosphate, or magnesium–ammonium–calcium phosphate)	Urinary tract infection (chronic or recurrent) by urease-producing bacteria such as *Proteus, Providencia, Klebsiella, Pseudomonas, Serratia,* and *Enterobacter* species

4. **Abdominal pain, tenesmus,** and **rectal pain** may occur with a stone in the renal pelvis and often are accompanied by nausea and vomiting.

5. **Renal colic,** with flank pain radiating to the inguinal ligament, urethra, labia, testis, or penis, is typical of a stone in the midureter.

C Diagnosis

1. **Patient history** should identify other family members with stone disease as well as the patient's past and present use of drugs and vitamins (particularly vitamins A, C, and D).

2. **Physical examination** is necessary to differentiate acute renal colic from other causes of abdominal, pelvic, and back pain.

3. **Urinalysis** is often useful.
   a. Urine pH is inappropriately high in renal tubular acidosis, favoring calcium phosphate stone formation. Low urine volume with low urine pH is a risk factor for uric acid stones.
   b. Crystals may be seen with characteristic morphologies, which indicate the composition of stones.

4. **Urine** and **blood chemistries** are critical to the metabolic evaluation of the patient with nephrolithiasis.
   a. A blood sample should be examined for levels of electrolytes, creatinine, BUN, calcium, phosphate, and uric acid.
   b. A 24-hour urine collection should be studied for urine volume and pH, as well as levels of calcium, phosphate, uric acid, oxalate, creatinine, sodium, citrate, and cystine, in patients with recurrent stone disease.

5. **Radiography** often confirms the diagnosis. Ultrasonography (Figure 7–3) and non–contrast-enhanced CT have become the modalities of choice for the diagnosis of nephrolithiasis.

6. **Cystoscopy** is indicated for the detection and removal of bladder calculi and for the removal of ureteral stones lodged near the ureterovesical junction.

7. **Stone analysis** is the definitive tool for ascertaining the status of the stone (passed or retained) and its composition. Efforts should be made to strain urine and capture stones for chemical analysis.

D Therapy

1. **Acute episodes** of nephrolithiasis should be treated with rigorous volume administration and pain control with NSAIDs or narcotics.

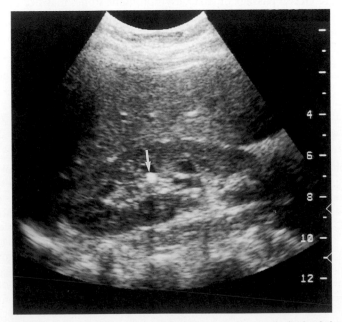

FIGURE 7–3 Ultrasound image demonstrating a renal calculus (*arrow*). Notice the shadowing below the stone.

2. Medical therapy varies, depending on stone composition. In all cases, adequate daily fluid intake to maintain a urine volume of more than 2 L/day is essential. For **calcium oxalate stones** (the most common type), therapy includes dietary restriction of oxalate-rich food, elimination of large doses (i.e., >500 mg/day) of ascorbic acid, and administration of hypocalciuric diuretics (thiazides or amiloride) or oral neutral potassium phosphate. Oral administration of potassium citrate may be useful in increasing the urinary excretion of citrate, a major urinary chelator of ionized calcium and an inhibitor of calcium oxalate crystal growth. Calcium phosphate, uric acid, and struvite stones are covered 🖰 online.

3. Extracorporeal or surgical removal may be required if stone size exceeds 5 mm.
   🖰 **a. Calcium phosphate stones**
   🖰 **b. Uric acid stones**
   🖰 **c. Cystine stones**
   🖰 **d. Struvite stones**

VIII URINARY TRACT OBSTRUCTION

A **Introduction**   An obstruction in the urinary tract may occur at any point between the renal tubules and the urethra. Urinary obstruction may be acute or chronic, unilateral or bilateral, and partial or complete. Chronic urinary obstruction often is partial and may be asymptomatic, particularly in slowly progressive cases. The consequences of urinary obstruction include structural changes in the lower urinary tract as a result of increases in pressure opposing normal urine flow **(obstructive uropathy),** gross dilation of the calyces and collecting system of the affected kidney **(hydronephrosis),** and, ultimately, renal parenchymal damage **(obstructive nephropathy).**

B **Etiology**   The causes of urinary obstruction can be divided into **mechanical** causes, which may be intrinsic or extrinsic, and **functional** causes.

1. **Intrinsic mechanical causes**
   a. **Intrarenal tubular obstruction** results from precipitation of uric acid, sulfonamide, or paraprotein crystals. Drugs such as indinavir and acyclovir may lead to intratubular precipitation of crystals.
   b. **Extrarenal pelvic** or **ureteral obstruction** is caused by calculus, thrombus, papillary necrosis, or tumor.
   c. **Structural lesions of the ureter or bladder** include stricture, tumor, urethral valves, ureteroceles, and foreign body.

2. **Extrinsic mechanical causes**
   a. **Compression** may be caused by:
      (1) Prostatic hypertrophy or carcinoma
      (2) Uterine prolapse or tumor
      (3) Ovarian abscess, cyst, or tumor
      (4) Endometriosis
      (5) Pregnancy
      (6) Retroperitoneal tumor, infection, lymphadenopathy, or fibrosis
   b. **Surgical errors** include accidental ureteral ligation.

3. **Functional causes.** Ureteral or bladder dysfunction results from myelodysplasia; injury or congenital defect of the spinal cord; tabes dorsalis; diabetes mellitus; multiple sclerosis (MS); and autonomic neuropathy, including drug-induced neuropathy (e.g., due to disopyramide).

C **Clinical features**   Signs and symptoms vary, depending on the site of the obstruction and the speed with which the obstruction develops.

1. An **absence of symptoms** often occurs in chronic, slowly advancing obstructive disease. The clinical picture often is overshadowed by signs of the primary disease (e.g., in a case of metastatic tumor or surgical complications) until biochemical evidence of renal impairment develops.

2. **Pain and renal enlargement** (abdominal or flank mass) usually are present in acute obstruction. The pain characteristically is a steady crescendo, is most severe in the flank, and radiates toward the ipsilateral testis or labium.

3. **Urinary symptoms** predominate in obstructive disease of the bladder or urethra. Hesitancy, decreased force of urinary stream, urinary frequency, and dribbling are common in the context of obstruction.

4. **Renal functional impairment** typically is expressed as tubular defects in acid and potassium transport as well as defective tubular responsiveness to hormone action. Clinically, hyperkalemia, mild acidemia, and polyuria precede azotemia, which may progress to renal failure.

D Diagnosis

1. **Urinalysis** varies but may reveal inappropriately dilute urine, hematuria (in cases of obstruction due to calculus or tumor), or bacteriuria. Because infection often complicates obstruction, causing serious detriment to renal function, urine culture is essential. Examination of the urinary sediment often shows no abnormality but may reveal crystals of uric acid or sulfonamide.

2. **Blood chemistries** usually are not diagnostic but are helpful in assessing the severity of impaired renal function.

3. **Radiography** provides the clinical essential evidence of obstruction. Ultrasonography or CT reliably detects evidence of hydronephrosis, such as calyceal blunting and dilation of the renal pelvis, ureter, or both (Online Figure 7–4). Doppler ultrasonography may be effective in demonstrating the rate of urine flow from each ureter. Intravenous urography may fail to visualize the kidneys if the GFR is decreased substantially. Retrograde urography occasionally may help identify unilateral (particularly partial) ureteral obstruction. Nuclear scanning of the kidney often is specific enough to confirm the diagnosis.

E Therapy

1. **Relief of obstruction** is paramount and should be appropriate to the structural nature of the occluding lesion. Methods include placement of a transurethral (Foley) catheter, surgery, percutaneous nephrostomy, ureteral stent, and nephroscopic stone removal.

2. **Medical management** following relief of obstruction is aimed at correcting postobstructive diuresis. Contributing factors include the excretion of solute (urea) that was retained during the period of obstruction and the impaired concentrating ability that usually exists in the recently obstructed kidney. Management involves careful, adequate fluid replacement with frequent assessment of body weight, intravascular volume, and blood and urine electrolyte concentration.

F Complications

1. **Infection,** particularly in the context of obstructing calculi, must be detected and promptly treated to prevent extensive pyelonephritis, perirenal abscess, and sepsis.

2. **Hypertension** occurs secondary to both intravascular volume expansion and ischemic stimulation of renin secretion.

3. **Polycythemia** has been reported in association with hydronephrosis and is purportedly due to increased erythropoietin release.

4. **Persistent tubular defects** may continue beyond 1 year following relief of obstruction. Impaired concentrating ability and limited excretion of a potassium load are the most common defects.

5. **Chronic renal failure** can develop from obstructive disease, most commonly with longstanding obstruction or with complicating urinary tract infection.

IX URINARY TRACT INFECTION

See Chapter 9 V F for coverage of urinary tract infections.

X GLOMERULAR DISEASE

A Hereditary nephritis (Alport's syndrome)

1. **Inheritance and incidence.** Hereditary nephritis is inherited as an X-linked or autosomal dominant trait with variable penetrance. Recent studies have shown that the disease is caused by a defect in one of the genes encoding the subunits of type IV collagen, a basement membrane protein.

2. **Clinical features**
   a. **Hematuria, RBC casts, pyuria, proteinuria,** and **progressive renal failure** occur with variable severity. Renal failure is more common in men.
   b. **High-frequency sensorineural hearing loss,** often without clinically significant deafness, is characteristic.

3. **Therapy and prognosis.** No treatment is successful in slowing or preventing the renal failure, and prognosis is variable. Occasionally, affected patients who undergo renal transplantation develop anti–glomerular basement membrane (anti-GBM) antibody disease (Goodpasture's syndrome) if the Alport host recognizes the normal type IV collagen of the transplanted kidney as a "foreign" antigen.

B Minimal change disease

1. **Incidence.** Minimal change disease accounts for 75% of cases of idiopathic nephrotic syndrome in children but only 25% of cases in adults.

2. **Pathology.** Information is scant and nonspecific. Fusion of epithelial foot processes is seen with electron microscopy, but this lesion is common to all proteinuric states.

3. **Clinical features**
   a. **Nephrotic syndrome** is the typical presentation by patients of all ages.
   b. Hypertension occurs in 10% of children and in 35% of adults.
   c. Hematuria is uncommon.
   d. Azotemia develops in 23% of children and in 34% of adults.

4. **Therapy**
   a. **Glucocorticoids.** The remission rate with adequate steroid treatment is 90% for both children and adults. Prolonged remission is seen in 10%–60% of patients; however, relapse is common and is multiple in 25%–50% of patients. Relapses typically are responsive to steroids, with only 5% of initially steroid-responsive patients developing steroid resistance or dependence. Recent studies have demonstrated that adults may have a poorer response to glucocorticoids than previously believed.
   b. **Cytotoxic agents.** Drugs such as cyclophosphamide and chlorambucil have been effective in steroid-resistant and multiple relapsing cases. Occasionally, steroid-resistant patients develop steroid sensitivity following treatment with cytotoxic alkylating agents. The possibility of gonadal (chromosomal) damage caused by these drugs must be carefully considered.
   c. **Other immunosuppressive agents.** Current research demonstrates that the use of agents such as cyclosporine and mycophenolate mofetil is effective in refractory cases.
   d. ACE inhibitors and ARBs are also necessary for the reduction of proteinuria.

5. **Prognosis.** Minimal change disease is associated with low mortality rates (i.e., 10% among adults and 1.5% among children), with only 10% of deaths caused by renal failure.

C Membranous glomerulonephritis (or glomerulopathy)

1. **Etiology**
   a. **Primary (idiopathic) membranous glomerulonephritis** accounts for 30%–50% of cases of idiopathic nephrotic syndrome in adults but less than 1% of cases in children.
   b. **Secondary membranous glomerulonephritis** may occur with a variety of underlying conditions, including the following:
      (1) **Infection** (e.g., chronic hepatitis B virus [HBV] infection or hepatitis C virus [HCV] infection, syphilis, malaria, schistosomiasis, and filariasis)
      (2) **Rheumatic disease** (e.g., SLE)
      (3) **Neoplasm** (e.g., carcinoma of the lung, colon, stomach, breast, and kidney; non-Hodgkin's lymphoma; leukemia; Wilms' tumor)
      (4) **Drug therapy** (e.g., mercury, gold, D-penicillamine, captopril)

2. **Pathology.** The findings presented in Online Table 7–7 characterize the stages of membranous glomerulonephritis. Characteristic electron microscope findings can be seen in Figure 7–5.

3. **Clinical features.** More than 85% of adults present with proteinuria (>3 g/day/1.73 m^2 body surface area). The GFR usually is normal at diagnosis and often remains normal for 4–5 years thereafter.

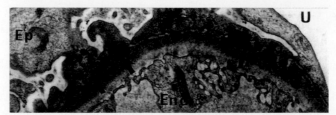

FIGURE 7–5 Electron microscopic findings of subepithelial dense deposits in basement membrane in a patient with membranous nephropathy.

4. **Clinical course.** Membranous glomerulonephritis has a variable course. About 20%–30% of patients achieve a lasting spontaneous remission, 20%–30% develop variable degrees of persistent proteinuria and nonuremic azotemia, and the rest advance to end-stage renal disease, usually over a 5-year period. Male patients, those with heavy proteinuria (>10 g/day), and those who do not respond with a remission in proteinuria have a worse prognosis.

5. **Therapy.** A combination of steroids and cytotoxic agents in addition to ACE inhibitor and ARB therapy has proved effective, but the unpredictable outcome of the disease makes the evaluation of therapy difficult. Recent randomized trials find that steroids alone should not be used as primary therapy. The use of alternating cycles of chlorambucil or cyclophosphamide and prednisone is effective in halting progression to end-stage renal failure in patients with nephrotic syndrome and mild renal insufficiency. Patients treated with cytotoxic drugs are more likely to experience remission of proteinuria.

6. **Complications.** Problematic conditions may intervene, causing an abrupt decrease in renal function.
   a. A **hypercoagulable state** exists in nephrotic patients. Renal vein thrombosis is a recognized problem; pulmonary embolism and arterial thrombosis also have been described.
   b. **Intravascular volume depletion** secondary to vigorous diuretic administration leads to decreased renal blood flow.
   c. **Hypertension, obstruction,** or **infection** may impair filtration.

D **Mesangial proliferative glomerulonephritis**

1. **Etiology.** The cause is unknown.

2. **Pathology**

3. **Clinical features.** Asymptomatic proteinuria or hematuria may occur. Although 24-hour urinary protein excretion can exceed 3.0 g, the complete nephrotic syndrome is inconsistently seen. One third of patients are hypertensive at the time of diagnosis. Creatinine clearance is reduced in only 25% of patients at presentation. Serum complement component levels are normal.

4. **Clinical course.** The disease has an extremely variable course.

5. **Therapy.** High-dose (1–2 mg/kg/day) glucocorticoids are reportedly effective in remission induction. Some steroid failures respond to treatment with cyclophosphamide or chlorambucil.

E **Membranoproliferative glomerulonephritis**

1. **Incidence and etiology**
   a. Collectively, the disorders in this group account for 41% of cases of idiopathic nephrotic syndrome in children and 30% of cases in adults. Males and females are affected equally.
   b. Membranoproliferative glomerulonephritis may be idiopathic or secondary to SLE, cryoglobulinemia, or chronic viral or bacterial infection (e.g., hepatitis C, syphilis, tuberculosis).

2. **Pathology.** The three pathologic types of membranoproliferative glomerulonephritis, each with distinct features, are described in Online Table 7–8.

3. **Clinical features.** The presentation is highly variable. Hypocomplementemia is the most characteristic laboratory finding but is not universally present. The degree of complement C3 depression may be used as a rough guide to disease activity.

4. **Clinical course.** Chronic glomerulonephritis with end-stage renal disease develops in most cases. Rapid progression to renal failure with edema and severe hypertension (acute nephritis) has been described.

5. **Therapy.** Treatment is not predictably effective, although occasional reports claim some therapeutic benefit. In children with proteinuria or impaired renal function, high-dose steroid therapy should be tried and maintained for 6–12 months. In adults with heavy proteinuria (>3 g/day), the **antiplatelet agents** dipyridamole and aspirin may be used. However, evidence does not definitively support the effectiveness of this regimen.

F Focal glomerulosclerosis

1. **Incidence and etiology**
   a. Focal glomerulosclerosis accounts for 30% of cases of idiopathic nephrotic syndrome in adults and is the most common cause of steroid-resistant nephrotic syndrome in children.
   b. This condition is reported to recur in 30%–40% of renal allografts within 3 weeks to 1 year following transplantation.
   c. The etiology is unknown. Focal glomerulosclerosis is seen occasionally in the context of AIDS, heroin and other intravascular drug use, and chronic vesicoureteral reflux, but the causal relationships are uncertain.

2. **Pathology.** The hallmark lesion of focal and segmental glomerulosclerosis evolves through several stages, including mild mesangial prominence, loss of glomerular cellularity, and collapse of capillary loops.

3. **Clinical features and diagnosis**
   a. **Nephrotic syndrome** is the most common clinical presentation. Hypertension and renal failure occur infrequently in childhood but become more prevalent with advancing age.
   b. There are no specific laboratory findings. Proteinuria tends to be heavy (i.e., >15 g/24 hours), and the biochemical derangements of nephrotic syndrome are accordingly severe.

4. **Therapy**
   a. Recent studies suggest that prolonged glucocorticoid therapy (i.e., >6 months) may lead to remission of proteinuria, although no randomized trials support this recommendation.
   b. Cyclosporine as well as ACE inhibitors and ARBs may be effective in reducing proteinuria.

G Goodpasture's syndrome

1. **Definition.** Goodpasture's syndrome refers to a group of illnesses defined by the following triad of findings: **glomerulonephritis** (usually crescentic), **pulmonary hemorrhage,** and **anti-GBM antibody** in serum. The renal and pulmonary components may be severe or clinically silent. The presence of the anti-GBM antibody, however, has become the essential feature of the diagnosis.

2. **Clinical features and diagnosis**
   a. **Clinical presentation** is highly variable.
      (1) **Generalized, systemic symptoms** may precede organ-specific complaints. Fever and myalgia are common.
      (2) **Renal involvement** usually is in the form of rapidly progressive renal failure. Proteinuria usually is mild, and the urinary sediment contains erythrocytes and RBC casts. This "nephritic" picture may be mild or severe.
      (3) **Pulmonary manifestations** include radiographic infiltrates, hemoptysis, cough, and dyspnea. The lung disease usually precedes kidney disease by a period of days to weeks.
   b. **Laboratory findings**
      (1) The most important finding is evidence of circulating immunoglobulin G (IgG) anti-GBM antibody, which is present in more than 90% of patients.
      (2) The pathologic appearance of the kidney is typically that of a crescentic, proliferative glomerulonephritis. Crescents involve 80%–100% of glomeruli and are highly cellular.

3. **Clinical course.** Like the clinical presentation, the course of disease is variable, ranging from a minor recurrent pulmonary hemorrhage that occurs for years—until an abnormal urinary sediment prompts measurement of anti-GBM antibody—to abrupt-onset, fulminant disease, complete renal failure, and asphyxiation by massive pulmonary bleeding over a period of hours to days.

4. **Therapy.** Several treatment methods appear to benefit patients. Poor prognostic indicators include oligoanuria, serum creatinine greater than 6 mg/dL for many weeks, and advanced histopathologic lesions.

    a. High-dose prednisone should be given as an initial therapy. Cyclophosphamide should also be administered to patients younger than 55 years of age. A variety of successful but uncontrolled clinical trials have involved combinations of corticosteroids and alkylating immunosuppressive agents.

    b. Intensive, daily plasmapheresis should be administered for 14 days or until anti-GBM antibody disappears.

H **Idiopathic crescentic glomerulonephritis** Individuals with this pathologically defined entity typically present with rapid, progressive deterioration of renal function. It is imperative to recognize that other lesions may induce the clinical syndrome of **rapidly progressive glomerulonephritis (RPGN)** (Table 7–9). This section considers only the idiopathic cases (i.e., those cases not due to other crescentic glomerular diseases). Idiopathic crescentic glomerulonephritis may be classified into three entities: **anti-GBM antibody disease** [see Part I: X G], **immune complex RPGN,** and **pauci-immune RPGN,** in which glomerular inflammation and necrosis are present but without immune deposits.

1. **Incidence and etiology.** Idiopathic crescentic glomerulonephritis accounts for about one third of all cases of crescentic glomerulonephritis. Males are affected twice as often as females.

2. **Clinical features.** Patients present with abrupt-onset renal failure, with rapid loss of renal function (in less than 3 months), frequently normal blood pressure, and normal kidney size. Nonspecific symptoms (e.g., weakness, nausea, cough, weight loss, fever, myalgia, arthralgia) often announce the disease. Extrarenal involvement, with the exception of lung involvement, is rare.

    a. Renal manifestations. Approximately 50% of patients are oliguric and azotemic at the time of presentation.

    b. Pulmonary manifestations. Transient, mild pulmonary infiltrates or hemoptysis is seen in one half of patients.

TABLE 7–9   **Causes of Acute Kidney Injury with Crescentic Glomerulonephritis**

In Primary Glomerular Diseases
Primary (idiopathic) diffuse crescentic glomerulonephritis
    Type I: anti-GBM antibody disease **without** pulmonary hemorrhage
    Type II: immune complex disease
    Type III: pauci-immune glomerulonephritis (ANCA associated)
Mesangiocapillary glomerulonephritis (especially type II)
Membranous glomerulonephritis with or without superimposed anti-GBM antibody disease
IgA nephropathy (Berger's disease)

In Association with Infectious Diseases
Poststreptococcal glomerulonephritis
Infective endocarditis
Occult visceral bacterial sepsis
Other infections (e.g., hepatitis B)

In Association with Multisystem Diseases
SLE
Goodpasture's syndrome (anti-GBM antibody disease with pulmonary hemorrhage)
Henoch–Schönlein purpura—disseminated vasculitis
ANCA-associated vasculitis
Microscopic polyarteritis (hypersensitivity angiitis)
Other variants
Cryoimmunoglobulinemia (mixed, essential)
Relapsing polychondritis
Lung cancer, lymphoma

ANCA, antineutrophilic cytoplasmic antibody; anti-GBM, anti–glomerular basement membrane; IgA, immunoglobulin A;
  SLE, systemic lupus erythematosus.

3. **Diagnosis.** There are no diagnostic laboratory findings. However, when intrarenal vasculitis (i.e., pauci-immune glomerulonephritis) is the underlying cause, the **antineutrophilic cytoplasmic antibody (ANCA)** test is positive. The diagnosis is based on the discovery of epithelial crescents in a majority of glomeruli in the renal biopsy specimen.

4. **Clinical course and prognosis.** The prognosis may be very bleak, depending on the level of renal function at the time of presentation. Renal failure requiring renal replacement therapy develops in 3–6 months in more than 50% of patients. However, recent data on the use of aggressive immunosuppressive regimens have demonstrated that 50%–75% of patients may enter remission.

5. **Therapy.** In anti-GBM disease, plasmapheresis and immunosuppressives should be used as described for Goodpasture's syndrome [see Part I: X G]. In immune complex glomerulonephritis, treatment depends on the individual causative disorder. In pauci-immune deposit disease, treatment involves pulse methylprednisolone and cyclophosphamide.

I **Postinfectious glomerulonephritis** This acute glomerulonephritis occurs with a variety of local or systemic infections. (Glomerulonephritis associated with infective endocarditis and visceral abscess is discussed in Part I: X Q.) Postinfectious glomerulonephritis has been described as a sequela of disease caused by viruses, fungi, protozoa, and helminths. However, the prototypical postinfectious glomerulonephritis is **poststreptococcal glomerulonephritis.**

1. **Incidence and etiology**
   a. The disease primarily affects school-aged children. The disease is rare before 2 years of age but has been reported in adults. Males are affected twice as often as females.
   b. Preceding infection with nephritogenic strains of group A β-hemolytic streptococci (particularly type 12) is the rule, although positive culture of the organism is demonstrated in less than 20% of cases at the time of renal disease. The site of infection (i.e., skin or pharynx) appears to vary with the geographic area of study. The latent period between infection and clinical glomerular disease is 7–15 days; rarely, it is as long as 3 weeks.

2. **Pathology.** Poststreptococcal glomerulonephritis is a diffuse proliferative disease with mesangial and endothelial hypercellularity. Electron-dense deposits (subepithelial "humps") and foot process fusion are seen by electron microscopy (Figure 7–6). Immunofluorescence often identifies granular deposits of complement C3 along the capillary basement membrane.

3. **Clinical features and diagnosis**
   a. The typical clinical presentation is a sudden onset of hematuria and edema. Nephrotic syndrome develops in fewer than 15% of patients.
   b. The characteristic, but not diagnostic, laboratory profile is azotemia, hypocomplementemia (CH_{50} or C3), hematuria, leukocyturia, and proteinuria. Supporting data include elevated titers of anti–streptolysin O, antihyaluronidase, and anti–deoxyribonuclease B antibodies, all of which suggest preceding streptococcal infection.

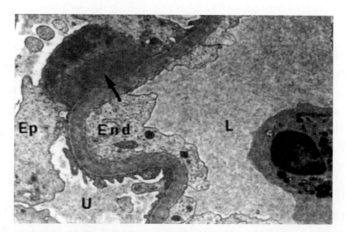

FIGURE 7–6 Electron microscopic findings of dense subepithelial deposits (humps) in a patient with poststreptococcal glomerulonephritis.

4. **Clinical course and diagnosis**

   a. The typical course of acute disease is recovery, particularly among children. The acute nephritis resolves with amelioration of edema and hypertension 1–3 weeks after onset. Proteinuria may persist for several months, exacerbated by erect posture and exercise. Microscopic hematuria similarly disappears slowly over a period of several months.

   b. Long-term prognosis is controversial. Some patients advance to end-stage renal disease. Factors associated with this poor prognosis are severe oliguria or anuria, crescents in the biopsy specimen, persistent heavy proteinuria, and relatively older age. Persistence of hypocomplementemia and progressive renal failure may, however, indicate an alternative diagnosis (e.g., membranoproliferative glomerulonephritis).

5. **Therapy.** Hypertension must be treated aggressively, particularly in children, who develop florid hypertensive encephalopathy at normal adult blood pressures. Furosemide or bumetanide may likely be required for the underlying edema-inducing disease. Antibiotic use is controversial, although a 10-day course of penicillin in nonallergic patients is safe enough for routine use. Prophylaxis following poststreptococcal glomerulonephritis is not indicated because recurrences are exceedingly rare. Immunosuppressive agents or corticosteroids have no therapeutic role.

J **IgA glomerulonephritis (Berger's disease)**

1. **Definition and incidence.** The disease is characterized by mesangial deposits of IgA in renal biopsies from patients with recurrent hematuria but normal renal function. The incidence of this disease varies remarkably with geographic location, and men are affected three to four times more often than women.

2. **Pathology.** Findings are characteristic.

   a. Diffuse, sometimes irregularly distributed IgA deposits are seen in the mesangium. IgM or IgG also may be present.

   b. Focal and segmental glomerulonephritis with mesangial proliferation is common. Mesangial prominence may be the only pathologic finding.

3. **Clinical features and diagnosis.** Affected patients, who usually are between 20 and 40 years of age, most commonly present with recurrent, often macroscopic hematuria but a normal GFR and normal tubular function. Biopsy specimens from normal-appearing skin have immunofluorescent positivity for IgA in 50% of cases. Measuring serum IgA levels is not useful.

4. **Clinical course and prognosis.** Course and outcome are variable. The 20-year survival rate is about 50%. A minority of patients progress to renal failure. Factors that predict a poor prognosis include advanced age at disease onset, heavy proteinuria, hypertension, and the presence of crescents or segmental sclerosis on renal biopsy.

5. **Therapy.** Patients with mild histologic changes and proteinuria of more than 3 g/day should receive prednisone for 4–6 months, as well as ACE inhibitor or ARB therapy. Recent data suggest that fish oil containing a number of anti-inflammatory fatty acids may be useful in some patients with slowly progressive disease.

K **Henoch–Schönlein purpura**

1. **Definition.** This systemic disease is characterized by purpura (which may be slight and go unnoticed), arthritis, abdominal pain, bloody diarrhea, and nephritis.

2. **Incidence.** Henoch–Schönlein purpura primarily affects children. Clinical nephritis affects 30% of patients, but almost all patients have an abnormal kidney biopsy.

3. **Pathology.** The histopathology ranges from mild, diffuse mesangial prominence to focal and segmental proliferative glomerulonephritis on a background of diffuse mesangial proliferation. The hallmark of Henoch–Schönlein purpura is the invariable immunofluorescent positivity for IgA in the mesangium.

4. **Clinical features and diagnosis**

   a. The clinical presentation often is preceded by an infection [caused by a virus (e.g., herpes zoster), *Mycoplasma*, or *Streptococcus*], vaccination, insect bite, or drug administration. Rash usually develops early and evolves from morbilliform to purpuric. The legs and buttocks are affected most commonly. Arthritis typically is mild and nondeforming. Gastrointestinal bleeding and pain may dominate the presentation.

b. Laboratory findings are exceedingly nonspecific, although elevated serum IgA is reported frequently. Serum complement component levels usually are normal.

5. **Clinical course and prognosis**
   a. The clinical course is variable. Patients with recurrent purpura, heavy proteinuria, and clinically severe nephritis at the time of presentation and patients whose biopsies show epithelial crescent formation tend to fare poorly.
   b. Among all children with Henoch–Schönlein purpura, the 15-year survival rate is 90%. By 10 years, however, 15% of these patients have persisting disease and 8% have renal impairment. Among adults, 50% heal completely, 15% progress to renal failure, and approximately 35% have persistent disease.

6. **Therapy.** Several treatment methods have been attempted (e.g., immunosuppression, steroid therapy, anticoagulation) but without proven benefit.

L Diabetic nephropathy

1. **Incidence.** End-stage renal disease develops in 30% of all patients with diabetes. Among patients with juvenile-onset diabetes, 30% develop renal disease within 20 years of the onset of diabetes. Among new patients considered for maintenance renal replacement therapy (largely chronic hemodialysis), at least 40% have chronic renal failure secondary to diabetes. African American, Hispanic, and Native American individuals have a higher likelihood of developing diabetic nephropathy than white patients who have diabetes.

2. **Pathogenesis**
   a. The evolution of diabetic nephropathy is symptomatically quiet until late in the disease process. Early in diabetes, the GFR often is above normal. This early hyperfiltration may be most striking in those patients who subsequently develop glomerular damage.
   b. Initially, **microalbuminuria** [the loss of small amounts of protein (range: 30–300 mg/day)] occurs, which progresses to macroproteinuria, followed by azotemia, and ultimately end-stage renal disease. The rapidity of this course is highly variable.

3. **Pathology.** Two major pathologic lesions are associated with diabetes.
   a. **Diffuse glomerulosclerosis** is uniformly present in patients with diabetic nephropathy. It is characterized by an eosinophilic thickening of the mesangium and basement membrane due to accumulation of extracellular matrix proteins.
   b. **Nodular glomerulosclerosis,** also known as **Kimmelstiel–Wilson syndrome,** consists of round nodules that are homogeneous at the center and have circumferential layering of nuclei (Online Figure 7–7). These nodules often are multiple within a given glomerulus and may be confluent. Nodular glomerulosclerosis is specific for diabetes but it is found in only 50% of patients with diabetic nephropathy.

4. **Laboratory findings.** Results are indicative of a slowly declining GFR.

5. **Clinical course.** Factors that accelerate renal deterioration include hypertension, poor glycemic control, urinary obstruction, infection, the administration of nephrotoxic drugs, and the use of intravenous radiocontrast material.

6. **Therapy**
   a. **Diabetic nephropathy** should be aggressively treated.
      (1) Tight control of blood glucose retards progression of renal disease, especially in those patients with the earliest lesions (microalbuminuria).
      (2) Restriction of dietary protein (i.e., to <0.8 g/kg body weight/day) may slow the development of renal failure once proteinuria occurs and should be initiated early.
      (3) Strict control of hypertension is crucial to slowing the progression of renal failure. Studies indicate that ACE inhibitors and ARBs play an important role as primary therapy for diabetic patients with renal dysfunction (including any degree of albuminuria, hypertension, or a reduced GFR).

(4) Avoidance of nephrotoxins and surveillance for urinary infection or obstruction (neurogenic bladder) are prudent conservative measures.

b. End-stage renal disease is treated using renal replacement therapy when the GFR is <15 mL/minute.

(1) Hemodialysis is the most common form of renal replacement employed and is the mainstay of management of end-stage renal disease.

(2) Good results may be achieved using continuous ambulatory peritoneal dialysis in patients with diabetes. Insulin may be given intraperitoneally, and improved diabetic control may be possible.

(3) Patients who undergo transplantation of a kidney from a living relative have a better 5-year survival rate than those who undergo chronic hemodialysis.

M **Lupus nephritis**   The most widely accepted classification in use for lupus nephritis is the World Health Organization (WHO) classification. It combines the use of light microscopic (LM) findings with immunofluorescence (IF) and electron microscopic (EM) findings to present a uniform classification system (Table 7–10).

1. WHO classes

a. WHO class II (mesangial glomerulonephritis) may occur as the earliest form of lupus nephritis.

(1) Pathology. Biopsy shows mesangial prominence with an increase in matrix and in the number of mesangial cells.

(2) Clinical features and diagnosis

(a) The complete spectrum of clinical findings is not fully known. Many patients are asymptomatic or present with only mild urinary abnormalities.

(b) Serologic findings include positive fluorescent antinuclear antibody (ANA), mild anti-DNA antibody elevations, and normal or mildly decreased C3 and C4 levels.

(3) Clinical course and prognosis

(a) Urinary abnormalities may remit, and transition to diffuse proliferative or membranous lupus nephritis occurs in 15% of patients.

(b) This mesangial lesion is associated with clinical progression only if there is transition to a less favorable histology.

b. WHO class III (focal proliferative glomerulonephritis) develops during the first year of clinical lupus in 50% of patients.

(1) Pathology. The lesion is sharply delineated segmental endothelial and mesangial cell proliferation, which usually affects less than 50% of all glomeruli.

(2) Clinical features and diagnosis

(a) Proteinuria is seen in almost all cases; however, nephrotic syndrome is rare. Hematuria is common, and mild renal insufficiency is seen occasionally. Hypertension is not present.

(b) Serologic findings include positive fluorescent ANA and modest elevations in anti-DNA antibodies. Complement components (C3 and C4) are at normal or decreased levels.

TABLE 7–10	Original World Health Organization (WHO) Classification of Lupus Nephritis
Class	**Description**
I	Normal glomeruli (by LM, IF, EM)
II	Mesangial glomerulonephritis
	Normocellular mesangium by LM but mesangial deposits by IF or EM
	Mesangial hypercellularity with mesangial deposits by IF or EM
III	Focal segmental proliferative glomerulonephritis
IV	Diffuse proliferative glomerulonephritis
V	Membranous glomerulonephritis

EM, electron microscopy; IF, immunofluorescence; LM, light microscopy.

      (3) Clinical course and prognosis

          (a) Remission, as measured by cessation of proteinuria, is seen in about 50% of patients. Relapses commonly occur with extrarenal flares of systemic lupus. Transition to other forms of the disease (e.g., diffuse proliferative or membranous lupus nephritis) occurs in at least 20% of patients.

          (b) Renal failure is rare unless the disease progresses to diffuse proliferative lupus nephritis.

          (c) The 5-year mortality rate is 10%.

  c. WHO class IV (diffuse proliferative glomerulonephritis) most commonly develops within the first year of clinical lupus.

      (1) Pathology. Mesangial and endothelial cell proliferation affect most glomeruli with varying severity. Capillary lumina are obliterated, and crescents affect up to 30% of glomeruli. Deposits of IgG, C3, C4, and C1q are diffuse. IgA and IgM deposits also are seen frequently.

      (2) Clinical features and diagnosis

          (a) Proteinuria and hematuria are universal; more than 50% of patients present with nephrotic syndrome. Azotemia, which is common early in the course of the disease, may be severe. Hypertension occurs commonly.

          (b) Serologic findings include positive fluorescent ANA, highly elevated anti-DNA antibodies, and depressed levels of C3 and C4. Cryoglobulinemia develops in some cases.

      (3) Clinical course and prognosis

          (a) Remission of the nephrotic syndrome, which is seen in 33% of patients, is sometimes sustained. Transition to mesangial lupus nephritis occurs occasionally in association with clinical remission.

          (b) The 5-year mortality rate is 50%. Death results from uremia or active systemic lupus, which frequently is complicated by infection. Hypertension and renal failure may occur as sequelae even after long periods of clinical remission.

  d. WHO class V (membranous glomerulonephritis) develops during the first year of clinical lupus in about 50% of patients.

      (1) Pathology. The histopathologic pattern of membranous lupus nephritis is very similar to that of idiopathic membranous glomerulonephritis [see Part I: X C 2].

      (2) Clinical features and diagnosis

          (a) Proteinuria is seen in all patients, and hematuria is common as well. Nephrotic syndrome is seen at presentation in 50% of patients and ultimately occurs in 80% of patients. Hypertension and renal insufficiency are rare at the outset of membranous lupus nephritis.

          (b) Serologic findings include positive fluorescent ANA, normal or only mildly elevated anti-DNA antibodies, and normal or decreased levels of C3 and C4.

      (3) Clinical course and prognosis

          (a) Remission from nephrotic syndrome is seen in 33% of patients, but relapses are common. Transition to focal or diffuse proliferative lupus nephritis has been reported but is rare.

          (b) The 5-year mortality rate is 10% for patients who develop hypertension and renal insufficiency during persistent nephrotic syndrome.

2. Superimposed lesions. In addition to the major lesions described in the WHO classification system, several superimposed (secondary) lesions may be seen.

  a. Glomerulosclerosis is a secondary lesion that is seen most commonly in diffuse proliferative lupus nephritis with a protracted course. Progressive glomerulosclerosis may be a cause of renal failure in patients whose systemic lupus remits.

  b. Interstitial lupus nephritis usually coexists with glomerular disease but may develop alone.

      (1) Pathologically, this lesion is characterized by intense, mononuclear interstitial infiltration, tubular damage, and interstitial fibrosis.

      (2) IgG and C3 are identified in peritubular capillaries and in tubular basement membranes. Parallel electron-dense deposits are seen.

      (3) Clinical disorders of tubular function (e.g., disorders of potassium excretion, acid excretion, and urine concentration and dilution) are seen in addition to variable, nonselective proteinuria.

  c. Necrotizing vasculitis usually complicates diffuse proliferative lupus nephritis and presents as rapidly accelerating hypertension and renal failure. Histopathologically, an acellular necrosis of vessel walls is seen with proteinaceous occlusive thrombi.

3. **Therapy.** Criteria for therapy are not rigidly established. The response of membranous lupus nephritis to therapy varies among reported series. Because of the poor prognosis associated with diffuse proliferative lupus nephritis, this lesion currently is treated—even in cases with few clinical signs or symptoms of renal disease.

  a. **Glucocorticoid therapy** involves various regimens. Induction therapy with oral prednisone (1–2 mg/kg/day) and pulse intravenous methylprednisolone (1–2 g/day) has been described.

  b. **Cytotoxic drugs** (e.g., cyclophosphamide), when added to steroids, often induce remission, preserve or improve renal function, or both.

N Vasculitis

1. **Introduction.** The kidney frequently is involved in systemic vasculitis, although the actual incidence is unknown. The spectrum of renal syndromes associated with vasculitis ranges from modest "microscopic" involvement of arterioles, venules, and capillaries (a syndrome referred to as **hypersensitivity vasculitis**) to extensive "classic" involvement of medium-sized vessels (a syndrome referred to as **polyarteritis nodosa**).

2. **Polyarteritis nodosa**

  a. **Etiology.** This type of vasculitis may be primary (idiopathic) or secondary to drugs, viral infections (e.g., HBV), or rheumatic diseases (e.g., lupus, rheumatoid vasculitis).

  b. **Pathology.** The kidneys show a focal necrotizing arteritis in vessels ranging in size from the renal artery to the interlobular veins.

  c. **Clinical features and diagnosis**

    (1) The clinical presentation often is vague, consisting of low-grade fever, myalgia, arthralgia, and weight loss.

    (2) The laboratory findings are numerous and, although nonspecific, frequently suggest the diagnosis of polyarteritis nodosa when considered collectively.

    (3) The diagnosis can be confirmed by renal angiography, which shows multiple small aneurysms with segmental infarctions (Figure 7–8). Positive serum ANCA titers have become a major diagnostic aid in vasculitis.

  d. **Clinical course and prognosis.** Progression to organ destruction or death is the expected outcome.

  e. **Therapy.** Use of daily high-dose glucocorticoids and daily cyclophosphamide (1–3 mg/kg/day) has increased the 1-year survival rate to greater than 80%.

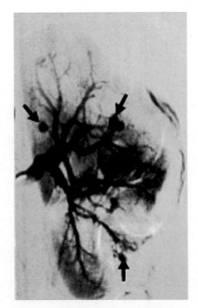

FIGURE 7–8   Angiographic demonstration of multiple microaneurysms characteristic of polyarteritis nodosa.

3. **ANCA-associated vasculitis,** which affects patients of all ages but is more common in middle-aged men, is a special kind of vasculitis (necrotizing granulomatous vasculitis) with renal involvement.

    a. **Pathology.** The characteristic and diagnostic lesion of necrotizing vasculitis and granulomatous inflammation is most reliably discovered in pulmonary or upper airway biopsy material. Often, a focal and segmental necrotizing vasculitis and glomerulitis are found with few (if any) immune deposits.

    b. **Clinical features and diagnosis**

        (1) The disease affects the kidney and upper respiratory tract, including the nose, throat, and bronchi. Ulcerative vasculitic lesions, including nasal septal perforation, are the most recognizable presenting signs.

        (2) The hematologic and serologic features of ANCA-associated vasculitis extensively overlap those of polyarteritis nodosa. ANCAs are present in the serum of most patients and may help in diagnosing the disease and in monitoring response to therapy.

    c. **Clinical course.** ANCA-associated vasculitis has a variable course. Long-term remissions are seen occasionally with therapy. Death usually results from renal failure, sepsis, hemorrhage, or disseminated intravascular coagulation (DIC).

    d. **Therapy.** Treatment with daily high-dose glucocorticoids and monthly cyclophosphamide has increased the 1-year survival rate from less than 20% to greater than 80%. Anecdotal reports indicate that trimethoprim–sulfamethoxazole may reduce the rate of recurrence.

O Cryoglobulins and cryoglobulinemia

1. **Cryoglobulins** are proteins that precipitate at low temperatures and dissolve on rewarming. Three types of cryoglobulins may be defined (Table 7–11).

2. **Cryoglobulinemia** (i.e., presence of cryoglobulins in the blood) occurs in a variety of clinically dissimilar conditions. Renal disease is associated primarily with types I and II and probably has an immune complex–mediated pathophysiology. Many patients with mixed cryoglobulinemia have an underlying infection with HCV.

    a. **Clinical features** (see Table 7–11)

    b. **Diagnosis** involves the detection, characterization, and quantitation of cryoglobulins in serum.

    c. **Therapy** in idiopathic cases is not standardized. Immunosuppressives and steroids are occasionally effective. Encouraging results have been obtained with plasmapheresis, particularly in patients with mixed cryoglobulinemia. Antiretroviral therapy may be effective in patients with HCV-caused mixed cryoglobulinemia.

P Multiple myeloma (see Chapter 4 VII E)

1. **Definition.** Multiple myeloma represents a neoplastic transformation of a monoclonal B lymphocyte into a plasma cell, which produces excessive quantities of immunoglobulin or immunoglobulin fragment (paraprotein). More than 50% of affected patients die of complications of

TABLE 7–11	**Cryoglobulins and Cryoglobulinemia**
Type	**Clinical Features**
I Monoclonal cryoglobulins	Associated with hematologic malignancies Heavy proteinuria, hematuria, and occasionally anuria Histologic lesion: usually membranoproliferative glomerulonephritis
II Mixed cryoglobulins that include a monoclonal component with antibody activity against polyclonal immunoglobulin G	Associated with a syndrome of immune-complex vasculitis Approximately 50% of patients have renal disease Wide spectrum of clinical signs that vary greatly in severity Hypertension, azotemia, and anuria, which are poor prognostic signs Endocapillary proliferation and mesangial prominence (common pathologic features)
III Mixed cryoglobulins in which both components are polyclonal	May be associated with a variety of other diseases, with or without renal disease, including , systemic lupus erythematosus, hepatitis B or C, and systemic infections

renal failure, and a much higher percentage of patients with multiple myeloma have some form of renal involvement.

2. **Pathology.** The many mechanisms of renal injury in multiple myeloma have different effects on the kidney (🖱 Online Table 7–12).

3. **Clinical features and diagnosis**

   a. The clinical presentation of renal disease in multiple myeloma often is subtle. Anemia and bone pain in the presence of any form of abnormal urinary finding should prompt evaluation for myeloma. Slowly progressive renal insufficiency is typical; however, acute kidney injury may be seen in certain circumstances (e.g., in the presence of hypercalcemia).

   b. Many chemical abnormalities commonly occur. Pseudohyponatremia develops secondary to the presence of large quantities of paraprotein, altering the nonaqueous phase of plasma. The anion gap is low and occasionally is negative because of the positive charges on the immunoglobulin molecules. Urine protein concentration is increased, reflecting excretion of the huge paraprotein burden. As mentioned previously, dipstick measurement for protein is insensitive to immunoglobulin and often yields false-negative results. Thus, acid precipitation with sulfosalicylic acid is required.

4. **Therapy and prognosis.** Although no specific therapy exists for the renal disease, chemotherapy for the malignancy, meticulous regulation of intravascular volume and electrolyte status, and dialysis (when necessary) may prolong life. Plasmapheresis may be useful in improving renal function in patients with acute kidney injury and circulating light chains.

🖱 Ⓠ **Glomerulonephritis in infective endocarditis**

XI **RENAL CYSTIC DISEASE**

Ⓐ **Adult polycystic kidney disease**

1. **Definition, etiology, and incidence.** Adult polycystic kidney disease represents the most common cause of renal failure and death in adults with renal cystic disease. It accounts for approximately 5% of all patients on maintenance dialysis.

   a. Inherited as an autosomal dominant trait, adult polycystic kidney disease achieves 100% gene penetrance by the time the patient is 80 years of age. In the majority of cases, the affected gene (polycystin-1) is on chromosome 16 (PKD1); however, in a minority of families, the genetic defect (polycystin-2) resides on chromosome 4 (PKD2).

   b. Men and women are affected equally. Family history is positive in more than 75% of cases.

   c. Adult polycystic kidney disease must be distinguished from **childhood (autosomal recessive) polycystic kidney disease** (which is universally fatal by the third decade of life) and the **congenital multicystic variant of renal dysplasia.**

2. **Clinical features**

   a. The typical presentation of enlarging flank or abdominal masses, abdominal pain, and slowly progressive renal failure becomes clinically evident by the fourth decade of life, and renal replacement therapy becomes necessary within 10 years of the onset of symptoms. Associated clinical findings may include hypertension, polyuria and nocturia, erythrocytosis, and nephrolithiasis.

   b. The onset of renal failure occurs later in the minority of patients who have the genetic defect on chromosome 4 (about 67 years as opposed to about 54 years) compared with the majority, who have the defect on chromosome 16.

   c. Hepatic cysts occur in 33% of cases. However, liver insufficiency is rare, unlike in the childhood form.

   d. Intracranial (berry) aneurysms occur in 12% of patients. In some series, 6% of all patients with berry aneurysms have adult polycystic kidney disease.

3. **Diagnosis.** Diagnosis is made most easily on the basis of specific ultrasonographic findings. Coincident findings include hematuria, impaired urine-concentrating ability, and low-grade proteinuria. Heavy proteinuria, persistent hematuria, and pyuria should be investigated because they rarely occur in uncomplicated adult polycystic kidney disease.

4. **Therapy.** Treatment is restricted to the therapy of end-stage renal disease as it develops. Genetic counseling is important because 50% of offspring are affected. Women with adult polycystic kidney disease are not at an increased risk for fetal demise or hypertension during pregnancy except as contributed by existing renal insufficiency.

B Nephronophthisis (medullary cystic disease)

C Medullary sponge kidney

D Simple renal cyst

1. **Definition and incidence.** The simple cyst is the most common renal cystic disease; at least one half of all individuals older than 50 years of age have one or more macroscopic renal cysts. Renal cysts may be solitary or multiple and unilateral or bilateral.

2. **Clinical features.** Symptoms are rare; simple cysts usually are diagnosed during patient evaluation for other problems. Bleeding and infection stimulate the cyst wall to thicken, and calcareous plaques often form within the cyst wall.

3. **Clinical course.** Simple cysts usually are static, although regression may occur from one radiographic assessment to the next. Solitary cysts may undergo malignant degeneration, although this finding is rare. Hemorrhagic cysts are more likely to contain a neoplasm than nonhemorrhagic cysts (i.e., in up to 30% of cases as compared with less than 1% of cases). **Multiple simple cysts** may develop in end-stage renal disease in patients who have undergone hemodialysis for longer than 7 years.

4. **Diagnosis** may be made by CT, ultrasonography, urography, or angiography. Cyst puncture (for fluid aspiration and cytology) and contrast radiology should be performed in patients with large cysts with abnormal ultrasonographic appearance.

5. **Therapy.** In the absence of infection or tumor, no specific therapy is indicated for this benign disease.

XII TUBULOINTERSTITIAL DISEASE

A Acute interstitial nephritis

1. **Definition.** Acute interstitial nephritis appears to be a kidney-based hypersensitivity reaction, usually caused by a drug. Although the true incidence of acute interstitial nephritis is unknown, several hundred cases have been formally reported, and an increasing awareness of this disease has come with increased case recognition.

2. **Etiology.** Drugs implicated in the pathogenesis of acute interstitial nephritis include β-lactam antibiotics (e.g., methicillin, oxacillin, and cephalothin) and other antibiotics (e.g., sulfonamides), NSAIDs (e.g., ibuprofen, indomethacin, fenoprofen, and tolmetin), diuretics (e.g., thiazides and furosemide), and many other unrelated drugs (e.g., phenytoin, cimetidine, sulfinpyrazone, methyldopa, and phenobarbital).

3. **Clinical features.** The **classic** presentation is development of acute kidney injury with fever, rash, and eosinophilia, yet only a minority of patients present with this symptom triad.

4. **Diagnosis**
   a. **Urinalysis** classically shows mild or no proteinuria, microscopic hematuria, pyuria, and eosinophiluria. Urine must be examined microscopically with appropriate staining methods for the presence of eosinophiluria. Some patients with acute interstitial nephritis due to NSAIDs present with nephrotic syndrome characterized by urinary protein excretion exceeding 3.0 g/24 hours.
   b. **Biopsy** shows patchy, irregular interstitial infiltration with inflammatory cells. Monocytes and lymphocytes are constant findings. Eosinophils may be abundant or completely absent. Fibrosis is extremely unusual and should suggest underlying or preexisting renal disease. Rarely, acute interstitial nephritis may progress to chronic interstitial nephritis, and fibrosis may be prominent. Glomeruli are normal or show only mild mesangial prominence.

5. **Therapy.** Treatment includes discontinuation of the etiologic drug and initiation of supportive measures (e.g., dietary restrictions, blood pressure management, and acute dialysis). The value

of glucocorticoid therapy is unclear; however, the use of steroids may be justified in patients with severe or rapidly progressive renal insufficiency. In such patients, the addition of immunosuppressive agents such as cyclophosphamide is warranted. When interstitial nephritis is associated with circulating antibodies (a rare occurrence), the addition of plasmapheresis is indicated.

6. **Prognosis.** Outcome is excellent, provided that the offending drug is promptly withdrawn. Recovery time varies and may be prolonged in patients with oliguria and in those with extensive interstitial cellular infiltrates. Temporary dialysis may be needed. Rarely, patients progress to end-stage renal disease.

B **Chronic interstitial nephritis** In general, the clinical features common to these interstitial diseases include a relative preservation of glomerular function until late in the disease but an impairment of tubular functions (e.g., urine concentration, dilution, acidification, and potassium excretion) early in the course of the disease.

1. **Drug-related nephropathy**
   a. **Analgesic nephropathy** is the prototypical drug-related chronic interstitial nephritis.
      (1) Analgesic nephropathy occurs more commonly in women than in men. Patients usually are older than 45 years of age and from low socioeconomic classes. Patients often complain of frequent headaches or have coincident psychiatric disease.
      (2) Intravenous urography reveals abnormality in more than 90% of cases, and papillary necrosis is seen in more than 50%. Half of the patients are hypertensive, and anemia is common and often out of proportion to the degree of clinically apparent renal disease.
      (3) Several agents have been implicated (e.g., acetaminophen, phenacetin, and aspirin), but none has been specifically proven culpable. The risk of analgesic nephropathy appears to be increased in patients who use more than 3 g/day of such agents.
      (4) Treatment of progressive analgesic nephropathy is supportive. Removal of the inciting agent may arrest the deterioration of renal function.
      (5) NSAIDs can also be associated with other renal disorders (Table 7–13).
   b. **Gold nephropathy** is a frequent and important complication of parenteral gold therapy for rheumatoid arthritis. Gold accumulation leads to immune-complex membranous glomerulonephritis and nephrotic syndrome. Cessation of gold therapy at the first sign of proteinuria is recommended and often results in regression of signs of renal disease. It is not known whether oral gold preparations are equally nephrotoxic.
   c. **Lithium nephrotoxicity** may be important. Lithium carbonate, used in the treatment of bipolar disorder, is filtered freely and undergoes significant (i.e., 60%–70%) reabsorption in the proximal tubules. Lithium toxicity results in antidiuretic hormone (ADH)–unresponsive nephrogenic diabetes insipidus, incomplete distal renal tubular acidosis, and, rarely, azotemia.

2. **Toxin-related nephropathy**
   a. **Lead nephropathy (saturnine gout)** is a well-recognized sequela of chronic lead intoxication.
      (1) The earliest cases of lead intoxication involved miners, paint manufacturers, and distillers of "moonshine" liquor. Lead poisoning also has been reported in children who have ingested lead-based paint. Individuals who recover from acute lead poisoning occasionally are found later to be victims of chronic lead–related renal disease.

TABLE 7–13   Mechanisms for Nonsteroidal Anti-inflammatory Drug–Induced Disorders

Disorder	Mechanism
Nephrotic syndrome	Severe interstitial nephritis; histologically normal glomeruli
Decreased glomerular filtration rate	Renal vasoconstriction, especially in patients with preexisting renal disease, congestive heart failure, or cirrhosis; patients treated with triamterene at particular risk
Papillary necrosis	Unknown
Edema	Primary renal sodium retention due to prostaglandin inhibition, especially in patients with underlying congestive heart failure
Hyperkalemia	Hyporeninemic hypoaldosteronism

(2) Clinical manifestations of lead nephropathy include a reduced GFR, reduced renal plasma flow (RPF), minimal or no proteinuria, normal urinary sediment, gouty arthritis due to hyperuricemia and low urate clearance, and, occasionally, hypertension, hyperkalemia, and acidemia.

(3) Treatment includes removal of lead exposure and chelation therapy with sodium or calcium **ethylenediaminetetraacetic acid (EDTA)** or **D-penicillamine** (in appropriate cases).

b. Cadmium nephropathy may lead to interstitial disease.

c. Copper nephrotoxicity

d. Mercury nephropathy

3. Crystalline nephropathy

a. Uric acid produces renal injury in three ways.

(1) Uric acid stones may develop in concentrated acid urine.

(2) Acute uric acid nephropathy (acute crystalline obstruction of renal tubules) may accompany sudden or extreme elevations in serum uric acid (i.e., serum levels >25 mg/dL), as occurs in **tumor lysis syndrome.**

(3) Gouty nephropathy, a syndrome of interstitial fibrosis and decreased renal function, may be related to cortical microtophi and a nephrotoxic influence of hyperuricemia in some gouty patients. Lead nephropathy (saturnine gout) may account for a significant percentage of patients with renal insufficiency and gout.

b. Oxalic acid also produces tubulointerstitial disease. Elevated urine levels of oxalic acid may lead to the formation of calcium oxalate stones or may mimic the syndrome of acute uric acid nephropathy (acute crystalline obstruction). **Primary hyperoxaluria** is an inherited disease of oxalate overproduction, which terminates in renal failure with extensive deposition of oxalate crystals throughout the body (a condition termed **oxalosis**). **Ethylene glycol poisoning** may lead to renal failure in part by the hyperoxaluria that results from the metabolism of ethylene glycol to oxalate. The use of **methoxyflurane** in anesthesia has been linked to an increased oxalate production with resultant nephrotoxicity. Increased oxalate absorption often is seen following ileojejunal bypass surgery for obesity and may lead to nephrocalcinosis. Mild hyperoxaluria may result from pyridoxine or thiamine deficiency.

c. Antiviral agents. High-dose **acyclovir** and **ganciclovir** may lead to intratubular crystal deposition and acute kidney injury. **Indinavir,** an antiretroviral agent, may also produce this lesion because its crystals are highly insoluble. High-dose **methotrexate** may induce intratubular crystal deposition as well, and high-dose **sulfadiazine** may lead to a similar complication when urine is particularly acidic.

4. Miscellaneous nephropathies

a. Amyloidosis (Online Figure 7–9)

b. Sarcoidosis [see also Chapter 3 XIII G]

C Renal papillary necrosis

1. Definition. Renal papillary necrosis results from ischemic necrosis of the renal medulla or renal papillae. There are two forms. The papillary form involves the entire papilla, whereas the medullary form begins with focal areas of infarction in the inner medullary zone.

2. Etiologic factors. Conditions associated with renal papillary necrosis include diabetes mellitus, urinary tract obstruction, severe pyelonephritis, analgesic abuse, sickle cell hemoglobinopathy, extreme hypoxia and intravascular volume depletion in infants, and renal allograft rejection.

3. Clinical features. The clinical presentation of renal papillary necrosis varies with the stage and extent of disease. Patients with sickle cell trait may have completely asymptomatic renal papillary necrosis, which is discovered incidentally during urography for unrelated complaints. Infection frequently complicates renal papillary necrosis and leads to clinical pyelonephritis. The necrotic papillae may be sloughed and produce typical ureteral colic or ureteral obstruction. Azotemia is an uncommon presenting sign.

4. Clinical course. The course of renal papillary necrosis is a function of the underlying disease. End-stage renal disease may develop, particularly among diabetics.

5. **Diagnosis.** Intravenous urography can establish the diagnosis of both forms of renal papillary necrosis. Radiographically, the affected calyces appear irregular and fuzzy early in the disease process. As the lesion progresses, sequestration of the necrotic tissue leads to sinus formation and the appearance of a sinus tract or arc shadow on the urogram. In advanced renal papillary necrosis, the sequestrum may be sloughed and surrounded by contrast material—the so-called ring sign. Calcification, calicectasis, and medullary cavities may be present in this stage.

6. **Therapy.** Treatment includes relief of obstruction, prevention and prompt eradication of infection, and control of pain (colic). Surgery occasionally is necessary to control hemorrhage or to relieve obstruction.

XIII RENAL TRANSPORT DEFECTS

A Meliturias

B Aminoacidurias

C Fanconi's syndrome

1. **Definition.** Fanconi's syndrome refers to a collection of proximal tubular defects that may exist in varying number and degree of severity and may be inherited or acquired.

2. **Etiology**
   a. **Inherited causes** include cystinosis, Lowe's syndrome, Wilson's disease, tyrosinemia, galactosemia, glycogenosis, and fructose intolerance.
   b. **Acquired causes** include transplant dysfunction, myeloma, Sjögren's syndrome, hyperparathyroidism, potassium depletion, amyloidosis, nephrotic syndrome, interstitial nephritis, heavy metal toxicity, and outdated tetracycline. **Ifosfamide,** a cyclophosphamide-related drug, can induce a Fanconi-like syndrome when it is used as an antineoplastic agent. Glycosuria and aminoaciduria have been reported in virtually all children treated with this agent.
   c. An **idiopathic** form of Fanconi's syndrome also exists.

3. **Clinical features and course**
   a. Symptoms and signs include glycosuria, aminoaciduria, phosphaturia, bicarbonaturia, vasopressin-resistant polyuria, rickets or osteoporosis, short stature, and uremia.
   b. The natural history of Fanconi's syndrome depends heavily on the course and prognosis of the underlying disease or diseases.

4. **Therapy.** Treatment is designed to replace lost urinary solutes and to correct the underlying disease or diseases. Phosphate, vitamin D, and bicarbonate should be given when indicated by laboratory and clinical data.

XIV RENAL VASCULAR DISEASE

A **Ischemic nephropathy** Occlusive disease of the renal arterial system encompasses a broad spectrum of clinical syndromes and pathophysiology. Arterial blood flow may be interrupted by in situ thrombosis or by embolism from distant endovascular sites. Occlusion may be sudden and complete or gradual, with resultant functional renal artery stenosis.

1. **Etiology**
   a. **Renal arterial thrombosis** may develop spontaneously in the context of atherosclerosis, aneurysm, arteritis, hypercoagulable states, sickle cell disease, and thrombotic microangiopathy. Thrombosis also may develop as a complication of external trauma, instrumentation with angiography catheters, arterial surgery, and renal allograft transplantation.
   b. **Renal arterial embolism** may be caused by a clot, tumor fragment, or infectious coagulum.
      (1) **Cardiac conditions** that may lead to renal arterial embolism include a dilated left atrium, artificial heart valves, myocardial infarction, infective endocarditis, marantic endocarditis, and myxoma.
      (2) **Noncardiac conditions** that may cause renal arterial embolism include atheromatous plaques and paradoxical, fat, or tumor embolism.

   c. Cholesterol emboli may occur spontaneously or follow vascular surgery or angiography. Acute kidney injury may be the only manifestation of disease, or there may be associated eosinophiluria. Occasionally, skin lesions such as petechiae or livedo reticularis may be seen. Pathology of the skin or kidney reveals cholesterol clefts in small and medium-sized vessels. There is no specific therapy, but the disorder may spontaneously regress, leaving the patient with adequate residual kidney function.

   d. Progressive renal atherosclerosis affects a large number (perhaps >20%) of individuals with end-stage renal failure; they have angiographically significant renal artery stenosis. The risks of contrast-dye–associated acute kidney injury, cholesterol embolization, and acute renal artery dissection have prevented many clinicians from suggesting an aggressive approach in most patients. Intervention is indicated in patients with severe, uncontrollable hypertension and in those with diffuse vascular disease with clearly progressive renal insufficiency.

2. Clinical features and diagnosis

   a. Acute, complete renal arterial occlusion usually manifests as flank pain, hematuria, fever, nausea, tissue necrosis (as evidenced by elevated lactate dehydrogenase [LDH] and aspartate transaminase (AST)], and acute kidney injury. The diagnosis is confirmed using radionuclide scanning or angiography. Bilateral occlusion and occlusion of a solitary functioning kidney produce severe anuric acute kidney injury.

   b. Chronic or **segmental occlusion** produces symptoms and signs commensurate with the degree of ischemic damage, including progressive renal failure.

3. Therapy

   a. Therapy for renal arterial thrombosis is surgical removal of the clot to restore renal blood flow. Best results are obtained when the operation is conducted within 48–72 hours following the onset of disease.

   b. Therapy for renal arterial embolism, which usually is diffuse and involves large numbers of smaller arterial branches, is anticoagulation with heparin and resolution of the underlying focus of emboli.

   c. Therapy for ischemic nephropathy may involve angioplasty, stent placement, or surgical revascularization. While the role of each of these therapies continues to be explored, there is little evidence that kidney function can be substantially preserved or that acute renal insufficiency due to ischemic nephropathy can be reversed.

B **Renal vein thrombosis**   Obstruction of renal venous drainage by a clot may be caused by extension of clots in the vena cava, invasion of the renal vein by tumor, severe dehydration in infants, renal amyloidosis, and certain glomerular diseases associated with nephrotic syndrome, particularly membranous glomerulonephritis. Renal vein thrombosis generally is not a cause of glomerular disease. Renal vein thrombosis may develop during nephrosis because of loss of anticoagulant proteins and procoagulant deactivators in the urine protein.

1. Clinical features and diagnosis. Slowly evolving renal vein thrombosis may be completely asymptomatic, whereas acute renal vein thrombosis may produce pain, hematuria, costovertebral angle tenderness, and, ultimately, signs of worsening renal function. The affected kidney appears to be enlarged when visualized with the aid of intravenous urography. Selective venography is diagnostic. New techniques such as Doppler ultrasonography may be particularly useful as a noninvasive approach to diagnosis.

2. Therapy. Treatment is controversial, as is the belief that renal vein thrombosis predisposes to pulmonary embolism. Current therapy is long-term (3–6 months) anticoagulation with warfarin sodium or low–molecular-weight heparins. Longer treatment is recommended if embolic phenomena occur.

C **Renal artery stenosis**   In experimental animals, it has been clearly shown that partial reduction in the luminal size of one or both renal arteries produces renovascular hypertension, which is mediated in most cases by increased renin production with resultant activation of angiotensin and aldosterone. In humans, renal artery stenosis is a recognized cause of renovascular hypertension. However, the coincidence of radiographically demonstrated renal artery stenosis and clinically demonstrated renovascular hypertension does not establish a causal relationship.

1. **Etiology**
   a. **Medial fibromuscular dysplasia** occurs more commonly in young women.
   b. Adults older than 50 years of age have **renal artery atherosclerosis,** which is twice as common in men as in women.
   c. Rare causes include **Takayasu's arteritis, arterial wall disease** (e.g., hematoma, dissecting aneurysm, and tumor), and **external arterial compression** due to tumor, fibrosis, or cyst.

2. **Clinical features.** Signs and symptoms include a nearly continuous abdominal or flank bruit, hypokalemia, mild metabolic alkalosis, and asymmetric kidney size. None of these is a constant finding, and often there is no feature to distinguish renal artery stenosis from essential hypertension.

3. **Diagnosis.** Diagnostic strategies vary according to clinical suspicion.
   a. **Magnetic resonance angiography (MRA),** or rarely, traditional angiography is the method of choice for a definitive diagnosis. Stenotic segments are reliably identified by this study.
   b. **Duplex ultrasonography** allows noninvasive determination of renal blood flow. This procedure is operator dependent and may not be technically feasible in all patients.
   c. **Renal vein renin studies.** Angiographic proof that renal artery stenosis is etiologically important is difficult to obtain. Finding that the renal vein renin from the affected side is 1.5 times greater than that from the unaffected side is helpful, but patients may respond to treatment without this biochemical finding.

4. **Therapy.** Therapeutic options are antihypertensive drugs, percutaneous transluminal angioplasty (PCTA) with or without stenting, and surgical repair of the affected vessel. Current research is evaluating the long-term effectiveness of renal artery stent placement.

D **Microangiopathy: hemolytic–uremic syndrome and thrombotic thrombocytopenic purpura** As members of the disease group termed microangiopathic hemolytic anemia, hemolytic–uremic syndrome (HUS) and thrombocytopenic purpura (TTP) are similar clinical syndromes that share features with disseminated intravascular coagulation, malignant hypertension, postpartum renal failure, sepsis, and systemic sclerosis.

1. **Clinical features**
   a. **TTP** characteristically manifests as fever, microangiopathic hemolytic anemia, thrombocytopenia, fluctuating neurologic signs, purpura, and renal failure. Gastrointestinal involvement (e.g., mucosal bleeding and jaundice) is common. In some cases, the etiologic agent is an autoantibody directed toward a protease, which cleaves von Willebrand's factor.
   b. **Hemolytic–uremic syndrome** is primarily a pediatric disorder characterized by microangiopathic hemolytic anemia, thrombocytopenia, and acute kidney injury. The disorder may occur in epidemics and has been reported to follow shigellosis. Hemolytic–uremic syndrome usually has a sudden and dramatic onset, with renal failure the dominant clinical feature. As in TTP, other organ systems may be involved. Renal function returns in most patients who recover from systemic disease, but relapses have been reported.

2. **Diagnosis**
   a. **Laboratory findings** are similar in both disorders.
      (1) Anemia is a constant finding, occurring in association with a variety of structurally damaged RBCs in the peripheral circulation. The reticulocyte count, fibrin split products, and indirect bilirubin levels are elevated. Serum LDH is also elevated and is the most useful clinical marker for following disease progress. Leukocytosis is common, and thrombocytopenia is severe (i.e., <20,000 platelets/mm^3). The bone marrow shows erythroid hyperplasia with adequate or increased megakaryocytes. Azotemia is common, and the degree of renal failure is characteristically severe. Recently, microangiopathic hemolytic anemia has been found in association with the antiphospholipid antibody syndrome.
      (2) Urinalysis shows hematuria, pyuria, hemoglobinuria, and granular cysts.
      (3) Microbiologic studies may reveal verotoxin-producing *Escherichia coli* (serotype O157:H7) as the cause, particularly in epidemics.
   b. **Renal biopsy findings** also are similar. Arterioles and small arteries are occluded by eosinophilic, hyaline thrombi containing fibrin and platelet aggregates, which cause impressive vascular dilation. Microinfarcts commonly occur, but without inflammatory infiltrates or signs of vasculitis. Renal lesions are focal and are almost completely confined to the arterial side.

3. **Therapy.** Controlled trials comparing individual treatment programs have not been performed. Therapeutic methods in use include antiplatelet drugs (e.g., aspirin, sulfinpyrazone, and dipyridamole), glucocorticoids, exchange transfusion, plasmapheresis, and, rarely, splenectomy. Most recent trials have suggested that plasma exchange therapy gives the best therapeutic outcome.

4. **Prognosis.** Outcome has improved with modern therapy. Untreated TTP is almost universally fatal within 1 year. However, with the institution of early therapy, 1-year survival rates may exceed 80%. Fewer than 5% of patients with hemolytic–uremic syndrome die within 1 month.

E **Systemic sclerosis (scleroderma)** This generalized disturbance of connective and vascular tissue leads to fibrosis of the affected tissue. Systemic sclerosis may be a localized disease (called **morphea**) or a lethal, systemic disease. Renal involvement is a common cause of morbidity and death. The incidence of renal involvement in systemic sclerosis is not solidly established but, based on autopsy series, is estimated to range from 42% to 80%. Clinical evidence of renal involvement (i.e., azotemia, hypertension, and active urinary sediment) is seen in about 45% of systemic sclerosis patients. In one study, subtle vascular and hemodynamic abnormalities were seen in 80% of patients.

1. **Clinical features and course**
   a. **Acute renal disease** occurs in the context of rapidly accelerating generalized disease activity, with prominent malignant hypertension. This is commonly referred to as "scleroderma crisis." Renal failure can ensue precipitously if the blood pressure is uncontrolled. Pathologically, acute renal disease is similar to other microangiopathic diseases. The interlobular arteries show marked intimal thickening and mucoid proliferation, which may lead to cortical necrosis. Glomerular changes usually are mild and nonspecific, often consisting of only mesangial prominence. Interstitial edema with some mononuclear infiltrate is common. Unlike isolated malignant hypertension, systemic sclerosis does not primarily affect arterioles but does produce adventitial fibrosis.
   b. **Chronic renal disease** may be present in patients with systemic sclerosis and little or no clinical signs of renal involvement. Kidney size usually is normal, and the earliest sign of disease is proteinuria, which is noted in 30% of patients. Nephrotic syndrome is rare, and hematuria, urinary casts, and pyuria usually are absent. Hypertension complicates chronic renal disease frequently (i.e., in 25%–50% of patients) and is a harbinger of impending deterioration of renal function. Renal failure occasionally develops in systemic sclerosis patients who have neither proteinuria nor hypertension.

2. **Therapy**
   a. **Treatment of acute renal disease** involves, to a large degree, the control of accelerated hypertension. ACE inhibitors, ARBs, minoxidil, and nitroprusside may be required. However, recent data suggest that overly aggressive lowering of diastolic blood pressure to less than 85 mm Hg may actually increase the risk of acute kidney injury in patients with scleroderma.
   b. **Treatment of chronic renal disease** is less clear-cut. It is not known whether some vasoactive therapy during early, nonazotemic, nonhypertensive stages of the disease is protective. Similarly, the role of treatment for patients with abnormal renal biopsy specimens but no clinical renal disease is unclear.

F **Sickle cell nephropathy**

1. **Pathology**
   a. Sickle cell trait and sickle cell disease are associated with a variety of renal complications. The renal medulla is relatively anoxic and hyperosmolar—factors that favor erythrocyte sickling. Most damage occurs in the renal papillae.
   b. Medullary infarction resulting from occluded (sickled) vessels produces a spectrum of tubular disorders, including impaired urine concentration. Because the injury is located in the renal papillae, these patients behave as though they have been papillectomized. Papillary necrosis also is seen. Patients with sickle cell trait are affected less severely than those with sickle cell disease.

2. **Clinical features**
   a. Impaired secretion of potassium and hydrogen ion occurs, and a frequent biochemical finding is hyperkalemia with a hyperchloremic (normal anion gap) metabolic acidosis [see Part II: IV D 2].

  b. Hematuria represents the most dramatic of the renal abnormalities in sickle cell disease. Although it is usually self-limited, life-threatening exsanguination occurs in rare cases.

  c. Glomerular disease, including nephrotic syndrome, has been documented in sickle cell disease. Membranoproliferative-like lesions have been reported, as has typical membranous glomerulonephritis.

3. Clinical course. Although frequently the GFR is supranormal early in the course of sickle cell nephropathy, gradual deterioration of renal function is common. Progression to end-stage renal disease occurs in some cases.

4. Therapy

  a. Careful fluid management to maintain adequate intravascular volume, both during crises and at other times, clearly is important. Volume depletion is injurious to renal function and is more likely to occur because of the urine-concentrating defect.

  b. Patients who are prone to hyperkalemia or acidosis should be advised to reduce their dietary intake of potassium and protein.

  c. Hemodialysis is useful and does not increase the number or severity of crises or alter the transfusion requirement in most patients.

  d. Kidney allografts are susceptible to sickle cell damage.

G Radiation nephritis

XV THE KIDNEY IN PREGNANCY

A General physiologic effects

B Urinary tract infections

C Acute kidney injury

D Hypertension

E Preeclampsia–eclampsia (toxemia of pregnancy)

  1. Definition
  2. Pathology
  3. Clinical features and diagnosis
  4. Therapy

PART II FLUID AND ELECTROLYTE DISORDERS

I WATER METABOLISM

A Normal physiology

1. Regulation of water intake. Increased thirst is the normal response to water loss. The neural center that controls the release of **ADH** is anatomically close to the thirst center. ADH release is stimulated by increased body fluid tonicity or decreased effective circulating volume.

  a. Tonicity refers to the shift of water through biomembranes produced by osmotically active particles such as glucose and sodium. Urea exerts virtually no tonicity because it easily crosses all membranes and produces no osmotic shift of water.

  b. Osmolality is a function of the number of molecules in solution independent of effects on water movement.

2. Regulation of water output

  a. Proximal tubular reabsorption. Of the 200 L/day of water that is filtered at the glomerulus, 125 L is reabsorbed in the proximal tubule.

    b. Osmotic gradient formation in the medulla. Glomerular filtrate not reabsorbed in the proximal tubule enters the loop of Henle, where, in the thick ascending limb, active sodium chloride reabsorption without water reabsorption causes dilution of the urine and increases the concentration of solutes in the medullary interstitium.

    c. Collecting tubular transport. Water that reaches the collecting tubule either is excreted (if ADH is absent, causing the tubule to be impermeable to water) or is reabsorbed (if ADH is present, causing the tubule to be permeable to water). Thus, ADH affects the osmolality of urine, which may range from 50 to 1200 mOsm/L.

B **Hyponatremia**

1. Definition. Hyponatremia refers to serum sodium concentration of less than 135 mEq/L. The name, however, is somewhat misleading because hyponatremia is usually a problem of too much water, not too little sodium. In fact, the sodium content of the body may be increased, decreased, or relatively unchanged. Hypotonicity always implies hyponatremia. The opposite is not always true: Hyponatremia can coexist with isotonicity, hypertonicity, or hypotonicity.

    a. Pseudohyponatremia (isotonic hyponatremia) is a laboratory artifact that occurs in the setting of extreme hyperlipidemia or hyperproteinemia. If the laboratory uses an instrument that reports sodium content per unit volume of total plasma rather than sodium content per volume of the aqueous phase, then significant elevations in plasma lipids or γ-globulins can cause the reported sodium concentration to be artificially low. This artifact can be obviated by using an ion-selective electrode that measures sodium ion concentration in the aqueous phase.

    b. Hypertonic hyponatremia results from the shift of water from the intracellular fluid to the extracellular fluid, which is caused by the presence of osmotically active particles (e.g., glucose) in the extracellular fluid space. Serum sodium concentration is reduced, but the osmolality of the extracellular fluid is above normal.

    c. True hyponatremia (hypotonic hyponatremia) occurs when there is excess total body water relative to solute content and is clinically significant when the serum sodium concentration is less than 125 mEq/L and the serum osmolality is less than 250 mOsm/kg.

2. Etiology

    a. Decreased renal water excretion

      (1) Decreased GFR. A decrease in the filtered load of water to less than 10% of normal results in a clinically significant decrease in the ability of the kidney to excrete water.

      (2) Increased proximal tubular reabsorption. An increase in proximal tubular reabsorption of filtered fluid from the normal 65% to more than 90% may impair the capacity of the kidney to excrete water. Increased proximal tubular reabsorption occurs when the kidney is hypoperfused (e.g., in states of excessive fluid loss from diarrhea or vomiting). Decreased effective renal perfusion in diseases such as CHF, cirrhosis, or nephrotic syndrome also stimulates proximal tubular reabsorption. This group of disorders is characterized by a low urine sodium concentration, indicating increased renal absorption of sodium, high BUN, and the physical finding of either true volume depletion or one of the edematous conditions.

      (3) Increased collecting tubular reabsorption of water. Nonosmotically stimulated ADH secretion induces such reabsorption. Characteristics of this condition include relatively normal urine sodium excretion (if intake is normal), a high urine osmolality, and signs of body water expansion resulting from excessive retention of ingested water.

    b. Increased fluid intake. Fluid intake in excess of 1 L/hour exceeds normal excretory capacity and leads to hyponatremia. This situation is seen in patients who are given excessive hypotonic intravenous fluids and in psychiatric patients who drink excessively.

    c. Syndrome of inappropriate ADH secretion (SIADH) results from ADH release in the absence of increased body fluid tonicity or decreased effective circulating volume. Causes of SIADH are listed in Table 7–14.

3. Clinical features. Central nervous system (CNS) dysfunction may develop as the tonicity of the extracellular fluid falls and water diffuses down an osmotic gradient into the brain cells, leading to cellular edema. Acute hyponatremia with a decrease in serum sodium concentration below 125 mEq/L over a period of hours almost always is associated with acute CNS disturbances such as obtundation, coma, seizures, and death if untreated.

TABLE 7–14 Causes of Syndrome of Inappropriate Antidiuretic Hormone Secretion (SIADH)

Cause	Mechanism
Tumor	Several tumors produce an ADH-like peptide, most notably small cell carcinoma of the lung
CNS disease	Excessive ADH release may occur secondary to seizures, cerebral trauma, brain tumors, or psychiatric disturbances; nausea and vomiting also may produce excessive ADH release
Pulmonary disease	SIADH may be seen with pulmonary tumors, infections, and bronchospastic disease; thought to be mediated by J receptors in the pulmonary circulation that stimulate pituitary ADH release
Adrenal insufficiency	The loss of glucocorticoid inhibition of ADH release results in excessive secretion of ADH; in addition, primary adrenal insufficiency involving both glucocorticoid and mineralocorticoid production may result in renal sodium wasting, exacerbating the hyponatremia
Drugs	Medications may act to produce SIADH by increasing ADH release or by sensitizing the renal tubule to the effects of ADH; examples include chlorpropamide, clofibrate, thiazide diuretics, and many CNS-active drugs
Idiopathic	Some patients, especially elderly patients, may have no apparent reason for SIADH, and increased ADH release in these patients may be due simply to advancing age
Reset osmostat	This is a variant of SIADH occurring in chronically ill and malnourished patients in whom the serum sodium is reset at a low value (typically about 125 mEq/L); these patients are able to maintain water balance and appropriately excrete a water load

ADH, antidiuretic hormone; CNS, central nervous system; SAIDH, syndrome of inappropriate antidiuretic hormone secretion.

4. **Diagnosis**
   a. **Physical findings.** Examination may reveal the following:
      (1) Volume depletion (e.g., in cases related to drugs such as diuretics)
      (2) Edema (e.g., in cases related to cirrhosis or CHF)
   b. **Laboratory data**
      (1) **Urine osmolality:** >50–100 mOsm/kg in the presence of plasma hypotonicity
      (2) **Urine sodium concentration:** high when plasma volume is expanded in SIADH but low when effective arterial blood volume is reduced, as in edematous conditions. A urine sodium concentration less than 20 mEq/L strongly argues against SIADH.
   c. **Water loading test.** When an intravascularly volume-expanded individual is given 20 mL water/kg orally or intravenously over a period of 20–40 minutes, the normal response is excretion of 80% of this water load within 4 hours and reduction of urine osmolality to less than 100 mOsm/kg. Failure to achieve these results suggests impairment in the kidney's ability to excrete water.

5. **Therapy**
   a. **Fluid restriction.** All patients who are severely hyponatremic should reduce free water intake to approximately 800 mL/day.
   b. **Inhibition of water reabsorption**
      (1) **Demeclocycline.** This agent has been shown to alter ADH-induced water flow in the collecting tubule. This drug must be given in doses of 600–1200 mg/day and requires 4–5 days to achieve its peak action. Demeclocycline cannot be administered to patients with liver disease, heart failure, or kidney disease because it may accumulate to toxic levels in these conditions.
      (2) **Furosemide.** Acute administration of this agent in combination with large amounts of saline may lead to increased water excretion.
      (3) **Tolvaptan.** This agent is an oral vasopressin with relative affinity for the V2 receptor, which has been shown to induce a diuresis with proportionally more free-water than sodium loss.
   c. **Hypertonic infusions.** The infusion of 3% sodium chloride rapidly raises the tonicity of the extracellular fluid. This is rarely done due to the risk of deleterious effects, including pulmonary or cerebral edema, pontine demyelination, and severe neurologic damage. When used, serum sodium concentration should not increase faster than 0.5 mEq/L/hour.

6. **Complications**
   a. **Acute hyponatremia.** Acute reduction of serum osmolality can produce intracranial hypertension and brain damage, particularly if the serum sodium concentration falls below 125 mEq/L over a period of hours.

b. Chronic hyponatremia. Brain cells adapt to chronic hyponatremia by loss of net intracellular solute (primarily potassium chloride and organic molecules, termed osmolytes). This adaptation, which can occur over a period of a few days, leads to marked reduction in the degree of cell swelling.

C Hypernatremia

1. **Definition.** Hypernatremia refers to serum sodium concentration that is above normal. Clinically significant effects are produced at serum sodium levels greater than 155 mEq/L. Hypernatremia always implies hypertonicity of all body fluids because the rise in the extracellular fluid osmolality obligates movement of water from the intracellular space, producing increased intracellular osmotic activity and cell dehydration.

2. **Etiology**
   a. **Extrarenal causes**
      (1) **Decreased fluid intake.** Adequate water intake is required to maintain the tonicity of body fluids in the face of continuous water losses through the skin as well as losses through the urine and gastrointestinal tract. In cool environments, this intake equals approximately 700 mL/day. If intake is less than external losses, body fluid osmolality rises.
      (2) **Increased skin losses.** Profuse sweating may lead to excess water losses through the skin. In addition, burns and other widespread inflammatory lesions of the skin may cause marked fluid losses.
      (3) **Increased gastrointestinal losses.** Diarrhea and protracted vomiting also may result in water deficits.
   b. **Renal causes**
      (1) **Osmotic diuresis.** The presence of osmotically active, nonreabsorbable solute in the glomerular filtrate prevents water and sodium reabsorption and leads to increased renal water losses. Hyperglycemia with glycosuria is a common cause of osmotic diuresis. Because water losses are relatively greater than sodium losses, the serum sodium concentration rises progressively during osmotic diuresis.
      (2) **Decreased ADH effect**
         (a) **Central diabetes insipidus** (i.e., failure of ADH synthesis or release) may occur in the following settings:
            (i) **Tumor.** ADH deficiency may occur either through direct invasion of the neurohypophysis or through increased intracranial pressure compressing the brainstem.
            (ii) **Histiocytosis.** Hand-Schüller-Christian disease, in particular, has a predilection for neurohypophyseal involvement, producing ADH deficiency.
            (iii) **Sarcoidosis.** The neurohypophysis may be involved, producing diabetes insipidus.
            (iv) **Trauma.** Classically, after resection of the pituitary stalk, a phase of acute ADH release is followed by a prolonged period of central diabetes insipidus.
         (b) **Nephrogenic diabetes insipidus** (i.e., failure of renal water conservation despite high levels of plasma ADH) may occur in the following settings.
            (i) **Renal disease.** Structural disease impairs the integrity of the renal medulla and, thereby, the urine-concentrating ability.
            (ii) **Hypercalcemia.** Elevation of serum calcium concentration greater than 12 mg/dL may impair urine-concentrating ability, most likely as a result of inhibition of sodium chloride reabsorption in the thick ascending limb of Henle's loop, increased medullary blood flow, dissipation of medullary hypertonicity, and interference with ADH-mediated water flow in the medullary collecting tubule.
            (iii) **Hypokalemia.** Reduction of serum potassium concentration to less than 3.5 mEq/L leads to a direct stimulation of thirst and a mild impairment of urine-concentrating ability.
            (iv) **Lithium ingestion.** This action blocks ADH-stimulated osmotic water flow in the collecting tubule.
            (v) **Demeclocycline.** This tetracycline antibiotic alters ADH-induced water flow through a direct effect on the cell membrane.

(vi) **Sickle cell anemia.** Reduced medullary blood flow produced by sickling erythrocytes within the vasa recta also may impair urine-concentrating ability.

(vii) **Urinary tract obstruction** and the **postobstructive state.** These conditions are associated with nephrogenic diabetes insipidus.

3. **Clinical features**

a. **CNS disorders.** Generalized CNS depression, including obtundation, coma, and seizures, develops in young children and elderly patients. Intracerebral and subarachnoid hemorrhage may occur if shrinkage of brain volume leads to tears in the bridging veins.

b. **Extracellular volume depletion.** Excessive water loss in hypernatremic states may lead to this condition. Although the intracellular fluid accounts for two thirds of water deficits, the extracellular fluid volume also contracts mildly. If loss of water as well as solute occurs, the contraction is more pronounced. However, if the etiology of the hypernatremia is due to excess salt intake (e.g., hypertonic sodium bicarbonate infusion or seawater drowning), the extracellular fluid volume increases.

c. **Abnormal urine output.** If the kidneys cause water losses, polyuria (i.e., urine output that is inappropriately high, given the level of plasma osmolality or extracellular fluid volume) may be present. If the kidneys are normal and water losses are extrarenal, urine volume typically is reduced.

4. **Diagnosis**

a. **Dehydration test.** Urine-concentrating ability may be tested after overnight dehydration to determine whether a patient has renal water wasting.

(1) Water deprivation begins at 8:00 p.m. and lasts 14 hours, after which the urine osmolality should exceed 800 mOsm/kg. The patient then is given a subcutaneous dose of ADH (5 units of aqueous vasopressin). The urine osmolality should not be further increased by this maneuver.

(2) If the urine osmolality is less than 800 mOsm/kg after water deprivation or if it increases by greater than 15% after ADH administration, some degree of ADH deficiency is present.

(3) If the urine osmolality does not exceed 300 mOsm/kg after water deprivation and there is no further increase after ADH administration, some form of nephrogenic diabetes insipidus is present.

b. **Plasma ADH assay.** In nephrogenic diabetes insipidus, the urine osmolality may not be a true reflection of ADH release, and, thus, plasma ADH levels should be measured.

c. **Assay of urine osmolality and composition**

(1) It is useful to measure the solute composition of the urine in the evaluation of polyuria. Urine osmolality less than 200 mOsm/L suggests a primary defect in water conservation. Urine osmolality greater than 200 mOsm/L during polyuria suggests an osmotic diuresis.

(2) After measuring urine osmolality, the urine should be analyzed for sodium, glucose, and urea to determine the etiology of the diuresis. A urine pH greater than 6 may indicate bicarbonate diuresis.

d. **Physical examination.** Although examination may be helpful in determining if hypovolemia or hypervolemia is present, it is generally not useful in determining the etiology and pathogenesis of polyuria.

5. **Therapy**

a. **Free water** may be administered orally, which is the preferred route, or intravenously as a 5% dextrose solution (D_5W). The dextrose is readily metabolized, leaving behind free water. Infusion of a fluid with an osmolality less than 150 mOsm/L is dangerous and may lead to acute hemolysis at the infusion site.

b. **Vasopressin** may be administered in several different forms. Currently, the agent of choice for treatment of ADH deficiency is **1-deamino-8-D-arginine vasopressin (DDAVP** or **desmopressin),** which may be administered orally or as a nasal spray every 12 hours.

c. **Thiazide diuretics** impair dilution in the distal nephron and stimulate proximal tubular reabsorption of sodium and water as a result of volume depletion. The latter action reduces the delivery of fluid to the distal nephron, thereby reducing the degree of polyuria. Thiazides are useful as adjunct therapy in patients with nephrogenic diabetes insipidus.

    d. Other drugs such as clofibrate, carbamazepine, and chlorpropamide, enhance the renal tubular effects of ADH and possibly contribute to the stimulation of ADH release in certain settings.

  6. Complications. Diseases of water conservation are dangerous only if patients are not allowed access to water. In such settings, cellular dehydration, CNS depression, and severe volume depletion may occur. The serious manifestations of acute hypernatremia are primarily due to brain cell shrinkage. Brain cells adapt to chronic hypernatremia by net gain of intracellular solute (mainly sodium chloride and organic osmolytes such as *myo*-inositol, taurine, betaine, and other methylamines). This adaptation, occurring over several days, leads to marked reduction in the degree of cell shrinkage.

II   SODIUM METABOLISM

A **Normal physiology** Sodium is the primary osmotic component of the extracellular fluid and determines the volume of that space and the effective volume of the systemic circulation. A less than 1% change in renal sodium excretion can produce major changes in extracellular fluid volume.

  1. Renal handling. Sodium is freely filtered at the glomerulus, and the majority must be reabsorbed to maintain sodium homeostasis. Although only 10%–15% of the glomerular filtrate is reabsorbed in the distal tubule and collecting duct, this site is the major regulator for determining final urine sodium composition.

  2. Hormonal regulation. Many hormones may alter tubular handling of sodium, but none is as well studied as aldosterone, which is regulated by the **renin–angiotensin system.**

    a. Renin secretion by the kidney is stimulated by renal hypoperfusion, adrenergic stimulation, and circulating catecholamines. Renin is released from the **juxtaglomerular apparatus,** which is located between the afferent and the efferent arterioles of the glomeruli.

    b. Renin is an enzyme that catalyzes the conversion of **angiotensinogen** to the decapeptide **angiotensin I** (in plasma). Angiotensin I is converted to the octapeptide **angiotensin II** (in the lung and kidney) by ACE. Angiotensin II is a potent vasoconstrictive agent as well as a potent stimulus for increased aldosterone release from the adrenal gland.

    c. Aldosterone stimulates sodium reabsorption in the cortical collecting duct.

    d. Other hormones that regulate sodium handling are listed in 🌐 Online Table 7–15.

B **Edema**

  1. Definition

    a. Edema generally is defined as an increase in the interstitial compartment of the extracellular fluid.

      (1) Normally, the extracellular fluid volume equals approximately 14 L and accounts for one third of the total body water. About 25% of the extracellular fluid is represented by plasma volume and is contained within the circulation. The other 75%, or 11 L, is represented by the interstitial fluid between cells.

      (2) If the interstitial fluid volume increases by approximately 2 L, clinically evident edema may result; edema may be **observable** (as **swelling**) or **palpable** (as **pitting**).

    b. Although edema generally is a function of increased extracellular fluid volume, in some instances increased transcapillary hydrostatic pressure (e.g., as occurs in the portal circulation in cirrhosis) also may contribute to edema.

  2. Pathophysiology. Edema, or the pathologic increase in extracellular fluid volume, primarily is a function of excessive renal tubular reabsorption of sodium. Decreased renal perfusion (e.g., as occurs in CHF with reduced cardiac output, in cirrhosis with reduced effective arterial blood volume, and in the nephrotic syndrome) is the proximate cause of the increased renal sodium reabsorption, which represents the body's attempt to maintain adequate effective arterial blood volume.

  3. Etiology

    a. CHF. When cardiac output is reduced, effective arterial blood volume is decreased as well. The decrease in effective arterial blood volume triggers the release of renin and aldosterone, leading to stimulation of distal tubular reabsorption of sodium. In addition, alterations in renal hemodynamics stimulate an increase in the proximal tubular reabsorption of sodium.

    b. Cirrhosis. The primary cause of sodium retention in liver disease may be ascites formation as a result of high pressure in the portal circulation. Portal hypertension leads to intravascular fluid volume depletion and secondary renal sodium retention. When hypoalbuminemia occurs, effective arterial blood volume drops, stimulating renal sodium retention. Secondary hyperaldosteronism is common and is caused by intravascular volume contraction as well as impaired hepatic clearance of aldosterone; these factors lead to stimulation of distal tubular reabsorption of sodium. A primary increase in renal sodium reabsorption may occur in cirrhosis.

    c. Nephrotic syndrome. Hypoalbuminemia leads to reduced effective arterial blood volume as a result of renal protein losses, which stimulates renal tubular reabsorption of sodium.

    d. Chronic renal failure. When the GFR falls to less than 10 mL/minute, the capacity of the kidney to excrete the typical dietary sodium load is limited, and edema may result.

    e. Excessive mineralocorticoid activity. Tumors of the adrenal gland and pituitary tumors that secrete large amounts of adrenocorticotropic hormone (ACTH) may be associated with marked sodium retention.

4. Clinical features

    a. Peripheral edema. Sodium retention may manifest as swelling in the dependent regions of the body.

    b. Pulmonary edema. If pulmonary venous pressure acutely rises above 18 mm Hg, pulmonary edema may develop.

5. Diagnosis

    a. On **physical examination,** peripheral edema may be identified by the persistence of an indentation following palpation of the soft tissues in the dependent areas. Pulmonary edema is identified by the physical findings of rales or wheezes or by chest radiography.

    b. Urine sodium assay reveals a urine sodium level that is less than sodium intake and usually less than 20 mEq/L.

6. Therapy

    a. Dietary sodium restriction is essential. A sodium intake of 2 g/day is the lowest practical intake level that can be achieved.

    b. Diuretics are useful for increasing sodium excretion.

        (1) Loop diuretics such as furosemide, torsemide, and bumetanide are particularly effective. Side effects of these drugs include intravascular volume depletion with azotemia, hyperuricemia, hypokalemia, metabolic alkalosis, and hypomagnesemia.

        (2) Thiazide diuretics such as hydrochlorothiazide inhibit sodium reabsorption in the distal convoluted tubule. They can be used effectively, although they are less potent than loop diuretics. Side effects are similar to those of loop diuretics.

        (3) Potassium-sparing diuretics such as amiloride and triamterene act primarily to block sodium reabsorption and secondarily to block potassium secretion in the distal tubule. Use of these agents may lead to potassium retention and increased sodium excretion.

        (4) Aldosterone antagonists such as the competitive agent spironolactone or eplerenone also lead to potassium retention and increased sodium excretion.

III   POTASSIUM METABOLISM

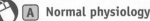

A Normal physiology

B Hypokalemia

    1. Definition. Hypokalemia is defined as serum potassium concentration of less than 3.5 mEq/L. Because most of the potassium content of the body is within cells and cellular potassium concentration is about 155 mEq/L, cellular potassium can be severely depleted without causing large changes in serum potassium.

    2. Etiology. Hypokalemia can result from extrarenal or renal causes.

        a. Extrarenal causes

(1) Dietary deficiency and gastrointestinal losses

    (a) Inadequate dietary intake. Because potassium conservation in the kidney is limited, a severe reduction of intake to less than 10 mEq/day for many days or weeks can lead to a large negative potassium balance and hypokalemia.

    (b) Diarrhea. Because the potassium content of diarrheal fluid may be as high as 100 mEq/L, diarrhea can lead to severe potassium depletion.

    (c) Vomiting. Although the potassium content of vomitus is relatively small, the secondary effect of intravascular volume depletion, which produces secondary hyperaldosteronism, stimulates renal potassium excretion.

(2) Potassium redistribution

    (a) Insulin administration. A therapeutic or replacement dose of insulin can drive potassium into cells, producing acute hypokalemia.

    (b) Epinephrine infusions. Epinephrine also can produce acute hypokalemia by an independent action involving β_2-receptors.

    (c) Folic acid and vitamin B_{12} therapy. In patients with megaloblastic anemia, folic acid and vitamin B_{12} stimulate cell proliferation, thus producing acute hypokalemia, because potassium is used in cell synthesis. This effect also may be seen in patients with rapidly growing tumors.

    (d) Alkalemia. In the presence of excess base, hydrogen ions shift out of cells in exchange for potassium.

    (e) Hypokalemic periodic paralysis.

b. Renal causes. Any hyperactivity of the normal components of renal potassium excretion can produce a negative potassium balance via increased renal losses.

(1) Drug-induced renal losses

    (a) Diuretics. Agents that act proximal to the site of potassium secretion stimulate urinary excretion of potassium by increasing the delivery of sodium and fluid to the distal tubules.

    (b) Penicillins. Carbenicillin, ticarcillin, and related drugs act as nonreabsorbable anions in the distal tubule and thereby stimulate potassium secretion. Significant hypokalemia is commonly seen.

    (c) Aminoglycosides. Tubular defects with magnesium wasting and secondary potassium wasting occasionally may be seen in patients treated with large doses of gentamicin or related compounds.

    (d) Amphotericin B. This antifungal agent causes damage to the apical membrane of the renal tubular cell, thus increasing potassium loss from the cell.

(2) Hormone-induced renal losses

    (a) Primary hyperaldosteronism

        (i) Primary adrenal adenomas are associated with hypokalemia, hypertension, and metabolic alkalosis.

        (ii) Diffuse bilateral adrenal hyperplasia may be associated with a milder hypokalemia than is seen with primary adrenal adenoma.

        (iii) In **ectopic ACTH syndrome,** massive mineralocorticoid increase and renal potassium wasting may occur in patients with small cell lung carcinoma (a tumor that produces and secretes ACTH).

        (iv) Exogenous mineralocorticoid. Licorice produced in Europe (anise) contains **glycyrrhetinic acid,** which prevents conversion of cortisol to cortisone in the renal distal tubule, thereby stimulating mineralocorticoid receptors and producing an aldosterone-like action. Ingestion of this agent may lead to hypokalemia with hypertension and metabolic alkalosis. Certain **tobacco** compounds also contain glycyrrhetinic acid and may cause hypokalemia.

    (b) Secondary hyperaldosteronism

        (i) Renin-secreting tumor. This rare entity, diagnosed by arteriography, is characterized by intrarenal tumors of the juxtaglomerular apparatus. Severe hypertension and hypokalemia may occur.

        (ii) Renal artery stenosis may be associated with hypokalemia and hypertension as a result of secondary hyperaldosteronism produced by hyperreninemia.

      (iii) In **malignant hypertension,** severe underperfusion of the kidney may occur and may lead to hyperreninemia, secondary hyperaldosteronism, and hypokalemia.

      (iv) Disorders with reduced effective arterial blood volume produce only mild hypokalemia despite hyperreninemia and hyperaldosteronism. Reduced tubular flow rate reduces potassium secretion. In **CHF,** secondary hyperaldosteronism may develop, causing mild hypokalemia even in the absence of diuretic use. In **cirrhosis,** severe hypokalemia is common because of low intake of potassium and secondary hyperaldosteronism.

   (3) Potassium loss due to primary renal tubular disorders

     (a) Renal tubular acidosis is often associated with potassium wasting, which may be secondary to sodium depletion and metabolic acidosis or directly attributable to tubular defects in potassium conservation. Potassium wasting is a feature of distal (type I) as well as proximal (type II) renal tubular acidosis of any etiology.

     (b) Bartter's syndrome and **Gitelman's syndrome** are characterized by renal potassium wasting, metabolic alkalosis, and polyuria. Blood pressure usually is normal or reduced, but renin and aldosterone levels are very high. In **Bartter's syndrome,** the primary defect lies in one of the epithelial transport proteins involved in the reabsorption of sodium chloride, most commonly the furosemide-sensitive Na^+–K^+–$2Cl^-$ cotransporter in the ascending limb of Henle's loop. In **Gitelman's syndrome,** the primary defect involves the thiazide-sensitive Na^+–Cl^- cotransporter in the distal convoluted tubule.

     (c) Chronic magnesium depletion produces a syndrome of renal tubular potassium wasting without other associated defects in ion transport. The potassium wasting can be severe and is unresponsive to potassium repletion until magnesium deficits have been corrected.

   (4) Potassium loss due to surreptitious diuretic use is associated with a clinical presentation identical to that of Bartter's or Gitelman's syndrome, including hypokalemia, magnesium wasting, metabolic alkalosis, hyperreninemia, and hyperaldosteronism.

3. Clinical features

  a. Neuromuscular disorders. Potassium depletion may cause weakness and paralysis.

  b. Cardiac disorders. Arrhythmia, particularly in the presence of digitalis intoxication, is a hallmark of severe hypokalemia.

  c. Endocrine disorders. Hypokalemia is associated with abnormalities in pancreatic insulin release. Glucose intolerance has been shown to worsen as a result of diuretic-induced hypokalemia.

  d. Polyuria. The polyuria of hypokalemia is a function of polydipsia as well as impaired ADH action.

4. Diagnosis

  a. Physical examination. The presence or absence of hypertension is a useful differentiating feature in the approach to the patient with hypokalemia.

   (1) If the patient is hypertensive, the hypokalemia may be caused by excessive mineralocorticoid activity. Because many hypertensive patients are treated with diuretics, any hypokalemia could be a side effect of such therapy.

   (2) If the patient is normotensive, the hypokalemia represents either a gastrointestinal or a primary renal loss of potassium.

  b. Serum electrolyte assay. This test rarely is useful for evaluating the specific cause of hypokalemia. However, the finding of combined acidosis and hypokalemia, which suggests renal tubular acidosis, is an exception.

  c. Urine potassium assay. Urine potassium levels below 20 mEq/L suggest extrarenal potassium losses, whereas levels exceeding 30 mEq/L suggest renal losses.

  d. Renin–aldosterone axis assay

   (1) Noninvasive tests. Several noninvasive texts can be used to determine whether excessive mineralocorticoid activity is due to excessive renin production or to a primary adrenal disorder (Table 7–16).

   (2) Invasive tests include measurement of bilateral renal venous renin as well as adrenal venous aldosterone and cortisol concentrations. However, these tests are rarely performed, as the diagnosis can usually be made by noninvasive means.

TABLE 7–16 Renin–Aldosterone Axis Assay

Test	Method	Significance
Renin stimulation test	40 mg of furosemide is administered; then plasma renin is measured in both supine and upright positions	Absence of stimulation of renin levels in upright position indicates renin suppression
Aldosterone suppression test	1–2 L of saline are infused; then plasma aldosterone is measured in both supine and upright positions	Lack of aldosterone suppression to below normal may indicate primary aldosterone overproduction
Plasma aldosterone-to-renin ratio	Serum renin and aldosterone levels are measured	Value greater than 15 is highly suggestive of primary hyperaldosteronism
Bilateral renal venous renin; adrenal venous aldosterone and cortisol concentrations	See first column	Hypertension of aldosteronoma is responsive to tumor removal (hypertension associated with bilateral disease is not)

   e. Urine chloride assay. In cases of mineralocorticoid excess, Bartter's or Gitelman's syndrome, and diuretic abuse, urine chloride levels tend to be elevated in the presence of metabolic alkalosis and hypokalemia. The absence of elevated urine chloride levels is highly suggestive of gastrointestinal potassium losses such as surreptitious vomiting.

   f. Diuretic assay. If Bartter's or Gitelman's syndrome is suspected, the urine must be analyzed for chloride and diuretics, including loop-active agents and thiazides, before a diagnosis of a primary tubular disorder can be established. Such diuretic assays are commercially available.

5. **Therapy.** In many cases, hypokalemia can be corrected by administration of potassium salts.

   a. Forms of potassium salts. Potassium may be administered with a variety of anions. Potassium chloride is the preferred form of therapy because many patients have concurrent chloride deficits. In cases of hypokalemia with coincident renal tubular acidosis, potassium citrate, potassium lactate, or potassium gluconate may be given.

   b. Routes of administration. Potassium may be given intravenously or orally.

   (1) Intravenous potassium solutions should not exceed a concentration of 60 mEq/L, and the rate of administration should not exceed 60 mEq/hour. Normally, potassium deficits are on the order of 300–1000 mEq. These deficits should be replaced slowly, over days, except when digitalis intoxication or life-threatening arrhythmias are present.

   (2) Oral potassium is absorbed effectively and should be substituted for intravenous potassium whenever possible.

   c. Chronic potassium therapy. Hypokalemic patients receiving diuretics should be given potassium supplementation to maintain the serum potassium level greater than 3.5 mEq/L. This level may be accomplished with oral potassium supplementation. Although some foods are high in potassium, it is difficult to overcome these deficits solely by ingesting potassium-rich food.

C **Hyperkalemia**

1. **Definition.** Hyperkalemia is defined as serum potassium concentration greater than 5.5 mEq/L.

2. **Etiology. Pseudohyperkalemia** may be caused by release of potassium from coagulated cells and platelets after blood is withdrawn for analysis. It can also occur if the platelet or white blood cell (WBC) count is extremely high, as in myeloproliferative disorders. Measurement of plasma potassium is required to eliminate this artifact. **True hyperkalemia** may result from extrarenal or renal causes.

   a. Extrarenal causes

   (1) **Insulin deficiency.** Hyperkalemia in diabetic patients may be due to a lack of insulin and to the presence of associated renal and adrenal abnormalities.

   (2) **Cell lysis syndromes.** Acute cell necrosis following either chemotherapy or a massive crushing injury (**rhabdomyolysis**) produces hyperkalemia by rapid cellular release of potassium.

   (3) **Succinylcholine therapy.** The muscle relaxant succinylcholine may produce hyperkalemia in susceptible individuals with generalized muscle or neurologic disease.

   (4) **Hyperkalemic periodic paralysis.**

(5) **Hyperosmolality.** Acute increases in extracellular fluid osmotic activity may produce a transcellular shift of potassium and result in hyperkalemia. This may occur with administration of intravenous contrast or glucose.

(6) **Acidosis.** Mineral acidosis, not organic acidosis, may be associated with an acute shift of potassium from the intracellular to the extracellular fluid as hydrogen ions enter cells.

b. **Renal causes.** The renal capacity to excrete potassium is approximately 500–1000 mEq/day, which is 10–20 times the normal intake. An impairment of the normal components of renal potassium excretion may reduce this excretory capacity so that normal intake may produce hyperkalemia.

(1) **Severe renal failure.** When the GFR falls to less than 10 mL/minute, hyperkalemia may occur, even with normal intake. At a GFR greater than this level, hyperkalemia is not a result of glomerular insufficiency per se but is the result of a specific disorder in tubular potassium transport or an extrarenal potassium disturbance.

(2) **Aldosterone insufficiency.** Aldosterone is the major hormonal determinant of renal potassium secretion.

(a) **Acquired aldosterone deficiency.** This condition may result from renal disease associated with reduced renin production. (Recall that renin is an enzyme that cleaves precursor molecules to produce the aldosterone secretagogue angiotensin II.) Primary adrenal disease also may be associated with reduced aldosterone production. Aldosterone deficiency due to impaired renin production or adrenal disease may be produced by the following:

(i) Interstitial renal disease

(ii) Lead nephropathy

(iii) Diabetic nephropathy (insulin deficiency in this condition may potentiate hyperkalemia)

(iv) Obstructive uropathy

(v) Angiotensin antagonist therapy

(vi) Addison's disease

(b) **Inherited aldosterone deficiency.** Several adrenal enzyme defects associated with deficiency of the 17- or 21-hydroxylase enzymes may be associated with aldosterone deficiency.

(c) **Drug-induced aldosterone deficiency.** NSAIDs and heparin act to reduce renin secretion or induce resistance and may produce hyperkalemia through aldosterone deficiency.

(3) **Aldosterone resistance.** The following conditions are characterized by tubular defects associated with elevated aldosterone levels but impaired potassium secretion.

(a) Sickle cell nephropathy

(b) SLE

(c) Amyloidosis

(d) Interstitial renal disease

(e) Obstructive uropathy

(f) Hereditary aldosterone resistance

(g) Use of triamterene, amiloride, or spironolactone

3. **Clinical features**

a. **Neuromuscular disorders.** By altering transmembrane electrical potential, severe hyperkalemia may alter muscle function or neuromuscular transmission, leading to severe weakness or paralysis.

b. **Cardiac disorders.** Cardiac arrhythmias may occur at any level greater than normal but generally are noted only when serum potassium concentration exceeds 6 mEq/L. As serum potassium level rises, a series of electrocardiographic (ECG) changes may be seen, including the following:

(1) Prolongation of the P-R interval

(2) T-wave peaking

(3) Prolongation of the QRS interval

(4) Ventricular tachycardias, ventricular fibrillation, and asystole

4. **Diagnosis**
   a. **Elimination of pseudohyperkalemia.** In vitro lysis of erythrocytes, leukocytes, or platelets can produce hyperkalemia as a result of intracellular potassium release (pseudohyperkalemia). All hyperkalemic patients should be checked for pseudohyperkalemia by measuring both plasma and serum potassium concentrations and by inspecting the serum for discoloration suggesting hemolysis. The presence of a myeloproliferative disorder may also produce pseudo-hyperkalemia.
   b. **Urine potassium assay.** Although only a rough correlation exists between urine and serum potassium levels, hyperkalemia induced by increased intake or increased cell lysis should be associated with urine potassium levels exceeding 50 mEq/L. Values less than 30 mEq/L in the setting of hyperkalemia suggest impaired renal secretion of potassium.
   c. **Renin–aldosterone axis assay.** In certain patients, evaluation of aldosterone and renin levels may help define the etiology of hyperkalemia.

5. **Therapy.** Treatment is divided into acute and chronic phases.
   a. **Acute antagonism and redistribution**
      (1) **Calcium.** The intravenous administration of one to two ampules of calcium chloride acutely antagonizes the cardiac effects of hyperkalemia. ECG changes may transiently improve, but serum potassium level remains elevated.
      (2) **Glucose and insulin.** The intravenous infusion of 25 g (one ampule) of dextrose plus 15 units of insulin lowers serum potassium within 10–15 minutes.
      (3) **β_2-Adrenergic agonists,** given by inhalation or intravenously, rapidly induce potassium uptake into cells, but they are not uniformly effective.
   b. **Acute removal**
      (1) **Diuretics.** Furosemide, bumetanide, and, especially, acetazolamide increase potassium excretion in individuals with adequate renal function.
      (2) **Cation-exchange resins.** The administration of sodium polystyrene sulfonate binds potassium in the gastrointestinal tract. About 2 mEq of sodium are exchanged for every 1 mEq of potassium removed, so that a substantial sodium load may result. Sorbitol is administered orally to prevent severe constipation. Cation-exchange resins can remove 50–100 mEq of potassium over a 6-hour period and may be given orally or rectally.
   c. **Chronic removal.** After the acute removal of potassium, potassium homeostasis may be maintained with any of the following agents.
      (1) **Diuretics.** Furosemide or acetazolamide may be used in combination with fludrocortisone acetate to increase potassium excretion.
      (2) **Cation-exchange resins** may be given on a chronic basis to increase gastrointestinal excretion of metabolism.

IV ACID–BASE METABOLISM

A Normal physiology

B Respiratory acidosis

1. **Definition.** Increased partial pressure of carbon dioxide in the arterial blood ($PaCO_2$) (i.e., >40 mm Hg) and **decreased blood pH** (i.e., acidemia) are characteristic.

2. **Etiology.** Respiratory acidosis is associated with a reduced capacity to excrete **carbon dioxide** via the lungs. Causes include all disorders that reduce pulmonary function and carbon dioxide clearance.
   a. **Primary pulmonary disease** that is associated with alveolar–arterial mismatch may lead to carbon dioxide retention, usually as a late manifestation.
   b. **Neuromuscular disease.** Any weakness of the pulmonary musculature that leads to reduced ventilation (e.g., myasthenia gravis) may produce carbon dioxide retention.
   c. **Primary CNS dysfunction.** Any severe injury to the brainstem may be associated with reduced ventilatory drive and carbon dioxide retention.
   d. **Drug-induced hypoventilation.** Any agent that causes severe depression of CNS or neuromuscular function may be associated with respiratory acidosis.

3. **Clinical features**
   a. **CNS disorders.** Because blood flow to the brain is regulated by blood $PaCO_2$, respiratory acidosis is associated with increased blood flow to the brain and increased cerebrospinal fluid (CSF) pressure. These effects may lead to a variety of symptoms of generalized CNS depression.
   b. **Cardiac disorders.** The acidemia in respiratory acidosis is associated with reduced cardiac output and pulmonary hypertension (effects that may lead to critically reduced blood flow to vital organs).

4. **Diagnosis**
   a. **Acute respiratory acidosis.** Acute carbon dioxide retention leads to an increase in blood $PaCO_2$ with minimal change in plasma bicarbonate content. For each 10 mm Hg rise in $PaCO_2$, the plasma bicarbonate level increases by approximately 1 mEq/L and the blood pH decreases by approximately 0.08. Serum electrolyte levels are close to normal in individuals with acute respiratory acidosis.
   b. **Chronic respiratory acidosis.** After 2–5 days, renal compensation (i.e., increased hydrogen ion secretion and bicarbonate production in the distal nephron) occurs; that is, the plasma bicarbonate level steadily increases. Arterial blood gas analysis shows that in the chronic phase of respiratory acidosis, for each 10 mm Hg rise in $PaCO_2$, the plasma bicarbonate level increases by 3–4 mEq/L and the blood pH decreases by 0.03.

5. **Therapy**
   a. **Correction of the underlying disorder.** Attempts should be made to correct muscular dysfunction or reversible pulmonary disease if either is the cause of the respiratory acidosis. In the case of drug-induced hypoventilation, vigorous attempts should be made to clear the offending agent from the body.
   b. **Respiratory therapy.** A blood $PaCO_2$ of greater than 60 mm Hg may be an indication for assisted ventilation.

C **Respiratory alkalosis**

1. **Definition.** Decreased blood $PaCO_2$ and an **increased blood pH** (alkalemia) are characteristic.

2. **Etiology.** Respiratory alkalosis is associated with excessive elimination of carbon dioxide via the lungs. Causes include any disorder associated with inappropriately increased ventilatory rate and carbon dioxide clearance.
   a. **Anxiety (hysterical hyperventilation).** This condition is the most common cause of respiratory alkalosis.
   b. **Salicylate toxicity.** Initially, salicylate excess causes overstimulation of the respiratory center, resulting in respiratory alkalosis. Metabolic acidosis may develop from the salicylate load, which enhances the hyperventilation.
   c. **Hypoxia.** Any disorder associated with decreased oxygen tension (PaO_2) of blood may lead to an increased respiratory rate and, thus, respiratory alkalosis.
   d. **Intrathoracic disorders.** Any inflammatory or space-occupying lesion in the lung may be associated with primary stimulation of ventilatory rate, leading to a low $PaCO_2$. Such conditions include the following:
      (1) Pulmonary embolism
      (2) Pneumonia
      (3) Asthma
      (4) Pulmonary fibrosis
   e. **Primary CNS dysfunction.** CNS disorders that may be associated with inappropriate stimulation of ventilation include the following:
      (1) Cerebrovascular accident (CVA)
      (2) Tumor
      (3) Infection
      (4) Trauma
   f. **Gram-negative septicemia.** An early manifestation of gram-negative septicemia or bacteremia is a primary stimulation of ventilation with respiratory alkalosis. The mechanism is unknown.
   g. **Liver failure.** The most common acid–base disorder in liver disease is primary respiratory alkalosis through a direct CNS effect of hyperammonemia.

h. Pregnancy. Primary stimulation of ventilation is typically seen throughout pregnancy.

3. **Clinical features.** Acute alkalemia may be associated with several organ system disorders.

   a. CNS disorders. A generalized feeling of anxiety may be present and may progress to more severe obtundation and even precoma.

   b. Neuromuscular disorders. Acute alkalemia may produce a tetany-like syndrome, which may be indistinguishable from that of acute hypocalcemia.

4. **Diagnosis**

   a. Acute respiratory alkalosis. Increased respiratory rate leads to a loss of carbon dioxide via the lungs, which in turn increases the blood pH. For each 10 mm Hg decrease in blood $PaCO_2$ acutely, the plasma bicarbonate level decreases by 2 mEq/L and the blood pH increases by 0.08.

   b. Chronic respiratory alkalosis. Within hours after an acute decrease in arterial $PaCO_2$, hydrogen ion secretion in the distal nephron decreases, leading to a decrease in plasma bicarbonate. For each 10 mm Hg decrease in blood $PaCO_2$ chronically, the plasma bicarbonate level decreases by 5–6 mEq/L and the blood pH increases by only about 0.02. Serum chloride level also is elevated.

5. **Therapy.** The primary goal of therapy is to correct the underlying disorder. Use of carbon dioxide–enriched breathing mixtures or controlled ventilation may be required in cases of severe respiratory alkalosis (pH >7.6).

D Metabolic acidosis

1. **Definition.** Metabolic acidosis is characterized by a decreased blood pH and a decreased plasma bicarbonate concentration. This condition may be caused by one of two basic mechanisms: the loss of bicarbonate or the accumulation of an acid other than carbonic acid (e.g., lactic acid).

2. **Etiology.** The causes of metabolic acidosis may be divided into those associated with a normal anion gap and those associated with an increased anion gap. **The anion gap reflects the concentrations of those anions that actually are present in serum but are not routinely assayed,** including negatively charged plasma proteins (mainly albumin), phosphates, sulfate, and organic acids (e.g., lactic acid). The anion gap, measured in mEq/L, represents the difference between the concentration of unmeasured anions and cations. It can be calculated as follows (the square brackets denote concentrations):

$$\text{Anion gap} = [Na^+] - ([Cl^-] + [HCO_3^-])$$

The normal value of the anion gap is 8 ± 4 mEq/L. An increase represents an increase in one moiety, usually the organic acids. No change with decreases in both plasma bicarbonate concentration and serum pH suggests a primary loss of bicarbonate or the addition of mineral acid.

   a. Metabolic acidosis with an increased anion gap

   (1) **Ketoacidosis.** This condition refers to a state of increased ketoacid formation, which leads to titration of bicarbonate and consequent metabolic acidosis. Ketoacidosis occurs as a complication of diabetes mellitus, prolonged starvation, and prolonged alcohol abuse.

   (2) **Lactic acidosis.** Decreased oxygen delivery to tissues results in increased lactate production, with accompanying severe metabolic acidosis. Lactic acidosis is a characteristic feature of many conditions associated with low tissue perfusion (e.g., shock and sepsis).

   (3) **Renal failure.** Metabolic acidosis results from the inability of the kidney to excrete the daily hydrogen ion load, derived from food and metabolism, as a result of a decline in ammonium excretion resulting from decreased renal mass. The acidosis of renal failure is characterized by either a normal or an elevated anion gap, depending on the severity of the decline in renal filtering function. In either case, the serum bicarbonate is reduced due to the titration by the retained hydrogen ions.

   (a) The anion gap is elevated only when the GFR is severely reduced (<25 mm^3/min) because the anions (sulfates and phosphates) that accompany the retained hydrogen ions cannot be filtered.

   (b) In mild-to-moderate renal failure (GFR = 25–60 mm^3/min), these anions are freely excreted and do not accumulate, resulting in metabolic acidosis with normal anion gap.

(4) Intoxication. The ingestion of a variety of chemical agents may result in the accumulation of organic acids (e.g., lactic acid). Such intoxicants include the following:

  (a) Salicylate

  (b) Methanol

  (c) Ethylene glycol

b. Metabolic acidosis with a normal anion gap (hyperchloremic metabolic acidosis) is the result of either renal or gastrointestinal losses.

  (1) Renal loss of bicarbonate may result from the following conditions.

   (a) Proximal tubular acidosis. Characteristics include decreased proximal tubular reabsorption of bicarbonate leading to excessive urinary excretion of bicarbonate. Causes include multiple myeloma, heavy metal poisoning, and Wilson's disease.

   (b) Distal tubular acidosis. Characteristics include a decreased distal tubular capacity for hydrogen ion secretion and inability to maintain an acidic urine (urine pH often is >6.0). This defect leads to an inability to generate "new" bicarbonate through elimination of protons buffered by ammonia. Causes include hereditary disorders, amphotericin B toxicity, SLE, obstructive uropathy, Sjögren's syndrome, and other hyperglobulinemic conditions.

   (c) Hyperkalemic renal tubular acidosis. Hyperkalemia, particularly that associated with hyporeninemic hypoaldosteronism, is characterized by reduced ammonia excretion, reduced bicarbonate production, and, thus, the inability to buffer nonvolatile acids derived from the diet. Acidosis (i.e., reduced plasma bicarbonate) is due to reduced ammonia production and, therefore, reduced capacity to excrete hydrogen ion and to generate "new" bicarbonate [Online Part II: IV A 5 a (3), b (2)].

   (d) Moderate renal insufficiency. The decline in ammonium excretion resulting from decreased renal mass causes a decrease in net acid excretion and, therefore, a decrease in serum bicarbonate concentration. Recall that when the GFR is greater than 25 mL/min, anions such as sulfate and phosphate are freely excreted in the urine and do not accumulate, resulting in a normal anion gap.

   (e) Carbonic anhydrase inhibition. Drugs such as acetazolamide (a diuretic) inhibit the action of carbonic anhydrase and thereby reduce proximal tubular reabsorption of bicarbonate.

  (2) Gastrointestinal loss of alkali also produces this syndrome and may occur because of the following:

   (a) Diarrhea

   (b) Pancreatic fistulas

   (c) Ureterosigmoidostomy

3. Clinical features. Signs and symptoms usually are related to the underlying disorder. A blood pH of less than 7.2 may lead to reduced cardiac output. Acidosis also may be associated with resistance to the vasoconstrictive action of catecholamines, resulting in hypotension. Kussmaul's (deep and rhythmic) respiration may be prominent as the ventilatory rate increases in response to the fall in serum pH.

4. Diagnosis

  a. Serum electrolyte assay shows decreased bicarbonate and variable chloride content, depending on whether the acidosis is associated with a normal or an increased anion gap.

  b. Arterial blood gas analysis also demonstrates a decreased bicarbonate level, with a compensatory decrease in blood $PaCO_2$. **Winters' formula** predicts that in pure metabolic acidosis the $PaCO_2$ should be 1.5 times the bicarbonate concentration plus 8 ± 2 mm Hg. Variance from this predicted response to pure metabolic acidosis suggests a complicating respiratory dysfunction. (A lower-than-predicted $PaCO_2$ suggests primary respiratory alkalosis; a higher-than-predicted $PaCO_2$ suggests a disorder of pulmonary function, leading to inappropriate carbon dioxide retention.)

5. Therapy. Metabolic acidosis may be treated with alkali when the blood pH is less than 7.2, with intravenous therapy aimed at elevating the pH above this point. Sodium bicarbonate is the preferred alkali.

   a. The required amount of bicarbonate can be calculated on the basis that bicarbonate occupies a space that accounts for approximately 50% of body weight. Thus, the amount of sodium bicarbonate needed to raise the plasma bicarbonate from 13 to 20 mEq/L is calculated as follows: 7 mEq/L $\times$ 0.5 $\times$ kg of body weight. This number is an approximation, and measurements of plasma bicarbonate and blood pH must be repeated in patients so treated. This space is much larger if the metabolic acidosis is more severe.

   b. Underestimation of bicarbonate requirements can occur if bicarbonate losses persist (e.g., diarrhea) or if ongoing acid production is sufficiently rapid to consume administered bicarbonate in a buffering reaction (e.g., lactic acidosis).

   c. In the presence of distal tubular acidosis or renal insufficiency, the chronic bicarbonate requirement is 1 mEq/kg/day, which is equivalent to the nonvolatile acid production daily. However, in proximal tubular acidosis, the bicarbonate requirement is much greater (2–4 mEq/kg/day) because of the ineffective reabsorption of filtered bicarbonate.

E Metabolic alkalosis

1. **Definition. Increased blood pH** and **increased plasma bicarbonate concentration** are characteristic.

2. **Etiology.** Increased plasma bicarbonate levels result from either **increased endogenous production of bicarbonate** (in the stomach or kidney), with reduced renal excretion, or **exogenous administration of bicarbonate or other alkali.** Metabolic alkalosis depends on both the factors that initiate alkalemia (generation phase) and those that maintain it (maintenance phase). Because the renal capacity for bicarbonate excretion is several thousand mEq/day, it is clear that some impairment in renal bicarbonate excretion is mandatory for the maintenance of metabolic alkalosis and a sustained rise in plasma bicarbonate.

   a. Excessive mineralocorticoid action on the distal convoluted tubule and collecting tubule stimulates hydrogen ion secretion, thereby raising the plasma bicarbonate level. This occurs in all cases of primary or secondary hyperaldosteronism.

   b. Vomiting generates and maintains metabolic alkalosis by several mechanisms. Loss of gastric hydrochloric acid raises plasma bicarbonate, and the concomitant decrease in extracellular fluid volume produced by vomiting reduces the GFR and increases the rate of proximal tubular reabsorption of sodium and bicarbonate to maintain the metabolic alkalosis. Secondary hyperaldosteronism due to extracellular volume depletion also contributes to urinary potassium wasting.

   c. Diuretics. Inhibition of renal sodium chloride reabsorption leads to increased flow rate and, therefore, increased hydrogen ion secretion in the distal convoluted tubule and collecting tubule. Increased hydrogen ion secretion causes increased generation of bicarbonate. The volume depletion produced by the sodium deficits following diuretic use reduces the GFR, stimulates proximal tubular reabsorption of bicarbonate, and maintains metabolic alkalosis. Secondary hyperaldosteronism due to volume depletion causes urinary potassium wasting and also contributes to maintenance of metabolic alkalosis by stimulating hydrogen secretion in the distal segments of the nephron.

   d. Administration of alkali, either as sodium bicarbonate (e.g., during cardiac resuscitation) or as organic ions (e.g., lactate, citrate, and acetate, which are metabolically converted to bicarbonate by hepatic action), results in an increased plasma bicarbonate level. However, unless renal reabsorption of bicarbonate is stimulated, plasma bicarbonate is not sustained at an elevated level.

   e. Rapid correction of hypercapnia. Following sustained respiratory acidosis, renal bicarbonate production is elevated as a compensatory event by a stimulation of hydrogen ion secretion. If arterial PCO_2 is then acutely reduced by mechanical ventilation, a transient state of hyperbicarbonatemia and elevated blood pH ensues (a condition termed **posthypercapnic metabolic alkalosis**).

3. **Clinical features.** Signs and symptoms generally are dominated by the underlying disease state. However, symptoms of tetany may be the most pronounced clinical features.

4. **Diagnosis**

   a. Serum electrolyte assay shows an increased bicarbonate level and a decreased chloride level. Hypokalemia is a frequent finding.

b. **Arterial blood gas analysis** reveals an elevated bicarbonate level and a compensatory increase in PaCO$_2$ value. Because a decrease in ventilation is required to elevate PaCO$_2$, hypoxia also may result.

c. **Urinary chloride** is useful in the diagnosis of metabolic alkalosis. If extracellular fluid volume contraction is not present (e.g., due to excessive mineralocorticoid activity) or if renal reabsorption of sodium chloride is inhibited (e.g., due to diuretic use), urine chloride levels are >15 mg/dL. If extracellular fluid volume depletion is present (e.g., due to vomiting), urine chloride level typically will be <15 mg/dL.

5. **Therapy.** Treatment involves correction of the underlying disease state as well as reduction of renal avidity for bicarbonate. The latter effect is accomplished by extracellular volume expansion with sodium chloride–containing solutions.

a. The metabolic alkalosis caused by excessive mineralocorticoid activity is highly dependent on potassium depletion. Administration of potassium chloride corrects this disorder.

b. In individuals who have posthypercapnic metabolic alkalosis, judicious administration of acetazolamide or other inhibitors of proximal tubular bicarbonate reabsorption is an adjunct to therapy.

V CALCIUM METABOLISM

 A Normal physiology

B **Hypocalcemia** is defined as a serum calcium concentration less than 8.5 mg/dL. **Hypoalbuminemia** lowers the total serum calcium by reducing the protein-bound component. Generally, the total serum calcium level is decreased 0.8 mg/dL for each 1-g/L decrement in serum albumin. However, **parathyroid hormone (PTH) deficiency** is the primary determinant of hypocalcemia. For a more complete discussion of hypocalcemia, see Chapter 10 V B.

C **Hypercalcemia** results from disorders that cause either increased gastrointestinal absorption or increased bone resorption of calcium. Normal serum calcium level may reach 10.5 mg/dL in men and 10.2 mg/dL in women. Higher values may indicate true hypercalcemia, but serum protein level also must be monitored to confirm that an increased level of protein does not explain the increased total serum calcium. **Hyperparathyroidism** is the result of oversecretion of PTH, which in turn causes hypercalcemia. A full discussion of hypercalcemia can be found in Chapter 10 V A.

VI PHOSPHATE METABOLISM

A Normal physiology

B Hypophosphatemia

1. **Etiology.** Hypophosphatemia can result from extrarenal or renal loss of phosphate. One of the most common causes of hypophosphatemia is **chronic severe alcoholism,** which leads to most of the following features.

a. **Extrarenal causes**

(1) **Dietary deficiency and gastrointestinal losses**

(a) **Inadequate dietary intake.** Most food contains some phosphate. Inadequate dietary intake of phosphate is unusual and occurs only under specific iatrogenic circumstances.

(b) **Antacid abuse.** Large amounts of calcium salts (e.g., acetate, carbonate) and aluminum- or magnesium-containing antacids bind phosphate in the gastrointestinal tract, increase gastrointestinal phosphate losses, and may produce hypophosphatemia.

(c) **Starvation.** During prolonged starvation, cell breakdown liberates phosphate into the extracellular fluid. The amount of phosphate in remaining, intact cells, however, is preserved at normal levels. As urinary plus stool loss of liberated, extracellular phosphate exceeds dietary intake, negative phosphate balance occurs. Although hypophosphatemia does not follow immediately, severe phosphate deficits may develop on refeeding as cellular uptake of phosphate is stimulated by new cell growth and macromolecule synthesis.

(2) **Redistribution of body phosphate**
   (a) **Increased glycolysis.** Any condition associated with increased glycolysis within cells causes organic phosphate compounds to accumulate as the phosphorylated carbon residues in the Embden–Meyerhof pathway, with depletion of intracellular inorganic phosphate. Serum phosphate level falls as phosphate diffuses into cells, causing hypophosphatemia. Reduction of intracellular inorganic phosphate through this mechanism may be drastic and lead to adenosine triphosphate (ATP) depletion and cell dysfunction, such as rhabdomyolysis.
   (b) **Respiratory alkalosis.** Hyperventilation is associated with reduced serum phosphate because of increased cellular uptake of phosphate.
   (c) **Sepsis.** Hypophosphatemia is a known concomitant of gram-negative sepsis and may coexist (although independently) with hypophosphatemia because of respiratory alkalosis.

b. **Renal causes**
   (1) **Excess PTH.** Any form of hyperparathyroidism results in renal phosphate wasting and hypophosphatemia, provided that GFR is not markedly reduced.
   (2) **Primary renal tubular defects.** Conditions such as cystinosis, heavy metal poisoning, multiple myeloma, and Wilson's disease may be associated with generalized proximal tubular defects (Fanconi's syndrome) and renal phosphate wasting.
   (3) **Specific transport defects for phosphate.** These defects have been designated as **hypophosphatemic vitamin D–resistant rickets,** which may be familial or sporadic and exist in both child-onset and adult-onset forms. In each of these conditions, decreased phosphate transport in the proximal tubule produces excessive renal phosphate wasting.
   (4) **Glycosuria.** Phosphate and glucose compete for transport in the proximal tubule. All glycosuric conditions are associated with excessive renal losses of phosphate.

2. **Clinical features**
   a. **Neurologic disorders.** Cellular ATP deficiency may produce an encephalopathy characterized by obtundation, coma, and seizures. Peripheral neuropathy and Guillain–Barré syndrome also have been described.
   b. **Hematologic disorders.** Hemolytic anemia, a rare complication of profound hypophosphatemia, is due to cellular ATP depletion and abnormal membrane integrity.
   c. **Muscular disorders.** Dysfunction of skeletal muscle has been described and attributed to ATP deficits. Acute rhabdomyolysis may be particularly prevalent in alcoholic patients who are acutely hypophosphatemic. Paralysis of respiratory muscles with respiratory failure also may be seen.
   d. **Bone disorders.** Increased bone resorption with abnormal mineralization occurs in chronic hypophosphatemia.

3. **Diagnosis.** Hypophosphatemia, unless due to renal phosphate wasting, causes near-complete elimination of phosphate from the urine. A urine phosphate level of greater than 100 mg/L strongly suggests renal **phosphate wasting.** A low urine phosphate level suggests antacid-induced phosphate depletion, gastrointestinal losses, or increased cellular uptake of phosphate. Glucose infusion with secondary insulin release is the cause of hypophosphatemia in most hospitalized patients.

4. **Therapy.** All hypophosphatemic patients should be treated. In general, therapy involves correction of the underlying condition, such as discontinuation of glucose infusions. In individuals with severe hypophosphatemia and preexisting phosphate depletion (e.g., alcoholic patients), symptomatic hypophosphatemia should be treated with phosphate supplementation. Oral phosphate is preferred, and 1500–2000 mg/day may be given in divided doses. If a patient is comatose or is unable to take oral phosphate, intravenous phosphate may be administered twice daily in 250-mg doses, if serum phosphate is less than 1 mg/dL, provided that serum phosphate measurements are taken at 12-hour intervals. Infusion of phosphate must be discontinued if the serum phosphate level rises to 1.5 mg/dL.

5. **Complications.** The greatest danger of hypophosphatemia lies in the injudicious administration of intravenous phosphate. Acute hypocalcemia due to the formation of calcium phosphate may lead to shock, acute kidney injury, and death. For this reason, intravenous phosphate should be administered only when specific clinical disturbances are clearly attributable to hypophosphatemia.

C Hyperphosphatemia

1. **Etiology**
   a. **Renal failure.** Because the kidney is the main regulator of serum phosphate level, renal failure commonly is associated with hyperphosphatemia. This disorder is not seen until the GFR has decreased to at least 25% of normal. Serum phosphate level generally does not exceed 10 mg/dL in renal failure. Values exceeding 10 mg/dL suggest an additional etiologic factor.
   b. **Cell lysis syndromes**
      (1) **Rhabdomyolysis.** Acute muscle breakdown of any etiology is associated with the release of cellular phosphate and, therefore, hyperphosphatemia. Severe hyperphosphatemia (i.e., serum phosphate concentration >15 mg/dL) may be seen in cases associated with acute kidney injury.
      (2) **Tumor lysis syndrome.** Malignant disorders associated with a high sensitivity to chemotherapy or radiotherapy result in rapid cell death from such treatments. This syndrome may lead to massive release of phosphate and other intracellular substances into the extracellular fluid. Severe hypocalcemia, cardiovascular collapse, and renal failure due to calcium, urate, and phosphate deposition in the kidney have been described.
   c. **Exogenous phosphate administration.** Any route (i.e., via intravenous infusion, by mouth, or via phosphate enemas) may result in severe and unpredictable hyperphosphatemia, especially if the GFR is reduced.
   d. **Hypoparathyroidism.** Because the level of PTH is a key determinant of the rate of renal phosphate handling, any condition associated with parathyroid insufficiency or a lack of renal response to PTH may be characterized by hyperphosphatemia.
   e. **Miscellaneous causes.** Growth hormone (GH) excess, hyperthyroidism, sickle cell anemia, and tumoral calcinosis may be associated with hyperphosphatemia.

2. **Clinical features.** Hypocalcemia, hypotension, and renal failure may be seen in severe hyperphosphatemia. Milder cases, typically seen in chronic renal failure, are associated with secondary hyperparathyroidism and renal osteodystrophy.

3. **Diagnosis.** Hyperphosphatemia in the absence of renal insufficiency is due to hypoparathyroidism, cell lysis, or tumoral calcinosis. The etiologic diagnosis of hyperphosphatemia is made on the basis of the patient history, physical examination, and laboratory data.

4. **Therapy.** Acute hyperphosphatemia may be a medical emergency that requires immediate therapy. In cases of tumor lysis syndrome, acute hemodialysis may be necessary and is an effective treatment. Administration of large amounts of phosphate-binding resins may be useful in the long-term treatment of hyperphosphatemic conditions.

VII   MAGNESIUM METABOLISM

A Normal physiology

B Hypomagnesemia

1. **Definition.** Clinically important hypomagnesemia occurs when serum magnesium concentration falls to less than 1.0 mg/dL, although it has been proposed that even mild degrees of hypomagnesemia may be associated with a variety of clinical disorders.

2. **Etiology**
   a. **Extrarenal causes**
      (1) **Dietary deficiency and gastrointestinal losses**
         (a) **Inadequate dietary intake.** Nutritional hypomagnesemia may develop after prolonged starvation as well as postoperatively.
         (b) **Malabsorption.** Generalized malabsorption syndrome, chronic diarrhea, diffuse bowel injury, and chronic laxative abuse all are associated with reduced gastrointestinal absorption of magnesium.
      (2) **Redistribution of body magnesium.** Acute cellular uptake of magnesium has been described in individuals who are in alcohol withdrawal.

b. **Renal causes**

(1) **Primary tubular disorders.** A number of tubular disorders, including Bartter's syndrome, renal tubular acidosis, and postobstructive diuresis, are characterized by a defect in renal magnesium conservation and hypomagnesemia. Hypomagnesemia also may develop in patients following renal transplantation. In a familial form of renal magnesium wasting, the molecular mechanisms involved have been identified.

(2) **Drug-induced tubular losses.** Diuretics such as thiazides and furosemide typically produce varied degrees of hypomagnesemia. Even small doses of the chemotherapeutic agent cisplatin produce marked renal magnesium wasting and clinically severe hypomagnesemia. Gentamicin and amphotericin B also may produce a toxic injury to the renal tubule, with magnesium and potassium wasting occurring in the absence of reduced GFR.

(3) **Hormone-induced tubular losses.** Hyperaldosteronism or hypoparathyroidism can be associated with renal tubular magnesium wasting and hypomagnesemia.

(4) **Ion- or nutrient-induced tubular losses.** Because calcium and magnesium compete for transport in the ascending limb of the loop of Henle, hypercalcemia is associated with reduced renal magnesium transport. Phosphate depletion, alcohol consumption, or both are associated with decreased renal reabsorption of magnesium, but the mechanisms are unknown.

3. **Clinical features.** Muscle twitching, tremor, and muscle weakness are commonly seen. These physical signs are due to the direct effect of magnesium on neuromuscular function as well as the hypocalcemic effect of hypomagnesemia. Severe chronic hypomagnesemia leads to decreased glandular secretion of PTH as well as impaired bone response to PTH, and both of these effects lead to hypocalcemia. In addition, hypomagnesemia produces a defect in renal potassium reabsorption, which eventually produces potassium depletion. Thus, all of the clinical signs of hypocalcemia and hypokalemia may be seen in hypomagnesemic patients. The clinical presentation of hypokalemia and hypomagnesemia includes cardiac arrhythmias, particularly in patients taking digitalis.

4. **Therapy.** In most patients, a normal diet makes up for magnesium deficits. If ongoing losses occur, magnesium supplementation is necessary. Even in severe magnesium deficiency, however, 50% of an administered dose of magnesium is excreted in the urine. Symptomatic deficits usually amount to 1–2 mmol/kg of body weight.

a. If **oral magnesium therapy** is required, magnesium oxide generally is tolerated and has 25%–50% absorption. It is given four times daily in doses of 250–500 mg.

b. In cases of severe hypomagnesemia, **parenteral magnesium therapy** may be necessary.

C **Hypermagnesemia**

1. **Etiology.** Because the kidneys can excrete several thousand milligrams of magnesium each day, hypermagnesemia usually is iatrogenic and occurs in a sustained fashion only in patients who have impaired renal function and ingest magnesium as either laxatives or antacids. Acute magnesium intoxication may occur in women who are treated for toxemia of pregnancy with intravenous magnesium salts that are administered at an excessive rate. Muscular paralysis can develop at serum magnesium levels of 10 mg/dL.

2. **Therapy.** Calcium ion is a direct antagonist of magnesium and should be given to patients who are seriously ill with magnesium intoxication. Hemodialysis may be required following cessation of magnesium therapy.

PART III ▢ HYPERTENSION

I   GENERAL CONSIDERATIONS

A **Definition**   Hypertension is present when the systolic blood pressure constantly exceeds 140 mm Hg or the diastolic blood pressure exceeds 90 mm Hg. Many studies suggest that systolic blood pressure elevation is as significant as diastolic blood pressure elevation as a risk factor for a variety of cardiovascular and renal diseases.

1. **Primary hypertension** is hypertension that has no known cause. Primary hypertension accounts for 90%–95% of cases of hypertension.

2. **Secondary hypertension** is attributable to a diagnosable disease and accounts for the remainder of cases of hypertension.

B **Diagnosis**

1. Blood pressure should be measured with a **loosely fitting cuff.** The width of the cuff should equal at least 50% of the length of the upper arm. Initially, blood pressure should be **determined in each arm** to be sure that arterial obstruction in the upper extremity is not falsely lowering the distal arm arterial pressure.

2. Blood pressure may be elevated at times of stress; in fact, in some patients, merely being in a physician's office may induce transient hypertension. **Multiple determinations over several visits** and some form of **home** or **workplace monitoring** should be conducted prior to initiating pharmacologic therapy in hypertensive patients.

C **Consequences of hypertension** In general, the mortality rate over 20 years among patients with a systolic blood pressure of greater than 160 mm Hg or a diastolic blood pressure of greater than 100 mm Hg increases 100% in those who are untreated.

1. **Stroke.** Patients with a systolic blood pressure of greater than 160 mm Hg have a fourfold increased risk of stroke if untreated.

2. **Coronary artery disease.** Patients with a diastolic pressure of greater than 95 mm Hg have a more than twofold increased risk of coronary artery disease as compared with normotensive patients.

3. **CHF.** Patients with blood pressure of greater than 160/95 mm Hg have a fourfold increased incidence of CHF. In 75% of patients with CHF, hypertension occurs at some time during the course of their illness. Thickening and hypertrophy of the left ventricle as a result of hypertension may produce CHF as a result of diastolic dysfunction.

4. **Chronic kidney disease.** Hypertension significantly increases the risk of chronic kidney diseases and end-stage renal disease. There is unequivocal evidence that blood pressure reduction slows the progression of renal disease.

II MECHANISMS OF HYPERTENSION

The major mechanisms of hypertension are listed in 🔎 Online Table 7–17.

A **Primary hypertension**

1. **Abnormal cardiac and peripheral hemodynamics.** Blood pressure is the product of cardiac output and total peripheral resistance; therefore, for hypertension to occur, there must be an elevation in cardiac output, total peripheral resistance, or both.
   a. An abnormality in peripheral resistance is a contributing factor in most cases of hypertension.
   b. Many patients with hypertension have either persistently elevated cardiac output or elevated total peripheral resistance early in the course of the disease.

2. **Impaired pressure natriuresis**
   a. In normal individuals, an elevation in blood pressure leads to an alteration in intrarenal hemodynamics and physical forces, resulting in natriuresis. This, in turn, causes a diuresis, a decrease in total extracellular volume, and a fall in blood pressure.
   b. In patients with essential hypertension, the kidney fails to respond normally to elevated arterial pressure and natriuresis is impaired. The homeostatic abnormality may either cause or help sustain the elevated arterial pressure.
   c. The cause of the failure of normal pressure natriuresis is unknown. Hormonal factors, abnormalities in the structure and activity of transport proteins (e.g., the sodium–hydrogen exchanger in the renal tubule), and autonomic nervous system activity have all been implicated experimentally and on a clinical basis.

3. **Baroreceptor resetting.** In hypertensive patients, baroreceptors in the carotid arteries and aorta are "reset" so that higher pressures are required to exert an influence toward lowering blood pressure.

4. **Abnormalities in the renin–angiotensin–aldosterone system.** Abnormalities in each component of this complex system may contribute to the pathogenesis of hypertension in many patients with hypertension.

5. **Abnormalities in other vasoregulatory systems**
   a. **Endothelin,** a peptide produced in many organs and tissues, is a vasoconstrictor with potency several times greater than that of norepinephrine.
   b. **Atrial natriuretic peptide (ANP),** derived from cardiac muscle, may play a role in normal vascular regulation as a vasodilator and may contribute to extracellular volume homeostasis and blood pressure control in states of mineralocorticoid excess by enhancing sodium excretion.
   c. **Endothelium-derived relaxation factor (EDRF) (nitric oxide)** is a gas derived from arginine metabolism that is crucial in a number of vasoregulatory phenomena. Defects in this system are thought to contribute to the hypertension associated with pregnancy.

B **Secondary hypertension** In 5%–10% of patients with hypertension, this condition is secondary to an identifiable disorder in the endocrine system or the autonomic nervous system.

1. **Renovascular hypertension** (see also Part I: XIV C) is an important cause of secondary hypertension. In this disorder, hypertension is the result of a complex interplay between activation of the renin–angiotensin–aldosterone system and the sympathetic nervous system. The pattern of endocrine stimulation may also depend on whether the vascular lesions are unilateral or bilateral.
   a. Initially, high angiotensin II levels lead to vasoconstriction and expanded extracellular fluid volume as aldosterone release is stimulated.
   b. With time, volume expansion may lead to suppression of total renal renin production so that circulating renin values may be normal despite the elevated blood pressure. This may explain why unstimulated plasma renin levels are not a good index of the presence of renovascular hypertension in all cases and why some patients (e.g., those with unilateral vascular lesions) may not even demonstrate increased renin secretion.
      (1) The normal levels of renin, which are inappropriate in the presence of hypertension and an expanded extracellular fluid volume, sustain the hypertension.
      (2) In addition, during this chronic phase, increased sympathetic nervous system activity resulting from chronic angiotensin II stimulation contributes to hypertension.

2. **Renal parenchymal diseases.** Hypertension frequently accompanies a variety of renal diseases, highlighting the important contribution of renal endocrine and excretory function in the regulation of blood pressure.
   a. **Altered excretory function.** Defects in the renal excretion of salt and water no doubt contribute to the pathogenesis of hypertension in patients with advanced renal failure. In patients maintained on hemodialysis or peritoneal dialysis, modest reductions in extracellular fluid volume can produce a striking reduction in arterial blood pressure.
   b. **Altered renin–angiotensin–aldosterone activity.** Ischemic changes resulting from intrarenal scarring may activate the renin–angiotensin system and contribute to hypertension in patients with early or advanced renal failure.

3. **Endocrinologic causes**
   a. **Oral contraceptives.** These agents cause hypertension in approximately 5% of patients who use them. Hypertension occurs as a result of estrogen-induced increases in angiotensinogen synthesis in the liver. Reduced estrogen levels or the addition of progesterone may ameliorate this complication.
   b. **Mineralocorticoid excess syndromes.** Mineralocorticoid excess leads to hypertension by inducing sodium and water retention, leading to expansion of the extracellular fluid volume. The hypertension is often accompanied by hypokalemia because mineralocorticoids promote renal potassium excretion in the collecting duct of the nephron. A variety of disorders produce mineralocorticoid excess states.
      (1) **Primary hyperaldosteronism.** Tumors of the adrenal gland, which are common on autopsy, are functionally active in 1%–3% of patients, leading to mineralocorticoid excess. Tumors may be unilateral or bilateral, or the excess may result from a diffuse bilateral hyperplasia of the adrenal zona glomerulosa.

(2) **Glucocorticoid-remediable hyperaldosteronism.** In rare patients, a defect in adrenal development leads to the synthesis of aldosterone in the adrenal gland under the influence of ACTH. A gene rearrangement allows expression of ACTH-responsive aldosterone synthase in the zona fasciculata rather than the zona glomerulosa, leading to the production of large amounts of mineralocorticoid hormone. Treatment with dexamethasone suppresses this abnormal pathway. This disorder should be suspected in patients with a family history of hypertension and hypokalemia.

(3) **Exogenous hypermineralocorticoidism.** Some patients may develop striking mineralocorticoid excess hypertension from the ingestion of **glycyrrhetinic acid,** a substance found in European licorice and in some forms of chewing tobacco. Glycyrrhetinic acid blocks the action of 11-beta-hydroxysteroid dehydrogenase (an enzyme that prevents glucocorticoid binding to receptors in the renal distal tubule), resulting in a high mineralocorticoid state. Patients present with hypertension, hypokalemia, and low renin and aldosterone levels.

(4) **Cushing syndrome.** Glucocorticoid excess resulting from exogenous glucocorticoid therapy, a pituitary tumor, or an adrenal adenoma produces hypertension in approximately 80% of patients with Cushing syndrome. Hypertension may occur because cortisol has mineralocorticoid-like effects and, therefore, leads to the retention of sodium and water. However, many patients with Cushing syndrome and hypertension do not manifest a low renin state as would be expected in primary mineralocorticoidism, implying that other mechanisms may contribute to the hypertension as well.

(5) **Liddle syndrome.** This familial disorder is transmitted as an autosomal dominant form of hypertension. It manifests as hypertension and hypokalemia with low renin and aldosterone levels. The cause is a genetic defect in the beta subunit of the sodium channel in the apical membrane of the distal renal tubule. This defect mimics the action of mineralocorticoid hormones to enhance sodium entry in the distal nephron, thereby enhancing sodium absorption, increasing potassium excretion, and expanding the extracellular fluid volume, leading to an elevated arterial blood pressure.

c. **Pheochromocytoma.** This tumor of the adrenal medulla increases the secretion of catecholamines, leading to hypertension. Approximately 50% of patients have episodic hypertension; the remainder have constant hypertension.

d. **Miscellaneous causes. Acromegaly, hyperparathyroidism,** and **hyperthyroidism** also may produce hypertension. **Coarctation of the aorta,** as noted in Chapter 2 VII D, is a correctable cause of hypertension.

III — APPROACH TO THE HYPERTENSIVE PATIENT

The majority of patients with hypertension have primary hypertension; no further evaluation is required. Secondary hypertension should be suspected in patients who develop hypertension at the extremes of age, patients without a family history of hypertension, or patients with hypertension refractory to medical therapy.

A Renovascular hypertension

1. Renovascular hypertension **secondary to atherosclerosis of the renal artery** should be suspected in patients with the following conditions:
   a. Severe hypertension associated with advanced hypertensive retinopathy
   b. Hypertension and severe peripheral vascular disease
   c. Hypertension and sudden deterioration in renal function (with or without the recent introduction of ACE inhibitor therapy)
   d. Known disparity in renal size or function

2. Renovascular hypertension **secondary to fibromuscular dysplasia** should be suspected in young women with severe hypertension, systolic and diastolic abdominal bruits, or a strong family history of hypertension. **Magnetic resonance angiography** is a useful screening test in those patients with a high prior probability of disease (see Part III: III A 1).

B **Hypermineralocorticoid states** should be suspected in patients with persistent hypokalemia and hypertension. There is no doubt that these disorders are underdiagnosed because many patients with proven mineralocorticoid excess states are normokalemic. Nevertheless, persistent and unexplained hypokalemia remains the most typical sign.

1. **Primary hyperaldosteronism.** The diagnosis rests on finding patients with hypokalemia and hypertension and proving that hyperaldosteronism causes both disorders.
   a. Patients who have unexplained hypokalemia and hypertension should have their **24-hour urinary excretion rate for aldosterone** measured while consuming a 150-mEq sodium diet. If the aldosterone value is elevated and plasma renin is low, an **abdominal CT scan** should be performed to determine whether a surgically correctable (i.e., adenomatous) form of hyperaldosteronism is present. Recent studies suggest that a plasma aldosterone–to–plasma renin ratio of greater than 50 is highly specific for primary hyperaldosteronism.
      (1) Surgery relieves hypertension and hypokalemia in greater than 70% of patients if adenoma is the cause. Although surgery does not cure hypertension in patients with bilateral hyperplasia, the hypokalemia does remit.
      (2) Although hypokalemia may not be found in some patients with primary hyperaldosteronism, patients with hypokalemia are more likely to have a positive response to surgery, so the finding of spontaneous hypokalemia remains a reasonable screening tool.
   b. Patients with a family history of hypertension should undergo a **trial of glucocorticoid therapy** to determine whether glucocorticoid-remediable hyperaldosteronism is present [see Part II: III B 2 b (2)].
   c. **Selective adrenal venography and sampling for lateralizing aldosterone levels** may be performed in some patients.

2. **Pheochromocytoma** should be suspected in hypertensive patients who experience episodes of flushing, diaphoresis, weight loss, and diarrhea.
   a. **Measurement of urinary catecholamines and catecholamine metabolites** is useful in making the diagnosis.
   b. **CT** or **magnetic resonance imaging (MRI)** should be used to locate the tumor in the adrenal medulla.
   c. An ^{131}I-metaiodobenzylguanidine (MIBG) scan may be performed when the suspicion of diagnosis is high but the CT or MRI is negative.

3. **Coarctation of the aorta** should be suspected in any young patient with hypertension when the blood pressure in the leg is at least 20 mm Hg lower than that in the arm.

IV   THERAPY FOR HYPERTENSION

A **Goals of therapy**   Treatment of hypertension is aimed at reducing the diastolic blood pressure to less than 90 mm Hg and the systolic blood pressure to less than 140 mm Hg.

B **Indications for therapy**   It is believed that almost all patients with a blood pressure of greater than 140/90 mm Hg should be treated. In patients with borderline hypertension, controversy exists about the risks versus the benefits of therapy, but most clinicians believe that the benefits of therapy predominate and that all patients with an elevated blood pressure should receive treatment to restore the values to less than 130/80 mm Hg.

C **Types of therapy**

1. **Nonpharmacologic measures**
   a. **Sodium restriction** alone may be sufficient to lower blood pressure in many hypertensive patients, particularly those with a high sodium intake. Limitation of sodium intake to no more than 2 g/day has been shown to reduce blood pressure significantly in susceptible patients.
   b. **Weight reduction** in obese patients also significantly reduces blood pressure.
   c. **Limitation of alcohol consumption** may be beneficial. Alcohol potentiates the action of catecholamines and may exacerbate hypertension in susceptible individuals.

2. **Pharmacologic measures.** Patient compliance often is best with therapeutic regimens that are simple to follow. In choosing an antihypertensive regimen, consideration should be given not only to side effects, but also to the number of medications and doses per day that the patient must take.
   a. **Diuretics,** which often are the first line of antihypertensive therapy, initially reduce extracellular fluid volume. After several months, a continued reduction cannot be measured, yet

blood pressure is maintained at a lower level primarily due to decreased vascular resistance. The exact mechanism by which diuretics reduce peripheral vascular resistance is unknown.

(1) Agents

(a) Thiazide diuretics (e.g., **hydrochlorothiazide, chlorthalidone, chlorothiazide,** and **metolazone**) are more effective antihypertensive agents than **loop diuretics** (e.g., furosemide, bumetanide, torsemide, and ethacrynic acid) if serum creatinine is <2 mg/dL.

(b) Potassium-sparing diuretics (e.g., **amiloride** and **triamterene**) act in the distal nephron and collecting tubule and are useful in the treatment of hypermineralocorticoid states.

(c) Spironolactone and **eplerenone** are competitive inhibitors of aldosterone.

(2) Side effects. Hypokalemia, hyperglycemia, hyperlipidemia, hyperuricemia, hypercalcemia (thiazides only), and prerenal azotemia may occur. Therefore, periodic laboratory determination of potassium and BUN levels is indicated. Uric acid should be monitored periodically in patients with a history of gout. Some studies implicate hypokalemia caused by diuretics as an important risk factor for unexplained sudden death, a catastrophic complication that can be avoided by potassium supplementation or use of potassium-sparing diuretics.

b. β-Adrenergic blocking agents reduce cardiac output and renin release. However, it is not clear that these are the primary mechanisms by which β-blockers reduce blood pressure. The combination of a β-blocker and a diuretic agent reduces the diastolic blood pressure to less than 90 mm Hg in approximately 80% of patients with mild-to-moderate hypertension.

(1) Agents. Propranolol, nadolol, metoprolol, atenolol, timolol, betaxolol, carteolol, pindolol, carvedilol, acebutolol, and **labetalol** are among the β-blockers that are currently approved for the treatment of hypertension. (Labetalol is also an α-adrenergic antagonist.)

(2) Side effects. Bronchospasm, bradycardia, a worsening of existing CHF, occasional impotence, fatigue, depression, and nightmares may occur.

c. Centrally acting adrenergic antagonists inhibit sympathetic outflow from the CNS by stimulating central α-adrenoreceptors, reducing peripheral resistance and blood pressure.

(1) Agents. Methyldopa and **clonidine** are the commonly used centrally acting drugs.

(2) Side effects. Somnolence, orthostatic hypotension, Coombs'-positive hemolytic anemia, impotence, and hepatic injury are side effects of methyldopa. With clonidine, the major side effect is a rebound phenomenon that produces severe hypertension after withdrawal of the drug.

d. Peripherally acting sympathetic nerve antagonists cause blood pressure to fall by reducing catecholamine release from peripheral sympathetic nerves.

(1) Agents. The most commonly used drugs in this category are reserpine and guanethidine. **Reserpine** depletes nerve storage vesicles of norepinephrine and, thus, limits norepinephrine secretion. **Guanethidine** directly inhibits the release of norepinephrine from adrenergic neurons.

(2) Side effects. The major side effect of reserpine is depression; it also may increase the incidence of gastric ulceration. Orthostatic hypotension is the most common side effect with guanethidine therapy.

e. α-Adrenergic blocking agents pharmacologically antagonize norepinephrine's stimulation of adrenergic receptors, reducing blood pressure by reducing total peripheral resistance. **Prazosin, doxazosin, terazosin,** and **phenoxybenzamine** are the most commonly used α-blockers.

f. Calcium channel antagonists reduce smooth muscle tone, thereby acting to produce vasodilation, by modulating calcium release in smooth muscle. The subsequent reduction in total peripheral resistance reduces blood pressure. Calcium channel blockers may also reduce cardiac output by decreasing venous return and the inotropic state.

(1) Agents. Currently, both dihydropyridines (i.e., **nifedipine, nicardipine, isradipine, felodipine, nimodipine, amlodipine,** and **nitrendipine**) and nondihydropyridines (e.g., **diltiazem** and **verapamil**) are approved for antihypertensive therapy.

(2) Side effects. Dihydropyridines may cause headache, flushing, and peripheral edema. Verapamil and, to a lesser extent, diltiazem have cardiodepressant actions (unlike the dihydropyridines), making their use problematic in patients with CHF.

g. **Direct vasodilators** dilate arteries and arterioles, reducing blood pressure by reducing total peripheral resistance. They are particularly effective when used with a β-blocker that inhibits the reflex tachycardia caused by direct vasodilation.

   (1) **Agents. Hydralazine** and **minoxidil** are the most commonly used direct vasodilators.

   (2) **Side effects.** The major side effects of hydralazine are headache and a lupus-like syndrome; the latter is reversed when the drug is discontinued. The major side effects of minoxidil are orthostatic hypotension and facial hirsutism.

h. **ACE inhibitors** block the conversion of angiotensin I to angiotensin II (a vasoconstrictor), thus reducing total peripheral resistance. In addition, aldosterone production is decreased, reducing the retention of sodium and water.

   (1) **Agents. Captopril, enalapril, fosinopril, benazepril, quinapril, ramipril,** and **lisinopril** are useful ACE inhibitors.

   (2) **Side effects.** The most common side effect of ACE inhibitors is cough, which typically disappears with discontinuation of the drug. Hyperkalemia may occasionally occur as a result of reduced aldosterone secretion. Other severe but uncommon side effects include leukopenia, rash, and angioedema. Because angiotensin II maintains the GFR during states of reduced renal blood flow (by maintaining a high vascular resistance in the postglomerular vessels), the use of ACE inhibitors in patients with compromised renal blood flow may lead to a form of acute kidney injury. Reduction in dose or discontinuation of drug is usually sufficient to reverse the fall in GFR.

i. **Angiotensin II–type 1 receptor antagonists** (ARBs) are a class of drugs that provide the benefits of blockade of the angiotensin system without some of the annoying side effects, particularly cough. These agents appear to offer all of the benefits of ACE inhibitors with fewer side effects.

   (1) **Agents. Losartan, valsartan, irbesartan, candesartan, telmisartan, eprosartan,** and **olmesartan** are available.

   (2) **Side effects.** These are similar to those of ACE inhibitors, except that cough has not been seen with receptor blockers.

j. **Direct renin inhibitors** are a new class of drugs that decrease plasma renin activity and inhibit conversion of angiotensinogen to angiotensin I, thereby resulting in similar initial therapeutic effects as ACE inhibitors and ARBs. Long-term use of ACE inhibitors or ARBs may lead to a compensatory increase in renin production, while direct renin inhibitors are not associated with this problem.

   (1) **Agents. Aliskiren** is the first direct renin inhibitor to be approved by the Food and Drug Administration.

   (2) **Side effects.** Diarrhea is the most common side effect of the direct renin inhibitors. Angioedema and rash may also occur. Patients on both a direct renin inhibitor and an ACE inhibitor or an ARB may be at increased risk of hyperkalemia and should have their potassium levels monitored closely.

D **Therapeutic strategies**

1. **First-line therapy.** Various agents are now considered appropriate for initial antihypertensive therapy. Many physicians still begin therapy with a diuretic, but β-blockers, ACE inhibitors, angiotensin-receptor blockers, or calcium channel blockers are also appropriate initial drugs. At the very best, monotherapy produces optimal control of blood pressure in only 75% of patients.

2. **Second-line therapy.** Submaximal doses of two or three antihypertensive agents added in a stepwise fashion have been advocated as a successful approach. The addition of 12.5 or 25 mg of hydrochlorothiazide will potentiate the action of a number of antihypertensive agents, particularly the ACE inhibitors and the angiotensin II–receptor antagonists. If the blood pressure is still uncontrolled, the use of multiple drug regimens or the addition of direct vasodilators is indicated.

V **HYPERTENSIVE CRISIS**

This condition is defined as severe hypertension characterized by a diastolic blood pressure of greater than 140 mm Hg. Blood pressure elevation to this degree can cause vascular damage, pulmonary edema, encephalopathy, retinal hemorrhages, renal damage, and death.

A **Diagnosis** A diastolic blood pressure of greater than 140 mm Hg, funduscopic findings of papilledema, changes in neurologic and mental status, and an abnormal renal sediment are the hallmarks of hypertensive crisis.

B **Therapy** Immediate lowering of the blood pressure is indicated.

1. Infusion of **sodium nitroprusside** is a mainstay of therapy.
   a. The patient's blood pressure should be monitored constantly so that the dose can be adjusted to maintain the blood pressure within the desired range. An excessive reduction in blood pressure can be reversed rapidly by reducing the dose of the infusion.
   b. Long-term administration of high-dose nitroprusside can lead to cyanide intoxication. The likelihood of this complication increases in patients with renal dysfunction or after 3 days of therapy.
   c. β-Blockers should be used in conjunction with nitroprusside to avoid reflex tachycardia.

2. **Labetalol, nicardipine,** and **nitroglycerin** are also effective intravenous therapeutic agents.

3. **The use of sublingual nifedipine has been shown to be dangerous (precipitating coronary ischemia or stroke), and it should not be a part of therapy.**

Study Questions

1. A 60-year-old man develops new-onset nephrotic syndrome. A percutaneous renal biopsy is contemplated to determine the nature of the glomerular disease. In which of the following situations is the renal biopsy absolutely contraindicated?

- [A] The patient has a diastolic blood pressure of 120 mm Hg.
- [B] The patient has a serum creatinine level of 2.5 mg/dL (normal = 0.8–1.4 mg/dL).
- [C] The patient has diabetes mellitus.
- [D] The patient has heavy proteinuria but no other urinary abnormality.
- [E] The patient has undergone a previous renal biopsy.

2. A 71-year-old man in the surgical intensive care unit is seen for acute kidney injury. After an operation for removal of gallstones, he had a persistent drainage from his biliary catheter associated with spiking fevers to 38.9°C. He has been taking gentamicin and ampicillin/sulbactam for the last 10 days. Over the last 4 days, his serum creatinine level has increased at a rate of 1 mg/dL/day, but his urine output of 1.5 L/day has not diminished. At no time has he had any hypotension during this hospitalization.

Physical examination shows normal blood pressure and vital signs. Results of laboratory studies indicate a creatinine level of 7.1 mg/dL, and renal ultrasonography reveals no evidence of obstruction. Which of the following is the most likely cause of the acute kidney injury?

- [A] Sepsis
- [B] Trauma to the ureter during surgery
- [C] Gentamicin nephrotoxicity
- [D] Acute glomerulonephritis
- [E] Cephalothin-induced acute kidney injury

3. A 39-year-old man who is experiencing labored breathing and mental obtundation comes to the emergency department. Physical examination is unremarkable. Laboratory studies show the following: serum sodium = 144 mEq/L, serum potassium = 3.7 mEq/L, serum chloride = 97 mEq/L, plasma bicarbonate concentration $[HCO_3^-]$ = 16 mEq/L, arterial pH = 7.38, and $PaCO_2$ = 21 mEq/L. These findings indicate which of the following acid–base disturbances?

- [A] Respiratory alkalosis
- [B] Metabolic acidosis
- [C] Metabolic acidosis and respiratory alkalosis
- [D] Metabolic acidosis and metabolic alkalosis
- [E] No acid–base disturbance

4. A 48-year-old man with a history of obesity, hypertension, and type 2 diabetes returns to your office for a routine follow-up visit. His body mass index (BMI) is 32, he consumes a low-fat diet but does not follow the low-sodium recommendations, and he gets little exercise. On physical examination, his blood pressure is 162/92 mm Hg, his pulse is 88 bpm, and he is comfortable. With the exception of mild retinopathy, his physical examination is normal. His hemoglobin A1c is 8, his blood urea nitrogen (BUN) is 24, and his serum creatinine is 1.5 mg/dL. His spot urine protein-to-creatinine ratio is 1.3. In addition to lifestyle modification, which of the following hypertensive agents should be initiated?

- [A] Hydrochlorothiazide
- [B] Lisinopril
- [C] Felodipine
- [D] Hydralazine
- [E] Clonidine

5. A 45-year-old man enters the hospital because of acute flank pain and red urine, which began at night and awakened him. Until this point, the man has been in good health. Physical examination in the emergency department is normal, but he does have hematuria, with essentially normal laboratory studies. Radiography of the abdomen reveals a stone in the right kidney. An abdominal CT scan shows the stone to be nonobstructing. Further laboratory studies demonstrate normal serum calcium and phosphate, and a subsequent urine culture is negative. Which of the following types of kidney stone is most likely to have caused this condition?

- (A) Calcium oxalate stone
- (B) Uric acid stone
- (C) Xanthine stone
- (D) Struvite stone
- (E) Cystine stone

6. A 70-year-old man with longstanding hypertension has developed more severe hypertension over a 6-month period. Despite antihypertensive medication, his blood pressure has risen from 140/90 mm Hg to 175/105 mm Hg. In addition, he had an episode of "flash pulmonary edema" that led to his hospitalization for 1 week. He has continued to take his antihypertensive medication faithfully, but he has developed some intermittent claudication in his left leg. Although he has a long history of smoking, he has had no other medical problems. Which of the following is the most likely cause of this clinical disorder?

- (A) Renal artery stenosis
- (B) Pheochromocytoma
- (C) Hyperaldosteronism
- (D) Primary worsening of hypertension
- (E) Coarctation of the aorta

7. A 68-year-old woman with end-stage renal disease and a history of hypertension and systemic lupus erythematosus presents to the emergency department with complaints of sweats and palpitations, shortness of breath, and dizziness. Physical examination is remarkable for an anxious-appearing woman with a blood pressure of 148/62 mm Hg, a pulse of 120 bpm, and a temperature of 36°C. She has mild carotid bruits, a soft systolic ejection murmur with a regular rate and rhythm, and a few scattered crackles on examination. Laboratory studies are sent. Her electrocardiogram is shown in the accompanying figure.

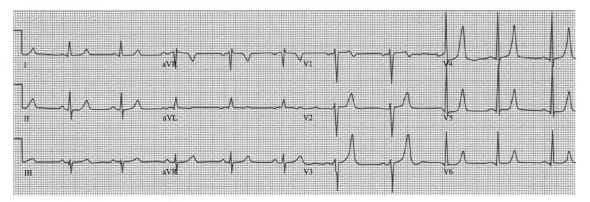

- (A) Start hemodialysis
- (B) Administer insulin and glucose
- (C) Administer calcium gluconate
- (D) Give epinephrine nebulizers
- (E) Administer oral Kayexalate resin

8. A 78-year-old man enters the hospital because of abnormalities of urination. Today he is passing large amounts of urine; however, some days he passes no urine at all. He now has a blood pressure of 180/90 mm Hg, and otherwise his physical examination is normal. Laboratory studies show a BUN of 120 mg/dL and a serum creatinine of 4.2 mg/dL. Urinalysis reveals a specific gravity of 1.010; urine that is negative for protein, glucose, ketone bodies, and blood; and an occasional WBC per high-power field on microscopic examination. Which of the following is the most likely cause of the renal insufficiency?

- (A) Obstructive uropathy
- (B) Acute glomerulonephritis
- (C) Acute interstitial nephritis

[D] Acute tubular necrosis
[E] Chronic renal failure of unspecified nature

9. A 47-year-old man enters the hospital with nephrotic syndrome. He reports that he initially experienced edema of his feet in the morning, but this condition rapidly progressed until the edema extended to his midcalves and lasted throughout the day. He has been in good health all his life and has not seen a physician in the last 5 years.

On physical examination, blood pressure is 155/100 mm Hg, pulse is 88 bpm, respiratory rate is 15 breaths per minute, and temperature is 37.0°C. Examination of the heart and lungs reveals no evidence of CHF, examination of the abdomen indicates mild ascites with normal hepatic size, and examination of the extremities reveals 4+ edema to the midcalf. Laboratory studies show a BUN of 10 mg/dL and creatinine of 1.0 mg/dL. The rest of the laboratory studies are unrevealing. Urinalysis reveals 4+ protein and one RBC per high-power field. No RBC casts or other cellular elements are seen on urinalysis. The 24-hour urine contains 9.6 g of protein. Which of the following is most likely to account for this clinical condition?

[A] Membranous nephropathy
[B] Poststreptococcal glomerulonephritis
[C] Lupus nephritis
[D] Amyloidosis
[E] Diabetes mellitus

10. A 31-year-old man enters the hospital with acute onset of edema and hematuria. He had been well until 3 weeks earlier, when he had a sore throat and was treated with oral penicillin. Since that time, he has felt generally good but has noted the onset of dark, tea-colored urine and swelling of his legs. He denies any other symptoms, including rash, joint pain, chest pain, and the use of any medication but the penicillin.

On physical examination, blood pressure is 160/110 mm Hg, pulse is 85 bpm, respiratory rate is 15 breaths per minute, and temperature is 37.0°C. Other findings include marked peripheral edema extending to the midleg. Laboratory studies reveal a BUN of 20 mg/dL, creatinine of 1.3 mg/dL, and normal electrolytes. The serum complement level, including CH_{50} and C4, is reduced by 50%, the anti–deoxyribonuclease B antibody and the anti–streptolysin O titer are increased, and the anti–glomerular basement membrane (anti-GBM) antibody assay and ANCA level are within normal limits. Urinalysis reveals 4+ protein, 4+ blood, and no glucose. Microscopic examination reveals three to four RBC casts per high-power field, as well as many RBCs and WBCs. No bacteria are visible. Which of the following is the most likely cause of this acute renal syndrome?

[A] Poststreptococcal glomerulonephritis
[B] Systemic lupus erythematosus
[C] Goodpasture's syndrome
[D] Immunoglobulin A nephropathy
[E] Allergic reaction to penicillin

11. A 64-year-old man enters the hospital because of renal insufficiency. Until 6 months earlier, when he developed persistent back pain, he was in good health. At that time, he was found to be severely anemic, and his BUN and creatinine levels were elevated (42 and 4.6 mg/dL, respectively).

He now undergoes further evaluation. He denies the use of any medications, any past history of renal injury, and any difficulty in voiding. He does complain of persistent weakness and easy fatigability, and his back pain has become more severe over the last 2 weeks.

On physical examination, blood pressure is 120/80 mm Hg, pulse is 70 bpm, respiratory rate is 15 breaths per minute, and temperature is 37.0°C. Major physical findings include severe pallor, as well as clear evidence of muscle wasting. Urinalysis reveals 1+ protein on dipstick testing and 4+ on sulfosalicylic acid testing. Microscopic examination of the urine reveals an occasional broad cast and an occasional granular cast. Laboratory studies give the following results: BUN = 61 mg/dL, creatinine = 5.1 mg/dL, serum sodium = 141 mEq/L, serum potassium = 5.6 mEq/L, serum chloride = 101 mEq/L, serum bicarbonate = 14 mEq/L, serum calcium = 11.7 mg/dL, and serum phosphorus = 6.0 mg/dL. Which of the following is the most likely cause of this condition?

[A] Renovascular disease
[B] Thrombotic renal disease

C Multiple myeloma

D Systemic lupus erythematosus

E Analgesic nephropathy

12. A 21-year-old woman enters the hospital because of severe anemia and acute kidney injury. Three weeks prior to admission, she had delivered a normal, full-term infant and had felt extremely weak and fatigued following delivery. Her physician notes that she is extremely pale. A complete blood count reveals severe anemia as well as thrombocytopenia. Further laboratory screening reveals elevated BUN and creatinine, and she is referred for admission. She denies any medication use postpartum and any previous medical problems similar to this one. Her laboratory studies were normal at the time of discharge from the hospital following delivery.

On physical examination, vital signs are normal, and the only physical findings aside from her pallor are petechiae on the skin and multiple ecchymoses on the lower extremities. Laboratory studies reveal hemoglobin of 6.3 mg/dL, hematocrit of 18%, platelet count of 23,000/mm^3, BUN of 94 mg/dL, and creatinine of 9.1 mg/dL. The serum ANCA and serum ANA levels are normal. A peripheral blood smear reveals multiple schistocytes. Urinalysis reveals many RBC casts. Which of the following is the most likely diagnosis?

A Hemolytic–uremic syndrome

B Goodpasture's syndrome

C Systemic lupus erythematosus

D Idiopathic thrombocytopenic purpura

E A drug reaction

13. A 69-year-old woman complains of easy fatigability, weight loss, and dizziness. Her medical history includes a remote history of tuberculosis. Physical examination reveals a blood pressure of 100/62 mm Hg and increased skin pigmentation. Laboratory studies reveal the following: serum sodium = 129 mEq/L, serum potassium = 6.1 mEq/L, serum chloride = 100 mEq/L, plasma bicarbonate concentration [HCO_3^-] = 21 mEq/L, glucose = 88 mg/dL, and BUN = 30 mg/dL. Which of the following diagnoses best fits these findings?

A Adrenal insufficiency

B Chronic renal failure

C Adrenocorticotropic hormone–secreting tumor

D Distal (type I) renal tubular acidosis

E Syndrome of inappropriate secretion of antidiuretic hormone

14. A 27-year-old man is referred for evaluation of hematuria. For the last 6 years, he has experienced painless gross hematuria two to three times per year. The condition has always remitted spontaneously within 1–2 days, but on this occasion, bright-red blood has appeared in his urine for the last 8 days. He denies any trauma to his kidneys or any other recent illnesses. Although he has a younger brother with sickle cell anemia, the man has been free from any symptoms of this abnormality. He has no other known family history or evidence of any other renal disease, including kidney stones and infection.

Urinalysis reveals red-to-pink urine, with numerous RBCs per high-power field, and no proteinuria on orthotoluidine dipstick test. Which of the following is the most likely diagnosis at this point?

A Nephrolithiasis

B Carcinoma of the kidney

C Renal vein thrombosis

D Prostatitis

E Sickle cell trait

15. A 21-year-old man enters the hospital complaining that he has been passing dark reddish urine. He has recently recovered from a football-related knee injury incurred 3 months before, and the day before entering the hospital he engaged in vigorous physical activity for the first time since his knee injury. This morning he awoke with sore, painful muscles and the aforementioned change in the character of his urine.

Physical examination is essentially normal except for the painful muscles. Findings on urinalysis include red-brown color; pH of 5.0; specific gravity of 1.02; 3+ dipstick test for blood; and no evidence of glucose, ketones, or bilirubin. Microscopic examination of the urine reveals occasional amorphous debris and three or four granular casts but no RBCs. Which of the following conditions most likely accounts for the urinalysis?

A Myoglobinuria
B Hemolyzed blood in the urine
C Ingestion of foodstuffs containing red dye
D Urinary tract infection
E Renal trauma

16. A 37-year-old man enters the hospital with a history of recent onset of hemoptysis and acute kidney injury. Until 6 weeks ago, when he noted the onset of a cough that, over the ensuing 3 days, produced streaky, blood-tinged sputum, he had been in good health. His local physician ordered laboratory studies, which revealed a serum creatinine of 1.2 mg/dL. A chest radiograph taken at that time revealed bilateral fluffy infiltrates. The patient was treated with antibiotics and followed over the next 3 weeks; during that time, the lung picture worsened and the serum creatinine rose to 2.5 mg/dL.

Now he appears ill and in moderate distress. His blood pressure is 120/80 mm Hg, his pulse is 110 bpm, his respiratory rate is 22 breaths per minute, and his temperature is 37.2°C. Examination of the chest shows bilateral rales and a few scattered wheezes, and examination of the heart reveals tachycardia but is otherwise normal. A chest radiograph reveals bilateral fluffy alveolar infiltrates. Laboratory examination shows a BUN of 65 mg/dL, a creatinine of 4.3 mg/dL, and electrolytes within normal limits. The hemoglobin level is 8.3 mg/dL and the hematocrit is 28%. Examination of the sputum reveals blood. Urinalysis reveals many RBC casts. Serum ANCA levels are negative, as are serum complement levels. The serum anti–glomerular basement membrane (anti-GBM) antibody titer is elevated to 1:64. Which of the following represents the most likely cause of this disorder?

A ANCA-associated vasculitis
B Goodpasture's syndrome
C Systemic lupus erythematosus
D Microscopic polyarteritis nodosa
E Idiopathic crescentic glomerulonephritis

17. A 60-year-old man enters the hospital complaining of nausea, weakness, and confusion of 1 week's duration. He has a long-standing history of hypertension and CHF that has been treated with increasing amounts of diuretics and digoxin without apparent benefit.

Physical examination indicates a blood pressure of 145/90 mm Hg (without orthostatic changes), jugular venous distention, bilateral basilar rales, and +2 bilateral ankle edema. Laboratory studies reveal the following: serum sodium = 120 mEq/L, BUN = 93 mg/dL, glucose = 135 mg/dL, plasma osmolality = 252 mOsm/kg, and urine osmolality = 690 mOsm/kg. Which of the following is involved in the treatment of hyponatremia in this patient?

A 3% sodium chloride infusion
B 0.9% sodium chloride infusion
C 50 mg of hydrochlorothiazide daily
D Salt and water restriction
E Demeclocycline

18. A 27-year-old woman presents with a 6-month history of polyarthritis, facial rash, and proteinuria. Urinalysis shows red blood cell casts and white blood cells. Which of the following findings are likely with further testing?

A Nodular glomerulosclerosis
B Positive fluorescent antinuclear antibody
C Glomerular capillary endotheliosis
D Necrotizing granulomatous vasculitis
E Positive Congo red staining for amyloid

19. A 57-year-old patient with a 13-year history of poorly controlled diabetes mellitus has developed a slow rise in serum creatinine and proteinuria over the last 18 months. Which of the following pathologic or laboratory findings is likely in this setting?

   [A] Nodular glomerulosclerosis
   [B] Positive fluorescent antinuclear antibody
   [C] Glomerular capillary endotheliosis
   [D] Necrotizing granulomatous vasculitis
   [E] Positive Congo red staining for amyloid

20. A 17-year-old woman in the third trimester of her first pregnancy has a blood pressure of 145/95 mm Hg and 2+ proteinuria. Further testing is most likely to reveal which of the following laboratory or pathologic findings?

   [A] Nodular glomerulosclerosis
   [B] Positive fluorescent antinuclear antibody
   [C] Glomerular capillary endotheliosis
   [D] Necrotizing granulomatous vasculitis
   [E] Positive Congo red staining for amyloid

21. A 34-year-old man who is a heavy smoker develops hematuria with red blood cell casts and 2+ proteinuria along with a chest x-ray that shows a nodular, cavitating lesion in the right middle lobe. He also has a necrotic-appearing lesion in his nares. Further testing is most likely to reveal which of the following laboratory or pathologic findings?

   [A] Nodular glomerulosclerosis
   [B] Positive fluorescent antinuclear antibody
   [C] Glomerular capillary endotheliosis
   [D] Necrotizing granulomatous vasculitis
   [E] Positive Congo red staining for amyloid

22. A 68-year-old man was diagnosed with multiple myeloma 1 year ago. Over the last 3 months he has developed severe lower extremity edema. Urinalysis shows 4+ proteinuria but no other abnormalities. The serum creatinine is 1.7 mg/dL. Further testing is most likely to reveal which of the following laboratory or pathologic findings?

   [A] Nodular glomerulosclerosis
   [B] Positive fluorescent antinuclear antibody
   [C] Glomerular capillary endotheliosis
   [D] Necrotizing granulomatous vasculitis
   [E] Positive Congo red staining for amyloid

Answers and Explanations

1. The answer is A [Online Part I: I D 2]. Hypertension is an absolute contraindication to performing a renal biopsy because the incidence of subclinical bleeding at the site is high (75%). In a hypertensive patient, this bleeding may lead to a major, life-threatening hemorrhage. Mild renal insufficiency (as evidenced by a small decrease in creatinine clearance), nephrotic syndrome without urinary casts, and moderately advanced age are not contraindications to performing a renal biopsy. Multiple renal biopsies may be performed in the same patient. A previous renal biopsy is not a contraindication for subsequent biopsies.

2. The answer is C [Table 7–1]. Approximately 5%–10% of patients treated with gentamicin develop a nonoliguric form of acute kidney injury. Although the patient has received normal doses of gentamicin, its accumulation in the kidney has produced a late form of acute kidney injury. The serum creatinine level then rises while an inappropriately high dose is maintained. This rise exacerbates the renal insufficiency and prolongs the course of acute kidney injury. The nonoliguric nature of this patient's clinical condition also is a typical finding in gentamicin nephrotoxicity. Although the patient could have obstructive uropathy, the negative results of ultrasonography strongly indicate otherwise. Cephalothin can produce an acute interstitial nephritis, but the patient's clinical course is much more compatible with the more common drug-induced disease of gentamicin nephrotoxicity. Acute glomerulonephritis usually is associated with hypertension and an active urinary sediment containing casts, protein, and red blood cells.

3. The answer is C [Part II: IV C, D]. Although the arterial pH is within the normal range, the patient has two separate acid–base disturbances (metabolic acidosis and respiratory alkalosis) which, together, tend to offset their effects on pH. The low $PaCO_2$ in this case is much lower than would be expected if the patient had only respiratory compensation. Thus, if the patient has a single acid–base disturbance, namely metabolic acidosis, then the expected $PaCO_2$ is calculated using Winters' formula:

$$\text{Expected } PaCO_2 = 1.5 \times [HCO_3^-] + 8 \pm 2$$
$$= 1.5 \times 16 + 8 \pm 2$$
$$= 32 \pm 2$$

The measured $PaCO_2$ of less than 32 mm Hg indicates that the patient also has a primary respiratory disturbance, namely respiratory alkalosis.

4. The answer is D [Part I: X L]. It is critical to recognize that in a patient with diabetes and proteinuria, inhibitors of the renin–angiotensin–aldosterone system (ACEs and ARBs) are the mainstay of therapy. Although the other agents are likely to lower blood pressure, they will not provide additional renal protection. It is likely that this patient will require more than one blood pressure medication, and the next agent selected should be a thiazide, as it acts synergetically with the ACE inhibitors and ARBs.

5. The answer is A [Part I: VII A; Table 7–6]. The patient most likely has idiopathic calcium oxalate stones. This conclusion is based on the fact that it is the most common form of kidney stone, the stone is radiopaque, and many of the findings suggest that the other answers are wrong. First, uric acid stones are radiolucent, so a stone would not have been seen on the radiographic flat plate prior to the intravenous urogram. Second, xanthine stones are extremely rare and are also radiolucent. Third, struvite stones are found only in the setting of a urinary tract infection. The absence of a positive urine culture strongly suggests that struvite stones are not present. Fourth, although cystine stones could present in this fashion even though the patient is middle-aged, cystine stones typically present much earlier and represent less than 1% of the stones analyzed in large studies. Thus, on a purely statistical basis, the patient is unlikely to have cystine stones. However, all patients with kidney stone formation who have not had their stone crystallography analyzed should have a 24-hour cystine determination to be certain that cystinuria is not present.

6. The answer is A [Part III: III A]. Renal artery stenosis is a common complication in patients with longstanding hypertension and peripheral vascular disease. As many as 80% of patients with this combination of disorders have renal artery stenosis. It is typically atherosclerotic in nature and involves the ostia of the renal arteries. "Flash pulmonary edema" commonly accompanies this condition and probably represents acute changes in hemodynamic status induced by an increased sensitivity to the adrenergic nervous system. Other features of this disorder are worsening of hypertension as well as development of azotemia. This constellation of findings often necessitates intervention with either percutaneous transluminal angioplasty or surgery.

7. The answer is C [Part II: III C]. This patient has ECG changes and symptoms consistent with hyperkalemia as the result of missed dialysis. Although each of the individual responses is acceptable, the most important first step is to administer intravenous calcium gluconate, which will stabilize the myocardial membranes. This has an immediate effect. Insulin and glucose, as well as epinephrine, act rapidly, but the effect dissipates quickly. Kayexalate takes time to work to reduce the potassium load. Hemodialysis for an existing patient would be an acceptable alternative if the dialysis could be initiated rapidly.

8. The answer is A [Part I: VIII A, C]. The incidence of prostatism in elderly men is so great that it must be considered the primary cause of renal insufficiency until proven otherwise. This patient's history is classic, in that he had 1 or 2 days on which he seemed to pass no urine, followed by days of high urine flow, a pattern that is caused by the gradual accumulation of large amounts of urine in the collecting system under pressure, which eventually may overcome some degree of obstruction. The high pressure is transmitted back to the kidneys and results in renal insufficiency. Acute glomerulonephritis and acute interstitial nephritis are ruled out by the normal results of urinalysis. The possibility of acute tubular necrosis (ATN) should be considered, but no information in the history suggests recent surgery or nephrotoxic drug intake that would have produced ATN. The best way to screen for obstructive uropathy is renal ultrasonography, which would demonstrate dilated upper tract calyces.

9. The answer is A [Part I: X C; XII B 4]. This patient most likely has membranous nephropathy, which is the most common cause of nephrotic syndrome in patients in this age group. It is characterized by an absence of evidence for a high degree of glomerular inflammation. Thus, the urinalysis, which reveals little in the way of cellular elements and heavy proteinuria, supports this diagnosis. Poststreptococcal glomerulonephritis and lupus glomerulonephritis are much more likely to demonstrate active urinary sediments with RBCs and RBC casts. In addition, these conditions are often associated with systemic manifestations of the underlying disease; none are present in this patient. Amyloidosis could give a clinical picture similar to that described, but the vast majority of patients with systemic amyloidosis have systemic signs such as peripheral neuropathy, autonomic neuropathy, or cardiac disease at the time that they develop nephrotic syndrome. Diabetic nephropathy is unlikely because of the absence of history. Failure to find abnormal retinal findings on ophthalmoscopic examination would also make diabetic nephropathy an unlikely diagnosis.

10. The answer is A [Part I: X I]. The most likely etiology of this patient's acute renal syndrome is poststreptococcal glomerulonephritis. The finding of a reduced serum complement and elevated anti–streptolysin O titer in the clinical setting of a streptococcal infection strongly suggests this cause. Although SLE may produce some aspects of the clinical picture, particularly the nephritic renal syndrome, the absence of other systemic signs of SLE makes this condition highly unlikely. However, an ANA assay should be performed to fully exclude this diagnosis. Goodpasture's syndrome is unlikely in the absence of a history of pulmonary abnormalities or hemoptysis. IgA nephropathy can present as a severe, acute nephritic picture but should not produce the other serologic abnormalities seen in this patient. A reaction to penicillin can result in an acute renal injury; however, like IgA nephropathy, it is not associated with the complement and antistreptococcal antibody titers that are seen. Furthermore, nephrotic syndrome would be an uncommon consequence of penicillin reaction, which much more typically presents as an acute interstitial injury to the kidney, with renal insufficiency, eosinophils and other white cell elements in the urine, and minimal proteinuria.

11. The answer is C [Part I: X P]. Multiple myeloma is the most likely etiology. The combination of hypercalcemia and acute kidney injury raises the possibility of multiple myeloma as the bone breakdown secondary to tumor involvement releases large amounts of calcium to the extracellular fluid and hypercalcemia ensues. The renal failure in myeloma is primarily related to hypercalcemia combined with proteinaceous cast formation within the renal tubules, producing a form of intratubular obstruction as well as a tubular inflammatory lesion. The major diagnostic clue is the finding of a urinary dipstick that is mildly positive for protein in the urine but a sulfosalicylic acid test that is strongly positive. Dipstick testing does not detect the negatively charged light-chain proteins, only the albumin. The sulfosalicylic acid test detects all forms of proteins. Renovascular lesions and thrombotic renal disease could present with this picture, although they should not be associated with hypercalcemia and severe back pain, and findings on examination of the urine would not include proteins. SLE can, of course, be associated with severe anemia and joint manifestations, but hypercalcemia is not part of the picture.

12. The answer is A [Part I: XIV D 1 b]. The most likely cause of this condition is hemolytic–uremic syndrome. This syndrome is associated with platelet consumption, as well as acute renal insufficiency. This condition may occur postpartum and can be diagnosed only by examining the entire clinical picture. Patients with SLE can present with thrombocytopenia and acute kidney injury, but the negative ANA level in the absence of other systemic manifestations makes this answer unlikely. The finding of schistocytes on the peripheral smear also strongly supports the diagnosis of the microangiopathic picture, which explains to a greater extent the anemia seen. The only drug-associated cause of renal insufficiency that manifests as severe thrombocytopenia of this degree as well as severe microangiopathic hemolytic anemia is cyclosporine or penicillamine treatment. Idiopathic thrombocytopenic purpura is not associated with concurrent renal disease. The correct therapy for this condition would be to perform plasma exchange, plasma infusions, or both as the best way of limiting the injury associated with hemolytic–uremic syndrome. The etiology of this syndrome remains unclear, although it can be associated with bacterial infections, particularly when it occurs in epidemic form in children.

13. The answer is A [Part II: I B]. The findings of low blood pressure, increased skin pigmentation, hyperkalemia, and hyponatremia all point to the likely diagnosis of adrenal insufficiency. ACTH-secreting tumors, while they may produce skin pigmentations, are usually associated with hypertension and hypokalemic alkalosis due to excess mineralocorticoid secretion. Hyperkalemia due to renal failure is seen when the GFR is less than 10–15 mm^3/min. The patient's BUN of 30 mg/dL suggests only mildly impaired renal function. Distal (type I) renal tubular acidosis is characterized by hypokalemia (although occasional cases of hyperkalemia have been described).

14. The answer is E [Part I: Table 7-5; XIV F 2 b]. Sickle cell trait, nephrolithiasis, carcinoma of the kidney, renal vein thrombosis, and prostatitis all may be associated with hematuria. The finding of gross hematuria in a young man with a family history of sickle cell anemia, however, strongly suggests that, in the absence of other stigmata of sickle cell disease, he suffers from sickle cell trait. This abnormality commonly is associated with hematuria and is caused by sickling of RBCs in the vessels on the surface of the renal pelvis and papilla, leading to small areas of infarction and bleeding. Renal tumor can produce bleeding, but it is rarely so persistent in the absence of other symptoms. Renal vein thrombosis can produce hematuria but usually in the setting of severe pain and proteinuria. Nephrolithiasis also may produce relatively silent hematuria if the stone has been present for a long period, but pain typically is associated with this condition. Urinary tract infection also can be associated with hematuria, but symptoms of infection (e.g., dysuria, fever) should be present.

15. The answer is A [Part I: 🅟 Online I A 1 b, 2 a, f; and II C 3 a (5).] The finding of dark reddish urine suggests a number of underlying conditions. However, the absence of RBCs on microscopic examination of the urine combined with the positive dipstick test for blood strongly suggests the possibility of myoglobinuria. Myoglobin is a pigment that is detected by the orthotoluidine reagent on the dipstick. Although hemolyzed blood could be present in the urine, a few RBCs should be noted, whereas none are seen in this patient's urine. Although foodstuffs do contain dyes that may color the urine, these dyes do not produce positive dipstick tests for blood. This clinical picture is most consistent with myoglobinuria caused by sudden, extreme physical exertion by an individual who is not well conditioned. Such activity leads to muscle cell breakdown and the release of myoglobin into the circulation, with its ultimate filtration by the kidney and appearance in the urine.

16. The answer is B [Part I: X G]. The most likely etiology of this disorder is Goodpasture's syndrome. ANCA-associated vasculitis can present with a pulmonary bleeding syndrome associated with acute glomerulonephritis, as seen in this patient and as evidenced by the hemoptysis as well as by the active urinary sediment. However, the negative ANCA level and the absence of a destructive upper airway lesion on physical examination argue against ANCA-associated vasculitis, and the finding of positive anti–glomerular basement membrane (anti-GBM) antibodies strongly points to Goodpasture's syndrome. SLE and microscopic vasculitis can present with pulmonary hemorrhage and renal insufficiency, but neither is associated with the serologies seen in this patient. Idiopathic crescentic glomerulonephritis describes an entity similar to that seen in this patient, but the finding of positive serum anti-GBM antibody titers eliminates glomerulonephritis as an "idiopathic" entity.

17. The answer is D [Part II: I B 5]. Water restriction should help produce a negative water balance. Salt restriction is also needed because the patient has excess total sodium burden; this change should also optimize the response to diuretics. Hyponatremia in the setting of an expanded extracellular volume (e.g., CHF) develops because of diminished renal ability to excrete water in the face of continuing water ingestion. The renal diluting defect is the result of impaired delivery of tubular fluid to distal diluting nephron segments and is precipitated by enhanced proximal tubular reabsorption. The latter is caused by decreased renal perfusion as a result of impaired cardiac output. A decrease in effective arterial volume also stimulates ADH release, which further impairs urinary dilution. Ideally, treatment should be directed at improving cardiac function. Digoxin and diuretics have been administered without significant benefit. The patient certainly cannot tolerate any saline infusions because this treatment would aggravate his congestive symptoms. Hydrochlorothiazide added to his regimen may not be sufficiently potent to improve the refractory congestive symptoms; besides, hydrochlorothiazide itself impairs urinary dilution and may aggravate the hyponatremia. Demeclocycline for the treatment of hyponatremia is reserved for the chronic management of the syndrome of inappropriate antidiuretic hormone. Because of its potential nephrotoxicity, demeclocycline is contraindicated in all states of azotemia, as in this case.

18. The answer is B [Part I: X M 1 a (2) (b)]. The patient has SLE. The glomerular abnormalities of SLE form a disease spectrum, with four associated major lesions: focal proliferative, diffuse proliferative, membranous, and mesangial forms of lupus nephritis. Serologic studies of the four lesions determine differing levels of anti-DNA antibodies and complement components, but common to all four are immunofluorescent findings for ANA. Nodular glomerulosclerosis is a pathologic lesion characteristic of diabetic nephropathy. Glomerular capillary endotheliosis is the pathologic finding in the kidney of patients with preeclampsia. Necrotizing granulomatous vasculitis is characteristic of ANCA-associated vasculitis but may be seen in other vasculitic conditions as well. Congo red staining for amyloid is seen in primary and secondary forms of amyloidosis, which can cause the nephrotic syndrome if there is kidney involvement.

19. The answer is A [Part I: X L 3 b]. All lesions in the kidneys of individuals with diabetes mellitus are grouped under the term diabetic nephropathy. The foremost clinical feature of diabetic glomerular disease is overt proteinuria, which develops after a prolonged course of diabetes mellitus. Although diffuse glomerulosclerosis is the most common lesion (found in 90% of all diabetic individuals with overt nephropathy) and is correlated with the degree of proteinuria and the renal failure, it is neither specific for nor diagnostic of diabetes. In contrast, the other major renal lesion associated with diabetes—nodular glomerulosclerosis (Kimmelstiel–Wilson syndrome)—is both specific for and diagnostic of diabetic glomerulopathy. A positive ANA is a typical feature of systemic lupus erythematosus. Glomerular capillary endotheliosis is the pathologic finding in the kidney of patients with preeclampsia. Necrotizing granulomatous vasculitis is characteristic of ANCA-associated vasculitis or other vasculitic conditions. Congo red staining for amyloid is seen in primary and secondary forms of amyloidosis, which can typically cause the nephrotic syndrome.

20. The answer is C [Online Part I: XV E]. Preeclampsia is the toxemia of pregnancy; this syndrome includes hypertension, edema, and proteinuria. Eclampsia includes the preeclamptic spectrum of symptoms combined with associated maternal convulsions and coma. The primary pathologic renal feature is glomerular capillary endotheliosis. A positive ANA is a typical feature of systemic lupus erythematosus. Necrotizing granulomatous vasculitis is characteristic of ANCA-associated vasculitis or other vasculitic conditions. Congo red staining for amyloid is seen in primary and secondary forms of amyloidosis, which can cause the nephrotic syndrome if there is kidney involvement.

21. The answer is D [Part I: X N 3]. Necrotizing granulomatous vasculitis (ANCA-associated vasculitis) is characterized by upper or lower respiratory tract symptoms of necrotizing vasculitis and granulomatous inflammation. The kidneys are involved in approximately 50% of patients. Individually, the vasculitis and granulomatous inflammation are not specific for ANCA-associated vasculitis; both must be histologically evident for diagnosis. The most recognizable presentation of the condition is the occurrence of necrotizing lesions. A positive ANA is a typical feature of systemic lupus erythematosus. Glomerular capillary endotheliosis is the pathologic finding in the kidney of patients with preeclampsia. Congo red staining for amyloid is seen in primary and secondary forms of amyloidosis, which can cause the nephrotic syndrome if there is kidney involvement.

22. The answer is E [Part I: X P 2; Online Table 7–12]. One of the main associations of multiple myeloma is the development of primary amyloidosis with light-chain restriction. Congo red staining is rather specific for identifying amyloidosis. Primary amyloidosis (AL) or secondary amyloidosis (AA) forms often affect the kidneys and typically cause the nephrotic syndrome with progressive renal insufficiency. A positive ANA is a typical feature of systemic lupus erythematosus. Glomerular capillary endotheliosis is the pathologic finding in the kidney of patients with preeclampsia. Necrotizing granulomatous vasculitis is characteristic of ANCA-associated vasculitis or other vasculitic conditions.

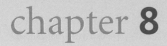

chapter **8**

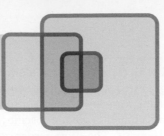

Allergic and Immunologic Disorders

JANELL A. SHERR • ROBERT HABICHT • MARY E. BOLLINGER

I OVERVIEW OF THE IMMUNE SYSTEM

II PATHOGENESIS OF THE IMMUNOGLOBULIN E–MEDIATED ALLERGIC REACTION

Antigen-stimulated release of mediators by cross-linking immunoglobulin E (IgE) molecules onto IgE-sensitized mast cells is an **IgE-mediated hypersensitivity reaction.** These reactions are the cause of many allergic disorders, including allergic rhinitis, urticaria, generalized anaphylaxis, insect sting sensitivity, food allergy, and some drug reactions (see III–VII). These reactions all require prior exposure (sensitization) to the antigen, and sometimes several exposures are needed for the allergic response to occur.

A **The IgE-mediated allergic response** can be divided into an early phase and a late phase. The early phase occurs soon after antigen exposure and is dominated by mast cells and histamine release. The late phase can occur hours later without additional exposure to antigen and, in addition to mast cells, involves neutrophils, lymphocytes, and eosinophils and release of additional mediators.

B **Initial exposure to antigen** stimulates the production of specific IgE molecules, which bind to high-affinity Fc receptors on the surface of mast cells. On reexposure, antigen cross-linking of these membrane-bound IgE molecules results in the release of inflammatory mediators from the mast cell and the recruitment of helper T cells. Examples of inflammatory mediators include histamine, prostaglandins, and leukotrienes.

III RHINITIS

A **Definition** Rhinitis is a disorder of the nasal mucosa that is characterized by nasal blockage, rhinorrhea, sneezing, and pruritus. Inflammation is usually present. Rhinitis can be divided into the following two categories:

1. **Allergic rhinitis:** This involves mast cell degranulation initiated by antigen cross-linking of IgE on the surface. There are two major classes of allergic rhinitis:
   a. **Seasonal allergic rhinitis** has periodic symptoms that occur only during the pollinating season of the antigen to which the patient is sensitive.
   b. **Perennial allergic rhinitis** has continuous or intermittent symptoms that occur year-round.
2. **Nonallergic rhinitis:** Symptoms may be periodic or perennial and are not IgE mediated. Examples include vasomotor rhinitis, infectious rhinitis, nonallergic rhinitis with eosinophilia syndrome (NARES), and hormonal rhinitis.
   a. **Vasomotor rhinitis** is a syndrome characterized by nasal blockage and rhinorrhea without evidence of immunologic or infectious nasal disease. Response to medical therapy often is poor.
   b. **Infectious rhinitis** can be an acute or chronic condition. The vast majority of acute infectious rhinitis is viral; however, secondary bacterial infections involving the sinuses can occur. No diagnostic value has been found in routine nasopharyngeal cultures. Infectious rhinitis often occurs in patients with underlying allergic rhinitis and usually is associated with reddened nasal mucosa, thick nasal secretions, sore throat, cervical adenopathy, and low-grade fever.

    c. NARES causes perennial symptoms that are similar to those of vasomotor and allergic rhinitis; however, in eosinophilic nonallergic rhinitis, nasal eosinophilia is present, nasal polyps are common, and allergy testing is usually negative. Symptoms usually respond to medical management. NARES may be a precursor of the **aspirin triad,** which includes nasal polyps, asthma, and chronic sinus disease. Symptoms are exacerbated after administration of aspirin or other nonsteroidal anti-inflammatory drugs (NSAIDs).

    d. Hormonal rhinitis can be caused by pregnancy, menstruation, or hormonal therapy. Pregnancy-induced rhinitis is characterized by significant congestion. Symptoms usually begin in the second month of pregnancy and usually resolve within 2 weeks of delivery. Rhinitis can also be found in patients with **hypothyroidism.**

    e. Anatomic abnormalities such as deviated septum may cause nasal obstruction. When unilateral discharge with a foul odor is present, obstruction by a foreign body should be suspected.

B **Prevalence**   Most studies suggest a pure nonallergic to allergic rhinitis ratio of 1:3, with the prevalence of allergic rhinitis increasing worldwide. Although accurate estimates are difficult to obtain, it is believed that 10%–30% of adults and up to 40% of children have allergic rhinitis, making this the most common chronic disorder of the respiratory tract. There is no apparent male or female predilection for allergic rhinitis, and no ethnic or racial patterns have been identified. Symptoms may begin at any age but develop in most patients before age 20 years. A history of allergic disorders in the immediate family is common. It is estimated that mixed rhinitis, with both allergic and nonallergic features, occurs in 44%–87% of patients diagnosed with allergic rhinitis, making it the most common form of rhinitis.

C **Etiology of allergic rhinitis**   Various aeroallergens (e.g., spores, pollens, and animal allergens) trigger the IgE-mediated hypersensitivity reaction that underlies allergic rhinitis.

  1. Specific seasonal allergens have typical calendar patterns, although this can vary depending on a location's altitude, latitude, and predominant vegetation. For example, in the northeastern United States:

    a. Tree pollen season runs from February to May.

    b. Grass pollen season is heaviest in May and June.

    c. Ragweed pollen season runs from mid-August until the first frost.

    d. Mold spores are high during damp weather, especially with wet leaves on the ground in the autumn.

  2. Specific perennial allergens

    a. Dust mites live primarily in bedding and feed on desquamated skin. They produce allergenic feces, which can be a significant cause of chronic symptoms.

    b. Epidermal antigens are produced primarily by furry pets such as cats, dogs, and rabbits.

    c. Indoor molds (i.e., spores found in homes) include *Aspergillus* and *Penicillium*.

    d. Other allergen sources include cockroaches and mice.

  3. Nonspecific irritants, which are not true allergens, include cigarette smoke, air pollution, perfumes, cooking odors, and chemical fumes.

D **Clinical features of allergic rhinitis**

  1. Characteristic symptoms

    a. Sneezing—often with paroxysms of 15–20 sneezes in quick succession—is characteristic and likely to occur in the early morning hours but can vary throughout the day and night depending on the trigger.

    b. Pruritus of the nose, palate, and pharynx is common and may lead to the "allergic salute" sign, characterized by repeatedly pushing up on the end of the nose, often causing a transverse nasal crease.

    c. A **thin, watery nasal discharge** usually is present and is associated with varying amounts of nasal obstruction and postnasal drainage. Mouth breathing is common due to nasal obstruction.

    d. Excess lacrimation as well as ocular pruritus and soreness are common.

    e. Loss of olfaction and **taste** may result from chronic severe nasal congestion.

    f. Otitis media, resulting from impaired drainage of the eustachian tube, and **sinusitis,** resulting from impaired drainage of the paranasal sinuses, sometimes occur.

2. **Characteristic physical findings** usually are seen at the time of maximal exposure to the offending antigens (e.g., during the height of the pollen season).
   a. **Nasal findings**
      (1) The nasal cavity characteristically contains thin nasal secretions, and the mucosal surface is edematous, boggy, and usually pale or bluish.
      (2) Nasal polyps may be seen but are **not** common in allergic rhinitis. If they are present, a workup of cyatic fibrosis in children and aspirin/NSAID sensitivity in adults and children should be considered.
      (3) Evidence of recent epistaxis in the anterior nasal vault may be seen if a patient's nasal congestion has led to frequent nose rubbing.
   b. **Allergic conjunctival findings** are often also found in patients with allergic rhinitis and include injection and swelling, excess lacrimation, granularity, and, occasionally, chemosis. Infraorbital "shiners" (infraorbital venous congestion) may develop.
   c. **Oropharyngeal findings** include mucus streaming down the posterior pharynx and cobblestoning of the lymphoid tissue of the same area.
   d. **Possible findings in children who have severe chronic nasal congestion** include broadened bony dorsum of the nose, narrowed high palatal arch, halitosis, retrognathic facies, excess gingival and pharyngeal lymphoid tissue, and dental abnormalities.

E Evaluation

1. **Diagnostic tests**
   a. Accurately applied **skin tests** with potent and specific antigens are the best diagnostic procedures to identify the antigens causing IgE-mediated allergic rhinitis.
   b. The **radioallergosorbent test (RAST)** is a serologic test for antigen specific IgE. Its sensitivity and specificity have improved dramatically, and for many allergens it is as accurate as skin tests. It is routinely used for patients with extensive eczematoid dermatitis, significant dermatographism, or a complicated history without corroborative skin tests.
   c. An **elevated IgE level** is present in only 30%–40% of patients with allergic rhinitis and is not a good screening test for this disorder. Clinicians also must consider other possible causes of elevated IgE levels, such as immunodeficiency disorders (see VIII). Total serum IgE should not be routinely used in the diagnosis of allergic rhinitis.
   d. **Peripheral eosinophilia** may be seen but is an **inconsistent** finding in patients with allergic rhinitis.
   e. A **stained smear of nasal secretions** at the time of clinically active disease often shows a higher number of eosinophils, but this finding also may be seen in patients with eosinophilic nonallergic rhinitis [III A 2 c], in hyperplastic sinusitis, and in normal infants younger than 6 months of age.

F Therapy Management is stepwise and involves avoidance of any offending allergens and provocative substances, administration of selective pharmacologic agents, and, in some instances, initiation of allergen immunotherapy.

1. **Avoidance.** *A first-line therapy.* This aspect of management is most successful when a single antigen (e.g., animal dander) is responsible for symptoms. In patients with multiple sensitivities, sensible environmental precautions are recommended and appear to limit severe exacerbation of symptoms. Environmental control measures can be utilized to decrease allergen exposure. Examples include use of air conditioning to minimize pollen exposure within buildings, removal of carpet to decrease the reservoir for dust mite and pet allergens, fixing leaks/drainage problems, use of bleach to remove mold, and use of pillow and mattress encasements to reduce dust mite exposure.

2. **Pharmacologic agents**
   a. **H_1-receptor antagonists** (i.e., **antihistamines**) are useful in controlling rhinorrhea and pruritus but have little clinical effect on nasal congestion. Sedation with impaired school or job performance is an undesirable side effect of first-generation H_1-receptor antagonists. Because second-generation antihistamines are not associated with these side effects, they are usually considered first as the initial pharmacologic treatment for allergic rhinitis.
      (1) **First-generation H_1-receptor antagonists**
         (a) Ethanolamines (e.g., diphenhydramine) are effective but often produce significant sedation and atropine-like side effects.

        (b) Ethylenediamines (e.g., pyrilamine) also are effective, produce less sedation than ethanolamines, and have minimal gastrointestinal side effects.

        (c) Alkylamines (e.g., chlorpheniramine) are effective and produce minimal to modest sedation.

    (2) Second-generation H_1-receptor antagonists

        (a) Loratadine, desloratadine, cetirizine, levocetirizine, and fexofenadine can be administered once daily and have not been associated with adverse cardiovascular effects.

        (b) All second-generation H_1-receptor antagonists lack anticholinergic side effects but may produce mild sedation if given at higher-than-usual doses. Cetirizine will produce sedation in some patients at recommended doses.

    (3) Intranasal H_1-receptor antagonists. Azelastine hydrochloride, which is approved for use in the United States, has an efficacy equal to that of oral H_1- and H_2-receptor antagonists. It also may reduce nasal blockage. Twenty percent of patients perceive a bitter taste.

  b. Adrenergic agonists (also known as **sympathomimetic medications or decongestants**)

    (1) Oral administration of an α-adrenergic agent (e.g., pseudoephedrine) is effective in reducing nasal congestion but not rhinorrhea. Central nervous system (CNS) stimulation may occur leading to insomnia, irritability, and palpitations, as well as hypertension and loss of appetite. Short-term use is preferable (<10 days).

    (2) Topical application of short-acting phenylephrine or long-acting oxymetazoline decreases nasal congestion, but regular administration for more than 3–4 days results in severe rebound nasal congestion (rhinitis medicamentosa).

  c. Cromolyn sodium. A 4% solution of cromolyn sodium is available for topical nasal use. It must be administered frequently (three to six times daily) but is effective in treating both seasonal and perennial allergic rhinitis. Because side effects are minimal, cromolyn sodium may at times be preferred to topical nasal steroids, but it is less effective. Pretreatment before allergen exposure may significantly reduce nasal allergic response.

  d. Corticosteroids

    (1) Topical agents. Highly effective and rapidly metabolized topical steroid preparations (e.g., mometasone furoate monohydrate, budesonide, flunisolide acetate, triamcinolone acetonide, fluticasone propionate, and ciclesonide) are the most effective medications to treat seasonal and perennial allergic rhinitis. This class of medications is considered the treatment of choice. These preparations have minimal systemic side effects; irritation and bleeding rarely occur, and *Candida* overgrowth is very uncommon.

    (2) Systemic agents. Systemic corticosteroids significantly improve symptoms during the height of a specific pollen season. This treatment is rarely indicated, however, and use of long-term oral corticosteroid therapy for perennial allergic rhinitis is ill advised because of the deleterious side effects.

  e. Intranasal anticholinergics. Ipratropium bromide nasal spray (0.03% and 0.06%) is available for topical use. Rhinorrhea but not other nasal symptoms are effectively reduced. Side effects, although minimal (5%), include dryness and transient epistaxis.

  f. Oral antileukotriene agents. Data suggest that these medications may be helpful when used alone or in combination with antihistamines. Montelukast sodium has been approved for this indication. Further studies are needed to define the role of these agents in the treatment of allergic rhinitis.

3. Immunotherapy. Such treatment may be indicated if patients continue to experience clinically significant symptoms after appropriate environmental avoidance and pharmacologic measures have been taken. Although treatment is time consuming and does not provide complete relief for all patients, increased cost of other medications makes immunotherapy relatively cost-effective.

4. Surgery. There is no effective surgical treatment for allergic rhinitis.

IV   URTICARIA AND ANGIOEDEMA

A **Definitions**

1. Urticaria (commonly known as **hives**) is a pruritic and sometimes painful or burning transient skin eruption involving superficial layers of the skin, with individual lesions presenting as

TABLE 8-1 Clinical Classification of Chronic Urticaria and Angioedema

Type	Subtype	Eliciting Factors
Physical urticarias (reproduced by stimulus in a predictable manner)	Dermatographism	Minor trauma/stroking the skin
	Delayed pressure	Sitting, lying, wearing tight clothing, running
	Vibratory	Prolonged occupational exposure to vibration
	Cold contact	Sudden exposure to cold
	Localized heat	Exposure to hot surfaces and objects
	Cholinergic	Emotion, states of increased body temperature
	Aquagenic	Hot or cold water exposure
	Solar	Exposure to sun or ultraviolet light
	Exercise induced	Physical exertion
Angioedema without wheals	Idiopathic	Stress, viral infection
	C1-esterase deficiency	Stress, infection
	Drug induced	Angiotensin-converting-enzyme inhibitors, nonsteroidal anti-inflammatory drugs, statins
Contact urticaria	IgE-mediated response	Latex, food, chemicals
Vasculitis	Urticarial vasculitis	Infection, drugs, autoimmune processes, malignancy
Rare hereditary syndromes	Cryopyrin-associated periodic syndromes (CIAS1 mutations)	Cold temperatures
Rare acquired syndromes	Schnitzler's syndrome	Cold temperatures

erythematous circumscribed papules, or wheals, often with white edematous centers. Lesions are annular, round, figurate, or confluent. Repeated scratching often results in a thickening of the skin known as **lichenification.**

2. **Angioedema** may occur alone or jointly with urticaria. Angioedema is usually of longer duration than urticaria and involves swelling of the deeper subcutaneous tissue—particularly in areas of loose connective tissue around the mouth, eyelids, and male genitalia. Angioedema in the submucosa of the upper respiratory tract may lead to laryngeal obstruction, an airway emergency. Clinically significant causes of angioedema include angiotensin-converting-enzyme (**ACE**) **inhibitors, NSAIDs,** and hereditary deficiencies in the complement systems (also known as **hereditary angioedema**).

B **Clinical classification of urticarias and angioedema (Table 8–1)**

1. **Urticaria** can be categorized as **acute** (lasting up to 6 weeks), **chronic** (lasting for 6 weeks or more), or **episodic** with acute intermittent or recurrent activity.
   a. **Acute urticaria** usually results from exposure to food products or medications or contact with an environmental allergen such as latex. It is the result of an IgE-mediated reaction and can frequently be diagnosed by obtaining a good history of exposures. Investigations are typically not needed but may include skin-prick testing and immunoCAP fluoroimmunoassay to evaluate in vitro allergen-specific serum IgE.
   b. **Chronic urticaria** may result from a number of conditions, including cancer and immunologic disorders like systemic lupus erythematosus; however, the etiology remains unknown in most cases.

2. **Angioedema** commonly occurs in the setting of urticaria but may present separately. Angioedema without urticaria is a classic feature of **acquired** or **hereditary angioedema (HAE).** Both disease processes result from C1 esterase inhibitor (C1 inh) deficiency but can be differentiated based on testing for levels and activity of C1 inh as well as for C4 and C1q. Further evaluation may involve genetic testing.

C **Therapy**

1. **Prevention of further episodes** involves avoidance of known evocative agents (e.g., foods, medications, and physical factors) and identification and management of underlying medical disorders, including autoimmune and endocrine processes, lymphoreticular neoplasms, and connective tissue disorders.

2. **Drug treatment of urticaria** usually proceeds in a stepwise fashion.
   a. **H₁-receptor blockers** alone often are effective. Second-generation antihistamines (e.g., loratadine, desloratadine, cetirizine, levocetirizine, fexofenadine) are effective treatments for urticaria and are typically preferred over first-generation antihistamines because of lower sedation side-effect profiles. First-generation antihistamines (e.g., cyproheptadine, hydroxyzine, diphenhydramine) may be preferred, however, for reducing the pruritis associated with urticaria and may be used in conjunction with second-generation antihistamines for more resistant cases.
   b. **Adding an H₂-receptor blocker** such as ranitidine or cimetidine often has a synergistic effect because H₂ receptors make up approximately 15% of the histamine receptors in cutaneous blood vessels. H₂-receptor blockers alone, however, are not effective. Doxepin, which blocks both H₁ and H₂ receptors, is sometimes useful in treating refractory urticaria.
   c. **Systemic steroids** are reserved for severe cases. A skin biopsy is suggested before maintenance steroid therapy is started to rule out underlying causes such as vasculitis.

3. **Drug treatment of angioedema** usually proceeds in a stepwise fashion.
   a. **Limited androgens** such as danazol are effective in treating C1 esterase inh deficiency, a cause of hereditary angioedema (HAE).
   b. **Berinert,** a plasma-derived C1-esterase inhibitor concentrate, was approved by the Food and Drug Administration in 2009 for acute treatment of abdominal attacks and facial edema associated with HAE.
   c. **Ecallantide** (Kalbitor), a plasma kallikrein inhibitor, is also approved for acute treatment of HAE.
   d. **Intramuscular epinephrine** can be life saving in severe laryngeal angioedema and anaphylaxis but may not be effective in HAE.

V GENERALIZED ANAPHYLAXIS

A Definition Anaphylaxis is an acute life-threatening hypersensitivity syndrome mediated by IgE. It affects multiple organ systems and results from the precipitous and massive release of inflammatory mediators from both mast cells and basophils. Symptoms usually begin within minutes of exposure to the causative factor and peak within 1 hour but can take up to 4 hours for the most severe symptoms (see V D). **Anaphylactoid reactions** have a similar clinical picture; however, they are not IgE mediated. Common practice is to use the term "anaphylaxis" for both types of reactions, given the similar clinical course and treatments.

B Incidence Exact incidence rates are unknown, probably because of inconsistent diagnoses of the anaphylaxis syndrome. Multiple studies have shown a deficiency in physician knowledge regarding signs and symptoms of anaphylaxis, leading to underreporting. Studies suggest an increase in the prevalence of anaphylaxis in children younger than 5 years of age and an increase in deaths from medication-induced anaphylaxis in the elderly.

C Etiology A variety of mechanisms, summarized in Table 8–2, can initiate "anaphylactic" reactions in which both IgE- and non–IgE-mediated etiologies may play a role.

1. **IgE-mediated (anaphylaxis).** The binding of IgE antibodies either to complete antigens or to antigenic determinants on hapten–carrier complexes can precipitate the release of inflammatory mediators. The most common causes of IgE-mediated anaphylaxis include **food** (most notably **peanuts, tree nuts, shellfish,** and **scaled fish**), **latex** (especially in **health care workers, medications, insect venoms,** and **inhaled allergens.** In children, foods are the most common cause of anaphylaxis. In adults, insect stings and medications are the most common cause.

2. **Non–IgE-mediated (anaphylactoid)**
   a. Certain substances [e.g., opiate analgesics, radiocontrast media, NSAIDs (aspirin)] can stimulate degranulation of effector cells directly without cross-linking of IgE.
   b. **Anaphylatoxin mediated.** Human blood products (plasma, immunoglobulins, and cryoprecipitates) can cause significant complement activation through the formation of immune complexes. This generates large amounts of the complement degradation products C3a and C5a. These protein fragments act as anaphylatoxins, binding to mast cell receptors and triggering mediator release.

TABLE 8–2 Etiologic Mechanisms of Anaphylaxis	
Mechanism	**Typical Allergens**

IgE-mediated mediator release	Drugs
	  Sulfonamides
	  Tetracyclines
	  Penicillins
	  Cephalosporins
	  Local anesthetics
	Insect venoms
	Allergen extracts
	Chymopapain
	Streptokinase
	Insulin
	(Any food can cause a reaction)
	Food
	  Shellfish/scaled fish
	  Peanuts/tree nuts
	  Eggs
	  Milk

Direct mast cell mediator release	Drugs
	  Polymyxin B
	  Opiates
	  Vancomycin
	  Radiocontrast media

Anaphylatoxin-induced mediator release
  (via complement activation)
	Human blood products
	  Plasma
	  Immunoglobulins
	  Cryoprecipitates

Other mechanisms	Nonsteroidal anti-inflammatory agents Sulfite additives Exercise Hormones

   c. Other triggers of anaphylaxis include NSAIDs (cyclooxygenase blockade leading to overproduction of leukotrienes), hormones, and exercise (the last two with unknown mechanisms).

D **Clinical features and diagnosis**   Clinical and laboratory findings characteristic of extensive mediator release are the basis for diagnosis (Table 8–3).

   1. **Diagnostic findings and symptoms** may include the following:
      a. Bronchial obstruction
      b. Upper airway obstruction
      c. Acute hypotension
      d. Urticaria
      e. Angioedema
      f. Vomiting, diarrhea, and/or abdominal pain
         Any heart, lung, or blood (e.g., hypotension) symptoms and/or **two or more organ systems** involved (e.g., skin and gastrointestinal symptoms) warrant immediate treatment with epinephrine.

   2. **Risk factors** for developing difficult-to-treat anaphylaxis include underlying **asthma** or **cardiac disease** and **nut allergy.**

   3. **Clinical course**
      a. Uniphasic: Symptoms occur within minutes to less than 1 hour from exposure and usually dissipate within 4–6 hours if appropriate treatment is initiated.

TABLE 8–3   Signs and Symptoms of Anaphylaxis

Organ or Organ System Affected (% Individuals Involved)	Characteristic Signs and Symptoms
Skin (88%)	Pruritus
	Flushing
	Urticaria
	Angioedema
Eyes (16%)	Ocular pruritus
	Excess lacrimation
	Conjunctival injection
Respiratory system	Nasal congestion
Upper airway edema (56%)	Rhinorrhea
Dyspnea and wheezing (47%)	Cough
	Hoarseness
	Stridor
	Wheezing
	Laryngeal edema
Cardiovascular system (33%)	Weakness
	Palpitations
	Tachycardia
	Hypotension
	Arrhythmias
	Shock
	Cardiac arrest
Gastrointestinal system (30%)	Cramping
	Nausea
	Diarrhea
	Vomiting
	Abdominal distention
	Metallic taste

    b. Biphasic: Up to 50% of cases may exhibit a biphasic (early and late phase) pattern. The appearance of new signs and symptoms, or the recurrence of symptoms, is noted several hours after the initial onset of the reaction. The signs and symptoms seen with the late phase may be similar or worse than those of the early phase.

    c. Protracted: Anaphylaxis can last several hours to days. Given the variations in clinical course, it is important that clinicians be particularly vigilant, as death can occur at any time during this period.

E **Therapy**

    1. Epinephrine. This is the most effective therapy and should be given immediately to treat anaphylaxis. Intramuscular injection of epinephrine in the lateral thigh is the most effective method of medication delivery. Timing is critical—delays in epinephrine injection are associated with increased mortality. In some cases repeated dosing is needed, and in more severe (protracted) cases, intravenous drips of epinephrine may be required. Patients at risk of anaphylaxis should carry self-injectable epinephrine kits with them at all times.

    2. Diphenhydramine (25–50 mg or 1-mg/kg pediatric dose) is given intravenously. This therapy will not stop an anaphylactic reaction but is used as adjunctive therapy to epinephrine.

    3. Corticosteroids (1–2 mg/kg) are administered intravenously. Corticosteroids are used to decrease the late-phase inflammatory response [II A].

    4. Intravenous fluids, volume expanders, and **pressor agents** are used to maintain blood pressure. **Supplemental oxygen** and even **mechanical ventilation** may be needed for respiratory support.

    5. Patients on **β-blockers** may be refractory to treatment of anaphylaxis. In this case, **glucagon** can be given in addition to epinephrine to provide both inotropic effects and chronotropic effects on the heart by increasing intracellular levels of cyclic adenosine 3′5′-monophosphate, independent of the β-adrenergic receptors.

6. Given the biphasic and protracted clinical course that can occur with anaphylaxis, **close monitoring** for 4–6 hours (or longer in severe cases) after the initial reaction is recommended. Patients with allergies at risk for anaphylaxis should wear a medical alert device.

VI · FOOD HYPERSENSITIVITY

A **Definition and Prevalence**   Food allergy refers to an immunologic response to a food protein and impacts approximately 12 million people in the United States. Prevalence rates are about 8% in children and up to 4% in adults. Food reactions can be IgE mediated (e.g., acute urticaria, angioedema, anaphylaxis), non-IgE mediated (e.g., allergic colitis), or combined (e.g., eosinophilic esophagitis). Up to one half of anaphylaxis cases are food induced.

B **Diagnosis** is by detailed history, skin testing, and/or serologic testing for food-specific IgE; in some cases definitive diagnosis requires double-blind, placebo-controlled food challenge. Delayed-type reactions such as seen with eosinophilic esophagitis may also require patch testing for foods to identify triggers. The most common foods in children are egg, milk, soy, wheat, peanut, tree nuts, scaled fish, and shellfish, and the last four are most common in adults.

C **Treatment** is strict avoidance of the offending food(s), requiring vigilant reading of labels. Food-allergic patients should have an emergency plan, self-injectable epinephrine, and medical alert identification. Treatment of allergic reactions is as previously noted [III E].

D **Natural history**   Most food allergies, such as those to egg, milk, soy, and wheat, are outgrown (about 50% by age 6 years). Peanut allergy is outgrown in about 20% and tree nut in about 9% of cases. Seafood allergy is less commonly outgrown.

E **Future directions**   Current studies are investigating desensitization procedures and use of anti-IgE monoclonal antibody in food-allergic patients.

VII · INSECT STING SENSITIVITY

Stings by a **honeybee, yellow jacket, wasp, hornet,** or **fire ant** may lead to sensitization and subsequent IgE-mediated hypersensitivity reactions.

A **Incidence**   Population studies show that up to 25% of people with no history of a systemic reaction after an insect sting nonetheless may be sensitized, as judged by positive skin tests and the presence of venom-specific IgE antibodies. As many as 20% of these individuals may have a systemic allergic reaction if stung again. It is estimated that 75–100 deaths occur in the United States each year from insect sting reactions. One study found that up to 50% of people with fatal reactions to insect stings had no prior systemic reactions.

B **Clinical features**   A **nonallergic reaction** to an insect sting consists of transient swelling, pain, and redness surrounding the injection site, all of which usually subside in 1–2 hours but can last up to 48 hours. **Allergic reactions** vary from scattered patches of urticaria to severe and fatal anaphylaxis.

1. **Large local reactions** extend a significant distance from the sting site (>8 cm), peak in 24–48 hours, and often take 5–7 days to resolve. Between 5% and 15% of patients who experience large local reactions may later develop a systemic reaction.

2. **Anaphylactic reactions** usually occur within a few minutes of the sting and may involve the skin (urticaria, angioedema, and pruritus), the respiratory tract (laryngeal edema and bronchospasm), the vascular system (hypotension), and the gastrointestinal system (diarrhea, abdominal cramps, and nausea). About 60% of systemic reactions in children are mild with just cutaneous manifestations, whereas in adults, respiratory or cardiovascular symptoms occur in about 70% of systemic reactions.

3. **Delayed reactions** include serum sickness, vasculitis, Guillain-Barré syndrome, glomerulonephritis, and myocarditis. The etiology of these reactions is unclear. Insect stings may also initiate biphasic anaphylactic reactions, which may be confused with a delayed reaction if symptoms in the initial phase are mild and therefore not appreciated.

C **Risk factors for severe reactions to insect stings**

1. Repeat stings may cause similar but more severe symptoms, especially if the interval between stings is short.

2. The risk of recurrence of systemic reactions increases with more severe initial reactions.

D **Diagnosis**

1. An accurate **history** of the symptoms and signs of a systemic allergic reaction after a sting is necessary.

2. **Specific antivenom IgE antibodies** are detected by prick or intradermal tests and/or serologic testing. In patients with large local reactions to insect stings, allergy tests are positive in up to 80% of cases. In adults with systemic reactions, studies have shown that serum IgE and/or skin tests are positive in 50%–100% of cases.

E **Therapy**

1. **Immediate therapeutic measures** are similar to those used in the treatment of anaphylaxis from any cause [see V E].

2. **Prophylactic therapy**
   a. **Avoidance** of insects that induce sensitivity.
   b. All at-risk individuals should own and know how to use a **self-injectable epinephrine kit.** Even in the absence of positive allergy testing, patients with a history of severe allergic reactions should carry these devices. Individuals should also wear a medical alert device.
   c. Individuals who have had an anaphylactic reaction to an insect sting require **specific venom immunotherapy (VIT)** if allergy tests are positive, which would then decrease their risk of anaphylaxis to that of the general population. Without immunotherapy, roughly 30%–60% of patients with a history of anaphylaxis to an insect sting and positive testing for specific IgE will experience a severe reaction if stung again. Currently, the duration of VIT is under debate. Most allergists consider discontinuing VIT when skin testing is negative or approximately 3–5 years after initiating treatment. VIT should be continued indefinitely in those patients with a history of severe systemic reactions with previous stings. VIT is not currently recommended for patients with only large local reactions.

VIII ADVERSE DRUG REACTIONS

A **Definitions** Adverse drug can be classified as either immune mediated or non–immune mediated. Adverse drug reactions account for approximately 106,000 deaths in the United States each year.

1. **Non–immune mediated**
   a. Known pharmacologic reactions, or **predictable responses,** are most often dose dependent and occur in normal individuals. Nearly 80% of adverse drug reactions are predictable responses, which include side effects, overdose/toxicity secondary drug effects, and drug–drug interactions. The effect of ciprofloxacin on warfarin use [increasing international normalized ratio (INR)] and dyspepsia resulting from erythromycin use are both examples of predictable responses.
   b. **Idiosyncratic** reactions are unexpected and qualitatively abnormal responses as seen, for example, with isoniazid-induced neuritis and angioedema as a result of ACE inhibitors. Idiosyncratic reactions may have a hereditary basis—for example, hemolytic anemia precipitated by quinolones in a patient with glucose-6-phosphate dehydrogenase (G6PD) deficiency.
   c. **Drug intolerance** refers to an adverse reaction that occurs at a subtherapeutic dose. Vomiting at low doses of theophylline is an example of this type of non–immune-mediated adverse drug reaction.
   d. **Pseudoallergic (anaphylactoid)** reactions are caused by direct mast cell and basophil mediator release. These reactions do not require prior sensitization and do not involve IgE antibody. Examples include reactions to opiates and radiocontrast media.

2. **Immune mediated.** Drug hypersensitivity results from an immunologic reaction that triggers an abnormal response to the drug, as seen, for example, with penicillin-induced urticaria. Hypersensitivity, or allergic reactions, constitute 7%–10% of all adverse drug reactions. Drug hypersensitivity reactions are categorized according to etiology, typically into four types using Gell and Coombs classification.

   a. **Type I** or **IgE-mediated** reactions occur when a pharmacologic agent or one of its metabolites binds with drug-specific IgE antibodies on mast cell or basophil membranes, triggering release of mediators, which can lead to symptoms such as urticaria and angioedema. As noted previously, these reactions can be severe, progressing to anaphylaxis.

   b. **Type II** or **cytotoxic** reactions result from complement-mediated damage to cell membranes precipitated by the binding of IgM or IgG antibodies to drug antigens on cell surfaces. These reactions usually involve blood cells; for example, drug-induced thrombocytopenia, granulocytopenia, and hemolytic anemia from treatment with quinidine, α-methyldopa, or penicillin, among others.

   c. **Type III** or **immune complex–mediated** reactions develop when soluble complexes of IgM or IgG antibodies and drug antigens are deposited in tissues. Complement activation occurs in the soluble phase or when the complex attaches to vessel walls, leading to inflammation and subsequent tissue injury. Rash and fever are the most common clinical manifestations, but lymphadenopathy and arthralgia may also occur. An example is serum sickness caused by injection of a foreign protein or serum.

   d. **Type IV** or **cell-mediated** reactions require sensitized T lymphocytes that recognize a drug or its metabolite. The antigen–T cell interaction leads to a lymphokine-induced inflammatory response occurring 24–72 hours after drug administration. **Contact dermatitis,** for example, from neomycin is the most common clinical example of a cell-mediated reaction. Another example is **drug-induced interstitial nephritis** from methicillin.

B **Clinical features**   Organ-specific syndromes resulting from drug allergy include the following:

1. **Dermatologic reactions** are the most common manifestations of drug sensitivity.

   a. **Urticaria,** occasionally progressing to anaphylaxis, can be precipitated by a variety of medications; the most common offenders are penicillin, sulfonamides, cephalosporins, and allergen extracts. Most urticarial reactions are the result of IgE-mediated or direct histamine release.

   b. **Fixed drug eruptions,** which are most likely attributable to a cell-mediated reaction, may develop after ingestion of tetracycline, sulfonamides, and penicillin. In this reaction, discrete, **nonpruritic** lesions with a macular-to-bullous appearance occur at the same place each time the medication is taken.

   c. **Photodermatitis** is characterized by a bright erythematous eruption or eczematoid lesions in areas exposed to ultraviolet light. Two presentations are recognized:

      (1) **Phototoxicity** as a result of ultraviolet light exposure occurs early in drug treatment. Drugs implicated in phototoxic reactions include doxycycline, coal tar derivatives, and psoralens.

      (2) **Photoallergy** occurs 4–21 days after the ingestion of the causative agent. It appears to be a cell-mediated process in which ultraviolet light induces a chemical alteration of the drug, leading to tissue sensitization and subsequent injury. Phenothiazines, griseofulvin, and sulfonamides are common offenders.

   d. **Contact dermatitis** develops 48–72 hours after topical application of the implicated medication and is characterized by a vesicular T cell–mediated inflammatory reaction. Common preparations causing these skin lesions are *para*-aminobenzoic acid (PABA), neomycin, and antihistamines.

   e. **Febrile mucocutaneous reactions** are uncommon but may be severe. Cytotoxic, immune complex, and cell-mediated reactions all contribute to the pathogenesis of these syndromes.

      (1) **Stevens–Johnson syndrome** may manifest as papular, urticarial, vesicular, or purpuric lesions involving two or more mucosal surfaces.

      (2) **Toxic epidermal necrolysis (TEN)** manifests as epithelial bullae with subsequent desquamation. TEN is often on a disease continuum with Stevens–Johnson syndrome. The main

difference between the two is the extent of skin affected, with TEN involving >30% of the skin. Fever and visceral involvement are common.

    (3) Drugs implicated in both syndromes include rifampin, phenobarbital, phenytoin, trimethoprim–sulfamethoxazole, and penicillins.

2. Hepatic syndromes result primarily in hepatocellular changes, granuloma formation, or cholestasis. Hydantoin and halothane, for example, can cause hepatocellular damage, as can aspirin when administered to children with juvenile rheumatoid arthritis. Allopurinol, methyldopa, or sulfonamides may cause granulomatous changes. Phenothiazines, azathioprine, and erythromycin estolate have been linked to cholestasis and painless jaundice.

3. Renal involvement most often takes the form of acute interstitial inflammation. Methicillin, sulfonamides, and cephalosporins have been implicated in this reaction. Membranous glomerulonephritis may occur after administration of captopril, gold, penicillamine, or probenecid.

4. Pulmonary reactions include pulmonary infiltration and bronchospasm. Pulmonary infiltration has been reported with use of nitrofurantoin, gold compounds, and methotrexate. Drug-induced bronchospasm may occur in asthmatic patients after administration of aspirin or other NSAIDs. Excess leukotriene production, resulting from inhibition of the cyclooxygenase pathway, presumably is responsible for this reaction.

C   **Diagnosis**   Because so few specific diagnostic laboratory tests are available to confirm drug allergy, obtaining an accurate history is essential. Drug allergy should be considered as the possible cause of almost any clinical symptom or sign because drug allergy reactions may mimic so many other clinical conditions.

1. Clinical features that suggest drug hypersensitivity

    a. Prior exposure to the drug.

    b. Onset of symptoms within 48 hours with previous exposure or 7 or more days after initiating drug treatment if there is no prior exposure.

    c. Administration of the drug at the recommended dose.

    d. Symptoms and signs commonly associated with known allergic reactions.

    e. Prompt disappearance of the symptoms after discontinuation of the implicated drug.

2. Specific diagnostic tests

    a. Immediate skin tests for IgE-mediated reactions (e.g., penicillin, insulin, and chymopapain). However, standardized skin testing materials are limited.

    b. Delayed skin tests or **patch testing** for cell-mediated, delayed-type hypersensitivity reactions (e.g., PABA, nickel, or other topical drugs causing contact dermatitis). A presumed antigen is placed on the skin, covered, and then reassessed for a reaction at 48 hours after application.

    c. Radioallergosorbent testing (RAST) serologic testing for specific IgE antibodies (e.g., penicillin). Sensitivity and specificity can vary.

    d. Coombs' antiglobulin test for cytotoxic reactions causing hemolytic anemia.

D   **Reactions to selected drugs and biologic agents (Table 8–4)**

E   **Prevention of drug reactions**

1. The concurrent administration of several medications should be avoided.

2. A detailed history of any previous drug reactions should be obtained for all patients to guide selection of a medication that is unlikely to cross-react.

3. Patients with documented allergic drug reactions should be instructed to carry identification (e.g., a medical alert bracelet). Medical records for such patients should be clearly marked.

4. Oral administration, when possible, is preferable to parenteral administration because the incidence of reactions after oral administration is much lower.

5. Allergic reactions are unlikely to be discovered during premarketing trials because the number of patients is small compared with the incidence of reactions, so particular vigilance is indicated when administering any new drug.

TABLE 8–4 Reactions to Selected Drugs and Biologic Agents

Drug/Biologic Agent	Clinical Features	Diagnosis/Cause	Treatment
Penicillin	Allergic reactions occur in 1%–10% of patients; monobactams rarely cross-react with penicillin; carbapenems do cross-react; up to 2% of patients have a cross-reaction to cephalosporins (first generation have a greater risk than second or third generation)	**Skin testing** is recommended when treatments are limited, but skin testing materials are limited	90% of sensitized individuals outgrow this allergy after 10 years; desensitization (for high-risk cases): administer penicillin in increments of increasing strength over several hours in a controlled setting; oral is safer then intravenous; maintain the desensitized state by administering the drug at least every 12 hours; once penicillin is discontinued, protection is lost
Radiographic contrast dye	Reactions occur in 4%–8% of patients; significantly increased risk of anaphylactoid reactions with repeat exposure; **lower-osmolarity contrast dyes** currently used decrease anaphylaxis risk; symptoms include bradycardia, hypotension, nausea, or vomiting, possibly shock	Diagnosis is based on symptoms; **there is no association between these reactions and shellfish or iodine sensitivity**	Treatment of an anaphylactoid reaction is identical to that for anaphylaxis from other cause; vagal reactions can be treated with atropine; pretreatment with prednisone and diphenhydramine and use of lower-osmolarity dyes decreases the likelihood of a repeat reaction; some experts also recommend ephedrine and an H_2-specific antihistamine
Insulin allergy and resistance (Composition: human insulin is produced by recombinant DNA technology and is less allergenic than animal preparations [bovine or porcine])	As many as 50% of people exhibiting insulin allergy also have experienced allergic reactions to other drugs; **local allergic reactions:** pruritus, swelling, and mild erythema; usually during the first few months of therapy; prolonged local reactions may result in lipoatrophy; **systemic allergic reactions:** much less common than local reactions (they occur in <0.1% of patients)	**Nonimmunologic** causes of **insulin resistance:** infection, stress, pregnancy, obesity, Cushing's syndrome, acromegaly, and leprechaunism; **immunologic insulin resistance:** mediated by IgG anti-insulin antibodies; manifested by a need for increasing daily doses; presence of high-titer IgG antibodies to insulin or to the insulin receptor	**Local allergic reactions:** often subside completely after a few weeks; antihistamines may be given alone or mixed with the insulin; divide the dose among two or more injection sites; **systemic allergic reactions:** treated similarly to generalized anaphylaxis; if insulin is restarted <24 hours after the systemic reaction, the next dose should be 1/3–1/6 the original and increased slowly; if >24 hours have passed since the reaction, a desensitization protocol must be implemented; lapses in insulin therapy increase risk of sensitization and loss of desensitized state
Protamine sulfate sensitivity (Use: A low–molecular-weight protein used to neutralize heparin prior to surgery and to prepare neutral protamine Hagedorn [NPH] insulin)	Flushing, urticaria, hypotension or hypertension, ventricular fibrillation, wheezing, noncardiac pulmonary edema, transient elevations in pulmonary artery pressure, thrombocytopenia, or neutropenia may develop	Allergic reactions to protamine sulfate have been attributed to IgE-mediated anaphylactic and complement-mediated anaphylactoid mechanisms; skin test not always reliable; higher risk of allergy in those with insulin allergy, status post vasectomy, and salmon allergy	Pretreatment with antihistamines and corticosteroids may be helpful for patients at high-risk for anaphylaxis; for high-risk surgical patients (e.g. during cardiopulmonary bypass procedures), alternative reversal agents should be used; desensitization can be performed

TABLE 8–4   Reactions to Selected Drugs and Biologic Agents (*Continued*)

Drug/Biologic Agent	Clinical Features	Diagnosis/Cause	Treatment
Angiotensin-converting-enzyme (ACE) inhibitors (Mechanism: These agents exert their effects by blockage of kininase II, which leads to elevated levels of bradykinin and substance P)	**Chronic cough:** develops in 5%–20% of patients, starts within 1 week to 6 months, most often nocturnal, nonproductive; **angioedema:** occurs in 0.1%–0.2% of patients, often develops by 24 hours or within 5–7 days; **anaphylaxis:** increased risk for those on dialysis	Based on symptoms	Chronic cough subsides 1–4 weeks after the medication is stopped; substitution of another ACE inhibitor is *not* useful; moderate symptoms resolve gradually when the drug is discontinued
Sulfonamides and HIV-infected patients	A maculopapular eruption occurs in up to 3% of sulfonamide recipients, sometimes followed by erythema multiforme or Stevens–Johnson syndrome; in HIV-infected individuals on sulfonamides, ≥50% develop a maculopapular eruption	Thought to be related to reduced levels of glutathione reductase; no reliable skin or in vitro tests are available	Oral desensitization protocols have sometimes been used successfully
Minocycline-induced lupus (Use: Minocycline is now frequently used in the long-term management of acne vulgaris)	Musculoskeletal complaints, fever, weight loss, and pleuropulmonary involvement are characteristic, with symptoms developing an average of 2 years after initiation of drug therapy; neurologic, renal, and vasculitic changes are unusual	Hepatic transaminase levels are commonly elevated; a positive antinuclear antibody (**ANA**) titer is uniformly present; **anti–double-stranded DNA** and antineutrophilic cytoplasmic antibody (**ANCA**) tests are also sometimes positive	Symptoms are self-limited once treatment with minocycline is stopped
Mumps, measles, rubella, influenza, and **yellow fever vaccines**	Grown on chick embryos; anaphylaxis after vaccination in egg-sensitive individuals has been reported but is extremely rare	In the extremely sensitive egg-allergic patient (e.g., patient who has anaphylaxis), testing using both the prick and intradermal methods should be considered before vaccination	The current recommendation is that the egg-allergic patient can be given the vaccine without concern unless anaphylactic reactions have occurred in the past; if a patient tests positive, the vaccine should be administered using a desensitization program
Aspirin reactions	**Urticaria and/or wheezing** are common; chronic rhinitis, sinusitis, and often-intractable steroid-dependent asthma develop in a small group of individuals between 30 and 60 years of age; in these individuals, life-threatening bronchospasm may occur after aspirin ingestion	Because there are no in vivo or in vitro tests for aspirin allergy, diagnosis can be made only from the medical history and by aspirin challenge	Although oral desensitization has been successful in some individuals, it is rarely indicated unless chronic treatment is needed (e.g., rheumatoid arthritis)

(continued)

TABLE 8–4 Reactions to Selected Drugs and Biologic Agents (*Continued*)

Drug/Biologic Agent	Clinical Features	Diagnosis/Cause	Treatment
Allergic reactions to latex	Health care workers and atopic individuals are particularly susceptible; children with spina bifida and genitourinary problems have a high incidence of latex allergy; **urticaria on contact, rhinitis, conjunctivitis, and bronchospasm** after inhalation are suggestive of latex allergy; severe anaphylaxis may ensue during surgery, barium enema, or dental procedures	Latex allergy is IgE mediated, and the diagnosis is best confirmed by serologic IgE assays, although they can miss up to 50% of allergic individuals; skin test not available in United States	Avoidance: natural latex is found in surgical gloves, catheters, balloons, condoms, and dental elastic adhesives; nonlatex gloves and tubing are available and should be used during surgery in patients with known latex allergy; premedication with antihistamines and corticosteroids is used to prevent severe reactions but may not prevent reactions

IX IMMUNODEFICIENCY DISORDERS

These disorders may be either **hereditary** or **acquired** and represent **four distinct abnormalities** of immune function. The genes that encode for many of the defects responsible for these disorders have now been mapped to specific chromosomes.

A **Complement system defects (Table 8–5)** may affect either the nine complement components or their associated regulatory proteins. This is the rarest of the immunodeficiencies, accounting for ≤2% of all primary immunodeficiencies.

TABLE 8–5 Complement System Defects

Defective Component (Inheritance)	Phenotypic Expression	Clinical Features	Diagnosis	Treatment
C3 (autosomal recessive)	Impaired opsonization of organisms	Recurrent severe bacterial infections, particularly with encapsulated organisms;	Assessment of total hemolytic complement (CH_{50})*	Cannot replace complement proteins, as they degrade too rapidly; prompt treatment of developing infection; routine vaccination for pneumococcus and meningococcus critical; occasionally prophylactic antibiotics
C2 (autosomal recessive)	Impaired activation of C3	increased prevalence of autoimmune diseases (e.g., systemic lupus erythematosus as early manifestation, rheumatoid arthritis), membranoproliferative glomerulonephritis in C3 deficiency		
C4 (autosomal recessive)	Impaired activation of C3			
C5–C9 (autosomal recessive)	Impaired formation of the membrane attack complex, which mediates bacteriolysis	Particularly susceptible to recurrent meningococcal and gonococcal infections; genitourinary tract infections; increased susceptibility to some viruses; rheumatic disorders		
Properdin (X-linked recessive)	Impaired opsonization	Recurrent infections due to pyogenic organisms and fulminant meningococcemia		Alternate pathway hemolytic complement titer (APH_{50}); properdin level

*CH_{50}: Assay to assess the classical complement pathway (amount of serum required to lyse 50% of sheep red blood cells sensitized with rabbit IgG antibody)

TABLE 8–6 Phagocytic Cell Immune Defects

Disorder (Inheritance)	Phenotypic Expression	Clinical Features	Diagnosis	Treatment
Chronic granulomatous disease (usually X-linked, may be AR)	Abnormal NADPH oxidase function, resulting in absence of respiratory burst by stimulated phagocytes	Onset of symptoms by age 1 year; recurrent abscesses and pneumonias; granulomas (e.g., hepatic, pulmonary, lymph nodes); osteomyelitis; recurrent infections with selected group of bacteria and fungi (*Klebsiella* spp., *Serratia* sp., *Staphylococcus aureus, Burkholderia cepacia, Nocardia* spp., *Aspergillus* spp., *Candida* spp.)	NBT (nitroblue tetrazolium test) or dihydrorhodamine 123 (DHR) flow cytometry assay confirmed by chemiluminescence; normal IgE to exclude hyper-IgE syndrome; prenatal diagnosis by fetal blood sampling	Early diagnosis and treatment of infection; surgical drainage/removal of infected lymph nodes; prophylactic antibiotics with trimethoprim-sulfamethoxazole and sometimes antifungals with itraconazole; IFN-γ three times weekly may reduce infections; BMT is curative
Chédiak–Higashi syndrome (AR)	Impaired chemotaxis, intracellular bacteriolysis, and movement of neutrophils from bone marrow	Frequent viral and cutaneous skin infections; enteric bacterial infections; partial oculocutaneous albinism; mild neutropenia; bleeding tendency	Presence of giant lysosomal granules in granulocytes and melanosomes in hair shafts; genetic testing for mutations in the CHS1/LYST gene; prenatal diagnosis by fetal blood sampling	Early diagnosis and treatment of bacterial and viral infections; BMT
Leukocyte adhesion deficiency (AR)	Reduced neutrophil chemotaxis and spreading	Delayed umbilical cord separation, with subsequent omphalitis; impaired wound healing; necrotizing deep soft tissue abscesses; periodontal disease later in life; leukocytosis	Sustained granulocytosis; decreased expression of CD11/CD18 on leukocytes by flow cytometry	Early diagnosis and treatment of bacterial infections; good oral hygiene; BMT in severe phenotype

AR, autosomal recessive; BMP, bone marrow transplant; IFN-γ, interferon gamma; NADPH, reduced form of nicotinamide–adenine dinucleotide phosphate; NBT, nitroblue tetrazolium.

B **Phagocytic cell immune defects (Table 8–6)**

1. **Common clinical features.** Recurrent cutaneous and sinopulmonary infections, as well as chronic cutaneous and oral inflammation (oral ulcers), may occur. Although the inflammatory response may be delayed, successive infections with *Staphylococcus aureus, Pseudomonas* species, *Haemophilus influenzae,* and *Aspergillus* are common and may be life threatening.

2. **Therapy.** Management consists primarily of the diagnosis, treatment, and prevention of pyogenic infections. However, such infections are often refractory to treatment despite appropriate antibiotic therapy.

3. **Genetic counseling** should be offered to families of affected individuals.

C **Antibody production defect disorders (Table 8–7)** are characterized by an inability to produce antigen-specific antibodies. These disorders have a variety of causes, including abnormalities of the structural genes for the heavy chain of IgA, congenital infections, and medications.

1. **Common clinical features.** Most patients with these disorders present with recurrent infections caused by encapsulated bacteria such as *Streptococcus pyogenes, Streptococcus pneumoniae,* and *H. influenzae.* These patients have primarily sinopulmonary infections.

TABLE 8–7   Antibody Production Defects

Disorder (Inheritance)	Phenotypic Expression	Clinical Features	Diagnosis	Treatment
X-linked agammaglobulinemia/ Bruton's (X-linked)	Dysfunctional gene product: [cytoplasmic tyrosine kinase (Btk)]	Recurrent mucocutaneous infections; severe infections due to pyogenic organisms, starting after 6 months of age; chronic meningoencephalitis due to enterovirus; autoimmune arthritis; reduced size or absence of tonsils and lymph nodes	Total immunoglobulin <100 mg/dL; severely reduced IgG, IgM, and IgA levels; confirmed by absence of Btk protein on monocytes/ platelets or detection of Btk mutant DNA; marked decrease in mature B cells bearing surface immunoglobulin; absence of plasma cells in lymphoid tissues	IVIG; sometimes prophylactic antibiotics; avoid live vaccines (e.g., measles, mumps, rubella, polio)
Late-onset hypogammaglobulinemia/ common variable immunodeficiency (unknown)	Abnormal B cell terminal differentiation to plasma cells; half of patients also have abnormal T cell activation and decreased IFN-γ	Variable presentation, infections due to pyogenic organisms, usually starting between ages 20 and 40 years (but can occur infancy to old age); giardiasis; sprue-like syndrome; bronchiectasis; nodular lymphoid hyperplasia; lymphoreticular malignancy; pernicious anemia; late development of autoimmune disorders	Reduced IgG, IgM, and IgA levels (total immunoglobulin may be <100 mg/dL); possible slight decrease in B cells bearing surface immunoglobulin; impaired antibody responses, and some may have combined T cell defects	IVIG; prompt treatment of infections; vigilance for neoplasm development
Selective IgA deficiency (unknown)	Arrested maturation of IgA-bearing cells; terminal block in B cell differentiation to plasma cells capable of secreting IgA	Recurrent respiratory or gastrointestinal bacterial infections; autoimmune disorders including SLE, RA, and ITP; allergic disorders; celiac disease; no symptoms in 60%–65% of cases; transient deficiency may be seen with certain medications; increased risk of anaphylaxis with blood products	Reduced serum IgA levels (<5 mg/ dL); reduced IgG2 or IgG4 levels in 20% of cases; occasional mild abnormalities of T cell function	Most are asymptomatic and do not require treatment; treat sequelae of IgA deficiency (e.g., infections with antibiotics, autoimmune disorders with NSAIDS/steroids, allergic disorders with typical allergy medications)
X-linked hyper-IgM (X-linked, AR, other)	Defective production of CD40 ligand on CD4 T lymphocytes prevents binding to CD40 receptor on B lymphocytes, resulting in impaired IgM isotype switching to IgG, IgA, and IgE	Recurrent sinopulmonary infections with encapsulated bacteria; gastrointestinal infections (including *Giardia*), opportunistic infections especially by *Pneumocystis jiroveci*; myelosuppression; malignancy; autoimmune disorders; neutropenia	Significant number of peripheral lymphocytes express IgM but decreased or absent IgG, IgA and IgE; DNA analysis for defective genes	IVIG; trimethoprim–sulfamethoxazole prophylaxis for *Pneumocystis jiroveci*; granulocyte colony-stimulating factor for significant neutropenia
Hyper-IgE/Job's syndrome (unknown)		Eczema; noninflamed abscesses; recurrent pneumonia and upper respiratory infections; recurrent *Candida* spp. infections; characteristic skeletal abnormalities and facies; retention of primary teeth	Extremely elevated levels of IgE (>2000 IU/mL); eosinophilia; characteristic skeletal abnormalities and facies	Early diagnosis and aggressive treatment of infections; meticulous skin care; topic and oral prophylactic antibiotics

AR, autosomal recessive; IFN-γ, interferon gamma; ITP, idiopathic thrombocytopenic purpura; IVIG, intravenous immunoglobulin; MHC, major histocompatibility complex; NSAIDs, nonsteroidal anti-inflammatory drugs; RA, rheumatoid arthritis; SLE, systemic lupus erythematosus.

TABLE 8–8 Cellular or Combined Defects

Disorder (Inheritance)	Phenotypic Expression	Clinical Features	Diagnosis	Therapy
DiGeorge syndrome (sporadic, deletion of 22q11.2)	Developmental field defect affecting structures of the third and fourth pharyngeal pouches, leading to thymic, parathyroid, and conotruncal cardiac defects; wide variation in phenotypic expression	Anomalies of the cardiac outflow tract; neonatal tetany from hypoparathyroidism and hypocalcemia; hypoplastic mandible; hypertelorism; short philtrum; bacterial, viral, or opportunistic infections (occasional or recurrent); autoimmune diseases; developmental delay	Genetic testing for 22q11.2 deletion (present in >90%); combination of clinical features if no genetic deletion but have clinical phenotype	Dependent upon phenotypic expression (e.g., calcium if hypoparathyroid, cardiac surgery if conotruncal defects); PCP prophylaxis if T cells profoundly decreased; most will reconstitute without treatment; rarely BMT or thymic transplant
Severe combined immunodeficiency syndrome (SCID) (X-linked most common, AR; 12 known genetic defects)	Absence of all adaptive immune mechanisms, including B cells, T cells, and frequently natural killer (NK) cells; absent or vestigial thymus; few thymocytes or Hassall's corpuscles; classic type: mutation of the γ chain of the IL-2 receptor	Overwhelming infections with typical childhood organisms; onset typically by age 3 months; diarrhea with marked failure to thrive; severe opportunistic infections (e.g., *Pneumocystis, Candida*, varicella, cytomegalovirus); hypoplastic peripheral lymphoid tissue	Profound lymphopenia; cutaneous anergy; heterogeneous abnormalities of lymphocyte subpopulations; impaired in vitro lymphocyte proliferative response; prenatal diagnosis by chorionic villous sampling or amniocentesis	BMT in first 3 months highly successful; IVIG; PCP prophylaxis; experimental gene therapy trial in progress; most die before age of 2 years without initiation of treatment
	Adenosine deaminase (ADA) deficiency: second-most-common type of SCID (AR)	Accumulation of toxic metabolites within lymphocytes leading to cell death	Lowest T lymphocyte counts with depressed T, B, and NK cell counts	BMT; modified bovine ADA enzyme (PEG-ADA)
Wiskott–Aldrich syndrome (X-linked)	Disorganization of actin cytoskeleton and lack of membrane-associated glycoproteins; accelerated synthesis and catabolism of all immunoglobulin isotypes; intrinsic platelet abnormality	Eczema; microcytic thrombocytopenia; recurrent pyogenic and fungal infections, starting by age 1 year; *Pneumocystis* and herpes virus infections, starting in late childhood; autoimmune disease; malignancy (lymphoma) in 15% of cases	Thrombocytopenia with small platelets (decreased mean platelet volume on CBC); low isohemagglutinins; normal IgG levels; impaired humoral response to polysaccharide antigens/vaccines; confirmation by decrease or absence of WASP in blood or WASP gene mutation; marked lymphopenia by 6 years of age	Early BMT or cord blood stem cell transplant; IVIG (especially if history of splenectomy); splenectomy in patients with bleeding disorders; treatment of iron deficiency secondary to blood loss; avoid live virus vaccination
Ataxia-telangiectasia (AR)	Hypoplastic thymus; lack of Hassall's corpuscles; intrinsic CD4 and B cell defects; T cell chromosomal translocation after x-ray irradiation	Progressive cerebellar ataxia; oculocutaneous telangiectasias (later finding); regression in motor milestones in early childhood; recurrent sinopulmonary infections; increased incidence of malignancy	Persistently elevated serum AFP; detection of ATM protein by Western blot; ATM gene sequencing; postradiation (e.g., x-ray) cellular death measurements; absent IgA in 70% of cases; IgG2 subclass deficiency in 35% of cases	IVIG in IgG deficiency; limit exposure to x-ray radiation

AR, autosomal recessive; ADA, adenosine deaminase; AFP, alpha-fetoprotein; ATM, ataxia-telangiectasia mutated; BMT, bone marrow transplantation; IL-2, interleukin-2; IVIG, intravenous immunoglobulin; PCP, *Pneumocystis jiroveci (carinii)* pneumonia; WASP, Wiskott–Aldrich syndrome protein.

2. **Therapy.** The treatment of choice for most antibody deficiency syndromes is **replacement therapy** with intravenous immunoglobulin.

D **Cellular or combined defect disorders** include those limited to defects in T cell function and combined disorders affecting both cellular and humoral immunity (**Table 8–8**).

1. **Common clinical features.** T cell deficiencies, whether partial or complete, typically result in recurrent infections of greater severity than those observed in the antibody deficiency syndromes and infections by opportunistic organisms like cytomegalovirus (CMV), *Pneumocystis jiroveci*, and *Candida* species.

2. **Therapy.** Bone marrow transplant and intravenous immunoglobulin are mainstays of therapy in many of the combined deficiencies.

E **Initial evaluation of suspected primary immunodeficiency**

1. **When to suspect a primary immunodeficiency:**
   a. Recurrent or unusually severe infections
   b. Persistent infection despite appropriate treatment
   c. Infections with classically less virulent organisms
   d. Infections with atypical and/or opportunistic organisms
   e. Unexplained abnormalities in blood cell counts (e.g., cytopenias)
   f. Autoimmune diseases (e.g., rheumatoid arthritis, lupus)
   g. Chronic diarrhea and failure to thrive

2. **Laboratory evaluation**
   a. **Initial evaluation**
      (1) Complete blood count with manual differential
      (2) Immunoglobulins (IgG, IgA, IgM)
      (3) Antibody titers (pneumococcal, *H. influenzae* type B, tetanus)
   b. **Additional evaluation** may include the following:
      (1) CH50, especially if considering encapsulated organisms or autoimmune disease (if considering complement deficiency)
      (2) T and B cell markers
      (3) Alpha-fetoprotein (if considering ataxia-telangiectasia)
      (4) Nitroblue tetrazolium test or dihydrorhodamine (DHR) test (if considering chronic granulomatous disease)
      (5) Immunofixation electrophoresis (to rule out monoclonal gammopathy if elevated immunoglobulins)

F **Human immunodeficiency virus** (**HIV**) selectively infects Th cells, leading to progressive deterioration of the immune system and, ultimately, **acquired immunodeficiency syndrome** (**AIDS**). For a detailed discussion of AIDS, refer to Chapter 9 VIII. **Acquired immunodeficiency** may also be secondary to severe malnutrition, diabetes, nephrotic syndrome, or malignancy/chemotherapy.

Study Questions

1. A 12-year-old boy is playing in the park near a trash can. He is stung by what he believes is a yellow jacket. He immediately has symptoms of urticaria and wheezing. These symptoms are treated in a local emergency department. He is followed up in his primary care provider's office 1 week later. There is a question about the proper diagnosis of insect allergy. Which of the following findings provides the best evidence of insect sting hypersensitivity?

- [A] Positive prick or intradermal skin test
- [B] Extensive local reaction lasting 5–7 days
- [C] Documented evidence of a systemic allergic reaction
- [D] Specific antivenom immunoglobulin E (IgE) antibodies
- [E] Generalized urticaria in this patient

2. A 25-year-old man presents to his primary care office with the following symptoms. He has clear rhinorrhea, ocular and nasal pruritus, nasal congestion, and sneezing. He knows that it is tree pollen season but has also recently acquired a pet cat for the first time. Which of the following tests is most useful in the diagnosis of the trigger for his allergic rhinitis?

- [A] Environmental cat challenge
- [B] Measurement of total serum immunoglobulin E (IgE) levels
- [C] Peripheral blood smear for eosinophils
- [D] Immediate hypersensitivity puncture skin test
- [E] Stained nasal smear for eosinophils

3. A 4-year-old boy in your practice has been having many infections. You suspect that he may have an immune dysfunction. Quantitative immunoglobulins were sent and were normal. Which of the following immunodeficiency disorders is associated with normal immunoglobulin G (IgG) levels?

- [A] X-linked agammaglobulinemia (Bruton's)
- [B] DiGeorge syndrome
- [C] Late-onset hypogammaglobulinemia
- [D] Ataxia-telangiectasia
- [E] Severe combined immunodeficiency

4. A 55-year-old woman comes into the emergency room complaining of a hoarse voice and states, "My mouth feels funny." On history, she reports that she was diagnosed with hypertension several months ago. After an unsuccessful attempt at lifestyle modification to reduce her blood pressure, her doctor started her on some medication a few weeks ago, but she cannot remember the name of the medication. On exam, she has swollen lips, periorbital edema, and a definite hoarseness to the voice. What would be the most appropriate next step?

- [A] Discontinue blood pressure medications; discharge to home, and advise her to obtain alternate medications from her primary doctor.
- [B] Recommend loratadine and follow-up with her primary doctor within 1 week to evaluate her symptoms.
- [C] Albuterol and Atrovent nebulizer therapy with intravenous steroids; admit to medicine floor for observation.
- [D] Intramuscular or subcutaneous epinephrine 0.5 mg 1:1000, intravenous diphenhydramine, ranitidine, and steroids; admit to intensive care unit for possible airway emergency.
- [E] None of the above.

5. Which one of the following adverse reactions is mediated by immunoglobulin G (IgG) autoantibodies?

- [A] Insulin resistance
- [B] Anaphylaxis after ingestion of peanuts
- [C] Latex reaction
- [D] Systemic reaction to an insect sting
- [E] Ragweed-induced rhinitis

6. A 33-year-old man has an acute anaphylactic reaction to an intravenous drug while in the hospital. He is taking a β-adrenergic blockade drug. Which of the following therapeutic choices may be most useful in treating resistant hypotension?

- A Subcutaneous aqueous epinephrine
- B Intravenous terbutaline
- C Intravenous glucagon
- D Intravenous aminophylline
- E Intravenous diphenhydramine

7. A 28-year-old woman with bronchial asthma is about to start a new job in a health care facility. She hears that health care workers are at a greater risk for developing a latex allergy. She is wondering whether any of her medical conditions make her at a higher risk. Which of the following clinical conditions is most commonly associated with latex allergy?

- A Bronchial asthma
- B Fibrosing alveolitis
- C Diabetes mellitus
- D Spina bifida
- E Inflammatory bowel disease

QUESTIONS 8–11

Directions: *The response options for Items 8–11 are the same. Select one answer for each item in the set.*

- A Antigen avoidance/environmental controls
- B Immunotherapy against known offending antigens
- C Antihistamine preparation
- D Topical nasal steroid

For each of the following patients with allergic rhinitis, select the most appropriate therapeutic intervention.

8. A 34-year-old-woman with severe perennial allergic rhinitis loses 10–15 days of work each year as a result of secondary sinusitis. Immediate skin tests show significant positive reactions to house dust mite, *Cladosporium,* and grass and ragweed pollens. Various medications have been only partially successful in controlling symptoms.

9. A 20-year-old man has mild but persistent year-round symptoms of nasal congestion, rhinorrhea, and watery eyes. He has recurrent epistaxis. Immediate skin tests show positive reactions to house dust mite, *Alternaria,* and grass and ragweed pollens.

10. A 10-year-old girl has rhinorrhea and nasal pruritus after visiting a friend who has a kitten.

11. An 8-year-old boy regularly experiences moderately severe sneezing spells and watery eyes in May and June, September and October, and occasionally during January through March. Immediate skin tests show positive reactions to *Alternaria, Cladosporium*, house dust mite, and grass and ragweed pollens. He has used antihistamines with some persistent symptoms.

QUESTIONS 12–14

Directions: *The response options for Items 12–14 are the same. Select one answer for each item in the set.*

- A Acute arthritis
- B Acute anaphylaxis
- C Chronic cough
- D Bronchospasm

E Interstitial nephritis
F Photoallergic reaction

For each of the following patients exhibiting an adverse drug reaction, select the most likely clinical expression.

12. A 22-year-old man who is in good health except for recurrent sinusitis elects to take 81 mg of aspirin as antithrombosis therapy.

13. A 54-year-old woman with newly diagnosed hypertension starts enalapril at an appropriate dose.

14. A 34-year-old woman is diagnosed with a dental infection and is started on penicillin. She has a history of a severe allergic reaction to an unknown antibiotic for a sexually transmitted disease (STD) in college.

Answers and Explanations

1. The answer is C [VII C]. Clinical documentation of a systemic allergic reaction is essential to the accurate diagnosis of insect sting hypersensitivity. Typically, signs of anaphylaxis develop within minutes after the sting. Subsequent prick or intradermal skin testing, supplemented as necessary by antivenom immunoglobulin E (IgE) levels [determined by radioallergosorbent test (RAST)], provides confirming evidence of hypersensitivity. A large local reaction alone, whether of short or prolonged duration, does not provide sufficient evidence of IgE-mediated hypersensitivity. Generalized urticaria in a child younger than 12 years of age is not considered anaphylaxis, and these children do not have a greater risk than the general population of an anaphylactic reaction on their next sting. The only objective test is a serum β-tryptase. This test measures tryptase released from mast cells. When elevated, it is useful, but it is not elevated in all anaphylactic reactions.

2. The answer is D [III E 1]. An accurately applied skin test is the most valuable tool for identifying the causative antigen in allergic rhinitis, yielding results in approximately 15–20 minutes. Environmental challenge tests are neither practical nor available to most patients and may lead to severe symptoms. Radioallergosorbent test (RAST) has almost equal accuracy but is more expensive. Elevated immunoglobulin E (IgE) levels are observed in only 30%–40% of patients with allergic rhinitis and may be secondary to other unrelated disorders. Peripheral eosinophilia seen in a peripheral blood smear is an inconsistent finding. Although eosinophils are usually identified in nasal secretions from patients with allergic rhinitis, they are also detected in eosinophilic nonallergic rhinitis and hyperplastic sinusitis.

3. The answer is B [Tables 8–6 and 8–7]. Although reduced levels of immunoglobulin A (IgA) or IgE may be seen in patients with DiGeorge syndrome—a T cell deficiency disorder—the total serum immunoglobulin level usually is normal and IgG levels are normal. In X-linked agammaglobulinemia (Bruton's) and late-onset hypogammaglobulinemia, IgG, IgM, and IgA levels are all reduced, and the total immunoglobulin level is less than 100 mg/dL. Patients with ataxia-telangiectasia have a defect in their DNA repair mechanism. One of the clinical features is low IgA and IgG. Severe combined immunodeficiency results in a decrease in all immunoglobulins.

4. The answer is D [IV]. This patient has angioedema, most likely from an ACE inhibitor prescribed recently to control her blood pressure. The swollen lips and periorbital edema are classic symptoms of angioedema. The hoarseness of the patient's voice is especially concerning since it suggests laryngeal edema, which could lead to an airway emergency. Given the airway involvement, epinephrine should be given, although this is most likely non–IgE mediated. In addition, H₁- and H₂-blockers should be administered, the latter providing a synergistic benefit in improving angioedema. Intravenous steroids should be used in severe cases such as this one. The potential airway emergency warrants extremely close observation, and admission to an intensive care unit would be most appropriate.

5. The answer is A [VIII D]. Insulin resistance is caused by immunoglobulin G (IgG) autoantibodies that bind to insulin receptors, thereby inhibiting their function. This problem usually occurs in women with Sjögren's syndrome, systemic lupus erythematosus (SLE), or a less well-defined clinical syndrome also suggestive of autoimmunity. Food-related anaphylaxis, reactions to latex, systemic reactions to insect stings, and ragweed-induced rhinitis are all IgE-mediated hypersensitivity responses.

6. The answer is C [V E 5]. Intravenous glucagon has a positive inotropic and chronotropic effect. In those patients taking β-blocker medications, an even greater increase in blood pressure may occur. Although subcutaneous epinephrine is always the first line of therapy, it may not be effective in patients using a β-adrenergic blockade drug. The other therapeutic agents are relatively ineffective in the face of β-adrenergic blockade.

7. The answer is D [Table 8-4]. The highest prevalence of latex allergy occurs in children with spina bifida. This appears to be related to early surgical intervention with constant exposure to the natural latex in catheters and tubing. Surgeons and operating room nurses are at increased risk of developing latex allergy. Bronchial asthma, fibrosing alveolitis, diabetes mellitus, and inflammatory bowel disease are not commonly associated with the occurrence of latex allergy.

8–11. The answers are as follows: 8—B [III F 3], 9—C [III F 2 a–c], 10—A [III F 1], 11—D [III F 2 d (1)]. Immunotherapy, which significantly ameliorates symptoms and is used when allergic rhinitis is severe, when medical complications or intolerance to medication occurs, and when various types of medications have been only partially successful, would be recommended for the 34-year-old woman.

Intranasal steroids are the most effective form of therapy, but they not an option here due to recurrent epistaxis. Therefore, antihistamine preparations are the drugs of choice for the treatment of allergic rhinitis. These preparations usually control mild-to-moderate symptoms such as those experienced by the 20-year-old man and the 8-year-old boy; however, some patients experience intolerable side effects such as drowsiness. A second-generation antihistamine such as fexofenadine is less likely to cause such sedation.

If an antihistamine preparation does not relieve symptoms or is not well tolerated, then intranasal therapy with corticosteroids or an H$_1$-blocker could be considered for the 8-year-old boy. Nasal cromolyn sodium, which in some cases is as effective as a decongestant in treating seasonal allergic rhinitis, could have been recommended for the 8-year-old boy with seasonal symptoms.

Topical nasal steroids are the most effective preventive treatment of allergic rhinitis if symptoms persist despite environmental controls and as-needed antihistamines.

Antigen avoidance is most successful when a single antigen can be identified as the causative agent. Because the 10-year-old girl developed symptoms only after being exposed to her friend's kitten, it is likely that avoiding cats will alleviate her symptoms. Antigen avoidance is not feasible for all patients, however. For example, although a patient may be able to avoid animal dander indoors, the avoidance of multiple outdoor antigens is likely to prove difficult, if not impossible. Nonetheless, sensible environmental precautions help limit the exacerbation of symptoms.

12. The answer is D [III A 2 c and Table 8-4]. This man, an individual with recurrent sinusitis, also may have underlying chronic rhinitis and perhaps undiagnosed nasal polyposis. Bronchospasm, which may be prolonged and severe, typically begins within 30 minutes after aspirin ingestion. The combination of asthma, nasal polyposis, and sinusitis is known as the aspirin triad. However, aspirin-induced anaphylaxis does not occur in patients with underlying sinusitis or polyposis and starts after two or more exposures to aspirin.

13. The answer is C [Table 8-4]. Chronic cough has been reported in 5%–20% of patients who take angiotensin-converting-enzyme (ACE) inhibitors. The cough is usually nonproductive and nocturnal. Symptoms may begin as early as 1 week or as late as 6 months after drug use. ACE inhibitors also lead to development of angioedema in 0.1%–0.2% of patients, and in certain clinical situations, this group of medications is known to exacerbate anaphylaxis.

14. The answer is B [VII D 1]. Penicillin can cause anaphylaxis, which is an acute life-threatening hypersensitivity reaction. In the past, the diagnosis of a penicillin allergy could be by history and skin testing; however, penicillin skin test materials are not available other than Pen G. If alternative antibiotics cannot be used, the patient should undergo penicillin desensitization in a monitored unit. Cephalosporins should be used with extreme caution in such patients because up to 2% of patients who are allergic to penicillin can have a cross-reaction.

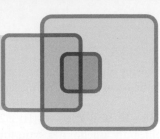

chapter 9

Infectious Diseases

LEROY VAUGHAN · DEVANG PATEL · JANAKI KURUPPU

I GENERAL PRINCIPLES OF HUMAN–MICROBE INTERACTION

The normal human body normally harbors a complex microbial ecosystem. These **commensal** organisms (referred to as the **indigenous flora**) are generally nonpathogenic and may even be necessary to normal human physiology and function. Infection and disease may result, however, when the body is challenged by a pathogenic organism that is not part of the normal flora or when the body's defense system is disturbed, allowing uncontrolled growth or invasion by the indigenous flora.

A Normal human–microbe ecology   Microorganisms can interact with humans in the following ways.

1. **Most indigenous organisms seldom cause disease.** Many of the organisms normally found on the skin and mucous membranes (e.g., *Staphylococcus epidermidis*, *Corynebacterium* species) are ubiquitous but may cause disease in unusual settings (e.g., when host defenses are significantly impaired or when artificial material such as a catheter or a prosthetic joint is present).

2. **Some indigenous organisms may cause disease in other body sites.** Many bacteria that normally exist in one body site may cause disease elsewhere. For example, α-hemolytic (viridans) streptococci are commensals in the oropharynx but can cause endocarditis if they enter the bloodstream and settle on a previously damaged heart valve.

3. **Transient organisms may cause disease.** The body's normal flora may allow the temporary growth of certain microbes that disappear spontaneously but may cause disease while present. For example, patients with invasive meningococcal disease first have pharyngeal carriage of *Neisseria meningitidis*, but only a tiny fraction of individuals with meningococci in the pharynx ever develop systemic disease.

4. **Pathogenic organisms usually cause disease.** Most viruses, as well as *Chlamydia* and *Rickettsia*, rarely are isolated from humans except during or following an acute illness. Pathogenic bacteria include *Brucella* and *Salmonella* species, *Neisseria gonorrhoeae*, and *Mycobacterium tuberculosis*.

B Host defense mechanisms   The human body has many ways of defending itself from potentially pathogenic microorganisms.

1. **Anatomic barriers** are integral in preventing infection. These include physical barriers such as intact skin and mucous membranes, as well as functional barriers such as the muscular protection of the glottis and bladder neck.

2. **Cellular immunity** is explained in Table 9–1.

3. **Humoral immunity** is explained in Table 9–1.

C Fever   One of the most recognized features of infectious diseases, regardless of the site of infection, is the elevation of body temperature.

1. **Normal regulation of body temperature.** The normal core body temperature is approximately $37° ± 1°C$ ($98.6° ± 1.8°F$) and varies diurnally. Monocytes secrete a polypeptide called **interleukin-1** (IL-1), which stimulates the hypothalamus to increase the body's temperature **set point.** The rise in set point causes alterations in circulation, metabolism, and perspiration, which ultimately lead to a rise in body temperature. Temperature readings greater than $38.3°C$ are considered abnormal. **Hypothermia** (body temperature $<36°C$) is sometimes a response to overwhelming infection, especially in neonates and the elderly.

TABLE 9–1 The Human Immune System

Component	Source	Function	Causes of Diminished Function	Opportunistic Organisms
Cellular Immunity				
Neutrophils	Bone marrow	Phagocytosis; acute inflammation	Genetic disorders: chronic granulomatous disease, myeloperoxidase deficiency. Acquired causes: cytotoxic therapy, leukemia, aplastic anemia, drug reaction	Endogenous flora, enteric bacilli, *Pseudomonas aeruginosa*, *Candida* spp., *Aspergillus* spp.
Eosinophils	Bone marrow	Modulate hypersensitivity reactions to multicellular parasites	Idiopathic, corticosteroid therapy	None known
Monocytes/ macrophages	Bone marrow	Release cytokines, interact with lymphocytes, phagocytosis	Cytotoxic therapy, lymphoreticular malignancy	
T lymphocytes	Thymus, bone marrow	Modulate activity of B lymphocytes, macrophages, and T lymphocytes	Genetic disorders, autoimmune disease, lymphoreticular malignancy, AIDS, organ transplantation, corticosteroid therapy	*Mycobacterium* spp., fungi, *Listeria* spp., *Nocardia* spp.
Humoral Immunity				
Antibodies	Plasma cells	Facilitate phagocytosis, inactivate toxins	Genetic disorders, multiple myeloma, splenectomy	Viruses, pyogenic bacteria
Complement	Liver	Enhances phagocytosis, direct cell destruction	Genetic disorders, severe liver disease	*Neisseria* spp. (especially with deficiency of complement components (C5–C9)

2. **Conditions associated with fever.** Almost any infectious process may be accompanied by fever; however, absence of fever does not rule out an infectious process. Fever also may occur with noninfectious disease states such as myocardial infarction (MI), pulmonary embolism, drug reactions, autoimmune disease, cancer (e.g., lymphoma and renal cell carcinoma), and a variety of inflammatory conditions (e.g., inflammatory bowel disease and sarcoidosis). Certain fever patterns are classically associated with specific diseases (e.g., tertian fever with *Plasmodium vivax* malaria), and sometimes charting the fever curve can help identify drug fever or other temporal associations. In many cases, however, the temperature pattern does not aid in identifying the cause.

3. **Fever management. Antipyretic drugs** (e.g., aspirin, acetaminophen, nonsteroidal anti-inflammatory drugs [NSAIDs]) can modify a fever, but they seldom completely suppress a fever caused by infection. When fever is extreme (i.e., >42°C) or when the accompanying tachycardia and circulatory changes are poorly tolerated, it is wise to try to reduce body temperature.

4. **Beneficial effects of fever.** Many infectious microbes prefer the normal range of body temperature for optimal survival and growth, and, thus, fever probably plays a role in host defense against infection. Some elements of the immune system function more efficiently at higher temperatures, whereas others are less efficient. Although the net effect of fever on recovery from infection is not clearly defined, several studies have shown that lowering fever in septic patients has no survival benefit, and some studies have shown a survival advantage associated with presence of fever in patients in the intensive care setting.

D **Microbial virulence factors** contribute to the likelihood that a pathogen will cause infection.

1. **Some microbes invade host cells or breach barriers** to reach susceptible body sites and, along the way, avoid or overcome host defenses. To invade a host, microorganisms must adhere to host tissue and may use specific receptors or general factors to accomplish this step. In some situations (e.g., chickenpox or measles), microbes can easily infect otherwise healthy individuals who have normal host defenses but no prior exposure to the microbe.

2. **Some microbes produce toxins** that result in disease. For example, a toxin elaborated by some strains of *Staphylococcus aureus* (toxic shock syndrome toxin-1 [TSST-1]) is responsible for **toxic shock syndrome** (TSS) [see VII D 1 a]. A second example is *Clostridium difficile,* which elaborates a toxin that causes diarrhea.

3. **In some situations, microbes can only cause disease in the presence of another pathogen.** An example is **delta hepatitis virus (HDV),** which cannot infect humans except in the presence of ongoing hepatitis B virus (HBV) infection but, when present, worsens the disease course of HBV hepatitis.

4. Because of the selective pressures induced by using antimicrobial agents to treat or prevent infections in humans and animals, **microorganisms that are resistant to antibiotics may have a propensity for causing infections.** This selection process plays an important role in infections occurring in settings where antibiotic use is widespread, such as in hospitals and nursing homes. This phenomenon also occurs in outpatient settings, where antibiotic use has been increasingly widespread. Children who receive repeated courses of antibiotics (e.g., for recurrent otitis media, which is usually viral in origin) harbor a more resistant microbial flora as a result.

E **Epidemiologic considerations** In addition to host and microbial characteristics, environmental factors contribute to defining the nature and severity of an infection.

1. **Contagious spread.** Some infectious agents are spread from person to person through direct physical contact (e.g., syphilis) or by infectious aerosols (e.g., tuberculosis).

2. **Vectors and fomites**
   a. **Vectors** are animals that act as hosts or carriers of a disease without becoming ill themselves. Most vectors are insects or arthropods. In general, infections that are related to animals or their products (e.g., meat, milk, or eggs) are called **zoonoses.**
   b. **Fomites** are inanimate objects capable of spreading infection. Fomites are most commonly identified in hospitals, where enhanced patient susceptibility and a high concentration of virulent organisms coexist, but they may also play a role in settings such as day care facilities and other public places.

3. **Geography.** Certain diseases may occur exclusively or with substantially higher frequency in specific countries, regions, or climates. For example, mosquito bites almost never result in the transmission of malaria in the United States, whereas a mosquito bite in sub-Saharan Africa, Southeast Asia, or South America confers a higher risk of acquiring malaria. Duration of exposure can also be important. For example, filariasis leads to elephantiasis only after repeated exposure to the mosquito vector over a period of months to years.

4. **Season.** Infections often occur more commonly during a particular time of the year. This may be because of certain activities that might expose an individual to risk and that are seasonal in nature (e.g., hunting and fishing) or to environmental factors that favor the growth of the microbe or its insect vector.

5. **Institutions.** Certain settings that bring together susceptible individuals may alter the risk of infection. Hospitals and nursing homes can amplify and alter the nature of infections among the sick and the elderly, whereas day care centers can have a similar effect on the young.

II   USE OF ANTI-INFECTIVE THERAPY

A **General principles** Appropriate use of antibiotics can be life saving, and therefore it is important to recognize when to initiate treatment. However, any type of medical intervention presents potential hazards, and the indiscriminate use of antibiotics is no exception. In general, four circumstances prompt antimicrobial therapy.

1. **Organism-based treatment**
   a. When cultures or stains from a patient demonstrate a credible microorganism, appropriate antibiotic treatment is initiated. Note the following examples:
      (1) A wet mount of vaginal secretions showing *Trichomonas vaginalis*
      (2) Blood cultures that are positive for *Streptococcus sanguis* in a patient with a history of mitral valve disease and a fever

   b. Techniques for recognizing specific antigens of microorganisms also may be used to help initiate therapy. An example is the finding of cryptococcal antigens in the cerebrospinal fluid (CSF) in a patient with chronic meningitis.

   c. Isolation of an organism allows in vitro testing of antibiotic susceptibility. In many cases, resistance patterns of identified pathogens are predictable enough to permit treatment without these further tests.

2. **Syndrome-based treatment** is initiated when all three of the following conditions apply:
   (1) The clinical picture strongly suggests specific organ disease.
   (2) The tests needed to make a microbiologic diagnosis are not available or practical.
   (3) The most likely causative organisms all respond to the same treatment.

   a. For example, if an otherwise healthy young woman has painful urination and a positive test for white blood cells (WBCs) in the urine, treatment can be initiated for a urinary tract infection without even submitting a urine specimen for culture.

   b. However, patients with a poor response to initial treatment, relapse, or complicating concomitant medical illness cannot be optimally managed without further diagnostic evaluation.

3. **Empiric therapy** is given when the diagnosis is uncertain but clinical experience suggests that the patient outcome in a particular setting is improved with antimicrobial therapy.

   a. Generally, empiric therapy is initiated while awaiting the results of diagnostic tests to identify a specific causative organism.

   b. Fever often develops as the first sign of infection in patients with severe neutropenia from cancer therapy. These patients may succumb to their infection before final reports are received from the laboratory. Thus, antimicrobial therapy should begin at the first sign of fever.

4. **Prophylaxis** is used when a specific infection or complication is anticipated and can be prevented. Generally, this form of empiric therapy is restricted to a fixed and brief period during which there is a risk of infection. Examples include the use of penicillin before dental procedures in patients with heart valve disease and the use of perioperative antibiotics in surgery. Longer duration of the prophylaxis leads to higher likelihood of developing antimicrobial toxicity or acquisition/selection of resistant flora.

B **Dosage and route**   (Online Figure 9–1)

C **Cost**

D **Specific antibiotic spectrum**

E **Concentration- or time-dependent effect**

F **Interpreting antimicrobial susceptibility tests**

G **Toxicity and side effects**   Although life-threatening toxicity rarely occurs with antibiotic treatment, physicians should be familiar with the specific risks of each drug administered so that side effects can be anticipated and minimized.

1. **Allergic reactions,** sometimes fatal, can occur with almost any pharmaceutical agent but are more common with the β-lactam antibiotics and sulfonamides than with other antimicrobials.

2. **Bone marrow suppression,** e.g., with chloramphenicol, which is seldom used in the United States, can cause irreversible aplastic anemia. Linezolid, an agent increasingly used for treatment of methicillin-resistant *Staphylococcus aureus* (MRSA) infections, is associated with thrombocytopenia.

3. **Renal dysfunction** is commonly seen with aminoglycosides. This toxicity is reversible and usually of minor clinical significance, but full recovery may take weeks or months. In rare instances, dialysis may be needed. Amphotericin B, used in the treatment of fungal infections, can also impair kidney function.

4. **Abnormalities in blood coagulation** (e.g., changes in the levels of clotting factors or in the number or function of platelets) have been associated with several β-lactam antibiotics and sometimes result in clinically significant bleeding.

5. **Ototoxicity** is an infrequent but potentially debilitating side effect of **aminoglycosides.** Either auditory or vestibular impairment can occur; often it is irreversible.

6. **Phototoxicity, or photosensitivity,** is an exaggerated response of the skin to sun exposure. This can result in severe "sunburn" and is associated with use of tetracyclines.

7. **Cardiotoxicity, particularly affecting cardiac conduction,** can arise from any number of drugs (including nonantibiotic compounds). The most common arrhythmia is associated with QT prolongation. At the extreme end of QT prolongation is a self-sustaining arrhythmia called torsades de pointes, which can be life-threatening. A number of antibiotics (macrolides and fluoroquinolones) have been associated with QT prolongation, and their actions are more likely to be serious if other medications also prolong the QT interval or if the patient has a predisposition to a long QT to begin with.

H Adult immunization

III EFFECTIVE USE OF THE MICROBIOLOGY LABORATORY

To maximize the usefulness of any microbiology laboratory, it is necessary to be familiar with its specific capabilities and procedures. The following are general guidelines.

A **Obtaining and handling specimens**

1. **Fresh specimens are superior to old ones.** This is especially true when quantitative results are important (e.g., colony counts of urine cultures) or when the target organism is fragile (e.g., protozoal trophozoites in stool). If immediate delivery of a specimen is not possible, proper maintenance of the specimen should be ensured until it can be processed.
   a. Some bacteria (e.g., *N. gonorrhoeae*) are sensitive to cold, and specimens should not be refrigerated.
   b. Specimens to be cultured for anaerobes should be maintained in a prereduced, oxygen-free environment or in a syringe without any air and without a needle. They should be transported to the laboratory for immediate plating.

2. **Large specimens are better than small ones.** When collecting specimens for microbiological culture and staining, submit as much material as can be obtained. When culturing a wound, use pressure on the wound to express as much purulent fluid as possible from any fluctuant areas, or aspirate fluid using aseptic technique. Sometimes, multiple specimens are needed to identify microorganisms (e.g., *M. tuberculosis*) that are shed infrequently or in small numbers.

3. **Biological hazards should be labeled and handled properly.** Laboratories have instituted **universal precautions** and treat all specimens as potentially infectious. Some bacteria and fungi may be especially hazardous in pure culture (e.g., *Brucella*, *Francisella*, and *Coccidioides*), and the laboratory should be notified if these organisms are suspected clinically so that appropriate care can be taken.

4. **Newer techniques may bypass or accelerate culture results.** Direct DNA probe test for *C. trachomatis* and *N. gonorrhoeae* can now be done without concern for maintaining bacterial viability (necessary for culture), and results are available much faster than with culture results. Similarly, culture testing for mycobacteria is now faster than before (positive results back in 10 vs. 30 days), and DNA probes can identify mycobacteria in less than a day once cultures are positive.

B Interpreting negative and positive culture results

IV RISK FACTORS FOR INFECTION

Sometimes it is possible to identify patient characteristics that modify the likelihood or severity of an infection. In general, the intensity or frequency of exposure and the degree of susceptibility correlate with potential hazard of infection.

A **Diabetes** In general, patients with diabetes are more prone to certain infections than individuals without glucose intolerance.

1. **Foot and lower leg ulcers,** which may become infected, are more likely to occur in patients with diabetes due to neuropathy or peripheral vascular disease. Such soft tissue infections are more likely to involve Gram-negative rods, and they are more difficult to cure than those occurring in nondiabetic individuals.

2. *Candida* **infections,** especially vulvovaginal candidiasis or thrush, are more likely to occur in patients with diabetes.

3. **Urinary tract infections** may be more common and more severe in diabetic patients, and the increased morbidity probably is related to bladder dysfunction in those patients with diabetic neuropathy. It is often recommended that urinary tract infections be more vigorously treated in patients with diabetes.

4. Some **rare diseases** occur almost exclusively in diabetic patients.
   a. **Malignant otitis externa** is a painful, rapidly progressive, and locally destructive disease of the external auditory canal that may extend to the temporal bone and the brain. *Pseudomonas aeruginosa* is the causative agent [see V B 1 a].
   b. **Rhinocerebral mucormycosis,** a fungal infection that starts in the nose or paranasal sinuses, is locally destructive. It is found in patients with severe metabolic acidosis (e.g., in patients with diabetes and ketoacidosis).
   c. **Synergistic gangrene** is a soft tissue infection that often is attributable to streptococci and obligate anaerobes. It may involve the skin or the underlying fascial structures and tends to progress relentlessly unless treated with extensive surgical débridement.
   d. **Emphysematous cholecystitis** is a rare but severe infection of the gallbladder. Unlike ordinary cholecystitis, it requires urgent antibiotic administration and may require surgery. The clinical clues are similar to those of cholecystitis, but there is often high fever, tachycardia, hypotension, and other evidence of sepsis. X-rays, computed tomography (CT) scan, and other imaging studies show gas in the gallbladder wall.

B **Alcoholism** Acute and chronic alcohol use can impair neurologic function and decrease the efficacy of neutrophils. In addition, chronic alcohol use can result in severe organ damage, especially to the liver.

1. **Pneumonia.** The incidence of pneumococcal, aspiration, and gram-negative bacillary is greater in alcoholics than it is in the general population. Tuberculosis, anaerobic lung abscess, and empyema also are more common.

2. **Spontaneous bacterial peritonitis (SBP).** When ascites is present, due to cirrhosis, the ascites fluid can become infected by bacteria, usually gram-negative aerobic bacilli or enterococci. SBP also occurs in nonalcoholic patients with ascites (e.g., nephrotic syndrome).

C **Injection drug use**

1. **Infections related to unsterile techniques.** Injection drug users (IDUs) are prone to a variety of suppurative complications because, in most cases, the preparation of the drug is not aseptic, equipment is not sterile, and skin cleansing is inadequate.
   a. **Bacterial endocarditis,** often involving the tricuspid valve (a valve rarely infected in non-IDU populations), is the most serious infection. Usually, the bacterium responsible is *S. aureus.*
   b. **Superficial skin infections** are common, and infectious arthritis, usually caused by *P. aeruginosa* or *S. aureus,* is seen frequently.
   c. **Tetanus,** although rare, occurs more frequently because injection drug users are more likely to have improperly cleaned wounds.

2. **Infections related to needle sharing.** Some contagious diseases can be transmitted efficiently via the small amount of blood in used needles and syringes. The incidence of HBV, HCV, and HIV infection is increased in injection drug users who share needles.

D **Occupational exposure**

1. The risk of occupation-related infection may be **unpredictable,** as in the outbreaks of **Pontiac fever,** which were related to the aerosolization of *Legionella pneumophila*–contaminated water via air-conditioning ducts throughout an office building.

2. The risk of infection also may be influenced by factors outside the immediate work environment. For example, the risk of brucellosis among slaughterhouse workers is determined largely by the number of livestock infected and to a lesser extent by the degree of the worker's exposure to the blood of infected livestock.

3. When an increased risk is **predictable,** certain preventive measures can be instituted (e.g., immunization of health care workers against hepatitis B).

E **Internal prostheses**   When a prosthesis (such as artificial hip or knee joints and heart valves, either mechanical or biologic material) is inserted into the body, there is a possibility that an infection will develop at the site of insertion. Because the immune system reacts to any foreign material, a prosthetic organ is susceptible to infection by a greater number and variety of organisms than is the native organ, even if that organ is damaged. In addition, the clinical presentation of these infections may be atypical, and the interval between surgery and any manifestation of sepsis may be long (e.g., many years). In most cases, bacteria are inoculated at the time of surgery, although secondary hematogenous or percutaneous spread also occurs.

F **Indwelling catheters**

1. Like internal prostheses, catheters such as intravenous or intra-arterial lines, bladder catheters, and endotracheal tubes offer sites of diminished host responsiveness. Furthermore, they provide communication between the external environment and the ordinarily sterile internal environment of the body.

2. In addition to intrinsic host factors, **two important factors determine the likelihood of catheter-related infection: the duration of catheterization and the degree of cleanliness maintained during catheterization.** Duration is the most important factor in tracheal and urethral catheterization. Both factors are important in vascular catheterization. (🖱 See online for more information.)

G **Granulocytopenia**   A specific risk that has been identified and carefully studied is related to granulocytopenia, the absence of adequate numbers of circulating neutrophils. The risk of infection is inversely related to the duration and degree of granulocytopenia. Neutrophil counts greater than 500/mm^3 are adequate protection against most infections.

1. In most patients with granulocytopenia, the **underlying disease is a hematologic malignancy,** although reduced neutrophil levels can be seen in association with aplastic anemia, drug-induced agranulocytosis, and cytotoxic chemotherapy for nonhematologic malignancies. Patients with hematologic malignancy have an additional infection risk when they receive chemotherapy, which also disrupts the lining of the gastrointestinal tract and permits bacterial and fungal invasion.

2. The indigenous flora of patients with granulocytopenia is likely to be altered during hospitalization and with the administration of antibiotics. The microflora most commonly associated with infections in affected patients is derived from their indigenous flora. Bacteria such as *Escherichia coli* and *P. aeruginosa,* as well as fungi such as *Candida albicans,* are most often found.

3. Molds such as *Aspergillus* species may cause serious, often fatal, infections in patients with granulocytopenia.

4. Persistent **fever** is the hallmark of infection in patients with neutropenia. Because uncontrolled infection can result in rapid clinical deterioration, **empiric** antimicrobials are given immediately after appropriate culture specimens are obtained.

5. Granulocytes released into the circulation after the use of **colony-stimulating factors** such as filgrastim are fully functional. Thus, granulocytopenia after chemotherapy of solid tumors is often brief and unaccompanied by serious infection.

H **Immunosuppressive agents**   These agents are used to treat a variety of medical problems, such as prevention of rejection of transplanted organs and control of autoimmune disorders.

1. The expression of this immunodeficiency is seen mostly in the increased incidence of infection usually controlled by **cellular immunity** (e.g., mycobacterial, fungal, nocardial, and cytomegaloviral infections). Steroids also alter some diagnostic tests, most notably the expression of delayed hypersensitivity.

2. Steroids are used widely in transplantation procedures involving the kidney, heart, lung, liver, and bone marrow. Infections experienced by these patients are related to corticosteroids in addition to other immunomodulators (i.e., cyclosporine, tacrolimus, azathioprine, and mycophenolate mofetil) used to prevent organ rejection. These latter drugs are sometimes referred to as "steroid sparing," but this refers to their use in reducing risk of steroid-associated side effects such as diabetes mellitus and osteopenia.

3. Injectable **tumor necrosis factor (TNF)–inhibiting drugs** are useful in the treatment of **rheumatoid arthritis** and **inflammatory bowel disease.** However, these drugs (especially infliximab) have been associated with an excess of cases of tuberculosis (TB), including extrapulmonary TB.

I **Neurologic deficits**   Neurologic dysfunction may predispose patients to infection if such deficits cause body defenses to be more easily breached. The following are examples.

1. Elimination of the gag reflex, whether by stroke or coma, predisposes patients to aspiration of oral or gastric contents, resulting in **pneumonia.**

2. Secondary infection of a hypoesthetic limb. **Diabetic neuropathy** can result in skin ulceration and infection.

3. Loss of neuromuscular control of the bladder. **Long-term catheterization** (with its attendant complications, such as infection) may be necessary.

J **Age**   The likelihood of acquiring certain infections varies considerably with age. In general, the maturation of the immune system is responsible for the changing pattern of infections in early childhood, and the presence of other medical illnesses accounts for most of the changes in late adulthood. Diminished immune response in the elderly may predispose them slightly to infection. For example, lower titers of antibody to influenza virus are found after immunization in the elderly than in younger adults.

K **Nosocomial infection**   Although nosocomial infections (i.e., infections acquired after 2 or more days in the hospital) can involve any body site, they have some important common characteristics.

1. **Etiology and pathogenesis**
   a. **Residence in the hospital** predisposes patients to skin and mucosal colonization by microbial flora different from that found in ambulatory patients. Specifically, enteric gram-negative rods (e.g., *E. coli, Klebsiella*) or *P. aeruginosa* in the alimentary tract may spill over onto the skin or into the respiratory tree. The degree of illness influences the likelihood and rapidity of acquiring hospital flora.
   b. **Antimicrobials** given to prevent or treat infection may predispose patients to colonization and subsequent infection by hospital flora.
   c. **Instrumentation** (e.g., endotracheal tubes and intravenous catheters) may bypass some of the natural host defenses.
   d. **Failure to observe appropriate infection control measures** may permit the dissemination of hospital flora. The most important route for such dissemination is on the hands of health care workers.
   e. **Environmental factors,** such as those that permit colonization of water by *Legionella* or imperfect air filtration that allows for fungal spores, may permit infection to occur at excess rates because of the inherently decreased resistance to infection of some patients.

2. **Therapy.** The duration of hospitalization and the likelihood that the infection was acquired nosocomially influence the use of empiric antibiotics to treat suspected infections. Knowledge of the antimicrobial susceptibility patterns of nosocomial microbes in one's institution can be especially helpful.

3. **Prevention.** See online for details, including respiratory precautions.

V   SPECIFIC INFECTIONS ACCORDING TO BODY SITE

A Central nervous system (CNS) infections
1. **Meningitis**
   a. **Acute meningitis** is an inflammatory disease involving the arachnoid layer of the meninges and the fluid that circulates in the ventricles and the subarachnoid space—the **CSF.**

TABLE 9–2   Examination of Cerebrospinal Fluid in Suspected Meningitis

	Glucose	Protein	White Blood Cells (cells/mL)
Bacterial	Low	Increased	100 to >1000 with neutrophil dominance
Fungal	Low to normal	Normal to increased	1–500
Tubercular	Low	Increased	5–100
Viral	Normal	Normal	5–300 with lymphocyte predominance

(1) **Classification** (Table 9–2). There are two major classifications of meningitis: **bacterial** and **aseptic.** In both forms, fever, headache, and stiff neck occur.

(2) **Etiology** (Table 9–3)

    (a) **Bacterial meningitis.** The **causes vary with the age of the patient.** *E. coli* and *Streptococcus agalactiae* occur most frequently in infants; *Haemophilus influenzae,* which used to predominate in young children (2 months to 6 years), has been practically eradicated by universal vaccination; *N. meningitidis* is most common in adolescents and young adults; and *Streptococcus pneumoniae* is most common in adults older than 25 years. *Listeria monocytogenes,* which enters the body through the gastrointestinal tract, is found most commonly in cancer patients, the elderly, and immunosuppressed individuals.

    (b) **Aseptic meningitis.** Usually a **viral disease,** aseptic meningitis may also reflect an **inflammatory process adjacent to the meninges** (e.g., cerebritis, brain abscess, sinusitis, or otitis). In partially treated bacterial meningitis, the CSF usually has a pyogenic nature, although antibiotics may modify the disease in such a way as to create an aseptic pattern. Drug hypersensitivity also may cause an aseptic meningitis (usually with a predominance of neutrophils in the WBCs) and may occur rarely with ibuprofen or a variety of other agents.

(3) **Clinical features.** When bacteria cause meningitis, this manifestation usually is part of a **systemic, bacteremic infection.** An exception occurs when bacteria gain access to the meninges after trauma or surgery or via a bony defect (usually in the temporal area or the cribriform plate). Typical presentation includes fever, nuchal rigidity, and altered mental status.

    (a) With disease due to *H. influenzae* or *S. pneumoniae,* focal infection such as **pneumonia** or **otitis** also may be apparent.

    (b) With disease due to *N. meningitidis,* there may be a characteristic systemic infection consisting of a **petechial** or **purpuric skin rash and hypotension,** which can develop rapidly.

    (c) With aseptic meningitis due to echoviruses or coxsackieviruses, there may be a characteristic **rash resembling rubella** or a **vesicular** or **petechial rash.**

(4) **Therapy**

    (a) **Bacterial meningitis. Antibiotics** have a significant impact on the outcome of this disease. Without treatment, death is almost certain; with treatment, however, the

TABLE 9–3   Organisms in Bacterial Meningitis

Organism	Age	Predisposing Factors	Important Points
Neisseria meningitidis	Children and young adults		Fatal if not treated early, diffuse purpuric rash, requires prophylaxis for exposed contacts
Group B *Streptococcus, Escherichia coli*	Neonates	Maternal infection	
Listeria monocytogenes	Neonates, elderly	Immunosuppression	
Streptococcus pneumoniae	All ages, elderly	Chronic illness, asplenia	Most common cause in adults
Haemophilus influenzae	Adults		Predominated in children until universal vaccination
Staphylococcus aureus	All ages	Bacteremia, foreign body, endocarditis	
Gram-negative rods	All ages, elderly	Sepsis, neurosurgery	

mortality rate is reduced to approximately 20% of those patients who are not moribund at the time of diagnosis. Bactericidal antibiotics should be given in doses that permit the drug to achieve killing levels in the CSF. Because the blood–brain barrier blocks virtually all drugs and reduces drug penetration from the blood into the CSF, maximum tolerated systemic doses should be given even at the end of the treatment course (usually a total of 2 weeks).

(i) In adults, initial therapy with a combination of a broad-spectrum cephalosporin and vancomycin is used initially. Frequently, this can be simplified once the results of cultures and sensitivities have been obtained. Ampicillin is added if *Listeria* is considered to be a possible etiology.

(ii) If resistant organisms are found, the appropriate drug (e.g., cefotaxime or vancomycin) is begun or continued, and other agents are stopped. *S. pneumoniae* resistant to penicillin (and sometimes cephalosporins) is being isolated more frequently. In critically ill patients with suspected or established pneumococcal meningitis, vancomycin should be added to the regimen until susceptibility information is available.

(iii) If pneumococcal meningitis is present, a short course of corticosteroids such as dexamethasone starting **before or with** the antibiotics can change morbidity outcomes.

(b) Aseptic meningitis. There is **no specific chemotherapy** for this condition. Any underlying disease should be treated. If drug hypersensitivity is suspected, the offending agent should be stopped.

b. Chronic meningitis

(1) **Etiology.** The most common causes of chronic meningitis are tuberculosis, cryptococcal disease, malignancy, and sarcoidosis. **Mollaret's meningitis is a benign recurrent lymphocytic meningitis that represents a rare complication to herpes simplex infection.**

(2) **Clinical features.** Chronic meningitis may have an indolent presentation, with symptoms similar to those of acute meningitis or with altered mentation with or without fever. CSF abnormalities may progress if the underlying disease is untreated. In many of these diseases, the CSF glucose level is low. Chronic meningitis should be considered when a low CSF glucose level is noted in patients who are found not to have acute bacterial meningitis.

(3) **Therapy.** Treatment is directed at the underlying disease. [See VII C 3 and VIII G 1 c (1) (c) for TB and cryptococcal treatment.]

2. Encephalitis

a. Etiology. Most encephalitides are caused by viruses, several of which are transmitted by the bites of infective mosquitoes.

b. Clinical features. Patients with encephalitis usually present with altered mentation, seizures, or both. The CSF may be normal or have an aseptic pattern.

c. Diagnosis. Diagnosis involves measuring rising titers of antibody to one of the encephalitis viruses in patients with a compatible clinical syndrome. When **herpes simplex encephalitis** is suspected (e.g., temporal lobe involvement on brain imaging), early antiviral treatment is recommended. Measurement of herpes simplex virus–specific nucleic acid in CSF has largely supplanted brain biopsy for diagnosis. Successful treatment of herpes encephalitis depends on initiation of medications before neurologic deterioration becomes extensive. West Nile virus was first described as a cause of encephalitis in New York in 1999, but since then this mosquito-borne infection has been found through much of North America. Patients with West Nile encephalitis can have a complete recovery of function, but many patients have severe weakness during the infection and may recover only partially if at all.

d. Differential diagnosis. *Toxoplasma gondii* can cause encephalitis in patients with diminished T cell function (e.g., due to AIDS or posttransplantation immunosuppressive therapy). Some intoxications and immune diseases (e.g., systemic lupus erythematosus [SLE]) may have a presentation indistinguishable from encephalitis. Endocarditis also should be considered. Other viruses to consider include cytomegalovirus (CMV), varicella-zoster virus (VZV), Epstein–Barr virus (EBV), HIV, and the zoonotic encephalic viruses such as Western equine encephalitis and St. Louis encephalitis virus. Syphilis, drug toxicity, and SLE should also be considered in an individual with acute encephalitis.

e. Therapy. Treatment of viral encephalitis is **supportive,** with the exception of acyclovir for herpes simplex encephalitis. Drug intoxication and immune diseases are treatable, and patients with associated encephalitis usually respond.

3. **Intracranial abscess.** Suppurative infections can involve the contents of the calvarium, usually by direct spread from an infected sinus or ear.

a. **Etiology.** The causative organism of an intracranial abscess (e.g., streptococci or anaerobic) usually reaches the CNS by superficially infected contiguous structures. Abscesses can be localized to the extradural (also called epidural) or subdural spaces or in the brain parenchyma. Rarely, hematogenous spread of bacteria can give rise to intracranial abscesses. Less common agents are *Toxoplasma*, *Nocardia*, and *Cryptococcus* species, which usually are seen in immunocompromised patients with reduced helper T cell numbers or function.

b. **Diagnosis. Magnetic resonance imaging (MRI)** (more sensitive) or **CT** (more widely available and less expensive) of the brain is helpful in making the diagnosis. Early scans may be equivocal, but studies repeated within a few days are almost always positive, especially with the use of contrast. Definitive diagnosis requires aspiration for stain and culture.

c. **Therapy.** Bacterial abscesses are treated with appropriate **antibiotics** that penetrate brain tissue well. These may include penicillin, chloramphenicol, and metronidazole. The treatment is given for the specific infection: for *Toxoplasma*, pyrimethamine, sulfadiazine; for *Cryptococcus,* amphotericin B, flucytosine; and for *Nocardia*, a sulfa drug with or without trimethoprim. Surgical excision or decompression is not always needed, but some patients, especially those with large lesions or slow response to treatment, require **serial aspirations** or more aggressive surgical débridement.

B Head and neck infections

1. **Otitis.** Infections of the ear can involve any of the ear's three major anatomic areas—the outer, middle, or inner ear.

a. **Outer ear infections,** also called "**swimmer's ear,**" tend to be minor irritations of the external auditory canal. Topical antibiotic treatment is used for external otitis. An exception is **malignant otitis externa,** a destructive process most commonly found in diabetic patients [see IV A 4 a]. Malignant otitis externa requires antibiotics that are effective against *P. aeruginosa* infection plus surgical débridement and drainage.

b. **Middle ear infection,** or **otitis media,** typically is a disease of children and manifests as ear pain and reduced auditory acuity. Otoscopy shows a dull, poorly mobile tympanic membrane with or without pus behind it. The most common causes are pneumococci, *Streptococcus pyogenes*, *Moraxella catarrhalis*, and *H. influenzae*. In chronic cases, especially if multiple courses of antibiotics have been given, enteric gram-negative rods and anaerobes may be involved. Treatment of otitis media is recommended primarily to prevent severe complications such as mastoiditis, which are decreasing in occurrence. Therapeutic options include amoxicillin, amoxicillin with clavulanic acid, trimethoprim with sulfamethoxazole, a macrolide such as azithromycin or clarithromycin, or an oral cephalosporin. Cultures and appropriate therapy are suggested for chronic otitis media.

c. **Inner ear infections** rarely are caused by bacteria. However, several viruses may be associated with a syndrome of **vertigo** with or without **tinnitus.** No treatment is helpful.

2. **Sinusitis** (Figure 9–2). The paranasal sinuses have continuous exposure to the external environment via the ostia in the nose. Under normal conditions, host defenses maintain the sterile environment of the sinuses. However, when mucociliary clearance is interrupted because of structural or functional abnormalities, infection can supervene. In addition, patients with mid- to late-stage HIV infection are prone to recurrent or chronic sinusitis.

a. **Etiology.** As in middle ear infections, **virulent bacteria** such as pneumococci and *H. influenzae* are most likely to cause acute disease, and anaerobic or enteric organisms are associated with more chronic infections. Bacterial sinusitis may follow and mimic viral upper respiratory infections; however, only the bacterial infections go on to develop suppurative complications of the CNS.

b. **Diagnosis. Sinus radiography** shows mucosal thickening or opacification or air–fluid levels in sinusitis. Tenderness and edema help localize disease to the sinuses but are not present in

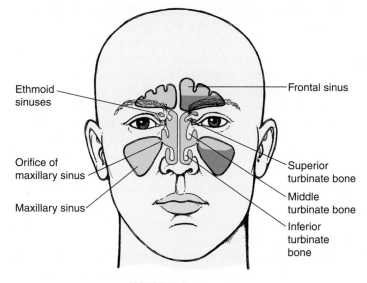

FIGURE 9–2 Sinsusitis.

all patients. **CT scanning** is more sensitive than sinus radiography, but it should not be performed in the early stages of "colds" because minor sinus abnormalities are commonly seen on CT scan in patients without significant ongoing sinusitis. Most cases of sinusitis are diagnosed clinically, and imaging is reserved for patients with refractory or recurrent disease.

  c. Therapy

  (1) In mild cases decongestants alone are adequate.

  (2) Functional **endoscopic sinus surgery** can be useful in patients with repeated or persistent infection.

3. Odontogenic infections, the most common infections occurring in the oral cavity, usually are local and respond to simple measures such as draining abscesses, restoring carious teeth, and maintaining good oral hygiene. Sometimes, however, soft tissue infections in the mouth can dissect through tissue planes and involve deeper structures of the face or neck. Examples are **Ludwig's angina,** which is an infection extending to the floor of the mouth, and **retropharyngeal abscess,** which can track down to the mediastinum. The involved bacteria are streptococci and indigenous oral anaerobes.

4. Eye infections. Normally, the eyes are resistant to infections.

  a. Conjunctivitis. Superficial infections of the conjunctiva usually are bacterial or viral and resolve spontaneously. An exception is **gonorrheal conjunctivitis,** a rare adult disease that must be treated vigorously.

  b. Keratitis. Because the transparency of the cornea is crucial for vision, diagnostic tests such as bacterial and viral smears and cultures are warranted. Initial therapy is guided by the clinical picture because a variety of organisms can cause keratitis, including *S. aureus, P. aeruginosa,* streptococci, numerous fungi, and herpes simplex and varicella-zoster viruses. It is important to recognize keratitis caused by **herpes simplex virus** so that appropriate antiviral therapy is started to prevent blindness.

  c. Endophthalmitis. Bacteria most commonly cause this infection of the internal structures of the eye, which may follow eye surgery or infection elsewhere in the body. Systemic and topical antibiotics, selected on the basis of clinical findings and Gram stain of ocular material, are administered to prevent irreversible destruction of the eye. However, the prognosis for normal visual acuity after endophthalmitis is poor. Mycotic (fungal) endophthalmitis should be considered in the setting of fungemia, penetrating eye trauma, and infection due to soil-contaminated foreign body.

C Respiratory tract infections

1. Upper respiratory infections. Infections involving the nose, throat, larynx, airways, and adjacent structures are the most common causes of morbidity in the United States.

  a. Etiology. Upper respiratory infections almost invariably are viral.

b. **Clinical features.** These "colds" and "flus" involve rhinorrhea, coryza, cough, a slight fever, and, sometimes, sore throat. During seasons when influenza is epidemic in a community, headache, cough, myalgia, and higher and often sustained fever may suggest the diagnosis.

c. **Therapy.** Treatment for "colds" is symptomatic. Influenza A virus infections may resolve more quickly when an antiviral such as amantadine, rimantadine, oseltamivir, or zanamivir is administered within 24–48 hours. Though resistance to these agents is increasing, patients with risk of severe complications warrant antiviral prophylaxis in certain situations. These medications can be useful in preventing influenza in high-risk patients when immunization is not feasible or is performed too late to offer meaningful protection.

d. **Prevention.** Seasonal vaccination against the most probable strains with pandemic potential offers the best strategy at curbing infection rates. However, there is no substitute for using proper hand hygiene and minimizing sick contacts during outbreaks.

2. **Pharyngitis**

a. **Etiology.** The major etiologic agents of pharyngitis, a common illness, are viruses and *S. pyogenes* (group A streptococci).

b. **Clinical features. Sore throat** that occurs with or without objective findings of erythema or exudate on the oropharynx or tonsils is characteristic.

c. **Therapy**

(1) Treatment for group A streptococcal pharyngitis may accelerate healing and reduce symptoms, but the major purpose of treating this disorder is **prevention of subsequent rheumatic fever,** a rare sequela.

(2) Viral pharyngitis does not improve with any known chemotherapy.

(3) Whether treatment of mycoplasmal or chlamydial pharyngitis is beneficial is not known.

3. **Tracheobronchitis** is an infection of the airways.

a. **Etiology.** Most cases of tracheobronchitis are associated with infection by mycoplasma or by **viruses,** such as influenza or parainfluenza virus (in adults) or respiratory syncytial virus (in young children). However, bacteria may play a role in patients with chronic obstructive pulmonary disease (COPD) and cystic fibrosis. *H. influenzae, S. aureus,* and *P. aeruginosa* are believed to be pathogenic in patients with cystic fibrosis [see Chapter 3 V B].

b. **Clinical features and laboratory findings.** Cough with abundant, thick sputum is characteristic of tracheobronchitis. Fever, chest pain, and wheezing also may occur. If rales or consolidation is found, pneumonia is suggested. The WBC count and chest radiograph are unchanged from baseline in uncomplicated tracheobronchitis.

c. **Therapy.** Simple supportive measures usually suffice. Antibiotics usually are given to patients with COPD exacerbation, although the benefit of such therapy is modest and most pronounced when all three elements of exacerbation are present: dyspnea, increased volume of sputum, and increased purulence of sputum. Patients with cystic fibrosis undergo chest physical therapy and receive antimicrobial agents according to sputum bacteriology [see Chapter 3 V B 6 b].

4. **Pneumonia**

a. **Etiology.** Causes include bacteria, viruses, fungi, and parasites. Although identification of the specific cause of pneumonia is ideal, many patients can be treated initially on the basis of clinical and demographic features.

b. **Clinical features and diagnosis**

(1) **Patient history** may indicate an underlying condition. For example, the incidence of bacterial pneumonia is increased in association with COPD or alcoholism. Fever is usually but not always present. Air space disease is evidenced by rales or signs of consolidation on physical examination and infiltrate on chest radiograph

(2) Because of the **vast differential diagnosis,** it is helpful to consider pneumonia in two ways (recognizing that a considerable overlap is possible):

(a) Whether it developed at home (**community acquired**) or in a hospital or institution (**health care associated** or **nosocomial**)

(b) Whether it had a rapid onset with chills, fever, and cough (**classical**) or a more indolent onset (**atypical**)

c. **Pneumonia syndromes** (Table 9–4)

TABLE 9–4   Classification of Pneumonias

	Community-acquired Pneumonias			Aspiration Pneumonia	Hospital-Acquired Pneumonia
	TYPICAL	**ATYPICAL**	**VIRAL**		
Etiology	Most common: *Streptococcus pneumonia* Also: *Haemophilus influenzae, Moraxella catarrhalis*	*Mycoplasma pneumoniae* (walking pneumonia) *Chlamydia pneumoniae*	Adenovirus, parainfluenza virus, respiratory syncytial virus	Gram-negative organisms from gut, anaerobes from mouth flora	*Pseudomonas* and typical pathogens with higher resistance patterns
Clinical considerations	Classically with shaking chills, fever, productive cough, pleuritic pain	More indolent course; myalgia, arthralgia more prominent		Related to ethyl alcohol use, altered mental status seizures, cardiovascular accident	Includes nursing homes
Gram stain	Large number of neutrophils with predominance of one organism	Less diagnostic	No organisms observed	Mixed microbial	Similar to community-acquired pneumonias
Chest x-ray	Generally lobar consolidation	Patchy bilateral infiltrates	Patchy bilateral infiltrates	Lobar consolidation most likely in right middle or lower lobe	Lobar or multilobar consolidations
Therapy	Macrolide or fluoroquinolone as an outpatient; if hospitalized, azithromycin ± ceftriaxone or intravenous fluoroquinolone	Macrolide or fluoroquinolone	Supportive care	Clindamycin to cover anaerobes in addition to macrolide or fluoroquinolone	Broad-spectrum antipseudomonal (cefepime, imipenem, piperacillin, tazobactam) ± macrolide for coverage of atypicals

(1) **Classic** community-acquired pneumonia (CAP)

   (a) **Etiology.** This syndrome most frequently is caused by *S. pneumoniae.* However, *H. influenzae, M. catarrhalis,* and *S. aureus* can also can cause this clinical picture.

   (b) **Diagnosis.** Gram staining of expectorated sputum shows large numbers of neutrophils (i.e., >25 per low-power field) and few squamous cells (<10 per low-power field). The bacterial flora may be mixed, but often there is a predominance of one morphologic type, such as paired lancet-shaped gram-positive cocci seen in pneumococcal pneumonia.

   (c) **Therapy.** When the presentation is truly classic, with shaking chills, rust-colored sputum, and a moderate fever accompanied by a Gram stain suggesting pneumococci, penicillin used to be the drug of choice. Due to high incidence of pneumococcal penicillin resistance, an alternative agent such as a macrolide or fluoroquinolone active against gram-positive bacteria (e.g., gatifloxacin, moxifloxacin, or levofloxacin) is preferred as initial treatment.

      (i) A macrolide or fluoroquinolone is used in penicillin-allergic patients when symptoms blend into those seen in the atypical form or when the Gram stain is inconclusive.

      (ii) If the Gram stain shows gram-negative rods, therapy appropriate for *Haemophilus* or enteric gram-negative bacilli is given, usually in the hospital.

      (iii) If gram-negative cocci appear singly or in pairs, treatment should be directed toward *M. catarrhalis* with trimethoprim–sulfamethoxazole or a macrolide.

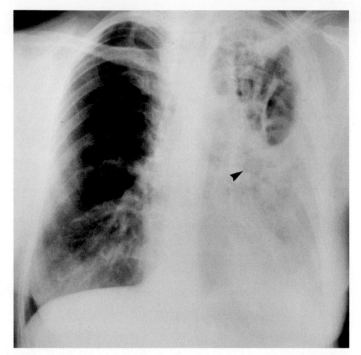

FIGURE 9–3 Pneumonia caused by *Klebsiella pneumoniae*. Chest x-ray reveals extensive consolidation of the left lower lobe. Cavity formation is apparent within the involved area (*arrow*).

(2) **Atypical community-acquired pneumonia**

(a) **Etiology.** This syndrome usually is caused by *M. pneumoniae* or *C. pneumoniae*, although a variety of viruses may be responsible, including adenovirus, parainfluenza virus, and respiratory syncytial virus.

(b) **Diagnosis.** Atypical CAP is less severe than the classical form, and sputum is typically nondiagnostic. Systemic symptoms (e.g., myalgia, arthralgia, and skin rash) are more prominent, and chest complaints (e.g., pleuritic pain and productive cough) are less marked in atypical pneumonia than in classical pneumonia. Gram stain shows some neutrophils and a variety of bacterial forms. Cultures seldom are diagnostic. Chest radiographs usually show patchy, bilateral infiltrates and little or no pleural effusion (Figure 9–3).

(c) **Differential diagnosis**

(i) **Aspiration pneumonia** may result from pulmonary aspiration of oral secretions, especially with diminished protection of the airways (e.g., after unconsciousness, a seizure, or vocal cord paralysis).

(ii) **Tuberculosis** is also a consideration in a case of a slowly evolving pulmonary infection. However, there usually is other evidence of tuberculosis (e.g., radiographic findings, an exposure history, or a positive acid-fast smear of the sputum) [see VII C].

(iii) **Legionnaires' disease** also may occur in this way [see VII E].

(d) **Therapy.** Patients with atypical pneumonia often present after they have had many days or more than a week of symptoms. Effective treatment may not bring immediate relief but may further shorten the course of the illness. Any of the macrolides or fluoroquinolones is appropriate, and the oral route is adequate. Therapy for other nonclassic pneumonias involves the following measures:

(i) When **aspiration pneumonia** is suspected, an antibiotic with activity against gram negatives, oral anaerobes, and streptococci is suggested (e.g., third-generation cephalosporin plus metronidazole, respiratory fluoroquinolone, or ampicillin–sulbactam).

(ii) **Tuberculosis** always is treated with combinations of antibiotics [see VII C 3].

(iii) **Legionnaires' disease** usually responds to macrolides or fluoroquinolones, although some severely ill patients may require hospitalization [see VII E 5].

(3) Classic (acute) hospital-acquired pneumonia

    (a) Etiology. This syndrome can be caused by a variety of bacteria. Patients often are granulocytopenic, postoperative, or intubated. Because these patients usually have pharyngeal colonization by enteric gram-negative aerobes, the pneumonia is likely to involve these organisms. All risk factors should be taken into consideration when assessing these patients.

    (b) Diagnosis. Gram stain and culture of sputum are important in determining the organisms involved in this infection. Even though good respiratory specimens can be hard to obtain, it is worth the effort to make a microbial diagnosis for pneumonia patients either in or recently discharged from the hospital. More-invasive tests such as bronchoscopy and lung biopsy may be needed to confirm the diagnosis.

    (c) Therapy. When the Gram stain suggests inflammation and shows abundant gram-negative rods, recommended treatment is a β-lactam antibiotic with activity against a wide variety of enteric gram-negative organisms, with or without an aminoglycoside. Knowledge of susceptibility patterns in the hospital can help in choosing empiric therapy. When culture results are available, more specific therapy can be given. In patients with neutropenia, broad coverage (including activity against *P. aeruginosa*) is used. If *Legionella* is seriously considered, a macrolide or fluoroquinolone should be added. Hospitals with significant rates of infection caused by methicillin-resistant *S. aureus* are settings where the use of vancomycin or linezolid is prudent if the Gram stain suggests a staphylococcal infection.

5. Lung abscess

    a. Etiology. This infection may be the result of a pyogenic pneumonia caused by pathogens such as *S. aureus* or *S. pyogenes*. More commonly, however, lung abscess occurs as a late stage in the evolution of untreated anaerobic or mixed-flora pneumonia. Neurologic impairment of normal glottal reflexes predisposes patients to aspiration and lung abscess.

    b. Clinical features. Approximately half of patients are afebrile, and some have longstanding constitutional complaints such as weight loss. Foul-smelling sputum is highly suggestive of anaerobic infection.

    c. Therapy. Most lung abscesses drain into the tracheobronchial tree and can be cured with appropriate antimicrobial therapy, although the duration of therapy often is long.

6. Thoracic empyema

    a. Etiology. This infection also is related to underlying pneumonia. Any pyogenic pneumonia may give rise to a pleural effusion, which may become infected. Rarely, anaerobic empyema is the only manifestation of thoracic infection; presumably, this occurs as a sequela to an anaerobic pneumonia or lung abscess, which may not be apparent at the time of the empyema.

    b. Therapy

        (1) Noninfected parapneumonic effusions with a relatively low WBC count and a pH greater than 7.2 usually resolve with systemic antimicrobial therapy.

        (2) Infected (complicated) effusions or those with a very low pH or a high WBC count usually require thoracostomy drainage.

D **Gastrointestinal infections**

1. Food poisoning. These syndromes represent a diverse collection of intoxications or infections associated with ingestion of food or beverage that has been contaminated with pathogenic organisms, toxins, or chemicals. Disregarding the purely chemical entities such as heavy metal poisoning, mushroom poisoning [see Chapter 6 Online IV C 3], and polychlorinated biphenyl (PCB) poisoning, food poisoning syndromes can be divided into those causing **gastrointestinal symptoms** and those causing **neurologic symptoms.** In all cases of suspected food poisoning, some epidemiologic assessment should be done to identify other infected individuals and to report outbreaks to public health authorities.

    a. Gastrointestinal food poisoning is the most familiar type of food poisoning (see Chapter 6 IV D 5 and Table 6–1). Diarrhea, nausea, vomiting, and abdominal pain are the most common manifestations.

(1) **Clinical categories** usually are based on the incubation period, the food vehicle, and the nature of the gastrointestinal complaint.

(a) Preformed toxins give rise to the shortest-onset syndromes. For example, the enterotoxin-mediated syndromes caused by staphylococci, *Bacillus cereus*, and *Clostridium perfringens* manifest within a few hours after ingestion of the contaminated food.

(b) Diseases that depend on the growth of bacteria require a period of hours to days to manifest, and it may be difficult to relate the illness to a specific exposure. Sometimes cultures of various leftover foods are helpful; in other cases, careful recall of foods consumed is diagnostic.

(2) **Therapy.** Almost all forms of gastrointestinal food poisoning are self-limited and remit spontaneously within 1–2 days. Careful replacement of fluid and electrolytes may be needed for young children or those adults with significant underlying medical disease, but watchful waiting is usually sufficient.

b. **Neurologic food poisoning** is rare. However, it is important to establish the diagnosis so that appropriate therapy can be instituted immediately.

(1) **Botulism.** This syndrome is an intoxication caused by a preformed toxin of *Clostridium botulinum*. Although the toxin is destroyed by heating, the duration or degree of heating may be inadequate. Often, a gastrointestinal prodrome occurs before the classic flaccid paralysis sets in. Infants have the highest rate of botulism, and it is characterized by the germination *of C. botulinum* spores inside the baby and elaboration of the toxin directly into the gastrointestinal tract. When adults develop botulism from this mechanism of endogenous production of toxin, it is called **hidden botulism.**

(2) **Fish poisoning** (see Chapter 6 🅟 Online IV C 2)

(a) **Consumption of contaminated shellfish** can result in two types of poisoning: paralytic and neurotoxic.

(i) **Paralytic shellfish poisoning** results from contamination by neurotoxin-producing dinoflagellates of the genus *Gonyaulax*. This syndrome includes paresthesias followed by muscle weakness.

(ii) **Neurotoxic shellfish poisoning** results from shellfish contamination by dinoflagellates of the genus *Gymnodinium*. This syndrome is characterized by paresthesias without muscle weakness. Consumption of fleshy fish can give rise to a similar neurologic syndrome called **ciguatera** [see Chapter 6 🅟 Online IV C 2 b].

(b) **Consumption of certain contaminated fish** such as tuna and bonito can result in an illness resembling a histamine reaction. This syndrome is called **scombroid.**

(3) **Monosodium glutamate intoxication** (sometimes called **Chinese restaurant syndrome**) is characterized by a burning and tightness in the upper body accompanied by systemic symptoms such as flushing, diaphoresis, cramps, and nausea.

(4) **Therapy.** Neurologic food poisoning syndromes usually resolve completely but require patient reassurance and supportive medical care. Supportive measures may include tracheal intubation for patients with botulism or paralytic shellfish poisoning. Identifying the vehicle is crucial to prevent further occurrences. Specific antitoxin therapy is available for botulism and should be administered as soon as possible if clinical suspicion is high.

2. **Peptic ulcer/gastroesophageal reflux disease (GERD).** Causative agent is often *Helicobacter pylori* and must be eradicated with appropriate therapy [see Chapter 6 I B 1 d].

3. **Infectious diarrhea.** Acute diarrhea often can be attributed to microorganisms. The occurrence of any infectious diarrhea suggests a break in optimal hygienic measures. The disease is transmitted either through fecal contamination of food or water or from human to human via fomites or by sexual contact [see Chapter 6 IV D 4].

a. **Etiology and pathogenesis.** Determining the specific etiologic agent of infectious diarrhea can be laborious and is often unsuccessful. It may be useful to distinguish invasive from noninvasive processes.

(1) **Invasive processes.** Certain agents of acute diarrhea (e.g., *Shigella*, *Salmonella*, *Entamoeba*, and *Campylobacter*) invade the terminal ileum and colon, where they destroy mucosal cells and cause inflammation. A bloody diarrhea has been associated with some strains of *E. coli* that bear a toxin. Most of these strains belong to the O157:H7 serotype

of *E. coli* and can be cultured by a clinical laboratory if they are alerted to the suspicion of this organism.

    (2) Noninvasive processes. Other agents of acute diarrhea [e.g., enterotoxigenic *E. coli*, *Vibrio cholerae* (rarely found in the United States), *Cryptosporidium*, *Giardia intestinalis*, rotavirus] are enterotoxigenic and adhere to mucosal cells in the small intestine, where they produce diarrheal toxins.

b. Clinical features. Manifestations vary with respect to the presence of abdominal pain, cramps, and blood or mucus in the stool, as well as to the frequency and nature of the bowel movements.

    (1) Diarrhea due to invasive agents generally is associated with rectal bleeding, fever, and systemic symptoms such as headache.

    (2) Diarrhea due to noninvasive agents usually occurs without fever and is associated with fewer systemic complaints. However, substantial fluid loss from watery diarrhea in these patients may occur.

    (3) Diarrhea due to enterohemorrhagic *E. coli* (O157:H7) is usually self-limited, but it can lead to hemolytic–uremic syndrome (HUS). This is a serious illness that tends to occur mostly in children and has a substantial mortality rate.

c. Diagnosis. It is important to distinguish among the various infectious diarrheal diseases because their therapies are different.

    (1) Microscopic examination

        (a) Fecal leukocytes. A useful test is to examine the stool for WBCs using Gram stain or preparations stained with methylene blue.

            (i) Invasive agents may secrete cytotoxin or penetrate the mucosal wall of the bowel. Either mechanism may lead to the presence of leukocytes in the stool. (The diarrhea associated with *Clostridium difficile*, sometimes called pseudomembranous colitis [see Chapter 6 V I], also is associated with pus in the stool, as are several of the sexually transmitted proctitides and **inflammatory bowel diseases**, e.g., ulcerative colitis and regional enteritis or Crohn's disease.)

            (ii) Noninvasive agents do not cause the migration of leukocytes into the bowel wall and the stool. However, special techniques are needed to identify microsporidia or *Cryptosporidium* in the stool, and the laboratory may not perform these tests routinely.

        (b) Trophozoites or **cysts** in the stool suggest the presence of protozoa such as *Entamoeba histolytica* or *G. intestinalis*.

    (2) Stool culture

        (a) The presence of fever or the identification of fecal leukocytes suggests an invasive pathogen. When the clinical severity or the epidemiologic setting makes the precise diagnosis important, the stool can be cultured for the most common of these pathogens (i.e., *Shigella*, *Salmonella*, and *Campylobacter*). Stool cultures take at least 2 days to process, so therapeutic decisions are often made clinically.

        (b) Evaluation of the stool for protozoa (i.e., the **ova and parasite test**) also is recommended.

        (c) *C. difficile* produces an enterotoxin leading to diarrhea, fever, and stool leukocytosis. (In severe cases, a pseudomembrane may be present in the rectum or colon.) Disease occurs during or shortly after the administration of antibacterial agents and is especially common in **nosocomial diarrhea**. Culture and toxin assays are available to diagnose *C. difficile* infection.

    (3) Proctosigmoidoscopy or colonoscopy. These techniques may aid in the diagnosis of inflammation-related diarrhea, especially by allowing differentiation of infectious from noninfectious causes.

    (4) Biopsy. In cases of persistent diarrhea in which less invasive techniques have failed to provide a diagnosis, **biopsy** of the large bowel (for *E. histolytica*) or the small bowel (for *G. intestinalis* or *Cryptosporidium*) may be diagnostic.

d. Therapy

    (1) Fluid and electrolyte replacement is paramount, regardless of the causal agent, and should be adjusted according to the patient's degree of depletion.

(2) Specific **antimicrobial therapy** may be necessary.
  (a) Among the bacterial causes of acute diarrhea, only *Shigella* infections are routinely treated. The inherent delay in diagnosis makes it unnecessary to treat most *Campylobacter*, *Salmonella*, and *E. coli* infections except in severely ill patients or those with impaired immunity. Most cases in previously healthy people resolve without incident within a few days to 1 week. When treatment is indicated, fluoroquinolones are usually effective, although increasing resistance to fluoroquinolones has been noted. Treatment of enterohemorrhagic *E. coli* (O157:H7) is not indicated, and, under some conditions, it may exacerbate the disease and lead to an increased risk of HUS.
  (b) Antiprotozoal agents usually are indicated for giardiasis and amebiasis.
  (c) Disease associated with *C. difficile* is treated with cessation of the causative antibiotic (when possible) and oral metronidazole. If this therapy fails, oral vancomycin may be used. Approximately 20% of patients will have recurrence after apparently successful treatment, and they can be retreated with the same regimen. A small number of patients have frequent recurrences despite good therapy.

  e. **Prognosis.** The prospect for complete recovery from infectious diarrhea is excellent for all patients except those who are severely immunocompromised. In most cases, a cause is not established or even investigated. Diarrhea associated with *C. difficile* can have poor outcomes, such as toxic megacolon and resultant perforation. These complications are often associated with significant underlying disease, including prior organ transplantation and immune suppression.

E **Intra-abdominal infections**

1. **Peritonitis** is covered in the chapter on gastrointestinal diseases [see Chapter 6 X A 2].

2. **Postoperative intra-abdominal abscesses.** Diagnosis of these infections is often difficult and needs to be considered in situations of occult fever.
  a. **Etiology and pathogenesis**
    (1) Postoperative abscesses develop most frequently when the bowel has been breached in an operative procedure. However, they may occur when nonviable tissue or accumulations of blood, serum, urine, or bile are present in the abdominal cavity.
    (2) Although these infections usually occur within several days of the operative procedure, they may be delayed by weeks or months. They tend to develop near the anatomic site of the surgery, although the contour of the abdomen may allow infected fluid to move to other locations.
  b. **Diagnosis.** CT and ultrasonography are the most commonly used techniques for locating these abscesses. Most important, there must be a high index of suspicion for patients who have prolonged fever, abdominal pain, or both after surgery.
  c. **Therapy.** Once intra-abdominal abscesses have been identified, **they should be evacuated,** either by repeat surgery or through a temporary flexible drainage catheter. **Antimicrobial therapy** should be administered based on the results of Gram stain and cultures. Anaerobes play a major role in intra-abdominal abscesses and should be suspected when the fluid is foul smelling or shows polymicrobial morphology on Gram stain. In selecting antimicrobial treatment, antibiotic choice should cover anaerobes and enteric gram-negative organisms.

3. **Hepatic and splenic abscesses**
  a. **Etiology and pathogenesis.** Bacterial (pyogenic) abscesses may develop in the liver and spleen, although these sites are relatively protected from infection. They may be single or multiple and often are multibacterial. Hepatic abscesses usually are associated with biliary disease or portal vein bacteremia. Splenic abscesses are associated with systemic bacteremia, hemoglobinopathy, trauma, endocarditis, or intravenous drug use.
  b. **Clinical features.** Fever, chills, and pain near the affected organ are common. However, clinical findings may be subtle, making localization and diagnosis difficult.
  c. **Diagnosis.** Cross-sectional anatomic imaging such as CT scanning, MRI, or ultrasonography are usually used to make the diagnosis. Blood cultures should always be obtained. In travelers to areas endemic for amebiasis or for immigrants from those areas, an evaluation for amebic abscess using serologic tests or a cytologic analysis of the abscess fluid can be very helpful.

d. Therapy. Treatment is primarily surgical, with excision of abscesses from the liver or splenectomy. Catheter drainage is another option for selected patients. **Systemic antimicrobial therapy is mandatory.** Sometimes small liver abscesses can be treated with antibiotics alone and have a good outcome.

4. **Cholecystitis and cholangitis.** For further details see Chapter 6 VIII B, C, G.

F **Urinary tract infections**

1. **Incidence.** These are the most common bacterial infections encountered in clinical practice and occur much more frequently in women than in men. Infections in men, pregnant women, or children should be considered complicated. Urinary tract infection (UTI) in sexually active women is generally considered uncomplicated.
   a. **UTIs** are **defined** in terms of the inflamed urinary structure:
      (1) **Cystitis:** the bladder
      (2) **Urethritis:** the urethra
      (3) **Pyelonephritis:** the renal tubules and interstitium
      (4) **Prostatitis:** the prostate (men).

2. **Etiology.** Most UTIs are caused from simple inoculation by gram-negative bacteria during instrumentation or during sexual intercourse.
   a. Agents of infection
      (1) Common agents include *E. coli* (most commonly), *Klebsiella*, and *Proteus*.
      (2) Less common causes include *Staphylococcus saprophyticus* and enterococci. Rare agents: *Nocardia*, actinomycetes, *Brucella*, adenovirus, and *Torulopsis*.
   b. **Urethral inoculation** is very common in women, particularly those with vaginal or periurethral colonization by virulent bacteria. Surgery, particularly cytoscopy, can contaminate the bladder urine.
   c. **Risk factors** include obstruction with resultant urinary stasis, vesicoureteral reflux (may lead to ascending infection), instrumentation (especially Foley catheter), pregnancy (altered smooth muscle function), diabetes mellitus, and immune deficiency.

3. **Clinical features**
   a. In general, symptomatic UTIs are characterized by the irritative symptoms of urinary frequency, urgency, and suprapubic pain. Lower tract (bladder and urethra) infection also includes dysuria, burning, malodorous or cloudy urine, and continence difficulties. Flank pain and fever suggest upper tract (kidney or ureter) involvement.
   b. Symptoms of **acute pyelonephritis** (parenchymal renal infection) include flank pain, fever, malaise, and symptoms of lower tract infection.
   c. In elderly or institutionalized patients, **septic shock associated with UTIs** presents with hypothermia, mental status alterations, syncope, and coma.
   d. The composition of the urinary sediment in urinary infections is characterized by a large number of neutrophils and a variable number of red cells. WBC casts may be observed in kidney infections (Online Figure 6–1).

4. **Clinical syndromes**
   a. There is standard agreement that a bacterial count exceeding 10^5 organisms per milliliter of urine combined with irritative voiding symptoms and pyuria indicate significant disease, not simple contamination. However, two clinically important situations are not covered by this definition of urinary tract infections.
      (1) Patients **with symptoms** of true urinary tract infection but with fewer than 10^5 bacteria per milliliter of urine may reflect early infection and should be treated with antibiotics.
      (2) Patients with no symptoms of urinary tract infection but a urine bacterial count exceeding 10^5/mL have a condition termed **asymptomatic bacteriuria,** which is not rare and occurs most often in women and in older patients and should not be treated with antibiotics.
   b. **Catheter-related bacteriuria** is an inevitable complication of prolonged bladder catheterization. It can be delayed by careful aseptic insertion, silver-impregnated catheters, and strict closed drainage. However, after 1–2 weeks, some degree of colonization is common, and, eventually, bacterial counts exceeding 10^5/mL of urine are reached.

    c. Prostatitis is a complication of many urinary tract infections in men. Acute prostatitis is characterized by perineal pain and irritative voiding symptoms.

    d. Urethritis is often a symptom of a sexually transmitted disease (e.g., gonorrheal or chlamydial infection). Copious urethral discharge is diagnostic, but mildly symptomatic urethritis can mimic a urinary tract infection.

5. Diagnosis

    a. Urinalysis of fresh, unspun urine should be performed. However, quantitative urine cultures do not distinguish between upper and lower tract infections.

        (1) Dipstick tests to examine presence of enzymes such as the leukocyte esterase may be useful. Identifying one bacterium per high-power field (400×) indicate colony growth on cultures greater than 10^5/mL.

        (2) Centrifuged sediment usually reveals leukocyturia (neutrophils) and bacteriuria.

        (3) Gram stain may characterize the organism, allowing more specific therapy.

    b. Routine urine culture is the definite method of diagnosis. Presence of greater than 10^5 colonies/mL signifies an infection that needs treatment.

    c. Examining the patient. When to examine patients for anatomic abnormalities to explain UTIs is controversial. Most evidence suggests that cystoscopy and urography seldom show treatable causes of infection; they are used only for patients with frequent recurrences and jeopardized kidney function. Men have a higher rate of anatomic complications (usually prostate related) than women. Rectal examination may indicate enlargement of the prostate leading to urethral obstruction and recurrent UTIs.

    d. When blood cultures are positive in the context of a UTI, involvement of the kidneys or prostate gland is implied. Fever also suggests renal involvement.

6. Therapy. Antibiotic treatment is usually directed at the agent most likely to be responsible for the infection. Corrective surgery is indicated to remove calculi or repair obstructive anatomic lesions.

    a. *E. coli–caused infections. E. coli* has a propensity for causing infections in otherwise healthy individuals, so one should administer antibiotics effective against *E. coli* in the absence of cultures. Oral trimethoprim and sulfamethoxazole can be used alone or together, as well as quinolones, tetracyclines, and some penicillin preparations such as amoxicillin with clavulanic acid. Ampicillin alone is likely to be ineffective because of the large number of ampicillin-resistant *E. coli*.

        (1) A 3-day course of therapy is adequate to cure most infections (especially cystitis), where urine drug levels seem to be the most important determinant of effectiveness.

        (2) Failure to cure infections rapidly does not alter the efficacy of future therapy. In rare instances, refractory infection may require a long course of therapy—sometimes up to several months—although briefer courses (e.g., 2 weeks) often are successful.

    b. Uncomplicated lower tract infection. Three-day treatment of trimethoprim–sulfamethoxazole (TMP-SMX) is effective and inexpensive. One needs to be aware of local patterns of bacterial susceptibility. Alternatives include nitrofurantoin and β-lactam antibiotics, such as amoxicillin or cephalexin.

    c. Relapsing UTI and **pyelonephritis are treated** for 14 days with TMP-SMX, if stable; alternatives include fluoroquinolones and amoxicillin or amoxicillin/clavulanic acid. In the presence of high fever, high white blood cell count, vomiting, dehydration, or evidence of sepsis, the patient should be admitted and treated with intravenous antibiotics until stable and then can complete therapy with oral agents as an outpatient.

    d. Asymptomatic bacteriuria. Treatment is indicated for patients with a known structural or functional abnormality of the kidneys (including renal transplant) and those who are pregnant.

    e. Catheter-related bacteriuria may occur in acutely catheterized patients and usually resolves when the catheter is removed. If not, or if symptoms develop within 12–24 hours, one should treat with the appropriate antibiotic. Frequent bladder catheterizations (several times daily) rather than use of an indwelling catheter may lessen the risk of this infection.

    f. Prostate infections. One should use antibiotics that penetrate and remain active in prostate tissue and fluid (e.g., trimethoprim, carbenicillin). Treatment is for at least 14 days.

    g. Recurrent UTI typically require TMP-SMX, methenamine mandelate, and sulfisoxazole. Using ciprofloxacin may result in sterile urine.

G **Skin and soft tissue infections**   Bacterial, fungal, and viral infections of the skin and related structures (e.g., hair follicles, sweat glands) are common. [See also Chapter 13 XI.]

1. **Bacterial skin infections** usually start in areas of trauma or previous disease.
   a. **Etiology.** In otherwise healthy individuals, gram-positive cocci such as *S. pyogenes* and *S. aureus* cause most skin infections. Immunocompromised individuals are subject to the usual gram-positive flora, as well as to a wider variety of pathogens, including enteric gram-negative bacilli and *P. aeruginosa*.
   b. **Clinical features**
      (1) **Cellulitis** is characterized by redness, warmth, and tenderness of the skin. It may involve a limited area or may spread widely and rapidly. Fever and leukocytosis are common. [In some patients, a rapidly progressive cutaneous infection (streptococcal toxic shock syndrome) caused by group A streptococci and characterized by significant systemic features can cause severe skin damage and even death.]
      (2) **Abscesses** represent deeper, circumscribed infections, which often start in accessory structures such as hair follicles. They may be warm or of normal skin temperature and frequently contain pus. Fever is most likely to be present in individuals with large, multiple, or deep abscesses. Hidradenitis occurs from inflammation of sweat glands with resultant abscess; often it can be treated with warm compresses.
      (3) **Ulcers** are not usually the result of bacterial infection alone but reflect tissue damage from ischemia or trauma. Invariably, ulcers are colonized by bacteria and may lead to deep soft-tissue or bone infection. They usually occur in dependent areas (e.g., the sacrum) or in areas of poor blood flow or decreased sensation (e.g., in the feet of a patient with diabetes).
   c. **Therapy**
      (1) **Cellulitis requires antibiotic management.** Agents active against streptococci and staphylococci usually are effective, including semisynthetic penicillins (e.g., nafcillin), cephalosporins, vancomycin, clindamycin, and linezolid. However, in many U.S. cities, MRSA represents the prevailing soft-tissue pathogen, and it is now recommended that antimicrobial therapy for these soft-tissue infections provide MRSA coverage.
      (2) **Abscesses should be drained,** although some rupture spontaneously. Antibiotics are seldom needed unless there is accompanying cellulitis.
      (3) **Ulcers** usually are managed by **débridement and antibiotic therapy** with broad-spectrum agents active against enteric gram-negative rods, gram-positive cocci, and anaerobes. Skin grafting may be beneficial.

2. **Fungal skin infections** usually are acquired by exposure of the skin to pathogenic fungi. Exceptions are cutaneous manifestations of blastomycosis or candidal fungemia.
   a. **Clinical features.** Fungal infections that start in the skin fall into three groups.
      (1) **Dermatophytosis** is a superficial infection of the epidermis due to dermatophytic fungi (e.g., *Trichophyton*, *Microsporum*, and *Epidermophyton* species). Athlete's foot and ringworm are examples. The skin usually is flaky and may be slightly discolored but is not frankly painful.
      (2) **Candidiasis** is a red, tender edematous rash occurring in moist body parts and is caused by *C. albicans*, often seen in diabetics and immunosuppressed patients. Intertrigo in the axillary or inframammary area is an example.
      (3) **Mixed bacterial flora and fungi** (usually *Candida* species) can be involved in superficial infection. This may be evident during or after administration of antibacterial therapy.
   b. **Diagnosis.** Potassium hydroxide preparations and fungal cultures are the foundation of diagnosis.
   c. **Therapy**
      (1) Dermatophytosis is treated with topical therapy for limited disease or with oral therapy for extensive infection. **Azoles** (e.g., ketoconazole, fluconazole) are most commonly used.
      (2) Candidiasis is treated topically, but special attention should be given to keeping the affected area clean and dry. Rarely, systemic azole therapy is required.
      (3) Mixed bacterial and fungal infections usually do not require specific antifungal therapy.

3. **Viral skin infections** may be cutaneously inoculated, as in the case of herpes simplex, but more commonly are a manifestation of systemic viral infection or an immune response to infection. An example of this is **varicella (chickenpox),** in which the virus is acquired via the respiratory tract and spreads to the skin after a viremia.

4. **Deep soft-tissue infections** are rare but serious infections usually caused by streptococci, anaerobes, and gram-negative rods. There may be comparatively little abnormality of the skin in some of these infections (e.g., **fasciitis**). Combinations of medical and surgical therapy usually are used, but even so, many patients succumb to these infections.

   a. **Gangrene** is an infection of the skin and soft tissues caused by a mixed anaerobic and aerobic bacterial flora that usually includes *C. perfringens.* It is characterized by cellulitis and gas in the soft tissues. Therapy involves surgical débridement and antibiotic therapy (e.g., with penicillin).

   b. **Fasciitis** is a rare infection between tissue planes. It usually occurs postoperatively, after rupture of an abdominal viscus, or in diabetic patients. Pathogenic bacteria include mixed anaerobes, streptococci, and, occasionally, gram-negative bacilli.

H **Osteomyelitis**   Bone infections can be classified according to their pathogenesis. In general, bone infections develop in three ways: by extension from a contiguous infection, by direct inoculation during surgery or as a result of trauma, and by hematogenous spread.

1. **Osteomyelitis due to contiguous infection or inoculation.** Bone infection should be suspected in patients with a history of **trauma** or **surgery** or with obvious **soft tissue infection** overlying bone, although the bone involvement may be difficult to prove.

   a. **Etiology.** Almost any bacterium can be responsible, including *S. aureus, P. aeruginosa,* or anaerobes.

   b. **Clinical features.** Symptoms and signs may simply be those of the adjacent infection. Pain is common, and fever is variable.

   c. **Diagnosis.** This process may be difficult. Radiographic evidence of osteomyelitis lags behind the symptoms and pathologic changes by approximately 7–10 days. Although bone scanning is sensitive for osteomyelitis, it may not distinguish bone infection from more superficial soft tissue infection. The definitive diagnosis rests on bone biopsy and bacterial culture. An expensive but useful test is the MRI scan, which shows changes in the bone marrow that can be detected well before change in plain x-rays (Figure 9–4).

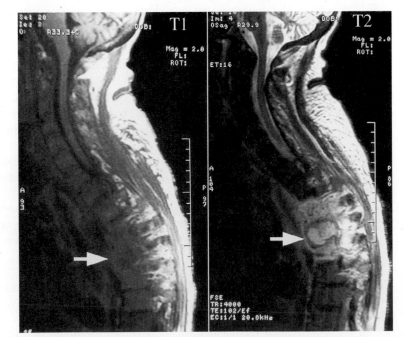

FIGURE 9–4   Magnetic resonance imaging (MRI) scan of osteomyelitis in the thoracic spine. In the T1 image **(left),** loss of bony structure in a vertebra is seen (*arrow*). In the T2 image **(right),** the high signal intensity due to water molecules shows edema and infiltrate in the same vertebra.

d. Clinical course and therapy. The clinical course guides the length of treatment, but, generally, **long courses of antibiotics** are necessary. Devitalized bone, poor blood supply, and adjacent infection may be reasons for extended (months) therapy and/or surgical débridement.

2. **Hematogenous osteomyelitis.** This type of disease should be suspected in febrile patients who experience pain and swelling over a bone but have no obvious source of infection.

   a. Etiology. The bacteriology involves largely *S. aureus.* However, *Salmonella* species seem to be more important in patients with sickle cell disease. Vertebral osteomyelitis also is somewhat different, in that gram-negative bacilli may be introduced from the urinary tract through venous channels.

   b. Diagnosis. Radiography and bone scanning are helpful. The erythrocyte sedimentation rate usually is elevated, but this is quite a nonspecific finding. Bone aspiration and culture are recommended for microbiologic diagnosis. Blood cultures also should be obtained.

   c. Therapy. Treatment is a prolonged course of **antibiotics.** Nonviable bone may need to be removed surgically because it provides a site for potential relapse.

I **Intravascular infections and endocarditis**   Intravascular infections manifest as **bacteremia,** or **fungemia,** depending on the type of infective organism demonstrated in the blood. Such infections may reflect **invasion or failure of containment at a localized site** (e.g., bowel or lung) or a **primary infection of the blood vessels or the heart** (e.g., endocarditis).

1. **Local infections** lead to positive blood cultures, with a frequency dependent on the site and severity of the infection and on the organism or organisms responsible for the infection.

   a. For example, among hospitalized patients with pneumococcal pneumonia, 10%–25% have bacteremia. The prognosis for these patients is worse than for those without bacteremia because those with bacteremia tend to have more diffuse lung involvement and more virulent organisms.

   b. Even when blood cultures do not demonstrate a particular organism, metastatic infection or dissemination (e.g., cryptococcal meningitis or miliary tuberculosis) strongly suggests blood-borne spread.

2. **Sepsis** is recognized as a systemic inflammatory response syndrome (SIRS) in the setting of an infection. SIRS is defined in a patient with two of the following criteria:

   1. Temperature $>38°C$ or $<36°C$
   2. Heart rate >90 bpm
   3. Respirations >20 breaths per minute or partial pressure of carbon dioxide in the arterial blood ($PaCO_2$) <32 mm Hg
      OR
   4. Leukocyte count $>12,000/min^3$, $<4000/mm^3$, or $>10\%$ immature (band) cells.

   a. Etiology. Sepsis can progress to septic shock, which includes organ dysfunction secondary to hypoperfusion. Septic shock can be multifactorial, but one identified cause is endotoxin (the lipopolysaccharide coat of gram-negative organisms). However, an indistinguishable clinical disease can be caused by gram-positive bacteria, viruses, and yeast.

   b. Therapy. Antibiotic treatment is critical for patient recovery. High-dose corticosteroid therapy to supplement usual supportive measures does not improve survival. Various immunomodulators such as tumor necrosis factor (TNF) inhibitors and antibody to endotoxin have failed to improve the prognosis of septic shock. Activated protein C (drotrecogin) has anticoagulant properties but also seems to block some of the destructive positive feedback loops that promote organ damage in shock. Some experts suggest using this agent in patients with sepsis-induced organ dysfunction that is clinically associated with a high risk of death.

3. **Catheter-related infections** are serious problems associated with hospitalization. Infection seldom is caused by the infusion of contaminated fluid. Rather, these infections most commonly occur at the **site of cannulation.**

   a. Diagnosis. Diagnosis involves demonstration of either local skin infection at the cannulation site or positive blood cultures and the presence of the same bacteria in significant numbers on a semiquantitative culture of the catheter. Sometimes a vein infection may not be apparent until after the catheter has been removed. Infected veins are almost always clotted at the site of the infection.

b. Therapy. Removal of the catheter when local infection is present is necessary. When vascular access is crucial and the catheter has been aseptically inserted into the vena cava (e.g., a **Hickman catheter**—a wide-bore silastic catheter used for chemotherapy, hyperalimentation, or drawing blood), conservative therapy with antibiotics alone may cure the infection. Fungal infections or those caused by highly resistant bacteria usually cannot be cured without removal of the catheter. Tunneled catheters that exhibit erythema and other signs of inflammation along the catheter tract also need to be removed. Rarely, an infected peripheral vein will require surgical management because pus needs to be drained.

4. Endocarditis usually results from infection of the cusp of a heart valve, although any part of the endocardium or any prosthetic material inserted into the heart may be involved.

a. Etiology. A variety of organisms may cause endocarditis, although bacteria account for almost all cases. The specific agent of endocarditis depends on which cardiac structures are affected.

(1) **Infection of normal valves,** which is rare, is usually associated with intravenous drug use. *S. aureus* is the most common pathogen.

(2) **Infection of previously damaged valves,** often from rheumatic heart disease, usually is attributable to viridans streptococci. Other agents of endocarditis in this setting are enterococci, *S. aureus,* and various small gram-negative rods constituting part of the normal oral flora known as the **HACEK** organisms:
- *Haemophilus parainfluenzae, Haemophilus aphrophilus*
- *Actinobacillus actinomycetemcomitans*
- *Cardiobacterium hominis*
- *Eikenella corrodens*
- *Kingella kingae*

(3) **Infection of prosthetic valves** involves staphylococci (both coagulase positive and coagulase negative) as the most common agents of early-onset disease (occurring <2 months postoperatively). Streptococci are the most common agents of late-onset disease (occurring >2 months postoperatively).

b. Clinical features. Signs and symptoms vary widely.

(1) **Fever** is almost universal. A **new heart murmur** is highly suggestive but not always present. Endocarditis is one of the most common causes of fever of unknown origin.

(2) Less commonly, **embolic disease** such as stroke or splenic artery embolism and infarction is evident. Most emboli are small and may give rise to uncommon but diagnostically helpful physical findings, including **Roth's spots, Osler's nodes, Janeway's lesions,** and **conjunctival hemorrhage.**

(3) A variety of constitutional symptoms such as myalgia, back pain, confusion, or fatigue may occur.

c. Diagnosis

(1) **Blood cultures** are critical and are positive in more than 90% of cases of endocarditis. (Previous use of antibiotics may suppress growth of cultures and lower the yield.) Because of the continuous bacteremia of endocarditis, virtually all cultures are positive, and it is rarely necessary to obtain more than three or four cultures.

(2) For patients with culture-negative endocarditis, there is little incremental value in collecting several additional blood samples for culture. Sometimes, the microbiology laboratory can enhance isolation by using **special culture techniques,** such as prolonged incubation to isolate slow-growing organisms (e.g., HACEK).

(3) Echocardiography should be performed in suspected endocarditis. Transthoracic echocardiography (TTE) may reveal vegetation or valvular insufficiency suggestive of endocarditis, but transesophageal echocardiography (TEE) has higher sensitivity.

(4) Immune complexes may cause **glomerulonephritis,** which is characterized by elevated serum creatinine, hematuria, and casts in the urine, or rheumatologic manifestations such as sterile arthritis. The role of immune complexes in other aspects of endocarditis is not well understood.

(5) **Moderate anemia** is associated with endocarditis that has been present for more than 2 weeks.

d. Therapy. Treatment has been carefully studied. When endocarditis is untreated, it is almost uniformly fatal. In general, prosthetic valve disease is more difficult to treat medically or surgically.

    (1) Antibiotic therapy alone provides an excellent chance of cure for streptococcal disease on a native valve and for staphylococcal disease on the tricuspid valve. The key is to provide an adequate dose for a long enough period, usually 4–8 weeks, depending on the organism.

    (2) In medical failures, **valve replacement** may be a necessary adjunct to antibiotic therapy. Other indications for valve surgery include the following:

        (a) Fungal endocarditis (an absolute indication)

        (b) Congestive heart failure (CHF)

        (c) Recurrent major emboli

        (d) Inability to sterilize the blood after 10–14 days

VI SEXUALLY TRANSMITTED DISEASES

A Modes of transmission Sexually transmitted diseases (STDs) usually affect healthy adults. Multiple STDs can be present at once. Microorganisms may be transmitted during intimate sexual relations in three ways.

1. Cutaneous inoculation is the most common route for the five "classic" STDs (syphilis, gonorrhea, chancroid, lymphogranuloma venereum, and granuloma inguinale), as well as for herpes simplex. Apposition of an infected site to a susceptible site in a partner results in a physical transfer of microorganisms. Abrasion or trauma may facilitate the infection of skin.

2. Blood-borne infection can be transmitted by sexual activity. HBV, HCV, CMV, and HIV are all transmitted by inoculation of microscopic amounts of blood or serum.

3. Enterically acquired infection may occur with sexual activity because the anal area is close to the genitals or is also used for sexual interaction. Infections due to *Shigella*, *Entamoeba*, and hepatitis A are examples of sexually transmissible enteric diseases.

B Urethritis

1. Etiology. Urethritis is classified as **gonococcal** or **nongonococcal.**

    a. Gonococcal urethritis is caused by *N. gonorrhoeae.* In almost all cases of gonococcal urethritis, Gram stain of the urethral discharge shows gram-negative intracellular diplococci.

    b. Nongonococcal urethritis is caused by *C. trachomatis*, *Ureaplasma urealyticum*, or some other, yet-unidentified, agent. (In 25% of cases of gonococcal urethritis, one of these organisms also is present, and patients may have recurrent symptoms after therapy for gonorrhea.)

2. Clinical features

    a. Dysuria is observed in most cases of urethritis, whether gonococcal or nongonococcal.

    b. Urethral discharge is observed more frequently in men than women and may be purulent (usually in gonococcal disease) or cloudy and mucoid (usually in nongonococcal disease).

3. Therapy

    a. A variety of **antibiotic regimens** can be used to treat gonorrhea. However, resistance patterns change, and up-to-date recommendations should be sought.

    b. Many clinicians recommend that treatment with a tetracycline or macrolide follow gonococcal therapy to eliminate possible simultaneous nongonococcal urethritis. A 7-day course of a tetracycline or erythromycin or a single dose of azithromycin is usually sufficient, although some patients experience a relapse within a few weeks. These patients usually respond to another course of antibiotics.

C Pelvic inflammatory disease (PID) PID refers to a complex of infections involving the uterus, fallopian tubes, or ligaments of the uterus.

1. Etiology

    a. *N. gonorrhoeae*, *C. trachomatis*, or a mixture of pelvic anaerobes may be involved, although it is difficult to determine which of these is responsible when instituting therapy.

    b. The presence of an intrauterine device (IUD) may predispose patients to PID.

2. **Clinical features and laboratory findings.** The symptoms may be contemporaneous with menstruation and usually consist of lower abdominal or pelvic pain and tenderness on palpation of the cervix, uterus, or adnexa. Fever is not necessarily a significant feature. A cervical discharge or pelvic mass may be present, and the WBC count may be normal or elevated.

3. **Diagnosis**

   a. It is important to obtain cultures or other diagnostic tests for *N. gonorrhoeae* and *Chlamydia*.

   b. Ultrasonography of the pelvis may demonstrate an adnexal mass or abscess, which should be followed carefully.

4. **Therapy.** No simple therapy is effective in all cases of PID. Hospitalization is suggested when pain is incapacitating or when parenteral therapy is given. Combinations of antibiotics are usually needed to cover the three major categories of possible pathogens.

5. **Complications.** The most serious long-term complications of PID are infertility, ectopic pregnancy, and the need for hysterectomy.

D **Infectious proctitis**

1. **Etiology.** Infectious proctitis can be caused by a variety of microorganisms. When anal sex is practiced, gonorrhea, syphilis, chlamydial infection, and herpes should be considered.

2. **Clinical features and diagnosis.** Proctalgia (rectal pain), a change in bowel habits, and a mucoid or bloody anal discharge between bowel movements suggest infectious proctitis. A sexual history should be obtained to aid in the diagnosis, and appropriate diagnostic studies (e.g., sigmoidoscopy, culture and Gram stain of the discharge, biopsy) should be performed.

3. **Therapy.** When specific agents of infectious proctitis can be identified, appropriate antibiotic treatment should be administered. In general, the same regimens used to treat these pathogens in other body sites are effective in proctitis. However, for gonorrheal proctitis, cure rates are lower than for gonorrheal urethritis, and posttherapy cultures should be obtained.

E **Syndromes of genital ulcers and lymphadenopathy**

1. **Incidence.** Ulcerative lesions of the genitalia are common outpatient problems.

2. **Etiology.** There are many causes, which vary in different parts of the world. In the United States, **genital herpes** is the most common cause of genital ulcers, followed by **syphilis**. Other causes include **lymphogranuloma venereum, chancroid,** and **granuloma inguinale (donovanosis),** all of which are uncommon in the United States.

3. **Clinical features** (Table 9–5). 🔗 See Online Figures 9–5 to 9–11 for color photos of these conditions.

TABLE 9–5 Sexually Transmitted Diseases

Disease	Causative Organism	Diagnostic Tests	Clinical Findings	
Genital herpes	Herpes simplex virus	Direct immunofluorescence; viral culture	Lesions: multiple, vesiculopustular, painful	
Syphilis	*Treponema pallidum*	Dark-field microscopy; rapid plasma reagin test	Lesions: usually solitary, indurated Painless nodes: rubbery, not fluctuant	
Lymphogranuloma venereum	*Chlamydia trachomatis*	Culture; serologic examination	Lesions: small papule or vesicle Nodes: large, suppurative	
Chancroid	*Haemophilus ducreyi*	Gram stain, culture (special media needed)	Lesions: ragged, soft, dirty looking Nodes: tender, suppurative	
Granuloma inguinale	*Calymmatobacterium granulomatis*	Biopsy with Giemsa or Wright's stain	Lesions: large, slowly advancing, rolled edges, not indurated Nodes: not prominent	Tetracycline, trimethoprim-sulfamethoxazole

    a. Genital herpes initially manifests as itching and soreness, followed by the appearance of erythema and, eventually, the development of herpetic vesicles. In immunocompromised patients (e.g., transplant recipients, patients with HIV), vesicles may be confluent and lead to large ulcers.

    b. Syphilis, in its primary form, manifests as a painless, often solitary chancre (ulcer) with a hard, indurated base. Oral and vulvar lesions may be subtle, and oral lesions may be painful.

    c. Lymphogranuloma venereum manifests as nodes that are disproportionately large compared with the ulcers characterized by a depression between the inguinal and femoral nodes (**groove sign**).

    d. Chancroid is characterized by multiple, painful ulcers with ragged, undermined edges and suppurative inguinal nodes.

    e. Granuloma inguinale is a more indolent infection characterized by a painless, beefy-red lesion with ragged edges and less prominent adenopathy. It is rare in the United States. The clinical characteristics and course of illness are more like genital cancer than are those other STDs.

4. Diagnosis (see Table 9–5)

    a. When a **genital ulcer** is noted, a **Tzanck smear** for herpes can help make a diagnosis. However, many labs use shell vials, which produce results in 1 day. Viral cultures are helpful especially with resistant viruses.

    b. In all cases of genital ulcers, serologic testing for syphilis should be performed.

    c. Diagnosis of **lymphogranuloma venereum** is difficult.

    d. Diagnosis of **chancroid** involves eliminating other causes of genital ulcers and isolating *Haemophilus ducreyi* from the ulcers or suppurative nodes.

    e. Diagnosis of **granuloma inguinale** is confirmed by demonstration of Donovan bodies in edge scrapings prepared with Giemsa or Wright's stain.

5. Therapy. Identification and treatment of sexual contacts is always desirable.

    a. Herpes infections are self-limited but recurrent. Acyclovir, famciclovir, or valacyclovir may shorten the course and reduce symptoms but do not affect the natural history of these infections. Patients with frequent recurrences can use lower doses of these same medicines as prophylaxis.

    b. Syphilis is treated with varying schedules of penicillin, depending on the stage. Tetracycline may be useful for patients with penicillin intolerance or other special requirements, but penicillin is clearly preferred even if it requires desensitization.

    c. Lymphogranuloma venereum is treated with a tetracycline or a macrolide.

    d. Chancroid is treated with azithromycin, ceftriaxone, fluoroquinolones, or erythromycin. However, resistance patterns of *H. ducreyi* are variable, and culture sensitivities should be obtained if possible.

    e. Granuloma inguinale is treated with a tetracycline or trimethoprim–sulfamethoxazole.

6. Late complications

    a. Herpes simplex recurrences tend to be most common early after acquisition but may continue to occur for many years and may become severe in immunocompromised patients. Herpes also can complicate parturition and cause devastating infection in neonates.

    b. Syphilitic chancres heal spontaneously after 1–2 weeks. However, in the secondary phase, syphilis can manifest as a multisystem disease including, but not limited to, lymphadenopathy, rash (especially on the palms and soles), fever, pharyngitis, and meningitis. The multisystem disease resolves spontaneously, and a latent, noninfective phase ensues. Most patients remain seropositive. In tertiary syphilis, approximately 10% of patients develop serious late complications of the aorta or the CNS. The neurologic lesions are varied but include pupillary disturbances, posterior spinal column problems, and major cognitive impairment. Treatment may halt progression but is unlikely to reverse damage, making early diagnosis and treatment critical.

    c. Lymphogranuloma venereum may rarely lead to genital or rectal scarring.

VII   OTHER INFECTIOUS DISEASES AND SYNDROMES

A **Infections associated with adenopathy and splenomegaly** Syndromes of adenopathy (both local and general), splenomegaly, and fever are common medical problems. The differential diagnosis should include tumors, rheumatic diseases, and vasculitis, as well as specific infectious processes.

1. **Generalized lymphadenopathy** and **fatigue** are the classic signs of **infectious mononucleosis.**
   a. Mononucleosis most commonly is caused by the **Epstein–Barr virus** (EBV) and is associated with splenomegaly, pharyngitis, and an atypical lymphocytosis.
   b. **CMV** causes a mononucleosis syndrome that is virtually indistinguishable from EBV-induced mononucleosis.
   c. Both infections tend to occur in adolescents and young adults and may be subclinical.
      (1) They are distinguished by serologic tests such as the **Monospot test,** which usually demonstrates the presence of heterophile antibody in EBV infection and the absence of heterophile antibody in CMV infection.
      (2) Specific antibody testing for the two viruses can confirm the diagnosis in equivocal cases.
      (3) Both viruses can be transmitted by intimate contact, including, but not limited to, sexual intercourse.
   d. Some cases of mononucleosis are caused by *Toxoplasma gondii,* but this infection usually is subclinical or presents as a mild "viral-type syndrome" in healthy adults.
   e. **Early HIV infection** may manifest as fever, lymphadenopathy, and fatigue, as well as rash, neck stiffness, or other features of a "viral infection." This set of symptoms occurs in 30%–60% of patients who experience acute HIV infection. (This is sometimes called seroconversion illness because antibodies to HIV become apparent at the end of this period.) Lymphadenopathy alone or with a variety of constitutional problems also occurs in middle to late stages of HIV infection.
2. Fever, adenopathy, and fatigue also may be **manifestations of secondary syphilis.**
3. **Splenomegaly out of proportion to adenopathy**
   a. This clinical presentation is characteristic of only a few infections, such as malaria, schistosomiasis, and kala-azar (visceral leishmaniasis).
   b. This syndrome also should suggest a **malignancy,** such as lymphoma or Hodgkin's disease; an **infiltrative disease,** such as Gaucher's disease; a **congestive disease,** such as hepatic cirrhosis; or a **connective tissue disease,** such as SLE.
   c. **Local infections** such as splenic abscess and left-sided subphrenic abscess may manifest as a palpable spleen.
4. **Localized adenopathy** helps pinpoint a potential **infection** or **tumor.**
   a. A few small (<8 mm) lymph nodes in the inguinal, axillary, or cervical region may be present in most healthy adults. If the nodes are nontender and firm but not rock hard and do not change over a period of weeks to months, they usually do not warrant attention.
   b. Lymphadenopathy in other areas is unusual without an obvious infection in the region drained by those nodes.
   c. Cutaneous inoculation with an infective agent may result in a local lesion and regional adenopathy. Examples are sporotrichosis (from exposure to *Sporothrix schenckii,* a plant-associated fungus) and cat-scratch disease (*Bartonella henselae* infection following cat bite or scratch).

B **Infections due to parasites**   These infections are more common in tropical climates and may be associated with eosinophilia.

1. Malaria is caused by a blood-borne parasite, *Plasmodium,* which is endemic to much of the tropical and subtropical world, resulting in nearly 3 million deaths per year. Of the four types of *Plasmodium* species (*P. falciparum, P. ovale, P. malariae,* and *P. vivax*), infection with *P. falciparum* is the most severe and is characterized by fever, chills, myalgias, nausea, vomiting, or diarrhea.
   a. **Diagnosis.** Blood smear should be performed in those with high clinical suspicion, such as individuals traveling from an endemic region. Smear should reveal parasites.
   b. **Treatment.** Due to high chloroquine resistance, agents such as quinine, sulfadine, and pyrimethamine are used in addition to a new class of antimalarial drugs classified as artemisinin derivatives.
   c. **Prophylaxis.** All travelers to malaria-endemic areas should take prophylaxis based on the resistance patterns of malaria in that region.
2. Protozoa such as *Entamoeba* and *Giardia* are associated with diarrheal illnesses.
3. Schistosomes (blood flukes) are helminths not limited to the lumen of the bowel and can produce eosinophilia.

4. ***Strongyloides.*** *Strongyloides stercoralis* is the most important helminth associated with eosino-philia in the United States. Strongyloidiasis should be suspected in persons who live or have lived in tropical areas (or in the southeastern United States) and who have persistent eosinophilia with or without cutaneous or gastrointestinal complaints. *Strongyloides* larvae can cross the bowel wall, so they may be associated with episodes of polymicrobial bacteremia involving typical bowel flora. Untreated disease can last for decades and worsen during periods of immunosup-pression.

C **Tuberculosis** This illness remains a major medical problem in certain immigrant and under-privileged groups in the United States as well as a widespread disease throughout the world.

1. **Clinical syndromes**
   a. **Pulmonary tuberculosis** is the most common form. In most adults, this condition is character-ized by an increased cough (possibly with altered sputum), weight loss, hemoptysis, and fatigue. Most cases of pulmonary tuberculosis are believed to be a reactivation of *M. tuberculosis* acquired months to years earlier rather than reinfection or initial infection by this bacterium. However, reinfection has been confirmed in patients both with and without HIV infection. Primary dis-ease may resemble bacterial pneumonia and should be especially suspected when a close contact has recently been discovered to have active tuberculosis.
   b. **Extrapulmonary tuberculosis** can develop in any organ, but the most seriously affected are the kidneys, bones, and meninges. Again, the diagnosis rests on finding *M. tuberculosis* in body fluid or tissue. Only approximately 40% of patients with extrapulmonary tuberculosis have clinical or radiographic evidence of lung involvement at the time of diagnosis of the extrapulmonary disease.

2. **Diagnosis.** The diagnosis is based on identification of acid-fast bacilli—specifically, *M. tuberculosis*—by microscopy, polymerase chain reaction (PCR), or culture. However, the diagnosis may be difficult to establish because many patients have too few bacteria to be seen on direct stain, and it takes several weeks of incubation for specimens to grow. The chest radiograph usually is abnor-mal and shows signs of a prior exposure to *M. tuberculosis* (e.g., calcified or enlarged intratho-racic lymph nodes and infiltrates in the posterior segment of the upper lobes).

3. **Therapy.** Treatment is aimed at curing the patient who has a definite diagnosis of tuberculosis. To be effective, the therapy must include **at least four antimicrobial agents for induction, fol-lowed by at least two drug combinations for the remainder of treatment.** Single-agent treat-ment has a high risk of failure because of the selection of drug-resistant strains of the infecting tubercle bacillus.
   a. Because of their potency and reliability, **isoniazid** and **rifampin** are the drugs of choice for tuberculosis. Other first-line drugs include ethambutol, pyrazinamide, and streptomycin. Most authorities recommend starting four drugs initially to provide adequate coverage, in view of possible isoniazid or rifampin resistance.
   b. Second-line drugs are used primarily for patients who are intolerant of the first-line agents or who have drug-resistant disease. These drugs include ethionamide, kanamycin, and cycloser-ine. Fluoroquinolones have activity against *M. tuberculosis*, which would make them seem to be reasonable first-line drugs, but the need for long courses and the concern about selecting a resistant bacterial flora pushes them to second-line status.
   c. The usual duration of treatment is 6–12 months, depending on the patient and the regimen. Shorter courses have an unacceptably high rate of failure.

4. **Prevention**
   a. **Skin testing.** The **tuberculin skin test** is used widely to screen certain high-risk populations, particularly those who have been exposed to an infectious individual. The test involves an intradermal injection of the **purified protein derivative (PPD)** of tuberculin (see online for details). Newer tests looking for direct immune responsiveness of lymphocytes to myco-bacterial components can be done in vitro and may yield less equivocal and more rapid results than skin tests.
   b. **Treatment of latent tuberculosis.** Individuals with a positive PPD and no evidence of active disease are considered to harbor latent tuberculosis, which must be treated to prevent reactiva-tion. In many cases, disease can be prevented by administering isoniazid alone for 6–12 months

at a dose of 300 mg/day. Pyridoxine is coadministered with isoniazid to prevent peripheral neuropathy.

c. **Immunization.** Vaccination of children and adults with bacille Calmette–Guérin (BCG) has been reported to reduce the risk of acquiring tuberculosis. BCG, a live bacterial vaccine, should not be used when there is known immunodeficiency. The PPD skin test can become positive after BCG administration. The BCG vaccine is seldom used in the United States, but it is widely used in other countries. Prior BCG vaccination does not alter the decision to use chemoprophylaxis.

d. **Isolation.** Because of the **potential hazard of transmission** of tuberculosis in the hospital, it is important to identify potentially infective patients and to ensure adequate containment of their infectious aerosols. Any patient suspected of active tuberculosis should be isolated with negative-pressure ventilation, and caregivers should wear masks until tuberculosis is ruled out (latent tuberculosis does not require isolation).

D **Infections associated with diffuse rash and fever**

1. **Toxin-associated diseases**

    a. **Toxic shock syndrome** (TSS) occurs when a susceptible individual is colonized or infected by a strain of *S. aureus* that produces a toxin (TSST-1). This toxin is a superantigen that can stimulate the immune system in a way that leads to severe hypotension and organ damage. Most adults have antibody to this toxin and are thus immune. Many cases have been associated with tampon use in young women, but current tampons seem to be safer, and menstrual TSS is considerably less common than it was in the early 1980s. Toxin-producing *S. pyogenes* (group A streptococci) can cause a very similar illness.

        (1) **Clinical features**

            (a) TSS is characterized by fever, hypotension, diarrhea, mucous membrane changes, and a diffuse erythematous rash with desquamation on the hands and feet. Multisystem involvement is the rule, with involvement of gastrointestinal, renal, hepatic, hematopoietic, and musculoskeletal organs.

            (b) TSS varies from a mild illness to a life-threatening disease. Hypotension from fluid loss and lack of vascular tone is the most ominous prognostic sign. There may be recurrences until protective antibody is formed.

        (2) **Therapy.** The treatment for acute illness is **supportive,** consisting of fluids and pressors. Antibacterial therapy is given to prevent recurrence.

    b. **Scarlet fever** is an illness caused by infection with toxigenic *S. pyogenes* (group A streptococci). It is characterized by fever, rough erythematous diffuse rash, mucous membrane erythema (including strawberry tongue), and local streptococcal infection (usually involving the skin). Less severe than TSS, scarlet fever usually responds to supportive measures and antistreptococcal therapy.

2. **Non–toxin-mediated illness with fever and rash**

E **Legionnaires' disease**

1. **Etiology.** Legionnaires' disease is a pneumonia caused by *Legionella pneumophila,* a gram-negative bacterium that dwells in warm aquatic environments. Several *Legionella*-like organisms have been discovered, which produce similar but distinct disease patterns.

2. **Epidemiology**

    a. Infection occurs when contaminated water is aerosolized and then inhaled (e.g., during nebulizer treatments). Some outbreaks of Legionnaires' disease have been connected to the airborne spread of contaminated fluid from air-conditioning cooling towers or from potable water.

    b. Individuals who are particularly vulnerable to infection include cigarette smokers, people with underlying lung disease, and immunosuppressed individuals (e.g., those receiving steroid therapy).

3. **Clinical features**

    a. Fever occurs in almost all cases, is abrupt, and usually is associated with shaking chills. A sudden headache may precede the rapid increase in temperature.

    b. Cough is a common symptom, which initially is nonproductive but progresses to a productive cough that may be associated with slight hemoptysis.

    c. Less common symptoms include diarrhea, nausea, vomiting, and pleuritic pain.

4. Diagnosis. The diagnosis is made by **culturing the bacterium** from infected body sites (e.g., lung tissue, pleural fluid, or sputum) or by demonstrating the bacterium by immunofluorescent, nucleic acid hybridization, or antigen detection techniques. Urinary antigen testing is available, but only for *L. pneumophila* type 1. When *L. pneumophila* infection cannot be confirmed by these methods, increasing titers of antibodies from the acute phase to convalescence can be diagnostic.

5. Therapy. The preferred therapy for all *Legionella* infections is a **macrolide** (e.g., azithromycin) or a **fluoroquinolone** (e.g., levofloxacin).

F Lyme disease

1. Etiology. Lyme disease is a multisystem infection caused by a spirochete, *Borrelia burgdorferi,* which is transmitted by tick bite.

2. Epidemiology. The incidence of Lyme disease is related to the presence of its vector (usually *Ixodes* ticks) and infected wild mammals such as deer and mice. In the United States, endemic foci have expanded from initial small areas in New England to include areas as far south as Georgia as well as areas in the Midwest and the Pacific states. Lyme disease is the most common tick-borne illness in the United States.

3. Clinical features. Lyme disease is divided into three phases. The phases may follow each other closely or be separated by periods without symptoms.

    a. The **first phase** is characterized by an enlarging erythematous rash (**erythema migrans**) at the site of the original tick bite. There may be central clearing or a few satellite lesions. Patients are often constitutionally ill with malaise, headache, and mild fever.

    b. The **second phase** involves the heart (conduction abnormalities, arrhythmias) or the nervous system (cranial or peripheral neuropathies or aseptic meningitis). **New onset of Bell's palsy** (paralysis of cranial nerve VII) should suggest the possibility of Lyme disease.

    c. The **third phase,** which affects only a few patients, consists of an oligoarticular arthritis or some persistent, mild neuropsychiatric disturbances.

4. Diagnosis. The diagnosis is difficult. In early illness, the production of antibody to *B. burgdorferi* may not be detectable. Conversely, people living in endemic areas may have antibody without any clinical illness. The organism may be demonstrated rarely in skin biopsies and can sometimes be cultured. High levels of immunoglobulin M (IgM) antibody and increasing levels of IgG antibody to one or more *B. burgdorferi* antigens corroborate clinical suspicions of Lyme borreliosis.

5. Therapy. Early **antibiotic therapy** seems to prevent disease progression for most patients. Tetracyclines are preferred for adolescents and adults; penicillin is an alternative. For later-stage disease, high doses of penicillin, tetracycline (especially doxycycline), and ceftriaxone have been shown to relieve symptoms. Some oral cephalosporins and azithromycin have also been shown to be useful. A vaccine that had been marketed to prevent Lyme disease is no longer available.

VIII RETROVIRUS INFECTION

A Etiology
Retroviruses are single-stranded RNA viruses characterized by the presence of **reverse transcriptase,** an enzyme that uses the viral RNA as a template to make a copy of complementary DNA for integration into the host cell.

1. Retroviruses known to cause disease in humans are the **human T cell lymphotropic viruses types I and II** (HTLV-I and HTLV-II) and HIV.

2. HIV comprises two types: type 1 (HIV-1) and type 2 (HIV-2). HIV-1 causes AIDS.

B Epidemiology
All of these agents can be transmitted from person to person via sexual activity or mingling of blood (as occurs via blood transfusion or sharing of blood-contaminated needles) and from mother to child in utero.

1. HTLV-I is found most commonly in the Caribbean basin and in southern Japan. Up to 10% of the population in certain villages may be infected.

2. HTLV-II is not known to have such marked geographic clusters, and incidence seems to be low worldwide.

3. HIV

    a. HIV-1 is found worldwide. Because it has a long latent period and one person may infect many others, this virus has spread explosively since 1981, when it was first identified. Male homosexual activity was the predominant mode of transmission in North America and Europe during the 1980s. Intravenous drug use and heterosexual transmission account for an increasing share of new infections, especially among women (one of the fastest-growing groups to be infected). In Africa, heterosexual transmission is predominant.

    b. HIV-2 is found primarily in West Africa.

C Clinical features

1. HTLV-I is the causative agent of adult T cell leukemia–lymphoma. This unusual malignancy, which is associated with skin involvement and hypercalcemia, is difficult to treat. HTLV-I also causes HTLV-I–associated myelopathy (HAM), also referred to as tropical spastic paraparesis (TSP). HAM presents with insidious onset of weakness or stiffness in one or both legs, back pain, and urinary incontinence, followed by slowly progressive and unremitting thoracic myelopathy. However, **most people** infected with HTLV-**I have no clinical illness** even after years or decades of infection.

2. HTLV-II has not been categorically associated with any illness.

3. HIV

    a. HIV-1 infection has traditionally been divided into three overlapping stages.

        (1) In **early illness** (seroconversion stage), within a few weeks or months after exposure to HIV, whole virus and viral antigens and nucleic acid can be found in the blood and body fluids. Although many patients are asymptomatic, approximately 40% of patients have a brief illness marked by headache, fever, skin rash, or lymphadenopathy, which resolves spontaneously within a few weeks. Most people who become infected with HIV-1 develop antibody within 1–6 months of exposure.

        (2) A clinical **latent period,** during which there is no clinical illness but virus can be detected and is replicating, occurs in almost all HIV-1–infected patients. Depending on host and viral factors, the viral load varies widely, from fewer than 50 to several million copies/mL. The virus alters the host immune response. The earliest indications may be declining numbers of T helper (Th) cells (CD4), which are targets of the virus, and normal to increased numbers of T suppressor (Ts) cells (CD8), leading to an abnormal CD4:CD8 ratio (normal ratio of Th to Ts cells is 2:1). Some patients have minor viral infections or more-frequent-than-usual recurrences of oral or genital herpes simplex, herpes zoster, oral hairy leukoplakia, mild fever, sweats, weight loss, and diarrhea. Common bacterial infections, such as streptococcal pneumonia and tuberculosis, may occur with increased frequency at any point in HIV-1 infection but tend to become more common as the disease progresses.

        (3) **Advanced symptomatic HIV-1 infection** is manifested as AIDS. HIV infection is best thought of as a continuum, with evidence of progressive immune depletion correlating with increased probability of specific infection or malignancy; nonspecific localized or generalized complaints such as fever, fatigue, or night sweats; or organ dysfunction such as renal failure or dementia. Older definitions of AIDS are mostly used to determine eligibility for disability insurance rather than to guide therapy.

    b. Monitoring of HIV-1 disease is helpful in establishing prognosis and adjusting treatment. Various quantitative assays of viral nucleic acid predict the rate of progression of disease; those patients with the lowest viral loads tend to remain symptom free and live longer than those with high viral loads. When treatment is effective, these assays show a drop to low or undetectable **viral load.** If viral load has been very low and then increases, treatment may be failing.

    c. HIV-2 infection follows the same general pattern as HIV-1 infection, but much less is known. The clinical course is usually milder or slower. Several well-described cases of AIDS have been associated with HIV-2 in the absence of HIV-1. It will probably be shown that determinants of immunosuppression are the most significant predictors of whether opportunistic infection or malignancy will occur.

D Therapy

1. **HTLV-I.** Treatment of HTLV-I–related malignancies with conventional cancer chemotherapy has been disappointing. However, the use of antiretrovirals directed against HIV-1 has resulted in some durable remissions. No treatment of asymptomatic HTLV-I infections is necessary.

2. **HTLV-II.** There is no need to treat HTLV-II infection at any stage.

3. **HIV**

   a. **HIV-1. At all stages of illness, the goal of therapy is to suppress viral replication as measured by viral load.** Improvement in clinical and immune parameters may be delayed but usually follows in a matter of weeks to months. Chemotherapy may influence the progression of HIV-1 infection. Careful evaluation and timely antiretroviral therapy may delay or prevent the development of significant complications. When to start therapy is a complex question that depends on a number of factors. For patients with **symptomatic** infection, therapy should be started as soon as possible. For patients with rapidly progressive infection (as determined by high viral loads and dropping CD4 counts), early therapy is also appropriate. What is most unclear is when to initiate therapy in a person with good immune function. Early intervention will preserve immune function but can be taxing in terms of side effects and cost. Interruptions of therapy are controversial, and recent studies have shown that interrupting antiretroviral therapy may increase the likelihood of morbidity and mortality. Therefore, structured treatment interruptions (STIs) should only be undertaken in the context of a research study.

      (1) A variety of drugs have been shown to be effective in reducing the viral load and improving immune function. Because recommendations change quickly, the decision about which therapy to use should be based on current studies. As of 2004, five classes of drugs for the treatment of HIV-1 are available: **nucleoside reverse transcriptase inhibitors (NRTIs), nucleotide reverse transcriptase inhibitors, nonnucleoside reverse transcriptase inhibitors (NNRTIs), fusion inhibitors,** and **protease inhibitors (PIs).**

      (2) Evidence indicating that **combinations** of agents are much more effective is very strong. Although single agents can be shown to have activity (as measured by reducing viral load and increasing CD4 counts), there is no occasion to use them alone due to almost universal development of resistant virus treated with monotherapy or dual therapy.

      (3) **Failure to adequately suppress viral replication** or rebound viral replication is a **poor prognostic sign.** A reevaluation of treatment is warranted in these cases.

      (4) **Resistance** to antiretroviral drugs occurs by mutational change in the viral genome. Exposure to any of the agents is predictably followed by resistance within weeks to months unless viral replication is successfully suppressed. Once resistance occurs, it is very stable and does not disappear even with drug cessation. Resistance to various antiretroviral drugs can be measured by genotypic analysis (looking for known mutations that confer specific resistance) or phenotypic analysis (akin to the tests to look for bacterial drug resistance). Both of these methods are expensive and somewhat inconclusive, although they can be helpful in guiding therapy.

      (5) **Drug–drug interactions** are common and potentially severe. Some antiretrovirals such as the protease inhibitors can have powerful effects on hepatic cytochrome enzymes. This may result in unexpectedly high or low levels of other drugs that depend on liver metabolism.

      (6) **Direct drug toxicity** is common although usually manageable. Akin to cancer chemotherapy, different agents tend to have different side effects and toxicities. Therefore when assembling a combination of HIV-1 medications one needs to take into account various toxicities. Some of the most severe toxicities include pancreatitis, peripheral neuropathy, severe hypersensitivity reactions, lactic acidosis, and dyslipidemia.

      (7) **Drug costs** are high, and the cost of monitoring is also considerable. Whereas effective HIV-1 care saves money in the long run (as compared with the cost of hospitalizations, decreased productivity, and early mortality), it can be difficult to afford good HIV-1 care.

   b. **HIV-2.** Treatment for HIV-2 infection tends to mirror that of HIV-1 and is much less extensively studied.

E **Prognosis**   The prognosis of HIV-1 infection has changed radically with the awareness that suppressing viral replication can allow for immune reconstitution. Before the widespread use of combination antiviral therapy (CART), also referred to as highly active antiretroviral therapy (HAART), individuals who contracted HIV-1 infection would survive on average 5–10 years without clinical symptoms (latent period). They would then experience a decline in immunocompetence, leading almost inexorably to death. Now, with careful medical management, HIV-1 can be controlled in many individuals, although the duration of this response is not yet known. This has considerably influenced the mortality rates of AIDS. Even for those patients who are unwilling or unable to follow the complex drug regimens needed to restore immune function, intermittent antiviral therapy may provide some benefit, although the long-term prognosis may not be good. With the many new treatment modalities in development for HIV-1–infected individuals, further prognostic changes may occur in the foreseeable future.

F **Prevention**

1. **Screening.** The Centers for Disease Control and Prevention (CDC) recently recommended HIV screening for patients in all health care settings after the patient has been notified that testing will be performed, unless the patient declines (opt-out screening). [Branson BM, Handsfield HH, Lampe MA, et al.; Centers for Disease Control and Prevention (CDC). Revised recommendations for HIV testing of adults, adolescents, and pregnant women in health-care settings. *MMWR Recomm Rep* 2006;55(RR-14):1–17.] Previously, due to concerns about stigmatization and discrimination, HIV testing has been presented on an "opt-in" basis, requiring explicit written consent and extensive pretest and posttest counseling. These requirements are loosened in the current guidelines, with the hope that more people will be encouraged to learn their HIV status and use appropriate protective measures to prevent transmission. HIV-1 screening tests are sensitive, specific, and widely available for HIV-1 infection, but they may not detect the antibody response to HIV-2. Home testing and point-of-use testing for HIV-1 are available and accurate, but standard tests should always be done to corroborate positive results.

2. **Controlling spread of infection.** Preventive measures for controlling the spread of HIV include **education** about risk factors, **sexual abstinence,** use of **barrier precautions** (condoms), **avoidance of childbirth** in women known to be HIV-1 infected, **needle-exchange programs,** and **universal testing of blood products.** Treatment of HIV-1–infected pregnant women with antiretrovirals substantially decreases prenatal and peripartum transmission of HIV, as does delivery by cesarean section. Breast-feeding should be avoided by women infected with HIV-1. Suppression of HIV-1 in the blood is accompanied by reduction of viral loads on mucosal surfaces, so it should also decrease infectivity. This in no way should be construed as a reason to reduce cautiousness with regard to safer-sex practices and needle sharing.

3. **Public health.** HIV-1 infection must be reported to the state or local department of health, which then reports total numbers to the CDC. Policies vary widely from state to state, and, therefore, health care professionals need to be familiar with the local regulations. Some states report using a name-based procedure, while others use anonymous or coded reporting. Partner notification requirements vary considerably among legal jurisdictions.

G **Complications**   Effects of HIV-1 infection can result from direct damage caused by the virus or from the opportunistic infections or malignancies that accompany the decline of the immune system in late-stage HIV-1 infection. In general, direct effects of HIV-1 infection include fevers, night sweats, weight loss, decreased libido, cognitive deficits, and muscle wasting (Figure 9–12).

1. **Types of complications**
   a. **Skin lesions**
      (1) Some lesions are rare in individuals without HIV infection but are relatively common in those with HIV-1 infection.
          (a) Kaposi sarcoma, which is caused by a herpesvirus (HHV-8)
          (b) Eosinophilic folliculitis
          (c) Disseminated molluscum contagiosum
          (d) Bacillary angiomatosis (*Bartonella*)
          (e) Thrush (*Candida*)

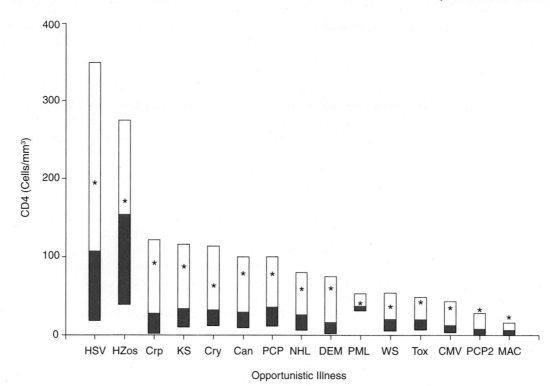

FIGURE 9–12 Boxplot of the median (line inside the box), first quartile (top of box), and mean (*asterisk*). CD4+ lymphocyte count at the time of the development of opportunistic disease. Can, *Candida* esophagitis; CMV, cytomegalovirus; Crp, cryptosporidiosis; Cry, cryptococcal meningitis; DEM, acquired immunodeficiency virus dementia complex; HSV, herpes simplex virus infection; HZos, herpes zoster; KS, Kaposi's sarcoma; MAC, *Mycobacterium avium-complex*; NH, non-Hodgkin's lymphoma; PCP, primary pneumonia; PML, progressive multifocal leukoencephalopathy; Tox, *Toxoplasma gondii* encephalitis; WS, wasting syndrome.

    (2) The following common disorders are more severe in individuals with HIV-1 infection.
        (a) Psoriasis (including psoriatic arthritis)
        (b) Seborrheic dermatitis
        (c) Alopecia
        (d) Onychomycosis (fungal infections of the nail beds)
        (e) Severe or recurrent genital candidal infection
  b. Lymphatic system. Lymph nodes are often enlarged, although usually this is not reflective of a specific infection or tumor. The enlarged nodes are characterized on biopsy as having reactive hyperplasia.
    (1) Lymphomas often occur as extranodal disease but may cause nodal enlargement later.
    (2) Several **infectious agents** can cause lymph node enlargement, including *T. pallidum*, *M. tuberculosis*, and *Histoplasma capsulatum*. Node aspirate or biopsy is useful in distinguishing among these organisms.
    (3) Kaposi's sarcoma may be found in lymph nodes.
  c. Nervous system. Such involvement may be diffuse or focal. Some cognitive or motor dysfunction is common and tends to become more severe. Usually there is evidence of cerebral atrophy, and no opportunistic agent can be found to explain the dementia.
    (1) Meningitis is caused most frequently by *Cryptococcus neoformans*, a ubiquitous yeast. Headache and neck stiffness range from mild or transient to severe, and the CSF is often normal or near normal with regard to cell count, protein level, glucose concentration, and general appearance. Cryptococci are seen on India ink preparations, and cryptococcal antigen can be demonstrated in serum and CSF. *Cryptococcus* is easily cultured from CSF and less commonly from blood.
        (a) Aseptic meningitis with headache, nuchal rigidity, and lymphocytic pleocytosis often occurs in the early stage of HIV-1 infection and occasionally in later stages.
        (b) Other forms of meningitis, although relatively uncommon, occur more often than in the general population.

(c) Cryptococcal disease can be prevented or delayed by the use of **fluconazole** in patients with late-stage HIV infection. Although fluconazole is safe and prevents or delays the occurrence of thrush, controlled studies show no survival benefit to this regimen as compared with treating fungal infections as they occur. Patients with cryptococcal meningitis should continue to receive antifungal therapy until their CD4 counts exceed 200/mm³.

(2) Neuropathy may be a part of HIV-1 infection, an opportunistic infection, or a side effect of treatment. For example, vincristine, which may be used for some AIDS-related malignancies, induces dose-related peripheral neuropathy, as do certain NRTIs such as zalcitabine (ddC) and didanosine (ddI).

(3) Space-occupying lesions of the CNS are found with some frequency in HIV-1 infection. The presentation is usually one of focal neurologic abnormality (often accompanied by seizures) and an abnormal CT or MRI scan.

(a) *T. gondii*, a protozoan parasite found worldwide, is the most common cause of **brain lesion** in patients who have AIDS. Many prophylactic regimens for *Pneumocystis carinii* **pneumonia** (PCP) also can prevent clinical toxoplasmosis from occurring. However, it is not usually advisable to add anti-*Toxoplasma* medications to the preventive regimen of an individual who is intolerant to the kind of PCP prophylaxis that also prevents toxoplasmosis.

(b) Lymphomas located in deep brain structures and **progressive multifocal leukoencephalopathy** (caused by the JC virus) are also disproportionately common.

(c) Syphilis can recrudesce in HIV-infected persons. **Standard treatments** are usually effective, but careful follow-up is indicated. When there is a question of whether a cure has been achieved, a more intensive regimen (e.g., that for the treatment of neurosyphilis) is recommended.

d. Eye. HIV-1 may be associated with some direct toxicity to the eye and optic nerve, but **CMV retinitis** is the most common and serious ocular complication of AIDS. The lesions are predominantly retinal and spare the choroid. They usually progress over weeks and can lead to blindness. Involvement of both eyes is the rule, and CMV retinitis is often part of a systemic illness including predominantly the gastrointestinal tract. Serious CMV ocular disease occurs in late-stage HIV infection when the CD4 count is very depressed. Treatment of HIV that results in increased CD4 counts often stops progression of disease.

e. Upper alimentary tract

(1) The upper gastrointestinal tract is most frequently affected by **local candidal** or **herpes simplex infections,** which can extend into the esophagus, or by **Kaposi's sarcoma,** which can be found throughout the intestine. Endoscopic esophageal brushes or biopsy can distinguish between the two most common opportunists.

(2) Visual examination of the oral cavity is sufficient for identifying **oral hairy leukoplakia,** an Epstein–Barr virus–related infection that predominantly involves the lateral tongue but may extend to other parts of the oral cavity.

(3) Aphthous ulcers of the mouth and esophagus are common, and esophageal ulcers can be large and painful.

f. Liver

(1) In the late stage of HIV-1 infection, the liver often is the site of **opportunistic infections** such as histoplasmosis, mycobacteriosis (due to *M. tuberculosis* and *Mycobacterium avium-intracellulare* [MAI]), cryptococcosis, and CMV. Hepatic candidiasis, which is sometimes seen in leukemia as part of systemic fungal disease, is not seen in AIDS.

(2) The same populations that are at risk for HIV-1 infection are also at risk for blood-borne hepatitis: **HBV, HCV, and HDV. HBV vaccine** is recommended for universal use. Because the vaccine is safe and the route of transmission of HBV is similar to that of HIV, vaccination of HIV-infected persons is logical. Peliosis hepatis is a treatable liver infection caused by *B. henselae,* the agent of cat-scratch disease.

g. Gastrointestinal tract distal to the esophagus

(1) HIV-1 can cause an **enteropathy** distinct from the infectious diarrheas. Because many meats and animal products such as milk and eggs can be contaminated with bacteria that cause enteric infection, HIV-infected persons should be advised to consume only pasteurized milk and to eat well-cooked eggs and meats.

(2) In addition, *Cryptosporidium* species, *Microsporidium, Cyclospora, Isospora,* and *G. intestinalis* are potentially causes of **watery diarrhea** and **diffuse abdominal pain** in HIV-1–infected patients. The discovery of *Cryptosporidium* in municipal water supplies is worrisome for patients with advanced HIV infection. It is not clear whether the use of water filters and bottled water can substantially reduce the risk of this infection.

(3) The stomach and small bowel also may be sites of origin of **extranodal lymphoma.**

(4) **CMV colitis** can be the cause of severe abdominal pain, diarrhea, and fever, and it occasionally can lead to perforation or megacolon.

h. Lungs. In AIDS, the lungs are the most common target organ for symptomatic disease.

(1) *Pneumocystis carinii pneumonia* develops in most patients who do not receive prophylaxis and whose CD4 cell count drops to less than 200/mm^3. In HIV-1–infected individuals, PCP has a subacute presentation that delays diagnosis, often for weeks. By the time patients come to medical attention, they have fever, dry cough, and hypoxemia. Chest radiographs may be normal or have interstitial markings or fluffy infiltrates. Usually, diagnosis is made by examining sputum, bronchoalveolar lavage fluid, bronchial washings or brushings, or lung biopsy specimens.

    (a) Even after initiation of treatment, PCP may progress temporarily but ultimately yields to effective therapy in 90% of patients. Short courses of steroids are often given to abort an early worsening with the initiation of therapy.

    (b) Every individual who has already had PCP should receive secondary prophylaxis. Because PCP is a common complication of middle- to late-stage HIV infection, and because preventive therapy is safe and effective, it has become general practice to offer PCP prevention to every HIV-infected person when the CD4 count falls to less than 300 cells/mm^3. First-line prophylaxis for PCP is trimethoprim–sulfamethoxazole. For patients intolerant of this medication, dapsone, clindamycin/primaquine, or atovaquone should be considered. Therapy is lifelong unless immune function is improved by HIV-1 suppression.

(2) **Bacterial pneumonias** also occur more commonly in HIV-1–infected patients than in otherwise healthy individuals. Although these pneumonias may be more severe than in immunocompetent patients, they usually respond to routine antimicrobial therapy. Pneumococcus is the most common cause of bacterial pneumonia in adult HIV-1–infected patients. Bacterial pneumonia can occur simultaneously with PCP. To prevent bacterial pneumonia in HIV, early administration of **pneumococcal vaccine** is recommended. A single dose should be adequate for a lifetime.

(3) **Fungal pneumonia** is less common and is usually a part of systemic cryptococcal, *Coccidioides*, or *Histoplasma* infection. Awareness of exposure to the agents of endemic mycoses (e.g., *Coccidioides* or *Histoplasma*) is crucial to make the diagnosis and to initiate appropriate therapy.

(4) **Viral pneumonia** can be severe in HIV-1–infected patients. CMV, a herpesvirus known to cause severe lung disease in other patients with Th cell deficiencies (especially bone marrow transplant recipients), may cause a fatal pneumonia alone or with PCP in HIV-1–infected patients.

(5) **Mycobacterial disease is common**

    (a) Infection with **M. tuberculosis** may appear relatively early in HIV-1 infection. Although it has a higher propensity to disseminate in patients who have Th cell (CD4) depletion, it usually responds to antimycobacterial therapy. Multiply resistant (to isoniazid and rifampin) *M. tuberculosis* is still uncommon, but these strains are difficult to treat. In immunologically competent individuals, the clinical response may be only 60%, whereas it is considerably lower in HIV-infected patients. Prevention of tuberculosis involves the following:

        (i) **Screening.** Early skin testing is most useful for identifying individuals at risk for recrudescence of previously acquired infection because many patients become anergic in the later stages of HIV infection. Only 5 mm of induration is needed to qualify as a positive skin test in a person with HIV infection. Aggressive contact tracing of persons who are known to be infectious with tuberculosis also can identify individuals at risk before they become ill with recently acquired tuberculosis.

      (ii) Prophylactic isoniazid reduces the risk of recurrent tuberculosis when administered for 6–12 months to patients who have had positive PPD skin tests.

    (b) Nontuberculous mycobacteria, usually MAI, may be found in sputum. In HIV-1–infected patients, the lungs are a fairly minor target organ for this pathogen, which usually infects the liver, spleen, blood, and bone marrow. **Macrolides** or **rifabutin** can be given when the CD4 count drops to less than 75 cells/mm^3.

  (6) A **noninfectious pneumonitis** characterized by lymphocytic infiltration of the lungs has been seen frequently in children with HIV-1 infection and is being recognized more commonly in adults.

i. Cardiovascular system. Cardiomyopathy may be found in HIV-1–infected patients.

j. Musculoskeletal system. This system is frequently involved in all stages of HIV-1 infection. Manifestations are seldom life threatening but do cause substantial morbidity. Except for AIDS-associated arthritis, most of these manifestations are clinically similar to entities in individuals without HIV-1 infection. However, the incidence and severity of these manifestations are greater in HIV-1–infected patients and tend to be worse in the late stage of HIV-1 infection.

  (1) Articular manifestations

    (a) Arthralgias occur in up to one third of HIV-1–infected individuals. The pain is intermittent and usually affects the large joints.

    (b) Reiter's syndrome has been reported to affect approximately 5% of HIV-1–infected men who have sex with men, although it seems to be rarer in individuals who acquire HIV-1 through needle sharing or heterosexual activity.

    (c) In patients with psoriasis, HIV-1 infection increases the risk of developing **psoriatic arthritis.**

    (d) AIDS-associated arthritis is severe and debilitating. It affects the large joints and produces only a mild synovitis. Intra-articular steroids may give considerable relief.

  (2) Muscular diseases

    (a) Myalgias are common in HIV-1 infection, especially in the early mononucleosis-like illness associated with seroconversion.

    (b) Polymyositis with proximal muscle weakness and elevated serum levels of muscle enzymes (e.g., creatine kinase [CK]) occurs in approximately 2% of HIV-1–infected individuals. It also may occur as a side effect of zidovudine therapy.

  (3) Bone and joint infections are fairly uncommon in HIV-1 infection, except among injection drug users. The causative agents are a mixture of common organisms (see V H) and opportunistic agents such as mycobacteria and fungi.

  (4) Various forms of **vasculitis** and **connective tissue disease** (e.g., Sjögren's syndrome) seem to occur with higher-than-expected frequency.

k. Hematopoietic abnormalities. These conditions are common in HIV-1 infection.

  (1) Immune thrombocytopenia may occur in middle- to late-stage HIV-1 infection and resembles idiopathic thrombocytopenic purpura (ITP) or thrombotic thrombocytopenic purpura (TTP).

  (2) Anemia is common in late HIV-1 infection. The pattern is usually one of chronic disease with normochromic, normocytic indices. Some antiretroviral therapies and antimetabolites used to prevent infections may induce macrocytic anemia. Serum levels of vitamin B$_{12}$ are often low, but vitamin B$_{12}$ therapy does not improve hematologic parameters. Many patients with low levels of erythropoietin respond to erythropoietin replacement therapy.

  (3) Neutropenia, along with the expected depletion of lymphocytes, may accompany HIV-1 infection. This may be a sign of disseminated bacterial or opportunistic infection, and blood and bone marrow culture (including mycobacterial cultures) can be helpful. Antiretroviral and antimetabolite therapies may contribute to neutropenia.

  (4) Immunoglobulin disorders are common. The most frequently described is a polyclonal increase in gamma globulin with an inability to produce novel immunoglobulins. Thus, patients with advanced HIV-1 infection may respond poorly to vaccination and may not demonstrate good serologic responses to acute infections, especially when challenged during the late stages of HIV infection.

TABLE 9–6   Treatment and Prevention of Infections Associated with HIV Infection

Organism	Clinical Manifestation	Treatment	Prevention/ Prophylaxis	Comments
Bacterial				
Streptococcus pneumoniae	Pneumonia	Appropriate antibiotic	Pneumovax	Higher rate than HIV
Mycobacterium tuberculosis	Pulmonary, extrapulmonary (central nervous system, gastrointestinal system, peritonitis, Pott's disease, etc.)	Standard therapy	Purified protein derivative test annually	Occurs at higher rates than in HIV, even with CD4 count >500
Mycobacterium avium-intracellulare; Mycobacterium avium-complex	Colitis, bacteremia, bone marrow, hepatitis	Clarithromycin + ethambutol	Azithromycin 1200 mg weekly	CD4 <50
Bartonella henselae, B. quintana	Bacillary angiomatosis, bacillary peliosis hepatitis	Erythromycin, other macrolides		Bacillary angiomatosis can be difficult to distinguish from Kaposi's sarcoma
Viral				
Hepatitis B virus (HBV)	Hepatitis, risk of cirrhosis/ hepatocellular carcinoma	Adefovir, lamivudine, tenofovir	Vaccination	Higher incidence in men who have sex with men
Hepatitis C virus (HBC)	Hepatitis, risk of cirrhosis/ hepatocellular carcinoma (>HBV)	Interferon-α/ribavirin	Avoid sharing needles	Higher incidence in intravenous drug users
Hepatitis A virus (HAV)	Acute self-limited hepatitis, no long-term sequelae	Supportive	Vaccination	HAV can cause aggravation of chronic HBV or HCV infection
Epstein–Barr virus	Oral hairy leukoplakia, B-cell lymphomas	None	None	
Cytomegalovirus (CMV)	Retinitis, colitis	Chemotherapy, ganciclovir	None	Check CMV immunoglobulin G to assess risk of reactivation; annual eye exams; CD4 count usually low (<50)
JC virus	Progressive multifocal leukoencephalopathy	Supportive; main treatment is HAART to restore immunocompetence	None	Diagnosis can be made by magnetic resonance imaging, polymerase chain reaction for JC in cerebrospinal fluid, brain biopsy
HHV-8	Kaposi's sarcoma (cutaneous or visceral)	Improved immune status with HAART; doxorubicin can be used	None	More common in men who have sex with men
Herpes simplex virus	Genital ulcers	Standard treatment	None	Outbreaks can be extensive and difficult to treat
Varicella-zoster virus	Herpes zoster, shingles	Acyclovir	None	
Human papilloma virus	Genital warts; cervical/ Rectal cancer	Standard treatment, excision	Frequent Pap smears, surveillance, "rectal Pap smear"	

(continued)

TABLE 9–6   Treatment and Prevention of Infections Associated with HIV Infection (*Continued*)

Organism	Clinical Manifestation	Treatment	Prevention/ Prophylaxis	Comments
Viral				
HIV	Dementia, eosinophilic folliculitis, renal disease, cardiomyopathy, vasculitis, arthritis, thyroid/adrenal insufficiency	HAART		
Fungal				
Candida	Thrush, vaginal candidiasis	Fluconazole	Mycelex troches, Nystatin swish-and-swallow	Common first indication of decreasing CD4 <200
Cryptococcus neoformans	Meningitis, cutaneous nodules	Amphotericin B, fluconazole	Fluconazole (for secondary prophylaxis)	
Pneumocystis jiroveci	Pneumonia	Bactrim	Bactrim for all patients with CD4 <200	
Histoplasma capsulatum	Pneumonia	Itraconazole	None	Suspect in patients from Ohio and Mississippi River Valleys
Coccidioides immitis	Pneumonia	Amphotericin B, fluconazole		
Parasitic				
Toxoplasma gondii	Central nervous system lesions, retinitis	Pyrimethamine + sulfadiazine	Bactrim	Clinical presentation can be confused with central nervous system lymphoma; ring-enhancing lesions on CT scan
Cryptosporidium, Microsporidium, Cyclospora, Isospora	Watery diarrhea	Paromomycin (although poor efficacy)		Occurs with advanced disease; best treatment strategy is HAART to improve immune status

HAART, highly active antiretroviral therapy.

l. **Endocrine system.** A variety of endocrine abnormalities, including thyroid and adrenal insufficiencies, have been reported in HIV-1 infection.

m. **Reproductive system**

(1) Carcinoma of the uterine cervix and dysplastic changes occur more commonly in HIV-1–infected women.

(2) Fungal (candidal) vulvovaginitis is more frequent and may be caused by antifungal drug-resistant strains.

(3) Herpes simplex infections can become very severe with the advanced immune depression associated with HIV-1. Patients with herpes genital infections can have large, confluent painful areas of involvement.

2. **Treatment of infections associated with HIV infection** (Table 9–6). Therapeutic regimens may be the same or more intensive than those for the same infection in immunocompetent individuals or patients with other causes of immune depression. Many of the infections associated with HIV are potentially chronic; lifelong secondary prophylaxis and close vigilance are necessary to control recurrences. Recommendations concerning the treatment of these conditions are revised constantly, and current information should always be sought.

3. **Prevention of complications**

a. **Immune reconstitution.** Prophylaxis can be stopped when immune function is restored. Some individuals experience transient worsening of infections as immune function improves.

This can be a fairly severe reaction that might require reinstitution of therapy for the previously quiescent infection. Most of the time it is most helpful to continue antiretroviral therapy despite the clinical worsening because immune reconstitution eventually goes away.

b. In general, prophylaxis against the common HIV-1–associated infections can be stopped when the CD4 count passes the level at which the risk of that infection begins to increase significantly. Usually this is done after at least two CD4 measurements have been high enough and when the patient is clinically stable. If the CD4 drops, it may be necessary to restart prophylaxis.

Study Questions

1. A 70-year-old man is admitted to the hospital for an elective hernia repair. The night before surgery, a nurse reports a rectal temperature of 38.1°C. After a careful examination shows no obvious source of infection, a single blood sample is sent for culture. The surgery is uneventful, but 3 days later, *Corynebacterium* is identified on blood culture. Which of the following best explains this finding?

- [A] The patient has bacterial endocarditis caused by *Corynebacterium*.
- [B] While taking the rectal temperature, the nurse inadvertently caused *Corynebacterium* bacteremia.
- [C] Tooth brushing just before the blood collection resulted in transient *Corynebacterium* bacteremia.
- [D] Inadequate skin preparation or careless handling resulted in contamination of the blood culture.
- [E] The laboratory mistook *Escherichia coli* for *Corynebacterium*.

2. A 19-year-old man with acute nonlymphocytic leukemia is admitted to the hospital 2 weeks after his first round of chemotherapy. His temperature is 39.2°C, and physical examination shows no localized abnormalities. Chest radiograph shows a Hickman catheter with its tip in the right atrium. The white blood cell (WBC) count is 300/mm³ with no polymorphonuclear or band cells in the differential count. Blood cultures are obtained. Which of the following is the next step?

- [A] Initiate antistaphylococcal treatment for the possibility of Hickman catheter–related bacteremia.
- [B] Administer broad-spectrum antibiotics with excellent activity for enteric gram-negative rods and *Pseudomonas aeruginosa*.
- [C] Await results of blood cultures and other diagnostic tests because infection could be caused by almost any microorganism.
- [D] Initiate oral prophylaxis to prevent bacterial and fungal infections.
- [E] Administer parenteral antifungal therapy.

3. A 20-year-old woman with a history of seizures for which she has taken phenytoin for 4 months has a fever of 38.7°C; she has felt febrile for 2 weeks. She has no respiratory or urinary symptoms. Physical examination findings are normal except for elevated body temperature. Chest radiograph, urinalysis, and complete blood count (CBC) findings are normal. Which of the following would be the best next step?

- [A] Admit the patient for toxic shock syndrome (TSS).
- [B] Administer acetaminophen.
- [C] Treat occult urinary tract infection with antibiotics.
- [D] Discontinue phenytoin and prescribe another anticonvulsant.
- [E] Cool the patient with a cooling blanket.

4. A sexually active 24-year-old woman known to be HIV-1 infected has had a fever for 2 days and has a productive cough. Chest radiographs show an infiltrate in the right lung. Two weeks earlier, her helper T (Th) cell (CD4) count was 510/mm³. Gram stain of sputum shows many white blood cells and squamous epithelial cells with a mixed bacterial flora. Testing for nontreponemal antigen (rapid plasma reagin) is positive at two dilutions, and treponemal antigen testing is also positive. Which of the following is the most likely cause of the pneumonia?

- [A] *Streptococcus pneumoniae*
- [B] *Pneumocystis carinii*
- [C] Cytomegalovirus (CMV)
- [D] *Mycobacterium avium-intracellulare* (MAI)
- [E] Syphilis

5. A 62-year-old man has right upper quadrant abdominal pain, nausea, and vomiting. Physical examination shows only guarding over the liver. Ultrasound examination confirms the diagnosis of gallstones without dilated bile ducts. The man is allergic to penicillin (a rash developed after penicillin therapy for a sore throat). In addition to dietary changes, which of the following treatments would be best?

- [A] No antibiotics
- [B] Erythromycin

C Oral quinolone

D Trimethoprim–sulfamethoxazole

E Amoxicillin

6. Two weeks after emergency surgery for a perforated duodenal ulcer, a 39-year-old woman complains of fever and vague abdominal pain. Her only medication is ranitidine. On physical examination, she appears a little pale, has a temperature of 38°C, and has a slight fullness in the epigastrium. Computed tomography (CT) scan of the abdomen shows an area of fluid collection measuring $3 \times 3 \times 8$ cm in the left paracolic gutter. Which of the following would be the most effective next step?

A Administer antibiotic therapy with an agent highly effective against aerobic gram-negative rods (e.g., aztreonam).

B Administer antibiotic therapy effective against abdominal anaerobes (e.g., clindamycin).

C Provide catheter drainage of the fluid collection and antibiotics appropriate for culture results.

D Administer no therapy unless blood cultures are positive or the collection changes in size.

E Order a magnetic resonance imaging (MRI) scan to confirm the CT findings.

7. A 64-year-old woman presents to the emergency department with abdominal pain and fever. She has had a long history of mild, intermittent dyspepsia that frequently has followed meals. She has had diabetes for 12 years, and although her response to oral hypoglycemic agents has been poor, she has refused to use insulin. At the time of presentation, she has been ill for 36 hours with vomiting, fever, and abdominal pain. On examination, she is febrile with a temperature of 38.9°C and has tachycardia of 124 bpm. She is mildly jaundiced. Bowel sounds are diminished, and tenderness and guarding are most marked in the right upper quadrant. Toward the end of the examination, rigor is evident, and she has broken into a sweat. Which of the following is most likely to be her problem?

A Pancreatitis with abscess

B Cholangitis

C Perforated peptic ulcer

D Splenic abscess

E Esophageal reflux

8. A 24-year-old man takes an exotic "around-the-world" vacation to Europe, Africa, India, and China. On his holiday, he has frequent sexual encounters and does not use condoms. In addition, he is bitten by mosquitoes many times. On his return, he notes fever, and his physician finds generalized lymphadenopathy. Which of the following is least likely to account for both these symptoms?

A Human immunodeficiency virus type 1 (HIV-1)

B Infectious mononucleosis

C Malaria

D Syphilis

E Cat-scratch disease

9. A 14-year-old girl from Pennsylvania goes to Wisconsin for a 2-week camping trip. Two weeks after she returns, she notices a solitary circular rash on her left calf just above the area normally covered by her socks. Overall, she feels well, and there is gradual progression of the rash over the next week. Which of the following diseases endemic in Wisconsin or Pennsylvania did she most likely acquire?

A Blastomycosis

B Lyme disease

C California encephalitis

D Rocky Mountain spotted fever

E Syphilis

10. Which of the following is the strongest indication to consider valve replacement surgery in a patient with infective endocarditis?

A Hematuria

B Positive cultures for *Staphylococcus aureus* on the second day of therapy

C Splinter hemorrhages and Osler's nodes

D Progressive congestive heart failure (CHF)

E Splenomegaly

11. An 18-year-old woman takes a summer job working in a day care center. A month after starting, she develops a rash over her whole body. The lesions are small vesicles on a slightly erythematous base. Except for a slight cough and fever of 38°C, she feels well. She has proof of having received her childhood immunizations before she started school. Which of the following statements is most correct?

A The patient probably has an elevated total white blood cell count and a differential with an abundance of neutrophils and band forms.

B Within 1 week, the patient will recover totally with lifelong immunity and no further sequelae.

C The patient probably developed an allergy to some of the fabric in the toys at the day care center.

D The patient may be infectious to other family members.

E If the patient becomes pregnant 1 year or more later, she will require close obstetric observation.

12. After a recent bad cold, an 18-year-old man has symptoms of sinusitis with nasal drainage and stuffiness. On examination, papilledema is evident. The physician is convinced that the patient has a brain abscess. Which of the following statements is correct?

A Magnetic resonance imaging scans are usually not helpful.

B The source of infection is usually cardiac.

C Antimicrobials active against *Pseudomonas aeruginosa* are usually a part of the treatment.

D Complete surgical excision is usually not needed.

E The patient is likely to develop bacterial meningitis in the next 5 years.

13. A 12-year-old boy has had fever and bloody diarrhea for 2 weeks and has lost 4 pounds of body weight. Three stool specimens have yielded no enteric pathogens on culture, and no ova or mature parasites are observed on direct examination. Which of the following is the best reason for his illness?

A Regional enteritis

B Giardiasis

C Travelers' diarrhea caused by enterotoxigenic *Escherichia coli*

D Cryptosporidiosis

E Jejunal infarction

14. A 26-year-old woman with no history of medical problems complains of 3 days of burning with urination and increased frequency. Urinalysis shows positive result for leukocyte esterase and nitrates on dipstick. The microscopic examination shows 5–10 white blood cells and no bacteria. Which of the following is the next step?

A Wait for results before starting therapy.

B Treat with Pyridium, a urinary analgesic, since there is no bacteriuria.

C Treat with 3 days of trimethoprim–sulfamethoxazole.

D Treat for 7 days with ciprofloxacin.

E Treat for 14 days with intravenous cephalosporin antibiotic.

15. A 70-year-old man has chronic lung disease. Which of the following immunizations should he receive annually?

A Influenza

B Tetanus

C Pneumococcal pneumonia

D Pertussis

E Hepatitis B virus (HBV)

16. A 49-year-old man reports recent sexual contact with a commercial sex worker. About 9 days later, he experiences dysuria and has a very modest urethral discharge. Which of the following infectious agents most likely accounts for his symptoms?

- A *Chlamydia trachomatis infection*
- B Syphilis
- C Trichomoniasis
- D Granuloma inguinale
- E *Escherichia coli*

17. A 41-year-old man with a history of weight loss and hairy leukoplakia reports that a recent HIV-1 blood test came back positive. His CD4 count is 204/mm^3, and his viral load is 58,000 copies/mL by reverse transcriptase polymerase chain reaction (moderately high). A purified protein derivative (PPD) skin test is negative for tuberculosis, and you find that he has already had a pneumococcal vaccination. Which of the following would be the next step?

- A Wait until he develops a more significant opportunistic infection before beginning antiretroviral therapy.
- B Begin zidovudine at standard doses and take the patient's CD4 count and a viral load in 6 weeks.
- C Begin a combination regimen with three active agents, such as zidovudine, lamivudine, and efavirenz.
- D Begin a course of fluconazole to prevent thrush and rifabutin to prevent *Mycobacterium avium-intracellulare* (MAI) infection.
- E Refer the patient to a dentist for management of the hairy leukoplakia.

18. When a patient needs a peripheral intravenous catheter for approximately 1 week, which of the following methods is the most important way of preventing catheter-related infections?

- A Using a powerful antimicrobial ointment at the junction of the hub and the skin
- B Changing the catheter site every 48–72 hours
- C Giving systemic antibiotics for the entire duration of catheter placement
- D Shaving the skin before cleansing it
- E Using the leg rather than the arm

Answers and Explanations

1. The answer is D [I A, III B]. Inadequate skin preparation or careless handling results in contamination of the blood culture. Even though all of the answers are possible, the most likely one is simple contamination; 2%–5% of blood cultures are contaminated by skin flora from the patient or the phlebotomist. *Corynebacterium* makes up a small fraction of oral and rectal flora and is less likely to enter the blood from these sites. Endocarditis caused by *Corynebacterium* is rare and almost never involves native valves. *Escherichia coli* and *Corynebacterium* are essentially impossible to confuse in the laboratory.

2. The answer is B [II A 3]. The next step is to administer broad-spectrum antibiotics with activity against enteric gram-negative rods and *Pseudomonas aeruginosa.* The heightened susceptibility of neutropenic patients to die quickly of overwhelming sepsis makes early intervention obligatory. Even though many clinicians include antibiotic coverage for staphylococci, the most common bacteria encountered are gram-negative rods. Antifungal treatment is used if antibacterial therapy fails to control the fever or if a specific fungal infection is found. Prophylaxis is started before having evidence of active infection.

3. The answer is D [Online VII D 2 a (1)]. The next best step is to discontinue the phenytoin and prescribe another anticonvulsant. Of the many drugs that cause fever as an unwanted side effect, anticonvulsant agents lead the list. Prolonged fever can have many causes other than medication reactions and may be difficult to diagnose. In ambulatory patients, common bacterial infections are fairly well excluded by normal findings on chest radiograph, urine, and blood tests. Toxic shock syndrome is a multisystem illness in which fever is only one component. Although juvenile rheumatoid arthritis affects patients in this age group, aspirin would be more appropriate than acetaminophen. Cooling blankets are used only in severely ill patients.

4. The answer is A [V C 4 b, c (1); VIII G 1 h (2)]. The most likely cause of the pneumonia is *Streptococcus pneumoniae.* Although *P. carinii* is the most common serious opportunistic infection in patients with HIV-1 infection, the productive cough, localized infiltrate, and brief duration argue against *P. carinii* pneumonia (PCP). In addition, the Th cell (CD4) count of more than 500 cells/mm^3 suggests that serious opportunistic infections such as PCP, cytomegalovirus, or *Mycobacterium avium-intracellulare* are unlikely for some time. Syphilis, which may have been present, almost never involves the lungs.

5. The answer is A [V E 4]. Uncomplicated cholecystitis without obstruction of the biliary ducts or empyema of the gallbladder is best managed conservatively. Although some bacteria may be found in the bile at the time of cholecystectomy, there is rarely progression to infection. Erythromycin essentially has no activity for any of the agents associated with cholecystitis or cholangitis. Amoxicillin is contraindicated for patients who are allergic to penicillin. Severely ill patients should be hospitalized to manage the possibility of serious complications.

6. The answer is C [V E 2 c]. Catheter drainage of the fluid collection and antibiotics appropriate for culture results would be the most effective step to take next. The most likely explanation for the clinical findings and the computed tomography (CT) abnormality is a postoperative intra-abdominal abscess. These rarely heal without drainage. Surgical drainage is effective, but a lesion that can be reached safely with a catheter may be drained equally effectively and more safely. Antibiotics are usually used as adjunctive therapy. The flora of these abscesses is usually mixed with enteric aerobes and anaerobes. Good cultures can be useful in refining the exact therapeutic regimen. Magnetic resonance imaging is a fine test, but the CT scan has already led to a diagnosis.

7. The answer is B [V E 4; Chapter 6 VIII G]. According to the patient, she has certainly had cholecystitis in the past. With gallstones in the gallbladder, there is always some risk of migration to the common bile duct and subsequent obstruction of the duct. The infection that may follow obstruction of the common bile duct may be very serious, with bacteremia and sepsis as common sequelae. Pancreatic abscess can manifest as abdominal pain, but it does not have the associated localized right upper quadrant findings as often as cholangitis. Perforated ulcers lead to peritonitis. Splenic abscesses are almost always the sequelae of bacteremia (e.g., with endocarditis). Reflux esophagitis can cause severe heartburn but does not result in sepsis.

8. The answer is C [VII A, B]. Malaria is characterized by lack of lymphadenopathy, although spleno-megaly and ever are characteristic. Although generalized enlargement of lymph nodes is a nonspecific finding, it often can lead to the diagnosis of a clinical entity. When the lymphadenopathy is coupled with fatigue and an atypical lymphocytosis, infectious mononucleosis is suggested. This syndrome most often is caused by Epstein–Barr virus, but a similar clinical picture is produced by cytomegalovirus infection. The infections can be distinguished by using serologic tests (e.g., Monospot test) or specific antibodies. Secondary syphilis also should be considered in patients with adenopathy of short duration; this can be confirmed on the basis of serologic tests and the finding of an appropriate rash. Reactive, hyperplastic lymph nodes are common in HIV-1 infection. For this patient, all of these are possibilities, but the malaria would not account for the enlarged lymph nodes. Cat-scratch disease usually causes enlarged lymph glands, with stellate microabscesses apparent histologically.

9. The answer is B [VII F]. Only Lyme disease and Rocky Mountain spotted fever (RMSF) occur with a rash as a common feature. California encephalitis (which is spread by mosquito) has few, if any, skin manifestations but does cause a syndrome of progressive neurologic deterioration that resolves sponta-neously in most cases. Blastomycosis, a disease that enters the body through the respiratory tract and may metastasize to other organs, almost never generates a circular rash. RMSF has a rash that usually begins peripherally but is rarely solitary. The course of disease is usually fairly rapid, in contrast to the indolent but progressive lesion that is typical of erythema migrans. Syphilis causes a rash but almost never involves only one spot on the leg.

10. The answer is D [V I 4 d]. Although all of the answers reflect aspects of endocarditis, the only abso-lute indications for valve replacement are fungal endocarditis, congestive heart failure, valve ring abscess, and failure to clear infection after a long course of antimicrobial therapy. Some authorities recommend valve replacement after multiple significant emboli. Minor emboli, an enlarged spleen, and immuno-logic phenomena are not cause for valve replacement.

11. The answer is D [🔍 Online II H 4]. Although a varicella vaccine does exist, its implementation has not been universal among older children or adults. Thus, many children and adults are still suscep-tible to varicella. Sequelae of varicella infection are rare and include pneumonia, meningitis, and hepa-titis, as well as herpes zoster (shingles). The white blood cell count is normal or slightly depressed in most of the childhood exanthems. Varicella in pregnancy can be severe, but this patient will be safe once her rash disappears.

12. The answer is D [V A 3 c]. Cross-sectional imaging studies (e.g., computed tomography and mag-netic resonance imaging) are critical to the diagnosis and management of intracranial abscess. Surgery is often undertaken to obtain a specimen for culture or to decompress the abscess. Total surgical exci-sion is rarely required in the patient who is responding well to medical therapy. Although occasional patients do have cardiopulmonary sources for infection, most patients have contiguous infection of the middle ear or, as in this case, the sinus. Meningitis can follow trauma to the cribriform plate but rarely follows a brain abscess.

13. The answer is A [V D]. Regional enteritis, ulcerative colitis, and a variety of invasive infectious pathogens can cause bloody diarrhea. A single stool specimen may miss any of these agents. *Giardia lamblia* and *Cryptosporidium* usually cause an upper small bowel lesion that leads to watery diarrhea without fever. Travelers' diarrhea is a toxin-mediated infection that also leads to minimal inflammatory changes in the bowel. Bowel infarcts are extremely rare in children.

14. The answer is C [V F 6 b]. The patient's presentation is consistent with uncomplicated acute uri-nary tract infection (UTI), and she should receive treatment. Cultures are not required to confirm the diagnosis, and absence of bacteria on microscopic examination does not rule out UTI. The presence of WBCs in the urine is strong suggestion of infection. Three days of therapy are adequate (and equivalent to a 7-day course), and trimethoprim–sulfamethoxazole is a good choice that is inexpensive and well tolerated. However, if rates of resistance in the community are high, using ciprofloxacin or another fluoroquinolone for 3 days would be advisable. Intravenous antibiotics are not indicated in the setting of uncomplicated UTI.

15. The answer is A [🄿 Online II H 1]. Immunity to pertussis is established by immunization in childhood. Tetanus immunity is maintained by boosters every 10 years. A single vaccination for pneumococcal infection should be given to all persons with chronic cardiopulmonary disease, to all adults older than age 60 years, and to all patients with HIV infection. Reimmunizations may not be needed at all, and certainly no more than once every 5–7 years. However, the immunity conferred by influenza vaccine is short lived and strain specific. Yearly immunizations for influenza are strongly recommended for the elderly and those with chronic cardiopulmonary diseases. Hepatitis B virus vaccine is not routinely indicated in the elderly, and vaccination is not needed for at least 5 years.

16. The answer is A [VI B 1 b, 2 b]. Chlamydial infection is one of the most common causes of urethritis and frequently manifests with dysuria. Syphilis and granuloma inguinale do affect the external genitals but tend to spare the urethral mucosa. Trichomonas is sometimes found in the male genitals, but it is almost always without symptoms. *Escherichia coli* can cause a urinary tract infection but not a sexually transmitted disease.

17. The answer is C [VIII D 3]. Symptomatic HIV-1 infection can be treated using combination therapy with exceedingly good results. With luck, the correct antiretroviral drug combination will lead to an improvement in this patient's immune function, and he might be able to avoid all chemoprophylaxis indefinitely. Delay in treatment now might spare him some drug side effects, but he is almost to the point of developing severe complications from HIV-1 itself. Treatment with a single drug such as zidovudine is not useful because of its limited impact on viral burden and the early emergence of resistance. Although prophylaxis for *Mycobacterium avium-intracellulare* and fungal infections may reduce the number of such infections, it need not be started until immune dysfunction has progressed considerably. Hairy leukoplakia is not serious and will subside with improved immune function.

18. The answer is B [🄿 Online IV F 2 b]. Assuming that all catheters are placed under the best possible conditions, keeping them clean and dry is all the daily care they need. Short plastic catheters are prone to infection over time, so routine replacement is recommended. This rule does not apply to central catheters (placed directly into a central vein or threaded up along the arm). There is no benefit to shaving the skin, except to provide a better surface for the adhesive tape used to secure the catheter. Intravenous lines in the leg, which are trickier to maintain and have a higher rate of infection, should be avoided whenever possible.

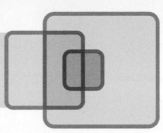

chapter 10

Endocrine and Metabolic Diseases

ELIZABETH LAMOS • EMILY FAIRCHILD

DISORDERS OF THE PITUITARY GLAND

A **General considerations**

1. The anterior pituitary gland produces several hormones [luteinizing hormone (LH), follicle-stimulating hormone (FSH), prolactin, thyroid-stimulating hormone (TSH), adrenocorticotropic hormone (ACTH) and growth hormone (GH)] that act at target organ sites throughout the body to promote growth and development or to stimulate the release of other hormones (Figure 10–1). The release of anterior pituitary hormones is controlled by positive and negative feedback loops that exert their influence on the pituitary itself, as well as on the production of releasing and inhibitory factors by the hypothalamus (Table 10–1). Anterior pituitary disease results from excessive production of pituitary hormones (hyperprolactinemia, acromegaly, Cushing's disease), from insufficient production of pituitary hormones (panhypopituitarism, insufficiency of selected hormones), or from the local mass effect of pituitary tumors.

2. The posterior pituitary gland produces antidiuretic hormone (ADH) and oxytocin. ADH is important for maintaining water balance. Its production is regulated by osmoreceptors in the hypothalamus, as well as by arterial baroreceptors in the carotid body and elsewhere in the body. Central diabetes insipidus and the syndrome of inappropriate ADH secretion (SIADH) are the major manifestations of posterior pituitary disease.

3. Evaluation of pituitary function involves measurement of the pituitary hormones themselves or measurement of the hormones produced by the target organ. In some cases, in order to diagnose pituitary disease, it is necessary to stimulate production of a hormone that is suspected to be deficient or to suppress release of a hormone that is suspected to be present in excess.

B **Pituitary tumors**

1. **Pituitary tumors** make up 10% of intracranial tumors. Most are benign, but their continued slow growth in the confined sellar and suprasellar areas may cause serious neurologic damage.
   a. **Types**
      (1) **Pituitary adenomas** are classified by cell type, based on electron microscopy and immunohistochemical staining. **Lactotroph tumors** produce prolactin, **somatotroph tumors** produce GH, and **corticotroph tumors** produce ACTH.
      (2) **Craniopharyngiomas,** the most common tumors of the hypothalamic–pituitary area in children, arise from remnants of cells from Rathke's pouch.
         (a) They are located above the sella turcica, but may produce changes within the sella itself.
         (b) They may be solid or cystic, may contain cholesterol-rich fluid, and often contain areas of calcification.
      (3) **Meningiomas** and **metastatic tumors** may involve the hypothalamic–pituitary area.
   b. **Clinical features**
      (1) **Excess hormone production** by pituitary adenomas may lead to **acromegaly, hyperprolactinemia,** or **Cushing's disease.**
         (a) In rare cases, these tumors may produce excess TSH, causing hyperthyroidism.

415

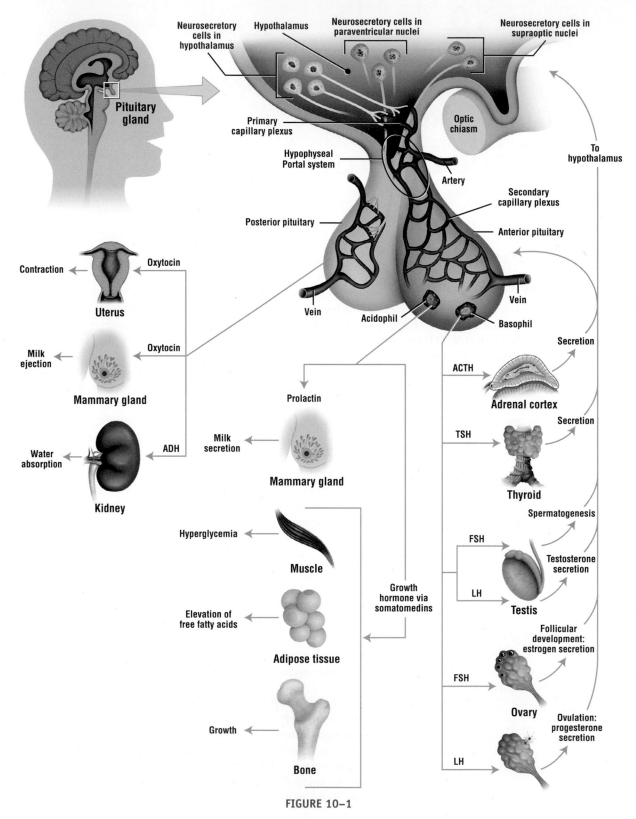

FIGURE 10–1

TABLE 10–1 Anterior Pituitary Hormones

Anterior Pituitary Hormones	Hypothalamic Hormones	Positive Feedback Influence	Negative Feedback Influence
Luteinizing hormone (LH), follicle-stimulating hormone (FSH)	Gonadotropin-releasing hormone (GnRH)	Low sex hormone levels	Elevated sex hormone levels
Thyroid-stimulating hormone (TSH)	Thyrotropin-releasing hormone (TRH)	Low triiodothyronine (T_3), thyroxine (T_4)	Elevated T3, T4
Adrenocorticotropic hormone (ACTH)	Corticotropin-releasing hormone (CRH)	Low cortisol	Elevated cortisol
Growth hormone (GH)	Growth hormone–releasing hormone (GHRH) Somatostatin (inhibitory)	Sleep, stress, hypoglycemia	Arginine, hyperglycemia
Prolactin	Prolactin inhibitory factor (PIF) (= dopamine)	Pregnancy	Dopamine agonists

  (b) FSH and LH are frequently produced in excess by pituitary tumors, but this usually does not result in a clear-cut clinical syndrome.

(2) Insufficient hormone production, due to compression or destruction of pituitary and hypothalamic cells, produces the syndrome of **hypopituitarism.**

(3) Neurologic effects

  (a) Optic nerve compression may occur. Pituitary tumors may press upward on the inferior surface of the optic chiasm. Vision loss typically occurs first in the superior temporal quadrants, with bitemporal hemianopia in more advanced cases.

  (b) Headache is common.

  (c) Other neurologic manifestations such as mental status changes, cranial nerve abnormalities, vomiting, papilledema, and pituitary apoplexy are less common.

(4) Multiple endocrine neoplasia type I (MEN I, Wermer's syndrome) is a syndrome consisting of tumors, often functioning, of the pituitary, parathyroids, and pancreatic islets.

c. Diagnosis

(1) Diagnostic imaging

  (a) Skull radiographs may show enlargement or distortion of the sella when tumors are 10 mm or more in diameter (**macroadenomas**). Suprasellar calcification suggests the presence of a craniopharyngioma.

  (b) Computed tomography (CT) will show macroadenomas, but more sensitive imaging techniques, such as **magnetic resonance imaging (MRI),** may be required to visualize microadenomas.

  (c) MRI can show pituitary **microadenomas** (tumors <10 mm in diameter) in 10% of normal individuals. If hyperprolactinemia or other hormone abnormalities are not present and if follow-up study shows no progressive enlargement, these tumors should be regarded as incidental findings of no clinical significance.

(2) Hormone studies. Pituitary adenomas that secrete excess GH, prolactin, or ACTH can be diagnosed by measuring the pituitary hormones, or in some cases the hormones produced by target organs, even if the adenoma is too small to be visualized by diagnostic imaging.

d. Therapy

(1) Surgery is indicated for pituitary adenomas that produce neurologic symptoms and for some tumors that cause syndromes associated with hormone overproduction.

  (a) Transsphenoidal pituitary microsurgery is used for intrasellar tumors that have minimal or no suprasellar extension. Small adenomas often can be removed without damage to normal pituitary tissue.

  (b) Transfrontal resection may be necessary for large tumors that extend far outside the sella turcica or compress the optic chiasm.

(2) Radiation therapy, used alone or in conjunction with surgery, may decrease the size of pituitary tumors and decrease hormone production.

(3) Medical therapy

    (a) Hormone replacement is required if hypopituitarism is present.

    (b) Dopamine agonists such as **bromocriptine** and **cabergoline,** as well as somatostatin analogs such as **octreotide,** may decrease the size and hormone production of certain pituitary tumors.

C Anterior pituitary disease—Excessive production

1. **Hyperprolactinemia.** As many as 50% of all pituitary adenomas have been found to secrete prolactin.

    a. Etiology

        (1) Prolactin-secreting pituitary adenomas (prolactinomas) are more common in women than in men, usually appearing during the reproductive years and causing menstrual abnormalities and galactorrhea **(galactorrhea–amenorrhea syndrome).** Men tend to have larger tumors at the time of diagnosis, which usually are suspected because of neurologic impairment and hypogonadism.

        (2) Damage to the hypothalamus or **pituitary stalk** by tumors, granulomas, and other processes may prevent the normal regulatory effect of hypothalamic dopamine on lactotrope activity, resulting in hypersecretion of prolactin.

        (3) Drugs that can inhibit dopamine activity and, thus, interfere with its regulation of prolactin secretion include psychotropic agents (e.g., phenothiazines, butyrophenones, tricyclic antidepressants), antihypertensives (e.g., methyldopa, reserpine), metoclopramide, cimetidine, and others.

    b. Clinical features

        (1) Amenorrhea or menstrual irregularity is due to the inhibition of hypothalamic gonadotropin-releasing hormone (GnRH) production by prolactin, as well as to the direct effects of the prolactin on the ovaries.

        (2) Galactorrhea is a direct result of prolactin excess.

        (3) Loss of potency and libido, with low testosterone levels, is the common endocrine manifestation in men.

    c. Diagnosis. Prolactin levels are elevated. A serum prolactin level greater than 300 ng/mL strongly suggests the presence of a prolactinoma. Functional causes of hyperprolactinemia such as drugs seldom elevate the level above 100–200 ng/mL.

    d. Therapy. Treatment of prolactinoma depends on the size of the tumor and its manifestations. A small, nonenlarging tumor in a woman with insignificant galactorrhea who does not desire pregnancy may not require treatment. If pregnancy is desired, if the galactorrhea or amenorrhea is unacceptable, or if the tumor is enlarging or causing local symptoms, therapeutic options include **administration of bromocriptine or another dopamine agonist, surgery,** and **radiation therapy.**

        (1) Dopamine agonists are remarkably effective in decreasing prolactin levels, usually to normal, which promptly relieves the galactorrhea and restores normal menses and fertility; it frequently reduces tumor size as well.

            (a) The side effects of bromocriptine include nausea, headache, dizziness, and fatigue.

            (b) Because of the poor surgical results in patients with large tumors, initial treatment with bromocriptine is given. If the tumor shrinks, there is a greater chance for successful surgery, or medical treatment alone may be continued indefinitely.

        (2) Transsphenoidal surgery is considered when patients cannot tolerate medical therapy or have evidence of compressive symptoms. Large tumors with suprasellar extension, however, usually are not cured by surgery.

        (3) Radiation therapy may be used in conjunction with surgery and dopamine agonists to further reduce tumor size and function.

2. **Acromegaly**

    a. Etiology. Acromegaly is caused by a pituitary adenoma that produces GH. Immunohistochemical staining shows that these adenomas are composed of somatotroph cells.

    b. Clinical features. Excess GH secretion may cause changes in bone, soft tissues, and metabolic processes.

(1) Bone and soft tissue changes
  (a) In children, excess GH secretion may cause increased linear growth of long bones, resulting in **gigantism.** After closure of the epiphyses at puberty, these changes cannot occur.
  (b) In adults, soft tissue growth and bone enlargement, especially in the acral areas of the skeleton, lead to diverse manifestations such as enlargement of the hands and feet, coarsening of the facial features, and enlargement of the mandible. One should consider comparing the patient's current features to those on an old photograph.

(2) Metabolic changes
  (a) Decreased glucose tolerance, a result of the anti-insulin actions of GH, is common, although overt diabetes occurs in only 10% of patients with acromegaly.
  (b) Hyperphosphatemia may develop secondary to increased tubular reabsorption of phosphate induced by GH.

c. Diagnosis. Clinical manifestations raise the suspicion of acromegaly. Abnormalities in the blood levels of GH, insulin-like growth factor I (IGF-I, formerly called somatomedin C), or both confirm the diagnosis.
  (1) Because glucose suppresses GH in normal subjects but not in acromegaly, **GH measurement after a glucose load** may best distinguish between normal and acromegalic subjects.
  (2) IGF-1 is a growth factor produced by the liver under the stimulation of GH. IGF-1 levels may be elevated in patients with acromegaly whose GH level is normal or equivocal. Elevated levels of IGF-1 provide an additional index of GH activity and further evidence of the diagnosis.
  (3) Initially, fasting levels of GH and IGF-1 should be measured. If the GH level is less than 0.4 μg/L and IGF-1 is normal, acromegaly is excluded.
  (4) If either the GH or the IGF-1 level is not low enough to exclude acromegaly, a 75-g oral glucose tolerance test should be performed, with GH measurements every 30 minutes for 2 hours. If the GH level does not fall below 1.0 μg/L, a diagnosis of acromegaly is suggested; an elevated IGF-1 level increases the likelihood of this diagnosis.
  (5) False-positive GH responses (i.e., failure of suppression) may occur after surgery and in patients with diabetes mellitus, liver disease, kidney disease, and malnutrition.

d. Therapy
  (1) Transsphenoidal pituitary adenomectomy causes prompt normalization of GH levels in most patients. Permanent cure is common when the adenoma is small, but it is uncommon when the tumor is large and extends beyond the sella turcica.
  (2) Conventional radiation therapy lowers GH levels slowly; normal levels may not be reached until 3–10 years after treatment, if at all.
  (3) Octreotide, an analog of somatostatin, can be given by subcutaneous injection. It lowers GH levels in many patients with acromegaly and may be useful in patients in whom surgery and radiation therapy have been unsuccessful.
  (4) Pegvisomant, an analog of GH that binds to GH receptors, blocks the binding of GH, thus inhibiting its actions. The result is a decrease in IGF-1 and lessening of the effects of excessive GH in acromegaly. Use of pegvisomant may be indicated in patients who have not responded adequately to other treatments.

3. Cushing's disease. Etiology, clinical features, diagnosis, and therapy are discussed in Section II.

D **Anterior pituitary/hypopituitarism**

1. Etiology
  a. Pituitary tumors, most commonly pituitary macroadenomas and craniopharyngiomas, may destroy normal hypothalamic–pituitary tissue.
  b. Sheehan's syndrome is hypopituitarism caused by infarction of the anterior pituitary gland during childbirth. The pituitary gland doubles in size during pregnancy, largely because of hyperplasia of the lactotrophs. The blood supply does not keep pace with the enlargement, however, and hypotensive episodes during a complicated delivery may lead to infarction.
  c. Surgery for the removal of pituitary or other brain tumors may damage the hypothalamus, the pituitary gland, or both.
  d. Less common causes of pituitary or hypothalamic destruction include **sarcoidosis, hemochromatosis, Hand–Schüller–Christian disease, tuberculosis, syphilis,** and **fungal infections.**

2. Clinical features

    a. GH deficiency has different effects in children and adults.

        (1) In children, **growth failure** occurs, leading to short stature in adulthood (**pituitary dwarfism**).

        (2) In adults, it is now recognized that GH deficiency causes undesired changes in body composition, with an **increase in body fat** and a **decrease in lean body mass.** These changes may be accompanied by decreased strength and exercise capacity.

        (3) Other adverse effects may include an increase in cardiovascular risk factors such as insulin resistance and hyperlipidemia, atherosclerosis, impaired quality of life, and perhaps shortened life expectancy.

    b. Gonadotropin (LH and FSH) deficiency causes **amenorrhea and genital atrophy in women** and **loss of potency and libido in men.** If adrenal androgens are deficient as well because of concomitant ACTH deficiency, pubic and axillary hair may be lost, especially in women.

    c. TSH deficiency results in the symptoms and physical changes of **hypothyroidism.**

    d. ACTH deficiency leads to **adrenal insufficiency.** Secondary adrenal insufficiency (caused by pituitary disease) differs in several clinical manifestations from primary adrenal insufficiency (caused by adrenal disease).

        (1) Hyperpigmentation of the skin and mucous membranes is characteristic of primary adrenal disease.

            (a) It is caused, indirectly, by the negative-feedback stimulation of ACTH by low plasma cortisol levels. (ACTH and melanocyte-stimulating hormone [MSH] are derived from the same large precursor molecule (pro-opiomelanocortin), so when ACTH is increased, MSH is increased as well. MSH stimulates melanocytes and causes pigmentation.)

            (b) ACTH (and, therefore, MSH) levels are low in secondary adrenal insufficiency; consequently, hyperpigmentation is not characteristic of this condition.

        (1) Electrolyte changes (i.e., decreased serum sodium and increased serum potassium levels) are minimal in secondary adrenal insufficiency because aldosterone production by the adrenal cortex (which promotes sodium retention) depends primarily on renin and angiotensin (which are undisturbed) rather than on ACTH.

    e. Prolactin deficiency may be responsible for the postpartum failure of lactation in Sheehan's syndrome but otherwise produces no clinical manifestations.

    f. With slow, progressive destruction of pituitary tissue, **failure of GH and gonadotropin secretion** occurs early. With continuing loss of tissue, TSH and finally ACTH and prolactin fall below normal levels.

    g. Deficiency of individual pituitary hormones may occur. Isolated GH deficiency and isolated gonadotropin deficiency are not uncommon, especially in children. Isolated deficiencies of TSH and ACTH are very uncommon.

3. Diagnosis

    a. Evaluation of target organ function is often the first step in the diagnosis of hypopituitarism. This condition is often suspected because of failure of more than one target organ (i.e., thyroid, adrenal glands, gonads). Tests of adrenal, thyroid, adrenal, ovarian, and testicular function are described in Sections II, III, VII, and VIII, respectively.

    b. Measurement of pituitary hormones. GH levels may be undetectable under basal conditions in normal individuals; therefore, provocative maneuvers may be needed to prove inadequacy of hormone production.

        (1) Insulin-induced hypoglycemia (the **insulin tolerance test**) is the most consistently effective test stimulus for GH and can also stimulate cortisol production. Regular insulin is given as an intravenous bolus, and GH levels are measured after 30, 60, and 90 minutes.

        (2) The patient must be observed closely during the test; central nervous system (CNS) symptoms of hypoglycemia require immediate intravenous administration of glucose. This test should not be performed in persons older than 65 years or persons with coronary disease or a seizure disorder. The next-most-effective stimulus for GH, after insulin-induced hypoglycemia, is the **intravenous (IV) infusion of arginine and GH-releasing hormone.**

        (3) In patients with panhypopituitarism, provocative tests may not be necessary to diagnose GH deficiency. If three or more other pituitary hormone deficiencies exist, the probability that GH is also deficient exceeds 95%. This probability is even higher if IGF-1 levels are low (although one third of GH-deficient patients may have normal levels of IGF-1.)

4. **Therapy**
   a. The **underlying cause** of the pituitary insufficiency (e.g., enlarging pituitary tumors, granu-lomatous diseases) should be sought and treated, if possible.
   b. **Hormone replacement**
      (1) **GH administration** can stimulate growth and increase the ultimate height in children with isolated GH deficiency or panhypopituitarism. Synthetic human growth hormone of recombinant DNA origin is available but must be given by injection and is expensive. GH replacement is given to some adults with GH deficiency; however, this treatment must be considered on a case-by-case basis.
      (2) **Thyroid hormone** is given in usual replacement doses [see III B 4].
      (3) **Cortisol** (hydrocortisone) is given in usual replacement doses.
      (4) **Estrogen–progesterone combinations** may be given to women, and testosterone to men, to prevent or treat the manifestations of hypogonadism.
      (5) Fertility is considerably more difficult to achieve because it depends on the precisely con-trolled administration of **gonadotropins** or **GnRH.**
         (a) GnRH has been successful in restoring ovulation in women and sperm production in men, but only in cases in which hypothalamic production of GnRH is impaired but the pituitary retains its ability to secrete LH and FSH in response to GnRH.
         (b) **GnRH** stimulates LH and FSH production only if it is administered in a way that mimics normal physiologic secretion; that is, it must be given by regular pulsatile injection every 90–120 minutes. (Constant rather than pulsatile administration of GnRH has the opposite effect. It decreases pituitary LH and FSH production.)

E **Posterior pituitary disease**

1. **Diabetes insipidus.** The term **central diabetes insipidus** is used to describe disease due to ADH insufficiency, and the term **nephrogenic diabetes insipidus** is used to describe disease due to renal unresponsiveness to ADH.
   a. **Etiology** of central diabetes insipidus
      (1) Approximately 50% of cases are **idiopathic.**
      (2) **Injury to the hypothalamic–pituitary area** may result from head trauma, brain tumors, and neurosurgical procedures.
      (3) **Less common causes** include **sarcoidosis, syphilis, Hand–Schüller–Christian disease,** and **encephalitis.**
   b. **Clinical features**
      (1) **Polyuria,** with urine volumes of 3–15 L daily, results from the inability to reabsorb free water and to concentrate urine in the absence of adequate ADH.
      (2) **Thirst** results, which leads to **increased fluid intake.** A conscious patient with a normal thirst mechanism and free access to water will maintain hydration; the disease in such a patient is an inconvenience rather than a threat to life. However, rapid and life-threaten-ing dehydration may occur in an infant or in an unconscious patient.
      (3) Laboratory abnormalities include a **dilute urine** (osmolality <200 mOsm/kg and specific gravity <1.005) and a high-normal or slightly **elevated plasma osmolality.**
   c. **Differential diagnosis.** In patients with polyuria and dilute urine, central diabetes insipidus must be differentiated from nephrogenic diabetes insipidus and compulsive water drinking.
      (1) **Nephrogenic diabetes insipidus** is a condition in which the renal tubules fail to respond to normal circulating levels of ADH.
         (a) The condition may be primary and familial, starting in infancy, or it may occur later in life as a secondary condition in association with hypokalemia, hypercalcemia, chronic renal disease, sickle cell anemia, amyloidosis, or the use of certain drugs (e.g., lithium, demeclocycline, and methoxyflurane).
         (b) The clinical features are the same as those caused by ADH deficiency. The difference is seen in the failure of nephrogenic diabetes insipidus to respond to administration of ADH.

TABLE 10–2   Response to Water Deprivation Test

Diagnosis	Increase in Urine Osmolality >280 mOsm/kg with Dehydration	Further Increase in Urine Osmolality in Response to Antidiuretic Hormone
Normal	+	−
Complete central diabetes insipidus	−	+
Partial central diabetes insipidus	+	+
Nephrogenic diabetes insipidus	+	−

       (2) Compulsive water drinking (psychogenic polydipsia) is a primary psychiatric abnormality that leads to polyuria and dilute urine. Differentiation from diabetes insipidus may be difficult. It is most common in young or middle-aged women who often have a history of psychiatric disorders.

   d. Diagnosis

      (1) Measurement of plasma osmolality. In untreated patients, this determination helps distinguish the causes of polyuria. In diabetes insipidus, the loss of free water is primary, and plasma osmolality tends to be high (280–310 mOsm/kg). In psychogenic polydipsia, excessive fluid intake is primary, and plasma osmolality tends to be low (255–280 mOsm/kg).

      (2) Water deprivation test (Table 10–2)

         (a) Method. Fluid intake is withheld until urine osmolality reaches a plateau (i.e., an hourly increase of <30 mOsm/kg for 3 consecutive hours). When urine osmolality is stable, plasma osmolality is measured. Desmopressin 2 µg (DDAVP, a synthetic analog of vasopressin) is then injected subcutaneously, and urine osmolality is measured again 1 hour later.

         (b) Response. The responses typical of normal individuals and of patients with partial, complete, and nephrogenic diabetes insipidus are shown in Table 10–2. Patients with partial diabetes insipidus show an increase in urine osmolality with dehydration, but the incompleteness of their response is demonstrated by a further increase after ADH is injected.

      (3) Administration of hypertonic saline. Infusion of a solution (2.5% sodium chloride given intravenously for 45 minutes at 0.25 mL/kg/min) after a water load (20 mL/kg in 30–60 minutes) causes a sharp decrease in urine flow in normal individuals because of stimulation of ADH secretion. Patients with diabetes insipidus cannot respond to this stimulus.

   e. Therapy

      (1) DDAVP can be administered orally, 0.1–1.2 mg daily in two or three doses. It also can be given as a nasal spray, and a parenteral preparation is available for use in acutely ill or postoperative patients.

      (2) Chlorpropamide, an oral hypoglycemic agent, has the additional effect of potentiating the action, the secretion, or both of endogenous ADH. This effect may be used in the treatment of diabetes insipidus.

         (a) Patients who have at least partial ADH production often become asymptomatic when 250–500 mg of chlorpropamide is taken daily.

         (b) Physicians and patients must watch for hypoglycemia, a possible side effect.

      (3) Thiazide diuretics have the paradoxical effect of decreasing urine output in patients with diabetes insipidus.

         (a) The volume depletion induced by diuretics increases sodium and water reabsorption in the proximal tubule, thus blunting the effect of the defective water absorption in the distal and collecting tubules.

         (b) Thiazides are only partially effective, decreasing urine volume by 30%–50%. However, unlike DDAVP, they are useful for treating nephrogenic diabetes insipidus because their action does not depend on distal tubular response to ADH.

2. SIADH

   a. Etiology

      (1) ADH production by **malignant tumors,** particularly oat cell carcinoma of the lung and carcinoma of the pancreas, was the originally recognized cause of SIADH.

(2) More commonly, excess ADH production by the neurohypophysial axis or by diseased tissue is caused by other disease processes through unknown mechanisms. These disease processes include **pulmonary diseases** (e.g., pneumonia, tuberculosis) and **CNS disorders** (e.g., stroke, head injury, encephalitis).

(3) **Drugs** (e.g., chlorpropamide, carbamazepine, vincristine, clofibrate) may stimulate hypothalamic–neurohypophyseal ADH production.

b. **Pathophysiology.** ADH excess causes water retention and extracellular fluid volume expansion, which is then compensated for by increased urinary sodium excretion. Clinically, significant volume expansion (i.e., edema or hypertension) is not present, because of the natriuresis. However, the water retention and the sodium loss both contribute to **hyponatremia,** which **is the hallmark of SIADH.** If water intake is minimized, this sequence of events does not occur, and serum sodium levels do not fall.

c. **Clinical features. Hyponatremia** refers to a serum sodium level less than 135 mEq/L.

(1) Symptoms of lethargy, confusion, agitation, headache, nausea and vomiting, and focal neurologic abnormalities are common when the sodium level declines rapidly or when it reaches a level less than approximately 125 mEq/L.

(2) Seizures and coma may occur with more severe hyponatremia.

d. **Diagnosis.** The following conditions are the basis of diagnosis.

(1) **Hyponatremia** is present, with low serum osmolality.

(2) **Urinary sodium concentration exceeds 20 mEq/L** despite the low serum sodium levels, and urine osmolality is higher than serum osmolality. (Other causes of hyponatremia, such as sodium depletion, cause renal retention of sodium, with urinary sodium concentration <20 mEq/L.)

(3) Conditions that might *appropriately* stimulate ADH secretion because of volume depletion must be excluded. These include adrenal insufficiency, fluid loss, edematous states (e.g., heart failure, nephrosis, cirrhosis), and renal failure.

e. **Therapy.** The cause of SIADH should be treated when possible.

(1) **Fluid restriction** to 500–1000 mL daily is effective in increasing the serum sodium level and is the mainstay of treatment. The limiting factor is patient adherence.

(2) If hyponatremia is severe, **hypertonic (3%) saline** should be cautiously administered to elevate the serum sodium level to greater than 120 mEq/L.

(a) Serum sodium must not be increased rapidly to a level exceeding 125 mEq/L, or CNS damage may result [see Chapter 12 XI B 1].

(b) Salt loading is of only temporary value because the additional sodium is soon excreted in the urine.

(3) If fluid restriction cannot be enforced, 300 mg of **demeclocycline** can be administered three or four times daily. Demeclocycline is an antibiotic with the useful side effect of inhibiting renal tubular response to ADH.

(4) **Conivaptan,** a vasopressin receptor antagonist, was recently introduced for the treatment of SIADH. In using this intravenous drug, precautions must be taken to avoid vein irritation and drug–drug interactions.

II DISORDERS OF THE ADRENAL GLAND

A **General considerations**

1. Diseases of the **adrenal cortex** are caused by the excessive production of cortisol (**Cushing's syndrome**), aldosterone (**primary aldosteronism**), and adrenal androgens (**congenital adrenal hyperplasia**), as well as by inadequate production of cortisol and aldosterone (**Addison's disease**).

2. Loss of the **adrenal medulla** does not cause illness, but **catecholamine overproduction by a pheochromocytoma** (a tumor of the adrenal medulla) causes a characteristic hypertensive syndrome.

B **Cushing's syndrome** is caused by excessive concentrations of cortisol or other glucocorticoid hormones in the circulation. Cushing's syndrome is a nonspecific designation that refers to increased glucocorticoid levels from any origin.

1. **Etiology**
   a. The most common cause of spontaneous Cushing's syndrome is **Cushing's disease,** which is caused by excessive production of ACTH by a pituitary adenoma, resulting in **bilateral adrenal hyperplasia.**
   b. **Adrenal adenomas** and **adrenal carcinomas** may cause Cushing's syndrome.
   c. **Ectopic ACTH** production by tumors such as oat cell carcinoma of the lung, carcinoma of the pancreas, bronchial carcinoid tumors, and others causes bilateral adrenal hyperplasia and Cushing's syndrome.
   d. **Iatrogenic Cushing's syndrome** is more common than the spontaneously occurring syndrome. It is an expected complication in patients receiving long-term glucocorticoid treatment for asthma, arthritis, and other conditions.

2. **Clinical features**
   a. **Central obesity** is caused by the effect of excess glucocorticoid levels on fat distribution. Fat accumulates in the face, neck, and trunk, while the limbs remain thin. The **"moon face," "buffalo hump"** (cervical fat pad), and **supraclavicular fat pads** contribute to the "cushingoid" appearance of affected individuals.
   b. **Hypertension** results from the vascular effects of cortisol, as well as other actions of the hormone, including sodium retention.
   c. **Impaired glucose tolerance** is common; 20% of patients have overt diabetes. This is a result of the increased hepatic gluconeogenesis and decreased peripheral glucose utilization caused by elevated levels of glucocorticoid.
   d. **Symptoms of androgen excess** (e.g., oligomenorrhea, hirsutism, and acne) may occur in women with Cushing's disease because of stimulation by ACTH of adrenal androgen production.
   e. **Purple striae** are linear marks on the abdomen where the thin, wasted skin is stretched by underlying fat.
   f. **Muscle wasting** and **weakness** reflect the catabolic effects of cortisol on muscle protein.
   g. **Osteoporosis** is a frequent result of cortisol excess. It is caused by increased bone catabolism and perhaps by the inhibitory effects of cortisol on collagen synthesis and calcium absorption.
   h. **Susceptibility to bruising** is probably caused by enhanced capillary fragility.
   i. **Psychiatric disturbances,** especially depression, are frequent results of cortisol excess.
   j. **Growth retardation** in children may be severe.

3. **Diagnosis.** Serum and urine cortisol levels are elevated in Cushing's disease and Cushing's syndrome, but overlap with normal values is common, and elevated levels are seen in normal persons at times of stress. Therefore, tests of the suppressibility of cortisol and other special tests are necessary. Figure 10–2 shows a scheme for the diagnosis of Cushing's syndrome that poses two questions. Is Cushing's syndrome present (Figure 10–2A)? If it is present, what causes its occurrence (Figure 10–2B)?
   a. **Nonspecific laboratory abnormalities** include leukocytosis, with a relatively low percentage of lymphocytes and eosinophils, and an elevation in the serum glucose level.
   b. The **serum cortisol** level in normal individuals is highest in early morning and decreases throughout the day, reaching a low point at about midnight. Although the morning level may be increased in patients with Cushing's syndrome, a loss of the normal diurnal variation and an increase in the evening level are more consistent findings. Salivary cortisol can be measured at midnight in the patient's home using commercially available kits.
   c. The **24-hour urinary free cortisol excretion rate** is increased in most patients with Cushing's syndrome. This test is the most useful indicator of daily cortisol secretion.
   d. **ACTH measurement** may help differentiate the causes of Cushing's syndrome.
      (1) ACTH levels are usually high-normal or slightly elevated in patients with Cushing's disease and may be markedly elevated in patients with ectopic ACTH production.
      (2) When an autonomously functioning adrenal tumor is the source of excess cortisol secretion, pituitary secretion of ACTH is suppressed by the high levels of circulating cortisol, and the ACTH level is extremely low or undetectable.
   e. **Low-dose dexamethasone suppression tests**
      (1) The **overnight low-dose dexamethasone suppression test** is recommended as an initial screening procedure for any patient suspected of having Cushing's syndrome. The patient

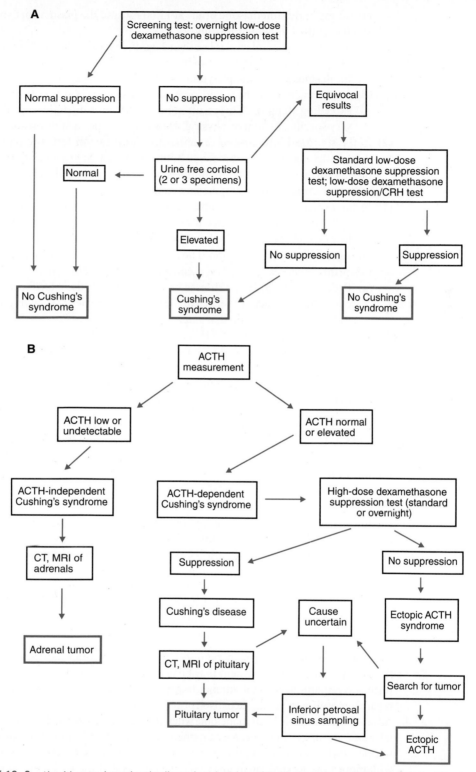

FIGURE 10–2 Algorithms to determine the diagnosis and etiology of Cushing's syndrome. **A.** Steps to take to determine whether a patient has Cushing's syndrome (of any cause). **B.** Steps to take to identify the cause of Cushing's syndrome (once the diagnosis has been made). ACTH, adrenocorticotropic hormone; CRH, corticotropin-releasing hormone; CT, computed tomography; MRI, magnetic resonance imaging.

takes 1 mg of dexamethasone orally at 11:00 PM, and the plasma cortisol level is measured at 8:00 AM the following morning.

    (a) The plasma cortisol level is less than 2 µg/dL in most individuals, indicating normal suppression of ACTH and cortisol by the dexamethasone. Because this test is very sensitive, the diagnosis of Cushing's syndrome is very unlikely in patients with a normal response.

    (b) Patients with Cushing's syndrome have cortisol levels greater than 3 µg/dL and usually exceeding 10 µg/dL. This result indicates that further study is needed. (The test is not very specific; mental or physical stress may produce a false-positive result.)

  (2) In the **standard low-dose dexamethasone suppression test,** the patient takes dexamethasone 0.5 mg every 6 hours for 48 hours, starting at 8:00 AM (eight doses). The morning plasma cortisol drawn after 48 hours is normally suppressed to less than 2 µg/dL.

f. High-dose dexamethasone suppression tests

  (1) In the **overnight high-dose dexamethasone suppression test,** plasma cortisol is measured at 8:00 AM on two consecutive days, and dexamethasone 8 mg is taken at 11:00 PM on the first day. A decrease in the plasma cortisol level of less than 50% on the second day indicates failure of suppression. The high-dose test is designed to distinguish between the two primary causes of ACTH-dependent Cushing's syndrome.

    (a) Patients with Cushing's disease behave as though their feedback response to glucocorticoids is intact but set at a higher-than-normal level; they respond to high but not to low doses of dexamethasone.

    (b) Patients with ectopic ACTH secretion produce ACTH autonomously; their cortisol levels are not suppressed even by high doses of dexamethasone.

  (2) In the **standard high-dose dexamethasone suppression test,** 2 mg of dexamethasone are taken every 6 hours for 48 hours (eight doses). A fall of 50% or more in the morning plasma cortisol at 48 hours indicates suppression.

g. Inferior petrosal sinus sampling

h. Combined standard low-dose dexamethasone suppression test and corticotropin-releasing hormone (CRH) test

i. Radiographic findings

  (1) Skull radiographs show enlargement of the sella turcica in the 10% of patients with Cushing's syndrome who have **macroadenomas,** but they do not reveal most of these tumors, which are **microadenomas** averaging 5–6 mm in diameter.

  (2) CT scans with injection of contrast medium detect approximately 50% of the pituitary adenomas that cause Cushing's disease. **MRI with gadolinium contrast,** however, reveals approximately 75% of these tumors and is the method of choice.

  (3) CT scans of the adrenal gland show most adrenal tumors. Uniform enlargement of both adrenal glands suggests an ACTH-dependent form of Cushing's syndrome—either Cushing's disease or the ectopic ACTH syndrome.

4. Therapy

a. Adrenal adenomas can usually be resected completely, often laparoscopically, with cure of the disease. Cortisol replacement may be needed for several months to a year postoperatively, until the remaining normal adrenal tissue, suppressed by the previous high cortisol levels, regains its ability to produce cortisol.

b. Adrenal carcinoma is often inoperable when first diagnosed because of metastases, usually to the liver and the lungs. Mitotane, metyrapone, and aminoglutethimide are drugs that block adrenal steroid production and may relieve the manifestations of excess cortisol production in patients with inoperable adrenal carcinoma. Prolonged survival of these patients is uncommon.

c. The **ectopic ACTH syndrome** can be cured by removal of the tumor, but this is not possible in many cases. The tumor causing the syndrome, rather than the Cushing's syndrome itself, is usually the primary problem.

d. Cushing's disease may be treated in several ways.

  (1) Transsphenoidal pituitary surgery is the treatment of choice. Even when tumors cannot be seen on CT scan or MRI, transsphenoidal exploration may disclose a microadenoma. Surgery is successful in 50%–95% of cases and is followed by normal pituitary and adrenal function as well as cure of Cushing's disease.

(2) Pituitary irradiation is effective in many children, but it cures fewer than one third of affected adults; the reason for the difference in response between children and adults is unclear.

(3) Bilateral adrenalectomy cures Cushing's disease but leaves the patient with **Addison's disease** and the need for lifelong steroid replacement. In addition, adrenalectomy is sometimes followed by the development of **Nelson's syndrome,** in which a pituitary adenoma undergoes rapid growth, perhaps because it is no longer inhibited by above-normal levels of cortisol.

(4) Medical therapy can be tried in a selective group of patients. Ketoconazole, mitotane, or aminoglutethimide (the latter two are more toxic) could be used.

C Adrenal insufficiency

1. **Etiology**
   a. **Primary adrenal insufficiency (Addison's disease)**
      (1) **Idiopathic atrophy of the adrenal cortex** due to an autoimmune process is the most common cause of adrenal insufficiency.
      (2) **Tuberculosis** may involve the adrenal glands, with destruction of both the adrenal cortex and medulla.
      (3) **Iatrogenic causes**
         (a) **Bilateral adrenalectomy** for Cushing's disease results in adrenal insufficiency.
         (b) **Adrenal suppression following prolonged steroid therapy** may persist for up to 1 year or longer.
      (4) **Acquired immunodeficiency syndrome (AIDS)** sometimes leads to adrenal insufficiency through cytomegalovirus (CMV) and other infections of the adrenal glands.
      (5) **Adrenoleukodystrophy** is an X-linked disorder caused by a deficiency of very long chain acyl CoA synthetase. This leads to an accumulation of very long chain fatty acids in the adrenal glands, causing adrenal insufficiency, and in the CNS, causing a demyelinating syndrome.
      (6) **Less common causes** of adrenal destruction include **amyloidosis, fungal infections, syphilis, bilateral adrenal hemorrhage** (especially in patients receiving anticoagulants), and **metastatic malignancy.**
   b. **Secondary adrenal insufficiency** is due to pituitary disease and results from any of the causes of hypopituitarism.

2. **Clinical features.** The symptoms of adrenal insufficiency are caused by both cortisol and aldosterone deficiencies.
   a. **Cortisol deficiency**
      (1) **Hyperpigmentation of the skin** is caused by increased MSH activity that accompanies the increased pituitary secretion of ACTH. The latter is a feedback response to the cortisol deficiency.
         (a) Hyperpigmentation is most noticeable over exposed areas, on mucous membranes, and in skin creases and scars.
         (b) In secondary adrenal insufficiency (which is caused by pituitary disease), ACTH levels are low rather than elevated, and hyperpigmentation is absent.
      (2) **Hypotension,** often orthostatic, is caused by the absence of the pressor effect of cortisol on vascular tone and by a decrease in cardiac output. In Addison's disease aldosterone deficiency also plays a role.
      (3) **Gastrointestinal symptoms** include anorexia, nausea and vomiting, and weight loss.
      (4) **Hypoglycemia** is related to decreased cortisol-induced gluconeogenesis.
      (5) **Mental symptoms** may include lethargy and confusion. Psychotic manifestations occur on occasion.
      (6) **Intolerance to stress** may occur. Patients who cannot increase their cortisol output in response to severe stress risk an acute exacerbation of the aforementioned symptoms, with life-threatening vascular collapse.
   b. **Aldosterone deficiency**
      (1) **Sodium loss** results from reduced aldosterone-mediated reabsorption of sodium in the distal renal tubules. **Hypovolemia, decreased cardiac output,** and **decreased renal blood flow with azotemia,** as well as weakness, hypotension, and weight loss, may be related to sodium depletion.

(2) Potassium retention caused by aldosterone deficiency may lead to **hyperkalemia** and **cardiac arrhythmias.**

(3) Because **angiotensin II,** rather than **ACTH,** has primary control of aldosterone production and the renin–angiotensin system is not affected by ACTH deficiency, there is usually no deficiency of aldosterone in secondary adrenal insufficiency.

3. Diagnosis

a. ACTH response

(1) The normal adrenal gland sharply increases its output of cortisol when stimulated by ACTH; absence of this response indicates adrenal insufficiency.

(2) ACTH test. The serum level of cortisol is measured before and 1 hour after an intravenous or intramuscular injection of 0.25 mg (25 U) of cosyntropin, a synthetic form of ACTH. The plasma cortisol should reach a level of 20 µg/dL or higher.

b. Laboratory findings

(1) Nonspecific laboratory abnormalities may include **hyponatremia, hyperkalemia, hypoglycemia,** and an **increased eosinophil count** (glucocorticoids lower the eosinophil count). Chest radiography may show a **small heart.**

(2) Plasma cortisol, urinary free cortisol, and urinary 17-hydroxycorticosteroid levels are low. Baseline levels, however, may overlap with the values in normal individuals, which is why ACTH testing is necessary for a definitive diagnosis.

4. Therapy

a. Glucocorticoid replacement is needed in all patients.

(1) The usual dose of cortisol is 10–30 mg daily. A higher dose is usually given in the morning and a smaller dose in the evening to mimic the normal diurnal variation. To avoid the potential harmful effects of excess cortisol, such as osteoporosis, the dose should be no more than is necessary to relieve the manifestations of cortisol deficiency.

(2) The dose must be increased during times of stress. Typical doses would be twice the usual dose during minor stress (e.g., common cold or dental extraction), three to five times the usual dose during moderate stress (e.g., influenza or minor surgery), and "stress doses" of 200–300 mg in a 24-hour period during severe stress (e.g., major surgery or a serious infection or injury).

b. Mineralocorticoid replacement is needed in patients with Addison's disease. **Fludrocortisone (Florinef)** is given in a daily dose of 0.05–0.2 mg. Persistence of low blood pressure, weakness, and low serum sodium and high serum potassium levels suggests that a higher dose of mineralocorticoid is needed; hypertension, edema, or hypokalemia suggest that the dose should be decreased.

5. Adrenal crisis (Addisonian crisis) is an acute, life-threatening complication of Addison's disease in which the manifestations of adrenal insufficiency are greatly exaggerated.

a. Clinical features. Fever, vomiting, abdominal pain, altered mental status, and **vascular collapse** may occur if Addison's disease remains undiagnosed, or it may occur in a treated patient during acute stress if additional glucocorticoid replacement is not provided.

b. Therapy. Immediate intravenous administration of 100 mg of cortisol over 5–10 minutes should be followed by an additional 300 mg in divided doses over the next 24 hours. Intravenous saline is also needed, and mineralocorticoid replacement should be provided if hypotension and volume depletion persist.

D **Primary aldosteronism**

1. Etiology. Excessive adrenal production of aldosterone is usually caused by a single **small** (0.5–3.0 cm) **adrenal adenoma.** Less often (i.e., in 20%–40% of cases), there is bilateral hyperplasia of the adrenal cortex.

2. Clinical features. Aldosterone increases the reabsorption of sodium and the excretion of potassium and hydrogen ions in the distal renal tubules.

a. Sodium retention causes blood pressure elevation, which is the chief clinical manifestation of this syndrome.

(1) The amount of sodium and water that are retained is limited by compensatory mechanisms that increase renal sodium excretion in response to extracellular fluid volume expansion; sodium balance is restored after 1–2 kg of fluid have accumulated.

        (2) Although this amount of volume expansion does not cause edema, the long-term increase in cardiac output and, perhaps, other effects of mineralocorticoid excess lead to hypertension.

  b. Hypokalemia may produce **muscle weakness, paresthesias,** and **tetany** in severe cases.

        (1) Hypokalemic nephropathy may cause polyuria.

        (2) Metabolic alkalosis is a result of the renal loss of potassium and hydrogen ions.

3. Diagnosis

  a. Laboratory diagnosis

      (1) Hypokalemia in a hypertensive patient is often the clue that triggers the search for primary aldosteronism, although not all patients with aldosteronism have low potassium.

      (2) Aldosterone must be measured under standardized conditions because it is affected by sodium balance, diuretics, and other factors.

         (a) Diuretics, angiotensin-converting-enzyme inhibitors, and vasodilators should be discontinued at least 2 weeks before studies of aldosterone (and renin) are undertaken.

         (b) Random aldosterone measurements in patients with primary aldosteronism may overlap those of normal individuals; sodium loading may be necessary to differentiate the aldosterone levels in affected patients (which are not suppressed by a sodium load) from the levels in normal individuals (which are suppressed by a sodium load). Two of the many ways that this procedure can be performed are as follows.

            (i) The **24-hour urinary aldosterone excretion rate** can be measured after the patient has ingested more than 250 mEq sodium daily for at least 3 days. (This can be ensured by giving sodium chloride tablets.) Sodium loading may further lower serum levels of potassium; therefore, caution is necessary if the patient is hypokalemic. An elevated aldosterone level in a 24-hour urine sample that contains more than 250 mEq of sodium indicates hyperaldosteronism.

            (ii) **Plasma levels of aldosterone** can be measured after 2000 mL of normal saline have been infused over 4 hours. In normal subjects, the plasma aldosterone concentration will fall to less than 6 mg/dL. Value greater than 10 mg/dL are consistent with primary aldosteronism. Severe hypertension and congestive heart failure (CHF) are contraindications to saline infusion.

      (3) Plasma renin activity is the most useful indicator of whether elevated aldosterone production is primary or secondary.

         (a) Secondary aldosteronism is caused by conditions that originate outside the adrenal gland and that reduce the effective arterial blood volume, thus diminishing the pressure or tension sensed by the juxtaglomerular cells.

            (i) Such conditions include heart failure, nephrosis, cirrhosis, volume depletion caused by diuretics, and renovascular disease.

            (ii) Decreased pressure on the juxtaglomerular cells stimulates renin release, which increases angiotensin II and, in turn, aldosterone. Thus, **the high aldosterone level is accompanied by increased renin activity.**

         (b) In **primary aldosteronism,** the enhanced aldosterone production is caused by an adrenal abnormality, not by increased renin activity; the resulting volume expansion suppresses renin production. This combination of **increased aldosterone production and reduced renin activity can be caused only by primary aldosteronism,** and it is a reliable indicator of this diagnosis.

         (c) Suppression of renin activity is diagnosed with certainty only if levels remain low after manipulations that are known to stimulate renin in normal individuals, such as dietary sodium restriction, several hours of upright posture, or furosemide administration.

      (4) The **best screening test for primary aldosteronism** is measurement of the ratio of plasma aldosterone (ng/dL) to plasma renin activity (ng of angiotensin I/mL/hour) in a blood sample drawn with the patient upright. This ratio is increased both by the elevated aldosterone level and the suppressed renin level characteristic of the disease. An aldosterone-to-renin ratio greater than 25 indicates need for further study.

  b. Adenoma versus hyperplasia. Primary aldosteronism due to an adenoma must be distinguished from primary aldosteronism due to hyperplasia because the distinction affects treatment, which is usually surgical in cases of adrenal adenoma and medical in bilateral hyperplasia.

(1) The biochemical changes of primary aldosteronism—the hypokalemia, the increased aldosterone level, and the low renin activity—are more pronounced in cases caused by a unilateral adenoma than in cases caused by hyperplasia.

(2) The plasma aldosterone concentration may be measured at 8:00 AM, after 8 hours of recumbency, and again at noon, after 4 hours of ambulation.

  (a) Levels are higher after ambulation in normal individuals and in patients with bilateral hyperplasia because renin and angiotensin are stimulated by the upright posture and sympathetic outflow.

  (b) However, patients with unilateral adrenal adenomas have a paradoxical fall in plasma aldosterone levels, presumably because when renin is profoundly suppressed, aldosterone is influenced mainly by the diurnal fall in ACTH.

(3) **Adrenal vein aldosterone concentrations** may be measured in blood samples obtained by selective catheterization. A very high level on one side indicates an adenoma; high levels on both sides indicate bilateral hyperplasia.

(4) **CT scans** and **MRI** sometimes show aldosterone-producing adenomas, but these tumors may be small and often cannot be visualized.

  c. **Ingestion of large amounts of natural black licorice,** which has mineralocorticoid effects, should be considered in the differential diagnosis of hyperaldosteronism.

4. Therapy

  a. Surgery

  (1) Removal of a unilateral adenoma results in cure of the hypertension in approximately 60% of cases and improvement in another 25%.

  (2) In contrast, only 20%–50% of patients with bilateral hyperplasia are improved by surgery, even if bilateral adrenalectomy is performed. Medical therapy is preferable.

  b. Medical therapy. Spironolactone inhibits the effects of aldosterone on the renal tubule. A dose of 200–400 mg daily corrects the hypokalemia and often corrects the hypertension. Eplerenone 50–100 mg daily can be used in patients who develop gynecomastia on spironolactone.

E **Congenital adrenal hyperplasia**

1. Etiology and pathophysiology. Congenital adrenal hyperplasia is caused by a defect in one of the enzymes (21-hydroxylase or 11-beta-hydroxylase) necessary for the synthesis of cortisol. Cortisol deficiency stimulates ACTH, which results in overproduction of steroid precursors in the early parts of the blocked pathway. One of these, 17-hydroxyprogesterone, is converted to adrenal androgens, resulting in virilization. Depending on the severity of the enzyme defect, patients with 21-hydroxylase deficiency may develop salt wasting due to decreased production of mineralocorticoids, and patients with 11-beta-hydroxylase deficiency may develop hypertension may due to accumulation of steroid precursors with mineralocorticoid effects (Figure 10–3).

2. Clinical features

  a. Androgen excess is caused by increased adrenal production of dehydroepiandrosterone, androstenedione, and testosterone.

  (1) If present during fetal development, this disorder may cause **ambiguous genitalia** in female infants. If androgen excess is manifested in the postnatal period, it may cause **virilization** in prepubertal girls or in young women.

  (2) In male infants, the consequence of androgen excess during fetal development is macrogenitosomia. In the postnatal period, the consequence is **precocious puberty.**

  b. The cortisol deficit usually does not cause major clinical manifestations, because the ACTH stimulation and adrenal hyperplasia maintain cortisol levels in the low-normal range, despite the enzyme deficiency.

  c. Other manifestations occasionally occur, depending on the specific enzyme affected.

  (1) **21-Hydroxylase deficiency** accounts for 95% of cases of adrenal hyperplasia.

    (a) In the mild (simple virilizing) form, only the androgen-excess symptoms are of importance.

    (b) In the severe (salt-losing) form, the production of aldosterone is impaired, as well as that of cortisol; mineralocorticoid deficiency leads to hyponatremia, hyperkalemia, dehydration, and hypotension.

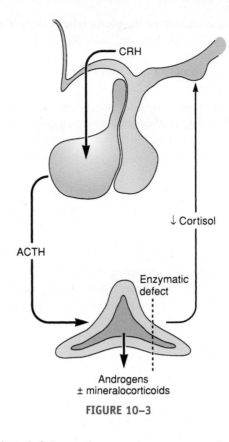

FIGURE 10–3

(2) In **11-hydroxylase deficiency,** deoxycorticosterone, a mineralocorticoid, as well as adrenal androgens are overproduced. This causes hypertension through mechanisms that are similar to those causing hypertension in primary aldosteronism.

(3) In **17-hydroxylase deficiency,** deoxycorticosterone is overproduced, resulting in hypertension. However, because 17-hydroxylase is necessary for sex steroid synthesis, there is androgen deficiency as well as estrogen deficiency. This causes the development of ambiguous genitalia in male infants and primary amenorrhea in women.

3. **Diagnosis.** Concentrations of adrenal androgens and precursors of cortisol are increased in blood and urine. The most useful measurements are of **blood testosterone, androstenedione, dehydroepiandrosterone,** and **17-hydroxyprogesterone** (a cortisol precursor), as well as **urinary 17-ketosteroids** and **pregnanetriol** (a metabolite of 17-hydroxyprogesterone).

4. **Therapy**
   a. **Medical therapy. Cortisol** administration suppresses the overproduction of ACTH and adrenal androgens. In the salt-losing syndrome, mineralocorticoid replacement with fludrocortisone may be necessary.
   b. **Surgery.** Reconstructive surgery of the external genitalia in female infants is done in the first few years of life.

F **Pheochromocytoma**   This tumor is derived from **chromaffin cells,** the cells that synthesize and store catecholamines. Located primarily in the adrenal medulla, they also are located in sympathetic ganglia and elsewhere. The cells in the adrenal medulla produce epinephrine and norepinephrine; the extra-adrenal chromaffin cells make only norepinephrine.

1. **Epidemiology**
   a. **Incidence.** Pheochromocytoma is found in approximately 0.5% of patients with severe hypertension and in less than 0.05% of all hypertensive patients. However, because this tumor may cause a dramatic and debilitating syndrome, often with fatal complications if undetected, diagnostic efforts and awareness are required out of proportion to the frequency of occurrence.
   b. **Familial occurrence.** Pheochromocytomas may occur sporadically or may occur as part of one of several familial syndromes.

      (1) Multiple endocrine neoplasia type II (Sipple's syndrome) is characterized by multiple pheochromocytomas and medullary carcinoma of the thyroid; hyperparathyroidism is often present.

      (2) Neurofibromatosis and **von Hippel–Lindau disease** may be associated with pheochromocytoma.

2. **Pathology.** Most pheochromocytomas are single tumors of the adrenal medulla. However, 10%–20% are located outside of the adrenal gland, and 1%–3% are in the chest or neck. Approximately 20% are multiple, and 10% are malignant.

3. **Clinical features.** The manifestations of pheochromocytoma are caused by increased levels of circulating catecholamines.

    a. Hypertension is paroxysmal in approximately 50% of cases and is sustained in the rest. The diagnosis is often suggested by the **paroxysmal nature of the symptoms,** caused by variations in the function of the tumor. Attacks typically last less than 1 hour and may be precipitated by exercise, induction of anesthesia, urination (suggesting a pheochromocytoma of the bladder), or palpation of the abdomen.

    b. Other features, also beginning with the letter H, that suggest the presence of a pheochromocytoma are headache, **hyperglycemia, hypermetabolism** (manifested by weight loss, tremor, palpitations, and sweating), and postural hypotension in a hypertensive patient.

4. **Diagnosis.** Pheochromocytoma is suspected far more often than it is diagnosed. Many patients with symptoms of catecholamine excess prove to have normal hormone levels. With the increased use of computed imaging, an increasing number of asymptomatic patients with pheochromocytomas have been diagnosed.

    a. The levels of **urine catecholamines** and their metabolites are elevated in most confirmed cases.

      (1) The **24-hour urinary metanephrine excretion rate** may be the most useful screening test, but tests of **urinary free catecholamines** (i.e., epinephrine and norepinephrine) and **vanillylmandelic acid** concentrations are also of value. Certain medications and stress can give false-positive results.

      (2) Stressful illness can raise catecholamine levels twofold; elevations greater than twofold are more suggestive of pheochromocytoma.

    b. Serum catecholamine levels are variable and are more difficult to interpret than the 24-hour urine measurements. Levels of **plasma free metanephrines** may prove to be a sensitive indicator of a pheochromocytoma.

    c. The **clonidine suppression test** is useful in patients with mild catecholamine elevation. Three hours after an oral dose of 0.3 mg clonidine, the plasma level of norepinephrine is lowered into the normal range in most normal individuals, but it remains elevated in patients with pheochromocytoma.

    d. CT scans or **MRI** of the abdomen detect as many as 90% of these tumors because they usually are greater than 1 cm in diameter.

    e. Adrenal scanning with ^{131}I-iodobenzylguanidine (**MIBG**) is especially useful for localizing extra-adrenal tumors.

5. **Therapy**

    a. Medical therapy

      (1) The α- and β-adrenergic blocking agents are useful for inoperable tumors and for preparation for surgery.

        (a) α-Adrenergic blocking agents relieve the hypertension and adrenergic symptoms.

          (i) Phenoxybenzamine is given orally, starting with 10 mg twice daily and increasing to 40 mg twice daily, if necessary.

          (ii) Phentolamine can be given intravenously to treat acute severe elevations in blood pressure.

          (iii) Prazosin, terazosin, or **doxazosin** also can be given to produce sustained α-adrenergic blockade.

        (b) β-Adrenergic blocking agents should not be used alone because unopposed α-adrenergic stimulation may lead to exacerbation of the hypertension. β-Blockers are sometimes useful in conjunction with α-blockers (see later discussion).

      (2) Metyrosine, which is an inhibitor of tyrosine hydroxylase, blocks the formation of norepinephrine and epinephrine and is an alternative agent for the relief of the symptoms of pheochromocytoma. It may be used when patients are intolerant of the adrenergic-blocking agents.

   b. Surgery. Surgical removal of the pheochromocytoma is the treatment of choice. Careful exploration of the adrenal glands and the periaortic sympathetic chain should be performed.

      (1) Complications that frequently occur during and after surgery are extreme swings in blood pressure, cardiac arrhythmias, and shock. These are caused by the sudden removal of the source of excess catecholamine production and by the low blood volume that results from long-term constriction of the vascular compartment.

      (2) To prevent vascular instability during removal of a pheochromocytoma, patients are treated with α-blockers to maintain normal blood pressure for at least 1 week before surgery. β-Blockers may be added for a few days before surgery, especially if tachycardia or another arrhythmia is present.

III   DISORDERS OF THE THYROID GLAND

A   Thyroid function studies

1. **Serum TSH measurement is** the standard screening test for the presence of thyroid dysfunction. TSH is produced by the pituitary gland in response to TRH secreted by the hypothalamus. TSH elevation is caused by the negative feedback effects of low thyroid hormone levels, as in primary hypothyroidism. Elevated thyroid hormone concentrations lead to suppression of serum TSH to levels below normal, as in primary hyperthyroidism.

2. **Serum total thyroxine (T_4) determination** measures the total bound (99.95%) and free (0.05%) T_4 in the circulation. The serum T_4 concentration is elevated in hyperthyroidism and decreased in hypothyroidism.

   a. In conditions that increase **thyroid hormone–binding globulin (TBG)** such as pregnancy, the total T_4 will be elevated due to an increase in the bound fraction. In conditions associated with a decrease in TGB (hypoproteinemia, androgen excess), the total T_4 will be low because of a decrease in the bound fraction, but the free T_4 will be normal.

   b. In order to be certain that a binding abnormality is not influencing the total T_4 result, it is necessary to order a **T_3 uptake** test along with the T_4. Both are elevated in hyperthyroidism, and both are reduced in hypothyroidism. They go in opposite directions when there is a TBG abnormality. Alternatively, one can simply order a **free T_4** (Table 10–3).

3. **Serum total T_3 determination** measures the concentration of the total bound and free T_3 in the circulation. The total T_3 measurement may give the same misleading results as the total T_4 measurement if there is an abnormality in binding proteins.

4. **T_3 uptake test**

5. **Free T_4 index**

6. **Radioactive iodine uptake and scan.**

   a. Uptake of the iodine isotope is increased in hyperthyroidism secondary to Graves' disease and in toxic multinodular goiter, in which hyperfunctioning nodule(s) produce excessive amounts of thyroid hormone.

   b. Uptake is decreased in hypothyroidism and in situations in which thyrotoxicosis is not due to primary hyperthyroidism, such as exogenous thyroid hormone administration, subacute thyroiditis, and ectopic hormone production (e.g., caused by struma ovarii).

   c. The scan portion will differentiate nodular disease and goiter.

TABLE 10–3   Relationship between Thyroid-Stimulating Hormone and Free Thyroxine

Thyroid-stimulating Hormone	Free Thyroxine	Clinical Picture
High	Low	Hypothyroid, thyroiditis
High	High	Pituitary hyperthyroidism
Low	High	Hyperthyroidism, thyroiditis
Low	Low	Pituitary Hypothyroidism

B Hypothyroidism

1. **Etiology**
   a. **Chronic autoimmune thyroiditis** is the most common cause of spontaneous hypothyroidism in the United States. This condition has a goitrous form (Hashimoto's disease) and an atrophic form; in both forms antithyroid antibodies are typically present in the serum.
   b. **Hypothyroidism frequently develops after the treatment of Graves' disease,** and the prevalence exceeds 50% after 15 years. Hypothyroidism may also occur after Graves' disease is treated by subtotal thyroidectomy or antithyroid drugs.
   c. **Secondary hypothyroidism** is caused by any of the conditions that may affect the hypothalamic–pituitary axis and cause hypopituitarism.
   d. **Less common causes** of hypothyroidism include congenital athyreosis, congenital biochemical defects that prevent thyroid hormone production, and insensitivity of the tissues to thyroid hormone. Iodine deficiency is an uncommon cause of hypothyroidism in most highly developed countries but is common in some areas of the world.

2. **Clinical features**
   a. **Symptoms** (Table 10–4)
   b. **Physical findings** (Table 10–4)
   c. **Cretinism** is severe **hypothyroidism beginning in infancy.** Cretinism is marked by mental retardation and impairment of physical growth and development.
   d. **Myxedema coma** may result if severe hypothyroidism goes untreated. This serious condition may occur gradually (over years) or more acutely in response to precipitating factors (e.g., infection, exposure to cold). The mortality rate is 50%–75%. Hypothermia, hypoglycemia, shock, hypoventilation, and ileus may be present in addition to the severely depressed state of consciousness.

3. **Diagnosis**
   a. **Overt hypothyroidism** is suggested in severe cases by the characteristic symptoms and physical findings; however, mild cases may escape detection unless laboratory tests are performed.

TABLE 10–4 Clinical Features of Hypothyroidism and Hyperthyroidism

	Hypothyroidism	Hyperthyroidism
Symptoms		
General symptoms	Weakness, lethargy, fatigue	Restlessness
	Cold intolerance	Sweating, heat intolerance
	Weight gain	Weight loss
Gastrointestinal	Constipation	Loose stools, diarrhea
Genitourinary	Menorrhagia	Amenorrhea, oligomenorrhea
Physical Findings		
Cardiovascular	Bradycardia	Palpitations, tachycardia
	Pericardial effusion	Wide pulse pressure
	Decreased cardiac output	Arrhythmia (atrial fibrillation, premature ventricular contractions)
Head, ears, eyes, nose, throat	Puffy eyelids	Stare and lid lag
		Exopthalmous
		Goiter, thyroid bruit
Pulmonary	Hypoventilation	
	Pleural effusion	
Hematology	Normocytic normochromic anemia	
Skin	Yellow, dry skin	Warm, moist
Extremities	Nonpitting edema	Muscle weakness fatigue
Neurologic	Slow return of deep tendon reflexes	Fine tremor
		Brisk deep tendon reflexes
Psychiatric	Psychosis	Emotional lability
	Depression	Nervousness

Routine laboratory screening is especially recommended for newborns and women older than 50 years of age. TSH levels should also be measured in elderly persons with nonspecific complaints because many hypothyroid symptoms, such as fatigue and constipation, may be mistaken for the changes of aging.

(1) Increased TSH is the earliest and most sensitive indicator of primary hypothyroidism, and a sensitive TSH assay should be used for screening. If the TSH level is elevated, the diagnosis may be confirmed by the finding of a decreased serum free T_4 or free T_4 index.

(2) Serum T_4 and T_3 levels, as well as T_3 uptake, are decreased.

b. **Subclinical hypothyroidism** is a common condition in which serum TSH is elevated but serum free T_4 or the free T_4 index is normal rather than decreased. Many affected patients progress to overt hypothyroidism. A greater degree of TSH elevation, the presence of symptoms that might be caused by hypothyroidism, and the presence of antithyroid antibodies are factors favoring a decision to treat.

4. **Therapy**

a. **Thyroid hormone preparations.** Thyroid extract derived from animal sources and synthetic preparations containing both T_4 and T_3 have been used in the past and are still available. However, synthetic L-thyroxine sodium is the agent of choice.

(1) The administered T_4 is slowly converted to T_3, and the proportions of circulating T_4 and T_3 approximate those of euthyroid individuals.

(2) The peaks and valleys of blood T_3 levels, which are seen when exogenous T_3 is given, are avoided.

b. **Initiation of treatment**

(1) Patients with severe hypothyroidism, older patients, and patients with cardiovascular disease may have an increased sensitivity to thyroid hormone and are at risk for acute cardiovascular and other complications if the hypothyroidism is corrected too quickly. Therefore, these patients should be given a very small dose of thyroid hormone initially (e.g., 25 µg of L-thyroxine), which is increased to a full maintenance dose during a 6- to 12-week period.

(2) Younger patients and patients with less severe hypothyroidism may be started on a slightly higher dose (50 µg of L-thyroxine) and advanced to a full replacement dose more quickly (e.g., the dose may be raised to 100 µg in 2 weeks and to 125 µg or 150 µg in another 2 weeks).

c. **Maintenance therapy.** Most patients require approximately 0.7–0.8 µg of L-thyroxine per pound of ideal body weight for physiologic replacement of thyroid hormone. When this dose is tolerated and symptoms of hypothyroidism have resolved, the dose should be further adjusted so that serum TSH is maintained in the normal range.

d. **Myxedema coma** has a high mortality rate and **must be treated rapidly,** despite the risk associated with sudden hormone replacement.

(1) Ancillary treatment includes respiratory support and temporary use of adrenal corticosteroids since concomitant adrenal insufficiency may accompany hypothyroidism on an autoimmune basis. To avoid development of adrenal crisis, stress doses of hydrocortisone should be administered after obtaining a random cortisol. The hydrocortisone may be discontinued if the random serum cortisol is found to be appropriately elevated.

(2) L-Thyroxine is given intravenously as a 500-µg bolus injection, followed by daily maintenance doses of 50–100 µg.

C Hyperthyroidism

1. **Etiology**

a. **Graves' disease (diffuse toxic goiter) is the most common cause of hyperthyroidism.** It is a form of autoimmune thyroid disease in which an abnormal immunoglobulin G (IgG) (thyroid-stimulating immunoglobulin) binds to TSH receptors on the thyroid follicular cells, causing diffuse enlargement of the gland and stimulation of thyroid hormone production. Graves' disease is most common in women between the ages of 20 and 50 years.

b. **Toxic nodular goiter (Plummer's disease)** and **toxic thyroid adenoma** are less common than Graves' disease and usually affect older individuals.

(1) Discrete areas of the thyroid function autonomously, secreting excessive amounts of thyroid hormone. The cause is unknown, but activating mutations in the TSH receptor gene

or in the stimulatory G protein that couple the TSH receptor to cyclic adenosine monophosphate (cAMP) formation have been found in many cases.

(2) The presence of both normal thyroid tissue and autonomously functioning abnormal tissue is the pathognomonic feature. **Radionuclide scanning** shows that the normal tissue is hypofunctioning; this occurs because TSH is suppressed by the excessive levels of thyroid hormone produced by the abnormal tissue.

c. **Subacute thyroiditis** may cause transient hyperthyroidism.

d. **Factitious hyperthyroidism** may be caused by surreptitious ingestion of thyroid hormone or inadvertent administration of excessive doses of replacement hormone in the treatment of hypothyroidism.

e. **Rare causes** of hyperthyroidism include excess TSH production by **pituitary tumors, teratomas of the ovary** that produce thyroid hormone (**struma ovarii**), and overproduction of hormone by the thyroid gland following iodine ingestion, which is called the Jod-Basedow phenomenon.

2. **Clinical features.** Thyroid hormone increases oxygen consumption by tissues, raising heat production and energy metabolism. It interacts with the sympathetic nervous system in a way that seems to increase tissue sensitivity to catecholamines and adrenergic stimuli. In addition, it affects protein, fat, carbohydrate, and vitamin metabolism.

a. **Presenting symptoms** (see Table 10–4).

b. **Physical examination** (see Table 10–4).

c. **Thyroid storm** is a sudden exacerbation of the signs and symptoms of hyperthyroidism. Precipitating events may include concurrent illness, trauma, surgery, or childbirth. Marked fever, tachycardia, and agitation are present and may progress to stupor and coma, with vascular collapse. The mortality rate is 20%–40%.

3. **Diagnosis**

a. **Family history** of thyroid disease is common.

b. **Laboratory studies** show an increase in the serum concentration of total T_4 and free T_4, serum concentration of total T_3 and free T_3, and T_3 resin uptake. Serum TSH levels are low.

c. **T_3 Thyrotoxicosis.** Early in the development of thyrotoxicosis, patients may have suppressed TSH levels associated with elevated T_3 levels but normal T4 levels. In a patient with a suppressed TSH level and a normal T_4 level, it is important to order a total T_3 level to exclude this condition.

4. **Therapy.** The **adrenergic manifestations of hyperthyroidism** (e.g., sweating, tachycardia, tremor) may be diminished by **β-blockers.** These drugs do not affect thyroid function but provide symptomatic relief until thyroid hormone levels can be lowered to normal.

a. **Treatment of Grave's disease.** The most common methods for treatment of Graves' disease are **antithyroid drugs, radioactive iodine,** and **subtotal thyroidectomy.**

(1) **Thionamides**

(a) **Mechanism of action. Methimazole (Tapazole)** and **propylthiouracil (PTU)** inhibit the oxidation of iodide and the coupling of iodotyrosines, thus decreasing the synthesis of thyroid hormone. In addition, PTU decreases the conversion of T_4 to T_3 in peripheral tissues.

(b) **Dosing.** Full doses (i.e., 30–40 mg of methimazole or 300–400 mg of PTU) are given daily until the patient is euthyroid.

(i) Although blockade of hormone synthesis is rapid, clinical improvement occurs only after a few weeks or months because a large pool of stored hormone continues to be released from the thyroid.

(ii) After clinical improvement, the dose is tapered to the lowest dose that maintains euthyroidism, and the drug is continued for 1–2 years. Treatment is then discontinued in the hope that a lasting or permanent remission has occurred.

(iii) PTU is the drug of choice in pregnancy.

(c) **Drug toxicity**

(i) **Skin rash** or **joint pain** occurs in 3%–5% of patients, necessitating a switch to the alternative drug.

(ii) **Agranulocytosis** occurs in fewer than 0.5% of patients but is life threatening. For early detection of agranulocytosis, patients should be instructed to stop the drug immediately if fever, sore throat, mouth ulcers, or other unexplained symptoms occur. Treatment should be resumed only after examination shows a normal white blood cell (WBC) count.

      (iii) Liver toxicity is rarely seen.

   (d) Advantages of medical treatment with antithyroid drugs

      (i) Hospitalization, surgery, and anesthesia are avoided.

      (ii) There is less likelihood of the occurrence of posttreatment hypothyroidism than in patients treated with radioactive iodine.

   (e) Disadvantages of antithyroid drugs

      (i) Permanent remission occurs in fewer than 50% of patients treated.

      (ii) Successful treatment depends on patient adherence, which is less of a problem when treatment is by surgery or radioactive iodine.

(2) Radioactive iodine

   (a) Method of treatment. A single dose of iodine-131 (^{131}I) causes a decrease in function and size of the thyroid gland in 6–12 weeks. Approximately 75% of patients with Graves' disease are made euthyroid by a single dose; those who are still thyrotoxic after 12 weeks are given a second dose. Additional doses can be given if needed. Eventually, almost all patients are cured in this way.

   (b) Advantages of radioactive iodine

      (i) Hospitalization, surgery, and anesthesia are avoided.

      (ii) The rate of cure approaches 100%.

      (iii) Little patient adherence is required.

   (c) Disadvantages of radioactive iodine

      (i) Multiple treatments may be needed.

      (ii) Hypothyroidism, the treatment of which requires long-term patient adherence, occurs in approximately 10% of patients after 1 year and continues to develop at a rate of 2%–3% each year. After 10–15 years, more than 50% of patients are hypothyroid. This complication is easily treated, however, with a single daily dose of L-thyroxine.

      (iii) There is a slight risk of genetic effects (comparable in magnitude to the effects of a barium enema or intravenous urogram) in future offspring. However, no increase in the risk of leukemia, thyroid cancer, or other malignancies has been found in patients treated with radioactive iodine.

(3) Subtotal thyroidectomy

   (a) Advantages of surgery

      (i) Cure of hyperthyroidism is rapid (once a euthyroid state has been produced by antithyroid drugs).

      (ii) The success rate is high; most patients are cured, and fewer become hypothyroid after surgery than after treatment with radioactive iodine.

      (iii) Patient adherence is required for a shorter period than it is in prolonged antithyroid drug treatment.

   (b) Disadvantages of surgery

      (i) Patients usually must be hospitalized, and surgical and anesthetic risks are incurred.

      (ii) Surgical complications include hypoparathyroidism and recurrent laryngeal nerve paralysis.

(4) Choice of therapy

   (a) Radioactive iodine is the treatment of choice for most patients older than 30–40 years and is frequently used in younger individuals.

   (b) In younger patients, the choice is more difficult. In patients with mild clinical manifestations, slightly to moderately elevated thyroid hormone levels, and an only moderately enlarged thyroid, a trial of antithyroid drugs is reasonable because patients with mild disease have a better chance for a lasting remission.

   (c) Surgery may be a better choice for patients with large goiters and severe disease and for patients who are unwilling to take antithyroid drugs for a prolonged period.

b. Treatment of toxic nodular goiter and toxic adenoma. Because antithyroid drug therapy does not lead to permanent remission in affected patients, the options for treatment are surgery and radioactive iodine.

        (1) Thyroidectomy or removal of a hyperfunctioning nodule rapidly cures the hyperthyroidism and relieves symptoms of pressure or tracheal or esophageal obstruction that may be caused by a large goiter.

        (2) Radioactive iodine treatment requires much larger doses in patients with toxic nodular goiter than in patients with Graves' disease because the affected thyroid cells are relatively radioresistant. However, because the unaffected thyroid cells are functionally suppressed, they do not trap ^{131}I and are spared the effects of radiation; therefore, hypothyroidism after radioactive iodine treatment is less common in these patients.

  c. Treatment of thyroid storm

        (1) Control the adrenergic stimulation with β-blockers. Traditionally propranolol has been used, which also decreases the peripheral conversion of $T_4 \rightarrow T_3$.

        (2) Thioamides are used first to block new synthesis of thyroid hormone.

        (3) Iodine may be given after thioamides are administered to inhibit the release of preformed hormones. If iodine is given prior to thioamides, it may provide substrate for further synthesis of the hormone.

        (4) Corticosteroids are also used to block conversion of $T_4 \rightarrow T_3$ in peripheral tissues.

D Thyroiditis

1. Chronic autoimmune thyroiditis (Hashimoto's thyroiditis)

  a. Etiology. Chronic thyroiditis is a common autoimmune disorder that primarily affects women. Antithyroid antibodies are present in most patients.

  b. Clinical features

        (1) Thyroid gland enlargement, the main clinical manifestation, is the result of autoimmune damage that leads to lymphocytic infiltration, fibrosis, and a weakened ability of the thyroid to produce hormone (🔘 Online Figure 10–4).

        (2) Hypothyroidism is present in many patients when the disease is first diagnosed and may affect additional patients as the disease progresses.

        (3) Pain and tenderness of the gland sometimes occur, as in subacute thyroiditis.

  c. Diagnosis. Chronic thyroiditis is suspected in any patient with a firm, nontoxic goiter. A high titer of antithyroid peroxidase antibodies or antithyroglobulin antibodies, or both, is confirmatory. Thyroid function tests usually are normal unless the patient has hypothyroidism.

  d. Therapy. Treatment with L-thyroxine sodium often decreases the size of the goiter and, therefore, is useful even in patients with normal thyroid function. If hypothyroidism is present, this treatment is, of course, essential.

2. Subacute thyroiditis (also called granulomatous thyroiditis or de Quervain's thyroiditis)

  a. Clinical features

        (1) Early symptoms. A prodrome of malaise, upper respiratory symptoms, and fever that lasts 1–2 weeks may occur. Then, the thyroid gland becomes enlarged, firm, and tender, with pain radiating to the ears, neck, or arms.

        (2) Hyperthyroidism. Leaking of thyroid hormone from damaged follicles into the circulation may lead to hyperthyroidism.

        (3) Disease course. The thyroid pain and hyperthyroidism subside in a few weeks or months. The gland usually returns to normal size; if enlargement persists, chronic autoimmune thyroiditis should be suspected. A self-limited period of **hypothyroidism** may occur after the released hormone has been metabolized but before new hormone production has resumed.

  b. Etiology. The cause of subacute thyroiditis generally is considered to be viral. Mumps and coxsackievirus, among others, have been suspected.

  c. Diagnosis. When the thyroid becomes acutely swollen, tender, and painful, especially if symptoms of hyperthyroidism are present, subacute thyroiditis is suspected. The diagnosis is confirmed by a **very low radioactive iodine uptake in the face of high serum T_4 and T_3 levels.** The radioactive iodine uptake is low because the follicular cells are injured and unable to trap iodine and because the high levels of circulating thyroid hormone suppress TSH.

  d. Therapy. Treatment is **symptomatic** because the disease is self-limited.

        (1) Aspirin, nonsteroidal anti-inflammatory drugs (NSAIDs), and adrenal corticosteroids (in severe cases) relieve the pain and tenderness.

        (2) β-Blocking drugs can be used to relieve symptoms of hyperthyroidism.

3. Painless thyroiditis (also called silent thyroiditis or postpartum thyroiditis). This syndrome resembles subacute thyroiditis in some ways and chronic thyroiditis in others.

  a. Like subacute thyroiditis, painless thyroiditis is associated with transient, self-limited hyperthyroidism, often with thyroid gland enlargement, and low radioactive iodine uptake. Thyroid pain and tenderness are absent, however.

   (1) Recognition of this cause of self-limited hyperthyroidism is important because, in the absence of thyroid pain to suggest thyroiditis, the syndrome could easily be mistaken for Graves' disease and be treated inappropriately.

   (2) The low radioactive iodine uptake is the most useful finding for distinguishing painless thyroiditis from Graves' disease.

  b. Like chronic thyroiditis, painless thyroiditis is characterized by lymphocytic infiltration of the thyroid and is considered to be an autoimmune disease. However, although antithyroid antibodies may be present, the titers are lower than in chronic thyroiditis.

  c. Painless thyroiditis is common after delivery; **postpartum thyroiditis** occurs after 5%–10% of pregnancies.

4. Rare forms of thyroiditis

E The **euthyroid sick** syndrome (nonthyroidal illness syndrome, low-T_3 syndrome) is a term used to describe the constellation of abnormal thyroid function tests seen in patients with severe illness.

1. Starvation and critical illness cause increased conversion of T4 to T3, increased formation of reverse T3, decreased levels of thyroid-binding globulin, and decreased TSH secretion by the pituitary. Critically ill patients typically demonstrate low T4 levels, low T3 levels, and normal or depressed TSH levels, giving the appearance of central hypothyroidism.

2. During the recovery phase of critical illness, mild TSH elevation may be observed. If the patient's thyroid function tests are first measured during the recovery phase of illness, the treating physician may suspect primary hypothyroidism. If the patient has recently been ill, has no history of thyroid disease, and has a mildly elevated TSH (not higher than 20 μIU/mL), recovery from nonthyroidal illness is more likely than primary hypothyroidism. Endocrinology consultation may be required to make the distinction.

F **Thyroid nodules** are present in 1% of individuals in their 20s and in 5% of individuals in their 60s; cancer is found in approximately 5% of these nodules. Thyroid nodules may be true adenomas, cysts, localized areas of chronic thyroiditis, colloid nodules, hemorrhagic necrotic tissue, or carcinoma.

1. Diagnosis

  a. Risk assessment

   (1) Radiation treatment of the head or neck in childhood is associated with an increased prevalence of thyroid nodules and thyroid cancer in adult life.

   (2) Gender. A higher percentage of nodules are malignant in men than in women (although nodules are much more common in women).

   (3) Age. A higher percentage of nodules are malignant in younger individuals (although nodules are much more common in older individuals). In children, 50% of nodules are malignant.

   (4) Disease course. Malignancy is suggested by recent growth of the nodule or by continuing growth despite suppressive therapy with L-thyroxine. Malignancy is less likely if the nodule disappears after aspiration of cyst fluid, if the nodule is visible as a "warm" or "hot" spot on scintiscan (i.e., as demonstrated by its uptake of radioactive iodine), or if the nodule shrinks with suppressive therapy.

   (5) Physical examination

    (a) Malignancy is suggested when the nodule is fixed in place and no movement occurs on swallowing.

    (b) Unusually firm consistency, irregularity of the nodule, or regional lymph node enlargement also suggest malignancy.

    (c) Malignancy is less likely if there are multiple nodules or if the nodule is less than 1 cm in diameter.

  b. Laboratory evaluation

   (1) Check **thyroid function tests.**

   (2) Obtain **ultrasound.** This can often be combined with fine-needle aspiration biopsy.

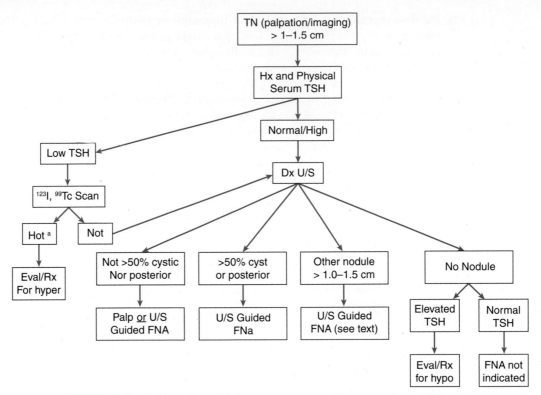

FIGURE 10–5   Algorithm for evaluation and management of patients with a thyroid nodule.

(3) **Fine-needle aspiration biopsy** is safe and easily performed in an office setting. Cells, not sections of tissue, are obtained and must be evaluated by a skilled cytopathologist.

(4) **Radionuclide thyroid scintiscanning** identifies the nodule as "hot," "warm," or "cold."

(a) Because most cancers appear on scan as cold areas, only cold nodules are considered to have a significant risk of malignancy.

(b) Of all nodules, 70%–90% are cold, and most of these are benign. Therefore, scanning may indicate a greatly reduced risk of malignancy in a nodule that is warm or hot, but it does not yield much additional information on the risk of malignancy in a nodule that is cold.

2. **Management.** The goal of management is surgical removal of the nodules with a high probability of malignancy and careful observation of the others, sometimes with attempted suppression by L-thyroxine. An algorithm for the management of thyroid nodules is shown in Figure 10–5.

G **Thyroid cancer**

1. **Epidemiology**

a. Thyroid cancer is common; it is found at autopsy in approximately 5% of patients with no known thyroid disease. However, death due to thyroid cancer is uncommon—approximately 1200 individuals die of this condition each year in the United States.

b. These contradictory observations are explained best by the behavior of thyroid cancer. It is usually indolent and tends to remain localized to the thyroid for many years, which is the reason for the low mortality rate.

2. **Etiology**

a. **Radiation exposure.** Incidence of thyroid cancer is increased in atomic bomb survivors and in individuals who received radiation therapy to the neck (e.g., for enlarged thymus or enlarged tonsils) in childhood.

b. **Genetic factors.** One form of thyroid cancer—medullary carcinoma—may be familial.

c. **TSH** can induce thyroid cancer in animals and may stimulate the growth of many human thyroid cancers.

3. **Types.** Thyroid cancer may manifest as a solitary thyroid nodule or, less commonly, as multiple nodules or a mass in the neck. These tumors occasionally cause hoarseness, symptoms of tracheal or esophageal compression (e.g., dyspnea, dysphagia), or pain.

    a. **Papillary carcinoma,** which accounts for 80% of all thyroid cancer, affects the youngest age group—50% of patients are younger than 40 years of age.

        (1) The neoplasm consists of columnar cells in folds (the papillae). It tends to grow slowly, often remaining localized to the thyroid for years, and eventually spreads via the lymphatic system to other parts of the thyroid and to regional nodes.

        (2) There are few recurrences after treatment, especially in young patients with small primary tumors.

    b. **Follicular carcinoma,** which constitutes 10% of all thyroid cancers, histologically may resemble normal thyroid tissue. Follicular carcinoma is more malignant than papillary cancer and often spreads to bone, the lungs, and the liver. The 10-year survival rate is 50%.

    c. **Medullary carcinoma,** which accounts for 5% of all thyroid cancers, arises from the parafollicular cells (or C cells) of the thyroid. It has a hyaline stroma, which may stain for amyloid.

        (1) Approximately 20% of these carcinomas are familial and may be a component of **MEN II** (Sipple's syndrome), a syndrome of medullary thyroid carcinoma and pheochromocytoma.

        (2) This tumor often produces calcitonin and occasionally produces other hormones.

        (3) It is more malignant than follicular carcinoma, with both local lymphatic and distant hematogenous spread.

    d. **Anaplastic carcinoma,** which accounts for 5% of thyroid cancers, usually affects patients older than 50 years of age and is highly malignant. It invades rapidly, metastasizes widely, and usually causes death within a few months.

4. **Therapy.** Papillary, follicular, and medullary carcinoma usually are treated with a combination of surgery, suppression with thyroid hormone, and radioactive iodine. Anaplastic carcinoma generally is treated palliatively. It may require surgery to relieve obstruction; chemotherapy may delay death.

    a. **Surgery**

        (1) Papillary carcinoma is often treated by total thyroidectomy.

        (2) Follicular carcinoma and more extensive papillary tumors usually are treated by near-total thyroidectomy; just enough tissue is left in association with the posterior capsule to spare the parathyroid glands. This more extensive procedure is more likely to be complicated by hypoparathyroidism, but it is followed by less tumor recurrence.

    b. **Radioactive iodine therapy.** Differentiated thyroid cancer (papillary and follicular) often accumulates radioactive iodine.

        (1) Radioiodine can be used to ablate any normal thyroid tissue that remains after near-total thyroidectomy; normal thyroid tissue has greater affinity for radioiodine than tumor tissue, and therefore limits the amount of radioiodine that would be taken up by tumor.

        (2) After all normal thyroid tissue has been ablated, whole-body scans with radioiodine will be more likely to reveal functioning metastatic tumor, which can be treated with subsequent large doses of radioiodine.

    c. **Suppression therapy.** Because many thyroid cancers grow more rapidly with TSH stimulation, TSH should be suppressed by treatment with L-thyroxine.

        (1) Because suppression of TSH produces a state of subclinical hyperthyroidism, which may decrease bone density, increase cardiac irritability, and have other deleterious effects, the extent to which TSH should be suppressed is not clear.

        (2) A reasonable approach may be to aim for full suppression (undetectable TSH) in patients with high-risk thyroid cancer (large tumor, known metastases, etc.) and to aim for TSH in the low-normal range in patients with low-risk cancer.

IV   DISORDERS OF GLUCOSE HOMEOSTASIS

A **Diabetes mellitus** This condition is **characterized by hyperglycemia** and other metabolic derangements that are **caused by inadequate action of insulin** on body tissues because of either reduced circulating levels of insulin or resistance of target tissues to its actions.

TABLE 10–5   Major Types of Primary Diabetes Mellitus

	Type 1 Diabetes Mellitus	Type 2 Diabetes Mellitus
Prevalence	0.2%–0.5%; men = women	2%–4%; women > men
Age at onset	Usually <25 years	Usually >40 years
Genetics	<10% of first-degree relatives affected; 50% concordance in identical twins	>20% of first-degree relatives affected; 90%–100% concordance in identical twins
Human leukocyte antigen (HLA)	Associated with HLA-DR3, HLA-DR4, HLA-DQ	None
Autoimmunity	Increased prevalence of autoantibodies to islet cells and other tissues	None
Body build	Usually lean	Usually obese
Metabolism	Ketosis prone; insulin production absent	Ketosis-resistant; insulin levels may be high, normal, or low
Treatment	Insulin	Weight loss; oral agents (e.g., sulfonylureas, metformin, thiazolidinediones) or insulin

1. **Classification** (Table 10–5). Diabetes mellitus is divided into two categories—**type 1 diabetes** (formerly called insulin-dependent diabetes) and **type 2 diabetes** (formerly called non–insulin-dependent diabetes). Syndromes with features from either of these categories may be related to the stage or severity of the disease or to other conditions. These syndromes include impaired fasting glucose, impaired glucose tolerance, gestational diabetes, previous abnormality of glucose tolerance, potential abnormality of glucose tolerance, and diabetes associated with certain other diseases.
   a. **Type 1 diabetes** affects 5%–10% of diabetic patients.
      (1) In type 1 diabetes, not only is insulin needed for optimal control of blood glucose, which also may be true for patients with type 2 disease, but **without exogenous insulin, patients are prone to the development of ketoacidosis.** This is thought to reflect a complete or almost complete absence of insulin in patients with type 1 diabetes, in contrast to the partial lack of insulin and the resistance to insulin characteristic of patients with type 2 diabetes.
      (2) Other key features of type 1 diabetes are its occurrence in children and young adults and its occurrence in individuals who are lean rather than obese.
   b. **Type 2 diabetes** commonly affects overweight individuals older than 40 years of age, although with the rising prevalence of obesity it is increasingly being diagnosed in children.
      (1) Because some insulin is produced by these patients, **ketoacidosis is unlikely to occur.**
      (2) However, insulin therapy may be necessary to prevent severe hyperglycemia.
   c. **Related syndromes**
      (1) **Impaired fasting glucose** or **impaired glucose tolerance** (Table 10–6). This is a disorder of glucose metabolism in which blood glucose levels are higher than those of normal individuals but lower than those of patients with diabetes. The risk of development of diabetes is increased in affected individuals.
      (2) **Gestational diabetes.** Diabetes or impaired glucose tolerance develops in 2%–3% of pregnant, previously nondiabetic women, most often in the last trimester of pregnancy.
         (a) β-Cell reserve is apparently inadequate for the increased insulin requirements of pregnancy.
         (b) Careful screening for gestational diabetes and intensive treatment are essential because of an increased risk of neonatal morbidity.
         (c) The glucose tolerance of most patients returns to normal within a few weeks after delivery, although diabetes develops in many patients as long as 5–15 years later.
      (3) **Previous abnormality of glucose tolerance.** This term refers to individuals with normal glucose levels who formerly were glucose intolerant or diabetic because of pregnancy, illness, obesity, or medications.
      (4) **Potential abnormality of glucose tolerance.** This refers to individuals with an increased risk of future diabetes because of a history of having had large babies (>9 pounds) or the presence of diabetes in an identical twin.

TABLE 10–6   Diagnostic Criteria for Diabetes Mellitus

Any one of the following criteria must be met to make a diagnosis of diabetes mellitus
The diagnosis should be confirmed by obtaining the same results (or finding another abnormality) on a different day
Fasting plasma glucose level ≥126 mg/dL (preferred test)*
Plasma glucose level ≥200 mg/dL at 2 hours after a 75-g glucose load (oral glucose tolerance test)†
Casual plasma glucose level (i.e., without regard to food intake) 200 mg/dL or greater (valid only if symptoms such as polyuria, polydipsia, or weight loss are present)
Recent recommendations now include the following:

- Further testing and closer follow-up if fasting plasma glucose of 100 mg/dL or greater, random plasma glucose of 130 mg/dL or greater, or HbA1c greater than 6.0%
- HbA1c of 6.5%–6.9% or greater, confirmed by a fasting plasma glucose level >126 mg/dL or a positive oral glucose tolerance test to establish the diagnosis of diabetes
- HbA1c of 7% or greater, confirmed by another HbA1c or fasting plasma glucose or oral glucose tolerance test to establish the diagnosis of diabetes

*A fasting plasma glucose level >110 mg/dL but <126 mg/dL indicates impaired fasting glucose.
†A plasma glucose level ≥140 mg/dL but <200 mg/dL at 2 hours after a 75-g glucose load indicates impaired glucose tolerance.
Saudek CD, Herman WH, Sacks DB, et al. Consensus statement. A new look at screening and diagnosing diabetes mellitus. *J Clin Endocrinol Metab* 2008;93:2447–2453.

(5) Diabetes or impaired glucose tolerance **may occur secondary** to certain diseases that affect the production or action of insulin, such as **chronic pancreatitis, Cushing's syndrome, acromegaly, insulin receptor abnormalities,** and others.

(6) The **metabolic syndrome** (insulin resistance syndrome, syndrome X). Some metabolic and pathophysiologic abnormalities tend to cluster in certain patients. Insulin resistance may be a common abnormality, perhaps the primary one. Components of this syndrome include diabetes mellitus, obesity, hypertension, dyslipidemia, and atherosclerosis.

2. Etiology. The cause of diabetes mellitus is unknown. Many etiologic factors are suspected, with major differences between those factors that are etiologic for type 1 and type 2 diabetes.

3. Pathophysiology

a. Levels of insulin

(1) In **type 1 diabetes,** some insulin may be produced for a few years after the disease is diagnosed, but insulin production eventually ceases totally.

(2) In **type 2 diabetes,** insulin levels vary and often are similar to the levels in nondiabetic individuals of similar weight. However, these insulin levels are low when considered in relation to the elevated blood glucose concentrations of diabetic patients, and these levels reflect a decrease in β-cell responsiveness to glucose.

b. Consequences of impaired insulin action. Impaired insulin action may be caused by inadequate insulin secretion, target-tissue resistance to the action of insulin, or both.

(1) Hyperglycemia. Insulin increases the synthesis of glycogen in the liver and in muscle and increases the uptake of glucose in muscle and adipose tissue. In the absence of adequate insulin action, hepatic glucose production increases (with increased glycogenolysis and increased gluconeogenesis) and peripheral glucose use decreases. The result is hyperglycemia.

(2) "Glucose toxicity." Hyperglycemia is thought to initiate a self-perpetuating cycle in which elevated glucose levels further impair both the ability of the β cells to produce insulin and the action of insulin on peripheral tissues, leading to a further rise in serum glucose levels.

(3) Other metabolic derangements

(a) Insulin normally acts as an anabolic, energy storage–promoting agent. In addition to the storage of glucose as glycogen, insulin stimulates the formation of fatty acids from glucose, the esterification of fatty acids to form triglycerides, and the storage of amino acids as protein.

(b) Inadequate insulin action on target tissues causes inadequate disposal of ingested nutrients and excessive consumption of endogenous metabolic fuels. Blood fatty acids and lipids are increased because of decreased lipogenesis and increased lipolysis; blood amino acids are increased because of decreased protein synthesis and increased catabolism of muscle protein.

   c. Levels of other hormones
      (1) **Glucagon** levels are often elevated in patients with type 2 diabetes. This may contribute to hyperglycemia through the action of glucagon in stimulating glycogenolysis.
      (2) **Epinephrine, cortisol,** and **GH** levels may be increased during periods of stress or poor diabetic control. This may contribute to hyperglycemia through the anti-insulin effect and diabetogenic action of these hormones.

4. Clinical features
   a. Polyuria and polydipsia usually occur. The most common symptom of hyperglycemia is increased urine volume, which is caused by glucose-induced osmotic diuresis. Increased fluid intake is a response to the resulting dehydration and thirst.
   b. Weight loss results from the loss of glucose in urine and the catabolic effects of the decrease in insulin action, despite increased food intake. Generalized weakness also reflects the metabolic derangements.
   c. Infections of the skin, vulva, and **urinary tract** are especially common in uncontrolled diabetes because hyperglycemia decreases resistance to infection.
   d. Blurring of vision is caused by changes in the shape and refractive qualities of the optic lens that result from hyperglycemia-induced osmotic alterations.

5. Diagnosis. Diabetes mellitus is often suspected because of typical clinical manifestations such as polyuria and unexplained weight loss; however, a definitive diagnosis is based on **elevated glucose levels.**
   a. Glucose levels. Diabetes mellitus is diagnosed if any one of the three abnormalities described in Table 10–6 is present. The diagnosis should be confirmed by repeating the fasting glucose on a different day.
   b. Urine glucose levels. Glucose appears in the urine only when the renal threshold of approximately 180 mg/dL is exceeded. This threshold varies widely and tends to increase with age. Therefore, urine glucose measurement is an insensitive and unreliable test for diabetes.

6. Acute complications of diabetes.
   a. Diabetic ketoacidosis occurs in patients with type 1 diabetes whose circulating insulin is insufficient to allow glucose use by peripheral tissue and to inhibit glucose production and tissue catabolism. Increased levels of glucagon and hormones that increase in response to stress (i.e., epinephrine, norepinephrine, cortisol, GH) contribute to the metabolic derangements. It can rarely occur in type 2 diabetes.
      (1) **Precipitating factors.** Ketoacidosis may occur after several days of worsening diabetic control or may appear suddenly within a few hours.
         (a) Precipitating factors include any event that decreases insulin availability or causes stress that increases the need for insulin.
         (b) Common factors are the omission of insulin doses, infections, injuries, emotional stress, excessive alcohol ingestion, and intercurrent illness.
      (2) **Pathophysiology** (Figure 10–6)
         (a) **Hyperglycemia.** Insufficient insulin reduces peripheral glucose utilization and, together with glucagon excess, increases hepatic production of glucose through the stimulation of gluconeogenesis and glycogenolysis and the inhibition of glycolysis. Protein breakdown in peripheral tissues provides a flow of amino acids to the liver as substrate for gluconeogenesis. Hyperglycemia is the result.
         (b) **Osmotic diuresis.** This condition, which results from the elevated serum glucose (and ketone) levels, produces **hypovolemia, dehydration,** and **loss of sodium, potassium, phosphate, and other substances in the urine.** Volume depletion stimulates catecholamine release, which further opposes insulin action in the liver and contributes to lipolysis.
         (c) **Ketogenesis.** The lipolysis that results from insulin lack and catecholamine excess mobilizes free fatty acids from their stores in adipose tissue. Instead of reesterifying the incoming fatty acids to form triglycerides, the liver shifts its metabolic pathways toward the production of ketone bodies.
           (i) Glucagon increases the hepatic level of carnitine, which enables fatty acids to enter the mitochondria, where they undergo β-oxidation to ketone bodies.

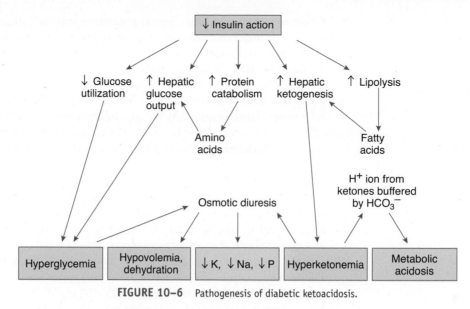

FIGURE 10–6 Pathogenesis of diabetic ketoacidosis.

    (ii) Glucagon decreases the hepatic content of malonyl coenzyme A, an inhibitor of fatty acid oxidation.

  (d) Acidosis. The increased hepatic production of ketone bodies (acetoacetate and β-hydroxybutyrate) exceeds the body's ability to metabolize or excrete them.

    (i) The hydrogen ions of the ketone bodies are buffered by bicarbonate, leading to a decrease in serum bicarbonate and pH.

    (ii) Arterial carbon dioxide tension ($PaCO_2$) also decreases because of ventilatory compensation.

    (iii) The anion gap increases because of the elevated plasma levels of acetoacetate and β-hydroxybutyrate.

    (iv) The result is metabolic acidosis that is associated with an increased anion gap.

(3) Clinical features and diagnosis

  (a) Physical findings

    (i) Rapid, deep breathing (Kussmaul's respirations) occurs as the body tries to compensate for metabolic acidosis by increasing carbon dioxide excretion.

    (ii) An **odor of acetone** is often detected on the breath.

    (iii) Marked dehydration is common, with **dry skin and mucous membranes** and **poor skin turgor. Orthostatic hypotension** may be present because of intravascular volume depletion.

    (iv) Clouding of consciousness is present in most cases, and approximately 10% of patients are **comatose.**

  (b) Laboratory abnormalities

    (i) Hyperglycemia. Serum glucose levels in ketoacidosis may be only slightly increased, but more often they are markedly elevated, averaging approximately 500 mg/dL. Renal function affects the degree of hyperglycemia; glucose levels are greatly elevated only when urinary excretion of glucose is limited by volume depletion or renal abnormalities.

    (ii) Hyperketonemia. Serum levels of acetoacetate, acetone, and β-hydroxybutyrate are greatly increased. The agent nitroprusside, in the form of tablets or reagent strips, is commonly used to measure serum and urine ketone bodies. It reacts only with acetoacetate. If the other ketone bodies are increased to a much greater or much lesser extent than acetoacetate, the results of the test may be misleading.

    (iii) Metabolic acidosis. The serum bicarbonate level is low (usually <10 mEq/L). The **blood pH is low,** and the **anion gap is increased.**

    (iv) Glycosuria and ketonuria. Urinary levels of glucose and ketone bodies are increased. The diagnosis of diabetic ketoacidosis can be made rapidly if marked glycosuria and ketonuria are present.

(v) Other laboratory findings. Serum potassium concentration may be increased initially in metabolic acidosis because of potassium ion movement from the intracellular to the extracellular space. Later, the serum potassium level is low because of both renal losses and the movement of potassium ions back into cells as the acidosis is corrected. **Serum sodium concentration** tends to be low, mainly because of dilution as the osmotic effect of the hyperglycemia increases extracellular water. **Serum osmolality** is high, usually greater than 300 mOsm/kg.

(4) Therapy. The treatment of diabetic ketoacidosis has four main components.

(a) Insulin is administered to increase glucose use in the tissues, to inhibit the flow of fatty acids and amino acids from the periphery, and to counter the effects of glucagon on the liver.

(i) Route of administration. If volume depletion and vascular collapse are present, poor tissue perfusion impairs the absorption of intramuscular or subcutaneous insulin, and insulin is usually administered intravenously. If no intravenous access is available, the intramuscular route can be used.

(ii) Dosage. A priming dose of 0.1 U/kg regular insulin is given intravenously and is followed by the infusion of 0.1 U/kg/hour or approximately 5–10 U/hour. If the serum glucose level does not decrease (75–100 mg/dL/hour), the serum level of ketone bodies does not fall, and serum pH does not increase in a few hours, then larger doses of insulin must be given.

(iii) After the acidosis and hyperglycemia have resolved and the urine has become free of ketone bodies, treatment with intermediate-acting insulin is resumed.

(b) Fluid replacement corrects the dehydration caused by glucose-induced osmotic diuresis. The fluid deficit in patients with diabetic ketoacidosis averages 3–5 L, which must be promptly replaced.

(i) Approximately 1 L of normal saline (0.9% NaCl) is given each hour for the first 2 hours, and then half-normal saline (0.45% NaCl) is given at a slower rate. When the serum glucose level falls to 200–300 mg/dL, 5% or 10% glucose is infused to prevent hypoglycemia. If the patient continues to demonstrate evidence of metabolic acidosis, the insulin infusion should continue. Once the acidosis has cleared, the dextrose infusion should be discontinued and the patient allowed to eat.

(ii) Fluid replacement lowers serum glucose levels, even without insulin, by increasing urine flow (and, hence, glycosuria) and by decreasing the levels of catecholamines and cortisol, which were increased by the stimulus of volume depletion. It also improves the acidosis by lowering the lactic acid.

(c) Minerals and electrolytes must be replaced because they are lost via osmotic diuresis.

(i) Potassium may be needed to replace low body stores. If initial serum potassium levels are elevated (due to severe acidosis), replacement is delayed; when the levels become normal or low, after therapy has been initiated, potassium chloride is infused at a rate of 20–40 mEq/hour. This can be given as potassium phosphate or potassium chloride, depending on the blood levels of calcium and phosphorus; too much phosphate replacement may cause hypocalcemia.

(ii) Phosphate replacement is recommended, although no benefit of phosphate administration has been demonstrated unless it is very low. Approximately 10–20 mmol over 6 hours may be given as potassium phosphate, for a total of 40–60 mmol in 24 hours.

(iii) Bicarbonate is given only when the arterial pH declines to less than 6.9 to maintain the pH greater than that level. Because diabetic ketoacidosis is corrected by fluids and insulin, excessive administration of bicarbonate may result in rebound alkalosis and hypokalemia. Some physicians recommend bicarbonate administration only when the pH decreases to less than 7.1, when the patient is hemodynamically unstable, or if hyperkalemia with electrocardiographic changes is present.

(d) Treatment of precipitating factors and complications

(i) Urinary tract infections, as well as other infections, must be investigated and treated.

(ii) Occult infection, stroke, and myocardial infarction should be considered because they may escape detection in patients whose sensoriums are clouded by ketoacidosis.

b. Hyperosmolar nonketotic coma is less common than ketoacidosis but has a much higher mortality rate. It occurs primarily in elderly patients with type 2 diabetes, often in previously undiagnosed individuals.

(1) Pathophysiology. Often a precipitating factor (e.g., infection, increased glucose ingestion, omission of insulin, intercurrent illness) causes increasing hyperglycemia within a few days or weeks. Osmotic diuresis, without adequate fluid intake, causes dehydration and progressive decline in mental status. Ketoacidosis is mild or absent, presumably because sufficient insulin is present to inhibit hepatic ketogenesis.

(2) Clinical features

(a) The **hyperglycemia** tends to be more marked than it is in ketoacidosis, with average plasma glucose concentrations of approximately 1000 mg/dL.

(b) In the absence of ketoacidosis, the osmotic diuresis continues for a longer time before the diagnosis is made and therefore produces more severe **dehydration.**

(c) Serum osmolality is very high, averaging approximately 360 mOsm/kg. The dehydration and hyperosmolality may cause **mental obtundation, seizures,** and **focal neurologic signs.**

(d) Lactic acidosis may be present because of the hypovolemia and indicates a worse prognosis.

(3) Therapy. Treatment is similar to that for diabetic ketoacidosis. Fluid replacement and reversal of the hyperglycemia with insulin are the main goals.

(a) Fluid replacement in elderly patients with cardiovascular disease requires care to avoid volume expansion, which might precipitate heart failure.

(b) Insulin should not be started until fluid replacement is underway; a fall in plasma glucose levels may worsen the hypovolemia and precipitate shock due to the loss of the intravascular volume-expanding effect of the hyperglycemia.

c. Hypoglycemic coma must be rapidly differentiated from diabetic ketoacidosis and hyperosmolar nonketotic coma because therapy is obviously quite different.

(1) Etiology

(a) Hypoglycemia in insulin-treated diabetic patients ("insulin shock") may be caused by **excessive insulin dose, delay in the ingestion of a meal,** and **excessive physical activity.** Sulfonylureas may cause hypoglycemic reactions but much less often than does insulin.

(b) Patients with type 1 diabetes may be susceptible to hypoglycemia because of **insufficient levels of the counterregulatory hormones** that normally limit the fall in serum glucose. The response of glucagon to hypoglycemia is frequently impaired in these patients, and epinephrine production may become impaired if autonomic neuropathy develops. (Epinephrine prevents severe hypoglycemia both by stimulating glucose production and by producing symptoms that alert the patient to hypoglycemia, prompting rapid glucose ingestion.)

(2) Pathophysiology and clinical features. Hypoglycemia produces symptoms through the following two mechanisms:

(a) A fall in the serum glucose concentration stimulates catecholamine production and sympathetic nervous system outflow. **Adrenergic stimulation** then causes sweating, tachycardia, palpitations, tremulousness, and muscular weakness.

(b) Prolonged hypoglycemia deprives the CNS of its main source of fuel, glucose. **CNS symptoms** of hypoglycemia usually occur later than the adrenergic symptoms, and they are potentially more serious. Mental changes may progress from **somnolence** and **confusion** to **coma.** Headache, slurred speech, focal neurologic signs, and seizures may occur.

(3) Diagnosis. The diagnosis of hypoglycemia is obvious if symptoms of sweating, palpitation, and tremulousness occur at the time of peak action of a recent insulin dose. Patients learn to recognize this reaction and treat it by drinking orange juice or eating candy. Less obvious is the cause of coma in diabetic patients who are brought to the emergency department. Clues that suggest hypoglycemia rather than ketoacidosis are the history of a missed meal or unusually vigorous exercise, the finding of profuse sweating rather than dehydration, and the absence of Kussmaul's respirations. A fingerstick blood glucose determination is useful for rapid confirmation of hypoglycemia.

(4) Therapy

(a) Patients who are unable to take glucose orally are given **50 mL of 50% glucose intravenously** over 3–5 minutes, followed by a constant infusion of 5% or 10% glucose.

(i) Some patients regain consciousness immediately; others do so more slowly.

(ii) Glucose infusion may have to be maintained during the expected duration of action of the insulin or oral agent responsible for the hypoglycemia. If the hypoglycemia is caused by **chlorpropamide,** this may be several days.

(b) An intramuscular injection of 1 mg of **glucagon** may increase the serum glucose level rapidly, allowing patients to regain consciousness and take oral glucose. Teaching patients' family members how to inject glucagon may decrease the frequency of emergency department visits.

(c) After an episode of insulin-induced hypoglycemia, the insulin dosage, diet, or both should be readjusted to prevent subsequent attacks.

7. Chronic complications of diabetes

a. Pathogenesis

(1) Microvascular complications. Patients with diabetes frequently develop microvascular disorders involving the small blood vessels of the eye, kidney, and nerves. The Diabetes Control and Complications Trial, a 10-year randomized controlled trial involving 1441 patients with type 1 diabetes, showed conclusively that better control of serum glucose levels reduces the incidence of retinopathy, nephropathy, and neuropathy. Several mechanisms have been proposed to explain how elevated glucose levels may cause these complications:

(a) Nonenzymatic glycosylation of proteins in capillary basement membranes and other tissues, similar to the process that produces glycosylated hemoglobin, may produce damage to these tissues that is related to the blood glucose levels.

(b) When glucose levels are elevated, the enzyme aldose reductase converts glucose to sorbitol, which may cause damage in nerve cells, the retina, and renal tissue.

(2) Macrovascular complications. Atherosclerotic disease of the medium and large vessels, leading to coronary, cerebrovascular, or peripheral vascular disease, is associated with diabetes mellitus. Unlike the microvascular complications, however, it is also associated with the lesser degree of glucose elevation known as impaired glucose tolerance.

b. Diabetic retinopathy. This condition is directly related to the duration and severity of diabetes. Prevalence increases from 3% at the time that diabetes is diagnosed to 20%–45% after 10 years. Of new cases of blindness in adults, 20% are caused by diabetes.

(1) Types

(a) Background (simple, nonproliferative) retinopathy makes up 90%–95% of all cases. Increased capillary permeability, vascular occlusion, and weakness of supporting structures lead to the findings on funduscopic examination of venous dilation, exudates, hemorrhages, and microaneurysms.

(b) Proliferative retinopathy makes up 5%–10% of all cases. In response to vascular occlusion and ischemia, new vessels form on the surface of the retina (neovascularization) and may grow into the vitreous body of the eye.

(i) Preretinal or vitreous hemorrhage may lead to clot retraction and scar formation, with retinal detachment.

(ii) Vitreous hemorrhage may cause sudden blindness.

(2) Therapy

(a) Background retinopathy is less likely to progress if diabetic control is good. Annual screening for retinopathy is recommended because blindness may be prevented by early treatment. Glucose and blood pressure control are very important.

(b) Proliferative retinopathy may be treated with **laser-beam photocoagulation,** which is effective in obliterating new vessels. **Vitrectomy** is beneficial in selected cases.

c. Diabetic nephropathy. The renal lesion that is specific for diabetes is **intercapillary glomerulosclerosis (Kimmelstiel–Wilson disease).** Other renal diseases associated with diabetes are papillary necrosis, chronic interstitial nephritis, and arteriosclerotic disease.

(1) Incidence. Significant renal disease develops in approximately 40% of patients with type 1 diabetes and 20% of patients with type 2 diabetes. Nearly all patients with severe glomerulosclerosis also have retinopathy. Almost 33% of new cases of end-stage renal disease are caused by diabetes.

(2) Pathogenesis. Hyperglycemia may cause increased intraglomerular pressure, leading to damage to the basement membrane, deposition of protein in the mesangium, glomerulosclerosis, and renal failure. **Pathologic features** of diabetic glomerulosclerosis include an increase in the mesangial matrix and increased width of the glomerular basement membrane, hyaline arteriosclerosis of the afferent and efferent arterioles, and IgG and albumin deposits lining the tubular and glomerular basement membranes. Diabetic kidneys tend to be large, even when end-stage renal disease is present.

(3) Clinical features

   (a) The first manifestation is usually **proteinuria,** which often progresses to the **nephrotic syndrome.**

      (i) Microalbuminuria, which can be detected by special tests, predicts the later occurrence of renal failure.

      (ii) The presence of **hypertension** is also associated with an increased risk of renal failure in diabetic patients.

   (b) When renal failure is associated with nephrotic range proteinuria, the progression to **end-stage renal disease** is rapid; transplantation or dialysis usually becomes necessary within 3 years.

(4) Prevention. Progression of diabetic nephropathy can be prevented or delayed by intensive glycemic control and by control of coexisting hypertension. Angiotensin-converting-enzyme (ACE) inhibitors and angiotensin-receptor blockers (ARBs) slow the progression of renal disease by their antihypertensive effect and probably by an action independent of blood pressure control. A low-protein diet (0.6–0.89 g protein/kg body weight) may also slow the progression of renal disease.

d. Diabetic neuropathy. Older patients with a relatively long history of diabetes and severe hyperglycemia have an increased incidence of this common complication. Accumulation of sorbitol in Schwann cells, with subsequent cell damage, may play a causative role. Slowing of nerve conduction velocity occurs, with changes in Schwann cell function and eventual segmental demyelination and axonal degeneration.

(1) Types

   (a) Peripheral polyneuropathy is the most common syndrome.

      (i) Distal, bilateral sensory changes in the lower extremities predominate. Weakness and upper extremity involvement are less frequent. Neuropathic ulcers of the feet are a common manifestation of diabetic neuropathy and are more common than ischemic ulcers.

      (ii) Symptoms include paresthesias and pain of the feet. Examination may show decreased reflexes, loss of vibratory sense, and loss of pain sensation.

   (b) Autonomic neuropathy is less common than peripheral polyneuropathy, but usually it is seen in patients who have peripheral polyneuropathy. **Postural hypotension** is a major manifestation. Other clinically important problems are sexual impotence in diabetic men and urinary retention with abnormal bladder function. Abnormal gastrointestinal motility may result in delayed gastric emptying (diabetic gastroparesis), constipation, and diarrhea. The adrenergic symptoms of hypoglycemia may be decreased or absent, leading to delayed recognition and treatment of insulin reactions.

   (c) Less common forms of diabetic neuropathy are **radiculopathy,** causing lancinating pain in a single dermatome, and **mononeuropathy,** involving cranial nerves or proximal motor nerves.

(2) Therapy

   (a) Improved diabetic control may lessen the symptoms of peripheral polyneuropathy.

   (b) Symptomatic treatment of painful neuropathy may be attempted with amitriptyline, phenytoin, carbamazepine, topical capsaicin, gabapentin, pregabalin, or duloxetine. Narcotics might be needed.

e. Atherosclerosis. The incidence of atherosclerosis is considerably increased in diabetic patients; that is, diabetes, like hypertension, smoking, hyperlipidemia, obesity, and a positive family history, is a major risk factor for the development of atherosclerosis.

   (1) Coronary artery disease is twice as common in diabetic patients as in nondiabetic patients. Small-vessel disease may contribute to myocardial ischemia.

   (2) Peripheral vascular disease, which is common in diabetic patients, is most likely to affect the legs and feet. Small-vessel disease may play a major role—ischemic changes in a foot with a normal pedal pulse on examination is typical of diabetes. Foot infections, poorly healing ulcers, and eventual gangrene, resulting in amputation, are frequent complications.

8. Treatment of diabetes
   a. Goals of treatment
      (1) Control of symptoms. The polyuria, weight loss, increased incidence of infections, blurring of vision, and other symptoms of diabetes are related to the hyperglycemia. Return of serum glucose levels to normal brings relief of these symptoms.
      (2) Prevention of acute complications. Diabetic ketoacidosis and nonketotic hyperglycemic coma are prevented by careful management of diabetes.
      (3) Prevention of long-term complications. The Diabetes Control and Complications Trial and the United Kingdom Prospective Diabetes Study clearly showed that intensive therapy, with lowering of blood glucose below the levels needed to control symptoms and prevent ketoacidosis, delays or prevents the onset of retinopathy, nephropathy, neuropathy, and macrovascular complications.

   b. Diet. Before insulin was available, severe restriction of carbohydrate intake was necessary to prolong life in patients with type 1 diabetes. In patients receiving insulin, the **regularity, timing of carbohydrate intake,** and its quantity are crucial. It is equally important to **avoid excessive fat intake,** which increases the risk of atherosclerosis. In seeking to balance these considerations, physicians recommend that caloric intake comprise 12%–20% protein, 50%–60% carbohydrate, and 20%–30% fat.

🔊 **(1) Specific objectives in the treatment of diabetes**

🔊 **(2) Diet calculation**

🔊 **(3) Additional suggestions in the treatment of diabetes**

   c. Oral antihyperglycemic agents (Table 10–7)
      (1) Sulfonylurea derivatives and meglitinides
         (a) Mode of action. These agents, which bind to receptors on the β-cell plasma membrane, result in closure of potassium channels, opening of calcium channels, and influx of calcium into the cell. The end result is an increase in insulin secretion by the β cell.
         (b) Side effects. The primary side effect is hypoglycemia, which may result from excessive dosing, drug interactions, renal or hepatic dysfunction, or inadequate food intake.
      (2) Metformin
         (a) Mode of action. The mechanism of action of the biguanide is not well understood, but metformin decreases hepatic glucose output and increase peripheral glucose utilization. The drug does not affect β-cell function directly.
         (b) Side effects. Hypoglycemia is not a side effect of metformin use.
            (i) Gastrointestinal symptoms of anorexia, nausea, abdominal discomfort, and diarrhea are common, but they usually disappear or can be tolerated if the initial dose is low and increased slowly.
            (ii) Lactic acidosis is a serious potential complication, but it is rare unless patients have a predisposing condition such as renal failure, liver disease, alcoholism, or any other condition that may cause tissue hypoxia (e.g., pulmonary disease or heart failure). Metformin should be stopped if radiocontrast dye for a procedure is anticipated and not resumed until normal renal function is documented 24–48 hours later.
      (3) Thiazolidinediones
         (a) Mode of action. Rosiglitazone and pioglitazone increase the sensitivity to insulin in muscle, fat, and, to a lesser extent, liver. They act by stimulating the peroxisome proliferator-activated receptor γ, a nuclear receptor that affects insulin-responsive genes.

TABLE 10–7   Oral Antihyperglycemic Agents

Drug/Brand Name	Usual Starting Dose (mg/day)	Maximal Daily Dose (mg)	Timing of Dose	Side Effects	Comments
Sulfonylureas (Second Generation)					
Glimepiride/Amaryl	1	8	Daily or BID	Hypoglycemia, weight gain	Glimepiride and glipizide are the preferred agents in renal impairment because they are shorter acting and less likely to cause hypoglycemia
Glipizide/Glucotrol, Glucotrol XL	5	20	Daily or BID		
Glyburide/Micronase, DiaBeta	2.5	20	Daily or BID		
Meglitinides					
Repaglinide/Prandin	1.5	16	15 minutes before each meal		Shorter acting and more expensive than sulfonylureas
Nateglinide/Starlix	180	360	15 minutes before each meal		
Biguanides					
Metformin/Glucophage, Glucophage XL	500	2500	BID to TID with meal	Nausea, diarrhea	Contraindicated if creatinine >1.6, avoid in elderly
Thiazolidinediones					
Rosiglitazone/Avandia	4	8	Daily or BID	Fluid retention, hypoglycemia	Potential for increased risk for cardiovascular events
Pioglitazone/Actos	15	45	Daily		Preferred agent
α-Glucosidase Inhibitors					
Acarbose/Precose	25	300	Divided doses at start of meals	Flatulence, diarrhea	
Miglitol/Glyset	25	300	Divided doses at start of meals		
DDP-4 inhibitors					
Sitagliptin/Januvia	50	100	Daily or BID	Low incidence of gastrointestinal symptoms	Adjust for creatinine clearance, avoid with hepatic dysfunction
Vidagliptin/Galvus	50	100	Daily or BID		
Saxagliptin/Onglyza	2.5	5	Daily		

BID, twice daily; DDP-4, dipeptidyl peptidase inhibitor 4; TID, thrice daily.

(b) **Side effects**
   (i) Hypoglycemia may occur, especially if thiazolidinediones are used with insulin or sulfonylureas.
   (ii) Other side effects associated with thiazolidinediones include weight gain that is partly attributable to fluid retention, increased plasma volume, edema, and possible exacerbation of congestive heart failure.
(4) **Dipeptidyl peptidase-4 (DPP-4) inhibitors**
   (a) **Mode of action.** In response to a meal, the gut releases different peptides (incretins) into the circulation. Glucagon-like peptide 1 (GLP-1) enhances glucose-dependent insulin stimulation, suppresses glucagon secretion (this decreases hepatic glucose production), and regulates gastric emptying. The half-life of GLP-1 is short because it is metabolized by the DPP-4 enzyme. By inhibiting the effect of this enzyme, the half-life and action of GLP-1 are increased. The dose needs to be adjusted for creatinine clearance.
   (b) **Side effects.** Abdominal pain, nausea, and diarrhea can occur in fewer than 4% of patients. The risk of hypoglycemia is very low.

TABLE 10–8 Insulin Preparations and Their Onset, Peak, and Approximate Duration of Action

Types	Onset of Action (hours)	Peak Effect (hours)	Duration of Action (hours)
Fast Acting			
Regular human insulin	½–1	2–4	5–8
Insulin lispro, insulin aspart, insulin glulisine	¼	½–1½	3–5
Inhaled insulin	¼	1–2	6
Intermediate Acting			
NPH human insulin	1–3	4–½	12–16
Lente insulin	1–4	8–½	14–18
70% NPH human, 30% regular human insulin	½–1	8	12–16
Long Acting			
Insulin glargine	—	Flat	24
Insulin detemir	2	11	24?
NPH, isophane insulin suspension			

    (5) α-Glucosidase inhibitors

        (a) Mode of action. These drugs inhibit the action of enzymes in the brush border of the small intestine, decreasing the conversion of disaccharides and oligosaccharides to monosaccharides. This delays the absorption of carbohydrates, allowing more time for insulin to act and blunting the postprandial rise in plasma glucose.

        (b) Side effects. The shifting of carbohydrate digestion to the distal small bowel and colon tends to cause symptoms of flatulence, abdominal discomfort, and diarrhea. To minimize these symptoms, these drugs are started at very low doses and increased very gradually.

  d. Insulin

    (1) Preparations

        (a) Insulin preparations are available with **short** (regular insulin, rapid-acting insulin analogs), **intermediate,** and **long durations of action** (Table 10–8).

        (b) Insulin lispro and insulin aspart have earlier onset of action and shorter duration of action than regular insulin. They therefore can be injected immediately before meals rather than 15–30 minutes before meals and are less likely to have prolonged action that could cause hypoglycemia before the next meal.

        (c) Insulin glargine and detemir are considered "peakless" insulins because there is little variability in insulin blood levels over 24 hours if the insulin is injected once daily. Some patients do not need to take them twice a day, but even if that is the case, there is less risk of hypoglycemia. This makes them excellent agents to provide basal insulin levels during an entire 24-hour period.

        (d) NPH and similar intermediate-acting insulins are available in **premixed combinations** with regular insulin and insulins lispro and aspart. These combinations are 70% or 75% intermediate insulin and 30% or 25% short-acting insulin.

    (2) Insulin regimens (Figure 10–7 and online content)

    (3) Factors affecting insulin requirements

    (4) Complications of insulin therapy

  e. Novel therapies

        (a) Incretin mimetics. These mimic the enhancement of glucose-dependent insulin secretion by GLP-1. The only one approved so far is **exenatide (Byetta).** It stimulates insulin release, decreases hepatic glucose production by lowering glucagon levels, suppresses appetite, slows gastric emptying, and may have a role in islet cell regeneration. It is given twice a day as a subcutaneous injection. It has been approved to be used in combination with metformin and sulfonylureas. Exenatide's major side effect is nausea, which usually decreases with time. Hypoglycemia can occur if it is used with sulfonylureas.

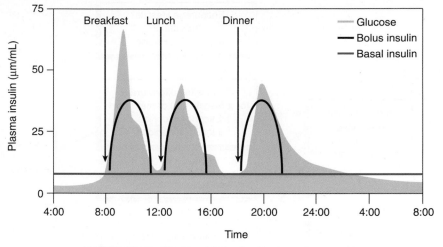

FIGURE 10–7 Ideal basal/bolus insulin absorption pattern.

(b) Pramlintide (Symlin). This is a human analog of amylin. Amylin is cosecreted with insulin from the β cell, and its secretion decreases with time. It slows gastric empty-ing, decreases glucagon secretion, and suppresses appetite. It is given as a subcutane-ous injection three times a day before meals. Its more common side effect is nausea, which decreases with time. It has been approved to be used in combination with insulin or oral agents.

f. Evaluation of glucose control

(1) Home monitoring of capillary glucose levels, using a glucose meter and test strips, is performed as often as necessary to evaluate glucose control. If satisfactory preprandial glucose levels are attained, the 2-hour postprandial glucose levels should be measured.

(2) Goals of treatment should be to achieve a fasting plasma glucose level less than 120 mg/dL, a postprandial glucose level less than 140–180 mg/dL, and an Hb_{A1C} level less than 6%–7%.

(3) Glycosylated hemoglobin measurements

(a) The free amino acid groups of hemoglobin and other body proteins combine with glucose to form a reversible compound (Schiff base), which can then become a stable glycosylated protein (Amadori rearrangement). The extent of this nonenzymatic gly-cosylation is dependent on the concentration of glucose in blood; that is, the percent-age of hemoglobin that is glycosylated depends on the blood glucose levels that were present during the life span of the currently circulating red blood cells (RBCs).

(b) The glycosylated hemoglobin level, therefore, reflects the degree of hyperglycemia during the preceding 6–12 weeks, and it may be useful in estimating the average con-trol of serum glucose levels during this time.

g. Pharmacologic therapy of diabetes (Figure 10–8)

B Hypoglycemia There is no simple definition of hypoglycemia. Glucose levels less than 45–55 mg/dL may be associated with hypoglycemic symptoms, but some normal individuals have glucose levels lower than this without symptoms after several days of fasting or several hours after a glucose load, with resultant stimulation of insulin secretion. If the diagnosis is in doubt, **Whipple's triad** (i.e., symptoms of hypoglycemia, low serum glucose levels, and relief of the symptoms when nor-moglycemia is restored) may be used as a criterion.

1. Insulinomas are rare tumors that arise from the β cells of the islets of Langerhans. Most are single, benign adenomas, but approximately 10% of these tumors are multiple, and 10% are malignant. They occur with equal frequency in the head, the body, and the tail of the pancreas. β-Cell hyperplasia occasionally may produce a similar syndrome.

a. Clinical features. Insulinomas produce excessive quantities of insulin, leading to **fasting hypoglycemia** (i.e., a category of hypoglycemia in which the lowest levels of serum glucose and the severest symptoms occur after prolonged periods without food intake).

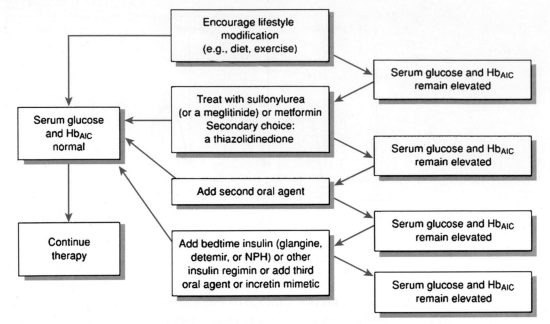

FIGURE 10–8 Pharmacologic therapy of diabetes.

(1) Symptoms are most likely to occur in the early morning or late afternoon or after fasting or exercise.

(2) The symptoms of hypoglycemia are the same as those that result from insulin overdose in diabetic patients.

(3) Patients may gain weight before the diagnosis is made because they learn to relieve or avoid hypoglycemic symptoms by frequently snacking on carbohydrates.

  b. Diagnosis (Table 10–9)

    (1) An **elevated serum insulin concentration** when the glucose level is low is strong evidence for the presence of an insulinoma if an exogenous insulin source or sulfonylurea use is excluded.

      (a) In normal individuals, insulin levels fall as glucose levels fall, and insulin levels become undetectable at glucose levels less than 30 mg/dL.

      (b) If the serum glucose concentration is less than 45 mg/dL, an insulin level greater than 10 mU/mL is abnormal.

    (2) A **prolonged fast,** extending for 24–72 hours, may be necessary to demonstrate fasting hypoglycemia with inappropriately high insulin levels. Some suggest the injection of 1 mg of glucagon intravenously at the end of the fast if no hypoglycemia developed. A rise in glucose of 25 mg/dL or more points to hypoglycemia-mediated by insulin.

    (3) **Proinsulin,** the large precursor molecule of insulin, is produced in increased amounts by insulinomas. Proinsulin normally makes up 5%–20% of the total insulin in blood that is measured by radioimmunoassay; in patients with an insulinoma, proinsulin usually exceeds 25%.

    (4) **Diagnostic imaging** with MRI, CT, ultrasonography (including endoscopic or intraoperative ultrasound), and selective arteriography may be used to identify and localize an insulinoma. These tumors may be small, however, averaging 1–2 cm, and they often cannot be visualized.

  c. Therapy

    (1) **Surgical removal** of an adenoma or partial pancreatectomy for multiple adenomas or β-cell hyperplasia is the treatment of choice.

    (2) **Medical therapy** is reserved for patients whose tumors cannot be completely removed because metastatic disease exists, previous surgical attempts have failed, or illness or patient refusal makes surgery infeasible.

      (a) **Diazoxide** inhibits the release of insulin from β cells. A dose of 200 mg daily, which can be raised as high as 800 mg if necessary, can prevent hypoglycemia in patients with an inoperable insulinoma.

TABLE 10–9   Diagnostic Interpretation of the Results of a 72-hour Fast

Diagnosis	Symptoms or Signs	Glucose* (mg/dL)	Insulin† (μU/mL)	C-Peptide‡ (pmol/L)	Proinsulin‡ (pmol/L)	Serum β-Hydroxy-butyrate (mmol/L)	Change in Serum Glucose¶ (mg/dL)	Sulfonyl in Serum
Normal	No	≥40	<3	<200	<5	>2.7	<25	No
Insulinoma	Yes	≤45	≥3§	≥200	≥5	≤2.7	≥25	No
Factitious hypoglycemia from insulin	Yes	≤45	≥3	<200	<5	≤2.7	≥25	No
Sulfonylurea-induced hypoglycemia	Yes	≤45	≥3	≥200	≥5	≤2.7	≥25	Yes
Hypoglycemia-mediated by insulin-like growth factor	Yes	≤45	≤3	<200	<5	≤2.7	≥25	No
Non–insulin-mediated hypoglycemia	Yes	≤45	<3	<200	<5	>2.7	<25	No
Inadvertent feeding during the fast	No	≥45	<3	<200	<5	≤2.7	≥25	No
Nonhypoglycemic disorder	Yes	≥40	<3	<200	<5	>2.7	<25	No

Measurements are made at the time the decision is made to end the fast.

*Sequential serum glucose measurements in the hypoglycemic range fluctuate. Serum glucose concentrations of 45 mg/dL at the time a decision in made to end the fast may rise to as much as 56 mg/dL when the fast is actually ended approximately 1 hour later. Serum glucose concentration may be as low as 40 mg/dL during prolonged fasting in normal women. To convert serum glucose values to mmol/L, multiply by 0.056.

†To convert insulin values to pmol/L, multiply by 6.0.

‡Serum C-peptide and proinsulin were measured by immunometric assay. In normal individuals serum insulin, C-peptide, and proinsulin concentrations may be higher if the serum glucose concentration is 60 mg/dL.

¶Refers to the change in serum glucose after the administration of intravenous glucagon.

§Serum insulin concentrations may be very high (>100 μU/mL) in factitious hypoglycemia from insulin.

Reproduced with permission from Service FJ. *N Engl J Med* 1995;332:1144. Copyright © 1995 Massachusetts Medical Society.

     (b) **Octreotide** inhibits insulin and glucagon release. **Streptozocin** is an antibiotic that specifically destroys β cells. It is used to treat malignant β-cell tumors. Systemic chemotherapy, interferon-α, or chemoembolization could be tired for malignant tumors.

2. **Factitious hypoglycemia** is caused by the surreptitious self-administration of insulin or an oral hypoglycemic drug, most often by an individual who is familiar with health care, such as a nurse or medical technologist, or by a diabetic or relative of a diabetic. Differentiation from hypoglycemia caused by an insulinoma may depend on special studies.

    a. **Serum C-peptide measurement** indicates the source of insulin secretion. The low glucose and high insulin levels that are pathognomonic of an insulinoma should be accompanied by increased C-peptide levels; if the latter are low, indicating an exogenous source of the high insulin concentration, the disease is factitious.

    b. Ingestion of a sulfonylurea, however, stimulates endogenous insulin production, and the C-peptide level is high; therefore, **screening of blood or urine for sulfonylureas** is also necessary to rule out factitious disease.

3. **Extrapancreatic tumors** may cause hypoglycemia. These usually are large, intra-abdominal tumors, most often of mesenchymal origin (e.g., fibrosarcoma), although they may be hepatic carcinomas or other tumors. The mechanism of hypoglycemia is poorly understood; increased use of glucose by some tumors and production by others of an insulin-like substance (IGF-II) have been observed.

4. **Ethanol-induced hypoglycemia** occurs in patients whose glycogen stores are depleted because of inadequate recent food intake, usually 12–24 hours after a bout of heavy drinking.

   a. The oxidation of ethanol to acetaldehyde and acetate generates reduced nicotinamide-adenine dinucleotide (NADH) and decreases the availability of nicotinamide-adenine dinucleotide (NAD), which is needed for gluconeogenesis. When neither glycogenolysis nor gluconeogenesis is available to maintain hepatic glucose production in the fasting state, hypoglycemia results.

   b. Prompt recognition and glucose administration are essential because the mortality rate is greater than 10%.

5. **Liver disease** may result in impairment of glycogenolysis and gluconeogenesis sufficient to cause fasting hypoglycemia. This is seen in fulminant viral hepatitis or acute toxic liver disease but not in the usual, less severe cases of cirrhosis or hepatitis.

6. **Other causes of fasting hypoglycemia** include cortisol deficiency, GH deficiency, or both, which may occur in **adrenal insufficiency** or **hypopituitarism.** Hypoglycemia may occur in patients with **renal failure** and **heart failure;** however, the causes are poorly understood.

7. **"Reactive hypoglycemia"** may occur as a result of another, smaller group of disorders, which cause hypoglycemia a few hours after the ingestion of carbohydrates. Insulinoma and the other conditions discussed previously most commonly produce hypoglycemia in the fasting state.

   a. **Alimentary hypoglycemia** occurs in patients who have had a gastrectomy or other surgical procedure that leads to abnormally rapid movement of food into the small bowel. Rapid absorption of carbohydrate stimulates excessive insulin secretion, causing hypoglycemia several hours after a meal.

   b. **Reactive hypoglycemia of diabetes** occurs in an occasional patient with early diabetes who may have a late but excessive release of insulin after a carbohydrate-containing meal. The glucose level is elevated after 2 hours but then decreases to hypoglycemic levels 3–5 hours after the meal.

   c. **"Functional" hypoglycemia,** although commonly diagnosed in patients with chronic fatigue and anxiety, is probably a rare condition. Hypoglycemia is not a cause of chronic fatigue, depression, and lack of energy.

      (1) **Clinical features.** Hypoglycemia, with adrenergic symptoms such as sweating and palpitations, occurs 2–5 hours after a carbohydrate-rich meal, presumably because of increased insulin production or insulin sensitivity.

      (2) **Diagnosis**

         (a) The overdiagnosis of functional hypoglycemia stems in part from misinterpretation of the 5-hour glucose tolerance test. One in four normal individuals has a serum glucose level less than 50 mg/dL at 3–5 hours after the nonphysiologic stimulus of 75–100 g of glucose, and some normal individuals have levels less than 35 mg/dL, without symptoms. These responses do not prove functional hypoglycemia, and the test should not be done to make the diagnosis of hypoglycemia.

         (b) The diagnosis depends on finding hypoglycemia that coincides with the patient's typical symptoms and on finding relief of symptoms by carbohydrate ingestion.

      (3) **Therapy** consists of eating four to six small meals daily that are low in carbohydrate and high in protein.

V DISORDERS OF THE PARATHYROID GLANDS

A **Primary hyperparathyroidism and hypercalcemia**   Primary hyperparathyroidism is the result of oversecretion of parathyroid hormone (PTH), which in turn causes hypercalcemia. PTH is important in maintaining normal calcium homeostasis (Figure 10–9).

1. **Epidemiology.** Primary hyperparathyroidism is common, affecting approximately 1 individual in every 1000 who are screened. The disease is especially common in middle-aged and elderly women.

2. **Etiology**

   a. A single **parathyroid adenoma** causes 80%–90% of cases, and **hyperplasia** of all four glands causes 10%–20% of cases of primary hyperparathyroidism. Parathyroid carcinoma is a rare cause.

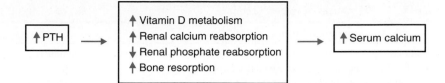

FIGURE 10–9 Actions of parathyroid hormone (PTH) in maintaining normal calcium homeostasis.

  b. Predisposing factors
   (1) Although most cases seem to arise without a known cause, a history of **radiation to the neck** is present in 10% or more of patients.
   (2) Familial occurrence of parathyroid hyperplasia and of the MEN syndrome, which often involves parathyroid adenomas or hyperplasia, indicates that **genetic factors** may be important.
 3. Pathophysiology
 4. Clinical features. The routine measurement of serum calcium levels in multichannel screening tests has led to early diagnosis of primary hyperparathyroidism. The disease commonly manifests as mild asymptomatic hypercalcemia, although occasionally patients are seen with the classic findings of advanced kidney and bone disease. Patients with serum calcium levels greater than 11–12 mg/dL often have gastrointestinal symptoms, neurologic symptoms, or both.
  a. Renal manifestations
   (1) Although PTH increases renal calcium reabsorption, the hypercalcemia and resulting increased glomerular filtration of calcium commonly lead to **hypercalciuria,** which may cause the formation of **urinary calculi.**
   (2) Chronic hypercalcemia may cause deposition of calcium within the renal parenchyma (nephrocalcinosis) and eventual **renal failure.**
  b. Skeletal manifestations. PTH excess increases the rate of osteoclastic bone resorption and can lead to the disorder of bone metabolism called **osteitis fibrosa cystica.**
   (1) Symptoms include bone pain, fractures, and areas of swelling and deformity localized to involved bones.
   (2) There are areas of **demineralization** in the skeleton. In severe cases, there may be **bone cysts** and "**brown tumors,**" which are localized lesions consisting of proliferating osteoclasts, osteoblasts, and fibrous tissue.
   (3) Radiographs may show **generalized osteopenia,** with demineralization of the skull and other areas. **Subperiosteal resorption** of bone occurs in the phalanges and distal portions of the clavicles. Loss of the lamina dura around the teeth is characteristic.
  c. Gastrointestinal manifestations. Symptoms related to the hypercalcemia of hyperparathyroidism include anorexia, weight loss, constipation, nausea and vomiting, and abdominal pain. Patients with hyperparathyroidism may have an increased incidence of peptic ulcer disease and pancreatitis.
  d. Neurologic manifestations. Emotional changes and abnormal mentation may occur, which also are related to the hypercalcemia of hyperparathyroidism. Fatigue and muscle weakness are common.
 5. Diagnosis
  a. Serum and urine chemistries
   (1) Blood chemistry
    (a) Elevation of the serum calcium level is the hallmark of primary hyperparathyroidism.
    (b) The serum phosphate level is lowered in many, but not all, cases.
    (c) The serum alkaline phosphatase level is elevated only in patients with significant bone disease.
   (2) Urine chemistry. Hypercalciuria is common, but, because of the calcium-reabsorbing action of PTH, approximately one third of patients have normal urine calcium levels. The finding of a low urinary calcium points toward the diagnosis of familial hypocalciuric hypercalcemia (see online description under 6c).

TABLE 10–10   Causes of Hypercalcemia

Primary Hyperparathyroidism	
Malignancy	Sarcoidosis
With bone metastases (e.g., breast cancer, myeloma, lymphoma)	Benign familial hypercalcemia
	Hypervitaminosis D
Without bone metastases (e.g., hypernephroma; pancreatic cancer; squamous cell carcinoma of the lung, cervix, and esophagus; head and neck tumors)	Milk–alkali syndrome
	Hyperthyroidism
	Thiazide therapy
	Immobilization

    b. PTH assay. An elevated blood PTH level in the presence of hypercalcemia is strong evidence for primary hyperparathyroidism because other causes of calcium elevation tend to suppress PTH levels. The **immunoradiometric assay for intact PTH** is more sensitive and specific than previously used assays.

    c. Diagnostic imaging. Noninvasive techniques such as **ultrasonography, CT scanning, MRI,** and **isotope scans** may demonstrate parathyroid adenomas in 60%–80% of cases (🅟 Online Figure 10–10).

🅟 6. Differential diagnosis. Hypercalcemia may be caused by entities other than primary hyperparathyroidism (Table 10–10).

7. Therapy of primary hyperparathyroidism

  a. Surgery

    (1) Indications. Asymptomatic patients with minimal elevation in serum calcium and no complications often have no progression of the disease for 10 years or longer. Such patients may be followed closely and considered for surgery only if they develop specific indications (Table 10–11).

    (2) Initial surgical exploration. In most cases, a **single adenoma** is found and removed. If **parathyroid hyperplasia** is found, the surgeon may remove three glands and part of the fourth, or remove all parathyroid tissue and transplant a portion to the muscles of the forearm or neck. The removal of additional parathyroid tissue from the transplanted portion may be accomplished more easily if necessary.

    (3) Repeat surgical exploration. Approximately 10% of initial neck explorations fail to indicate abnormal parathyroid tissue or cure the disease. After the patient is reevaluated, additional invasive and noninvasive localizing procedures are considered before a second operation is performed.

    (4) Postoperative course. Transient hypocalcemia is common after the removal of a parathyroid adenoma because the remaining normal glands are likely to have been suppressed by longstanding hypercalcemia.

      (a) Patients usually recover within a few weeks.

      (b) In the occasional patient with severe bone disease, marked intractable hypocalcemia may persist for several months because, when the excess PTH stimulus is suddenly removed, the demineralized bone becomes avid for calcium (the "hungry bones" syndrome).

TABLE 10–11   Indications for Surgery in Primary Hyperparathyroidism

Symptoms related to hypercalcemia
Serum calcium levels >1 mg/dL above normal range
Age <50 years
Renal manifestations
Renal calculi
Reduced creatinine clearance
Twenty-four–hour urine calcium excretion >400 mg/dL
Bone mineral density >2.5 standard deviations below peak bone mass (t-score)
Patient preference for surgery or unwillingness/inability to undergo prolonged follow-up

    b. Medical therapy may be used if no indications for surgery are present (see Table 10–11), if other illness contraindicates surgery, or if the patient refuses surgery.

      (1) Increased fluid intake and activity help to minimize hypercalcemia.

      (2) Oral phosphate in doses of 1–2 g daily often lowers the serum calcium level. The main complication—extraskeletal calcification—is uncommon if this dose is not exceeded.

      (3) Estrogen may lower mildly elevated serum calcium levels to normal, apparently by decreasing bone resorption. This treatment may be considered in postmenopausal women, who make up two thirds of the cases of primary hyperparathyroidism.

    c. Emergency treatment is necessary if the calcium level increases to greater than 13–15 mg/dL before the adenoma can be removed or if surgical treatment is refused or is unsuccessful. Hypercalcemia caused by diseases other than hyperparathyroidism (e.g., hypercalcemia due to malignancy) also may be treated by the following methods.

      (1) Hydration with sodium diuresis. From 4 to 6 L or more of intravenous saline daily, with large doses of furosemide, increase renal calcium excretion and reduce serum calcium levels.

      (2) Bisphosphonates such as **pamidronate** and zolendric acid (Zometa) bind to hydroxyapatite in bone and block dissolution of this mineral; they also inhibit osteoclast activity. The resulting inhibition of bone resorption produces a decline in serum calcium levels over 1–7 days. Pamidronate is given intravenously in a single dose over 24 hours; this can be repeated in 7 days if necessary.

      (3) Calcitonin lowers serum calcium levels by inhibiting osteoclastic bone resorption. It is the fastest-acting hypocalcemic agent and is very safe, but it is less potent than plicamycin, gallium nitrate, or pamidronate, and its effect tends to decrease after several days. Salmon calcitonin is given intramuscularly or subcutaneously every 12 hours.

      (4) Glucocorticoids lower serum calcium levels in patients with sarcoidosis and vitamin D intoxication and sometimes in those patients with myeloma and hematologic malignancy. However, glucocorticoids do not lower serum calcium levels in patients with hyperparathyroidism.

      (5) Plicamycin (formerly called mithramycin) is an antineoplastic agent that lowers serum calcium levels by inhibiting osteoclastic bone resorption. A single intravenous dose may lower the serum calcium levels for several days. This drug is commonly used in treating hypercalcemia due to malignancy.

      (6) Gallium nitrate is a potent inhibitor of bone resorption. It is given by continuous infusion for 5 days. Potential nephrotoxicity limits its use to patients without renal failure.

B **Hypoparathyroidism and hypocalcemia**

  1. Etiology

    a. Surgical removal of the parathyroid glands is the most common cause of hypoparathyroidism.

      (1) This may be an unavoidable result of radical neck dissection for cancer or a rare complication of subtotal thyroidectomy.

      (2) Temporary hypoparathyroidism after neck surgery is not uncommon and may be due to ischemic injury to the glands. Recovery usually occurs in a few weeks or months.

    b. Idiopathic hypoparathyroidism of autoimmune etiology is much less common. It usually is diagnosed in childhood, may be familial, and sometimes is associated with adrenal insufficiency and mucocutaneous candidiasis.

  2. Pathophysiology. PTH deficiency leads to hypocalcemia, the hallmark of hypoparathyroidism, through the same mechanisms by which increased secretion of PTH causes hypercalcemia.

  3. Clinical features and diagnosis. Hypocalcemia produces acute symptoms related to increased neuromuscular irritability. In addition, long-term changes may occur as a result of effects on ectodermal tissues and ectopic calcium deposition.

    a. Symptoms and signs

      (1) Latent tetany

        (a) Mild hypocalcemia may cause **muscular fatigue and weakness** as well as **numbness** and tingling around the mouth and in the hands and feet.

        (b) Chvostek's sign may be positive (i.e., a tap over the facial nerve in front of the ear elicits a contraction of the facial muscles and upper lip). However, Chvostek's sign may be positive in 10% of normal individuals.

(c) **Trousseau's sign** may be positive; that is, inflation of a blood pressure cuff on the arm to a pressure higher than the patient's systolic pressure for 3 minutes elicits carpal spasm (flexion of the metacarpophalangeal [MCP] joints and extension of the interphalangeal joints, with drawing together of the fingers and adduction of the thumb).

(2) **Overt tetany.** Severe hypocalcemia causes **twitching and cramps of the muscles with carpopedal spasm. Laryngeal stridor** and **seizures** may occur in severe cases.

(3) **Long-term effects of hypocalcemia**

    (a) **Ectodermal changes** include atrophy, brittleness, and ridging of the nails; dryness and scaling of the skin; and enamel defects and hypoplasia of the teeth.

    (b) **Calcification of the basal ganglia** may occur and is occasionally associated with parkinsonian signs and symptoms.

    (c) **Calcification of the optic lens may lead to cataract formation.**

  b. Laboratory abnormalities. Hypocalcemia and **hyperphosphatemia** are consistently present in hypoparathyroidism. PTH levels, of course, are low, but clinical assays may not be sufficiently sensitive to distinguish between low and normal levels. An albumin level should always be checked and the serum calcium corrected for a low albumin. The correction formula is 0.8(4.0 – measured albumin) + serum calcium.

4. Differential diagnosis

5. Therapy

  a. Hypoparathyroidism. PTH, which must be injected twice daily, is not commonly used for long-term therapy. Instead, treatment with **supplemental calcium,** combined with **vitamin D** to enhance its absorption, is effective in correcting the hypocalcemia and hyperphosphatemia of hypoparathyroidism, even in cases caused by end-organ unresponsiveness to PTH (e.g., pseudohypoparathyroidism).

    (1) **Calcium supplementation.** Usually 1–2 g of elemental calcium is given daily.

      (a) Commonly used preparations include calcium carbonate (each tablet of Os-Cal contains 500 mg of elemental calcium; each tablet of Caltrate contains 600 mg of elemental calcium) and calcium citrate (each tablet of Citracal contains 200 mg of elemental calcium, although higher-potency Citracal tablets containing up to 650 mg of elemental calcium are available). Calcium carbonate is more readily absorbed when taken with food. Calcium citrate is the preferred formulation for patients with reduced levels of stomach acid such as those on chronic proton pump inhibitor therapy.

      (b) The calcium is given in two or three divided doses with no more than 500–600 mg of calcium per dose.

    (2) **Vitamin D.** Vitamin D_2 **(ergocalciferol)** has been used for years in the treatment of hypoparathyroidism, but **calcitriol** has largely replaced it.

      (a) **Calciferol**

        (i) Because vitamin D_2 must be converted to 1,25-dihydroxyvitamin D_3 to be fully effective (a conversion that is greatly inhibited in the absence of PTH), large doses of vitamin D are necessary. The average daily dose is 50,000 IU, with a range of 25,000–150,000 IU.

        (ii) The onset of action is slow (1–2 weeks), but the effect may persist for months after administration is stopped.

      (b) **Calcitriol (1,25-dihydroxyvitamin D_3).** The main advantage of calcitriol over vitamin D_2 is the faster onset and cessation of action, which may lead to more precise control of blood calcium levels. Calcitriol is given in doses of 0.25–2.0 µg/day.

  b. Acute hypocalcemia. Treatment of this condition, which may occur shortly after parathyroid resection and may cause severe tetanic symptoms, consists of intravenous administration of calcium. Calcium gluconate (10%) in a dose of 1–2 g is given intravenously in approximately 10 minutes followed by slow infusion of 1 g of calcium gluconate over the next 6–8 hours.

VI   METABOLIC BONE DISEASE

The metabolic bone diseases include osteomalacia, osteoporosis, and osteitis fibrosa cystica. Osteitis fibrosa cystica is discussed briefly in the section on hyperparathyroidism [see V A 4 b].

A **Osteomalacia**

1. **Definition.** Osteomalacia is a **skeletal abnormality** in which there is **inadequate mineralization of bone matrix.** In children, this usually takes the form of rickets, caused by vitamin D deficiency. In adults, osteomalacia may be caused by various abnormalities of calcium, phosphorus, and vitamin D metabolism.

2. **Etiology**
   a. **Vitamin D deficiency** causes osteomalacia because its most active metabolite, 1,25-dihydroxyvitamin D_3, is essential for absorption of calcium from the gastrointestinal tract. Vitamin D deficiency may result from lack of dietary sources of vitamin D or lack of production of vitamin D in the skin.
      (1) **Vitamin D metabolism.** Exposure to sunlight converts 7-dihydrocholesterol, a precursor of vitamin D in the skin, to vitamin D_3 (cholecalciferol). In the liver, vitamin D_3 is converted to 25-hydroxyvitamin D_3, the storage form of vitamin D. In the kidney, 25-hydroxyvitamin D_3 is converted to 1,25-dihydroxyvitamin D_3, the active form of vitamin D.
      (2) Although the recommended daily allowance of vitamin D, set in 1997 by the National Academy of Sciences, is 400 IU/day, the average adult needs 800-1000 IU/day of vitamin D to maintain a 25-hydroxyvitamin D level of 30 ng/mL, the lower limit of normal. Important sources of vitamin D in the diet include fish, eggs, and fortified milk and cereals. Dietary deficiency of vitamin D can result from inadequate intake of vitamin D due to poverty, restrictive diets, or inadequate absorption of vitamin D as a consequence of gastric bypass surgery or other conditions associated with intestinal malabsorption
      (3) Since skin concentrations of 7-dihydrocholesterol diminish as a result of the aging process, it more difficult for elderly patients to manufacture vitamin D in the skin. Consequently elderly patient, especially those confined indoors, are dependent on dietary vitamin D in food or supplements to prevent deficiency.
   b. **Abnormal metabolism of, or response to, vitamin D**
      (1) **Liver disease,** when far advanced, may cause osteomalacia by interfering with the normal hepatic conversion of vitamin D to 25-hydroxyvitamin D_3.
      (2) **Anticonvulsant drugs** such as phenobarbital and phenytoin, if taken over a long period, may alter the metabolism of vitamin D by inducing hepatic microsomal enzymes. Osteomalacia and decreased serum levels of 25-hydroxyvitamin D_3 have been described in patients receiving long-term treatment with anticonvulsants.
      (3) **Vitamin D–dependent rickets type I** is an autosomal recessive disorder caused by impaired activity of renal 1α-hydroxylase, leading to inadequate conversion of 25-hydroxyvitamin D_3 to 1,25-dihydroxyvitamin D_3 (calcitriol). It is treated with small, physiologic doses (0.5–1.0 µg) of calcitriol.
      (4) **Vitamin D-dependent rickets type II,** also autosomal recessive, is caused by resistance to the action of vitamin D because of altered structure or function of the calcitriol receptors. To overcome this resistance, large, supraphysiologic doses of calcitriol, along with calcium supplementation, must be used.
   c. **Renal abnormalities**
      (1) **Renal osteodystrophy** may occur in patients with chronic renal failure of any cause. Both osteomalacia, caused by impaired renal production of 1,25-dihydroxyvitamin D_3, and osteitis fibrosa cystica, caused by the secondary hyperparathyroidism of renal failure, are present in varying degrees.
      (2) **X-linked hypophosphatemic rickets** and **autosomal dominant hypophosphatemic rickets** are X-linked dominant disorders in which the primary abnormality is renal loss of phosphate. They are caused by gene mutations that affect the proximal tubular reabsorption of phosphate. Relative deficiency of calcitriol production is also present. Supraphysiologic doses of calcitriol, together with phosphate, may raise the serum phosphate level, decrease the bony abnormalities of rickets, and increase growth.
      (3) In **Fanconi's syndrome,** renal tubular defects may lead to the loss of phosphate as well as calcium, glucose, and amino acids, with resulting osteomalacia.

d. Gastrointestinal disorders. Any disease or surgical procedure that leads to malabsorption and steatorrhea may reduce the absorption of calcium, phosphate, and vitamin D; osteomalacia may result.

e. Tumors such as hemangiopericytomas and giant cell tumors of bone may produce a humoral substance that causes phosphaturia and osteomalacia; the syndrome (**"oncogenic osteomalacia"**) is cured by removal of the tumor.

3. Pathophysiology

a. The **common defect** in the various diseases associated with osteomalacia is the **lack of calcium and phosphorus for mineralization of bone matrix.**

b. Rickets is caused by defective mineralization of bone before closure of the cartilaginous growth plates. Deformity occurs because of pressure on weakened growth plates and on the abnormally soft shafts of the long bones. After closure of the growth plates, only osteomalacia can occur, with defective mineralization of mature lamellar bone.

c. Histologically, bone biopsy shows an excess of unmineralized bone matrix, which is seen as an increase in the volume and thickness of osteoid seams covering the bone surfaces.

4. Clinical features

a. Pain and **tenderness** are common in affected areas of the skeleton, especially the spine, ribs, pelvis, and lower extremities.

b. Muscle weakness is common, affecting particularly the proximal muscles of the legs.

c. Skeletal deformities and fractures occur in severe cases.

(1) The long bones may bow because of the softening of the skeleton.

(2) Rickets in children is associated with widening of the epiphyses; swelling of the wrists, knees, ankles, and costochondral joints; bowlegs; and disturbances in growth.

5. Laboratory findings

a. Radiographs may show **decreased bone density** and coarsening of the trabecular pattern. **Looser's zones** are radiolucent bands that are perpendicular to the periosteal surface, caused by pseudofractures.

b. To evaluate for vitamin D deficiency a serum 25-hydroxyvitamin D level should be obtained (normal range 30–100 ng/mL).

c. Although laboratory abnormalities depend on the cause and the severity of the osteomalacia, they often include **low serum phosphate, low or normal serum calcium,** and **increased serum alkaline phosphatase levels.**

6. Therapy

a. Treatment of the primary disorder is sometimes possible (e.g., correction of a bowel disorder causing malabsorption or removal of a tumor causing osteomalacia).

b. Vitamin D is usually the mainstay of treatment (Table 10–12).

(1) Vitamin D deficiency can be replaced in a number of ways. One approach based on the 25-hydroxyvitamin D level is outlined in Table 10–12. Vitamin D toxicity has not been reported when vitamin D is replaced in this manner.

TABLE 10–12 **Treatment of Vitamin D Deficiency**	
25(OH) Level (ng/mL)	**Treatment**
<15	Vitamin D_2 50,000 IU 3 times/week for 6 weeks
16–25	Vitamin D_2 50,000 IU 2 times/week for 6 weeks
>25	Vitamin D_3 2000 IU daily or vitamin D_2 50,000 IU every other week

Goal: 25(OH) >30 ng/mL, 40 ng/mL ideal.
Vitamin D_2, ergocalciferol (vitamin D of plant origin); vitamin D_3 = cholecalciferol (vitamin D of animal origin).
After repletion, start maintenance vitamin D_3 2000 IU daily or vitamin D_2 50,000 IU every other week.
After last dose of pharmacologic vitamin D, wait 2 weeks and repeat 25(OH) vitamin D level.
Vitamin D_3 is the preferred replacement form because some, but not all, studies suggest that it increases serum
25-hydroxyvitamin D levels more efficiently than does ergocalciferol. Vitamin D_3 in a dose of 50,000 IU has recently
become available in pharmacies.
Used with permission from Dr. Elizabeth Streeten, University of Maryland.

(2) Patients with renal failure and hypoparathyroidism who have low 25-hydroxyvitamin D levels may need to be managed with both vitamin D_2 or D_3 (in order to replenish their 25-hydroxyvitamin D levels, the storage form of vitamin D) and calcitriol, the active form of vitamin D. This is because patients with renal failure may be unable to make the active form of vitamin D due to loss of renal mass, and patients with hypoparathyroidism may be unable to convert 25-hydroxyvitamin D_3 to 1,25-hydroxyvitamin D in the absence of PTH.

(3) Large doses of calcitriol may be needed to manage the uncommon syndrome caused by altered metabolism or action of vitamin D or renal wasting of phosphate.

B Osteoporosis

1. **Definition.** Osteoporosis is a decrease in total bone volume, with changes in bone microarchitecture, leading to an increased susceptibility to fractures. In the United States more than 1 million of osteoporotic fractures occur yearly. Both increased bone resorption and decreased bone formation have been observed.

2. **Etiology**
   a. **Decreased bone mass at maturity**
      (1) After reaching its peak at approximately 30 years of age, bone mass declines throughout the remaining years of life. A low total bone mass at maturity, a relatively rapid rate of bone loss, or both contribute to the development of "involutional" osteoporosis.
      (2) **Genetic factors** affect the bone mass at maturity.
         (a) Men and blacks have greater peak bone mass and less osteoporosis; women and individuals of northern European ancestry have less bone mass at maturity and more osteoporosis.
         (b) A familial tendency toward osteoporosis has been observed.
   b. **Calcium deficiency.** Evidence suggests that calcium intake in American women is less than is needed to maintain calcium balance. Associated vitamin D deficiency is very common.
      (1) More than 75% of women older than 35 years of age fail to ingest the recommended daily allowance of 1000 mg of calcium. In addition, calcium absorption decreases in later life.
      (2) The need to maintain normal serum levels of calcium may lead to increased bone resorption through the action of PTH. (The effect of PTH on bone is to increase the rate of calcium and phosphate resorption, and when serum calcium levels are low, the secretion of PTH increases.)
   c. **Hormone changes.** When estrogen levels decrease, whether because of ovarian disease, oophorectomy, or normal menopause, the rate of bone loss is accelerated.
      (1) Estrogen deficiency may result in less stimulation of osteoblastic activity and may increase the sensitivity of bone to the action of PTH.
      (2) The increased rate of bone loss persists for 5–10 years after menopause.
      (3) Hypogonadism in men is also a cause of bone loss and increased risk of fractures.

3. **Classification**
   a. **Two types** of osteoporosis have been described.
      (1) **Postmenopausal osteoporosis** primarily affects women within 15 years of menopause. The loss of trabecular bone is accelerated, and fractures of the vertebrae, which consist mainly of trabecular bone, are common.
      (2) **Senile osteoporosis** affects men and women older than 75 years of age, causing loss of both cortical and trabecular bone. Fractures of the hip, which is largely cortical bone, occur, as do vertebral fractures.
   b. **Secondary osteoporosis** may be associated with glucocorticoid therapy or spontaneous Cushing's syndrome, malabsorption syndromes or malnutrition, multiple myeloma, and prolonged immobilization, among other conditions.

4. **Clinical features**
   a. **Fractures**
      (1) **Vertebral compression fractures** typically affect T8 to L3 and occur more commonly in women. They may cause acute back pain that persists for several months or may occur gradually and painlessly.
      (2) **Hip fractures,** characteristically in the neck and intertrochanteric regions of the femur, are common in both men and women older than 65 years of age. Loss of function frequently

results, and, because of complications, mortality rates may be as high as 20% within 1 year.

(3) The **distal radius** and other areas also may be the site of fractures.

b. **Pain and deformity.** Back pain may persist long after an episode of vertebral fracture because of spinal deformity and alteration of spinal mechanics. Several inches may be lost from height, and severe kyphosis may be the result of multiple vertebral fractures.

5. **Diagnosis**

a. **Radiography of the spine** may indicate a decrease in bone density, with accentuation of the cortical outlines and prominence of the trabeculae.

(1) However, approximately 30% of bone tissue must be lost before these abnormalities appear on plain radiographs.

(2) Wedge-shaped deformities and compression fractures on spinal radiographs also suggest the diagnosis of osteoporosis.

b. **Dual-energy absorptiometry (DEXA),** the best method for evaluating bone mineral density, is the reference standard for the diagnosis of osteoporosis. The World Health Organization has suggested that a diagnosis of **osteopenia** be made when bone mineral density is reduced by more than 1 standard deviation (SD), but less than 2.5 SD, below the mean bone density of young adults, and **osteoporosis** when it is reduced by 2.5 SD or more. The World Health Organization Fracture Risk Assessment (FRAX) Tool is available online. On the basis of the patient's bone density result and risk factor profile, an estimate of fracture risk can be made. This fracture risk score in turn can be used to decide whether use of bisphosphonates or other therapy is appropriate for an individual patient.

c. **Screening for osteoporosis**

(1) Precise guidelines are not available, but many agree that DEXA of the spine and hip should be performed in women older than 65 years and in postmenopausal women younger than 65 years if they have additional risk factors for osteoporosis.

(2) **Risk factors for osteoporosis** are listed in Table 10–13.

6. **Therapy.** Weight-bearing exercise and adequate intakes of calcium and vitamin D should be encouraged in everyone to help prevent osteoporosis, and these measures remain important in the treatment of osteoporosis. The most potent pharmacologic agents are the bisphosphonates

---

TABLE 10–13   Risk Factors for Osteoporosis

Personal History of Fracture as an Adult

History of fragility fracture (defined as a fracture with low trauma such as a fall from standing height) in a first-degree relative

Low body weight (<58 kg [127 lb])

Current cigarette smoking

Female sex

Estrogen deficiency at an early age [menopause or bilateral oophorectomy before age 45 years, prolonged premenopausal amenorrhea (>1 year)]

White race

Advanced age (>age 65 years)

Lifelong low calcium intake

Alcoholism

Inadequate physical activity

Recurrent falls

Dementia

Impaired eyesight despite adequate correction

Poor health/frailty

Medical conditions: chronic obstructive pulmonary disease, gastrectomy, hyperparathyroidism, hypogonadism, multiple myeloma, celiac disease

Glucocorticoid therapy for >3 months

Other drugs: anticonvulsants, gonadotropin-releasing hormone agonists, lithium, excessive doses of thyroid hormone, chronic opioid use

and parathyroid hormone. Other treatments that may be of somewhat lesser value are estrogen replacement therapy, raloxifene, and calcitonin.

a. Calcium

(1) Patients with osteoporosis should ingest at least 1500 mg of elemental calcium daily.

    (a) Because the average American takes in only approximately 500 mg of calcium in food, calcium supplements should be given. Calcium carbonate tablets (e.g., 500 mg of Os-Cal two or three times daily) are usually well tolerated but may contribute to constipation.

    (b) Exogenous calcium may reduce the rate of bone loss and the fracture rate in patients with osteoporosis whose usual calcium intake is inadequate.

(2) Prevention of osteoporosis requires attention to calcium intake in healthy persons. Recommended daily calcium intake is 1000 mg in women who are premenopausal or taking estrogen replacement and in men younger than 65 years. A higher intake (1500 mg daily) is recommended in younger individuals who have not yet achieved their peak bone mass, in older men, and in estrogen-deficient women. Achieving these goals often requires calcium supplementation.

b. Vitamin D. Pharmacologic doses (>1000 U daily) have not proven to be effective in the treatment of osteoporosis, but physiologic doses (400–800 U daily) of vitamin D have decreased the fracture rate in elderly persons who may be deficient in vitamin D because of poor nutrition and lack of exposure to sunlight. Vitamin D supplementation of 400–800 U daily should be recommended in such individuals and in patients with osteoporosis. If vitamin D deficiency is documented based on a 25-hydroxyvitamin D level, higher doses of vitamin D may be necessary.

c. Bisphosphonates

(1) These agents bind to hydroxyapatite in bone and decrease osteoclastic bone resorption. Because osteoblastic bone formation continues for a time while resorption cavities in bone are filled in, bone density may increase by 5%–10% over the next 1–2 years. After this, the main effect of antiresorptive agents such as the bisphosphonates is to prevent the gradual decrease in bone density that might otherwise occur.

(2) **Alendronate (Fosamax)** is very effective in increasing bone mineral density and in decreasing the fracture rate.

    (a) The dose is 10 mg once daily or 70 mg once weekly, which is equally effective.

    (b) The primary side effects are gastrointestinal symptoms, especially esophageal irritation and in a few cases esophageal erosion. To prevent these complications and to maximize drug absorption, patients must take alendronate with a full glass of water on arising in the morning and 30 minutes before the first meal, beverage, or other medication, and they must not lie down for 30 minutes after they swallow the pill.

(3) **Risedronate (Actonel)** is similar in effectiveness to alendronate but may be less likely to cause gastrointestinal side effects. The dosage is 5 mg once daily, 35 mg once weekly, or 150 mg once monthly.

d. Parathyroid hormone. When the skeleton is exposed to constantly elevated blood levels of PTH, as in patients with primary hyperparathyroidism, bone density is lost and fracture risk is increased [see V A 4 b]. Paradoxically, when low doses of PTH are injected once every 24 hours, the opposite effect occurs: Bone density increases and fracture risk falls. Apparently the intermittent exposure of bone to PTH favors bone formation over bone resorption.

(1) It is possible that PTH initially causes resorption of bone, which releases growth factors such as IGF-1 and transforming growth factor beta, which then stimulate osteoblastic bone formation. This hypothesis is favored by the observation that PTH loses much of its bone-forming activity if given together with alendronate, an inhibitor of bone resorption.

(2) **PTH (teriparatide, Forteo)** is given once daily in a dose of 20 mg by subcutaneous injection. Side effects may include hypercalcemia (requiring dose reduction or discontinuation of PTH), dizziness, and leg cramps. It has been shown to prevent vertebral fractures, but its role in prevention of hip fractures is unclear.

(3) The role of PTH in the treatment of osteoporosis is not yet known. Its effects on bone density are quite favorable compared with other available agents, but it is expensive, requires daily injections, and long-term experience with its use is lacking. Its use should be considered in patients with severe osteoporosis who are at high risk for fractures and who have not responded well to other treatments.

    e. Estrogen. Estrogen replacement therapy after menopause has been an important measure for the prevention and treatment of osteoporosis. Recent findings, however, suggest that the risks associated with estrogen therapy, especially breast cancer, thromboembolism, and cardiovascular disease, are greater than previously thought. Because other effective treatments for osteoporosis are available, such as bisphosphonates and PTH, estrogen replacement therapy is assuming a secondary role in treatment of osteoporosis.

    f. Raloxifene. A group of compounds called selective estrogen receptor modulators (SERMs) have been developed. Raloxifene, one member of this group, has beneficial effects on the skeleton similar to estrogen (although less potent)—it reduces the risk of vertebral fractures, but without the undesired estrogenic effects on the breasts and uterus.

    g. Calcitonin. This hormone, which is secreted by the parafollicular cells of the thyroid, inhibits osteoclast activity and decreases the rate of bone loss and fractures in osteoporosis. It may be given by injection or nasal spray (Miacalcin). The nasal spray delivers 200 units of calcitonin, the daily dose, in one puff; the patient alternates nostrils each day because of possible nasal irritation. It is recommended in patients with significant pain from an acute osteoporotic fracture. Tachyphylaxis occurs with chronic use.

VII FEMALE REPRODUCTIVE DISORDERS

Endocrine disorders that affect the female reproductive system usually cause menstrual abnormalities and include those disorders in which menarche does not occur (**primary amenorrhea**) and those disorders that cause cessation of menstrual periods after menarche (**secondary amenorrhea**). Androgen-excess syndromes are a common cause of reproductive abnormalities that also are considered in this section.

    A Primary amenorrhea (Table 10–14)

        1. Gonadal dysgenesis (Turner's syndrome). This condition occurs in 1 in 2500 live female births.

            a. Etiology and pathophysiology. Gonadal dysgenesis is caused by a **chromosomal abnormality** that is not familial and is not related to the mother's age. Patients have a chromatin-negative buccal smear and a 45,X karyotype.

            b. Clinical features

                (1) Ovaries fail to develop; only bilateral streaks of connective tissue are present, without germ cells. Estrogen deficiency, caused by the absence of ovarian tissue, results in **sexual infantilism,** with absence of breast development and other secondary sexual characteristics, and increased levels of LH and FSH.

                (2) Somatic abnormalities are associated with gonadal dysgenesis.

                    (a) Most patients are short, between 48 and 58 inches in height.

                    (b) Other features, present in varying numbers of patients, include a short, webbed neck, epicanthal folds, low-set ears, a shield-like chest with widely spaced nipples, cubitus valgus (wide carrying angle), and renal and cardiac abnormalities.

            c. Therapy

                (1) Estrogen therapy induces the development of secondary sexual characteristics. If estrogen is given cyclically with progesterone, regular menstrual bleeding occurs, but fertility is not possible because of the absence of ovaries.

                (2) GH therapy, if started early enough, may add 2–4 inches to the adult height.

                (3) Removal of streak gonads may be necessary. Gonadal dysgenesis may occur in patients with sex chromosome mosaicism, in which one or more cell lines bear a Y chromosome.

TABLE 10–14 Causes of Primary Amenorrhea

Gonadal Causes	Extragonadal Causes
Gonadal dysgenesis (Turner's syndrome)	Hypopituitarism
Testicular feminization syndrome	Hypogonadotropic hypogonadism
Resistant ovary syndrome	Delayed menarche
	Congenital adrenal hyperplasia
	Abnormalities of the uterus or vagina

The frequency of gonadoblastoma and other gonadal tumors is increased in patients with these gonads, and their prophylactic removal is recommended.

2. **Testicular feminization syndrome.** Individuals with this syndrome are genetic males with a 46,XY karyotype, but they have normal female external genitalia and are raised as girls.
   a. **Pathogenesis.** The basic defect is resistance of target tissues to the action of androgens. The fetal testes produce testosterone, but because the Wolffian ducts and genital tissues cannot respond to testosterone, female differentiation of the external genitalia takes place. The fetal testes also produce Müllerian duct–inhibiting factor, which acts to inhibit the Müllerian anlage. As a consequence, the fallopian tubes, uterus, and upper vagina do not develop.
   b. **Clinical features.** The result is a phenotypic woman with a vagina that ends in a blind pouch, hypoplastic male ducts instead of the fallopian tubes and uterus, and testes located in the abdomen, inguinal canal, or labia majora. Endogenous estrogen stimulates normal breast development at puberty. The condition is suspected when menarche fails to occur or when a testis is felt as an abdominal mass, which is explored.
   c. **Therapy.** The testes are prone to malignant degeneration and should be removed. Estrogen treatment is then given to maintain secondary sexual characteristics.

3. **Resistant ovary syndrome.** Inability of the ovaries to respond to normal or increased stimulation by gonadotropins may be a result of autoimmune destruction of the ovaries or other conditions.

4. **Hypogonadotropic hypogonadism**
   a. **Panhypopituitarism** due to destructive lesions of the hypothalamic–pituitary area causes primary or secondary amenorrhea, depending on whether the problem is prepubertal or postpubertal in onset.
   b. **Isolated gonadotropin deficiency** is most often caused by defective hypothalamic production of GnRH, usually of unknown etiology. In **Kallmann's syndrome,** this defect is associated with anosmia.

5. **Delayed menarche.** This diagnosis should be considered when menstrual periods have not begun by 16 years of age.
   a. A diagnosis of delayed menarche, as opposed to that of primary amenorrhea, can only be made in retrospect, after spontaneous menstrual periods have begun. A family history of late pubertal development suggests that spontaneous menarche may yet be expected.
   b. If severe psychological stress is caused by the absence of sexual development, it may be necessary to give one or more 6-month courses of estrogen therapy, with long treatment-free periods to observe whether spontaneous puberty will occur.

B **Secondary amenorrhea (Table 10–15)**   Pregnancy should always be excluded as a cause.
1. **Hypothalamic** (also called **"psychogenic," "functional,"** and **"idiopathic"**) **amenorrhea** is the **most common form of nonphysiologic secondary amenorrhea.** Obvious psychological stress may or may not be present. LH and FSH levels are low in some cases and normal in others. If the

---

TABLE 10–15   Causes of Secondary Amenorrhea

Pregnancy	Ovarian causes
Menopause	Primary ovarian failure ("premature menopause")
Uterine causes	Oophorectomy
Intrauterine synechiae (Asherman's syndrome)	Radiation therapy, chemotherapy
Hysterectomy	Estrogen excess
Discontinuation of oral contraceptives	Ovarian tumors
Hypopituitarism	Prolactin excess
Hypothalamic ("psychogenic") amenorrhea,	Pituitary tumors
chronic opioid use	Androgen excess
Malnutrition, chronic illness	Polycystic ovary syndrome
Exercise	Overproduction of adrenal androgen

hypothalamic-releasing hormone GnRH is infused in physiologic fashion (pulse doses every 90–120 minutes), all abnormalities may be corrected—ovarian follicles mature, ovulation takes place, a corpus luteum develops and functions, and pregnancy may occur. This supports the clinical impression that most cases of functional or idiopathic amenorrhea are caused by abnormal hypothalamic GnRH production.

2. **Malnutrition** may play a role. Menarche seems to occur when a critical body weight is reached, and menstruation often ceases when the weight of a woman whose menstrual cycle was previously normal falls below this critical weight, whether because of food deprivation, chronic illness, excessive dieting, or anorexia nervosa.

3. **Exercise** may be a factor. Amenorrhea is present in up to 50% of female ballet dancers, runners, and athletes. Exercise-related weight loss is at least partially responsible; the risk of amenorrhea is much higher in women who have lost more than 10%–15% of their body weight. Levels of LH, FSH, and estrogen tend to be low, suggesting a hypothalamic abnormality.

4. **"Post-pill amenorrhea"** refers to a delay of more than 6 months in the return of menses after the discontinuation of oral contraceptive use. It occurs in fewer than 1% of oral contraceptive users. Other causes of amenorrhea must be excluded before contraceptive use is blamed.

5. **Primary ovarian failure ("premature menopause")** is similar to normal menopause; that is, ovarian function declines, estrogen levels decrease, and gonadotropin levels increase. However, primary ovarian failure occurs before 40 years of age. Autoantibodies against ovarian antigens have been found in some cases.

6. **Ovarian tumors** (e.g., granulosa–theca cell tumors) may inhibit normal menstrual cycling by producing excessive quantities of estrogen.

7. **Prolactin excess** is a common cause of secondary amenorrhea.

8. **Menopause**
    a. **Manifestations**
        (1) Menopause, or total cessation of menstrual periods, occurs in all women when the ovaries are depleted of follicles and ovulatory function and estrogen production cease. The average age of menopause in the United States is 51 years.
        (2) As follicular secretion of estradiol and inhibin (a suppressor of gonadotropins) falls at menopause, FSH and LH levels rise. Estradiol levels remain low, although some estradiol is formed by peripheral conversion of androstenedione produced by the adrenals and ovaries.
        (3) The most prominent symptoms of the menopause is the **hot flash,** a sensation of warmth that may last up to 5 minutes, sometimes followed by sweating and a cold sensation. Headache, palpitations, dizziness, and weakness may accompany the hot flash. These episodes occur irregularly and may interfere with sleep. Hot flashes usually disappear within a few years of menopause.
            (a) The hot flash seems to be related to a fall in estrogen levels. Feedback stimulation of GnRH-producing cells in the hypothalamus may affect nearby thermoregulatory centers.
            (b) Estrogen therapy is very effective in decreasing the frequency and severity of hot flashes.
        (4) Other symptoms associated with the menopause include genitourinary atrophy, vaginal dryness, urinary symptoms, insomnia, and depression.
    b. **Postmenopausal hormone replacement therapy.** For many years it was widely accepted that replacement of estrogen after menopause had benefits that greatly outweighed its drawbacks. Recent studies have changed this perception, and the indications for postmenopausal hormone replacement therapy are being reconsidered.

(1) **Effects of estrogen on cardiovascular disease**

(2) **Benefits of estrogen therapy**

(3) **Risks of estrogen therapy**

(4) **Indications for hormone replacement therapy**

(5) **Estrogen administration**

TABLE 10–16 **Diagnostic Criteria for Polycystic Ovary Syndrome: Rotterdam Criteria by the European Society of Human Reproduction and Embryology/American Society of Reproductive Medicine (2003)**

Two of three of the following findings are required for diagnosis:
Menstrual irregularity due to anovulation or oligo-ovulation
Evidence of clinical or biochemical hyperandrogenism:
 Clinical: hirsutism, acne, or male-pattern balding
 Biochemical: high serum androgen concentrations
Polycystic ovaries (by ultrasound)

C **Androgen excess syndromes**

1. **Polycystic ovary syndrome,** a disorder of unknown etiology, is characterized by a chronic lack of ovulation, associated with symptoms of androgen excess and often with obesity. It is present in 5%–10% of reproductive-age women and is one of the most common causes of infertility.

   a. **Pathophysiology** (see Online Figure 10–11).

   b. **Clinical features** (Table 10–16)

      (1) **Infertility** and **menstrual abnormalities** are the result of chronic anovulation. Most patients have amenorrhea or oligomenorrhea. The prolonged, noncyclic, unopposed estrogenic stimulation of the endometrium may cause functional bleeding and increased risk of endometrial carcinoma.

      (2) **Androgen excess** causes oiliness of the skin, acne, and hirsutism in most women with this syndrome. Signs of true virilization (e.g., deepening of the voice, enlargement of the clitoris) are rare.

      (3) **Obesity** is present in approximately 40% of patients.

   c. **Laboratory findings**

      (1) An **increased LH-to-FSH ratio** ($\geq$2) is a useful diagnostic finding. The LH level is usually elevated, and the FSH level is in the low-normal range.

      (2) **Serum testosterone and androstenedione levels** are usually elevated. Increased levels of the androgens of predominantly adrenal origin (i.e., dehydroepiandrosterone [DHEA], dehydroepiandrosterone sulfate, the storage form of DHEA) are found less often.

      (3) **Serum estrone levels** are usually high, and estradiol levels are normal.

      (4) **Prolactin** level can be high.

      (5) In patients with **abnormal fasting glucose,** an oral glucose tolerance test can be considered.

   d. **Therapy.** The **goals of treatment are the relief of symptoms of androgen excess, the induction of ovulation and fertility, and the prevention of endometrial hyperplasia** due to excess noncyclic estrogen stimulation.

      (1) **Androgen excess**

         (a) **Metformin** and **thiazolidinediones,** drugs that increase the sensitivity of tissues to insulin, have lowered testosterone levels and improved the symptoms of hyperandrogenism and menstrual dysfunction in individuals with polycystic ovary syndrome. The efficacy of **metformin** in this syndrome makes it a reasonable choice for initial therapy, although it does not cause improvement in all cases.

         (b) **Spironolactone,** an aldosterone antagonist that is used primarily for its diuretic and antihypertensive properties, has additional actions that make it useful in the treatment of hirsutism. This agent decreases ovarian and adrenal synthesis of androgens and inhibits androgen binding to receptors in hair follicles and other target tissues. A dose of 100 mg once or twice daily is often effective.

         (c) **Estrogen–progestin combinations** may decrease androgen levels by feedback inhibition of pituitary LH production and by stimulation of hepatic synthesis of sex hormone–binding globulin, which decreases the unbound fraction of testosterone.

         (d) **Glucocorticoids** (e.g., prednisone 5.0–7.5 mg daily) may decrease adrenal androgen production by suppressing ACTH. These agents may also lower ovarian androgen secretion, although the mechanism is unknown.

(e) The effects of medical therapy in diminishing the growth of unwanted facial and body hair are seldom dramatic and usually take place over a period of 3–6 months. **Mechanical methods of hair removal** are usually needed as well (e.g., shaving, electrolysis, laser treatment, bleaching, chemical depilatories, and wax treatments). **Vaniqa cream** (eflornithine hydrochloride) inhibits an enzyme in skin—ornithine decarboxylase—and may slow the rate of hair growth.

(2) **Infertility.** If metformin does not restore normal ovulatory menstrual cycles, other drugs may be used to treat infertility.

    (a) **Clomiphene citrate** blocks the binding of estrogen to receptors in target tissues. By blocking the negative feedback effects of estrogen on the hypothalamus and pituitary gland, this drug stimulates LH and FSH production.

        (i) If given on the fifth day through the ninth day after a menstrual period induced by progesterone, clomiphene citrate often stimulates follicle maturation and ovulation.

        (ii) Ovulation can be induced with clomiphene citrate in approximately 80% of patients.

    (b) **Human menopausal gonadotropin** has both FSH and LH bioactivity.

        (i) It is injected daily until increasing serum estrogen levels and ultrasonography of the ovary indicate that follicle maturation has occurred.

        (ii) Then human chorionic gonadotropin (hCG), which has primarily LH activity, is injected to induce ovulation. Because the risk of ovarian hyperstimulation and of multiple gestation is high, this therapy should be reserved for resistant cases of infertility.

    (c) **GnRH,** when given intravenously or subcutaneously in pulse doses every 90–120 minutes, may induce ovulation without causing ovarian hyperstimulation.

(3) **Chronic anovulation and abnormal menstrual bleeding.** Unopposed noncyclic stimulation of the endometrium by estrogen may cause dysfunctional uterine bleeding and may increase the risk of endometrial cancer. Persistent endometrial proliferation can be interrupted either with progestin treatment (e.g., 10 mg daily of medroxyprogesterone acetate for 10 days every 1–3 months) or with cyclic estrogen–progestin therapy.

2. **Androgen-producing ovarian tumors** are rare. Arrhenoblastoma, the most common of these tumors, makes up less than 1% of solid ovarian tumors; others are hilar cell tumors, adrenal rest tumors, and granulosa cell tumors.

    a. Testosterone levels tend to be higher than those in the polycystic ovary syndrome, and virilization occurs more frequently.

    b. Androgen levels are not suppressed by treatment with glucocorticoids or estrogen–progestin combinations, as they often are in the polycystic ovary syndrome.

    c. Diagnosis depends on detection of the tumor by pelvic examination (the majority are palpable) and on diagnostic imaging techniques.

3. **Hyperthecosis** of the ovary is probably a severe form of the polycystic ovary syndrome, but the androgen excess is more evident.

    a. **Diagnosis** depends on the histologic finding of luteinized thecal and stromal cells.

    b. **Medical therapy** is not effective, and oophorectomy may be necessary.

4. **Adrenal tumors,** either adenomas or carcinomas, may produce excess androgens with or without excess cortisol. High levels of adrenal androgens (urinary 17-ketosteroids, serum dehydroepiandrosterone) that cannot be suppressed by dexamethasone suggest this diagnosis; 24-hour urinary 17-ketosteroid levels greater than 50–100 mg strongly suggest adrenal carcinoma.

5. **Congenital adrenal hyperplasia** is discussed in the section on disorders of the adrenal gland.

6. **Idiopathic hirsutism** is a poorly understood but common condition in which hirsutism occurs in the absence of marked hormone abnormalities or menstrual dysfunction.

    a. The cause of idiopathic hirsutism is not known. It may have a familial occurrence, and it is more common in women of Mediterranean ancestry.

    b. Increased response of hair follicles to normal levels of testosterone is suspected.

    c. Patients may be managed with Vaniqa cream, spironolactone, or mechanical methods of hair removal discussed previously.

VIII **MALE REPRODUCTIVE DISORDERS AND GYNECOMASTIA**

A **Hypogonadism** in men affects two separate functions—the production of spermatozoa by the seminiferous tubules and the secretion of testosterone by the Leydig cells. The seminiferous tubule defect causes infertility; the testosterone deficiency leads to inadequate development and maintenance of secondary sexual characteristics.

1. **Physical and developmental effects**
   a. **Before puberty,** testicular failure prevents normal sexual development.
      (1) The penis and testes remain small, and spermatozoa are absent.
      (2) Facial and body hair are sparse.
      (3) The voice remains high pitched, and muscle mass and strength are diminished.
      (4) Increased growth of long bones (because of delayed epiphyseal closure) produces the "eunuchoidal habitus," in which the arm span is more than 2 inches greater than the height, and the floor-to-pubic symphysis distance is more than 2 inches greater than the symphysis-to-crown distance.
   b. **After puberty,** loss of libido and sexual potency may be the first symptoms of testicular failure. Partial regression of secondary sex characteristics may occur gradually, with slowing of facial and body hair growth and decreased muscle mass and bone density.

2. **Clinical syndromes**
   a. **Hypogonadotropic syndromes** (Table 10–17). The causes of hypogonadism are divided into **disorders of the hypothalamic–pituitary axis (hypogonadotropic hypogonadism)** and **disorders that originate with testicular damage,** with consequent feedback stimulation of LH and FSH **(hypergonadotropic hypogonadism).**
      (1) **Hypogonadotropic (secondary) hypogonadism** is characterized by deficiency of LH and FSH, with resulting testosterone deficiency and eunuchoidism. **Kallmann's syndrome** is a form of hypogonadotropic hypogonadism that is associated with midline defects such as agenesis of the olfactory lobes, anosmia, and cleft palate. It is more common in men than in women. The basic hormonal defect is in the hypothalamus rather than in the pituitary gland; this has been demonstrated by LH and FSH response to GnRH administration.
      (2) Chronic opioid use commonly results in hypogonadism in men. Opioids preferentially suppress LH production, resulting in low testosterone levels. Testosterone replacement should be considered to prevent bone loss.
      (3) **Delayed puberty** is a retrospective diagnosis. Puberty may occur spontaneously up to about 20 years of age; until this age, true hypogonadotropic hypogonadism cannot be diagnosed with certainty unless associated abnormalities such as anosmia are present. The diagnosis of delayed puberty is suggested by a family history of late maturation.
         (a) If delayed puberty is suspected, a course of therapy with low doses of testosterone can be initiated to induce pubertal changes; true puberty may be induced by this treatment.
         (b) Testosterone should be given for no more than 6 months at a time, with 6 months between courses, to avoid causing epiphyseal closure and limitation of ultimate height and to allow recognition of the onset of spontaneous puberty, if it should occur.

TABLE 10–17   Causes of Hypogonadism in Men

Hypogonadotropic Syndromes	Hypergonadotropic Syndromes
Hypopituitarism	Klinefelter's syndrome
Hypogonadotropic eunuchoidism	Testicular agenesis
Kallmann's syndrome	Cryptorchidism
Delayed puberty	Mumps orchitis, gonorrhea
Chronic opioid use	Surgery, trauma
	Radiation, chemotherapy
	Myotonic dystrophy

  b. Hypergonadotropic syndromes (primary hypogonadism)
   (1) Klinefelter's syndrome, in which the presence of two or more X chromosomes causes congenital testicular damage, occurs in approximately 1 in 400 male births.
    (a) Approximately 80% of patients have a **47,XXY karyotype.**
    (b) The testes are small (<2 cm in length), with hyalinization of the seminiferous tubules and **azoospermia.**
    (c) Leydig cell function is variable. Testosterone levels are deficient, and **eunuchoidism** is present in many, but not all, cases.
    (d) Gynecomastia is present, and LH and FSH levels are elevated, even (for unknown reasons) in patients without testosterone deficiency.
    (e) Mental deficiency is an associated finding in 25% of patients.
    (f) The only available treatment is **testosterone replacement** in those patients who require it.
   (2) Testicular agenesis is recognized by failure of pubertal development and absence of testes in the scrotum or in the inguinal canals. Loss of the testes occurs after 7–14 weeks' gestation, because absence of testicular hormones before this stage would result in a female phenotype.
   (3) Mumps orchitis affects mainly germinal cells; if the disease is bilateral, infertility may result, although this is uncommon. Testosterone production is usually unimpaired.
   (4) Cryptorchidism, especially if it is bilateral, may be associated with hypogonadism because the undescended testes are damaged by trauma or torsion.
    (a) An association between hypogonadism and cryptorchidism may exist because the cryptorchidism is sometimes a consequence of an intrinsic abnormality in the testes.
    (b) Treatment with hCG or GnRH may induce testicular descent in some cases.
   (5) Myotonic dystrophy is a syndrome consisting of myotonia, cataracts, and testicular atrophy.

 3. Therapy
  a. Testosterone deficiency. Although oral androgenic steroids are available, they do not provide fully virilizing blood levels of male hormones. Treatment of male hypogonadism is the injection of 200–400 mg of a long-acting testosterone preparation (e.g., Delatestryl or DEPO-Testosterone) every 2–4 weeks, or the use of skin patches (Testoderm, Androderm) or a gel (AndroGel, Testim) to provide transdermal testosterone absorption.
  b. Infertility. Sperm production and fertility cannot be induced in individuals with primary testicular injury. In hypogonadotropic hypogonadism, spermatogenesis can sometimes be brought about by providing the testes with adequate gonadotropic stimulation.
   (1) This can be done either by injections three times per week of hCG (which has LH activity) and human menopausal gonadotropin (which has FSH activity) or by administration via portable infusion pump of pulse doses of GnRH every 90–120 minutes.
   (2) Both of these methods are expensive and impractical for long-term use, but they have been used successfully in some highly motivated men for the several months that are necessary to induce spermatogenesis.

B **Gynecomastia** is enlargement of the male breast. In true gynecomastia, firm, sometimes tender, glandular tissue is present. The disorders that cause gynecomastia are usually associated with increased levels of estrogens, decreased levels of androgens, or both.

 1. Causes
  a. Pubertal gynecomastia is not uncommon. At 12–15 years of age, approximately two thirds of normal boys have some degree of gynecomastia, usually a small, firm subareolar nodule that disappears in most cases within 1–2 years.
   (1) In the occasional boy with persistent breast enlargement, medical treatment with the antiestrogen **tamoxifen** may be tried.
   (2) If this is ineffective, however, **reduction mammoplasty** must be considered if psychological stress is severe.
  b. Hypogonadism, either primary (hypergonadotropic) or secondary (hypogonadotropic), may be associated with gynecomastia.
  c. Refeeding after a period of starvation often leads to transient gynecomastia, which may last for several months. Renewed secretion of previously inhibited gonadotropins and sex steroids and decreased hormone inactivation by the starved liver may be contributing factors.

    d. Liver disease, especially alcoholic cirrhosis, is a common cause of gynecomastia.

      (1) Estrogen levels are increased because of accelerated conversion of androgenic precursors by peripheral tissues.

      (2) In addition, alcohol inhibits the testicular production of testosterone and the pituitary production of gonadotropins and increases hepatic metabolism of testosterone.

    e. Chronic renal failure is associated with gynecomastia, especially after the start of hemodialysis. The refeeding phenomenon may play a role, as may an increase in the ratio of estrogens to androgens in chronic renal failure.

    f. Drugs

      (1) Estrogens, commonly used to treat prostatic carcinoma, stimulate the breast directly.

      (2) Spironolactone, cimetidine, and **digitalis** also produce gynecomastia. They are believed to inhibit androgen action by displacing dihydrotestosterone from its intracellular receptor.

      (3) Marijuana binds to estrogen receptors and may cause gynecomastia through a direct estrogenic action.

      (4) Other drugs that may cause this problem include **phenothiazines, tricyclic antidepressants, methyldopa, reserpine,** and **isoniazid.**

    g. Tumors may cause gynecomastia.

      (1) Adrenal and **testicular tumors** may cause gynecomastia through the production of estrogen.

      (2) Testicular choriocarcinomas may cause gynecomastia through the secretion of hCG, which stimulates testicular estrogen production.

      (3) Other malignant tumors may cause the condition through the ectopic production of gonadotropins.

    h. Hyperthyroidism increases the conversion of androgens to estrogens in the peripheral tissues and increases the circulating level of sex hormone–binding globulin, which raises the estrogen-to-androgen ratio. These hormonal changes may cause gynecomastia in men with hyperthyroidism.

2. Evaluation and management of gynecomastia

    a. If the cause of gynecomastia is not evident from the history and physical examination, a series of hormone levels should be obtained to screen for hypogonadism (LH, FSH, total and free testosterone, prolactin), tumors of the adrenals and testicles (estradiol, HCG), and hyperthyroidism (TSH).

    b. Management may require removal of an offending drug or treatment of an underlying endocrine disorder.

Study Questions

1. A 23-year-old man with gynecomastia is found to have a 47,XXY karyotype. This patient probably also has which of the following conditions?

- A. Abnormal liver function tests
- B. Low blood levels of luteinizing hormone and follicle-stimulating hormone
- C. High blood levels of estrogen
- D. Azoospermia
- E. Enlargement of the testes

2. An 18-year-old woman is evaluated because she has never had a menstrual period. Pelvic examination is normal except that the vagina ends in a blind pouch. A karyotype is reported to be 46,XY. Which of the following diagnoses is most likely?

- A. Congenital adrenal hyperplasia
- B. Turner's syndrome
- C. Kallmann's syndrome
- D. Testicular feminization syndrome
- E. Polycystic ovary syndrome

3. A 55-year-old woman has been treated for type 2 diabetes with isophane insulin suspension (NPH), 35 U once daily before breakfast. Home glucose measurements on a typical day are as follows: 7:00 AM (fasting), 238 mg/dL; 11:00 AM, 155 mg/dL; 4:00 PM, 128 mg/dL; 8:00 PM, 125 mg/dL. Which of the following changes in insulin therapy would be reasonable?

- A. Increasing the dose of insulin
- B. Adding regular insulin to the dose of NPH
- C. Giving the dose in the evening instead of the morning
- D. Adding a dose of regular insulin before supper
- E. Adding a second dose of NPH insulin at bedtime

4. A 23-year old woman has noted a small amount of milk secretion from her nipples, and she has had no menstrual periods for the past 8 months. Serum prolactin is 78 ng/mL (normal, 5–25). Which test would be most sensitive for the diagnosis of a pituitary adenoma?

- A. Measurement of serum luteinizing hormone and follicle-stimulating hormone
- B. Visual field examination
- C. Computed tomography scan with contrast injection
- D. Magnetic resonance imaging with gadolinium injection
- E. Insulin tolerance test

5. Successful treatment of primary hyperparathyroidism in a 60-year-old woman involves surgery to remove a single parathyroid adenoma. After surgery, she has a prolonged period of hypocalcemia, which requires continuous treatment with large doses of vitamin D and calcium. After 2–3 months, the need for vitamin D and calcium subsides, and she remains normocalcemic without treatment. This woman probably had which of the following conditions?

- A. Accidental destruction of the other three parathyroid glands
- B. Removal of the wrong parathyroid gland
- C. Severe pancreatitis caused by her hyperparathyroidism
- D. Unrecognized pseudohypoparathyroidism
- E. Severe bone disease

6. A 32-year-old woman is found on gynecologic evaluation to have multiple ovarian cysts. Which of the following findings would lead you to make the diagnosis of polycystic ovary syndrome?

- A. Deepening of the voice, enlargement of the clitoris, and a high testosterone level
- B. Oligomenorrhea, obesity, a high luteinizing hormone level, and a low follicle-stimulating hormone level

C Amenorrhea, acne, a low luteinizing hormone level, and a low follicle-stimulating hormone level

D Facial hirsutism, acne, and increased urinary pregnanetriol and 17-ketosteroids

E Facial hirsutism, normal menstrual periods, and normal levels of follicle-stimulating hormone, luteinizing hormone, and testosterone

7. A 58-year-old woman complains of fatigue, weight gain, and constipation. Examination shows puffy facial features and a slow return phase of the ankle reflex. Serum TSH is 52 mU/L (high), and free T_4 is 0.3 ng/dL (low). Treatment should be started with which of the following preparations?

A Thyroid extract

B Thyroglobulin

C Thyroxine

D Triiodothyronine

E Thyroxine and triiodothyronine

8. A 45-year-old woman complains of nervousness, palpitations, and a 10-pound weight loss. Her thyroid gland is enlarged twofold, and her heart rate is 108 bpm. Free T_4 is 3.6 ng/dL (high), and TSH is undetectable. You recommend radioiodine therapy, and the patient asks you about possible complications. What is the most common complication of radioiodine therapy?

A Thyroid storm

B Subacute thyroiditis

C Thyroid cancer

D Hypothyroidism

E Leukemia

9. A 60-year-old woman complains of headaches, and an MRI of the head is performed. This study shows a 9-mm microadenoma of the pituitary gland. Which of the following hormones is most likely to be elevated?

A Growth hormone

B Adrenocorticotropic hormone

C Prolactin

D Thyroid-stimulating hormone

E Insulin-like growth factor I

10. A 19-year-old woman complains of nervousness, a 5-pound weight loss, tremors, palpitations, and sweating for the last 4 weeks. The thyroid gland is slightly enlarged but not tender. The total T_4 level is 15.3 µg/dL (normal, 4.5–12.5), and T_3 uptake is 38% (normal, 25–35), and the TSH is undetectable. The best way to differentiate between the syndrome of painless thyroiditis and Graves' disease involves which of the following findings?

A Thyroid enlargement

B Low blood thyroid-stimulating hormone levels

C Elevated blood thyroxine levels

D Low radioactive iodine uptake

E Tenderness and pain involving the thyroid gland

11. A 23-year-old man is evaluated because of a diagnosis of hypogonadism. Which of the following findings would suggest primary testicular disease rather than hypothalamic or pituitary disease?

A Anosmia

B Increased levels of follicle-stimulating hormone and luteinizing hormone

C Eunuchoidal habitus

D Loss of libido and sexual potency

E Decreased sperm number and motility

12. A 48-year-old man requires surgery to remove a tumor involving the hypothalamic area. The pituitary stalk is damaged by the surgery. Which pituitary hormone might be expected to increase rather than decrease in serum concentration?

[A] Adrenocorticotropic hormone
[B] Thyroid-stimulating hormone
[C] Growth hormone
[D] Prolactin
[E] Luteinizing hormone

13. A 35-year-old woman has an MRI of the abdomen because of abdominal pain. Unexpectedly a 1-cm adenoma is seen in the left adrenal gland. In your evaluation of the patient, which of the following findings would be most compatible with a diagnosis of primary aldosteronism?

[A] Hyponatremia
[B] Acidosis
[C] Hypotension
[D] Hyperkalemia
[E] Suppressed plasma renin activity

Directions: *The response options for Items 14–16 are the same. You will be required to select one answer for each item in the set.*

[A] Graves' disease
[B] Hypothyroidism
[C] Pregnancy
[D] Subacute thyroiditis
[E] Nontoxic goiter

For each result of thyroid function tests, select the clinical condition with which it is most likely to be associated.

14. A 31-year-old woman complains of inability to sleep, weakness, heat intolerance, and sweating. The free T_4 is elevated, and the radioiodine uptake is low.

15. A 26-year-old woman with some fatigue is found to have an elevated total T_4 level and a low T_3 resin uptake.

16. A 21-year-old woman has noted weight loss and palpitations. Her free T_4 is increased, and the radioiodine uptake at 24 hours is 62% (normal, 10%–30%).

Directions: *The response options for Items 17–21 are the same. You will be required to select one answer for each item in the set.*

[A] Stimulation of an endocrine gland by autoimmune mechanisms
[B] Destruction of an endocrine gland by tumor, trauma, or infarction
[C] Destruction of an endocrine gland by autoimmune mechanisms
[D] Excessive production of hormone by an endocrine tumor
[E] Impaired sensitivity of peripheral tissues to normal circulating levels of a hormone

For each case, select the primary pathologic process most likely to cause the patient's disorder.

17. A 55-year-old man complains of headaches, coarsening facial features, and increasing shoe size. His growth hormone and IGF-1 levels are increased.

18. A 25-year-old woman has lost 15 pounds recently and is irritable and tremulous. Her free T_4 level and radioiodine uptake are elevated.

19. A 40-year-old man has noticed darkening of his skin in the last year, as well as weakness and generalized aching of his joints. An ACTH test is performed: baseline plasma cortisol is 5 μg/dL, rising to 6 μg/dL at 1 hour after ACTH injection.

20. A 38-year-old woman has surgery to remove a pituitary macroadenoma that was causing visual impairment. Postoperatively she developed amenorrhea and fatigue, with low levels of LH, FSH, free T_4, and cortisol.

21. A 21-year-old woman presents to the emergency department complaining of abdominal pain. She states that she has been having increased urination, increased thirst, and a 10-lb weight loss. On exam she has a blood pressure of 80/60 mm Hg, rapid deep breaths, and dry mucous membranes. Which lab abnormality fit with the patient's clinical presentation?

- A Low potassium
- B Low hematocrit
- C Anion gap acidosis
- D Low serum osmolality
- E Elevated sodium

22. Match the following medications with the appropriate mechanism of action or side effect. Some may be used more than once.

- A Metformin
- B Sulfonyureas
- C Thiazolidinediones
- D α-Glucoside inhibitors

1 Increase insulin by the pancreatic beta cell
2 Decrease hepatic glucose output
3 Side effects include flatulence, abdominal discomfort, and diarrhea
4 Hypoglycemia might result
5 Increases sensitivity of muscle and fat to insulin
6 Lactic acidosis is a serious potential side affect

Answers and Explanations

1. The answer is D. The 47,XXY karyotype indicates Klinefelter's syndrome. Elevation of gonadotropin levels, small testes, and gynecomastia also are common findings in Klinefelter's syndrome.

2. The answer is D. Patients with the testicular feminization syndrome have a normal male karyotype and testes (located in the abdomen or groin) that produce testosterone. However, because there is resistance of the tissues to the effects of testosterone, the external genitalia develop as female during fetal life. Congenital adrenal hyperplasia is not associated with a short vagina and blind pouch, both of which are typical of testicular feminization. Turner's syndrome (gonadal dysgenesis) is characterized by a 45,X karyotype. Kallmann's syndrome is more common in men than in women and is often accompanied by anosmia and cleft palate. Polycystic ovary syndrome usually causes secondary, not primary, amenorrhea, and this patient has none of the other typical clinical features (e.g., oily skin, obesity, or hirsutism).

3. The answer is E. The pattern of glucose levels suggests that the dose of isophane insulin suspension (NPH) is effective during the day but does not retain its effect until the next morning. Giving more insulin in the morning or adding regular insulin would risk causing hypoglycemia in the afternoon and evening when glucose levels are already at a satisfactory level. However, a second dose of NPH at bedtime would be expected to have its maximal action in the early morning, which is the time that an increased glucose-lowering effect is desired.

4. The answer is D. MRI with gadolinium is the most sensitive test for the detection of pituitary adenomas. In fact, microadenomas may be seen in as many as 10%–20% of normal women. Oversecretion of LH and FSH is common, but many pituitary adenomas do not produce excessive amounts of these hormones. Impaired GH response to insulin-induced hypoglycemia or visual field changes would occur only in those tumors that are large enough to interfere with normal pituitary function or to compress the optic chiasm. CT scans show very small adenomas, but MRI with gadolinium is even more sensitive.

5. The answer is E. When primary hyperparathyroidism causes osteitis fibrosa cystica, the sudden correction of the primary hyperparathyroidism and consequent removal of the source of excessive PTH allows the skeleton to undergo rapid repair and remineralization, which creates a marked but self-limiting demand for calcium and phosphate. If the patient had hypoparathyroidism of this severity after surgery, the hypocalcemia would probably have been permanent, and the need for treatment would not have resolved.

6. The answer is B. Polycystic ovary syndrome is characterized by a chronic lack of ovulation associated with symptoms of androgen excess and often with obesity. Severe virilization and marked testosterone elevation are more likely to be caused by an ovarian tumor or hyperthecosis. Neither a low luteinizing hormone level nor an increased urinary pregnanetriol concentration is characteristic of the polycystic ovary syndrome. Hirsutism without other clinical or laboratory abnormalities usually is diagnosed as "idiopathic hirsutism."

7. The answer is C. Thyroxine (T_4) is the agent of choice. Thyroid extract and thyroglobulin contain varying proportions of the two thyroid hormones—T_4 and triiodothyronine (T_3)—making it difficult to adjust the dose precisely. Preparations containing T_3 must be given several times daily to maintain a normal blood level of T_3 because T_3 has a short half-life. However, T_4 has a long half-life and is converted to T_3 in the liver and elsewhere; hypothyroid patients taking the optimal dose of T_4 once daily have normal, stable blood levels of both T_4 and T_3.

8. The answer is D. Hypothyroidism is present in 50% or more of patients treated with radioiodine 10–15 years after treatment. Thyroid storm and subacute thyroiditis are rare complications. No increased incidence of thyroid cancer, leukemia, or other malignancies has been attributed to radioiodine therapy.

9. The answer is C. As many as 50% of all pituitary adenomas have been found to secrete prolactin, and blood prolactin levels should be measured in a patient suspected of having a pituitary tumor.

Acromegaly due to growth hormone excess and Cushing's disease due to adrenocorticotropic hormone excess are considerably less common, and overproduction of thyroid-stimulating hormone is rare. Insulin-like growth factor I is increased in acromegaly but is not elevated in most patients with pituitary tumors.

10. The answer is D. Low radioactive iodine uptake is the most useful finding for distinguishing painless thyroiditis from Graves' disease. Inflammation and injury to thyroid cells, as well as a lack of TSH, inhibit radioactive iodine uptake in painless thyroiditis, whereas the uninjured and immunoglobulin-stimulated thyroid cells in Graves' disease concentrate radioactive iodine at an increased rate. Enlargement of the thyroid gland and increased blood levels of thyroid hormone, with suppression of TSH, may occur in both Graves' disease and painless thyroiditis. The gland is not tender or painful in either condition.

11. The answer is B. Increased gonadotropin production indicates primary testicular failure with negative-feedback stimulation of the hypothalamic–pituitary axis. Anosmia is sometimes associated with hypothalamic failure to secrete gonadotropin-releasing hormone. Hypogonadism, whether caused by hypothalamic–pituitary disease or testicular disease, is associated with loss of libido and potency and abnormalities of sperm production. A eunuchoidal habitus results from continued growth of long bones due to delay in testosterone-induced epiphyseal closure; therefore, eunuchoidal habitus can result from either primary testicular failure or hypothalamic–pituitary disease.

12. The answer is D. Hypothalamic hormones reach the anterior pituitary gland through the portal vessels in the pituitary stalk, and injury to the stalk may remove the pituitary from the influence of the hypothalamus. Most of the hypothalamic factors are stimulatory: ACTH production is stimulated by corticotropin-releasing hormone, TSH by thyrotropin-releasing hormone, growth hormone by growth hormone–releasing hormone, and LH by gonadotropin-releasing hormone. However, the main effect of the hypothalamus on prolactin production is inhibitory, through the action of dopamine. When injury to the pituitary stalk prevents dopamine and other hypothalamic factors from reaching the pituitary gland in high concentration, prolactin production increases, in contrast to the fall in levels of other pituitary hormones.

13. The answer is E. Plasma renin activity suppression is a clinical feature of primary aldosteronism. Excess circulating levels of aldosterone increase the reabsorption of sodium, in exchange for potassium and hydrogen ions, in the distal tubules. The resulting expansion of extracellular fluid volume causes suppression of plasma renin activity and eventually causes hypertension. The loss of potassium and hydrogen ions causes a tendency toward metabolic alkalosis.

14–16. The answers are: 14—D, 15—C, 16—A. In subacute thyroiditis, injured thyroid follicular cells release thyroid hormone, raising the blood level of T_4. Radioactive iodine uptake is low, however, because the injured follicular cells are unable to trap iodine normally. In addition, thyroid-stimulating hormone is suppressed by the increased level of circulating thyroid hormone, and this further reduces the radioactive iodine uptake.

In pregnancy, the high estrogen levels cause increased production of T_4-binding globulin. This raises the serum level of total T_4 and lowers the T_3 resin uptake. However, patients remain euthyroid because the serum free T_4 level remains normal.

In Graves' disease, the follicular cells trap increased amounts of iodine and produce increased amounts of thyroid hormone. Therefore, both the radioactive iodine uptake and the serum T_4 level are elevated. This combination of findings indicates hyperthyroidism, caused either by Graves' disease or by toxic nodular goiter.

17–20. The answers are: 17—D, 18—A, 19—C, 20—B. The usual cause of acromegaly is a GH-secreting pituitary adenoma. Rarely, GH-releasing hormone production by an islet-cell adenoma may cause acromegaly.

Graves' disease is caused by abnormal stimulation of the thyroid gland by thyroid-stimulating immunoglobulin. This immunoglobulin G antibody binds to receptors for thyroid-stimulating hormone. This hormone then stimulates growth and hormone production by the thyroid follicular cells.

Addison's disease is most commonly caused by atrophy of the adrenal cortex. Antiadrenal antibodies are often present. Other evidence of autoimmunity such as antibodies against other tissues and the presence of other autoimmune diseases also are common findings. Hemorrhage into the adrenals and infectious agents (e.g., tuberculosis) are less common causes of Addison's disease.

Pituitary tumors may compress normal tissue, impairing its function. Surgical removal of the tumor may further damage the hypothalamus and pituitary gland. Ischemic infarction at childbirth (Sheehan's syndrome) and various destructive, infectious, and granulomatous lesions also cause hypopituitarism.

21. **The answer is C.** The patient most likely had diabetic ketoacidosis (DKA), a condition in type 1 diabetes characterized by a lack of insulin that led to hyperglycemia and other metabolic derangements. DKA results in anion gap metabolic acidosis. The liver produces more ketone bodies than the body can metabolize. The anion gap reflects an elevation of the acetoacetate and β-hydroxybutyrate in the plasma. Serum potassium levels may be elevated initially, but often patients have a low body store and require repletion. As the acidosis corrects, potassium will shift into cells in response to insulin. Patients may appear to have an elevated hematocrit secondary to hemoconcentration. Serum osmolality is often elevated and serum sodium is diluted secondary to osmotic pull of the glucose that shifts fluid into the intravascular space.

22. **The answers are: 1–B; 2–A; 3–D; 4–B and C; 5–C; 6–A.** Sulfonylurea derivative bind to receptors on the β cell in the pancreas, increasing insulin secretion. Binding of the β-cell receptors closes potassium channels, opens calcium channels, and creates an influx of calcium into the cell.

Metformin decreases hepatic glucose output. Hypoglycemia does not occur when metformin is used alone because it does not stimulate insulin secretion.

The α-glucosidase inhibitors delay absorption of carbohydrates until they reach the distal small bowel and colon. This results in the common side effects of these drugs: flatulence, abdominal discomfort, and diarrhea.

Both sulfonylureas and thiazolidinediones can cause hypoglycemia. Sulfonylureas stimulate insulin secretion, and thiazolidinediones increase sensitivity to insulin in the peripheral tissue.

Thiazolidinediones such as rosiglitazone and pioglitazone increase sensitivity to in insulin in muscle and fat.

Metformin is contraindicated in patients with renal failure, liver disease, and alcoholism, as it may potentially lead to lactic acidosis. There have also been cases of lactic acidosis in patients on metformin after administration of intravenous contrast dye for certain procedures. This may occur if the renal function of the patient declines after exposure to contrast. Metformin should be held 48–72 hours after a patient receives contrast to prevent this complication.

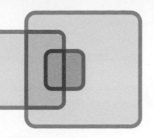

chapter 11

Rheumatic Diseases

ESTEBAN GALLEGO · TAREQ ABOU-KHAMIS · RAYMOND FLORES

I   APPROACH TO THE PATIENT WITH JOINT PAIN

A **A thorough history and physical examination** are the cornerstones in the evaluation of patients with joint complaints (Figure 11–1).

1. **Step 1.** Is the pain joint-centered or localized in the periarticular tissues involving muscle, nerve, bursa, tendons, or ligaments?

2. **Step 2.** Is the arthritis inflammatory or noninflammatory? An important clue in making this distinction is the duration of morning stiffness. Morning stiffness lasting more than 1 hour is suggestive of an inflammatory arthritis (e.g., rheumatoid arthritis), whereas stiffness lasting less than 30 minutes is suggestive of a noninflammatory arthritis (e.g., osteoarthritis).

3. **Step 3.** How many joints are affected? What is the pattern of joint involvement? The answers to these questions also provide important diagnostic clues. For example, if the pattern of joint involvement is asymmetric, it is more likely that the patient has a seronegative spondyloarthropathy, especially if there is associated inflammatory back pain. If the polyarthritis is symmetric, the differential diagnosis should include rheumatoid arthritis, systemic lupus erythematosus (SLE), polymyositis, and scleroderma.

B **Laboratory tests**   (Online Tables 11–1 and 11–2)

II   APPROACH TO THE PATIENT WITH LOW BACK PAIN

(Online Figure 11–2 and Online Table 11–3)

III   RHEUMATOID ARTHRITIS

A **Definition**   Rheumatoid arthritis (RA) is a chronic, immunologically mediated inflammatory disorder of unknown cause that is typified by synovial cell proliferation and inflammation with subsequent destruction of adjacent articular tissue. The presentation is characterized by polyarticular, symmetric joint involvement, as well as characteristic extra-articular involvement. **Rheumatoid factor** and **anti–cyclic citrullinated peptide (CCP)** frequently are present in the serum of affected individuals [Online I B 2].

B **Epidemiology**

1. **Prevalence and sex distribution.** As many as 1% of adults may have rheumatoid arthritis, depending on the criteria used for diagnosis. Clinically meaningful forms of disease are less common—0.5% of women and 0.1% of men have forms of the illness that require ongoing treatment.

2. **HLA associations.** There is an increased prevalence of the B cell alloantigen HLA-DR4 in patients with rheumatoid arthritis. Evidence also suggests that similar amino acid sequences coded by the third hypervariable region of the DR β chain may explain disease association with HLA-DR4, -DR1, -Dw4, -Dw14, and -Dw15. HLA-DR4 positivity also is a marker for more severe rheumatoid arthritis.

3. **Seropositivity for rheumatoid factor.** Patients who have rheumatoid factor in their serum appear to have a different illness from patients who are seronegative. Seropositive patients tend

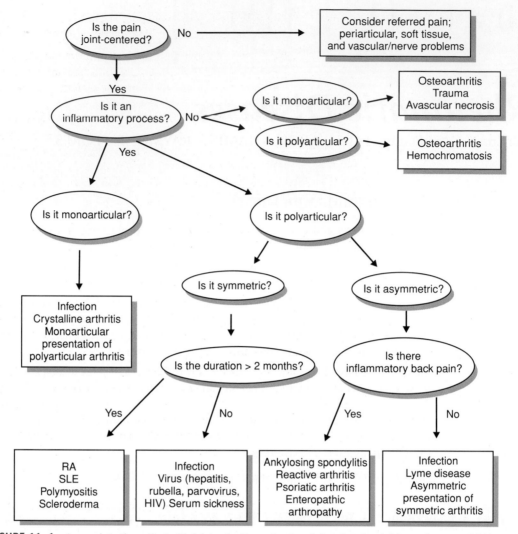

FIGURE 11–1 Approach to the patient with joint pain. The evaluation of chronic polyarthritis requires a careful history and physical examination for identification of systemic features typical of other illnesses that can cause arthritis. Selected laboratory and radiographic testing also can be helpful. RA, rheumatoid arthritis; HIV, human immunodeficiency virus; SLE, systemic lupus erythematosus.

to have more severe disease, more erosions, and more extra-articular features. Anti-CCP is more specific than rheumatoid factor and is more likely to be positive in early RA.

C Etiology   No single factor or agent is known to cause rheumatoid arthritis. Presumably, an initial insult (possibly infectious) interacting with the host's genetically established immune responses determines whether an initial synovitis is suppressed or perpetuated.

1. **Extra-articular agent.** The earliest inflammatory changes in the rheumatoid joint involve inflammation and occlusion of small subsynovial vessels, suggesting that the agent is carried in the circulation to the joint.

2. **Infectious agent.** An infectious etiology is suggested because virus-like particles often are present in synovial biopsies early in the disease course and because polyarthritis occurs in association with several human and animal bacterial or viral illnesses. However, no direct evidence of infection has been discovered. Symmetric inflammatory arthritis can occur in patients who have parvovirus or rubella virus infections, although the joint findings are not typically persistent.

3. **Genetic factors.** A genetic susceptibility to altered immune responses probably is important in rheumatoid arthritis. There is no known association of HLA-A or HLA-B haplotypes with the disease, but a significant association exists between rheumatoid arthritis and the presence of HLA-DR4 and related alloantigens of the major histocompatibility complex (MHC). The

TABLE 11–4 The 1987 American Rheumatism Association Revised Criteria for the Classification of Rheumatoid Arthritis

Criterion	Definition
1. Morning stiffness	Morning stiffness in and around the joints, lasting at least 1 hour before maximal improvement
2. Arthritis of three or more joint areas	At least three joint areas simultaneously have had soft-tissue swelling or fluid (not bony overgrowth alone) observed by a physician; the 14 possible areas are right or left PIP, MCP, wrist, elbow, knee, ankle, and MTP joints
3. Arthritis of hand joints	At least one area swollen (as defined above) in a wrist, MCP, or PIP joint
4. Symmetric arthritis	Simultaneous involvement of the same joint areas (as defined in No. 2) on both sides of the body (bilateral involvement of PIPs, MCPs, or MTPs is acceptable without absolute symmetry)
5. Rheumatoid nodules	Subcutaneous nodules over bony prominences, or extensor surfaces, or in juxta-articular regions, observed by a physician
6. Serum rheumatoid factor	Demonstration of abnormal amounts of serum rheumatoid factor by any method for which the result has been positive in <5% of normal control subjects
7. Radiographic changes	Radiographic changes typical of rheumatoid arthritis on posteroanterior hand and wrist radiographs, which must include erosions or unequivocal bony decalcification localized in or most marked adjacent to the involved joints (osteoarthritis changes alone do not qualify)

For classification purposes, a patient is said to have rheumatoid arthritis if he or she has satisfied at least four of these seven criteria. Criteria 1 through 4 must have been present for at least 6 weeks. Patients with two clinical diagnoses are not excluded. Designation as classic, definite, or probable rheumatoid arthritis is **not** to be made.

MCP, metacarpophalangeal; MTP, metatarsophalangeal; PIP, proximal interphalangeal.

Reprinted from Arnett FC, Edworth SM, Bloch DA, et al. American Rheumatism Association1987 revised criteria for the classification of rheumatoid arthritis. *Arthritis Rheum* 1988;31:315.

presence of these and other genetically coded immune response alloantigens may be important in modulating the host's cellular and humoral immune responses to potential etiologic agents.

4. Effects of Epstein–Barr virus on the immune response. Rheumatoid arthritis patients have a defect in their ability to regulate B cells infected with Epstein–Barr virus. The virus may act as a polyclonal activator of B cell autoantibody production in rheumatoid arthritis and, as such, may play a role in perpetuating (not initiating) the disease.

D Pathogenesis (Online III D and Online Figure 11–3)

E Clinical features

1. **Synovitis**
   a. **Articular involvement.** Fairly symmetric, bilateral joint involvement is typical, often sparing the distal interphalangeal (DIP) joints of the hands. Metacarpophalangeal (MCP), proximal interphalangeal (PIP), and wrist joint involvement are so common as to be part of the American Rheumatism Association (ARA) revised criteria for disease diagnosis (Table 11–4).
   b. **Tendon and ligament involvement.** Synovial linings outside joints can be involved as well.
      (1) **Palmar flexor tendinitis** can cause carpal tunnel syndrome.
      (2) **Rotator cuff tendinitis** can cause shoulder pain and limitation of motion.
      (3) **Atlantoaxial ligament involvement** in the cervical spine can lead to instability between the C1 and C2 vertebrae and potential neurologic complaints.

2. **Extra-articular features** (Table 11–5) more often exist in patients who are seropositive for rheumatoid factor and patients who have more severe and established disease.
   a. **Rheumatoid nodules** are the most common features of extra-articular disease and are found in 20%–25% of patients. These firm, subcutaneous masses typically are found in areas of repetitive trauma (e.g., the extensor surfaces of the forearm), although they also can appear in the viscera (e.g., lungs).
   b. **Eye involvement** also is common. **Keratoconjunctivitis sicca** is seen in 10%–15% of rheumatoid arthritis patients who have a secondary form of Sjögren's syndrome [see XI]. The often subtle inflammation of scleritis or episcleritis occurs less commonly.
   c. **Other organ involvement** is noted in Table 11–5.

TABLE 11–5	Extra-articular Features of Rheumatoid Arthritis	

Skin
Nodules (20%–25% of patients)
Vasculitis (purpura)

Eye
Sicca complex
(10%–15% of patients)
Episcleritis
Scleritis

Heart
Pericarditis
Myocarditis (rare)
Valve dysfunction (rare)

Lung
Pleural effusion
Interstitial fibrosis
Nodules

Nerve
Entrapment (carpal tunnel syndrome)
Vasculitis
Distal sensory neuropathy
Mononeuritis

Blood
Anemia of chronic disease
Thrombocytosis
Felty's syndrome

Metabolism
Amyloidosis

Vessels
Vasculitis
Skin
Nerve
Viscera (rare)

F **Diagnosis** Rheumatoid arthritis is a sustained, inflammatory polyarthritis that typically is symmetric in distribution. It is a diagnosis of exclusion of other forms of polyarthritis, which it may imitate. The patient must have arthritis for at least 6 weeks to eliminate viral syndromes or other causes of nonsustained polyarthritis. Finding rheumatoid factor in the serum is useful in patients who have other features of inflammatory polyarthritis, but as many as 40% of patients with rheumatoid arthritis do not have this marker initially. Anti-CCP antibody may be present earlier and is more specific than rheumatoid factor. New American College of Rheumatology (ACR) criteria regarding diagnosis and management of RA are anticipated within a year.

1. **History.** Patients with rheumatoid arthritis often have **prolonged** (>1 hour) **morning stiffness. Pain in involved joints** typically is worse in the morning. **Constitutional complaints** (weight loss, anorexia, and fatigue) are common.

2. **Physical examination.** Classically involved joints are the **wrists** and the **MCP** and **PIP joints of the hand;** DIP joints are typically spared, as is the axial skeleton except for the cervical spine. **Soft-tissue swelling,** rather than bony enlargement, is typical around involved joints, unless secondary degenerative changes have occurred; limitation of joint motion and warmth may be noted. **Rheumatoid nodules** often are present in highly expressed disease; they can be found over extensor prominences, especially near the olecranon (🔗 Online Figure 11–4).

3. **Laboratory findings.** The complete blood count (CBC) may reveal a **normocytic, normochromic anemia** of chronic disease, leukocytosis, and thrombocytosis. These findings along with an increased erythrocyte sedimentation rate (ESR) reflect chronic inflammation.

4. **Rheumatoid factor** and **anti-CCP antibody** (🔗 Online I B 2). Synovial fluid findings reflect mild-to-moderate inflammation; leukocyte counts are 5000–25,000/mm³ and consist mainly of neutrophils.

5. **Radiographic findings.** Early characteristics include **soft-tissue swelling** and loss of bone in periarticular areas (**periarticular osteopenia**). Signs of sustained inflammation include loss of bone at joint margins (**erosions**) and diffuse **joint space narrowing** as a result of cartilage loss (🔗 Online Figures 11–5 and 11–6A).

6. **Differential diagnosis** (see Figure 11–1). Because rheumatoid arthritis is one of many illnesses characterized by chronic polyarticular inflammation, diagnosis relies on excluding other such illnesses and searching for symmetric periarticular soft-tissue swelling and inflammatory characteristics of rheumatoid arthritis.

   a. **Nonarticular disorders.** Fibromyalgia is a syndrome of generalized aching and tenderness in specific soft tissue areas, without joint involvement or inflammation. Tendon, neurologic, and vascular complaints also may mimic joint pain.

b. Noninflammatory disorders
  (1) Osteoarthritis usually causes bony rather than soft-tissue swelling, and the involved joints typically are the DIP and PIP joints of the hand, the hips, and the knees. The lumbar and cervical spine can be involved as well. Constitutional and inflammatory complaints are absent, and synovial fluid leukocyte counts are less than 2000/mm^3.
  (2) Metabolic disorders (e.g., calcium pyrophosphate deposition [CPPD], hemochromatosis, and Wilson's disease) cause bony degenerative change in atypical joints (e.g., MCP joints).
c. Axial joint inflammation. Inflammation of the axial spine (especially the sacroiliac joints) is characteristic of the spondyloarthropathies, and inflammatory back pain due to **sacroiliitis** should be sought. Inflammatory back pain is insidious, day-after-day pain starting in the sacroiliac area and typically associated with prolonged morning stiffness. It is worsened with rest and improved by exercise, the opposite of mechanical low back pain. The absence of sacroiliac joint involvement does not rule out these disorders, but its presence makes spondyloarthropathy likely.
d. Oligoarticular presentations. Certain illnesses must be considered more strongly when the initial inflammatory presentation involves four or fewer joints and is asymmetric. These disorders include crystal diseases, infectious arthritis (e.g., Lyme disease, gonococcemia, endocarditis, and rheumatic fever), and spondyloarthropathies (e.g., reactive arthritis, psoriatic arthritis).
e. Polyarticular presentations. It also is important to consider inflammatory disorders that initially involve four or more joints and are fairly symmetric. Although rheumatoid arthritis is the prototype, many other illnesses must be distinguished, based on clinical features or organ involvement not typical of rheumatoid arthritis. Detailed history and physical examination with basic laboratory data are critical in distinguishing among disorders that feature polyarthritis.
  (1) Other rheumatic diseases (e.g., lupus, scleroderma, polymyositis/dermatomyositis, polymyalgic rheumatica [PMR], and vasculitis) are distinguished by the features of the primary illness.
  (2) Viral disorders (e.g., rubella, hepatitis B virus, and parvovirus infection) are distinguished by a typical rash, serologic markers, or organ involvement.
  (3) Malignancies may manifest as long-bone pain, digital clubbing, and periostitis mimicking polyarthritis (hypertrophic osteoarthropathy) or as paraneoplastic polyarthritis.
  (4) Sarcoidosis exhibits mediastinal adenopathy on chest radiograph and usually erythema nodosum when it includes a polyarthritis.
  (5) Amyloidosis is associated with Congo red–positive deposits in typical organs, subcutaneous tissue, and joints.

G Therapy   In all patients with rheumatoid arthritis, an attempt is made to control pain and reduce inflammation without causing undesirable side effects. Preservation of joint function and the ability to maintain lifestyle are important long-term goals.

1. Nonpharmacologic therapy
  a. Patient education. Educating patients about the disease process is particularly important in chronic diseases such as rheumatoid arthritis in which compliance with instructions and drug treatment is critical to the outcome.
    (1) Description of the illness. The various disease courses of rheumatoid arthritis must be described, emphasizing that most patients do well if they are treated appropriately. The chronicity and intermittency of symptoms must be discussed so that patients understand that spontaneous fluctuations in an extended disease course are normal. Patients must be educated about the systemic nature of the disease process so that both they and their families understand that fatigue, malaise, and weight loss often accompany this illness.
    (2) Rest and exercise. Patients should be advised to rest or splint acutely involved joints to reduce inflammation. Brief periods of bed rest may be useful in patients with severe polyarticular exacerbations, and regular naps may help patients deal with the fatigue of rheumatoid arthritis. Conversely, exercises to strengthen muscles surrounding involved joints should be encouraged when the arthritis is under good control. All joints should be put through a full range of motion once daily to prevent contractures.
  b. Physical medicine
    (1) Patients may benefit from coordination of their nonpharmacologic treatment by **physiatrists (rehabilitation physicians).**

    (2) Physical therapists can help patients strengthen weakened muscle groups to protect damaged joints. They can show patients range-of-motion exercises that prevent joint contractures.

    (3) Occupational therapists can help patients obtain devices to assist them, can construct splints for involved joints, and can aid in rehabilitating patients for activities of daily living and employment.

2. Pharmacologic therapy. Nonsteroidal anti-inflammatory drugs (NSAIDs) and corticosteroids are often used to provide relatively prompt control of pain and inflammation, but these drugs do not alter disease progression. Although the course of rheumatoid arthritis can be variable, most patients undergo a relentless progressive course requiring the use of disease-modifying antirheumatic drugs (DMARDs). Corticosteroids, which are not viewed as first- or second-line therapies, often are used intra-articularly for disease flare-ups or orally to help patients who are waiting for a DMARD to take effect.

  a. NSAIDs. Aspirin is the prototypic drug of this class. Nonacetylated salicylates also have been developed, which cause less suppression of prostaglandin synthesis.

    (1) Mechanism of action. The primary mechanism of action is the inhibition of cyclooxygenase, with a resultant decrease in prostaglandin production. More recent data have shown that cyclooxygenase exists in two isoforms: COX-1 and COX-2. COX-1 is expressed constitutively in monocytes/macrophages, the central nervous system (CNS), gastric mucosa, kidneys, and platelets, where it is responsible for many of the "housekeeping" activities. However, COX-2 is tightly regulated and produced during inflammation. Most of the available traditional NSAIDs inhibit both COX-1 and COX-2.

    (2) Use. NSAIDs are used to control pain and inflammation by the mechanisms explained previously. Most patients use them in combination with DMARDs.

    (3) Toxicity. Because the majority of NSAIDs inhibit both COX-1 and COX-2, they are more likely to produce gastrointestinal ulceration. Typical toxicities include dyspepsia, peptic ulcers (primarily of the stomach), hypertension, renal dysfunction, and bleeding. Some patients are placed on misoprostol or omeprazole to reduce the risk of ulcers. Clinical hepatitis and bone marrow toxicity are very rare. The COX-2 agents have been shown to have a lower incidence of peptic ulceration and do not inhibit platelet function.

    (4) COX-2 inhibitors. Celecoxib is a COX-2–specific inhibitor. This agent is purported to have a lower incidence of gastrointestinal ulceration than traditional NSAIDs and, because of the lack of effect on platelets, can be used in patients on anticoagulation. Celecoxib must be used with caution in patients with renal insufficiency, and it also may cause increased fluid retention. Recent data suggested an increased cardiovascular mortality in patients receiving rofecoxib and valdecoxib, leading to the withdrawal of these agents from the market by the U.S. Food and Drug Administration (FDA). Sulfa-allergic patients should not take celecoxib.

  b. Corticosteroids. These drugs have potent anti-inflammatory effects but equally potent and predictable toxicities. They are used most commonly in rheumatoid arthritis to control serious extra-articular manifestations (e.g., vasculitis).

    (1) Systemic administration. In rare situations such as severe progressive disease, prednisone doses no higher than 5–10 mg once daily in the morning may be used to allow continued functioning. Continual attempts to taper the dose should be made.

    (2) Local instillation. Injectable corticosteroid preparations can be instilled into one or two joints inflamed "out of phase" with other involved joints. These injections should be performed only occasionally because cartilage loss may result from frequent injections into the same joint.

  c. Traditional DMARDs. Disease-modifying antirheumatic drugs are critical in the armamentarium in the treatment of rheumatoid arthritis. These agents need to be started early in the course of disease (ideally within 3 months). The hallmark of these agents is their ability to halt progression of disease, such as the development of erosions. Commonly used DMARDs in the treatment of rheumatoid arthritis are listed in Table 11–6. Although side effects of many of these medications may be serious, in most instances they are mild, predictable, and can be managed. In most cases, the risk of ongoing progressive disease outweighs the potential risk of medication toxicity. Each of the agents may be used alone or in combination.

TABLE 11–6 Disease-Modifying Antirheumatic Drugs Used in the Treatment of Rheumatoid Arthritis

Agent	Mechanism of Action	Side Effects/Potential Toxicity	Monitoring
Hydroxychloroquine sulfate	Unknown, but likely inhibits lysosomal enzymes and macrophage function	Macular damage	Eye examination every 6 months to 1 year
Methotrexate	Inhibits dihydrofolate reductase, thereby inhibiting purine (DNA) synthesis	Myelosuppression, hepatic fibrosis/ cirrhosis, pulmonary inflammation/ fibrosis, stomatitis	CBC, AST, ALT, creatinine, albumin every month for 6 months then every 6–8 weeks; baseline CXR and hepatitis profile
Leflunomide	Inhibits dihydro-orotate dehydrogenase, thereby inhibiting pyrimidine (DNA) synthesis	Diarrhea, elevated liver enzymes, alopecia, teratogenicity requiring elimination protocol with cholestyramine	Same as MTX but no baseline CXR
Sulfasalazine	Inhibits prostaglandins and chemotaxis	Gastrointestinal intolerance, hematologic cytopenias, hepatotoxicity, contraindicated if sulfa allergic	CBC every 2–4 weeks for first 3 months then every 3 months Baseline G6PD testing
Azathioprine	A prodrug converted to 6-mercaptopurine, subsequently converted into thiopurine nucleotides, decreasing de novo synthesis of purines	Myelosuppression, hepatotoxicity, lymphoproliferative disorders; caution with concurrent use of allopurinol	CBC every 1–2 weeks with changes in dose and every 1–3 months thereafter
Cyclosporine	Inhibits T cell activation	Renal insufficiency, anemia, hypertension hypertrichosis, paresthesias, gingival hypertrophy; caution: multiple medication interactions	Creatinine every 2 weeks until stable then monthly, periodic CBC, LFTs

ALT, alanine aminotransferase; AST, aspartate aminotransferase; CBC, complete blood count; CXR, chest x-ray; LFTs, liver function tests; MTX, methotrexate.

(1) **Monotherapy**

(a) **Methotrexate** is considered the gold standard for the treatment of rheumatoid arthritis, usually given as a weekly oral dose. At higher doses, subcutaneous injections of methotrexate may be given to improve absorption and diminish side effects. Concurrent daily folic acid administration helps prevent common side effects, including mucosal ulcers, dyspepsia, and cytopenias. The use of leucovorin may be necessary if the side effects do not respond to the folic acid. The starting dose of methotrexate is 7.5–10 mg weekly, escalating to a maximum of 25 mg weekly. If a patient has underlying liver disease or pulmonary disease or uses alcohol, methotrexate may not be appropriate.

(b) **Leflunomide** acts similarly to methotrexate and requires essentially the same monitoring strategy except that there is no risk of pulmonary toxicity; thus, it is often used when methotrexate cannot be used, such as in a patient with underlying pulmonary disease.

(c) **Sulfasalazine,** although not approved by the FDA for use in rheumatoid arthritis, has been used because of its modest effectiveness and rather low incidence of toxicity. In Europe it is typically used as a first-line agent.

(d) Less commonly used agents as monotherapy in the treatment of RA include **gold, azathioprine,** and **hydroxychloroquine sulfate.**

(2) **Combination therapy** is used if patients have had a suboptimal response to monotherapy. Commonly used combinations are as follows.

(a) **Methotrexate and hydroxychloroquine sulfate**

(b) **Methotrexate and hydroxychloroquine sulfate and sulfasalazine**

(c) **Methotrexate and leflunomide**

(d) **Methotrexate and cyclosporine**

TABLE 11–7	Biologic Disease-Modifying Antirheumatic Drugs Used in the Treatment of Rheumatoid Arthritis		
Agent	**Mechanism**	**Dose and Routine**	**Side Effects**
Etanercept	Recombinant fusion protein binds to soluble TNF receptor and leukotriene (LT)	25 mg SQ twice weekly or 50 mg once weekly	Flu-like symptoms, injection-site reactions, infections, exacerbation of heart failure, possible demyelination, unknown long-term malignancy risk, autoimmune phenomena
Infliximab	Chimeric monoclonal antibody that binds TNF	3 mg/kg IV over 2 hours every 8 weeks	Infusion may be associated with fever, nausea, flushing, hypertension, or hypotension; infection, autoimmune phenomena, exacerbation of congestive heart failure, possible demyelination, unknown long-term malignancy risk
Adalimumab	Recombinant human IgG1 monoclonal antibody that binds TNF	40 mg SQ every other week	Injection-site reactions, infections, lupus-like symptoms, unknown long-term malignancy risk
Golimumab	Human monoclonal antibody that binds to TNF	50 mg SQ monthly	Injection-site reactions, infections, unknown long-term malignancy risk
Certolizumab pegol	Pegylated humanized antibody Fab' fragment of TNF monoclonal antibody selectively neutralizes TNF	Initial: 400 mg, repeat dose at 2 and 4 weeks Maintenance: 200 mg every other week	Injection-site reactions, infections, unknown long-term malignancy risk
Anakinra	Binds to interleukin–1 receptors (IL-1RA)	100 mg SQ daily	Injection-site reactions, infections, unknown long-term malignancy risk
Tocilizumab	Monoclonal antibody to interleukin-6 receptor (IL-6 RA)	Start 4 mg/kg every 4 weeks, may be increased to 8 mg/kg	Injection-site reactions, infections, unknown long-term malignancy risk, elevated liver function tests, elevated low-density lipoprotein, gastric perforations
Rituximab	Chimeric monoclonal antibody that binds CD20 on B cells	1000 mg IV on days 1 + 15, premedicate with a corticosteroid	Infections, hypotension, rash, malignancy
Abatacept	Recombinant fusion protein that modulates T cell activity by binding CD80 and CD86	IV dose by weight	Infections, infusion reactions such as dizziness and headache

IV, intravenous; SQ, subcutaneously; TNF, tumor necrosis factor.

    d. Biologic DMARDs. As the pathogenesis of rheumatoid arthritis and the various immune and inflammatory mediators have been identified, novel agents in the treatment of RA have been developed. These include the development of tumor necrosis factor (TNF) antagonists, anti-cytokine therapy, and B cell modulators. The common biologic DMARDs available for use are listed in Table 11–7.

    (1) TNF inhibitors. TNF is a proinflammatory cytokine that is synthesized by a variety of cell types. Normally, small amounts of TNF are present, but overproduction triggers a cascade of inflammatory reactions. **Etanercept, infliximab, adalimumab, golimumab,** and **certolizumab pegol** are FDA approved for the treatment of RA. Each of these agents has been shown to be effective in reducing signs and symptoms and inhibiting the progression of structural damage in rheumatoid arthritis.

      (a) Use. TNF inhibitors may be used alone or in combination (usually with methotrexate).

      (b) Safety considerations. Serious infectious and opportunistic infections (tuberculosis [TB]) have been seen with all of the TNF antagonists. TNF has been shown to be necessary in granuloma formation that is critical in the control of TB. Thus, inhibition of TNF has been associated with reactivation of TB. Screening for TB is recommended before initiating treatment with these agents.

    (2) Anticytokine therapy. IL-1RA (anakinra) and a newly released **IL-6 antagonist (tocilizumab)** control RA through a mechanism different from that of the TNF-blocking agents but have similar safety concerns, including increased risk of infections (not TB), neutropenia, and the potential development of malignancies. In addition, tocilizumab has been

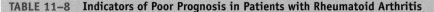

TABLE 11–8	Indicators of Poor Prognosis in Patients with Rheumatoid Arthritis

Many persistently inflamed joints
Poor functional status (ascertained from health-assessment questionnaires)
Low formal education level
Rheumatoid factor positivity
Human leukocyte antigen-DR4 positivity
Extra-articular disease
Persistently elevated acute-phase reactants (e.g., erythrocyte sedimentation rate)
Radiographic evidence of erosions

associated with increased risk of gastric perforations and lipid abnormalities. No data as yet suggest higher risk of demyelination or development of congestive heart failure.

(3) **Anti–B cell therapy.** B cells play a key role in the development of inflammation in RA, in addition to the destructive T cells. Therefore, an agent that can control the effects of B cells may be beneficial to these patients. Rituximab is a chimerical monoclonal antibody that binds CD20, a B cell surface antigen. This leads to a decrease in the B cell population and has shown beneficial effects at controlling inflammation in RA.

(4) **T Cell–targeted therapy.** CTLA4 Ig (abatacept) prevents CD28 from binding to its counter receptor CD80/CD86, causing inactivation of pathogenic T cells.

e. **Assessment of response.** The effectiveness of drug therapy is judged by assessing the reduction in a number of factors: morning stiffness, constitutional complaints, number of swollen and tender joints, and ESR. Sometimes, improvement in anemia of chronic disease and resolution of thrombocytosis occurs. Indices that measure a patient's disease activity (Disease Activity Score, DAS-28) or ability to perform activities of daily living (Health Assessment Questionnaire) also are used.

f. As new therapies are being introduced, the treatment strategy has been evolving. In 2008, the American College of Rheumatology revised the management guidelines.

3. **Surgery.** Arthroplasties or total joint replacements may be appropriate to relieve pain or help restore function in structurally damaged joints.

H **Prognosis**

1. **Prognostic factors** (Table 11–8). Inability to control disease activity and the presence of several of these indicators suggest a poor prognosis and the need for more aggressive therapy, perhaps including combinations of second-line agents and low-dose oral glucocorticoids.

2. **Mortality.** Many patients with rheumatoid arthritis have a reasonably good prognosis if they respond well to treatment. Adequate early response to the use of NSAIDs or antimalarials, with or without corticosteroids, is a favorable prognostic sign. However, recent epidemiologic studies suggest that patients with severe and persistent disease have increased mortality rates. In those with the most highly expressed forms of rheumatoid arthritis, mortality rates approach those found in stage IV congestive heart failure (CHF) or stage IV Hodgkin's disease. The increase in mortality appears to be the result of organ compromise caused by extra-articular features (e.g., interstitial lung disease, cardiac complications, and vasculitis), complications of drug therapy, and infection.

IV **SPONDYLOARTHROPATHIES**

A **Unifying characteristics** (see Table 11–9). The spondyloarthropathies are a group of inflammatory arthritides distinct from rheumatoid arthritis, including ankylosing spondylitis, reactive arthritis, psoriatic arthritis, and arthritis associated with inflammatory bowel disease. Typical distinguishing features include the following.

1. **Clinical features**
a. **Skeletal**
(1) **Axial.** As a group, the spondyloarthropathies prominently involve the axial skeleton, particularly the **sacroiliac joints.** With the exception of the cervical spine, the axial skeleton is not commonly involved in rheumatoid arthritis.

TABLE 11–9   Distinguishing Characteristics of Spondyloarthropathies

Axial skeleton inflammation
Enthesis inflammation, often asymmetric
Characteristic extraskeletal features
Uveitis or conjunctivitis
Urethritis
Inflammatory bowel lesions
Psoriasis-like rashes
Association with Human leukocyte antigen–B27
Absence of rheumatoid factor

      (2) **Appendicular.** Inflammatory arthritis of the appendicular skeleton also occurs in these disorders, but the involvement tends to be **oligoarticular** and **asymmetric.** In contrast, rheumatoid arthritis usually is polyarticular and symmetric.

      (3) **Enthesis.** In both the axial and appendicular skeletons, inflammation of tendon and ligament sites of attachment to bone is common (e.g., costochondritis, Achilles tendinitis, and plantar fasciitis). Tendon inflammation is less prominent in rheumatoid arthritis.

   b. Extraskeletal

      (1) **Nodules.** Rheumatoid nodules are not found in the spondyloarthropathies.

      (2) **Internal organ involvement.** The typical eye involvement in the spondyloarthropathies (conjunctivitis and anterior uveitis), cardiac involvement (aortitis), and genitourinary involvement (urethritis and prostatitis) are much different from the usual extra-articular features of rheumatoid arthritis.

   c. Laboratory findings. Several cardinal laboratory features of chronic inflammation (i.e., anemia, thrombocytosis, and elevated gamma globulin levels) are not commonly present in the spondyloarthropathies as they are in rheumatoid arthritis. Although the ESR may be increased, it is not a good measure of disease activity. Rheumatoid factor typically is absent.

   d. Radiographic findings. The characteristic changes seen radiographically are those of periosteal new bone formation at the site of the enthesopathic lesions [see IV A 3], both at axial locations (in the form of **syndesmophytes**) and appendicular locations. Although erosive changes can occur, they occur most typically in the axial skeleton (in the hips, sacroiliac joints, and shoulders).

   e. Therapeutic response. Several second-line agents commonly used in treating rheumatoid arthritis (e.g., gold and hydroxychloroquine) have no proven role in the treatment of spondyloarthropathy, with the exception of psoriatic peripheral arthropathy. Sulfasalazine and methotrexate are used for both rheumatoid arthritis and the appendicular arthritis of the spondyloarthropathies. TNF inhibitors (etanercept, infliximab, adalimumab, and golimumab) are now FDA approved for the treatment of ankylosing spondylitis.

  2. Genetic factors. The strong association of the histocompatibility antigen **HLA-B27** with clinical expression of the spondyloarthropathies provides evidence for genetic transmission of these disorders. However, HLA-B27 is found in 8% of whites, 3% of African Americans, and less than 1% of Asians, and all of these individuals do not develop spondyloarthropathies. Conversely, spondyloarthropathies are found in patients who are HLA-B27 negative (10%–20%).

   a. This relationship also is a major reason for grouping these disorders. The independent correlation of HLA-B27 with specific features of spondyloarthropathies (e.g., sacroiliitis, aortitis, and anterior uveitis) explains both the clinical overlap among these diseases and their familial clustering.

   b. The role of the antigen in disease causation is not understood. However, transgenic rats can express HLA-B27 on cell surfaces and develop clinical features of spondyloarthropathies, so this gene product is clearly involved in disease causation or perpetuation.

   c. Disease susceptibility is also associated with other unknown genes—perhaps T cell receptor genes—accounting for the 10-fold increase in risk associated with HLA-B27 positivity in spondylitis families.

3. Pathology

  a. The basic pathologic lesion in the spondyloarthropathies is an **enthesopathy**—an inflammation occurring at the site where ligaments and tendons attach to bone. This type of inflammation explains the frequency of sacroiliitis, ascending spinal lesions, and peripheral tendon lesions (e.g., Achilles tendinitis).

  b. Although inflammatory synovitis that is indistinguishable from rheumatoid synovitis can be seen in these illnesses, it is not typically as widespread, chronically active, and potentially destructive as it is in rheumatoid arthritis (psoriatic arthritis mutilans is a notable exception).

4. HIV-related spondyloarthropathic disease. Some HIV-positive patients have spondyloarthropathic illness, often with features of **reactive arthritis** or **psoriatic arthritis**. However, most commonly, they have skin, joint, and tendon features that prevent easy classification into one illness or the other, suggesting that these spondyloarthropathic illnesses have a common pathogenesis [see XIV A 1].

B **Specific disorders**

1. Ankylosing spondylitis

  a. Definition. Ankylosing spondylitis is the spondyloarthropathy that is most closely associated with inflammation of the axial skeleton. **Back pain** and **limited spinal mobility** caused by **sacroiliitis** and variable ascent of the inflammation up the spine dominate the clinical expression of this disease.

  b. Epidemiology

   (1) Prevalence. Ankylosing spondylitis may be as common as 1 in 1000 whites because the frequency of disease parallels the prevalence of the HLA-B27 antigen in the population [see IV A 2]. The frequency of ankylosing spondylitis is lower in African American and Asian populations, paralleling the prevalence of the antigen in these groups.

   (2) Gender distribution. Ankylosing spondylitis may be as prevalent in women as in men if radiographic findings of sacroiliitis are considered to be diagnostic of the disease. However, women tend to have somewhat milder disease with more peripheral joint manifestations.

   (3) Familial aggregation. The risk of ankylosing spondylitis in an HLA-B27–positive family member of an affected proband is 20%, as compared to 1%–2% for the general population of those with HLA-B27.

  c. Etiology

   (1) The major histocompatibility antigen HLA-B27 occurs in 90%–95% of white patients with ankylosing spondylitis, but the association is less marked in nonwhite populations (40%–50% of African Americans with ankylosing spondylitis have HLA-B27).

   (2) Because the gene coding for the expression of HLA-B27 resides on chromosome 6, autosomal transmission occurs. Thus, children of a proband who is heterozygous for the gene controlling HLA-B27 production have a 50% probability of eventual expression of the antigen on cell surfaces.

   (3) The **presence of HLA-B27 on cell membranes** is thought to be important in the causation of ankylosing spondylitis. The disease is somehow caused or perpetuated by the presence of a short amino acid sequence in the peptide-binding cleft of the HLA-B27 molecule that is able to bind a unique arthritis-causing peptide.

   (a) Receptor theory (see Online Figure 11–6A).

   (b) Molecular mimicry theory (see Online Figure 11–6B).

   (c) Thymic selection theory

  d. Clinical features

   (1) Disease onset. The disease usually develops in the second or third decade of life.

   (2) Disease course. The disease begins with the gradual onset of chronic sacral backache, which is associated with prolonged morning stiffness and improves with exercise. Most patients have prolonged, unremitting low back pain for years. The disease may be mild and cause minimal interference with function, or it may be severe and deforming.

   (3) Manifestations of disease

    (a) Axial skeletal involvement. Symmetric inflammation of the sacroiliac joints (sacroiliitis) is the most common presentation. Inflammation and consequent calcification of the spinal ligaments and the intervertebral zygapophyseal joints can cause limited spinal mobility, and intercostal ligament enthesopathy can cause limitation of chest wall expansion.

    (b) Peripheral joint involvement. This feature is typical of more severe ankylosing spondylitis. Erosive hip and shoulder involvement is not uncommon and may be severe. More distal synovitis is less common, although 35% of patients with ankylosing spondylitis have some evidence of peripheral joint disease.

    (c) Extraskeletal features. Constitutional complaints, fatigue, and weight loss are not as common in ankylosing spondylitis as in rheumatoid arthritis, but they may occur. Anterior uveitis occurs in 25% of patients with ankylosing spondylitis and sometimes occurs as an isolated clinical association of HLA-B27. Aortic root inflammation can occur, usually in patients with longstanding disease; this process can lead to aortic valve insufficiency or, if it extends into the conduction system, complete heart block. Upper lobe pulmonary fibrosis and chronic prostatitis are other uncommon extraskeletal features.

e. Diagnosis. Combining historical, physical, and radiographic evidence, as well as excluding mechanical low back pain, other spondyloarthropathies, and other inflammatory arthritides, allows for diagnosis.

  (1) Historical information

    (a) Inflammatory versus mechanical low back pain. Inflammatory sacroiliitis has a gradual onset in early adulthood and is persistent for more than 3 months; the pain is associated with prolonged early-morning back stiffness and is relieved by exercise and worsened by rest. In contrast, the onset of mechanical low back pain usually occurs later in life with sudden, self-limited episodes that are worsened by exercise and improved by bed rest.

    (b) Familial association. Patients with ankylosing spondylitis often have other affected family members.

    (c) Associated complaints. Evidence of prior inflammatory eye symptoms, recurrent oligoarthritis, and inflammatory tendinitis should be sought.

  (2) Physical findings

    (a) Musculoskeletal examination. Each sacroiliac joint should be evaluated for tenderness, lumbar spinal mobility should be assessed in all directions, and chest expansion should be evaluated to assess severity of chest wall enthesopathic lesions.

    (b) General physical examination. Evidence of associated abnormalities should be sought, including ocular erythema, aortic insufficiency murmurs, and peripheral arthritis and tendinitis.

  (3) Laboratory findings. The only characteristic laboratory abnormality in ankylosing spondylitis is the variable presence of HLA-B27 in different population groups. In general, testing for this antigen **is not necessary** for the diagnosis.

  (4) Radiographic findings. Sacroiliac involvement is best seen on an anteroposterior radiograph of the pelvis. Blurred joint margins, periarticular sclerosis, erosions, and joint-space widening are characteristic, but total joint obliteration is typical of longstanding disease. If the illness is more severe or longstanding, ascending spinal involvement can occur, with delicate flowing calcifications (syndesmophytes) that bridge the intervertebral disk, culminating in a **bamboo-spine** appearance on a radiograph (Figure 11–7).

  (5) Differential diagnosis

    (a) Nature of low back pain. As mentioned previously, mechanical low back pain must be differentiated from inflammatory low back pain [see IV B 1 e (1) (a)].

    (b) Other disorders. Sacroiliitis is highly unusual in nonspondylitic diseases. Characteristic skin lesions may suggest that a patient with sacroiliitis has psoriasis or reactive arthritis. Prominent urethritis in association with sacroiliitis may also suggest reactive arthritis, and prominent bowel complaints with sacroiliitis may suggest inflammatory bowel disease.

f. Therapy. Patient education and multidisciplinary treatment are important therapeutic components in ankylosing spondylitis, just as they are in rheumatoid arthritis. Short-term goals involve control of pain and reduction of inflammation without causing drug toxicity, and long-term goals are prevention of postural deformity and retention of employment.

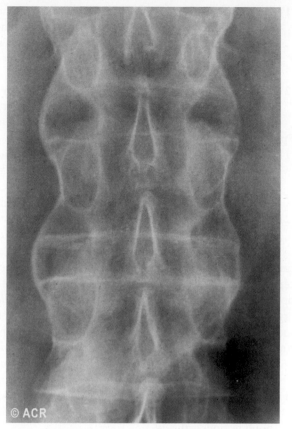

FIGURE 11–7   Extensive lateral bony bridges (syndesmophytes) connect all the lumbar vertebral bodies to produce a bamboo spine.

  (1) **Education**
    (a) **Cigarette smoking.** Individuals with enthesopathic chest wall restriction or fibrotic lung disease should be discouraged from smoking.
    (b) **Genetic counseling.** Patients should be made aware of the familial incidence of the illness so that it can be diagnosed early in children and treatment of spondylitic symptoms begun.
    (c) **Protection of brittle spine.** Patients with extensive spinal involvement must understand that minimal trauma can cause a spinal fracture. Wearing a hard or soft collar should be recommended for automobile driving.
  (2) **Exercise.** Spinal extension exercises and correct posture are important for prevention of deformity. Hard mattresses and small cervical pillows help prevent excessive spinal flexion during sleep.
  (3) **Drug therapy.** Although many patients require DMARDS, methotrexate, sulfasalazine, and NSAIDs are the mainstay of treatment. For persistent disease activity, TNF inhibitors (etanercept, infliximab, adalimumab, and golimumab) are now FDA approved for the treatment of ankylosing spondylitis. They alleviate symptoms, improve function, and may impact the natural progression of the disease. Local joint or peritendinous instillation of a corticosteroid sometimes is beneficial in patients with prominent peripheral disease manifestations not controlled by NSAIDs.
  g. **Prognosis.** Most patients with ankylosing spondylitis remain employable and continue to function well in society. The progression to severe, deforming disease cannot be predicted on the basis of HLA-B27 status or other criteria. Patients with severe spondylitis tend to have brittle spines, more cardiopulmonary disease, and other extraspinal complications; these patients may have shortened life spans.
2. **Reactive arthritis**
  a. **Definition.** Reactive arthritis is another spondyloarthropathy that is strongly associated with HLA-B27.

(1) Reactive arthritis initially referred to the classic triad of nongonococcal **urethritis, conjunctivitis,** and **arthritis** that occurred after a diarrheal illness or genitourinary infection, usually with *Chlamydia trachomatis.* Many patients still have the classic disease triad, but the use of HLA-B27 typing has allowed "incomplete" forms (without the urethritis or conjunctivitis) to be identified.

(2) Reactive arthritis is a predominantly lower extremity oligoarthritis triggered by **urethritis, cervicitis,** or **dysenteric infection.** The variable features of the typical syndrome include **mucocutaneous lesions, inflammatory eye lesions,** and **sacroiliitis** or **peripheral arthritis.**

b. Epidemiology

(1) Incidence. Reactive arthritis occurs in 1%–3% of patients after nonspecific urethritis and 0.2% of patients after dysentery outbreaks caused by *Shigella flexneri.* HLA-B27 is present in 75%–80% of cases. Patients with the marker who develop nonspecific urethritis or *S. flexneri* dysentery have a 20%–25% chance of developing reactive arthritis.

(2) Gender distribution. Reactive arthritis is diagnosed in men much more often than in women, in part because cervicitis is less symptomatic than urethritis. However, the arthritis tends to be less severe in women as well.

c. Etiology and pathogenesis. Specific infections trigger the clinical expression of arthritis in susceptible patients, including chlamydial and mycoplasmal urethritis, as well as dysenteric infections caused by certain serotypes of *Shigella, Salmonella,* and *Yersinia.* The presence of the organism may not be necessary for later exacerbations or chronic activity of the disease, although some polymerase chain reaction (PCR) and electron microscopic studies of inflamed synovium suggest the persistence of chlamydial organisms or fragments in reactive arthritis. The unusual severity of reactive arthritis in patients with acquired immunodeficiency syndrome (AIDS) suggests that the inflammatory response does not require functioning $CD4^+$ cells.

(1) Exaggerated immune response. Conceivably, infectious antigens cross-react with self antigens such as HLA-B27 and stimulate an exaggerated immune response that can include a noninfectious arthritis.

(2) Suppressed immune response. It is also conceivable that molecular mimicry between HLA-B27 and bacterial peptides prevents the host immune system from recognizing the pathogen, thus allowing dissemination and production of disease at widely varied sites. Evidence that suggests persistence of organisms or fragments at sites of chronic inflammation supports this theory.

(3) Protected site of infection. Persistent subclinical genitourinary or gastrointestinal infections (e.g., *Chlamydia, Shigella*) could cause recurrent shedding of organisms or bacterial antigens to joints. Persistent specific immunoglobulin A (IgA) responses to causative organisms and improvement with surgical stripping of the urethra in venereal onset of reactive arthritis support this theory.

d. Clinical features

(1) Disease onset. Reactive arthritis begins most often in young adulthood. From 1 to 3 weeks after an episode of urethritis or dysentery, any of the typical clinical features of the syndrome can occur. The disease often is misdiagnosed because these features tend to occur serially rather than simultaneously.

(2) Manifestations of disease

(a) Musculoskeletal

(i) Arthritis. A lower extremity oligoarthritis is the most common joint presentation. The arthritis may be acute and self-limited, but it is more commonly relapsing or chronic.

(ii) Enthesopathy. Inflammation of the tendons and ligaments is as much a part of reactive arthritis as it is of ankylosing spondylitis. Plantar fasciitis and Achilles tendinitis are most typical. **Dactylitis** (sausage digit), a lesion involving both joint and tendon inflammation in the same digit, is also a common feature.

(iii) Sacroiliitis. Asymmetric involvement of sacroiliac joints occurs in approximately 20% of patients. Less frequently, asymmetric ascending spinal disease occurs. The consequent back pain has typical inflammatory characteristics, but only rarely does the ascending spinal disease limit thoracic or cervical spinal mobility.

(b) Genitourinary. Symptomatic or asymptomatic **urethritis** is extremely common. Chronic **prostatitis** also is common, affecting as many as 80% of patients in some series.

(c) Ocular. Both **conjunctivitis** and **anterior uveitis** often occur. The conjunctival inflammation is an acute, usually self-limited manifestation, which may be recurrent. Anterior uveitis occurs in more established forms of disease; it may be chronic and require topical or systemic corticosteroids to prevent visual deterioration.

(d) Mucocutaneous. Fleeting and painless oral ulcers are the typical mucous membrane features. **Keratoderma blennorrhagica** is the characteristic scaling, plaque-like lesion found anywhere on the body, including the palms and soles. This lesion resembles pustular psoriasis clinically and pathologically. **Circinate balanitis** is a painless, erythematous erosion of the glans penis that may expand to surround the urethral orifice. Each of these skin lesions occurs in approximately 20%–30% of patients with reactive arthritis, although circinate balanitis is the most common.

(e) Cardiovascular. Early cardiovascular changes include transient **pericardial rubs** or **first-degree heart block.** In more severe, longstanding disease, an **aortitis** identical to that seen in ankylosing spondylitis can cause valvular insufficiency or conduction system lesions.

e. Diagnosis

(1) General considerations. Reactive arthritis can be difficult to diagnose when the onset of various clinical features is widely separated over time, but it is quite easy if **arthritis, dysentery** or **urethritis, conjunctivitis,** and **mucocutaneous lesions** appear simultaneously. A tentative diagnosis can be made when a seronegative asymmetric oligoarthritis is associated with any of these extra-articular features. Because this form of arthritis is, strictly speaking, a "reactive" arthritis, the temporal appearance of arthritis after urethritis or a dysenteric illness is especially convincing. The mucocutaneous lesions, urethritis, and cervicitis, which often are asymptomatic, must be sought specifically while taking the patient history and during the physical examination.

(2) Laboratory findings. Eighty percent of whites with reactive arthritis have HLA-B27. The synovial fluid typically is mildly to moderately inflammatory, with neutrophil predominance and no important distinguishing characteristics.

(3) Radiographic findings. Asymmetric, oligoarticular erosions, joint space narrowing, and periarticular osteopenia can be seen radiographically in established disease. Periosteal new bone formation is a characteristic feature of reactive arthritis, especially adjacent to the insertions of the Achilles tendon and plantar fascia. Sacroiliitis, if it occurs, typically is asymmetric, and the occasional patient with spondyloarthropathy has asymmetric, large syndesmophytes at scattered vertebral levels.

(4) Differential diagnosis

(a) Diseases most likely to mimic acute reactive arthritis are gonococcal arthritis and other infectious arthropathies, even Lyme disease. Thus, appropriate tissues should be cultured and serologies obtained. Crystal-mediated arthritis (i.e., gout and pseudogout) and the arthritis of rheumatic fever should be excluded.

(b) Diseases most likely to mimic chronic recurring reactive arthritis include other spondyloarthropathies, especially psoriatic arthritis and ankylosing spondylitis. Close attention to the symmetry and severity of sacroiliac and spinal involvement, to extraskeletal features, and to the presence or absence of infectious triggers may help differentiate these illnesses. Many cases of so-called **seronegative rheumatoid arthritis** may actually be cases of reactive arthritis. Typical clinical features, as well as radiographic evidence of sacroiliac joint and periostitis, should be sought. The presence or absence of HLA-B27 may be helpful in diagnosing particularly difficult cases.

f. Therapy

(1) Goals of treatment are essentially the same as in ankylosing spondylitis [see IV B 1 f].

(2) Exercise. Patients should be advised to rest to lessen inflammation and to perform appropriate exercises that allow preservation of joint function and prevention of contractures.

(3) Drug therapy

(a) NSAIDs. These agents are the mainstay of treatment. However, aspirin is relatively ineffective.

(b) Corticosteroids. Occasional intra-articular instillation may be useful in the management of particular joints that do not respond to treatment with NSAIDs.

(c) Second-line agents. Both azathioprine and methotrexate have been used to control particularly severe and chronic disease, and sulfasalazine is used for arthritis unresponsive to NSAIDs. The effects of these medications on disease course are not yet known. HIV testing should be considered for patients with reactive arthritis sufficiently severe to require immunosuppressive medications.

(d) Antibiotics. Trials of tetracycline-like drugs, used for 3-month periods early in disease associated with urethritis, suggest that antibiotic treatment may lessen the severity and chronicity of arthritis.

g. Prognosis. Chronic or recurrent disease appears to be common. In 60%–80% of patients with reactive arthritis, skeletal complaints, extraskeletal complaints, or both recur or become chronic. Perhaps as many as 25% of patients are functionally disabled by their illness. Long-term problems with aortic regurgitation and conduction disturbances are unusual but increase with the duration of the disease. Patients who have HLA-B27 antigen have more sacroiliitis and are more likely to have recurrent or chronic disease.

3. Psoriatic arthritis

a. Definition. Any form of inflammatory arthritis associated with psoriasis is called psoriatic arthritis. Rheumatoid factor generally is absent.

b. Epidemiology

(1) Psoriatic arthritis occurs much more commonly in patients who have a first-degree relative with the disorder.

(2) Psoriasis occurs two to three times more commonly in patients with arthritis than in the normal population. Conversely, as many as 10%–20% of patients with psoriasis may have an inflammatory arthritis.

c. Etiology. Although a hereditary etiology is apparent in psoriatic arthritis, its characteristics are not fully understood. HLA-B27 is highly associated with sacroiliitis in psoriasis, and HLA-B27, -B13, and -DR7 are independently associated with arthritis and psoriasis at an increased frequency. Unknown environmental factors also may be important in disease expression.

d. Clinical features

(1) **Disease onset.** Most patients with psoriatic arthritis develop the disease in their late 30s to early 40s. Most patients develop skin lesions before the arthritis, but as many as 16% develop inflammatory arthritis before the psoriasis.

(2) **Patterns of arthritis.** Five patterns of psoriatic arthropathy have been distinguished, although the typical patient often has the skeletal manifestations of several of these patterns. Peripheral joint and tendon involvement may be more severe in the upper than in the lower extremities.

(a) **DIP arthritis** is the classic form of psoriatic arthritis. It is strongly associated with typical fingernail abnormalities, as well as DIP joint redness, soft-tissue swelling, and erosive changes seen radiographically in a clinical picture resembling primary erosive osteoarthritis.

(b) **Asymmetric oligoarthritis.** Large- and small-joint oligoarthritis is another clinical form of psoriatic arthritis. **Sausage digits** are common in this form as a manifestation of joint and enthesis involvement of a single phalanx.

(c) **Symmetric polyarthropathy.** A fairly symmetric polyarthropathy can occur in conjunction with psoriasis, and it can be difficult to distinguish from rheumatoid arthritis. As many as 25% of these patients may be seropositive for rheumatoid factor.

(d) **Arthritis mutilans** is an unusually destructive form of psoriatic arthritis because of the severe periarticular bone resorption that occurs in the small finger joints. "Telescoping digits" characterize the end stage of this uncommon form of arthritis. Widespread joint ankylosis also can occur.

(e) **Sacroiliitis.** As many as 20% of patients with psoriatic arthritis can have clinical or radiographic evidence of sacroiliitis, usually asymmetric. Ascending spinal syndesmophytes occur in an asymmetric and patchy fashion.

(3) **Extra-articular features**

(a) **Skin** [see Chapter 13 VIII]. Arthritis is more likely to occur in patients with severe skin involvement than in those with mild psoriasis, although it can occur in the presence of localized cutaneous lesions. Skin and joint flares of disease can occur in association with each other or independently in individual patients.

    (b) Nails. Nail abnormalities most commonly occur in conjunction with DIP joint lesions; however, nail changes are noted more frequently in all of the peripheral forms of psoriatic arthritis in comparison to psoriasis uncomplicated by arthritis. Multiple **pitting,** transverse depressions, and **onycholysis** are the characteristic abnormalities found.

    (c) Ocular. The only other extra-articular features that occur commonly in patients with psoriatic arthritis are conjunctivitis (in 20% of cases) and anterior uveitis (in 10% of cases).

  e. Diagnosis

    (1) Clinical considerations. An association should be made between the typical skin and nail lesions and the joint and spinal involvement to diagnose psoriatic arthritis. The skin manifestations may be subtle, so particular care must be taken to check the elbows, scalp, groin, navel, and buttock cleft.

    (2) Laboratory findings. Laboratory indicators of chronic disease (e.g., anemia, thrombocytosis) typically are absent. Patients usually are seronegative for rheumatoid factor, although 25% of patients with symmetric polyarthritis are seropositive.

    (3) Radiographic findings

      (a) DIP joint erosions can lead to joint-space narrowing, and proximal phalangeal bone resorption can lead to a "pencil-in-cup" abnormality seen in arthritis mutilans. This severe destruction also can occur in more proximal joints.

      (b) Spinal involvement. Asymmetric sacroiliitis and asymmetric patchy syndesmophytes are seen and are similar to those seen in reactive arthritis.

      (c) Enthesopathy. Calcifications at tendon and ligament insertions occur.

    (4) Differential diagnosis

      (a) Reactive arthritis is distinguished from psoriatic arthritis by its characteristic extra-articular features and its tendency to involve the lower extremities more than the upper extremities. In psoriatic arthritis, upper extremity peripheral joint involvement is more common.

      (b) Rheumatoid arthritis. Patients with psoriasis who present with symmetric polyarthritis, seropositivity for rheumatoid factor, and rheumatoid nodules may be diagnosed with rheumatoid arthritis. Other overlapping presentations of the two diseases may be difficult to diagnose.

  f. Therapy. Drug treatment for psoriatic arthritis is similar to that for the other spondyloarthropathies, in that NSAIDs are the cornerstone of therapy. An important difference is that gold can be administered intramuscularly to treat sustained manifestations of peripheral arthritis. Sulfasalazine also is effective. Methotrexate is often the first agent used if NSAIDs are not sufficient; it has been particularly successful in controlling both the skin disease and refractory arthritis. Other cytotoxic drugs (e.g., azathioprine) also have been used in treatment of severe skin and joint disease. Biologic agents (TNF inhibitors) are now FDA approved for the treatment of psoriatic arthritis and plaque arthritis.

  g. Prognosis. Most patients with psoriatic arthritis, except for the 5% or so who develop arthritis mutilans, can avoid significant deformity and remain employed.

4. Enteropathic arthropathies

  a. Definition. Inflammatory arthritis associated with either Crohn's disease or ulcerative colitis is typified by a seronegative, migratory polyarticular involvement that waxes and wanes with the activity of the bowel disease. Sacroiliitis and spondylitis also can occur in affected individuals.

  b. Clinical syndromes

    (1) Peripheral arthritis. In 10%–20% of patients with severe ulcerative colitis or Crohn's disease—usually those with other extraintestinal manifestations—a predominantly lower extremity arthritis or tendinitis occurs in association with flare-ups of bowel disease. The arthritis often occurs abruptly and usually remits completely within weeks. There is no association with HLA-B27 in this peripheral arthritis. Treatment is directed at control of the bowel disease, although NSAIDs or local or systemic corticosteroids may help control the articular complaints.

(2) Spondylitis. The spondylitis of inflammatory bowel disease is associated with HLA-B27 in about 50% of patients. The radiographic findings are typical of those found in primary ankylosing spondylitis (i.e., symmetric sacroiliac joint changes and, less commonly, ascending symmetric spondylitis without skin lesions). Approximately 5% of patients with inflammatory bowel disease develop sacroiliitis or spondylitis, but the activity of these lesions and that of the bowel disease are independent of one another. NSAIDs usually are effective in controlling symptoms but can cause increased bowel complaints; sometimes only nonacetylated salicylates can be tolerated by these patients.

c. **Differential diagnosis.** Whipple's disease can be confused with enteropathic arthropathies because most patients manifest prominent bowel and joint complaints. In fact, sacroiliitis occurs in about 20% of cases. However, Whipple's disease is quite rare and most commonly manifests in middle-aged men as weight loss, skin hyperpigmentation, lymphadenopathy, fever, and symptoms of malabsorption.

V CRYSTAL-RELATED JOINT DISEASES

A Gout

1. **Definition.** Gout is a disorder of purine metabolism that is characterized by **serum uric acid elevation** (hyperuricemia) and **urate deposition** in articular or extra-articular tissues. Elevation of serum uric acid alone is not sufficient for the diagnosis of gout; in fact, only 10% of patients with hyperuricemia develop gout. Some unknown factor predisposes patients to urate deposition and articular inflammation in the setting of sustained hyperuricemia.

2. **Etiologic classification of hyperuricemia.** Gout is characterized by either episodic or constant **elevation of serum uric acid** concentration **greater than 7 mg/dL.** Patients with elevated serum uric acid can be classified as **overproducers** or **underexcreters** of uric acid, depending on the amount of uric acid excreted during a 24-hour period. Excessive dietary intake of purines can contribute to hyperuricemia in both types of patients.

   a. **Overproducers,** who make up approximately 10% of the gout population, excrete **more than 750–1000 mg** uric acid per day on an unrestricted diet. These patients synthesize greater-than-normal amounts of uric acid de novo from intermediates or via breakdown of purine bases from nucleic acids. The defect causing uric acid overproduction can be **primary** (associated with purine pathway enzymatic defects) or **secondary** (increased cell turnover associated with alcohol use, hematologic malignancies, chronic hemolysis, or cancer chemotherapy).

   b. **Underexcreters,** who constitute approximately 90% of the gout population, excrete **less than 700 mg** uric acid per day.

      (1) The most common causes of decreased uric acid excretion are **drug effects** (e.g., diuretics, alcohol, and low-dose aspirin interference with tubular handling of urate) and **renal disease** (e.g., chronic renal failure and lead nephropathy) [see Chapter 7, Part I: XII B 2 a]. Subtle renal tubular defects in urate handling also may be **inherited** and predispose to underexcretion.

      (2) This **group includes patients with combined defects** because overproducers of uric acid also may be underexcreters. The decreased renal excretion of uric acid is the basis for hyperuricemia in these individuals.

      (3) Multiple factors contribute to the occurrence of gout in **cardiac, renal, and liver transplant recipients.** Underlying renal insufficiency, use of diuretics, and cyclosporine immunosuppressive therapy are the most common predisposing factors. Affected patients tend to have a rapidly progressive form of gout with the formation of extensive tophi.

3. **Associated conditions.** The following conditions occur more commonly in patients with gout but are not known to be causal.

   a. **Obesity.** Serum uric acid level rises with body weight. Gout is significantly more common in individuals who are more than 15% overweight, partly because of decreases in urate excretion.

   b. **Diabetes mellitus.** Impaired glucose tolerance is common in gout and may be a function of obesity.

   c. **Hypertension.** Although hypertension is common in patients with gout, no independent correlation exists between blood pressure and serum uric acid level. Obesity probably is responsible for a high rate of hypertension in patients with gout.

d. Hyperlipidemias (types II and IV). Increased plasma concentrations of some lipids are common in patients with gout; however, diet, alcohol intake, and body weight seem to be more important associations.

e. Atherosclerosis. Death in patients with gout is commonly attributable to cardiovascular or cerebrovascular diseases. However, the previously mentioned risk factors that commonly occur in patients with gout seem to explain the tendency for accelerated atherogenesis.

4. Clinical stages of gout

a. Asymptomatic hyperuricemia is characterized by an increased serum uric acid level in the absence of clinical evidence of deposition disease (i.e., arthritis, tophi, nephropathy, or uric acid stones).

(1) Hyperuricemia. The risk of acute gouty arthritis or nephrolithiasis increases as the serum uric acid concentration increases. However, most patients do not develop either of these conditions.

(2) Hyperuricosuria. The risk of uric acid stone formation in patients with hyperuricemia is most closely related to a urinary uric acid excretion exceeding 1000 mg/day. These patients also are at risk for **acute obstructive uropathy,** a form of acute renal failure occurring most often following combination chemotherapy for cancer. Large purine loads lead to sudden increases in serum uric acid levels, with subsequent precipitation of uric acid crystals in the collecting tubules and ureters.

b. Acute gouty arthritis, the second stage and primary manifestation of gout, is an extremely painful, acute-onset arthritis.

(1) Typical patient. Most patients (80%–90%) are middle-aged or elderly men who have had sustained asymptomatic hyperuricemia for 20–30 years before the first attack. Women seem to be spared until menopause, perhaps via an estrogen effect on uric acid clearance. Onset of acute gouty arthritis in the teens or 20s is unusual and most often associated with a primary or secondary cause of uric acid overproduction.

(2) Typical attack

(a) Presentation. A monoarticular, lower extremity presentation is most common, with 50% of patients experiencing their first attack in the first metatarsophalangeal (MTP) joint (called **podagra**) (🖱 Online Figure 11–8). Many attacks occur suddenly at night, with rapid evolution of joint erythema, swelling, tenderness, and warmth. Intense joint inflammation can extend into the soft tissues and mimic cellulitis or phlebitis. Fever can occur in severe attacks.

(b) Course. Attacks usually resolve in a few days, although some can extend over several weeks. The joint usually returns to normal between attacks. Polyarticular involvement can occur in some cases, and a typical progression from monoarticular to polyarticular involvement occurs by extension to adjacent joints.

🖱 **(3) Pathogenesis of acute attacks** (🖱 Online Figure 11–9)

c. Intercritical gout, the third stage of gout, is an asymptomatic period after the initial attack. This stage may be interrupted by new acute attacks.

(1) Recurrence of monoarticular attacks. About 7% of patients never experience a new attack of acute gouty arthritis after the first episode. However, 62% experience a recurrence within 1 year. Typically, patients are asymptomatic between attacks, but attacks eventually become more frequent and abate more gradually if urate deposition remains untreated over time.

(2) Disease progression. Attacks tend to become polyarticular and more severe over time. Some patients develop a chronic inflammatory arthritis without asymptomatic intervals—a condition that may be difficult to distinguish from rheumatoid arthritis. Tophaceous gout typically occurs over a 10- to 20-year period of untreated urate deposition.

d. Chronic tophaceous gout, which develops in untreated patients, is the final stage of gout. The tophus is a collection of urate crystal masses surrounded by inflammatory cells and variable fibrosis. Tophi tend to develop in areas that are lower in temperature, which diminishes the solubility of the crystals.

(1) Typical locations of tophaceous deposits

(a) The **pinna of the external ear** is a potential site of tophus development, although deposition here is uncommon.

(b) Other common locations are the surfaces of chronically involved joints and subchondral bone, as well as extensor surfaces of the forearms, olecranon bursae, and the infrapatellar and Achilles tendons.

(2) Pathogenesis of tophaceous gout

5. **Renal complications** may arise at any stage of gout, but nephrolithiasis is the only common clinical presentation of renal involvement. Proteinuria and impaired ability to concentrate urine related to urate deposition in the renal interstitium have been described in gout patients (see Chapter 7, Part I: XII B 3).

6. **Diagnosis**
   a. **Acute gouty arthritis—laboratory findings**
      (1) **Serum findings.** The serum uric acid value often is not helpful in the clinical diagnosis of acute gout. Serum uric acid concentration is normal in at least 10% of patients at the time of an acute attack, and an elevated serum uric acid level is not specific for acute gout.
      (2) **Synovial fluid findings.** The demonstration of **urate crystals,** especially intracellular crystals, in synovial fluid is diagnostic. These **crystals characteristically are needle shaped and negatively birefringent** in red-compensated, polarized light, and they may be present in neutrophils during an acute attack. Synovial fluid white blood cell (WBC) counts of 10,000–60,000/mm^3 (predominantly neutrophils) also are common in acute attacks.
   b. **Chronic tophaceous gout**
      (1) **Physical appearance.** Tophi are firm, movable, and cream colored or yellowish if superficially located. If they ulcerate, a chalky material is extruded.
      (2) **Radiographic findings.** Tophaceous deposits appear as well-defined, large erosions (punched-out erosions) of the subchondral bone. These erosions are most common at the first MTP joint and at the bases and heads of phalanges; however, any articulation can be affected. Typical gouty erosions have an **overhanging edge** of subchondral new bone formation. Periarticular osteopenia is absent.
      (3) **Aspiration.** Tophi can be aspirated and crystals demonstrated by polarized microscopy.

7. **Therapy.** In all stages of gout, secondary causes of hyperuricemia (e.g., medications, obesity, excess dietary purine intake, alcohol intake, other disease) should be altered if possible.
   a. **Asymptomatic hyperuricemia.** In general, patients without evidence of urate deposition do not require treatment other than correction of underlying causes. Patients with uric acid elevations that chronically exceed 10 mg/dL have a greater than 90% chance of developing acute gout at some time, but most physicians wait for an acute attack to begin treatment.
   b. **Acute gouty arthritis.** Drug treatment of the acute attack is most effective when started very early after symptoms begin. As with any inflammatory arthritis, rest or immobilization of the involved joint is an important adjunct to treatment.
      (1) **Colchicine,** which inhibits neutrophil chemotaxis and inflammatory mediator release by suppressing phospholipase A$_2$, has been used intravenously to treat acute attacks. However, it is rarely used today, as it has been associated with irreversible bone marrow suppression. Caution is necessary in elderly patients and in those with renal or hepatic impairment due to increased bone marrow toxicity and neuromyotoxicity. Colchicine can be used orally for acute attacks, but nausea, vomiting, and diarrhea often appear before therapy is successful, so that NSAIDs and corticosteroids are usually preferred.
      (2) **NSAIDs** often are used in high but quickly tapered doses to treat acute attacks. Any of these agents can be used, although drugs that affect uric acid clearance (e.g., salicylates, diflunisal) should be avoided because any fluctuation in serum urate can prolong acute attacks. Caution is warranted when using NSAIDs in the presence of gastrointestinal, hepatic, or renal disease. Indomethacin, if tolerated, appears to be the most acutely efficacious agent.
      (3) **Corticosteroids,** oral and intra-articular, can be used to treat acute attacks, particularly when NSAIDs are contraindicated.
      (4) **Drugs that alter serum uric acid concentrations** (e.g., **allopurinol, probenecid**) should be avoided during acute attacks because raising or lowering serum uric acid can prolong attacks. In patients already taking such drugs, the dose should not be altered.
   c. **Intercritical gout.** Prophylactic treatment with small doses of colchicine (0.6 mg once or twice daily) or small doses of an NSAID can be used to forestall new attacks.

d. Chronic or tophaceous gout. Therapy for chronic gout centers on control of hyperuricemia. Drugs that increase renal uric acid excretion (uricosuric drugs) or that decrease uric acid production (xanthine oxidase inhibitors) are available. The aim of this treatment is to reduce serum urate to less than 6 mg/dL to allow reduction in serum supersaturation by urate and mobilization of tissue uric acid deposits. Patients who have had a recent acute attack should receive low-dose colchicine or an NSAID to prevent new attacks caused by fluctuation in serum urate.

   (1) Uricosuric drugs (e.g., **probenecid, sulfinpyrazone**) can be used in patients who excrete less than 700 mg uric acid daily, who have normal renal function, and who have no history of urinary stones.

   (2) Xanthine oxidase inhibitors include **allopurinol,** which is an analog of hypoxanthine. This drug inhibits de novo uric acid synthesis and competitively inhibits xanthine oxidase via enzymatic conversion to oxypurinol. Inhibition of uric acid synthesis with xanthine oxidase inhibitors is preferred in patients with urate excretion greater than 1000 mg/day, creatinine clearance less than 30 mL/minute, tophaceous gout, or a history of nephrolithiasis. Doses are reduced in the presence of renal failure to avoid toxicity. The most common side effects of allopurinol are dyspepsia, diarrhea, and rash, which occur in 3%–10% of patients. A full-blown hypersensitivity syndrome can occur rarely, with a mortality rate around 20%–30%.

     Febuxostat is a nonpurine selective xanthine oxidase inhibitor that works by noncompetitively inhibiting the active site on xanthine oxidase. In contrast to allopurinol, it is not a purine analog and should not inhibit other enzymes related to purine and pyrimidine synthesis. It is indicated in patients with allopurinol hypersensitivity, as well as patients with renal impairment who cannot take allopurinol. It should not be used in the setting of liver disease because it can cause elevations in liver enzymes.

   (3) Important treatment issues include the following:

     (a) It is important to use colchicine, NSAIDs, or steroids while instituting allopurinol therapy to avoid an acute attack of gout induced by fluctuation in serum urate levels.

     (b) Colchicine can be used chronically in patients unable to tolerate allopurinol.

     (c) Secretion of colchicine is reduced in patients with renal insufficiency and should be avoided in this group since severe toxicity may occur.

     (d) Chronic low-dose steroid treatment may be used in patients with chronic gout and chronic renal insufficiency.

B Calcium pyrophosphate dihydrate deposition disease

1. Definition. Deposition of CPPD crystals in cartilage and periarticular connective tissues can cause a gamut of articular manifestations, ranging from asymptomatic deposition to acute and chronic inflammatory arthritis. The acute form of CPPD deposition disease is commonly called **pseudogout.**

2. Etiologic classification

   a. Hereditary CPPD disease. A high prevalence of CPPD disease has been noted in many families, with autosomal dominant transmission the typical pattern. Secondary metabolic associations with CPPD disease typically are not present in these families.

   b. Osteoarthritis. Chondrocalcinosis and CPPD crystals can occur as a result of severe osteoarthritis. CPPD disease also can cause osteoarthritis by damaging cartilage.

   c. CPPD disease associated with metabolic disorders. Correction of underlying metabolic disorders, if possible, does not seem to alter the progression of CPPD disease.

     CPPD disease occurs at a higher-than-expected frequency in association with certain diseases and conditions. Potential abnormalities of calcium, phosphorus, or cartilage metabolism can explain the associations, which include the following:

   (1) Hyperparathyroidism

   (2) Hemochromatosis

   (3) Hypothyroidism

   (4) Hypophosphatasia

   (5) Hypomagnesemia

   (6) Wilson's disease

3. Pathogenesis (🖱 Online Figure 11–9)

🖱 **a. Crystal deposition**

🖱 **b. Crystal-mediated joint damage**

🖱 **4. Clinical syndromes**

    a. Pseudogout accounts for 25% of cases of CPPD disease. Acute swelling, pain, stiffness, and erythema develop in previously asymptomatic joints. The knee is most commonly involved (50% of cases), but almost any synovial joint, including the first MTP joint, can be involved. Spread to adjacent joints can occur, and precipitation of attacks by acute medical or surgical illness is common, occurring in 10%–20% of cases. Systemic findings such as fever and leukocytosis may be present, especially in elderly patients. Joints typically return to normal between attacks.

    b. Pseudo–rheumatoid arthritis accounts for 5% of cases of CPPD disease. In some patients, a smoldering chronic arthropathy can occur. Subacute episodes of pain and swelling in one or more joints can be superimposed on a more chronic picture of prolonged morning stiffness, fatigue, synovial thickening, and progressive deformities.

    c. Pseudo-osteoarthritis accounts for 50% of cases of CPPD disease. Affected patients present with a clinical and radiographic picture similar to that of degenerative joint disease, although about half have superimposed acute attacks of pseudogout. Flexion contractures are more common than in typical osteoarthritis, and bilateral knee varus deformities or isolated patellofemoral arthritis may occur more commonly than in osteoarthritis. A small percentage of these patients may have such severe joint destruction (e.g., of the shoulders or knees) that the clinical and radiographic appearance is that of a **neuropathic joint disorder,** even in the absence of underlying neurologic disease or apparent proprioceptive deficit.

    d. Asymptomatic CPPD disease occurs in 20% of cases. These patients do not have joint pain; the disease typically is uncovered by the finding of asymptomatic chondrocalcinosis on radiography. The prevalence of this asymptomatic disease, as well as other clinically evident forms of CPPD disease, increases with age.

5. Diagnosis. The finding of typical crystals on synovial fluid analysis is diagnostic of pseudogout. Chondrocalcinosis seen on radiography is evidence for a diagnosis of CPPD deposition. However, chondrocalcinosis may be present in patients who never develop acute pseudogout.

    a. Synovial fluid findings. Chunky, rhomboid **crystals that exhibit weakly positive birefringence** in red-compensated, polarized light are the hallmark of the acute arthritis syndromes associated with CPPD disease. These may be intracellular (in neutrophils) or extracellular, but they usually are much less prevalent than in a typical gout-involved joint. Synovial fluid leukocytosis of 10,000–20,000 cells/mm^3 (mostly neutrophils) is typical.

    b. Radiographic findings

        (1) Chondrocalcinosis. Calcification of articular hyaline cartilage, fibrocartilage (most commonly in the knee menisci, intervertebral disk annuli, symphysis pubis, and wrist triangular fibrocartilage), synovial membrane, tendons, and bursae can occur, usually in a stippled, linear fashion.

        (2) Osteoarthritis. Osteoarthritic changes in atypical joints (e.g., wrist, elbow, and shoulder and MCP joints) suggest CPPD disease. Subchondral bone cysts may be more extensive in radiographs of joints affected by CPPD disease, and hook-shaped osteophytes characteristically are present with MCP involvement.

        (3) Pseudoneuropathic joint. Radiographic findings typical of neuropathic joint disorders, including extreme joint disorganization and bone fragments, can be found in severe cases of CPPD disease.

    c. When to suspect CPPD

        (1) Clinical or radiographic evidence of osteoarthritis in joints not usually involved by osteoarthritis should suggest CPPD disease as an alternative diagnosis.

        (2) Attacks of acute inflammatory arthritis in a setting of apparent osteoarthritis should suggest CPPD disease.

        (3) Acute arthritis occurring shortly after a medical illness or surgical procedure should suggest a crystal-mediated arthritis such as gout or pseudogout.

        (4) Radiographic changes more typical of osteoarthritis in patients thought to have rheumatoid arthritis should suggest CPPD disease as an alternative diagnosis.

(5) The **presence of diseases commonly associated with CPPD disease** (e.g., hyperparathyroidism, hemochromatosis) should suggest CPPD disease as a possible cause of any joint manifestations. In people younger than 55 years of age or in those with recurrent polyarticular disease, an associated metabolic disease is more likely. In these patients, determinations of calcium, magnesium, alkaline phosphatase, ceruloplasmin, and ferritin levels as well as liver and thyroid function tests should be considered.

(6) **Neuropathic joint presentations** should prompt investigation for CPPD disease as well as potentially associated neurologic disorders.

6. **Therapy**
   a. **Acute attacks.** Typical treatment involves aspiration of inflammatory joint fluid, intraarticular injection of corticosteroid, and use of NSAIDs.
   b. **Prophylaxis.** No clearly effective regimen is available, although NSAIDs and, rarely, low-dose colchicine are used.

C **Hydroxyapatite arthritis**   Hydroxyapatite crystals, the typical complexed form of calcium in bone, also can cause several rheumatic syndromes.

1. **Clinical syndromes**
   a. **Crystal deposition in osteoarthritis.** Mineral formation in cartilage may be a result of abnormal cartilage metabolism in more severe forms of osteoarthritis. Joint effusions in these patients contain crystals of hydroxyapatite as often as they contain CPPD crystals.
   b. **Calcific periarthritis.** Hydroxyapatite deposition in bursae and tendon sheaths can cause episodes of acute inflammation (i.e., periarthritis and peritendinitis), with acute attacks of pain, swelling, and erythema. Discrete clumped deposits can be found radiographically around the shoulders, greater trochanters, wrists, elbows, and digits and in other periarticular areas. These deposits can be shown to disintegrate gradually on radiographs taken several weeks after the acute periarthritis.
   c. **Destructive arthritis.** Hydroxyapatite crystals can be associated with a chronic destructive arthropathy, which is characterized by erosive radiographic changes, large (usually noninflammatory) effusions, proliferative synovitis, synovial mineral deposition, and periarticular ligamentous instability. This syndrome occurs most often in the knee and shoulder (**"Milwaukee shoulder"**) of elderly patients. Synovial fluid analysis shows few WBCs (500–1000/mm^3), with monocytes predominating. High concentrations of neutral proteases and collagenases sometimes are present.

2. **Diagnosis.** Light microscopic examination of synovial fluid occasionally reveals brownish globules that are large clumps of hydroxyapatite crystals. Isolated crystals are too small to be seen with ordinary light or polarized light microscopy. A calcium stain, **alizarin red S,** can be used as a screening test for the presence of hydroxyapatite or CPPD crystals in effusions. Aspirates from bursae or tendon sheaths may yield milky or pasty material that contains high concentrations of these hydroxyapatite crystals.

3. **Associated conditions.** Disorders of calcium and phosphorus metabolism should be sought if multiple deposits are found.

4. **Therapy.** Mechanical splinting and NSAIDs are used to treat acute episodes of periarthritis. NSAIDs often are used in chronic hydroxyapatite arthropathy as well. Periodic aspiration of the large synovial effusions that occur in the Milwaukee shoulder may help preserve ligamentous integrity and remove destructive enzymes. Corticosteroid injections may help treat acutely symptomatic joints.

VI   **OSTEOARTHRITIS**

A **Definition**   Osteoarthritis is traditionally defined as a noninflammatory joint disorder characterized by deterioration of articular cartilage and formation of new bone at the joint surfaces and margins. Emerging evidence recognizes the importance of biomechanical, biochemical, and cytokine-mediated changes in the pathogenesis of osteoarthritis.

B **Etiology**   Both systemic and local factors contribute to the development of osteoarthritis. Systemic factors include age, sex, genetics, bone density, and nutritional elements, which may make the cartilage more vulnerable to injury and less efficient at repair. Local biomechanical components, in combination with systemic factors, have a synergistic effect on the process of cartilage breakdown.

1. **Age.** The prevalence and incidence of osteoarthritis in all joints correlates with increasing age. Aging is associated with the following changes:
   a. Decreased responsiveness of chondrocytes to growth factors that stimulate repair.
   b. Increased laxity of ligaments, which makes the joints more unstable and susceptible to injury.
   c. Failure of shock absorbers or protectors of the joint, which includes decreases in muscle strength and neurologic responses.
   d. Development of a thinner rim of noncalcified cartilage, which leads to an increased shear stress at the basal cartilage level.

2. **Race.** No clear racial predilection has been documented.

3. **Sex.** Gender appears to be particularly important in the development of **erosive osteoarthritis** of the DIP and PIP joints. This variant is 10 times more common in women than men; it is autosomal dominant in women and recessive in men.

4. **Genetics.** Researchers have discovered a defect in the gene coding for **type II collagen synthesis,** which allows for early degeneration of the type II collagen. The presence of this abnormal gene is associated with a type of premature polyarticular osteoarthritis and mild epiphyseal dysplasia seen in several families.

5. **Inflammation.** Despite the noninflammatory nature of the synovial membrane and synovial fluid in osteoarthritis, evidence indicates that inflammatory mediators produced by synovial tissues and cartilage play a significant role. Cytokines such as IL-1, as well as other inflammatory mediators such as nitric oxide and prostaglandins, are important in the autodestructive processes that promote cartilage degeneration. These mediators, sequestered within avascular and aneural hyaline cartilage, do not provoke the classic signs of inflammation.

6. **Obesity and abnormal stresses.** An association exists between obesity and osteoarthritis of the knee, but, of interest, the same association does not exist with osteoarthritis of the hip. Abnormal mechanical loading contributes to disease progression by altering the metabolism of osteocytes within subchondral bone and chondrocytes within articular cartilage. In addition, abnormal biomechanical forces can increase the expression of mechanoresponsive genes, with the resultant release of proteolytic enzymes, growth factors, and mediators.

7. **Neuropathy.** Muscle tone around a joint modulates the forces of joint impact loading. If proprioceptive input to the joint is impaired, abnormal muscle tone may result in osteoarthritis by transferring abnormal forces to the joint.

8. **Deposition diseases** (e.g., hemochromatosis, ochronosis, Wilson's disease, crystal deposition diseases). These conditions, which cause deposition of substances in the cartilage matrix, can result in direct chondrocyte injury and premature osteoarthritis.

C Pathogenesis
   1. **Initial insult**
   2. **Progression**
   3. **Factors involved**

D Pathology

E Classification (Table 11–10)
   1. **Primary osteoarthritis** has no underlying cause for joint damage. It typically involves the DIP and PIP joints and the first carpometacarpal joints. Knees, hips, and first MTP joints often are involved, as well as cervical and lumbar spine facet joints. The joint involvement may be **generalized** or it may occur in an isolated, **sporadic** fashion. **Erosive** osteoarthritis is a unique subset that occurs predominantly in middle-aged women and has autosomal dominant, sex-influenced characteristics. Episodic erythema, swelling, and tenderness occur in involved joints, especially the DIP and PIP joints of the hands. Characteristic radiographic abnormalities include bone erosions and ankylosis, which are unusual in typical osteoarthritis. **Diffuse idiopathic skeletal hyperostosis** is noninflammatory axial and peripheral enthesis hyperostosis manifested by

TABLE 11–10 Classification of Osteoarthritis	
Primary Osteoarthritis (Multiple Sites) Heberden's nodes Generalized osteoarthritis "Erosive" osteoarthritis Diffuse idiopathic skeletal hyperostosis **Primary Osteoarthritis (Local)** Cervical spine Hip First carpometacarpal joint Distal interphalangeal joints Lumbar spine Knee First metatarsophalangeal joint Proximal interphalangeal joints	**Secondary Osteoarthritis** Congenital (e.g., hip dysplasia) Deposition disease Ochronosis Wilson's disease Hemochromatosis Gout Calcium pyrophosphate deposition disease Neuropathic joint (e.g., diabetes mellitus, syphilis) Endocrine/metabolic (e.g., acromegaly) Osteonecrosis (especially hips, knees) Infection (tuberculosis) Inflammation (rheumatoid arthritis)

radiographic "whiskering" at tendon or ligament insertion and flowing osteophytes adjacent to vertebral disks.

2. **Secondary osteoarthritis** exhibits an underlying cause for degenerative joint disease and may involve joints not typically affected by primary osteoarthritis (e.g., elbow, wrist). A primary metabolic, inflammatory, or mechanical process leads secondarily to osteoarthritis (see Table 11–10).

F **Clinical features**

1. **Symptoms** vary with the joint involved and the severity of the disease.
   a. **Pain.** Most patients experience the gradual onset of a deep, aching pain, which worsens with activity and is relieved by rest. With more severe disease, pain can occur even at rest and interfere with sleep.
   b. **Morning stiffness** is brief (<30 minutes), in contrast to that occurring in inflammatory rheumatic conditions, which generally lasts much longer.
   c. **Gelling phenomenon** refers to the sensation of renewed stiffness in osteoarthritic joints after prolonged inactivity.

2. **Signs**
   a. **Tenderness.** Mild or moderate tenderness can be present in involved joints.
   b. **Painful range of motion** in large joints (e.g., knees, hips) is the equivalent of tenderness in small joints.
   c. **Crepitus** (i.e., a grinding sound or sensation) can be felt and sometimes heard when a joint is put through a full range of motion. Crepitus is caused by surface incongruities in the joint.
   d. **Warmth.** Involved joints usually are cool but can feel warm with flare-ups of disease activity.
   e. **Joint enlargement.** Soft-tissue swelling may occur if an effusion is present. More commonly, bone enlargement occurs in the form of osteophytes.
   f. **Deformity. Varus** (medial) or **valgus** (lateral) **angulation** of joints can occur late in the disease. Gross bone enlargement and joint subluxation also can occur in severe disease.
      (1) **Heberden's nodes** specifically refer to enlargement of the DIP joints of the hand.
      (2) **Bouchard's nodes** specifically refer to enlargement of the PIP joints of the hand (Online Figure 11–10).

G **Diagnosis**   Patient history combined with physical, laboratory, and radiographic findings forms the basis for diagnosis.

1. **Joint involvement**
   a. The **distribution of the involved joints** should suggest whether the osteoarthritis is primary or related to an underlying disorder [see VI E 1–2].
   b. **Joint swelling** is typically **bony,** sometimes with superimposed **fluid.**

2. **Laboratory findings**
   a. **Hematologic findings.** Results, including the ESR, are generally normal.

    b. Synovial fluid findings. Typical osteoarthritic synovial fluid is slightly turbid, contains no crystals, and has a WBC count that is only mildly inflammatory (i.e., <2000 cells/mm^3 and <25% neutrophils).

   3. Radiographic findings. Radiographic evidence is common after age 40 years in joints typically affected by osteoarthritis, and it often is asymptomatic (see Online Figure 11–6B).

    a. Findings typically present

      (1) Joint space narrowing (due to loss of cartilage)

      (2) Subchondral sclerosis (increased subchondral bone density)

      (3) Marginal osteophytes

      (4) Subchondral cysts

    b. Findings typically absent

      (1) Periarticular osteopenia

      (2) Marginal erosions (except in the distal DIP and PIP joints in the erosive osteoarthritis variant)

   4. Differential diagnosis

    a. Monoarticular problems

      (1) Periarticular abnormality. Patients may complain of pain in a joint yet have involvement of a periarticular structure such as a tendon, ligament, or bursa as the real cause of symptoms.

      (2) Other causes. Bacterial infections and crystal-mediated problems must always be considered if only one joint is involved. Trauma, hemorrhage, and monoarticular presentations of inflammatory diseases also can be confused with osteoarthritis.

    b. Polyarticular problems

      (1) Inflammatory rheumatic disease. Systemic complaints (e.g., anorexia, weight loss, fatigue, and fever), prominent morning stiffness, and findings of inflammatory rheumatic diseases should be sought.

      (2) Soft-tissue syndromes. Disorders associated with regional aching (regional myofascial pain) or generalized aching (e.g., fibromyalgia, PMR) also should be considered in polyarticular presentations.

H **Therapy**

   1. Nonpharmacologic therapy

    a. General advice to patients. Joint overuse or repetitive trauma must be avoided. **Weight loss** may be beneficial in arthritis of weight-bearing joints such as the knees. Osteoarthritic pain improves with rest, so **joint rest** is particularly important when pain is prominent.

    b. Supports

      (1) A **knee cage** or **brace** sometimes is used when knee ligamentous instability coexists with osteoarthritis.

      (2) A **soft cervical collar** may be used for symptomatic flare-ups of cervical spine osteoarthritis.

      (3) A **lumbar corset** (back brace) sometimes is used to buttress sagging abdominal or back muscles in patients with low back pain.

      (4) A **cane** may be helpful in supporting a patient with unilateral hip or knee osteoarthritis.

      (5) **Arch supports (orthotics)** or cushioned shoes may decrease the transmission of weight-bearing forces to the hips and knees.

    c. Exercise. Isometric strengthening of supporting muscles around joints may be helpful (e.g., quadriceps-setting exercises in knee arthritis). Swimming and water aerobics are the best form of **aerobic exercise** for a patient with osteoarthritis of the hips or knees; running should be avoided by these patients.

    d. Heat/cold modalities. Application of moist heat or heating pads, or even ice, often can temporarily lessen the pain of osteoarthritis.

   2. Pharmacologic therapy

    a. Analgesics

      (1) Topical. Direct application of **capsaicin** (substance P inhibitor) to the skin overlying a painful joint can relieve pain.

      (2) Systemic. Pain-relieving medications such as **acetaminophen** often are effective in moderate-to-high doses for mild-to-moderate osteoarthritis. Narcotics should be used only under extenuating circumstances.

b. NSAIDs. Pain relief with low-to-moderate doses of aspirin or other NSAIDs may be useful. Elderly patients have more gastrointestinal and renal side effects from these drugs and, thus, should be carefully monitored when receiving such treatment. The selective COX-2–blocking agents have been shown to have similar efficacy but with less gastrointestinal toxicity [see III G 2].

c. Corticosteroids. Oral steroids have no place in the management of osteoarthritis. Occasional **intra-articular** injections of corticosteroids may be of temporary benefit in flare-ups, but repeated use of steroids carries the risk of possible acceleration of the disease process.

d. Viscosupplementation therapy with intra-articular hyaluronic acid. Two formulations of intra-articular hyaluronic acid are available for use in the treatment of early (mild) osteoarthritis of the knee. Studies have shown these agents to be effective in modulating pain originating from the osteoarthritic knee joint and have demonstrated that these agents may have a positive effect on articular cartilage biology.

e. Nutritional supplements. Glucosamine sulfate and chondroitin sulfate have been shown in several studies to decrease symptoms of pain and stiffness in osteoarthritis. A recent National Institutes of Health (NIH)–supported multicenter trial of glucosamine hydrochloride and chondroitin sulfate failed to show symptom benefit. The role of these agents in slowing disease progression has not been established.

f. Ongoing research

3. Surgery. In advanced disease of the knee or hip, **total joint replacement** can be dramatically effective in alleviating pain and restoring function. **Angulation osteotomy** is still performed in osteoarthritis of the knee to treat unicompartmental disease. The development of new biomaterials and expanding knowledge on the biology of prosthesis loosening should help lower the failure rate.

VII · BACTERIAL (SEPTIC) ARTHRITIS

Bacterial arthritis is a serious inflammatory arthritis of one or more joints that can lead to rapid joint destruction if untreated. Numerous organisms can cause a septic arthritis syndrome.

A Epidemiology (Table 11–11) Otherwise healthy individuals can develop bacterial arthritis by direct inoculation or by blood-borne invasion of a joint, but certain people are at higher risk.

1. Joint damage. Patients with joints damaged by osteoarthritis, rheumatoid arthritis, or other destructive joint processes are more at risk for infection in the already damaged joints.

2. Immunosuppression. Patients with immune deficiencies are at greater risk for bacterial arthritis, particularly if those defects involve neutropenia or impaired phagocytosis.

3. Inoculation. Repeated septicemia (e.g., in the setting of intravenous drug abuse) presents the greatest risk. Most medical procedures involving potential direct inoculation (e.g., joint aspiration and injection) are performed aseptically and only minimally increase the risk of organism introduction into the joint.

4. Prosthetic joint. Replacement of a joint with a prosthesis removes the normal defenses against joint infection, and prosthetic materials are difficult to sterilize once infected.

TABLE 11–11 Epidemiology of Bacterial Arthritis

Risk Factor	Clinical Setting	Organism
Prior joint damage	Rheumatoid arthritis, osteoarthritis	*Staphylococcus aureus*
Immunosuppression	Diabetes mellitus, alcoholism, chronic renal failure, cytotoxic drugs, systemic lupus erythematosus; cancer, acquired immunodeficiency syndrome	*S. aureus*, gram-negative rods
Joint aspiration or injection	Damaged or inflamed joint (rare)	*Staphylococcus epidermidis, S. aureus*
Intravenous drug abuse	Axial joint (acromioclavicular, sternoclavicular, sacroiliac) involvement	*S. aureus*, gram-negative rods, *Pseudomonas aeruginosa*
Sickle cell arthropathy	Joint infection or osteomyelitis	*Salmonella* and *Staphylococcus* species, *Streptococcus pneumoniae*, gram-negative rods
Prosthetic joint	Perioperative period	*S. epidermidis*
	Postoperative period	*S. aureus*, gram-negative rods or anaerobes

B **Etiology**   Infectious arthritis is best classified as **gonococcal** or **nongonococcal.** Gonococcal infections account for at least half of cases of bacterial arthritis in adults, are much less destructive, and are very responsive to treatment.

1. *Neisseria gonorrhoeae.* This gram-negative intracellular diplococcus causes **disseminated gonococcal infection (DGI).** Typically sexually transmitted, *N. gonorrhoeae* can cause **septic arthritis** or a **periarthritis–dermatitis syndrome.**

2. *Staphylococcus* **species.** Clusters of gram-positive cocci on Gram stain suggest a staphylococcal infection.
   a. *Staphylococcus aureus* is the most common nongonococcal cause of septic arthritis, which typically arises from a skin source and can be especially rapid in causing joint destruction.
   b. *Staphylococcus epidermidis* also typically arises from a skin source. Although usually less virulent than *S. aureus, S. epidermidis* is becoming a more common cause of joint infection in prosthetic joints and in the setting of intravenous drug abuse.

3. *Streptococcus* **species**
   a. **Group A β-hemolytic streptococci** remain the most common cause of infection associated with gram-positive chains on Gram stain and arise from skin or respiratory tract sources.
   b. **Non–group A streptococci** arising from skin or urinary tract sources are being seen more often in immunocompromised patients, those with prosthetic joints, and those who use intravenous drugs.

4. **Nongonococcal gram-negative organisms**
   a. **Gram-negative enteric pathogens.** Skin colonization with gram-negative organisms is a potential source of joint infection in elderly or immunocompromised individuals, particularly those in hospitals or chronic care institutions. Urinary tract sources also are common in these patients.
   b. *Haemophilus influenzae.* This gram-negative coccobacillus remains a major respiratory pathogen in infants. The potential for dissemination to joints is greatest between 6 months and 2 years of age, when infants are without protective maternal antibodies and have not developed their own.
   c. *Neisseria meningitidis.* This gram-negative intracellular diplococcus, similar to *N. gonorrhoeae,* arises from an upper respiratory tract source. It is a much less common cause of a disseminated periarthritis–dermatitis infection, which is typically characterized by more skin lesions than are seen in DGI.

5. **Anaerobic and polymicrobial infections** are uncommon; they typically arise in the setting of prosthetic joint infection or in severely immunocompromised patients.

C **Pathophysiology**

D **Clinical features**

1. **Gonococcal arthritis.** Patients with DGI typically have genital infection without symptoms of arthritis or pelvic inflammatory disease; changes in the endometrium or cervical mucus may allow causative strains to disseminate during menses. The lack of genitourinary complaints delays treatment before dissemination.
   a. **Periarthritis–dermatitis syndrome.** Most patients exhibit **migratory or additive polyarthralgias** for several days, followed by **fever, tenosynovitis,** and often **dermatitis.** The skin lesions can be **maculopapular** or **vesicular,** with the vesicles becoming **vesiculopustular** over time.
   b. **Monoarthritis.** From 25% to 50% of patients with DGI develop an infectious monoarthritis or oligoarthritis with purulent joint effusions. These "septic joints" can occur with or without preceding **periarthritis–dermatitis syndrome.**

2. **Nongonococcal arthritis.** Patients typically present with acute pain, tenderness, swelling, and severe limitation of motion in the affected joint(s). Warmth and erythema are sometimes present, and some patients have evidence of a source (e.g., skin, urinary tract, pharynx, lung, cardiac valve) responsible for septicemic joint inoculation.

E **Diagnosis**

1. **Making a presumptive diagnosis**
   a. **Gonococcal arthritis.** History of recent sexual contact should be sought and cultures from appropriate sites (pharynx, skin lesions, joint fluid, blood, rectum, urethra, and cervix) taken

in patients who have suspicious skin lesions or tenosynovitis. A sexually active adult who has an acute monoarthritis without crystals or other known cause should be cultured and treated for DGI, until other information suggests a more appropriate course.

    b. **Nongonococcal septic arthritis.** Synovial fluid should be aspirated and sent for Gram stain, glucose, WBC count and differential, and culture and sensitivity. A synovial fluid WBC count greater than **50,000/mm³** with more than **90% neutrophils** is highly suggestive of bacterial infection. Infected fluids can sometimes have less striking WBC elevations (10,000–20,000/mm³).

2. **Differential diagnosis.** Other causes of infectious and noninfectious arthritis should be considered when making a presumptive diagnosis of bacterial arthritis. **Periarticular bone and soft-tissue infections** should also be sought.

    a. **Other infections.** Patients with monoarticular arthritis may have another infection.

        (1) **Lyme disease.** This condition should always be considered in patients living in endemic areas who have a monoarticular or oligoarticular inflammatory arthritis, particularly the knees. The arthritis may be accompanied by one or more of the dermatologic, cardiac, or neurologic features of the disorder.

        (2) **Tuberculous or fungal arthritis.** These infections generally are more indolent; they typically are associated with lower synovial fluid WBC counts and lower percentages of neutrophils than are seen in bacterial infections. Synovial biopsy may be required for diagnosis because joint fluid cultures are frequently negative.

    b. **Infection outside joints**

        (1) **Osteomyelitis** near a joint can cause fever and a sterile, inflammatory effusion mimicking septic arthritis.

        (2) **Subcutaneous bursae** next to joints (e.g., prepatellar, olecranon) can be inflamed or infected and mimic an infection of the adjacent joint. The physical appearance and location of the swollen bursa should be distinctive.

    c. **Inflammatory arthritis.** Disorders such as rheumatoid arthritis, acute rheumatic fever (ARF), reactive arthritis, and psoriatic arthritis can manifest as severe monoarticular involvement looking like an infection, sometimes with WBC counts exceeding 50,000/mm³ and more than 90% neutrophils. In some instances, patients with these diseases must be treated with antibiotics for 48 hours until joint fluid cultures are known to be negative. Gout and pseudogout can cause acute monoarthritis, so synovial fluid must be examined under polarized light microscopy for the causative crystals.

F **Therapy**

1. **Antibiotics**

    a. **Choice of therapy**

        (1) **Empiric treatment.** Because bacterial arthritis is so rapidly destructive, presumptive antibiotic therapy must be started before results of definitive cultures are known. The particular antibiotic regimen is tailored to the organisms most likely in a particular individual (see Table 11–11) and particular age group (Table 11–12). In adults, gonococcal coverage is appropriate unless sexual contact can be excluded. Otherwise, coverage for *S. aureus* and streptococci typically is included. Gram-negative coverage is added in patients who are immunocompromised or who are intravenous drug abusers.

TABLE 11–12	**Bacterial Arthritis: Age Groups and Common Organisms**
Age Group	**Organism**
<2 years	*Haemophilus influenzae,** *Staphylococcus aureus,* group A streptococci, Enterobacteriaceae
2–6 years	*S. aureus,* group A streptococci, *H. influenzae*
6 years to adult	Sexually transmitted: *Neisseria gonorrhoeae*†
	Non–sexually transmitted: *S. aureus,* group A streptococci, Enterobacteriaceae

*Young children are at risk after loss of maternal antibody.
†In adults, *N. gonorrhoeae* is implicated twice as often as all other agents combined.

   (2) Directed therapy. Positive results on synovial fluid Gram stain or positive culture results from blood, synovial fluid, or other sources allow more specific treatment of the causative organism.

   b. Route and duration of therapy

   (1) Gonococcal arthritis. The gonococcus is so sensitive that 3 days of intravenous antibiotic followed by 7 more days of oral antibiotic usually is sufficient treatment.

   (2) Nongonococcal arthritis. Antibiotics typically are given intravenously for at least 2 weeks in nongonococcal bacterial arthritis and longer if clinical improvement is slow. Oral medication is given for 2 additional weeks.

2. Drainage

   a. Closed-needle aspiration. Daily drainage of any effusion is imperative to remove organisms and inflammatory debris, which can destroy cartilage and subchondral bone. Closed-needle aspiration usually is appropriate because open surgical drainage prolongs immobilization and delays return of effective function.

   b. Open surgical drainage. Hip infections are best handled by immediate open drainage, especially in children. Joints that do not respond to needle drainage are treated either by open drainage or by arthroscopy.

   c. Arthroscopic drainage. Arthroscopy is an attractive alternative to open drainage because lysis of adhesions and removal of inflamed synovium can often be accomplished without the prolonged immobilization of open drainage.

3. Other ancillary measures. Continuous passive motion early in treatment is somewhat more effective than complete immobilization at preventing loss of cartilage and subchondral bone. The avascular cartilage depends on joint motion for nutrition. **Weight bearing and ambulation of involved joints should be avoided** until effusions are gone; otherwise, **postinfectious inflammatory arthritis** can delay recovery.

4. Response to treatment

   a. Trends in the following clinical and laboratory parameters allow assessment of therapeutic progress:

   (1) Resolution of fever

   (2) Resolution of synovial effusion

   (3) Improvement in joint pain, tenderness, and range of motion

   (4) Resolution of leukocytosis (blood, synovial fluid)

   (5) Sterility of synovial fluid cultures

   b. Failure of improvement should lead to reconsideration of diagnosis, reconsideration of choice or dose of antibiotic, and consideration of open or arthroscopic drainage.

VIII SYSTEMIC LUPUS ERYTHEMATOSUS

A Definition   SLE is a chronic autoimmune disorder characterized by multisystem involvement and clinical exacerbations and remissions. **Circulating immune complexes** and **autoantibodies** cause tissue damage and organ dysfunction. Manifestations involving the skin, serosal surfaces, CNS, kidneys, and blood cells are particularly characteristic.

B Epidemiology

1. The overall **prevalence** of SLE is approximately 15–50 cases per 100,000 population. The prevalence in young women of childbearing age is approximately 8–10 times that in men. African American women are affected approximately three times as often as white women.

2. The frequency of occurrence of lupus is higher in the relatives of affected individuals than in the general population, and the disease concordance rate in identical twins approaches 50%.

C Etiology   No single cause of lupus has been discovered. Complex interrelationships among environmental factors, genetically determined host immune responses, and hormonal influences probably are critical in the initiation as well as the expression of the disease.

1. Environmental factors. Viruses and drugs or toxins have been pursued as causative agents, but neither has been shown to cause idiopathic SLE. Microbial toxins and viral (particularly retroviral) products can function as **superantigens,** binding to the helper T cell receptors and MHC class II molecule complexes nonspecifically. Binding to B cell MHC class II molecules might activate helper T cells to generate **autoimmune responses.**

2. **Genetic factors.** Twin and family studies suggest a genetic predisposition to SLE. The disease occurs commonly in families with hereditary deficiencies of early complement components. The histocompatibility antigens HLA-DR2 and HLA-DR3 are present much more commonly in SLE patients than in controls. Some of the HLA-DR3 association may be due to linkage with a deletion for a C4a gene. Specific combinations of histocompatibility antigens may be associated with the production of specific autoantibodies (e.g., HLA-DR or HLA-DQ associations with Ro and La antibodies).

3. **Autoimmunity.** Loss of tolerance to autoantigens is central to the pathogenesis of SLE, and genetic tendencies toward the development of autoantibodies, B cell hyperactivity, and T cell dysfunction are evident in patients with the disease. The tendency to develop autoimmunity in SLE is not MHC linked but may be caused by genes outside the histocompatibility loci.

4. **Apoptosis.** Programmed cell death, or apoptosis, leads to the orderly replacement of old cells in all organs, including the B and T lymphocytes of the immune system. Defects in apoptosis genes have been discovered in lupus mouse kindreds, resulting in the development of autoimmunity, perhaps related to failure to delete autoreactive T cells or autoantibody-producing B cells.

5. **Hormonal influences.** Lupus is predominantly a disease of women of childbearing age, but hormonal factors probably are more important in modulation of the expression of disease than in causation. Estrogen may be a permissive factor in polyclonal B cell activation.

D Pathogenesis

E Pathology

1. **Characteristic microscopic changes**
   a. **Hematoxylin bodies.** Amorphous masses of nuclear material bound with immunoglobulin can be found in connective tissue lesions that become purple-blue when stained with hematoxylin. Neutrophils that ingest these bodies in vitro are called **LE cells.**
   b. **Fibrinoid necrosis.** In SLE, immune complexes of DNA, antibody to DNA, and complement may stain with eosin (which can stain immune complexes as well as fibrin) in vessel walls and connective tissue, demonstrating so-called "fibrinoid necrosis."
   c. **Onion-skin lesions.** Lesions characteristic of SLE in splenic arteries are called onion-skin lesions because of the concentric deposition of collagen around them, presumably formed as vasculitic lesions heal.

2. **Tissue changes**
   a. **Skin.** Although some of the milder skin lesions in SLE have only nonspecific lymphocytic infiltration in perivascular locations in the dermis, more typical lupus lesions show **dermal–epidermal junction deposits of immunoglobulins** and complement as well as necrosis. Classic discoid lesions show follicular plugging, hyperkeratosis, and the loss of skin appendages. Frank vasculitic lesions also can occur in small dermal vessels.
   b. **Kidney.** Immune complex deposition in the kidney can lead to various histologic pictures of inflammation. A cardinal characteristic of renal pathology in SLE is the tendency of these pathologic pictures to change over time, based on changes either in disease activity or therapy. Biopsy specimens are graded with regard to activity (active inflammation) and chronicity (glomerular sclerosis and fibrotic interstitial change); the most treatable lesions have high activity and low chronicity.
      (1) **Mesangial disease** refers to **mesangial hypercellularity** caused by the presence of immunoglobulin deposits and is the most common renal pathologic lesion in SLE.
      (2) **Focal proliferative nephritis** involves cellular proliferative change only in **segments of glomeruli** and in **less than 50% of glomeruli.**
      (3) **Diffuse proliferative nephritis** involves cellular proliferation in **most of the segments** of the glomerulus and in **more than 50% of glomeruli.**
      (4) **Pure membranous nephritis** consists of **subepithelial** glomerular basement membrane immunoglobulin deposits without glomerular hypercellularity (called **wire looping** on light microscopy), although patients may have overlapping combinations of proliferative and membranous forms on biopsy.

(5) **Interstitial inflammation** can also occur in all of the aforementioned pathologic pictures.

c. **CNS.** Large-vessel vasculitic lesions can occur (although they are uncommon) in focal presentations of the disease, but focal areas of perivascular small-vessel inflammation, microinfarction, or microhemorrhages are more typical and do not correlate well with abnormalities found on imaging studies (computed tomography [CT] or magnetic resonance imaging [MRI] scans) or the neurologic examination. The **phospholipid antibody syndrome** may be associated with the small-vessel occlusive lesions.

d. **Vasculitis.** Inflammatory lesions of capillaries, venules, and arterioles caused by immune complex deposition and variable cellular infiltration are responsible for much of the tissue destruction and damage seen in SLE.

e. **Other tissue lesions.** Nonspecific mild synovitis and lymphocytic infiltration of muscles occur frequently. Nonbacterial endocarditis often is present but typically is asymptomatic.

F **Clinical features and laboratory findings (Table 11–13)**

1. **Manifestations of SLE.** Fatigue, weight loss, and fever are prominent **systemic complaints.**

a. **Skin.** The **butterfly rash** (i.e., facial erythema over the cheeks and nose) and the chronic, potentially scarring, **discoid lesions** (i.e., coin-shaped lesions with hyperemic margins, central atrophy, and depigmentation) are the most classic. Less commonly, bullous and maculopapular eruptions can occur. Nonscarring, psoriasiform lesions (**subacute cutaneous lupus**) occur and are associated with the Ro antibody. Recurrent mucous membrane ulceration, generalized or focal alopecia, digital vasculitis, and photosensitivity also are potential dermatologic features (Online Figure 11–11).

b. **Nerve**

(1) **CNS.** Focal or diffuse neurologic disorders occur in approximately 50% of patients. **Generalized manifestations** include severe headache, reactive depressions, psychoses, cognitive disturbances, and seizures. Psychosis in some lupus patients correlates with the presence of antibody to ribosomal P protein. **Focal seizures** also have been described, and hemiparesis, cranial nerve deficits, transverse myelitis, and movement disorders may pinpoint discrete areas of involvement. Lumbar puncture (LP), electroencephalography (EEG), and CT scanning often are unrevealing. However, MRI scanning reveals CNS lesions in many patients, especially those with focal presentations.

(2) **Peripheral nervous system.** Some patients have sensory or sensorimotor neuropathies, and those with vasculitis of the vasonervorum may manifest as mononeuritis multiplex.

c. **Heart.** Symptomatic **pericarditis** occurs in approximately 20% of patients with SLE and pericardial effusions on echocardiography in as many as 50%, but tamponade is uncommon. **Myocarditis** (conduction abnormalities, arrhythmias, and CHF) is less common and may be reversible if treated promptly with corticosteroids. Although **coronary vessel vasculitis** can occur in fulminant cases, premature atherosclerosis in steroid-treated patients is a more common cause of myocardial infarction (MI) in patients with lupus. **Nonbacterial endocardial lesions** (Libman–Sacks endocarditis) can be associated with embolic CNS events, valvular dysfunction, the antiphospholipid antibody syndrome, or infective endocarditis.

d. **Lung.** At some time in the disease course, approximately 30% of SLE patients have symptomatic **pleuritis.** Diaphragmatic fibrosis or diaphragm dysfunction may manifest as "**shrinking lung syndrome,**" with a restrictive picture on pulmonary function testing. Parenchymal involvement (**lupus pneumonitis**) can be difficult to distinguish from acute infections; lupus infiltrates may be unilateral or bilateral, tend to be fleeting, occur with active disease, and lack purulent sputum. **Hemoptysis** occurs as a feature of pulmonary vasculitis and the **acute pulmonary hemorrhage syndrome. Diffuse interstitial lung disease** is recognized, albeit uncommonly. **Pulmonary hypertension** as a result of isolated pulmonary vascular involvement also occurs.

e. **Gastrointestinal tract.** Although symptoms of nausea, vomiting, and abdominal pain are common, diagnostic testing often is unrevealing. Overt **intestinal vasculitis** can lead to bowel infarction, perforation, and hemorrhage. Lupus- or corticosteroid-related **pancreatitis** and reversible gastric damage or hepatitis induced by NSAIDs can occur as well.

f. **Kidney.** Most lupus patients have some clinical and pathologic evidence of renal involvement. Active disease often is announced by abnormalities in the urinary sediment (i.e., red

TABLE 11–13   Criteria for the Classification of Systemic Lupus Erythematosus

Criterion	Definition
1. Malar rash	Fixed erythema, flat or raised, over the malar eminences, tending to spare the nasolabial folds
2. Discoid rash	Erythematous raised patches with adherent keratotic scaling and follicular plugging, atrophic scarring may occur in older lesions
3. Photosensitivity	Skin rash as a result of unusual reaction to sunlight, by patient history or physician observation
4. Oral ulcers	Oral or nasopharyngeal ulceration, usually painless, observed by a physician
5. Arthritis	Nonerosive arthritis involving two or more peripheral joints, characterized by tenderness, swelling, or effusion
6. Serositis	(a) Pleuritis—convincing history of pleuritic pain or rub heard by a physician or evidence of pleural effusion OR (b) Pericarditis—documented by electrocardiogram or rub or evidence of pericardial effusion
7. Renal disorder	(a) Persistent proteinuria greater than 0.5 g/day or greater that 3+ if quantitation not performed OR (b) Cellular casts—may be red cell, hemoglobin, granular, tubular, or mixed
8. Neurologic disorders	(a) Seizures—in the absence of offending drugs or known metabolic derangements; e.g., uremia, ketoacidosis, or electrolyte imbalance OR (b) Psychosis—in the absence of offending drugs or known metabolic derangements; e.g., uremia, ketoacidosis, or electrolyte imbalance
9. Hematologic disorder	(a) Hemolytic anemia—with reticulocytosis OR (b) Leukopenia—less than 4000/mm^3 total on two or more occasions OR (c) Lymphopenia—less than 1500/mm^3 on two or more occasions OR (d) Thrombocytopenia—less than 100,000/mm^3 in the absence of offending drugs
10. Immunologic disorder*	(a) Anti-DNA: antibody to native DNA in abnormal titer OR (b) Anti-SM: presence of antibody to SM nuclear antigen OR (c) Positive finding of antiphospholipid antibodies based on (1) an abnormal serum level of immunoglobulin G (IgG) or IgM anticardiolipin antibodies, (2) a positive test result for lupus anticoagulant using a standard method, or (3) a false-positive serologic test for syphilis known to be positive for at least 6 months and confirmed by *Treponema pallidum* immobilization or fluorescent treponemal antibody absorption test
11. Antinuclear antibody	An abnormal titer of antinuclear antibody by immunofluorescence or an equivalent assay at any point in time and in the absence of drugs known to be associated with "drug-induced lupus" syndrome

This classification is based on 11 criteria. For the purpose of identifying patients in clinical studies, a person must have SLE if 4 four or more of the 11 criteria are present, serially or simultaneously, during any interval of observation.

*The modifications to criterion number 10 were made in 1997.

Adapted from Tan EM, Cohen AS, Fries JF, et al. The 1982 revised criteria for the classification of systemic lupus erythematosus (SLE). *Arthritis Rheum* 1982;25:1271–1277, with permission from the American College of Rheumatology; and Hochberg MC. Updating the American College of Rheumatology revised criteria for the classification of system lupus erythematosus [Letter]. *Arthritis Rheum* 1997;40:1725, with permission of the American College of Rheumatology.

blood cells [RBCs], WBCs, or cellular casts formed in the absence of acute bacterial infection). Other clinical laboratory features typically associated with active renal disease are elevations in serum creatinine and blood urea nitrogen (BUN) levels, decreased levels of serum complement components, or increased titers of antibodies against double-stranded DNA. The renal biopsy often can aid in treatment decisions and the determination of prognosis, although the biopsy pathology may change with disease course or therapy.

(1) **Mesangial disease** is the most common and mildest form of renal involvement and may be asymptomatic. Many patients have mild proteinuria or RBCs or WBCs on urinalysis. Treatment usually is not required.

(2) Focal proliferative nephritis often has a good prognosis as well and typically requires treatment with corticosteroids alone; however, its more severe presentations blend with diffuse proliferative nephritis clinically and prognostically.

(3) Diffuse proliferative nephritis is the **most severe** pathologic lesion and usually is associated with hypertension, severe proteinuria, and some degree of renal insufficiency. The most severe cases can be associated with **crescents** and the rapid development of severe renal insufficiency. Corticosteroids and cytotoxic agents typically are required for preservation of renal function.

(4) Membranous glomerulopathy classically manifests as large amounts of protein in the urine and nephrotic syndrome, usually with relatively few cells in the urine. Corticosteroid therapy may help control protein loss. Slowly progressive renal insufficiency may develop over time; it is not clear whether the addition of cytotoxic agents retards this progression.

g. Muscle and bone. Arthralgia and **symmetric arthritis** often are features of acute SLE, but the rare joint deformities (**Jaccoud's arthropathy**) that occur are a function of tendon or ligament laxity rather than erosive joint disease. Inflammatory muscle involvement usually is subclinical, but clinical inflammatory myopathy can occur.

h. Other. Photosensitivity can trigger systemic symptoms as well as skin manifestations. Raynaud's phenomenon and secondary Sjögren's syndrome each occurs in approximately 25% of patients.

2. Laboratory findings

a. Hematologic findings. Anemia is common during active disease and more often is the anemia of chronic disease than hemolytic anemia. Antibodies to leukocytes also occur, with autoimmune lymphopenia a common feature of active disease; neutropenia is less common. Antibodies to platelets can cause chronic immune thrombocytopenia or more acute falls in the platelet count with active disease. Elevation of the erythrocyte sedimentation rate is common and correlates with disease activity in some patients.

b. Coagulation parameters. Antibodies to the phospholipid components of individual clotting factors can interfere with coagulation testing, causing prolongation of the partial thromboplastin time (PTT) not correctable by the addition of normal plasma. Paradoxically, patients with PTT prolongation (the **"lupus anticoagulant"**) have a higher frequency of thrombosis than bleeding.

c. Serologic findings. Phospholipid antibodies also can cause false-positive test results for syphilis, more often by interference with reagin (e.g., rapid plasma reagin [RPR] or Venereal Disease Research Laboratory [VDRL]) testing than with antitreponemal (e.g., fluorescent treponemal antibody absorption [FTA-ABS]) testing.

d. Immunologic findings. Patients with lupus commonly have **low complement component (C3 and C4) levels** as a result of immune complex activation; in many patients, falls in serum complement levels parallel disease flare-ups if complement synthesis is unchanged.

(1) Hypergammaglobulinemia reflects B cell hyperactivity. By far the most significant immunologic findings in SLE patients are **autoantibodies,** such as antinuclear antibodies (ANAs), anti-DNA, and anti-Sm.

(2) ANAs. Approximately 99% of patients with SLE have ANAs. These antibodies are detectable by an immunofluorescence technique that involves human epithelial cell lines (e.g., HEp-2 cells). When the test serum is applied to the epithelial cells that have been frozen and cut to expose nuclear components, the patient's ANAs interact with the nuclear material, and this interaction can be detected by fluorescence microscopy. A **diffuse** or **homogeneous** immunofluorescent staining **pattern** is most common in SLE, although **speckled, nucleolar,** and **rim patterns** also can be seen (Online I B 3).

G Diagnosis Careful consideration of the historical and physical findings that suggest this multisystem disease is necessary. Systemic illness with characteristic rash, polyarthritis, and serositis is a common presentation, but the possibility of lupus should be entertained even when patients present with seemingly isolated hematologic cytopenias, CNS disease, or glomerulonephritis. In suspicious settings, physicians should seek laboratory evidence of autoimmunity and attempt to exclude other illnesses.

1. Diagnostic criteria (see Table 11–13). The 1997 ARA revised criteria for the diagnosis of SLE are useful when the disease is suspected, and the presence over time of any **4** of the 11 criteria strongly suggests the diagnosis. Although findings such as alopecia, periungual vasculitis, and low serum complement levels are not among the criteria, they may be supportive evidence in individual patients.

2. **Differential diagnosis.** Physicians must be careful to exclude other chronic rheumatic diseases, especially rheumatoid arthritis, overlap syndromes (inflammatory myopathies or scleroderma overlapping with SLE), and vasculitic syndromes in arriving at the diagnosis of SLE. The following syndromes also should be considered in the setting of possible SLE:

   a. **Undifferentiated connective tissue disease (UCTD).** This disorder is used to describe patients with clinical features of several connective tissue diseases and high titers of antibody to U_1RNP. Patients with UCTD may have cutaneous features of SLE, dermatomyositis, or scleroderma; inflammatory muscle disease; and a destructive form of arthritis more typical of rheumatoid arthritis. Furthermore, the severe renal and CNS manifestations of SLE usually are not present. When followed for prolonged periods, most patients with this disease more closely resemble patients with scleroderma or SLE.

   b. **Drug-induced lupus.** Chronic ingestion of several drugs can precipitate a syndrome of **polyserositis, arthritis,** and **antihistone ANAs.** The drugs most commonly associated include hydralazine, procainamide, penicillamine, isoniazid, and phenytoin. Renal disease is rare in this syndrome, and dermal and CNS features are less common than in idiopathic SLE. Drug-induced SLE typically resolves on discontinuation of the drug. Hepatic acetylation of drugs such as hydralazine, isoniazid, and procainamide is apparently slow in patients who develop this syndrome. However, these drugs typically are tolerated well by patients with spontaneous SLE.

   c. **Discoid lupus.** Patients can have typical skin manifestations of SLE without systemic disease. Fifteen percent of these patients have positive ANAs. These patients should be considered to have SLE when other disease features are present.

3. **Associated syndromes**

   a. **Neonatal lupus syndrome** can develop in infants of mothers (who may not have SLE) who have high-titer **IgG antibodies** to **Ro.** The maternal antibodies apparently cross the placenta, bind to fetal tissue, and cause immunologic injury. The most typical features include evanescent lupus skin lesions, but transient thrombocytopenia or hemolytic anemia can occur. The most serious clinical presentation occurs in pregnant women when the antibody to Ro binds to fetal cardiac tissue and causes congenital heart block, which can require permanent pacing. Most mothers of affected infants develop a mild version of some autoimmune disease over time, often SLE.

   b. **Phospholipid antibody syndrome** can occur as a mimic of SLE or as part of the disease. One third to one half of lupus patients exhibit phospholipid antibody if tested, although the associated clinical syndrome occurs less commonly.

      (1) Manifestations most commonly include **venous or arterial thromboses,** sometimes of large vessels, and can also include **episodic thrombocytopenia. Pregnant patients may experience fetal death** after the first trimester or premature birth, and these problems may recur in successive pregnancies. Some of these patients exhibit placental thrombosis, infarction, or insufficiency, but the cause of fetal death is not always clear.

      (2) Testing for antibodies to phospholipids is involved [🔲 Online I B 6].

      (3) **Management** primarily involves **chronic anticoagulation therapy,** typically with warfarin, after the first episode of clinical thrombosis.

H **Therapy** Treatment must be individualized to the features that a particular patient exhibits, and it need not always include corticosteroids. Patients must understand that the prognosis in this chronic disease generally is better than they fear and that their compliance with medication regimens and avoidance of disease precipitants (e.g., ultraviolet light and emotional stress) often can favorably affect the disease course. Physicians must be alert to disease flare-ups related to surgery, antecedent infections, or the postpartum period.

1. Topical **sunscreens** containing *para*-aminobenzoic acid (PABA) or benzophenones are effective in protecting the one third of lupus patients who are photosensitive.

2. **NSAIDs** are used in full anti-inflammatory doses for fever, joint complaints, and serositis. Mild elevation in transaminase levels often develops in SLE patients on these drugs, and aseptic meningitis has been reported in lupus patients on ibuprofen, tolmetin, and sulindac.

3. **Antimalarial drugs** (e.g., hydroxychloroquine and chloroquine) often are used to treat fatigue, skin disease, and arthritis in SLE. Retinal pigmentary deposition leading to blindness is a rare complication of antimalarial treatment since hydroxychloroquine replaced chloroquine. Patients should be screened by an ophthalmologist every 6 months to 1 year.

4. **Corticosteroids**
   a. **Topical preparations.** Some of the skin manifestations are improved by treatment with topical glucocorticoids, although discoid lesions usually require additional treatment with antimalarial agents.
   b. **Systemic corticosteroids**
      (1) **Glucocorticoids** in varying doses are often required to control severe manifestations of SLE and less severe symptoms when they are persistent and disabling. These drugs should be used cautiously because long-term treatment usually is needed and typical side effects ensue. **Chronic arthritis** and **serositis** may require glucocorticoids if NSAIDs are not sufficient. Severe **hemolysis**, life-threatening **thrombocytopenia, pneumonitis, CNS** or **peripheral nervous system disease,** clinically evident **cardiac** or **skeletal muscle disease, renal disease,** and **vasculitis** are typical indications for systemic glucocorticoids. Usually the drug dose selected is proportionate to the severity of the illness; the dose is tapered as manifestations subside.
      (2) **"Pulse" corticosteroids** may be necessary. Large doses of corticosteroids sometimes are administered intravenously for particularly severe cases of SLE. Serious **renal** and **CNS manifestations** have been the typical indications for pulse treatment, but dangerous **cardiopulmonary** and **hematologic involvement** also might warrant this aggressive treatment.

5. **Cytotoxic agents** (e.g., azathioprine and cyclophosphamide) sometimes are used to treat severe, refractory features of lupus, particularly **renal disease.** Intravenous "pulse" cyclophosphamide is effective for the treatment of diffuse proliferative glomerulonephritis and other acute severe manifestations of lupus.

6. **Mycophenolate mofetil** is a reversible inhibitor of inosine monophosphate dehydrogenase and blocks proliferation of B and T cells. It has been used successfully in renal allograft rejection. It has currently gained momentum as an equivalent treatment to cyclophosphamide for treatment of lupus nephritis.

7. **Intravenous immunoglobulin** may be effective. Large doses of immunoglobulin have been given intravenously to treat refractory manifestations of lupus, particularly **immune-mediated thrombocytopenia** or **hemolytic anemia.** This therapy is expensive, often must be given monthly, and **cannot be given to IgA-deficient patients** because of the risk of anaphylaxis.

8. **Belimumab** is a monoclonal antibody against B cell activating factor, B lymphocyte stimulator (BLyS). Two large phase III trials showed clinical benefit in groups of patients who had no CNS or renal disease.

[I] **Prognosis** Outcomes are clearly better today than in the presteroid era; milder forms of disease are recognized, and, presumably, appropriate drug treatment improves morbidity and mortality rates. **Renal disease** and **infectious complications** are still major causes of death, and prominent **CNS disease** can lead to severe disability. The mortality rate is higher in patients of lower socioeconomic status and educational attainment, a characteristic common to many chronic illnesses. Steroid-related complications can be crippling (e.g., avascular necrosis of the femoral head and osteoporotic vertebral fractures) or fatal (e.g., premature coronary atherosclerosis).

IX   SYSTEMIC SCLEROSIS

[A] **Definition** Systemic sclerosis (scleroderma) (SSc) is a connective tissue disease characterized by widespread **small-vessel obliterative disease** and **fibrosis of the skin** (especially distal, digital skin) and **multiple internal organs,** including the heart, lungs, kidneys, and gastrointestinal tract. The description best fits the diffuse form, but localized forms also exist. These latter forms involve patches of skin and subcutaneous tissues but do not include digital skin involvement, Raynaud's phenomenon, or internal organ changes.

B **Epidemiology** SSc is a relatively rare disease; familial clustering is uncommon. The disease is three to four times more common in women than in men. Coal miners are at a higher risk for the disease, possibly as a result of exposure to silica dust.

C **Etiology** The etiology of SSc is unknown. In some cases it seems likely that an environmental agent (e.g., toxin or virus) causes vascular endothelial injury, with later immunologic responses leading to continued endothelial damage and tissue fibrosis. Supportive evidence includes the initiation of a fibrosing syndrome in patients with polyvinyl chloride exposure, Spanish "toxic oil" syndrome, and L-tryptophan–related eosinophilia myalgia syndrome. Whether the initiating event is environmental or immunologic, the early lesion in SSc seems to be one of **vascular endothelial damage,** especially in small vessels.

D **Pathogenesis** There is evidence of T cell activation in the blood, skin, and lungs. Unregulated immunologic processes appear to be responsible for continuing vascular damage and widespread **dermal** and **internal organ fibrosis.**

1. **Vascular endothelial damage**

2. **Tissue fibrosis**

3. **Autoantibodies**

E **Clinical features** The degree of skin change and the type and progression of internal organ involvement are different in the **limited form** as compared to the **diffuse form** of SSc. In addition, spontaneous fluctuations in disease activity can occur.

1. **Skin involvement.** Skin changes occur in **95% of patients** with SSc. An early **edematous phase** of small-vessel endothelial injury and increased permeability may progress through an **indurative phase** as increasing amounts of collagen are produced in the subcutaneous tissue. Epidermal and skin appendage atrophy may occur in late forms of the disease (**atrophic phase**) as the skin becomes progressively bound to underlying tissue.
   (1) **Distribution.** Changes most often begin in the fingers and hands and may spread to involve more proximal tissues, including the trunk and face. The lower extremities often are less severely involved (Online Figure 11–12).
   (2) **Associated features**
      (a) **Raynaud's phenomenon** occurs in **95% of patients** with SSc. Episodic vasospasm of the damaged small vessels in the digits results in a **triphasic color change** of the involved area as blood flow ceases (white), returns sluggishly (blue), and exhibits reactive hyperemia (red).
      (b) **Telangiectasias** can occur in involved areas as well as on mucous membranes.
      (c) **Subcutaneous calcifications** can occur, especially in finger tips.
      (d) **Salt-and-pepper changes may occur,** in which the skin can become taut, shiny, and immobile, and hyperpigmented areas can alternate with depigmented areas.
      (e) **Microcapillary abnormalities** may be present. The distal nail bed proliferates, and the capillary bed becomes visibly abnormal, with dilation, tortuosity, and loss of vessels. These abnormalities can be seen by examining the proximal nail beds with wide-field microscopy.
      (f) **Skin ulcers** are possible. Distal digital ulcers and finger tapering occur due to distal infarctions and consequent loss of digital pulp, sometimes resulting in infection.

2. **Gastrointestinal tract**
   (1) **Esophageal dysfunction** is the most common manifestation of internal organ involvement. **Esophageal motility dysfunction** and **reflux** develop as collagen replaces smooth muscle in the lower two thirds of the esophagus; striated muscle in the upper one third of the esophagus is relatively unaffected. **Esophageal strictures** can result from the constant reflux, and **ulceration** can occur at the gastroesophageal junction. Barium swallow and esophageal manometry may be helpful in documenting disease extent. Upper gastrointestinal endoscopy is helpful in evaluating the extent of involvement and possible Barrett's esophagus [see Chapter 6 I B 1 e (5)].
   (2) **Similar small bowel involvement** leads to intestinal hypomotility and intermittent cramping, diarrhea, and **bacterial overgrowth malabsorption syndrome. Wide-mouth**

diverticula can be seen in the transverse and descending colon in areas of patchy muscularis involvement. Lower gastrointestinal contrast radiographic studies or malabsorption testing may demonstrate small bowel or colonic involvement.

3. **Lung.** Widespread small pulmonary arterial narrowing and fibrotic change eventually can lead to **isolated pulmonary hypertension.** More commonly, a fibrotic proliferation in the peribronchial and perialveolar tissues leads to progressive **interstitial lung disease.** Patients with interstitial lung disease present with symptoms of progressive dyspnea on exertion and demonstrate a restrictive pattern on pulmonary function testing, a better disease indicator than chest radiographic changes. High-resolution CT (HRCT) scanning of the lung can reveal the character and distribution of fine structural abnormalities not visible on chest radiography. Studies with bronchoalveolar lavage (BAL) have shown that a significant proportion of patients with SSc have an alveolitis, and aggressive chemotherapy may be indicated in this subset of patients. Pleuritis is uncommon in SSc as compared with other rheumatic diseases (e.g., rheumatoid arthritis and SLE).

4. **Heart.** Clinical cardiac involvement can take several forms. Clinically, acute and chronic pericarditis are unusual, but effusions often can be seen on ultrasonography and are associated with myocardial involvement. If interstitial myocardial disease is extensive, frank **cardiomyopathy** can result, producing CHF, arrhythmias, and conduction disturbances. Angina can be a result of fibrotic involvement of small myocardial vessels. Ambulatory electrocardiogram (ECG) monitoring or exercise stress testing can help to uncover dangerous arrhythmias or subtle ischemia in need of treatment.

5. **Kidney.** Sudden renal failure (**scleroderma renal crisis**) can occur often as a combination of interlobular artery fibrotic damage and some vasoconstrictive stimulus (e.g., diuresis, blood loss, surgery). Massive renin–angiotensin release in response to decreased renal perfusion worsens the vasoconstriction, and acute renal failure can occur. **Malignant hypertension** and **microangiopathic hemolytic anemia** often accompany these renal events. **Chronic renal failure** and **death** occur unless emergent treatment restores renal perfusion. Some but not all patients demonstrate new hypertension, urinary protein, or elevated serum creatinine testing before acute renal decompensation, so these features should be monitored periodically.

6. **Muscle.** In many patients, a mild indolent myopathy manifested by minor enzyme elevations and perhaps mild weakness occurs but does not require treatment. In some patients, an overt **inflammatory myopathy** identical to polymyositis can occur (**"overlap" presentation**).

7. **Joint and tendon.** More than 50% of patients with scleroderma develop swelling, stiffness, and pain in finger, wrist, and knee joints. Mild, self-limited inflammatory arthritis can occur early in the disease, but typical joint involvement is limited to synovial fibrosis and impaired range of motion due to the generalized restriction of the fibrotic process. Tendon sheath involvement is not unusual; carpal tunnel syndrome can result from extensive tendon sheath fibrosis in the wrist.

8. **Nerve.** Neurologic involvement typically is limited to fibrotic **entrapment neuropathies** of the median and trigeminal nerves.

F **Clinical syndromes** Classification of the disease into **limited** and **diffuse forms** is important because of differences in organ involvement and, thus, prognosis. In general, the more widespread visceral involvement of the diffuse form gives it a poorer prognosis than the limited variant. Scleroderma can also exist in **overlap forms,** the most distinct of which is **UCTD.**

1. **Diffuse scleroderma** (SSc) is typified by **proximal skin involvement** (skin proximal to the MCP joints or forearms in various definitions) and the presence of **Scl-70 antibodies** or **antinucleolar ANAs.** Visceral organ involvement in this form typically occurs earlier than in the limited variant. Renal involvement is much more common than in the limited form, and pulmonary fibrosis occurs earlier and more quickly.

2. **Limited scleroderma** typically has skin involvement limited to the distal extremities and face, and also is known as the **CREST variant** (involving the coexistence of subcutaneous **calcinosis, Raynaud's phenomenon, esophageal motility dysfunction, sclerodactyly,** and **telangiectasia**). **Anticentromere antibody** is most closely associated with this form, and visceral involvement is usually more slowly progressive than in the diffuse form. One exception is the early development

of **pulmonary vascular hypertension** in this form due to obliterative changes in pulmonary arterioles. The pulmonary fibrosis so typical of the diffuse variant occurs more slowly in this form but can become severe after several decades of disease.

3. **UCTD** is a rheumatic syndrome that can include clinical features of scleroderma, SLE, and polymyositis in association with the presence of high titers of **antibody** to **U_1RNP.** Most cases evolve into more typical scleroderma or SLE over time.

G Diagnosis

1. **Clinical approach.** A diagnosis of scleroderma should be entertained in the presence of symptoms of **Raynaud's phenomenon, distal skin thickening,** and **visceral organ involvement.** Physicians should evaluate distal nail beds for the suggestive capillary abnormality and attempt to document the location and extent of the skin thickening to differentiate local from generalized forms. In addition, they should look for evidence of internal organ change. Characteristic ANA test results also may be useful in classifying patients.

   a. **Raynaud's phenomenon.** The abnormal vascular response to cold or emotional stimuli is present in most patients with the diffuse or limited form of scleroderma, but most patients with Raynaud's phenomenon do not have scleroderma or another form of connective tissue disease. As many as 5%–10% of nonsmoking women in population surveys may have Raynaud's phenomenon; typical screening procedures for scleroderma include examination for finger edema, finger nail–fold capillary abnormalities, and ANAs. Patients with none of these features are unlikely to develop scleroderma. Because patients can have Raynaud's phenomenon in association with other connective tissue diseases (SLE or polymyositis), a clinical search for these illnesses should be made as well.

   b. **Distal skin thickening.** Such epidermal thickening is a diagnostic feature of both the diffuse and limited forms of scleroderma. Patients with diffuse scleroderma also have more proximal involvement, typically of the upper arms, upper legs, or trunk. Fewer than 5% of patients may have visceral involvement typical of scleroderma without skin thickening (**scleroderma sine scleroderma**).

   c. **Laboratory findings.** Differences in ANA testing may discriminate between diffuse and limited forms of scleroderma. Patients with the diffuse form often have **Scl-70 antibodies** or **antinucleolar ANAs.** Patients with the more limited forms often have **anticentromere antibodies.**

   d. **Visceral involvement.** Typical internal organ involvement [see IX E 1] lends further support to scleroderma diagnosis and helps discriminate between diffuse and limited forms.

2. **Differential diagnosis.** Skin thickening can be seen in other illnesses besides scleroderma. Typically, Raynaud's phenomenon, characteristic distal hand involvement, and visceral organ changes of scleroderma are absent.

   a. **Local scleroderma.** Two forms of purely local disease, **morphea** and **linear scleroderma,** have similar clinical and pathologic appearance to sclerodermatous skin. These forms manifest as localized fibrotic plaques (morphea) or as longitudinal bands (linear scleroderma).

      (1) **Morphea** may occur at any age (it is more common in childhood) as a disease characterized by small circumscribed skin lesions (**guttate morphea**) or larger patches (**morphea en plaque**).

      (2) **Linear scleroderma** occurs most commonly in children and young adults. Facial involvement (**coup de sabre**) can be extremely disfiguring. The principal impact of linear scleroderma can be interference with function or growth of underlying muscle or bone, leading to extremity wasting or contractures.

   b. **Eosinophilic fasciitis.** Pain, swelling, and tenderness develop in one or more extremities, sometimes after an episode of vigorous exercise. Induration of involved skin and subcutaneous tissue develops, but without Raynaud's phenomenon or sclerodactyly. Patients often have marked peripheral blood eosinophilia, and a full-thickness skin biopsy (including underlying fascia and muscle) is required to demonstrate the deep fascial eosinophils and chronic inflammatory cell infiltrate.

   c. **Eosinophilia–myalgia syndrome.** A clinical syndrome related to the ingestion of ʟ-**tryptophan dietary supplements** can be confused with scleroderma (due to the skin thickening in some cases) and may be responsible for some cases of eosinophilic fasciitis. Patients who take L-tryptophan likely have ingested a toxic contaminant generated by the synthetic process, although some may metabolize L-tryptophan abnormally. The cornerstones of diagnosis are **eosinophilia (>1000/mm³) and severe myalgia** found in the absence of other possible causes. Variable features include skin rashes and induration, interstitial pulmonary infiltrates, and polyneuropathy. Elevation of muscle enzymes (aldolase, not creatine kinase [CK]) and hepatic enzymes also can occur.

    d. Nephrogenic systemic fibrosis. The administration of gadolinium-containing contrast media for magnetic resonance imaging in patients with advanced renal failure has been associated with the potentially severe syndrome of nephrogenic systemic fibrosis. It is characterized by involvement of skin that can mimic scleroderma. On histologic examination, there is marked expansion and fibrosis of the dermis, in association with CD34-positive fibroblasts. Free gadolinium, which is highly toxic, accumulates in patients with kidney failure who have not undergone dialysis and precipitates in tissues. This may initiate a cascade of events leading to increased production of transforming growth factor beta 1, which in turn regulates dendritic cell maturation and antigen presentation, leading to increased tissue fibrosis. An alternate theory suggests that this same toxin can stimulate bone marrow production of $CD34^+$ circulating fibrocytes, which accumulate in the affected tissue and produce collagen in the absence of tissue injury. Skin disease typically presents as symmetric, bilateral fibrotic indurated papules, plaques, or subcutaneous nodules that first develop on the ankles, lower legs, feet, and hands and then move proximally to involve the thighs, forearms, and, less often, the trunk or buttocks. The head is spared. A distinguishing feature of this disease is the absence of **Raynaud's phenomenon.** Systemic involvement may also occur and includes muscle induration, joint contractures due to periarticular skin thickening, fibrosis of the lungs, diaphragm, myocardium, pericardium, and dura mater.

H Therapy

    1. General. Disease expression in individual patients is extremely heterogeneous. Specific therapy should focus on extent of organ damage and rate of progression of disease.

    2. Specific disease features

        a. Skin involvement. There are no FDA-approved therapies for skin disease. **Mycophenolate mofetil** and **methotrexate** may be useful in rapidly progressing skin disease. Rituximab is being investigated for a potential role in skin disease. D-Penicillamine and colchicine are largely outdated therapies of the past.

        b. Raynaud's phenomenon. Patients should understand the need to cover their head, ears, hands, feet, and trunk in cold weather to minimize reflex vasoconstriction, and smoking should be discouraged. **Calcium channel blocking agents** are useful vasodilating agents in the treatment of scleroderma. Patients should avoid nonselective β-blockers that can also contribute to vasoconstriction. Agents used for the treatment of pulmonary hypertension [see d below] have also been used for refractory vasospastic episodes.

        c. Esophageal involvement. Reflux esophagitis, often severe, requires the use of proton-pump inhibitors (e.g., omeprazole, lansoprazole). Antireflux measures (e.g., head-of-bed elevation, frequent small feedings) are helpful as well.

        d. Pulmonary involvement. For interstitial pulmonary disease, daily **oral cyclophosphamide** may be the most effective therapy for alveolitis and progressive pulmonary fibrosis. Tobacco smoking may be synergistic in pulmonary injury. Treatment for the primary pulmonary hypertension–like syndrome include the endothelin-1 receptor antagonist bosentan; the phosphodiesterase-5 inhibitor sildenafil; and various prostaglandin analogs (e.g., iloprost, epoprostenol). Anticoagulation in combination with vasodilators improves survival, which probably relates to the high incidence of in situ microthrombi or pulmonary emboli.

        e. Lower gastrointestinal involvement. Bacterial overgrowth malabsorption may be improved by intermittent treatment with **broad-spectrum antibiotics** (e.g., tetracycline). **Prokinetic agents** (e.g., octreotide, cisapride) help constipation and bloating related to lower gastrointestinal motility dysfunction.

        f. Muscle involvement. When inflammatory myositis occurs in overlap syndromes, **corticosteroids** are used, as in polymyositis. Methotrexate may be helpful in treating myositis and joint disease. **NSAIDs** may be used in treating articular symptoms as well, taking care to monitor renal function closely.

g. **Renal involvement.** Aggressive control of hypertension is best. The **angiotensin converting enzyme (ACE) inhibitors** (e.g., captopril and enalapril) are major advances in controlling blood pressure in patients with scleroderma and may help reverse the angiotensin-dependent vasoconstrictive state of scleroderma renal crisis. The avoidance of hypovolemia in diuresis and in the perioperative state is important.

h. **Cardiac involvement.** Medications useful for control of angina, CHF, and arrhythmias are used when these complications occur.

X INFLAMMATORY MYOPATHIES (POLYMYOSITIS AND DERMATOMYOSITIS)

A Definition Polymyositis is an idiopathic inflammatory muscle disease associated with prominent proximal muscle weakness, muscle enzyme elevations, characteristic myopathic electromyogram (EMG) patterns, and inflammatory infiltrates on muscle biopsy. When this complex is accompanied by a characteristic rash it is called **dermatomyositis.** Dermatomyositis is much more common than polymyositis in children.

B Epidemiology Polymyositis is a rare disease, occurring in approximately 1 in 200,000 individuals, with a peak incidence in childhood and in late adulthood. It is twice as common in females as in males and may be associated with malignancy in the adult-onset form.

C Etiology The basic cause of polymyositis is unknown. However, it is believed that an initiating viral infection and altered immune responses are potentially important in causation and pathogenesis. Lymphocyte-mediated muscle cell damage is thought to be the central pathogenetic factor in this disease, although small-vessel damage is also an important factor in dermatomyositis.

1. **Infections** can cause acute myositis.

2. **Autoimmunity**

D Pathology The major sites of inflammation are skeletal muscle and, less commonly, cardiac muscle. Skin involvement is a minor pathologic feature.

1. **Inflammatory infiltrate.** Lymphocytes and plasma cells are the predominant inflammatory cells, although macrophages, eosinophils, and neutrophils also can be seen in muscle tissue. $CD8^+$ cells infiltrate muscle fibers in polymyositis. In dermatomyositis, $CD4^+$ cells and B cells often are clustered around small blood vessels within the muscle.

2. **Muscle fiber damage.** Spotty muscle fiber necrosis and degeneration occur, with loss of cross striations and variation in the size of surviving fibers. Increased numbers of muscle nuclei and enhanced basophilic staining of fibers indicate regeneration in the midst of cell death. Interstitial fibrotic infiltrates occur in chronic cases.

E Clinical features and laboratory findings Inflammatory myopathies are clinically grouped into specific syndromes, depending on specific organ manifestations and results of laboratory tests.

1. **Organ involvement**
   a. **Skin.** The rash of dermatomyositis consists of erythematous patches, which sometimes are scaling or atrophic and are distributed over the face, neck, upper chest, and extensor surfaces. Only scattered inflammatory infiltrates in the dermis are evident on biopsy.
      (1) Pathognomonic skin findings include **heliotrope rash** (a violet discoloration and swelling of the eyelids) and **Gottron's sign** (heaped-up erythematous papules over the MCP or PIP joints) (Online Figure 11–13).
      (2) Other significant findings include **mechanic's hands** (roughened erythematous skin and hypertrophic changes of the palms and fingers), as well as the erythematous **V sign** (anterior chest) and **shawl sign** (neck and upper back) (Online Figure 11–14).
   b. **Lung.** Chronic interstitial lung disease can occur, especially in association with antisynthetase antibodies. Aspiration pneumonitis and ventilatory insufficiency also can occur [see d (1) below].
   c. **Joint.** A mild, symmetric inflammatory arthritis occurs uncommonly and rarely is destructive; it is seen most often in patients with the synthetase antibodies [see X E 2 b (2) (a)].

d. Muscle. Most patients have gradual but steady progression of muscle weakness; however, some patients have such fulminant courses that **acute respiratory failure** or **myoglobinuric renal failure** can ensue.

  (1) Skeletal muscle weakness is the primary manifestation of polymyositis.

  (a) Symmetric, proximal, and **upper and lower extremity weakness** occurs, causing difficulty with rising from a chair, sitting up in bed, or combing hair.

  (b) Pharyngeal muscle involvement can lead to swallowing difficulties and aspiration, and respiratory muscle dysfunction can lead to respiratory failure.

  (2) Cardiac muscle involvement is not as common, but when it occurs it manifests as cardiomyopathy with CHF, arrhythmias, and conduction disturbances.

2. Laboratory findings

  a. Muscle enzymes. An increased concentration of enzymes typically present in skeletal muscle is prominent in polymyositis. **CK** and **aldolase** are routinely measured, and CK fractionation may suggest myocardial involvement if the **MB fraction** (i.e., the CK isozyme found mainly in myocardium but also in regenerating skeletal muscle) is increased. However, in most patients, CK elevation is caused by the **MM band** (i.e., the fraction most prevalent in skeletal muscle). Serum **myoglobin** levels are also elevated in most patients and may be more sensitive than CK levels in some myositis patients. Enzyme elevations usually correlate with activity of the muscle disease and are used as a parameter to evaluate treatment response.

  b. Autoantibodies. Most patients with polymyositis/dermatomyositis (80%–90%) have antibodies to nuclear or cytoplasmic antigens. Routine ANA testing against HEp-2 cells is performed; other myositis-specific antibodies require specialized testing (e.g., immunoprecipitation).

  (1) Nonspecific autoantibodies. ANAs, particularly **speckled-pattern ANAs,** are the most common autoantibodies in the inflammatory myopathies, occurring in more than 50% of patients. Other antibodies also can be seen, including **Ro antibodies, La antibodies, PM/Scl antibodies,** and **Ku antibodies.**

  (2) Specific autoantibodies. Several autoantibodies are formed only in inflammatory myopathies; they target cytoplasmic or nuclear constituents of myocytes. The appearance of these antibodies, which seem to correlate with clinical patterns of involvement, may be more useful in classifying patients.

  (a) Synthetase antibodies (anti-aminoacyl–tRNA synthetases) are directed against cytoplasmic enzymes involved in specific amino acid attachment to tRNA. **Jo-1 antibody,** found in 20% of myositis patients, is the most common, directed against histidyl–tRNA synthetase. Patients with these antibodies may be considered to have the "antisynthetase syndrome," which is associated with DR3 and DRw52 haplotypes. This condition, which usually occurs in the spring, is characterized by acute onset of arthritis, interstitial lung disease, fever, mechanic hands, and Raynaud's phenomenon. Affected patients have a 5-year survival rate of 70%.

  (b) Signal recognition particle antibodies (SRP antibodies) recognize one of the components of the SRP, a cytoplasmic protein complex involved in polypeptide transfer across the endoplasmic reticulum. Immunogenetic data indicate a DR5 and DRw52 association. Patients tend to have an acute onset of severe myalgia and significant cardiac problems such as palpitations. Prognosis is very poor, with a 5-year survival rate of only 25%.

  (c) Mi-2 antibodies target a nuclear protein of unknown function, in contrast to the cytoplasmic proteins of the other myositis-specific antibodies. This antibody pattern is found in patients with classic dermatomyositis. The 5-year survival is nearly 100%.

3. Clinical syndromes. The traditional classification scheme is as follows.

  a. Polymyositis. Characteristic features include upper and lower extremity proximal muscular weakness and elevated muscle enzymes. All organ manifestations listed in Section X E 1 can occur, except the skin findings. Patients with polymyositis tend to have disease that is less responsive than dermatomyositis to therapy. The treatment-resistant, acutely severe disease is often associated with cardiac muscle involvement, a finding more prominent in patients with **SRP antibodies.** Patients with polymyositis who have **PM/Scl antibodies** tend to do relatively well.

b. Dermatomyositis. Characteristic features include the muscle weakness, elevated muscle enzymes, and organ manifestations seen in polymyositis, but the distinct feature of this syndrome is the presence of **skin involvement.** In general, dermatomyositis patients respond reasonably well to therapy.

c. Polymyositis or dermatomyositis associated with malignancy. Visceral malignancies occur in approximately 10%–25% of cases, especially in elderly individuals with late-onset inflammatory myopathy. The incidence of malignancy is thought to be higher in patients with dermatomyositis than in those with polymyositis. The most common malignancies are those that are typical in middle-aged or elderly individuals (i.e., cancers of the lung, gastrointestinal tract, breast, uterus, and ovaries). Removal of the malignancy occasionally results in remission of the muscle disease, but the prognosis in general for these patients is poor; they die of their malignancy or uncontrollable muscle disease.

d. Juvenile dermatomyositis. Most children have dermatomyositis rather than polymyositis. Late in the disease course, young patients may develop muscle contractures from calcific deposits in the chronically damaged muscle. A widespread small artery and capillary vasculitis may lead to skin, muscle, and bowel ischemic lesions. Otherwise, prognosis is similar to that in adult forms of inflammatory myopathy.

e. Overlap syndromes. Muscle disease that is identical to polymyositis can occur in SLE, rheumatoid arthritis, systemic sclerosis, and Sjögren's syndrome. Patients often have milder muscle disease that is responsive to therapy, and prognosis is determined by the features of the underlying disease more than the muscle findings.

f. Inclusion body myositis. This syndrome is considered a subset of inflammatory myopathies because of the associated CD8$^+$ cell cytotoxicity directed against muscle fibers. The syndrome tends to affect **older men** and has a gradual disease onset and progression. Although patients have muscle weakness, CK elevations, and myopathic EMGs, they are distinguished from typical polymyositis patients by having **distal as well as proximal weakness,** typical **absence of autoantibodies,** and a **characteristic muscle biopsy** showing **vacuolar changes** and distinctive electron microscopic findings. The clinical features often are poorly responsive to immunosuppressive therapy, but patients have an excellent 5-year survival rate because of the slow progression of the disease.

F Diagnosis

1. **Approach**

   a. Distinctive muscle findings. A clinical diagnosis of inflammatory myopathy typically is considered when patients present with **proximal muscle weakness** or **increased muscle enzymes** (e.g., CK, aldolase). True proximal muscle weakness must be distinguished from generalized fatigue, distal weakness more typical of neuropathy, and pain-related weakness (i.e., joint or tendon pain that prevents full muscle contraction). Patients with true proximal muscle weakness complain of being unable to comb their hair or to rise from a squatting or sitting position. If true proximal weakness appears likely from the history and physical examination, CK testing is performed and EMG and biopsy of symptomatic deltoid or quadriceps muscle should be considered. MRI may also be useful in localizing the best biopsy site. The diagnosis of polymyositis is likely if a patient has three of the following muscle criteria:

   (1) Characteristic proximal muscle weakness

   (2) Inflammatory cell infiltrate and myofibril degeneration on muscle biopsy

   (3) Increased muscle enzyme levels

   (4) Myopathic EMG changes

   b. Supportive findings

   (1) The **characteristic skin findings,** if found, are supportive evidence and sometimes precede clinical evidence of muscle involvement.

   (2) Because 90% of polymyositis patients have autoantibodies when their serum is tested against HEp-2 cells, the presence of a positive test for autoantibodies also is supportive evidence for the disease, particularly if a **myositis-specific antibody** is found.

2. **Consideration of malignancy.** A search for a malignancy is warranted in middle-aged or elderly polymyositis/dermatomyositis patients. Thorough physical examination, including a careful pelvic evaluation in women, chest radiograph, routine hematologic and biochemical testing, urinalysis,

and stool testing for occult blood should be performed. Abnormalities found should be pursued through additional testing.

3. **Differential diagnosis.** Other entities should be considered in making a diagnosis of inflammatory myopathy, especially when the presentation is somewhat atypical. Some disorders can be eliminated on clinical grounds; others require laboratory testing, EMG, or muscle biopsy.

a. **Endocrine disorders**

(1) **Hypothyroidism** can manifest as proximal muscle aching, weakness, and mild-to-moderate CK elevation.

(2) **Hyperthyroidism** can manifest as diffuse weakness; CK levels typically are normal.

(3) **Patients with Cushing's syndrome** may have lower more than upper extremity proximal muscle weakness; muscle enzymes are normal.

b. **Drugs.** Numerous drugs and toxins can cause muscle weakness and sometimes CK elevation; these effects usually resolve when the agent is removed. Some of the most common of these agents include alcohol, cholesterol-lowering drugs (e.g., clofibrate, gemfibrozil, and lovastatin), colchicine, chloroquine, corticosteroids, D-penicillamine, and zidovudine.

c. **Muscle diseases.** Muscular dystrophies and metabolic muscle diseases can be distinguished by careful family history, distinguishing patterns of weakness, and lack of inflammation on muscle biopsy. Some require exercise testing with venous lactate determinations or electron microscopic examination of muscle.

d. **Neurologic diseases.** Early in the disease course, illnesses such as myasthenia gravis or amyotrophic lateral sclerosis (ALS) can mimic inflammatory myopathy. The presence of ocular muscle involvement or characteristic EMG or nerve conduction velocity (NCV) findings can help in diagnosing these diseases.

e. **Infections**

(1) **Bacterial.** Some cases of Lyme disease are associated with myopathy.

(2) **Viral.** Acute and convalescent serologies can distinguish viral illness. Common causes include coxsackievirus, echovirus, influenza virus, and HIV.

(3) **Parasitic.** Serologic testing can help distinguish toxoplasmosis or trichinosis from polymyositis.

f. **Sarcoidosis.** Inflammatory muscle involvement, which can be distinguished by characteristic organ involvement and finding of noncaseating granulomas on muscle biopsy, may occur.

G **Therapy**

1. **Corticosteroids.** Large doses of corticosteroids appear to be effective in controlling the muscle disease in most patients. Prednisone usually is begun at a dose of 60 mg/day and is reduced gradually over several months as muscle strength improves and CK level falls. Alternate-day regimens can be used to prevent steroid toxicity, but only after the normalization of CK level and return of muscle strength.

2. **Immunosuppressive agents.** Patients who do not respond to the previously mentioned corticosteroid schedules within 3 months are considered to be nonresponders to treatment. Frequently, the addition of methotrexate or azathioprine allows control of the muscle disease and gradual tapering of the steroids. The CD4$^+$ cell–specific drug cyclosporine also has been effective in some patients who do not respond to general immunosuppression. Tacrolimus and mycophenolate mofetil may be effective in treating interstitial disease and muscle inflammation. Rituximab, an anti-CD20 antibody, may be used in resistant cases.

3. **Physical therapy.** When the disease process has been clinically controlled (i.e., CK levels normalized and muscle strength improved), muscle strengthening exercise and aerobic training can be initiated. Mild exercise and passive stretching to prevent contractures should be used in active disease.

4. **Hydroxychloroquine.** This agent may help control the rash of dermatomyositis.

5. **Intravenous immunoglobulin.** This agent has been helpful in some steroid-resistant patients and in patients presenting with early, severe disease including respiratory involvement/respiratory failure.

XI   **SJÖGREN'S SYNDROME**

A   **Definition**   Sjögren's syndrome (SS) (also called **sicca syndrome**) is an idiopathic, autoimmune disorder characterized by dry mouth (**xerostomia**) and dry eyes (**keratoconjunctivitis sicca**). Variable **lacrimal** or **salivary gland enlargement** can occur (related to lymphocytic infiltration of lacrimal and salivary glands).

B   **Classification**   Sjögren's syndrome is divided into primary and secondary forms. The two forms can be distinguished on the basis of clinical features and HLA associations.

1. **Primary Sjögren's syndrome** has characteristic organ and exocrine glandular features and a significantly increased association with **HLA-DR3**. Patients can present with a variety of clinical manifestations that are uncommon in the secondary form, mainly due to a wider attack on exocrine glands in the primary form. Specific organ involvement is as follows:
   a. **Skin:** dry skin and vagina, Raynaud's phenomenon, and purpura (vasculitis)
   b. **Lung:** recurrent infections and interstitial fibrosis
   c. **Gastrointestinal tract:** angular cheilitis, oral candidiasis, beefy red tongue, recurrent parotitis, dysphagia, atrophic gastritis, chronic active hepatitis, biliary cirrhosis, and pancreatitis
   d. **Kidney:** renal tubular acidosis and interstitial nephritis
   e. **Muscle:** indolent myositis
   f. **Nerve:** CNS involvement (possibly vasculitis, with clinical manifestations similar to CNS lupus) and peripheral neuropathy
   g. **Hematologic system:** splenomegaly with neutropenia, lymphomas, and pseudolymphomas
   h. **Joint:** arthralgias or mild inflammatory arthritis
   i. **Endocrine system:** chronic thyroiditis (increased thyroid-stimulating hormone [TSH] levels and antithyroid antibodies, perhaps in as many as 50% of patients)
   j. **Vasculitis** (polyarteritis like)
2. **Secondary Sjögren's syndrome** occurs in the setting of another rheumatic disease (e.g., rheumatoid arthritis, SLE, and scleroderma) and has an increased association with **HLA-DR4**. Patients usually have symptoms that are limited to lacrimal and salivary gland abnormalities, although they also have typical features of a primary rheumatic disease.

C   **Diagnosis**

1. **Clinical approach.** Patients are most commonly evaluated for Sjögren's syndrome when they have complaints of **dry eyes, dry mouth,** or **salivary gland enlargement.** Primary Sjögren's syndrome also should be considered in the setting of **cutaneous vasculitis** (purpura), **CNS dysfunction** similar to that which occurs in SLE (either focal neurologic abnormalities or diffuse features such as depression, psychosis, or cognitive dysfunction), or the conspicuous presence of other clinical features listed in Section XI B 1.
   a. Complaints of **gritty eyes** and **dry mouth** can be investigated in the following way:
      (1) **Ophthalmologic slit-lamp examination** with fluorescein or Rose Bengal staining can be used to examine for the punctate staining of keratoconjunctivitis. The **Schirmer test,** which measures the degree of tear wetting on filter paper, is a supportive test; limited wetting suggests that keratoconjunctivitis found on staining is sicca related.
      (2) **Lip biopsy** of the lower lip mucosa can be used to search for characteristic lymphocytic infiltration of the minor salivary glands in that location.
   b. **Salivary gland enlargement** can be evaluated with an MRI of the parotid gland. A nonhomogeneous density, which can be distinguished from parotitis, tumor, and normal glandular tissue, may be evident.
   c. **Salivary flow rate tests (sialometry)** and **radiographic studies (sialography)** are sensitive but nonspecific tests and are not often used.
   d. Many **laboratory abnormalities** occur and may offer suggestive evidence; however, no specific laboratory test is diagnostic.
      (1) **Tests suggesting chronic inflammation.** Anemia of chronic disease, elevated ESR, hypergammaglobulinemia, and rheumatoid factor often are found in Sjögren's syndrome, whether primary or secondary.

    (2) Autoantibody findings. ANAs are seen frequently in Sjögren's syndrome; antibodies to the small RNA protein **Ro** are found in **70%** of patients and antibodies to the protein **La** are found in **40%** of patients. La antibodies rarely are found without Ro antibodies, and the presence of both is relatively specific for Sjögren's syndrome. Salivary duct antibodies are common only in the secondary form.

2. **Differential diagnosis**
   a. **Salivary gland enlargement** also may be caused by a lymphoid or parotid gland neoplasm, granulomatous infiltration (sarcoidosis), alcohol use, cirrhosis, starvation, diabetes, amyloidosis, graft-versus-host disease (GVHD), hyperlipidemias, or infection (e.g., bacterial infections, mumps, HIV).
   b. **Dry mouth** may be caused by the use of certain drugs, including tricyclic antidepressants, phenothiazines, and antihistamines.
   c. **Dry mouth** and **dry eyes** are common in the geriatric population, and they often are present without any other features of Sjögren's syndrome.

D **Therapy**
1. **General considerations**
   a. **Scrupulous oral hygiene** is important to prevent rampant dental caries.
   b. Patients with primary Sjögren's syndrome who demonstrate salivary gland or lymphoid tissue enlargement must be considered **at risk for lymphoma** because non-Hodgkin's lymphomas occur at 40 times the normal rate in these patients.

2. **Symptomatic treatment**
   a. **Xerostomia.** Avoidance of drugs that dry out the mouth and frequent drinks of water or other liquids to keep the mouth wet are the usual symptomatic measures for this condition. Artificial salivas are commercially available, which may help with mouth wetting and prevention of dental caries. Pilocarpine hydrochloride, a cholinergic agonist, is available for oral use and can increase secretion by the exocrine glands increasing salivary flow.
   b. **Keratoconjunctivitis sicca.** Artificial tears (methyl cellulose) are used as often as needed to keep the eyes lubricated. Refractory symptoms may respond to punctal insertion of silicone plugs.
   c. **Features of severe disease. Progressive pneumonitis, vasculitis, neuropathy,** and **CNS involvement** may require anti-inflammatory treatment with corticosteroids and immunosuppressive drugs.

E **Prognosis**   Outcome for patients with primary Sjögren's syndrome depends on the severity of involvement of organs other than the salivary glands, particularly the CNS. In addition, the risk of lymphoma is higher in more severe cases. Features of the primary rheumatic disease determine the prognosis for patients with secondary Sjögren's syndrome.

XII   VASCULITIS

A **Definition**   Vasculitic syndromes are a group of clinically disparate disorders characterized by **necrosis** and **inflammation of blood vessel walls.** Vasculitis can exist as the primary feature of an idiopathic condition or as a secondary manifestation of infectious, malignant, or rheumatic disease.

B **Etiology**   Most of the vasculitic syndromes are idiopathic. Hepatitis B surface antigen (HBsAg) and hepatitis C virus (HCV) have been found in immune complexes of several different syndromes, including some cases of polyarteritis nodosa and essential mixed cryoglobulinemia. HIV, parvovirus, and cytomegalovirus (CMV) have been associated with vasculitic diseases, particularly polyarteritis.

C **Pathogenesis**

D **Classification**   The current systems for classifying vasculitic syndromes use clinical features, size of the involved vessel, and type of cellular infiltrate to separate the syndromes (Table 11–14).
1. Pathologic classification by vessel size may be the most clinically useful:
   a. Large vessel
      (1) Giant cell (temporal) arteritis (GCA)
      (2) Takayasu's arteritis

TABLE 11–14   Major Vasculitic Syndromes: Clinicopathologic Distinctions

Syndrome	Clinical Features	Pathology		
		VESSEL SIZE	CELLULAR INFILTRATE	DIAGNOSIS
Hypersensitivity vasculitis (serum sickness; drug reactions; Henoch–Schönlein purpura; mixed essential cryoglobulinemia)	Skin involvement predominant. Visceral involvement typically minimal and self-limited	Small (capillaries, venules, arterioles)	Leukocytoclastic vasculitis with all lesions at the same developmental stage	Skin biopsy	
Polyarteritis nodosa	Multisystem illness. Major arterial ischemic lesions that spare lungs and spleen. Nodose skin lesions uncommon	Small and medium-sized arteries	Necrotizing arteritis at vessel branch points. Simultaneous lesions at various stages	Biopsy of involved organ. Visceral angiography	Corticosteroids; cytotoxic agents added if no response
Allergic angiitis (Churg–Strauss disease)	Prominent allergic, asthmatic history. Lung involvement. Blood eosinophilia common	Varying (capillaries, venules, small arteries)	Granulomatous infiltrates with eosinophils	Biopsy of involved organ, typically lung	
Wegener's granulomatosis	Upper and lower respiratory tract involvement. Prominent renal abnormalities	Small (arteries; veins)	Necrotizing granulomas in upper and lower airways. Focal necrotizing arteritis in lungs. Necrotizing glomerulonephritis in kidneys	Lung biopsy (sinus biopsy usually nondiagnostic). c-ANCA	
Giant cell arteritis (temporal arteritis)	Polymyalgia rheumatica in 50%. Occurs in patients >50 years. Signs and symptoms of cranial artery involvement. High erythrocyte sedimentation rate	Large arteries (especially temporal artery)	Giant cell and chronic mononuclear infiltrates in vessel walls	Temporal artery biopsy	
Takayasu's arteritis	Large-vessel claudication. Occurs in young (often Asian) women	Large arteries (aortic arch)	Giant cell and chronic mononuclear infiltrates in vessel walls	Angiography. Chest MRI. Neck ultrasonography	

ANCA, antineutrophil cytoplasmic antibody; c-ANCA, cytoplasmic ANCA; MRI, magnetic resonance imaging.

  b. Medium vessel
    (**1**) Polyarteritis nodosa (PAN)
    (**2**) Kawasaki's disease
  c. Small vessel
    (**1**) Immune-complex mediated
        (**a**) Hypersensitivity vasculitis
        (**b**) Serum sickness
        (**c**) Mixed essential cryoglobulinemia
        (**d**) Henoch–Schönlein purpura (HSP)
        (**e**) Urticarial vasculitis

    (2) ANCA associated (para-immune)
       (a) Wegener's granulomatosis
       (b) Churg–Strauss syndrome
       (c) Microscopic polyangiitis (MPA)

  2. Nonspecific hematologic and immunologic abnormalities (e.g., anemia, leukocytosis, elevated ESR, and hypocomplementemia) often exist in many of these syndromes, but these are not noted in Table 11–14 unless they are specifically important for the diagnosis of a particular syndrome. It is important to understand that these syndromes often blur and overlap in actual patients.

E **Vasculitic syndromes**

  1. Hypersensitivity vasculitis (🔊 Online Figures 11–15 and 11–16)

    a. Typical hypersensitivity vasculitis syndrome. Hypersensitivity vasculitis (also called **leukocytoclastic vasculitis** or **cutaneous vasculitis**) is immune complex–mediated inflammation of small vessels (arterioles, capillaries, and venules). The cause often is unclear. In many cases, hypersensitivity vasculitis seems to occur as an exaggerated immune response to a **drug** (e.g., penicillin) or **infection** (viral or bacterial antigen), causing a self-limited immune complex vasculitis. The skin almost always is involved, with palpable purpura, urticaria, or ulcers. Polyarticular arthritis is common. Distinct organ involvement may allow further classification.

    b. Distinctive subsets

      (1) Henoch–Schönlein purpura is a systemic, small-vessel vasculitis that occurs primarily in children, often following a streptococcal pharyngitis.

        (a) Clinical features. Palpable purpura, polyarticular arthralgias or inflammatory arthritis, abdominal pain or gastrointestinal bleeding due to mesenteric vessel involvement, and immune complex–mediated glomerulonephritis typically occur. A distinctive feature is **IgA deposition** in the vascular lesions.

        (b) Course. Most cases of Henoch–Schönlein purpura resolve spontaneously over a period of days to weeks. Patients with severe renal or gastrointestinal involvement may require steroids.

      (2) Serum sickness is an immune complex vasculitis that often follows a drug (e.g., penicillin or sulfonamide) or foreign protein exposure by 7–10 days. Antilymphocyte globulin now is one of the most common causes. Hepatitis B virus (HBV) arthritis–dermatitis syndrome is a serum sickness–like response to HBsAg.

        (a) Clinical features. Urticaria, purpura, arthritis, and arthralgias are characteristic, and lymphadenopathy and immune complex glomerulonephritis are common.

        (b) Course. Resolution is typical following removal of the inciting agent.

      (3) Hypocomplementemic urticarial vasculitis

        (a) Clinical features. Patients with this form of vasculitis exhibit urticaria, typically lasting longer than 24 hours and, sometimes, arthritis, glomerulonephritis, or gastrointestinal involvement. **Hypocomplementemia** is a consistent feature, apparently related to antibodies directed against C1q; the degree of complement depression typically parallels disease activity.

        (b) Course. The disease follows a relapsing, remitting course and may require corticosteroids for the more disabling manifestations.

      (4) Mixed essential cryoglobulinemia is an idiopathic disorder caused by **cold-precipitated immunoglobulin (cryoglobulin) complexes,** which produce a vaso-occlusive or inflammatory injury. The syndrome typically occurs in patients who have type II (mixed) cryoglobulin. Many patients have been found to have HCV or, less often, HBV in the immune complexes.

        (a) Clinical features. Recurrent attacks of palpable purpura, Raynaud's phenomenon, arthralgia, and immune complex glomerulonephritis may occur. Gastrointestinal, hepatic, and pulmonary dysfunctions are occasional features.

        (b) Course. Severe renal involvement is the most common reason for treatment, which may include corticosteroids, cytotoxic agents, or removal of the cryoglobulin by apheresis. Interferon-α (IFN-α) may help when the disease is associated with HBV or HCV.

2. **Polyarteritis nodosa** is a necrotizing vasculitis of small- and medium-sized arteries, which manifests as a multisystem illness. Ischemic arterial lesions are caused by vessel wall inflammation, in some cases associated with immune complex deposition. HBsAg is positive in up to 50% of patients.

   a. **Clinical features. Constitutional complaints** (e.g., fever, weight loss, and anorexia) are common, and **multiorgan ischemic dysfunction** is the rule. The lungs and spleen typically are spared.

   (1) **Renal involvement** is most common and manifests as severe hypertension, proteinuria and active sediment from glomerulonephritis, or renal insufficiency.

   (2) **Other common features** include arthralgias, myalgias, peripheral nervous system abnormalities (sensory polyneuropathies, mononeuritis multiplex), and skin lesions (infarctions, nodose lesions). Insidious CHF, diffuse or focal CNS dysfunction, and gastrointestinal involvement also can occur, depending on the size of the ischemic lesions.

   (3) **Microscopic polyarteritis** is a clinical variant typified by prominent lung involvement and segmental glomerulonephritis, sometimes rapidly progressive. The vessels involved tend to be smaller (capillaries, arterioles, and small arteries). **p-ANCA** is commonly found (50%–80% of patients), and abdominal angiography is typically negative (because the smaller vessels are involved).

   b. **Course.** Treatment with corticosteroids, cytotoxic agents, or both is necessary; the illness typically is fatal if untreated. IFN-α may help in HBV-associated cases.

3. **Allergic angiitis (Churg–Strauss disease)** is a granulomatous vasculitis that typically occurs in patients with asthma.

   a. **Clinical features.** Allergic angiitis is typically a triphasic disease. **Asthma** occurs first, often associated with **blood eosinophilia. Tissue infiltrates,** especially **pulmonary** ones, occur next; eosinophils are often present in these lesions, sometimes in granulomas. **Vasculitis** of small- or medium-sized vessels occurs last, commonly involving skin, nerve, or muscle lesions.

   b. **Course.** The farther apart in time the three phases of illness occur, the milder is the disease; the closer together, the more explosive. Catastrophic lung, gastrointestinal tract, cardiac, or nerve lesions may mandate aggressive intravenous corticosteroid and cytotoxic therapy, but more indolent forms are often easily controlled with moderate corticosteroid doses.

4. **Wegener's granulomatosis** is a granulomatous, small-vessel vasculitis that typically involves the upper and lower respiratory tract and kidney.

   a. **Clinical features**

   (1) **Respiratory tract.** Pulmonary features typically include upper airway complaints (e.g., sinusitis, rhinitis), as well as lower airway symptoms (e.g., cough, shortness of breath, hemoptysis). Cavitary or multiple infiltrates may be seen on chest radiography.

   (2) **Kidney.** Renal involvement is characterized by abnormal sediment or renal functional impairment.

   (3) **Organs.** Other, less classical features include skin lesions (palpable purpura), arthritis, ocular or orbital inflammation (typically with proptosis), cardiac lesions, and CNS or peripheral nervous system involvement.

   (4) **Presence of c-ANCA.** c-ANCA is often found in patients with active, multiorgan disease. In these patients, the presence of c-ANCA may be a relatively specific diagnostic test and may help monitor disease activity.

   b. **Course.** Although corticosteroids may be used initially, cytotoxic agents such as cyclophosphamide are uniformly required to prevent death. Methotrexate may play a role in maintaining disease remission or in limited forms of the disease.

5. **Giant cell (temporal) arteritis** usually is a granulomatous inflammation of the carotid artery and its branches, but it sometimes can involve the vertebral artery or other aortic branches. The pathology is indistinguishable from that of Takayasu's arteritis.

   a. **Clinical features.** The disease rarely occurs in patients younger than age 50 years.

   (1) Approximately 50% of patients have **PMR** (i.e., aching and stiffness of shoulder and hip girdles associated with an ESR of greater than 50 mm/hour, age greater than 50 years, and constitutional complaints such as fever, malaise, and weight loss), and most patients have features related to ischemia in the carotid artery region (i.e., headache, visual symptoms, jaw claudication, scalp tenderness, and neurologic complaints).

      (2) Superficial temporal artery involvement is common but often is clinically silent. Potential clinical features include tenderness, nodules, or erythema. Even when the artery is clinically normal, temporal artery biopsy typically reveals pathology.

  b. Course. Patients require steroids early and in high doses to prevent **blindness,** the most serious complication of this illness. Patients should be started immediately on at least 1 mg/kg prednisone to prevent blindness. A temporal artery biopsy may still be diagnostic up to 1 week after the initiation of steroids. A contralateral temporal artery is necessary for diagnosis if the original biopsy specimen is negative.

6. Takayasu's arteritis is a granulomatous inflammation of the vessels of the aortic arch that is characterized pathologically by a panarteritis containing mononuclear and giant cells. Young women, often Asian, are at highest risk for this disorder.

  a. Clinical features

      (1) Generalized aching similar to PMR often occurs early in the illness. Features of **large-artery ischemia** develop weeks to months later and may include upper extremity claudication, angina, and CHF from cardiac or aortic involvement. Pulmonary and mesenteric vessels also can be involved.

      (2) Findings on physical examination include arterial bruits, pulse deficits, and blood pressure differences between extremities.

  b. Course. Patients may require steroids early in the course of the illness; later, vascular reconstruction may be required for occlusive lesions. Cytotoxic agents are typically added if steroids do not control inflammatory disease.

7. Other vasculitic syndromes do not fit into the major categories of vasculitis due to distinct clinical or overlapping pathologic features.

  a. Vasculitis as a secondary feature of a primary disease. Certain diseases can exhibit vasculitic inflammation as a secondary feature. The vasculitis typically is small-vessel, cutaneous vasculitis but sometimes can overlap with polyarteritis-like vessel involvement, especially in **rheumatoid arthritis** and **lupus.** Dermal and CNS vasculitic lesions are recently recognized secondary features of **Sjögren's syndrome. Hematologic malignancies** and bacterial and viral **infections** also can include vasculitic features; usually the skin is the predominant organ involved.

  b. Behçet's syndrome. The presence of **recurrent oral and genital ulcers** defines this syndrome. Patients also may have eye inflammation, **pathergic skin lesions** (lesions occurring at sites of skin injury), and vasculitis of the CNS or other organs.

  c. Kawasaki's disease (mucocutaneous lymph node syndrome). This febrile illness of infants and young children is characterized by conjunctival injection; diffuse maculopapular rash with associated edema, erythema, and eventual desquamation of the hands and feet; cracked lips; "strawberry tongue"; and cervical adenopathy. Coronary vasculitis can develop in 25% of patients and lead to aneurysm, MI, and sudden death. However, the incidence of this vasculitis has greatly decreased since the advent of intravenous immunoglobulin therapy, which, along with aspirin, is the treatment of choice in this disease.

  d. Isolated CNS vasculitis. This condition is a granulomatous inflammation of small- or medium-sized arteries of the brain. It is a very rare condition and should be a diagnosis of exclusion. Other etiologies that need to be considered and ruled out include infection, malignancy, and drugs, such as amphetamines and cocaine. Typically, patients do not have clinical or laboratory evidence of inflammation elsewhere. Presenting features often are combinations of diffuse CNS complaints (headache, altered mental status, poor memory) and more focal ones (cranial nerve defects, hemiparesis). A chronic meningitis picture, with pleocytosis and increased protein, typically is found on LP. An enhanced MRI scan of the brain is a sensitive but nonspecific indication of possible involvement.

F **Diagnosis**

1. Why suspect an underlying vasculitic process? Combinations of clinical features suggest the possibility of a vasculitis.

  a. There is evidence of a multisystem disease.

  b. Infectious etiologies are thoroughly excluded.

  c. Laboratory data may suggest an inflammatory process.

  d. Distinctive clinical features or patterns are present (Table 11–15).

TABLE 11–15 Clinical Data Suggesting Vasculitis

History	Physical Examination	Laboratory Studies
Constitutional Complaints Malaise Anorexia Fever Weight loss	**Vessel Findings** Blood pressure/pulse deficits Hypertension (sudden onset) Vessel tenderness, nodules, 　bruits	**Nonspecific Tests** (chronic inflammation) Anemia (chronic disease) Thrombocytosis Increased erythrocyte sedimentation rate Increased gamma globulins
Drug Exposure 　(prescribed or illicit) **Infection** Human immunodeficiency virus 　(HIV) Hepatitis B or C virus	**Skin Findings** Palpable purpura Infarctions Ulcers **Muscle Findings** Tenderness, cramping	**Test Indicating Potential Ischemia** Abnormal renal function ($\uparrow$ creatinine, BUN) Abnormal muscle/liver enzymes ($\uparrow$ CK, AST, ALT) Electrocardiogram
Organ Ischemic Complaints Angina Extremity or jaw claudication Visual complaints Transient ischemic attacks Stroke	**Nerve Findings** Sensory/motor neuropathies Focal/diffuse CNS dysfunction **Testis** Tenderness	**Tests Pointing Toward Specific Diagnoses** HIV (several syndromes) HBsAg (20%–30% of polyarteritis patients) Hepatitis C RNA ANA (SLE more likely) c-ANCA (Wegener's granulomatosis) p-ANCA (microscopic polyarteritis) Cryoglobulins (mixed essential cryoglobulinemia) Anti-Ro (Sjögren's syndrome, SLE)

ALT, alanine aminotransferase; ANA, antinuclear antibody; ANCA, antineutrophil cytoplasmic antibody; AST, aspartate aminotransferase; BUN, blood urea nitrogen; CK, creatine kinase; CNS, central nervous system; SLE, systemic lupus erythematosus.

2. **Confirming the diagnosis.** If the clinical evaluation suggests a reasonable chance of vasculitis, the appropriate approach to making a diagnosis usually lies in biopsy of involved tissue or visceral angiography; ANCA testing may be helpful when microscopic polyarteritis or Wegener's granulomatosis is suspected.

   a. **Biopsy of a fresh lesion.** Biopsy from clinically involved tissues is the preferred method of diagnosing vasculitis; if involved, the skin often is the easiest tissue to obtain.

      (1) Diagnosis of **Wegener's granulomatosis** often relies on open lung biopsy demonstration of granulomatous vasculitis because paranasal sinus tissue typically shows nonspecific inflammation and renal tissue shows only glomerulonephritis.

      (2) Diagnosis of **temporal arteritis** requires examination of a 3- to 6-cm segment of the superficial temporal artery in multiple sections; biopsy of the contralateral side may be needed if the first biopsy is negative and clinical suspicion remains high.

      (3) Biopsy of leptomeninges and clinically involved brain tissue may be needed when **isolated CNS vasculitis** is strongly suspected.

   b. **Visceral angiography.** When polyarteritis is suspected and appropriate tissue cannot be obtained for biopsy or when the biopsy is unrevealing, abdominal three-vessel angiography may show aneurysms or arteriopathy (discrete narrowing) suggestive of small- to medium-sized artery vasculitis. Aortic arch and large-vessel angiograms, carotid ultrasonography, and MRI studies of the chest are useful in Takayasu's arteritis and giant cell arteritis because the involved vessels often cannot be safely subjected to biopsy. CNS angiograms may be warranted when isolated CNS vasculitis is suspected.

   c. **Presence of ANCA.** ANCAs are typically IgG antibodies directed against cytoplasmic components of neutrophils and monocytes [🔲 Online I B 5].

3. **Differential diagnosis.** Numerous conditions should be considered in the differential diagnosis of vasculitis. Important disorders and the tests used to eliminate them include the following:

   a. **Bacterial endocarditis** (blood culture)

   b. **Left atrial myxoma** (two-dimensional or transesophageal echocardiogram)

   c. **Cholesterol embolism** syndrome (biopsy showing refractile crystals)

   d. **Thrombotic diseases** such as **antiphospholipid syndrome** (antiphospholipid antibody) and **disseminated intravascular coagulation (DIC)** or **thrombotic thrombocytopenic purpura** (TTP) (prothrombin time [PT], PTT, platelet count, fibrinogen, and fibrin split products)

G **Therapy**   The management of patients with vasculitis is complex. In all patients with known vasculitic disease, it is important to record the extent of disease initially and to monitor organ involvement (in terms of clinical, biopsy, and angiographic evidence). The tempo of disease progression also should be gauged to determine the best treatment.

1. **Antigen removal.** Drugs that may be causing vasculitic processes should be stopped; plasmapheresis has been used in attempt to remove known antigens (HbsAg and HCV) and unknown antigens (cryoglobulin).

2. **Treatment of primary disease.** Control of any primary rheumatologic, infectious, or malignant process generally is the most effective way to control vasculitis that is a secondary feature.

3. **Immunosuppressive treatment.** Vasculitic syndromes that are not related to a removable antigen or treatable primary disorder often should be controlled with immunosuppressive agents—either **corticosteroids, cytotoxic drugs,** or a combination of both. **Cyclosporine,** working specifically on activated CD4$^+$ T cells, has been used in some vasculitis diseases, particularly to counteract eye involvement in Behçet's syndrome and some cases of refractory small-vessel vasculitis.

   a. **Corticosteroids** alone should be attempted as first-line pharmacologic treatment in all patients who require concomitant cytotoxic therapy, except those with Wegener's granulomatosis. Daily dosing usually is required, although alternate-day dosing may be sufficient once systemic features of the illness are controlled. **Low-dose aspirin therapy** is often added to treatment of vasculitic disorders to counteract the potential **vaso-occlusive** effects of glucocorticoids.

   b. **Cytotoxic drugs** (e.g., cyclophosphamide)

      (1) **Wegener's granulomatosis** almost always is fatal without cytotoxic therapy; therefore, patients should be started on a combination of one of these agents and corticosteroids.

      (2) **Polyarteritis nodosa** and **allergic angiitis** also often require cytotoxic drugs in addition to steroids for control of disease manifestations, although recent prospective studies have shown benefit in decreasing disease recurrences but not in preventing mortality.

      (3) In other disorders, cytotoxic drugs typically are added to corticosteroid therapy if the steroid doses cannot be easily lowered without the disease flaring.

4. **Other drugs** such as dapsone, colchicine, NSAIDs, hydroxychloroquine, and H$_1$- or H$_2$-blocking antihistaminic agents have been used, particularly in refractory small-vessel vasculitis.

5. **Plasmapheresis,** which removes antibodies and immune complexes from plasma, has not been shown to improve outcomes in systemic necrotizing vasculitis (e.g., polyarteritis and allergic angiitis). In **mixed cryoglobulinemia,** whether or not it is related to HBV or HCV infection, plasmapheresis may improve disease features, at least temporarily.

XIII   JUVENILE IDIOPATHIC ARTHRITIS

A **Definition**   Juvenile idiopathic arthritis (JIA) is a **chronic inflammatory arthritis** that begins before age 16 years. Before considering a diagnosis of JIA, arthritis should be present in one or more joints for more than 6 weeks, and other rheumatic diseases should be excluded.

B **Epidemiology**   Annual incidence may be as high as 0.01%. Although the apparent HLA associations suggest that the altered immune responses are genetically transferable, familial aggregation of cases is uncommon.

C **Etiology and pathogenesis**   The same factors important in the development of adult rheumatoid arthritis also apply to JIA [see III C]. Etiologic factors are unknown but may include infectious agents. **Immune system dysfunction** is apparent in the prolongation and maintenance of synovitis. A subset of patients with JIA have selective IgA deficiency, which may be important in disease pathogenesis.

D **Pathology**   The **synovial lesions** cannot be distinguished histologically from those in adult rheumatoid arthritis. Inflammatory changes contiguous to the growth plate may lead to premature epiphyseal closure and shortened limbs or digits. Chronically involved joints exhibit **fibrous ankylosis** more often than in adult rheumatoid arthritis. **Pannus formation** can occur, although typically later in the disease course than in adults with rheumatoid arthritis. As a consequence, destructive joint disease also is much less common in JIA.

E **Classification**   Three primary subtypes of JIA (i.e., systemic-onset juvenile arthritis, pauciarticular arthritis, and polyarticular arthritis) can be distinguished in the first 6 months of illness. It is important prognostically and therapeutically to distinguish between subtypes of illness. Important classification features are the **presence or absence of prominent systemic features** and the **total number of involved joints.**

1. **Systemic-onset juvenile arthritis,** also called **Still's disease,** occurs in approximately 10%–20% of patients and is characterized by an early pattern of **prominent systemic complaints** and **extra-articular involvement.** Boys are affected as commonly as girls, and a peak age of incidence is not evident.
   a. **Clinical features**
      (1) **Typical features of the early disease course** are **high spiking fevers** and marked **constitutional complaints.** Overt arthritis may not be part of the early course but develops within weeks to months of the onset of illness. A characteristic **nonpruritic, fleeting, maculopapular rash** occurs in 90% of patients and is most apparent with fever spikes.
      (2) **Common features of active disease** include lymphadenopathy, hepatosplenomegaly, and pericarditis. Accompanying myocarditis is rare.
      (3) The most serious manifestation of systemic-onset juvenile arthritis is macrophage activation syndrome. Activated macrophages in multiple organs lead to leukopenia, thrombocytopenia, CNS and liver dysfunction, and possible multiorgan failure and death.
   b. **Laboratory findings**
      (1) **Hematologic findings** include a strikingly elevated ESR, prominent leukocytosis, thrombocytosis, and moderate-to-severe anemia of chronic disease, although there often is striking microcytosis.
      (2) **Serologic findings** only rarely include rheumatoid factor and ANAs.
   c. **Disease course.** Disease flare-ups are punctuated by relatively symptom-free intervals. Polyarticular arthritis becomes evident at some point in the first 6 months of illness. Systemic symptoms most often decrease within 9 months after onset.
      (1) Approximately 50% of patients may begin to develop symptoms of disease that resemble the polyarticular arthritis subset, with progressive joint involvement determining disease outcome.
      (2) The remaining 50% of patients eventually recover completely.

2. **Polyarticular arthritis** occurs in approximately 30%–40% of patients and **involves five or more joints** in the first 6 months of illness. **Systemic features are not present.** Girls are affected much more often than boys. Polyarticular arthritis can be further separated into **rheumatoid factor–positive or –negative subsets.** Patients who are positive for rheumatoid factor present most often in late childhood; a peak age of incidence is not evident for patients who are negative for rheumatoid factor.
   a. **Clinical features**
      (1) Typically, inflammatory polyarticular arthritis may have an acute or a gradual onset similar to the presentation of adult rheumatoid arthritis. Symmetric large- and small-joint involvement also is typical. Prominent features may include cervical spine and temporomandibular joint (TMJ) disease.
      (2) Rarely, patients have symptoms and signs of anterior uveitis.
      (3) Patients who are positive for rheumatoid factor can have subcutaneous nodules as in adult-onset rheumatoid arthritis.
   b. **Laboratory findings**
      (1) **Hematologic findings** frequently include moderate elevation of erythrocyte sedimentation rate, leukocyte count, and platelet count. Patients usually develop a mild normochromic, normocytic anemia of chronic disease.
      (2) **Serologic findings** include rheumatoid factor in 10%–20% and ANAs in 20%–40% of patients.
   c. **Disease course.** Polyarticular arthritis can be chronic and persistent or can pursue a more intermittent, relapsing course.
      (1) Patients who are positive for rheumatoid factor are at greatest risk for chronic, erosive, and severe arthritis and significant disability. These patients have disease that is very similar to adult-onset rheumatoid arthritis.

(2) Patients who are negative for rheumatoid factor less often have severe disease or disease that lasts into adulthood.

3. Pauciarticular arthritis occurs in approximately 50% of patients and involves **four or fewer joints** in the first 6 months of illness. This patient group is composed of three subsets.

    a. Oligoarthritis and **anterior uveitis** affect girls more often than boys, and peak incidence is in early childhood.

        (1) Clinical features

            (a) Typically, the arthritis is asymmetric and mild and involves the knee. Other peripheral joints also can be involved, but the axial skeleton usually is spared.

            (b) Systemic symptoms and signs are mild or absent.

            (c) Potentially serious **anterior uveitis** unrelated to arthritis activity can develop in up to 25% of patients. This usually chronic eye lesion can be asymptomatic and can lead to **blindness** if unrecognized or inadequately treated.

        (2) Laboratory findings

            (a) Hematologic findings usually do not include anemia, thrombocytosis, and leukocytosis. The ESR is normal or only minimally elevated.

            (b) Serologic findings include ANA positivity in 60% of patients, which identifies those at higher risk for chronic uveitis. Rheumatoid factor typically is not present.

        (3) Disease course. Most patients have pauciarticular involvement that is manageable and not disabling. In approximately one third of patients, the disease eventually involves more than four joints and is further subdivided as extended pauciarticular arthritis.

    b. Axial skeleton oligoarthritis predominantly affects boys, with disease onset usually beginning in late childhood.

        (1) Clinical features. Asymmetric knee, ankle, or midtarsal arthritis is most common, followed by that of the sacroiliac hip joints. Acute anterior uveitis can occur as in adult spondyloarthropathies, but this feature is not the chronic and sight-threatening form seen in the other pauciarticular subset.

        (2) Laboratory findings

            (a) Hematologic findings are not distinct.

            (b) Serologic findings indicate that 50% of these patients have HLA-B27, but few have rheumatoid factor.

        (3) Disease course. Many of these patients develop features of ankylosing spondylitis, psoriatic arthritis, or reactive arthritis in later life.

    c. Oligoarthritis with prominent dactylitis is a third presentation seen most frequently in girls of any age. **Psoriasis** commonly affects these patients and their families.

F **Diagnosis**

1. Difficulties in diagnosis. Diagnosing arthritis in children may be difficult. Children may avoid using an involved joint instead of complaining of pain. They may respond to the pain of an inflamed joint by displaying irritability, regressive behavior, or emotional withdrawal. Once joint involvement has been discovered, disease should be present for at least 6 weeks before a diagnosis of JIA is seriously considered. Within the first 6 months, an attempt should be made to classify patients into a clinical subset.

    a. The **synovial fluid** usually is mildly inflammatory (i.e., a WBC count of 10,000–20,000/mm³); however, the number of WBCs present may not parallel disease activity. Joint fluid culture and analysis are especially important in more acute pauciarticular forms to exclude infection (bacterial or mycobacterial).

    b. Radiographic findings are nonspecific.

        (1) Early findings may include only soft-tissue swelling and periarticular demineralization.

        (2) Late findings include epiphyseal changes (either premature closure or overgrowth, depending on epiphyseal activity at the time of involvement) and articular erosion or joint-space narrowing.

        (3) Distinctive long-bone periosteal elevation in leukemia may allow differentiation from JIA. Localized joint abnormalities (e.g., osteonecrosis and osteochondritis) may have distinct radiographic presentations.

        (4) Cervical spine involvement, particularly with ankylosis at C2–C3, is common in JIA.

2. **Differential diagnosis**
   a. A variety of **genetic or inborn metabolic disorders** as well as nonrheumatic conditions can superficially resemble JIA. It is specifically important to rule out **infectious etiologies** (e.g., Lyme disease and tuberculosis) and **malignancies** (e.g., leukemia) as causes of childhood arthritis.
   b. **Other rheumatic diseases** (e.g., rheumatic fever, SLE, and undifferentiated connective tissue disease) may require a period of observation for characteristic extra-articular features to evolve.

G **Therapeutic approach**

1. **Education of patients and parents** about inflammatory arthritis is important, and the generally favorable course of JIA should be emphasized. Long-term goals of suppression of disease activity and prevention of deformity should be instituted, and children's psychological and emotional development should not be neglected.

2. The use of appropriate **therapy** is important in relieving pain and maintaining function. Parents should be urged to perform active roles in giving physical therapy and medications, encouraging school attendance, and maintaining children's ability to be self-sufficient.
   a. **Pharmacologic therapy**
      (1) **Salicylates.** These agents are no longer the primary drugs used in the treatment of JIA because of concerns about the potential precipitation of Reye's syndrome by aspirin.
      (2) **Other NSAIDs.** Currently, naproxen and ibuprofen are most often prescribed as initial treatment. Although indomethacin and nabumetone are not FDA approved for children, they are also effective.
      (3) **Second-line agents.** Methotrexate, the most commonly used second-line agent, is effective. Oral gold, hydroxychloroquine, and d-penicillamine also are now rarely used in the treatment of juvenile rheumatoid arthritis. Sulfasalazine is also used because it has rapid onset of effect, infrequent serious toxicity, and relatively good efficacy. A recent trial of leflunomide showed the agent to be effective.
      (4) **Biologic agents.** Etanercept, a genetically engineered fusion protein of recombinant TNF and human IgG, is approved for use in children. This agent is most often indicated in juvenile rheumatoid arthritis of a polyarticular course that is unresponsive to methotrexate.
      (5) **Corticosteroids**
         (a) In **patients with systemic complaints who have life-threatening manifestations** (e.g., pericarditis), moderate-to-high-dose systemic corticosteroids may be required.
         (b) In **nonambulatory children with polyarticular disease,** a small, every-other-day dose of corticosteroids may promote weight bearing. The consequences of being nonambulatory in childhood outweigh possible corticosteroid complications in this clinical situation.
         (c) Local corticosteroid injections often are effective in managing **pauciarticular disease** or more **severely involved joints in polyarticular disease.** In some children with limited pauciarticular disease, intra-articular steroid therapy at onset may lead to complete remission.
         (d) In the treatment of **chronic uveitis,** systemic corticosteroids may be needed if initial treatment with topical or local corticosteroids and dilating agents is not effective. Recent clinical trials with infliximab are very encouraging. Patients at high risk for chronic uveitis (oligoarticular subgroup) should be evaluated every 3 months to determine treatment effectiveness.
      (6) **Intravenous infusions of gamma globulin.** This agent has been used to control severe systemic-onset or polyarticular disease.
   b. **Surgery.** Correction of deformities and total joint replacements may be needed in chronic, severe disease. Jaw implants have been used for micrognathia.
   c. **Physical and occupational therapy.** Such treatment is especially important in JIA. Children must learn and practice exercises that maintain muscle tone and prevent joint contractures. Night splints may help minimize the evolution of joint contractures; serial splinting may improve existing joint contractures.

H **Prognosis**

1. **Disability.** Between 50% and 75% of patients recover completely by adulthood. Approximately 10% develop severe functional deformities.

2. **Specific complications**
   a. **Joint deformities.** Patients with polyarticular arthritis are most likely to develop chronic, erosive arthritis and subsequent joint deformities, especially children with rheumatoid factor, who resemble patients with adult rheumatoid arthritis.
   b. **Chronic uveitis.** As many as 15% of patients with oligoarticular disease who have chronic uveitis develop some visual impairment, even if the problem is carefully treated.
   c. **Growth retardation**
      (1) **General growth retardation** can occur in patients with persistent, widespread inflammatory activity and in those treated with systemic corticosteroids.
      (2) **Local growth abnormalities** from the inflammatory process can lead to **micrognathia** as well as to **leg and finger length discrepancies** in some patients.

3. **Death.** Macrophage activation syndrome may be life threatening, and, in rare cases, patients with particularly severe and protracted disease develop progressive **amyloidosis** or die of secondary infection. Rarely, overwhelming **myocarditis** in systemic-onset juvenile rheumatoid arthritis can lead to CHF and death.

XIV MISCELLANEOUS SYNDROMES

A **Rheumatic manifestations of human immunodeficiency virus (HIV)** Musculoskeletal complaints are relatively common during the course of HIV infection. The clinical spectrum is varied, ranging from arthralgias to distinct rheumatic disorders. Arthralgia and myalgias, the most common rheumatic manifestations, occur in 10%–20% of patients, usually with the initial infection. Other manifestations can be classified into the following groups:

1. **Spondyloarthropathy** (reactive arthritis, psoriatic arthritis, and undifferentiated spondyloarthropathy). In young persons with seronegative arthritis, it is important to consider HIV.

2. **HIV-associated arthritis.** The usual presentation is an oligoarticular asymmetric peripheral arthritis affecting the knees and ankles. A symmetric polyarticular erosive form, which can also occur, may be difficult to distinguish from rheumatoid arthritis. This form is usually responsive to treatment with NSAIDs.

3. **Painful articular syndrome.** This poorly understood syndrome, which affects 10% of HIV-infected patients, is characterized by severe joint pain of abrupt onset that lasts a few hours to 2 days. Laboratory studies and imaging results usually are normal.

4. **Septic arthritis.** This condition is usually seen more frequently in patients with a history of intravenous drug abuse and in hemophiliacs. Both the usual and opportunistic organisms are implicated. In intravenous drug abusers, the most common pathogens are *S. aureus* and *Streptococcus pneumoniae*. Of the opportunistic organisms, *Candida albicans* is the most common. Axial joints are affected more frequently than peripheral joints.

5. **Diffuse infiltrative lymphocytosis syndrome** (DILS). This syndrome consists of dry eyes and mouth with a positive Schirmer test and salivary gland enlargement. DILS differs from classic Sjögren's syndrome in that it usually affects males and is not characterized by arthritis or autoantibody production (SS-A, SS-B, and rheumatoid factor).

6. **Myopathies.** Significant muscle weakness may be the presenting complaint. Such conditions may be the result of HIV myopathy, zidovudine myopathy, HIV wasting syndrome, rhabdomyolysis, or pyomyositis.

7. **Avascular necrosis and osteopenia/osteoporosis.** Recently, avascular necrosis has been reported in HIV patients. The etiology is unclear. Osteopenia and osteoporosis also are newer findings in this patient group. HIV therapy may be implicated.

B **Hepatitis and cryoglobulinemia** Both HBV and HCV can be linked with arthritis. HBV is associated with sudden-onset symmetric arthritis, occasionally found with urticaria. HCV is often associated with type II cryoglobulinemia and can manifest as a combination of arthritis, palpable purpura, and cryoglobulinemia.

C **Acute rheumatic fever (ARF)** The disorder occurs following a group A streptococcal (*Streptococcus pyogenes*) pharyngeal infection. In one third of patients, the triggering infection is silent, but it can be identified serologically. The incubation period from pharyngitis to infection is 2–3 weeks. According to the revised Jones Criteria (1992) for the diagnosis of ARF, if a patient has supportive evidence of preceding infection, the presence of two major or one major and two minor manifestations suggests a high probability of ARF.

1. **Major manifestations** are carditis, polyarthritis, chorea, erythema marginatum, and subcutaneous nodules. The arthritis is usually migratory, preferentially affecting the large joints of the lower extremities. Pain in affected joints may be out of proportion to physical examination findings of inflammation.

2. **Minor manifestations** are arthralgias, fever, elevated ESR, and a prolonged P-R interval.

3. **Supporting evidence of preceding group A streptococcal infection** includes a positive throat culture, elevated or rising anti–streptolysin O titer, or rapid streptococcal antigen test.

D **Avascular necrosis**   This condition, which is also referred to as **osteonecrosis,** is used to describe the death of cellular components of bone as the result of diminished arterial blood supply. It may be idiopathic or occur in a variety of settings associated with certain medications (steroids and cytotoxic agents), underlying connective tissue diseases, hematologic disorders, infiltrative disorders, embolism, alcohol, and trauma. Involvement of the epiphysis of long bones such as the femoral heads is usually characteristic, but other bones can be affected. In the earliest stages, diagnosis can be made by MRI, but at later stages, findings can be identified on plain films. Blood stasis, hypercoagulability, and damage to endothelial cells are important.

E **Fibromyalgia**   This common noninflammatory condition is characterized by diffuse pain. The etiology remains unclear, but affected patients tend to have disruption of non–rapid-eye movement (REM) stage IV sleep. In addition to diffuse pain, patients often report problems with insomnia, irritable bowel, tension headaches, migraines, and depression. Examination reveals multiple tender points (pain on palpation) over the following muscle regions: suboccipital muscle insertion; trapezius; supraspinatus; gluteal; greater trochanter; low anterior cervical; second costochondral junction, 2 cm distal to the lateral epicondyles; and the medial fat pad of the knees, proximal to the joint line. Laboratory investigation should include studies to rule out metabolic disorders (e.g., hypothyroidism and hyperthyroidism); electrolyte disturbances (e.g., low magnesium, calcium, or phosphorus); liver disease (e.g., viral hepatitis); connective tissue disease (e.g., PMR and SLE); and primary myopathy as clinically indicated. Treatment is aimed at improving the quality of sleep. Amitriptyline or low-dose muscle relaxants, in addition to regular physical exercise, are commonly used. If depression is a major component, referral for psychiatric consultation is indicated.

F **Amyloidosis**   The three main forms of amyloid deposition disorders that present with an arthropathy are AL amyloid, B2 microglobulin amyloid, and AA amyloid.

1. **AL amyloid** usually manifests as **proteinuria/renal failure,** a **cardiomyopathy,** or a **variety of neuropathic symptoms.** Other findings include edema, hepatomegaly, macroglossia, and purpura. Periarticular amyloid deposition can present as pseudoarthritis, but joint effusions with amyloid fibrils may also be found. The characteristic finding may be a soft tissue "shoulder pad sign."

2. **B2 microglobulin** amyloid is the second-most-common form of amyloid deposition. Most patients who develop this form of amyloidosis have been on **renal dialysis** for prolonged periods and present with **joint pain, carpal tunnel syndrome,** and **osteonecrosis.**

3. **AA amyloid** is found in patients with **rheumatoid arthritis** and **familial Mediterranean fever.** It is also referred to as a secondary (reactive) amyloid because it can occur in any chronic inflammatory disorder, including infections, neoplasia, or other rheumatic conditions.

G **Parvovirus B19 infection**   Parvovirus or Fifth's disease is endemic in school-age children. It manifests as fever, constitutional symptoms, and a "slapped cheek" appearance with striking erythema on the child's face. Adults typically present with arthralgias or a symmetric arthritis that may mimic rheumatoid arthritis. Testing for parvovirus serology early in the course of the disease can be diagnostic (positive IgM antibody). The course is self-limited and responds to anti-inflammatory pain medications.

H **Relapsing polychondritis** is a condition characterized by inflammation of cartilage. It can affect any cartilage in the body but most commonly affects the cartilaginous portion of the nose and external ear, presenting as sudden pain, redness, and swelling with eventual destruction if untreated. The etiology is unclear, but autoimmune mechanisms may be involved. It is sometimes associated with other connective tissue disorders as well as malignancies.

I **Auto-inflammatory diseases** These disorders are delineated most often by cycles of clinical inflammation without the presence of antigen-specific T cells or characteristic autoantibodies. Several of these diseases previously had been categorized as periodic fever syndromes. Over the last 5 years, the genetic basis for most of these disorders has been determined, and DNA sequencing to detect specific mutations is available in commercial laboratories (Online Table 11–16).

1. **Familial Mediterranean fever (FMF).** This disorder usually presents before age 20 years with periodic 1- to 3-day episodes of fever, pleuroperitoneal pain, and arthritis. A majority of patients, particularly those not treated with colchicine, develop amyloidosis.

2. **Tumor necrosis factor–associated periodic syndrome (TRAPS).** This syndrome also presents primarily before age 20 years, but patients experience longer and less regular episodes of fever and also develop tender deep erythematous patches and painful conjunctival injection.

3. **Hyper IgD syndrome (HIDS).** Clinical symptoms usually start within the first 6 months of life. Along with fever, there is significant abdominal pain, often with diarrhea, cervical lymphadenopathy, maculopapular rash, and oligoarthritis.

4. **Familial cold autoinflammatory syndrome (FCAS).** Symptoms start during infancy with a short-lived (<24 hours) maculopapular rash, conjunctival injection, and irritability without fever, all of which is usually triggered by exposure to cold temperatures.

5. **Muckle–Wells syndrome (MWS).** Clinical manifestations include an urticarial-like but not pruritic eruption, severe distal limb pains, and the gradual development of sensorineural deafness.

6. **Neonatal-onset multisystem inflammatory disease (NOMID).** This disorder not uncommonly presents during the neonatal period with an urticaria-like rash, the gradual development of severe arthropathy with extensive cartilage overgrowth, chronic meningitis, and sensorineural hearing loss.

    FCAS, MWS, and NOMID are now considered to be a family of disorders with a spectrum of progressive clinical severity and common mutations of the *CIAS1* gene at the q44 locus of chromosome 1.

Study Questions

1. A 56-year-old women presents to your office with pain and stiffness in her hands. She states that the stiffness seems to last the entire morning. Which of the following joint findings is most suggestive of an inflammatory arthritis, rather than osteoarthritis, as the cause of her joint pain?

- [A] Painful range of motion
- [B] Crepitus
- [C] Bony articular enlargement
- [D] Swelling and warmth
- [E] Instability

2. A 45-year-old man with a history of hypertension complains of left great toe pain of 24 hours' duration. He has had a low-grade fever and chills. He has no history of joint problems. The examination is notable for a red, warm, swollen, left great toe. No other joints are involved. There are no tophi. How is a definitive diagnosis made?

- [A] Obtain an x-ray
- [B] Obtain fluid for synovial analysis
- [C] Obtain a serum uric acid level
- [D] Obtain blood cultures
- [E] Obtain HLA-B27

3. Which one of the following forms of juvenile idiopathic arthritis is most likely to be associated with serious eye complications?

- [A] Polyarticular arthritis that is seropositive for rheumatoid factor
- [B] Polyarticular arthritis that is seronegative for rheumatoid factor
- [C] Oligoarticular arthritis without axial spine involvement
- [D] Oligoarticular arthritis with axial spine involvement
- [E] Systemic-onset juvenile rheumatoid arthritis

4. An 18-year-old woman comes to the emergency department complaining of severe right knee, right wrist, and left ankle pain. She has several skin lesions on her arms and legs; some are petechial and others are vesiculopustular. Physical examination also reveals tenderness and swelling of tendons around the involved joints but no actual joint swelling. Which of the following tests is most likely to yield the diagnosis?

- [A] Pelvic examination and cervical culture
- [B] Joint fluid aspiration
- [C] Antinuclear antibody testing
- [D] Rheumatoid factor testing
- [E] Streptococcal enzyme testing

5. While awaiting results of laboratory testing, the patient in question 4 should receive which of the following treatments?

- [A] Corticosteroids
- [B] Nonsteroidal anti-inflammatory drugs
- [C] Antibiotics
- [D] Local care of skin lesions
- [E] Splinting of painful joints

6. A 50-year-old woman complains of a 2-month history of her hands becoming painful and turning white or blue in the cold; progressive skin tightness and thickening of fingers, hands, and forearms; shortness of breath on exertion; and a sensation of lower chest burning and food sticking on swallowing. Antibody testing shows the presence of antinuclear antibody and elevated titers of antibody to Scl-70. Which of the following pathogenetic explanations best fits this patient's illness?

- [A] Infiltration of mucopolysaccharides into underlying subepithelial tissues
- [B] Unregulated fibroblastic collagen synthesis

C) Raynaud's phenomenon leading first to ischemia and later to tissue fibrosis

D) Vascular endothelial damage and immunologically mediated tissue fibrosis

E) Carcinomatous paraneoplastic process

7. Which of the following manifestations is more likely to be found in the diffuse form of systemic sclerosis than in the CREST variant?

A) Esophageal motility dysfunction

B) Pulmonary involvement

C) Distal skin thickening

D) Renal disease

E) Telangiectasias

8. Which of the following therapies is essential for treating polymyositis?

A) Antimalarial drugs

B) Nonsteroidal anti-inflammatory drugs

C) Corticosteroids

D) Bed rest

E) Aerobic exercise

9. A 32-year-old man presents with back pain with prominent stiffness lasting several hours, in addition to a painful swollen left ankle. The examination shows limited motion of the spine and a left Achilles tendinitis. You are considering a spondyloarthropathy as a unifying diagnosis. Which of the following clinical features is typical of all spondyloarthropathies?

A) Enthesopathic inflammation

B) Urethritis

C) Skin lesions

D) Bowel inflammation

E) Oral ulcers

10. A 57-year-old previously well man has been ill for 2 months with fatigue, malaise, dyspnea on exertion, abdominal pain, and progressive numbness in his feet. He has lost 20 pounds during this period. Recently, he developed mild inflammatory polyarthritis of the hands and has physical signs suggesting a mononeuritis in the right median nerve distribution. Chest radiograph shows cardiomegaly and findings of early pulmonary edema. Which of the following is the most likely diagnosis?

A) Hypersensitivity vasculitis

B) Rheumatoid arthritis

C) Systemic lupus erythematosus

D) Polyarteritis nodosa

E) Churg–Strauss syndrome

11. A 64-year-old woman presents with gradually increasing right knee pain. The pain is worse with weight bearing and relieved with rest. The knee is cool to touch. There is marked crepitus on range of motion, with a trace effusion. Which of the following would help confirm the diagnosis?

A) Joint aspiration

B) Trial of oral corticosteroids

C) X-ray with weight-bearing views

D) CBC, ESR

E) Bone scan

12. A 70-year-old man complains of increasing back pain for more than 6 weeks. He has no other history of arthritis or preceding trauma. He can walk about two block and then has to stop because of the low back pain with an associated numbness and tingling extending into his buttocks and left thigh. His examination shows a well-appearing man. His peripheral pulses were normal. There was no spinal tenderness. His straight-leg test was negative. His left lower extremity strength, range of motion, sensation, and reflexes were normal. What is the most likely diagnosis?

- [A] Spondyloarthropathy
- [B] Herniated disk
- [C] Spinal stenosis
- [D] Osteoarthritis of the left hip
- [E] Muscular strain

Directions: *The response options for Items 13–15 are the same. You will be required to select one answer for each item in the set.*

- [A] Rheumatoid arthritis
- [B] Lyme disease
- [C] Gonococcal arthritis
- [D] Systemic lupus erythematosus
- [E] Polymyositis
- [F] Sjögren's syndrome
- [G] Polymyalgia rheumatica
- [H] Reactive arthritis (Reiter's syndrome)
- [I] Pseudogout

For each of the following case descriptions, select the most appropriate diagnosis.

13. A 20-year-old woman complains of 2 weeks of fever, pleuritic chest pain, stiffness and swelling in wrists and metacarpophalangeal and proximal interphalangeal joints, an erythematous rash over both cheeks, and bilateral pretibial edema.

14. A 50-year-old man complains of a gritty sensation in his eyes and dry mouth, which he has experienced for several months. He has vague arthralgias in his hands and knees but only bulge signs (small amount of synovial fluid) in the knees on physical examination. He has scattered purpuric lesions over both calves and ankles.

15. An 80-year-old man complains of right knee pain and swelling. He has bony enlargement of the second and third metacarpophalangeal joints bilaterally, as well as wrist, proximal interphalangeal, and distal interphalangeal joints. His knee is swollen, and his range of motion is moderately limited by pain. A radiograph shows only flecks of calcium in the meniscal cartilage of the knee.

16. A 25-year-old woman presents to your office with a month-long history of fatigue, generalized arthralgias, and photosensitivity. Her examination shows an erythematous rash sparing her nasolabial folds. Her lab tests indicated a normal CBC and comprehensive metabolic profile. Her ESR was elevated at 40, ANA was positive at 1:320 speckled, and SSA was borderline positive. Her urinalysis was normal. Which of the following is the best treatment now?

- [A] Hydroxychloroquine
- [B] NSAIDs
- [C] Steroids
- [D] Sunscreen
- [E] Cyclophosphamide

17. A 35-year-old preschool teacher presents with a 2-week history of malaise, low-grade fever, and a symmetric polyarthritis. Her examination shows synovitis affecting her wrists, MCPs, and PIPs bilaterally. Her CBC and comprehensive metabolic profile are normal. The ANA and RF are negative. Which of the following is the most likely diagnosis?

- [A] Parvovirus B19 infection
- [B] Polymyalgic rheumatica
- [C] SLE

D Scleroderma
E Osteoarthritis

18. A 56-year-old man presents with a several-month history of aching and stiffness of the neck, shoulder, and hip girdle; low grade fever; and malaise. Over the last few days, he has noted a persistent right frontal headache and jaw claudication. Examination of the right temporal artery reveals a diminished pulse and slight tenderness. A stat ESR returns 92 mm/hour (normal <20 mm/hour). Your most appropriate course of action would be which of the following?

A Trial of an NSAID
B Trial of prednisone 10 mg/day for 10 days
C Referral to ophthalmology clinic to schedule a temporal artery biopsy
D Immediately begin prednisone at 1 mg/kg per day and refer the patient for a temporal artery biopsy ASAP
E Immediately obtain an enhanced MRI scan of the brain

19. A 48-year-old woman with established rheumatoid arthritis (RA) is referred to you for a second opinion regarding therapeutic options. She is concerned about treatment of her RA because of a recent positive tuberculin test noted on her yearly physical. She has no symptoms, and her chest x-ray is clear. Reactivation of tuberculosis has been associated with which of the following disease modifying antirheumatic drug(s)?

A Methotrexate
B Leflunomide
C Hydroxychloroquine sulfate
D TNF inhibitors
E Methotrexate combined with sulfasalazine

Answers and Explanations

1. The answer is D [I A]. A swollen and warm joint is more likely to be affected by an inflammatory arthritis than by osteoarthritis. The presence of synovial fluid is more commonly associated with inflammatory arthritis than osteoarthritis, and warmth suggests some degree of inflammation. Osteoarthritis typically is associated with bony joint enlargement in response to cartilage and subchondral bone injury. Painful joint range of motion, joint crepitus, and joint instability could occur in either an inflammatory or osteoarthritic joint problem.

2. The answer is B [V A 6 a (2)]. The likely diagnoses are gout and pseudogout. The only way to make a definitive diagnosis is to perform a diagnostic arthrocentesis and evaluate the fluid under the polarized microscope for the presence of crystals. X-rays in patients with longstanding symptoms can show erosions characteristic of gout, but they are usually normal in this setting, with this being his first attack. Hyperuricemia can be a risk factor for gout, but not everyone with hyperuricemia develops gout. In addition, during an acute attack the uric acid level may be falsely low. Thus, in this patient with acute symptoms, the uric acid level would not be that helpful. The toes can be involved in the presentation of a spondyloarthropathy, but usually as a sausage digit. He has no other features of spondyloarthropathy. HLA-B27 testing would not be helpful.

3. The answer is C [XIII E]. Patients with oligoarticular arthritis without axial spine involvement are most likely to develop chronic and potentially severe anterior uveitis, which can be clinically quite subtle even as it leads to progressive visual loss. Up to 25% of patients in this subset may develop anterior uveitis, and the group that is antinuclear antibody positive appears to be at highest risk. Patients with axial spine involvement can also develop anterior uveitis, but this tends to be acute, self-limited, and easily treatable.

4–5. The answers are: 4—A [VII D 1], 5—C [VII F 1]. This patient has clinical features suggestive of gonococcal periarthritis–dermatitis syndrome. In this setting, the cervix would be the most likely site for a positive culture. Joint fluid aspiration could yield a positive culture, but the patient does not have joint effusions. Antinuclear antibody testing would be helpful if the findings were more consistent with systemic lupus erythematosus than with gonorrhea. A patient with rheumatoid arthritis would be unlikely to have the skin findings, so rheumatoid factor is not a helpful test. Different skin and articular findings would be present in rheumatic fever, so streptococcal enzyme testing would be unlikely to yield a diagnosis.

Because gonorrhea is the most likely diagnosis, antibiotic treatment is required. Corticosteroids are contraindicated. Nonsteroidal anti-inflammatory agents, local skin care, and splinting of joints may be useful ancillary measures but do not treat the primary problem of a bacterial infection.

6. The answer is D [IX E]. This patient presents with characteristic features of scleroderma, a chronic illness in which unregulated immunologic processes (perhaps triggered by unknown environmental antigens) cause small-vessel endothelial damage and widespread dermal and internal organ fibrosis. The small-vessel endothelial damage leads to secondary vascular reactivity (Raynaud's phenomenon) and, possibly, ischemic tissue damage. The increased collagen synthesis by tissue fibroblasts, which leads to widespread fibrosis, is not unregulated; rather, it is caused by cytokine and growth factor secretion from lymphocytes, mast cells, and platelets. There is no evidence that patients with scleroderma have tissue mucopolysaccharide infiltration or that there are tumors responsible for paraneoplastic dermal fibrosis.

7. The answer is D [IX E 5]. Of the clinical manifestations listed, only renal disease is more likely to be found in diffuse systemic sclerosis than in the CREST syndrome, which involves the coexistence of subcutaneous calcinosis, Raynaud's phenomenon, esophageal motility dysfunction, sclerodactyly, and telangiectasia. In addition, pulmonary interstitial fibrosis typically worsens faster in the diffuse form. Both forms are characterized by esophageal motility dysfunction, distal skin thickening, and Raynaud's phenomenon. Telangiectasias also can occur in both forms of scleroderma, although they are more common and widespread in the CREST syndrome.

8. The answer is C [X G 1]. Oral corticosteroids are the typical initial treatment for inflammatory myopathy. NSAIDs, antimalarial drugs, bed rest, and aerobic exercise are not recognized treatments for polymyositis, although NSAIDs might help with associated joint complaints, and antimalarial drugs have been used for the skin features of dermatomyositis. Aerobic exercise is appropriate for patients with controlled disease but might be detrimental to those with active disease.

9. The answer is A [IV A 3 a]. Enthesopathic inflammation (i.e., inflammatory lesions at ligamentous, cartilaginous, and tendinous attachments to bone) is a characteristic feature of all spondyloarthropathies. Urethritis and oral ulcers are typical of reactive arthritis (Reiter's syndrome), and skin lesions are seen in reactive and psoriatic arthritis. Some patients with inflammatory bowel disease also have skin lesions (e.g., pyoderma gangrenosum), but the most typical feature other than rheumatic complaints is bowel inflammation.

10. The answer is D [XII D]. This patient has constitutional complaints (fatigue, malaise, and 20-pound weight loss) and has clinical evidence of impaired functioning of multiple organs; these findings make vasculitis a distinct diagnostic possibility. Mononeuritis is an even more specific finding, suggesting a small to medium-sized vasculitis of vasa nervorum. The other clinical findings are compatible with vasculitic organ impairment as well and are typical of polyarteritis nodosa. Hypersensitivity vasculitis is unlikely because patients with this disorder of the very small vessels almost always have distinct skin findings (e.g., palpable purpura) to support the diagnosis. Both rheumatoid arthritis and systemic lupus erythematosus are systemic illnesses that can be complicated by a small to medium-sized vessel vasculitis, but the only findings supporting these diagnoses are the mild joint complaints. The absence of allergic history, eosinophilia, and chest radiograph infiltrate distinct from pulmonary edema makes Churg–Strauss syndrome unlikely.

11. The answer is C [VI G 3]. The patient has classic findings of osteoarthritis of her knee. The best test to confirm the diagnosis would be an x-ray, which usually shows joint space loss, bony sclerosis, and degenerative spurs. Although the patient does have an effusion, the knee has no associated warmth; thus, an aspiration in not necessary. If there is concern about a crystalline disease or infection, then joint fluid analysis would be helpful. Laboratory studies such as CBC and ESR would not be indicated in this patient because there are no constitutional symptoms or inflammatory signs or symptoms. A bone scan will likely show degenerative changes but is more costly and time consuming. Only if an occult fracture, avascular necrosis, infection, malignancy, or an inflammatory arthritis is suspected would a bone scan be helpful. Oral steroids have no role in the treatment of this disorder.

12. The answer is C [Online II C 2 a]. The patient presents with classic symptoms of spinal stenosis. Pseudoclaudication is the most common symptom, with pain worsened by erect posture and improved by forward flexion and with associated numbness and weakness. Spondyloarthropathies usually present in younger individuals with associated inflammatory back pain (pain lasting more than 1 hour). The lack of a positive straight-leg test helps eliminate sciatica/herniated disk. Although underlying osteoarthritis of his hip may be contributing to his left thigh discomfort, it does not explain his back symptoms. In addition, on examination he has good range of motion of his hip, making hip pathology less likely. His symptoms are not consistent with simple strain because most strain syndromes improve in 6–8 weeks.

13–15. The answers are: 13—D [VII F 1 and Table 11–13], **14—F** [XI C], **15—I** [V B 5 b]. This young woman has the sudden onset of a systemic febrile illness that includes findings suggestive of serositis (pleuritic chest pain), arthritis, and a facial skin rash (possibly a butterfly rash). New pretibial edema suggests the possibility of urinary protein loss from renal involvement (glomerulonephritis or nephrotic syndrome). Although laboratory data (including positive antinuclear antibodies) or radiographic support is necessary to confirm possible organ abnormalities, systemic lupus erythematosus is the most likely cause of these findings.

This man likely has primary Sjögren's syndrome. The dry eyes and dry mouth suggest lacrimal and salivary gland involvement in this disorder, and further ophthalmologic evaluation or labial salivary gland biopsy could confirm these suspicions. Arthralgias are a common feature of primary Sjögren's syndrome; the arthritis of rheumatoid arthritis should have more actual joint findings (tenderness, swelling, or limitation of motion) to be considered as a primary disease accompanied by a secondary form of Sjögren's syndrome. The purpuric lesions on the calves suggest the possibility of a small-vessel vasculitis, a common skin feature of primary Sjögren's syndrome.

The man's presentation is most consistent with a chronic degenerative arthritis and a superimposed acute inflammatory arthritis. The degenerative, bony changes involve unusual joints (wrist, metacarpophalangeals) and include an unusual feature (chondrocalcinosis on knee radiograph). These findings are most compatible with calcium pyrophosphate deposition (CPPD) disease causing atypical degenerative arthritis, and the superimposed acute knee inflammation (pseudogout) is likely caused by release of the CPPD crystals into the knee joint. Finding positively birefringent crystals under red-compensated, polarized light examination of synovial fluid would be diagnostic.

16. The answer is A [VIII H 3]. The patient has SLE, with the main manifestations being fatigue, arthralgias, and the malar rash and photosensitivity, all of which would respond to hydroxychloroquine. Although NSAIDs may improve her joint symptoms, they have no effect on the rash. Likewise, sunscreen would be helpful in controlling the skin disease and possibly preventing disease flares but would not directly improve her fatigue or arthralgias. There is no evidence of major organ involvement; thus, use of steroids or cytotoxic therapy has no role in this patient at this point.

17. The answer is A [XIV G]. Given that the patient is exposed to young children and has an acute (less than 6 weeks) symmetric polyarthritis, parvovirus B19 is the most likely diagnosis at this point. Polymyalgic rheumatica usually presents with proximal shoulder and pelvic girdle pain and stiffness and does not occur in this age group. SLE could be a consideration if her symptoms were to persist, but the fact that her ANA is negative makes SLE very unlikely. She has no features of scleroderma. Osteoarthritis would be unlikely based on her age and the fact that she has inflammatory joint findings on examination (synovitis).

18. The answer is D [XII E 5 b]. The patient presents with a classic presentation for PMR associated with giant cell arteritis (GCA), suggested by the persistent frontal headache, tender temporal artery, and, most specifically, jaw claudication. The most appropriate course of action is to treat the patient with high-dose prednisone (1 mg/kg) to prevent blindness and obtain a temporal artery biopsy as soon as possible to document the diagnosis. A temporal artery biopsy may still be diagnostic up to 1 week after initiation of steroids. A trial of an NSAID or low-dose prednisone would be appropriate for PMR alone, but the presence of headache and jaw claudication in this patient strongly suggests underlying GCA. Referring to ophthalmology clinic and waiting for the results of a temporal artery biopsy could lead to blindness while the patient remains untreated. An enhanced MRI has no role in the diagnosis of GCA in this patient with a classic history.

19. The answer is D [III G 2 d and Table 11–7]. Tumor necrosis factor has been shown to be necessary in granuloma formation that is critical in the control of TB. Thus, use of TNF inhibitors (etanercept, infliximab, and adalimumab) has been associated with reactivation of TB. Screening for TB is recommended before initiating therapy with these agents. Treatment with antituberculous medications is recommended for individuals who are purified protein derivative (PPD) positive prior to considering treatment with these agents.

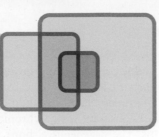

chapter 12

Neurologic Disorders

RALPH LEBRON • NEIL PORTER

I   **APPROACH TO THE PATIENT WITH A NEUROLOGIC COMPLAINT**

A **Patient history**   The patient history is the cornerstone of neurologic assessment.

1. **Key questions.** Questions that may help direct the patient interview include the following:
   a. Was the onset of symptoms gradual or sudden?
   b. Are the symptoms static, intermittent, or progressive?
   c. Has the problem remained limited in scope, or have new features been introduced over time?
   d. What concurrent problems does the patient have, and what medications or drugs are being used?
   e. Is there a family history of the disorder or predisposing conditions?
   f. What habits and toxin exposures might the patient have?

2. **Review of symptoms.** Depending on the clinical complaint, a patient should be asked whether there is any history of the following:
   a. Headache or trauma to the head, neck, or spine
   b. Loss of consciousness, convulsive activity, mood alterations, confusion, or memory disturbances
   c. Impaired or double vision, facial numbness or weakness, impaired hearing or swallowing, or abnormal speech
   d. Arm or leg weakness or heaviness, slowness of movement, altered limb sensation, discomfort or tingling in the extremities
   e. Clumsiness, falling, or dizziness
   f. Bowel or bladder disturbances or sexual dysfunction

B **Neurologic examination**   From the patient history, the physician can generate a series of diagnostic hypotheses that can be tested with a focused neurologic examination. Anatomic localization of the pathology within the nervous system is essential to this process (Figure 12–1).

1. **Mental status.** If the patient's mental status is abnormal, the history and those components of the physical examination that depend on patient cooperation must be approached within the proper context. For example, if the patient is confused, the sensory examination may be unreliable.
   a. The patient's level of arousal, orientation, short- and long-term memory, affect (i.e., mood), concentration and attention, fund of knowledge, insight, judgment, and constructional ability should be assessed.
   b. Language skills should be assessed by testing the patient's comprehension, repetition, fluency, naming, reading, and writing.
   c. The integrity of other cortical functions (e.g., graphesthesia, stereognosis, two-point discrimination, right–left orientation, and neglect) should be examined if parietal lobe dysfunction is suspected.

2. **Cranial nerves.** Examination of cranial nerves II–XII is necessary (Table 12–1).
   a. In particular, visual acuity and fields should be checked; the optic nerve should be examined, and abnormalities of ocular motility, including nystagmus and dysmetria, should be documented (Table 12–2).
   b. Abnormalities of facial sensation and movement also should be investigated.

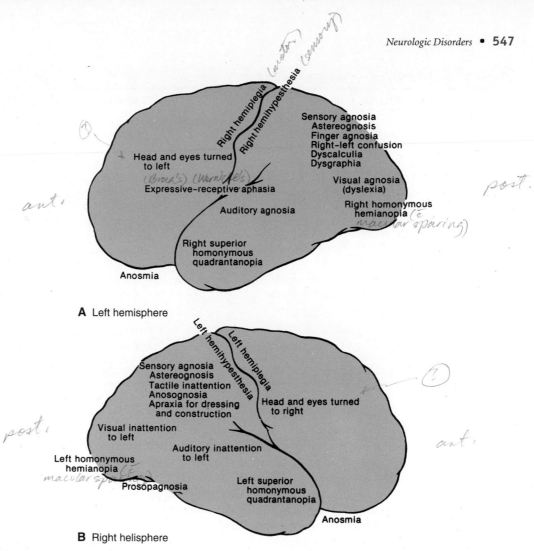

FIGURE 12–1   Summary of some of the outstanding neurologic signs and symptoms that occur with focal destructive lesions in the right or left cerebral hemisphere as detected on neurologic examination. **A.** Lateral view of the left cerebral hemisphere. **B.** Lateral view of the right cerebral hemisphere.

3. **Sensory system.** Regions of abnormal appreciation of light touch, pain (estimated by pinprick), temperature, vibration, and proprioception should be defined.

   a. Findings confined to one side of the body suggest a central disturbance, while "crossed findings on the face and body suggest a brainstem disturbance.

   b. Sensory changes found in a "stocking-glove" distribution suggest a peripheral neuropathy, while those restricted to a dermatome suggest a radiculopathy.

TABLE 12–1	Twelve Cranial Nerves	
Cranial Nerve	**Nerve**	**Function**
I	Olfactory	Smell
II	Optic	Vision
III	Oculomotor	Eye movements
IV	Trochlear	Eye depression (when adducted)
V	Trigeminal	Facial sensation
VI	Abducens	Eye abduction
VII	Facial	Facial movement
VIII	Vestibulocochlear	Hearing
IX	Glossopharyngeal	Palatal sensation
X	Vagus	Palatal movement
XI	Spinal accessory	Shoulder shrug
XII	Hypoglossal	Tongue protrusion

TABLE 12-2   Innervation of the Eye by Its Six Nerves

Number and Name of Nerve	Innervation	Clinical Effects of Interruption of Nerve
Efferent		
CN III (oculomotor nerve)	Striated muscle: superior, medial, and inferior recti; inferior oblique	Diplopia, eye abducted and turned down
	Levator palpebrae	Ptosis (paralysis of volitional lid elevation)
	Smooth muscle: pupilloconstrictor	Pupil dilated and fixed to light
	Ciliary muscle	Loss of lens thickening
CN IV (trochlear nerve)	Striated muscle: superior oblique	Diplopia, most severe on looking down and in; eye extorted; head tilted to side opposite paralyzed eye
CN VI (abducens nerve)	Striated muscle: lateral rectus	Diplopia, most severe on looking to side of paralysis; eye turned in (adducted)
Carotid sympathetic nerve	Smooth muscle; superior tarsal and pupillodilator	Horner's syndrome (ptosis, miosis, hemifacial anhidrosis, vasodilation)
Afferent		
CN II (optic nerve)	From retina	Blindness
CN V (trigeminal nerve)	Corneal/conjunctival afferents	Anesthesia of cornea with loss of corneal reflex

Adapted from DeMyer, W. *NMS Neuroanatomy.* Philadelphia: Lippincott Williams & Wilkins, 1988:219.

4. **Motor system**
   a. The patient's **strength** should be defined as it pertains to individual muscles or groups of muscles. The predominant method of grading muscle strength for purposes of comparison and description is shown in Table 12–3.
   b. A pronator drift can be assessed by having patients extend their arms (palm upward) with their eyes closed. Any depression or pronation is significant.
   c. The presence of **atrophy, fasciculations, spasticity,** and **rigidity** should be noted.
   d. The patient's ability to perform **rapid alternating and other complex maneuvers** should be determined.

5. **Coordination.** Finger-to-nose and heel-to-shin testing should be performed. The physician should look for **Romberg's sign** (i.e., falling to one side when standing with eyes closed and feet close together). Lastly, the patient's **stance** and **gait** should be evaluated.

6. **Deep tendon reflexes.** The activity and symmetry of the brachioradialis (C5, C6), biceps (C5, C6), triceps (C7, C8), knee (L3, L4), and ankle (S1, S2) reflexes should be determined. Hyperreflexia suggests a central disturbance, while reduced or absent reflexes suggest a peripheral disturbance. The presence of the **Babinski response** should be assessed with plantar stimulation.

C Neurodiagnostic studies

1. **Cerebrospinal fluid (CSF) evaluation**
   a. **Indications.** Study of the CSF can provide information about intracranial pressure (ICP) and infection, bleeding, malignancy, and sterile inflammation within the central nervous system (CNS).

TABLE 12-3   Medical Research Council of Great Britain Muscle Strength Grading Scale

Grade	Equivalent Patient Ability
5/5	Normal ability
4/5	Ability to overcome gravity and some resistance imposed by the examiner
3/5	Ability to overcome gravity only
2/5	Ability to move with gravity eliminated
1/5	Only a flicker of movement
0/5	Complete inability to move

b. Specific measurements and assays

    (1) Pressure. The opening pressure should be determined. Pressure exceeding 180–200 mm H_2O is abnormal when a patient is relaxed and in a lateral decubitus position.

    (2) Protein. An elevated CSF protein level is a nonspecific indicator of inflammation or breakdown of the blood–brain barrier.

    (3) Glucose. Hypoglycorrhachia (i.e., CSF glucose <40 mg/dL or a simultaneous CSF:blood glucose ratio of <0.6) suggests infection or sterile inflammation.

        (a) Relatively common causes of hypoglycorrhachia include bacterial, fungal, or tuberculous infection; carcinomatous meningitis; and hypoglycemia.

        (b) Less common causes include mumps, herpes simplex virus (HSV) or zoster infection, subarachnoid hemorrhage (SAH), sarcoidosis, syphilitic meningitis, and systemic lupus erythematosus (SLE).

    (4) White blood cell (WBC) count. A WBC count exceeding 5 cells/mm^3 is considered abnormal.

        (a) Excessive neutrophils suggest acute infection or, on occasion, sterile inflammation.

        (b) Excessive mononuclear cells suggest a viral infection, an indolent nonviral infectious process, or sterile inflammation.

    (5) Blood. Blood may appear in the CSF as a result of the local trauma of a lumbar puncture (LP) or by CNS hemorrhage from multiple causes.

        (a) A traumatic LP is suspected if gross blood exudes from the needle and then clears quickly or if a large discrepancy exists between the number of red blood cells (RBCs) in the first drops of CSF obtained and a later aliquot.

        (b) A traumatic LP should not appear xanthochromic (yellow) when spun down; xanthochromia is the result of red cell lysis, which requires some hours to occur.

    (6) Culture and Gram staining. These studies are indicated to evaluate the possibility of infection. A CSF Venereal Disease Research Laboratory (VDRL) test is indicated if CNS syphilis is being considered.

    (7) Cytology. Cytologic examination is useful if malignancy is suspected.

    (8) Intrathecal immunoglobulin production. This can be determined using the immunoglobulin G (IgG) index:

$$\frac{\text{CSF IgG/serum}}{\text{CSF albumin/serum albumin}}$$

or through CSF electrophoresis, which reveals the presence of oligoclonal bands (discrete immunoglobulin aggregates). An elevated IgG index or oligoclonal bands are found in CNS inflammatory disorders such as multiple sclerosis (MS) and infections.

c. Contraindications to the performance of an LP

    (1) Mass effect sufficient to cause distortion of the lateral or third ventricles or a midline shift on head CT

    (2) A **posterior fossa mass.**

    (3) A **coagulopathy** (e.g., a prothrombin time [PT] >3 seconds over control or a platelet count of <50,000/mm^3)

2. Electroencephalography (EEG) and **evoked potentials (EPs)**

a. EEG is indicated in the evaluation of **seizure disorders, encephalopathies, sleep disorders,** and sometimes **brain death.** Prolonged video EEG monitoring is the **gold standard** for evaluating seizure problems that are difficult to diagnose or treat.

b. Evoked potentials (EPs) are recordings of repetitive stimuli presented to the patient's eyes, ears, skin, or cerebral cortex that are averaged together and analyzed by computer.

    (1) Visual, brainstem auditory, and **somatosensory EPs** can detect lesions, which are often clinically silent, in the anatomic pathways subserving these sensory systems.

    (2) Motor EPs, which can be elicited by transcranial magnetic stimulation of the motor pathways, provide information about the integrity of the motor system.

3. Imaging studies

a. Computed tomography (CT) scanning provides an image of the brain that allows definition of **hemorrhage, edema, atrophy, mass lesions,** and **ventricular size.**

        (1) Intravenous contrast can be administered to define **regions where the blood–brain barrier has broken down.**

        (2) CT scanning can also visualize the **spinal cord** and **surrounding bony structures;** transverse images are especially well represented.

    b. Magnetic resonance imaging (MRI) provides excellent **anatomic depiction of the brain,** especially the posterior fossa, and the **spinal cord.** Disease of the cerebral white matter is particularly well defined. Intravenous contrast can detect sites of a disturbed blood–brain barrier. **Diffusion-weighted imaging** can detect regions of cerebral ischemia, as reflected by an area of decreased free water diffusion.

    c. Single-photon emission computed tomography (SPECT) provides an image-based estimate of **cerebral blood flow** after intravenous injection of a radioactive tracer.

    d. Noninvasive vascular studies

        (1) Duplex scanning provides an ultrasound image of the extracranial carotid and vertebral arteries together with a Doppler description of flow patterns.

        (2) Transcranial Doppler (TCD) defines intracranial large-artery flow patterns.

        (3) Magnetic resonance angiography (MRA) uses magnetic resonance technology to image the vascular anatomy.

        (4) Computed tomography angiography (CTA) uses computed tomography with intravenous contrast administration to image the vascular anatomy.

    e. Conventional angiography. The vascular anatomy is best defined with conventional cerebral angiography. This study is useful for identifying an aneurysmal source of subarachnoid hemorrhage, evaluating cerebral arterial stenosis (especially if surgery is contemplated), defining vasculitis, and assessing arteriovenous malformations. This technique, however, is associated with higher morbidity, given that it requires an arterial puncture and passing of a catheter through the major arteries.

4. Nerve conduction studies (NCS) and electromyography (EMG)

    a. NCS can help characterize a peripheral nerve disorder as being sensory, motor, or sensorimotor, as well as being primarily demyelinating or axonal in nature. NCS can also define specific sites of nerve compression or injury.

    b. EMG utilizes electrical responses from muscles to further characterize disturbances of the peripheral nervous system.

        (1) The **distribution of the observed changes** can help localize a problem to the nerve root (radiculopathy) versus the peripheral nerve.

        (2) Certain abnormalities can help one distinguish an acute versus a chronic process.

        (3) Disorders of the muscle (myopathies) can be classified into those involving muscle destruction versus simple dysfunction.

II   LOSS OF CONSCIOUSNESS

A   Syncope

1. Definition. Syncope refers to a transient loss of consciousness that typically follows insufficient blood supply to the brain for more than a few seconds.

2. Clinical signs. Patients are transiently unresponsive, with diminished muscle tone. A few generalized tonic spasms may occur, especially if patients are prevented from lying down.

3. Etiology. Cardiac and circulatory causes of syncope are discussed in Chapter 2 IX. Most patients with syncope have a cardiac or circulatory basis for the event, although neurologic conditions need to be considered if the diagnosis remains elusive.

    a. Circulatory disturbances are particularly common.

        (1) Vasovagal syncope, which is often seen in young people, is commonly associated with emotional stress, fear, or pain.

        (2) Postprandial syncope, which frequently affects the elderly, often occurs following meals in which alcohol has been consumed.

        (3) Syncope can occur in diverse settings that have in common a **preceding Valsalva** or **straining maneuver** that decreases venous return and promotes parasympathetic tone (e.g., micturition syncope).

b. Cardiac output disturbances, other than arrhythmia or mechanical obstruction, should be considered.

   (1) Vasodepressor (neurocardiogenic) syncope is caused by undue stimulation of afferent cardiac mechanoreceptors because of cardiac distention or strenuous contractions. This causes a decrease in sympathetic activity and an increase in parasympathetic activity that leads to vasodilation, bradycardia, and subsequent hypotension.

   (2) Carotid sinus hypersensitivity can lead to bradyarrhythmias and hypotension. Because carotid sinus hypersensitivity is present in many older men, it should be considered responsible for syncope only if other causes have been excluded.

c. Hypoglycemia causes a lack of nutrient supply to the brain and can lead to syncope. Hypoglycemia as a cause of syncope is particularly likely in patients with type 1 (insulin-dependent) diabetes. Therapy involves the administration of glucose.

d. Neurologic disorders are relatively uncommon causes of syncope. Several conditions are important because they can lead to unresponsiveness and are therefore often considered during the evaluation of a patient with transient unresponsiveness.

   (1) Seizures (see also IX A, B) are a cause of unresponsiveness that must be differentiated from syncope.

   (a) Patients are rarely limp during seizures. Many seizures cause sustained limb extension (tonic activity) or intermittent, relatively rhythmic limb contractions (clonic activity).

   (b) Atonic seizures are rare in adults but do cause sudden collapse. Absence seizures, conversely, do not result in falls.

   (c) Because some patients with syncope can exhibit involuntary movements, the possibility of a primary seizure is a consideration. However, in most cases, the tonic or myoclonic activity tends to occur several seconds after consciousness is lost and merely reflects cerebral hypoperfusion, not a primary seizure disorder.

   (2) SAH can transiently increase ICP, compromising global cerebral perfusion. Clues to the diagnosis include persistent, severe headache, meningismus, and papilledema.

   (3) Basilar artery migraine (a unique type of migraine with aura) is a rare cause of unresponsiveness. A history of recurrent headache, recurrent episodes of unresponsiveness, and associated symptoms (e.g., visual distortion and dizziness) should lead to consideration of this condition. In most instances, other causes of vertebrobasilar ischemia should be sought before assigning a diagnosis of basilar artery migraine.

   (4) Narcolepsy can cause episodes of sleep or cataplexy (loss of tone) that can be mistaken for syncope.

e. Psychogenic unresponsiveness can be associated with anxiety, panic attacks, or hyperventilation, as well as somatoform (conversion) disorder. In this case findings on the exam should allow one to confirm consciousness.

4. Diagnosis. A history and physical examination often can provide clues to the proper diagnosis. If no clues are evident, it is generally appropriate to proceed with a cardiovascular evaluation as outlined in Chapter 2 IX D.

a. Neurologic testing frequently includes an EEG. Rarely is a CT scan diagnostic. In some patients, an MRI or an imaging study of the vascular system can be informative.

b. Upright tilt testing, possibly with isoproterenol infusion, can provide evidence for a diagnosis of vasodepressor (neurocardiogenic) syncope, especially if the characteristic hemodynamic changes occur in less than 15 minutes without isoproterenol infusion.

5. Therapy. Treatment depends on the underlying diagnosis.

B **Coma**

1. Definition. Coma is a state in which a patient is unconscious and unresponsive to environmental stimuli. Coma is associated with extensive structural or physiologic damage to both cerebral hemispheres or to the ascending reticular activating system in the brainstem.

2. Etiology. The many causes of coma can be broadly grouped as shown in ⊕ Online Table 12–4.

3. Approach to the patient. Complete and rapid assessment is critical for optimal care.

a. Patient history. The physician should ascertain the time of onset of the loss of consciousness, as well as the following information from someone close to the patient:

    (1) Past medical history, especially of a preexisting neurologic, cardiac, pulmonary, hepatic, or renal condition

    (2) Prescription and **over-the-counter drugs** used by the patient

    (3) History of **drug abuse,** if applicable

    (4) Recent patient complaints

    (5) Details regarding the site where the patient was found (e.g., presence of empty drug vials, evidence of a fall)

  b. Physical examination. The **examination** should be thorough. Extremes of blood pressure, pulse, or temperature, abnormal breathing patterns, evidence of head or neck trauma, and the presence of meningismus should be noted carefully. The skin should be inspected for signs of trauma or needle tracks. Special attention should be directed to the following:

    (1) Pupils. Pupillary size and reactivity are dependent on sympathetic and parasympathetic innervation. Brainstem reflexes such as the pupillary reaction to light offer clues to the location of the lesion responsible for the coma.

      (a) Large, nonreactive pupils result from the disruption of the parasympathetic portion of the third cranial nerve but may also be seen with barbiturate overdose.

      (b) Small, reactive pupils result from the disruption of the sympathetic pupillodilatory impulses that arise in the hypothalamus and course caudally through the periaqueductal gray matter and cervical spinal cord before traveling rostrally with the internal carotid artery toward the eyes.

      (c) Pinpoint pupils that are nonreactive to light may be seen with narcotic overdose.

    (2) Ocular motility. Analysis of ocular motility allows assessment of damage to the brainstem and the cranial nerves that control eye movement.

      (a) The eyes should first be examined in the resting position for spontaneous motion of the eyeballs. Although the eyes of comatose patients may move spontaneously, they do not fixate or track in a purposeful manner.

      (b) If the eyes are immobile, movement can be elicited through the **vestibulo-ocular reflex** by moving the patient's head side to side (the **"doll's eyes"** or **oculocephalic maneuver**) or by elevating the patient's head 30 degrees and irrigating the external auditory canal with ice water (i.e., cold caloric testing). The former should only be performed after a cervical injury is ruled out.

        (i) Conjugate deviation of the eyes bilaterally toward the cold water implies intact brainstem circuitry.

        (ii) Failure of an eye to abduct in response to these maneuvers implies sixth nerve compromise.

        (iii) Failure of an eye to adduct implies dysfunction of the medial longitudinal fasciculus or oculomotor nucleus or nerve.

        (iv) Failure of either eye to respond implies an ipsilateral pontine lesion.

        (v) The presence of **conjugate nystagmus** away from the side of ice water irrigation suggests psychogenic coma.

    (3) Motor functions. Quadriparesis, hemiparesis, or monoparesis may occur in comatose patients.

      (a) Quadriparesis and flaccidity suggest pontine or medullary compromise or a high cervical spinal cord insult.

      (b) Decorticate posturing (i.e., leg extension with flexion of the arm, wrist, and fingers) can be unilateral or bilateral and suggests a hemispheric or diencephalic lesion.

      (c) Decerebrate posturing (i.e., leg and arm extension) also can be unilateral or bilateral and suggests midbrain or pontine compromise.

 4. Clinical features. Once global brainstem dysfunction has developed, differentiation between supratentorial and infratentorial causes of coma cannot be made without diagnostic testing unless a history and serial observations of the patient's clinical course can be documented.

  a. Supratentorial causes of coma are often characterized by pathologic processes that result in **swelling of a cerebral hemisphere.**

    (1) This mass effect causes a midline shift of the affected hemisphere toward the contralateral side, compression of the ipsilateral third nerve as it courses near the medial temporal lobe (uncus), herniation of the medial temporal lobe below the tentorial notch (uncal herniation), distortion of the mesencephalon, and herniation of the cingulate gyrus under the midline falx (subfalcial herniation).

(2) Typically, there is a progressive clinical deterioration characterized by increasing unresponsiveness, development of a third nerve palsy ipsilateral to the swollen hemisphere, and, ultimately, midbrain compromise (reflected by bilaterally nonreactive, dilated pupils).

b. Infratentorial causes of coma can be suspected if ataxia, multiple asymmetric cranial nerve palsies, and unilateral or bilateral limb weakness or sensory loss develop before the development of more global, severe impairment of brainstem function (characterized by nonreactive pupils, absent ocular motility, and absent corneal and gag reflexes).

c. Diffuse, toxic, or metabolic causes of coma can be suspected if pupillary responses are intact, ocular motility is preserved, corneal reflexes can be elicited, a gag reflex is present, and limb movement in response to noxious local stimuli is observed. If pupillary responsiveness persists in the absence of other brainstem and limb function, a metabolic cause of coma should be considered.

d. Psychogenic coma should be suspected if the patient has a history of psychiatric disease or if the findings on physical examination are nonphysiologic. Examples of nonphysiologic responses in a "comatose" patient include the following:

(1) The presence of **nystagmus** when the patient's ears are irrigated with ice water

(2) Adversive head and eye movements

(3) Failure of the patient's arm, when held by the examiner over the patient's face, to fall towards the face when released by the examiner

(4) Resistance to having the eyelids opened

5. **Therapy.** Ideally, care of the comatose patient is intertwined with the initial assessment and the development of etiologic hypotheses.

a. Initial therapy. The "ABCs": Maintaining an **adequate airway, optimal ventilation,** and **appropriate blood pressure** are priority concerns.

(1) If **cervical fracture** is a possibility, **immobilization of the neck** is of great importance.

(2) **Endotracheal intubation** may be indicated to protect the airway.

(3) **Blood samples** for a complete blood count (CBC), electrolytes, glucose, renal and liver function studies, coagulation profiles, blood gases, and toxicology should be obtained.

(4) **Intravenous thiamine** (100 mg), one ampule of **dextrose 50% in water ($D_{50}W$),** and **naloxone** (0.4 mg) are often administered. **Flumazenil** can be given if benzodiazepine or hepatic coma is suspected.

b. Management

(1) **Imaging.** If the patient's general medical condition permits, and if the cause of coma is not clearly cerebral anoxia after cardiopulmonary arrest or a drug overdose, most patients should have a brain **CT scan** to define the presence of an **intracranial mass, cerebral edema,** or **hydrocephalus.** Further management depends on the etiology of the coma.

(2) **ICP evaluation and management**

(a) **ICP evaluation.** Consideration of the patient's ICP is intimately tied to the evaluation of coma. The intracranial cavity has a finite volume and compliance.

(i) Normally, modest volume additions to the intracranial contents (e.g., from a small intraparenchymal hematoma) cause only a small rise in ICP.

(ii) With progressive incremental increases to the intracranial volume (e.g., from massive cerebral edema, a hematoma, or a tumor), the intracranial compliance decreases and the ICP markedly increases.

(iii) Because cerebral perfusion pressure is the result of the mean arterial pressure minus the ICP, an **excessive rise of the ICP** is associated with **impaired cerebral perfusion** and **progressive neurologic deterioration.**

(b) **ICP management.** If a pathologic process associated with elevated ICP is suspected, emergency management should include steps to decrease the pressure or, at the very least, avoid increasing it. If possible, the cerebral perfusion pressure (CPP), where CPP = mean arterial pressure (MAP) − ICP, should be kept at greater than 60 mm Hg and the ICP at less than 20 mm Hg. Optimal management of increased ICP often requires direct ICP monitoring, as well as determination of hemodynamic parameters.

(i) Patients can be hyperventilated with an Ambu bag before intubation. Intubation and endotracheal suctioning should be performed carefully to minimize elevation of ICP.

(ii) Fever and agitation should be minimized.

(iii) The patient's head should be elevated 30 degrees and kept in midposition to optimize venous drainage.

(iv) Osmotic therapy is used to dehydrate the brain and decrease the ICP. Patients are kept euvolemic, and intravenous mannitol or hypertonic saline is administered to achieve a hyperosmotic state.

(v) **Durotomy and hemicraniectomy can be used to decompress swollen brain.**

(c) **Prognosis.** The prognosis of coma is generally related to the cause of the coma, the depth of the coma, and the duration. In one series, the probability of good or moderate recovery was only 2% once the patient had remained in coma for 14 days.

C Vegetative state

1. Definitions

a. The vegetative state is characterized by the unawareness of self or external stimuli. Patients cannot interact with others in a meaningful fashion. Autonomic functions are relatively well maintained, and a sleep–wake cycle exists. Patients can survive with medical and nursing support.

b. A **persistent vegetative state** is defined as a vegetative state that persists for at least 1 month after the initial brain insult. If, with continued observation (usually 3 months for nontraumatic injury), there is no meaningful recovery, the likelihood of functional recovery can be judged to be nil; the patient can be said to be in a **permanent vegetative state.**

2. Therapy. The family and physician should determine the level of treatment appropriate for the patient in a persistent vegetative state.

D Brain death

1. Definition. Death is recognized as occurring when there is irreversible cessation of all brain function. A brain insult sufficient to cause complete loss of cerebral function should be documented, if possible.

2. Approach to the patient

a. Physical examination. Patients are completely unresponsive to external visual, auditory, and tactile stimuli and are incapable of communication in any manner.

(1) Pupillary responses are absent, and eye movements cannot be elicited by the vestibulo-ocular reflex or by irrigating the ears with cold water.

(2) The corneal and gag reflexes are absent, and there is no facial or tongue movement.

(3) The limbs are flaccid, and there is no movement, although primitive withdrawal movements in response to local painful stimuli, mediated at a spinal cord level, can occur.

b. Apnea test. Patients have no respiratory function. An apnea test should be performed to ascertain that no respirations occur at an arterial carbon dioxide tension ($PaCO_2$) of at least 60 mm Hg. The oxygenation should be maintained as the $PaCO_2$ is allowed to rise. The inability to develop respiration is consistent with medullary failure.

c. Exclusionary criteria. A diagnosis of brain death cannot be made in the setting of drug intoxication, hypothermia (defined as a core temperature of $<32°C$), or severe hypotension (i.e., shock).

d. Confirmatory tests. These tests are usually not necessary to diagnose brain death but can be used if doubt exists or if local statutes require them.

(1) An **EEG** does not demonstrate any physiologic brain activity.

(2) **Tests to assess cerebral blood flow** fail to show cerebral perfusion.

e. Period of observation. Periodic evaluation is necessary before a diagnosis of brain death can be made, unless there is gross evidence of a nonsurvivable insult to the brain.

(1) Two evaluations (6–12 hours apart) are usually sufficient to support a diagnosis of brain death.

(2) In the presence of anoxic brain damage, a period of 24 hours of observation is appropriate before declaring brain death.

III ALTERATION IN BEHAVIOR

A Delirium

1. **Definition.** Delirium is a disorder of brain function affecting behavior and causing impaired attention and cognition, motor hyperactivity or hypoactivity, altered sleep–wake cycles, and altered states of arousal. It is often acute, reversible, and secondary to a medical or neurologic disorder.

2. **Etiology.** Generalized or focal causes of cerebral dysfunction are potential causes of delirium.
   a. **Generalized brain dysfunction.** Causes include the following:
      (1) **Drugs,** including anticholinergics, antiparkinsonians, analgesics, cimetidine, digoxin, benzodiazepines, antidepressants, and illicit substances, may produce delirium. Withdrawal from alcohol, barbiturates, and benzodiazepines is associated with delirium as well. The **serotonin syndrome** consists of delirium and disordered motor and autonomic function; it results from overstimulation of serotonin receptors. The **neuroleptic malignant syndrome** causes delirium in association with fever, rigidity, tremulousness, and, occasionally, myoglobinuria.
      (2) **Metabolic alterations,** including hypoxia, hypercarbia, hyponatremia, uremia, hepatic failure, hyperglycemia, hypoglycemia, fever, dehydration, hypercalcemia, myxedema, hyperthyroidism, porphyria, antithyroid antibodies (Hashimoto's encephalopathy), and thiamine and niacin deficiencies, can cause delirium.
      (3) **Diffuse insults to the brain,** such as meningitis, encephalitis, fat emboli, and disseminated intravascular coagulation (DIC), are associated with cognitive impairment.
      (4) **Nonconvulsive status epilepticus,** including absence or complex partial seizures, may cause delirium. Postictal patients may also be delirious.
      (5) **Systemic infections,** such as a urinary tract infection, pneumonia, or sepsis
   b. **Focal cerebral disease.** Differentiating a global cerebral disorder from a focal brain disease that also may cause altered behavior presents a clinical challenge. For example, focal brain disease can cause a subtle aphasia, which may be misinterpreted as delirium. Appropriate laboratory and neurodiagnostic tests should be performed based on the clinical presentation.
      (1) **Focal cerebral disease,** typically caused by stroke, involves the nondominant temporoparietal area, frontal lobes, head of the caudate nucleus, thalamus (the top-of-the-basilar syndrome), or occipital lobes, which may cause blindness. Patients who have a focal cerebral disease may be agitated and experience hallucinations.
      (2) **Mass lesions** also can cause a confusional state, especially if they are located in the frontal lobes.

3. **Therapy.** The aim of therapy is identification and treatment, when possible, of the causes of delirium. An offending agent may have to be withdrawn. Adequate nutrition should be maintained and the safety of the patient ensured. If necessary, sedation with a low dose of haloperidol or a newer antipsychotic such as risperidone, quetiapine, or olanzapine can be helpful.

B Dementia

1. **Definition.** Dementia can be defined as a global decline in cognitive function in clear consciousness. One should be extremely cautious in making the diagnosis of dementia in a delirious patient.

2. **Etiology.** The causes of dementia are many. Identification of a treatable condition masquerading as a degenerative process is critical.
   a. **Causes of dementia** include Alzheimer's disease, Parkinson's disease, multiple cerebral infarcts, Huntington's disease, frontotemporal degeneration including Pick's disease, dementia with Lewy bodies, human immunodeficiency virus (HIV) infection, and Creutzfeldt–Jakob disease.
   b. **Potentially treatable conditions that can manifest as dementia** include depression (pseudodementia), normal-pressure hydrocephalus (NPH), subdural hematomas, tumor, adverse drug effects, thyroid disease, vitamin B_{12} deficiency, syphilis, heavy metal intoxication, conditions causing hypersomnia (e.g., sleep apnea syndrome), chronic meningitis, and Wilson's disease.

3. **Alzheimer's disease.** This condition is the **most common cause** of chronic dementia.
   a. **Definition.** Alzheimer's disease is a clinicopathologic entity characterized by progressive memory loss and other cognitive deficits. Onset commonly is late in life, although patients may be affected in middle age.

(1) The disease usually arises spontaneously, but genetic factors have been identified. Familial cases have been associated with mutations of the genes for amyloid precursor protein, presenilin 1, and presenilin 2.

(2) There is an association between the age of onset of Alzheimer's disease and the apolipoprotein E genotype. Patients with the APOE4/4 genotype have the greatest risk for Alzheimer's disease at a given age.

b. Prevalence. Alzheimer's disease is a burgeoning public health problem. It is estimated that 60%–80% of demented patients have Alzheimer's disease. The prevalence increases sharply with age, affecting 5%–15% of people older than age 65 years and about three times as many people older than age 85 years (the fastest-growing segment of the population).

c. Pathology. Although the cause and pathogenesis are unknown, Alzheimer's disease has a characteristic pathology consisting of **intracellular neurofibrillary tangles** and **extracellular neuritic plaques.**

(1) The tangles are composed primarily of abnormally phosphorylated, microtubule-associated **tau** protein.

(2) The amyloid protein, Aβ, is derived from amyloid precursor protein and is deposited in senile plaques and blood vessels. The gene for amyloid precursor protein resides on chromosome 21 and may be involved in familial cases.

(3) Associated pathologic processes disturb many neurotransmitters, particularly the **cholinergic system.**

d. Diagnosis

(1) The **clinical diagnosis** of **senile dementia of the Alzheimer's type (SDAT)** can be made if an otherwise alert patient exhibits progressive memory loss and other cognitive deficits such as disorientation, language difficulties, inability to perform complex motor activities, inattention, visual misperception, poor problem-solving abilities, inappropriate social behavior, and, occasionally, hallucinations.

(a) The **intellectual decline** should be present in two or more cognitive domains and be documented by clinical examinations such as the **Mini-Mental State Examination.** [For the original examination see Mini-Mental State. A practical method for grading the cognitive state of patients for the clinician. *J Psychiatr Res* 1975;12 (3):189–198.] Table 12–5 shows sample test items and where the test may be obtained.

(b) **Formal neuropsychological testing** can confirm the clinical impression and document progression of the disease. Tests that address recall (with or without cues) and delayed recall are especially sensitive for documenting early memory impairment.

(c) Other systemic and neurologic diseases that could produce cognitive decline should be absent.

(2) **Differential diagnosis**

(a) Patients with **pseudodementia (depression)** can exhibit many of the features of Alzheimer's disease. To complicate matters further, patients with Alzheimer's disease

---

TABLE 12–5   Mini Mental State Examination Sample Items

Orientation to time
  "What is the date?"
Registration
  "Listen carefully. I am going to say three words. You say them back after I stop. Ready? Here they are [. . .].
  Now repeat those words." Pause. "Now repeat those words back to me."
  Repeat up to five times, but score only the first trial.
Naming
  "What is this?" Point to a pencil or pen.
Reading
  "Please read this and do what it says." Show examinee the words on the stimulus form: "Close your eyes."

Reproduced by special permission of the publisher, Psychological Assessment Resources, Inc., 16204 North Florida Avenue, Lutz, Florida 33549, from the Mini Mental State Examination, by Marshal Folstein and Susan Folstein, Copyright 1975, 1998, 2001 by Mini Mental LLC, Inc. Published 2001 by Psychological Assessment Resources, Inc. Further reproduction is prohibited without permission of PAR, Inc. The MMSE can be purchased from PAR, Inc. by calling (813) 968-3003.

may present with depression. Identification of patients with pseudodementia is important because treatment of the depression can restore cognitive function.

  (i) A careful history and neuropsychological evaluation often can determine the proper diagnosis.

  (ii) If doubt remains as to the role of depression in the clinical presentation, appropriate treatment for depression may be warranted.

  (b) **Mild cognitive impairment**

  (i) Individuals with mild cognitive impairment have a memory impairment beyond that expected for normal aging. However, these individuals do not yet meet the criteria for Alzheimer's disease.

  (ii) People with mild cognitive impairment evolve to Alzheimer's disease at a rate of 10%–15% annually, compared with 1%–2% annually for normal individuals.

  (c) **Other types of dementia**

  (i) **Pick's disease** is a frontotemporal dementia characterized by personality changes, disinhibition, hyperorality, and frontotemporal atrophy on imaging studies. Hyperphosphorylated tau protein that accumulates in the cerebral cortex is associated with the disease.

  (ii) **Dementia with Lewy bodies** is characterized by fluctuating cognitive impairment, hallucinations, and early parkinsonian features.

  (iii) **Frontotemporal dementia with parkinsonism linked to chromosome 17 (FTDP-17)** is characterized by the same behavioral characteristics as the frontotemporal dementia described for Pick's disease. It is also associated with abnormal tau protein.

d. **Therapy**

  (1) **Medical therapy** is useful in treating insomnia, agitation, and depression.

  (a) In general, drugs should initially be given at a low dose; the dose can be adjusted upward slowly as clinically indicated.

  (b) Medications with a short half-life and few anticholinergic side effects are best tolerated.

  (c) Cholinesterase inhibitors such as donepezil, galantamine, and rivastigmine may improve cognitive and behavioral function.

  (2) **Day care centers** (including day hospitals) and **respite care** are useful adjuncts to family supervision of the patient with Alzheimer's disease and other dementing disorders.

4. **Normal-pressure hydrocephalus**

  a. **Definition.** NPH is a condition characterized by a triad of **cognitive impairment, urinary incontinence,** and **gait apraxia** (i.e., impaired ambulation without evidence of primary motor, sensory, or cerebellar dysfunction).

  b. **Etiology.** In most patients, the cause of NPH is unknown. However, NPH can follow SAH or meningitis, sometimes even years later.

  c. **Diagnosis.** NPH should be suspected in patients who present with the clinical features noted in III B 4 a. The following tests may help confirm the diagnosis.

  (1) **Imaging studies**

  (a) **CT** or **MRI** reveals ventricular enlargement with relatively little cortical atrophy (Figure 12–2).

  (b) **Cisternography** involves injecting a radionuclide into the lumbar thecal sac and then taking serial determinations of the flow pattern of the radioactive bolus. In the presence of NPH, cisternography demonstrates persistent activity of the radionuclide in the lateral ventricles after 48 hours. The validity of this test has been questioned.

  (2) In certain settings, **ICP monitoring** for 24–48 hours can reveal transient pressure increases if the diagnosis is in doubt.

  d. **Therapy.** Insertion of a **ventriculoperitoneal shunt** can improve the patient's condition, especially if performed within 6 months of the onset of the problem.

5. **Creutzfeldt–Jakob disease.** This progressive, degenerative illness is caused by **prions** (i.e., infectious proteinaceous particles) and is associated with a **spongiform encephalopathy.**

  a. **The gene for the prion protein is on chromosome 20;** approximately 10% of cases are hereditary. Illness can develop because of **infection** or **somatic** and **germ cell mutations.** The CSF 14-3-3

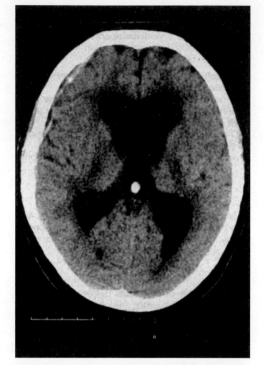

FIGURE 12–2 A nonenhanced computed tomography (CT) scan showing hydrocephalus consistent with normal-pressure hydrocephalus (NPH). Note the lack of cortical atrophy (sulcal effacement).

protein is a marker for Creutzfeldt–Jakob disease. **"Mad cow disease"** probably represents transmission of prion disease from infected cows to humans via ingestion of bovine food products.

   b. Patients may exhibit **myoclonus.** The **EEG** often demonstrates bilateral **periodic discharges** and an abnormal background rhythm.

   c. Death usually occurs within several months of the onset of the disease.

IV   HEADACHE

Headache is an extremely common complaint that in rare circumstances may portend a life-threatening process. Screening for certain "red flags" may allow one to identify high-risk individuals. Patients suffering from the worst or first headaches of their lives should always be considered for further evaluation. Similarly, elderly patients with new headaches or patients with changes in the character of their headaches should be seriously considered for further evaluation.

A Etiology

1. **Nonneurologic causes.** Before assuming that cephalic discomfort is caused by an intracranial disorder, the physician should consider the possibility of a nonneurologic cause. Disorders of the head and neck such as sinus disease, glaucoma, dental infections, temporomandibular joint (TMJ) disease, ear pathology, muscular injury, or cervical spine problems can cause headache.

2. **Intracranial stimulation of pain-sensitive structures.** Problems that affect the meninges or distort the larger blood vessels cause pain.

3. **Life-threatening causes**

   a. An **intracranial mass** causes a headache that typically develops insidiously and progressively worsens.

   (1) Clinical features. The **pain** is unlike any the patient has experienced and **may awaken the person** from sleep. Occasionally, the headache is worse in the morning. With time, **associated symptoms** (e.g., **nausea, vomiting, exacerbation with lifting** and **straining**) can develop. On examination, evidence of papilledema or **focal CNS disease** is typically apparent.

   (2) Therapy. Treatment is directed at the underlying lesion.

b. Subarachnoid hemorrhage typically produces "the worst headache of one's life." It causes the apoplectic onset of headache in previously healthy individuals or the sudden occurrence of headache that is of unique character in a chronic headache sufferer [see also VIII C 1].

    (1) Clinical features. The possibility that a headache is a result of SAH is strengthened if the cephalic discomfort cannot be easily attributed to any of the usual causes of head pain. No neurologic findings may be present on examination, and meningismus may be absent.

    (2) Diagnosis. Given the potential seriousness of the condition, patients should have a **cranial CT scan.** If this is unrevealing, an **LP** documents the presence of subarachnoid bleeding.

    (3) Treatment. Patients with SAH should undergo emergent clipping of any offending aneurysm. Nimodipine, a calcium channel blocker with specific action within the CNS, should be administered upon admission to prevent vasospasm. Supportive measures should be undertaken, if necessary, with regard to ventilation and nutrition.

B Headache syndromes

1. Migraine

  a. Etiology. The cause of migraine is unknown, but several common precipitants have been observed.

    (1) A **family history** of migraine often exists.

    (2) Headaches can be related to **stress, altered sleep patterns, menses, oral contraceptives, alcohol use, caffeine withdrawal, monosodium glutamate (MSG) intake,** and various **foodstuffs** (e.g., chocolate, nuts, aged cheeses, and meats containing nitrates).

    (3) Migraine can develop **after seemingly minor head trauma;** recognition and treatment may prevent prolonged disability.

  b. Pathophysiology. Hypotheses center around the idea that a migraine attack is brought on by neurovascular disturbances.

    (1) The classic **vasospasm–vasodilation theory** arose from clinical observations. Recent data suggest that oligemia, secondary to a slowly spreading area of **neuronal depolarization** (the cortical depression of Leão), occurs during a headache prodrome and persists into the headache phase. Hyperemia occurs subsequently and can persist after the headache subsides.

    (2) Current theory maintains that **dysfunction** of the **trigeminovascular system,** resulting in the perivascular release of substance P and other neurotransmitters and inflammatory markers, leads to migraine.

  c. Migraine syndromes

    (1) Migraine without aura (common migraine) is a syndrome characterized by recurrent unilateral or bilateral headache that is throbbing in character and worsened by movement. These headaches are often associated with nausea, vomiting, photophobia, phonophobia, and anorexia.

    (2) Migraine with aura (classic migraine) is a syndrome of recurrent unilateral headaches of similar nature, preceded by auras characterized by visual loss and flashing lights (i.e., scintillating scotoma and fortification spectra). Rarely, patients may suffer with transient neurologic deficits akin to stroke (e.g., complicated migraines).

  d. Therapy. Treatment should first involve the removal of inciting agents when possible.

    (1) Abortive therapy for migraine

      (a) Triptans, a family of serotonin 5-HT$_1$–receptor agonists, have become the first-line agents to abort migraines.

      (b) Aspirin and other nonsteroidal anti-inflammatory drugs (NSAIDs) are useful alternatives.

      (c) Ergotamine, a serotonin receptor agonist that is available orally and in intravenous (IV) formulations (e.g., dihydroergotamine [DHE 45]), is currently used much less frequently.

    (2) Symptomatic treatment of individual headaches is necessary if abortive measures fail. Often patients use NSAIDS for milder headaches but oral or parenteral narcotics for more severe instances, such as those requiring a visit to the emergency room. Metoclopromide is often used an antiemetic.

    (3) Prophylactic measures include medications and lifestyle modifications.

(a) **Medications** such as β-blockers, calcium channel blockers, tricyclic antidepressants, NSAIDs, and antiepileptic drugs such as gabapentin, topiramate, and valproic acid have been used to prevent migraines.

(i) The choice of medication is guided, in part, by the need to avoid or exploit a particular drug action (aside from the antiheadache effect).

(ii) Initially, a low dose should be administered, and the therapeutic benefits and undesirable side effects should be monitored as the dose is increased. The dose can be increased until either a beneficial response is achieved or adverse side effects develop. A maximal dose is best maintained for several weeks before concluding that an agent is not effective.

(b) **Biofeedback therapy** may enable patients to lessen migraine events by helping them deal more effectively with stress.

2. **Tension headaches are** characterized by a bandlike discomfort about the head; the pathophysiology is not well understood, but stress is often felt to play a role.

a. **Clinical features.** Tension headache often develops during the course of the day, involving the posterior cervical and occipital muscles. Distinguishing between this type of headache and migraine without aura can be difficult.

b. **Therapy.** Treatment involves reassurance, NSAIDs, muscle relaxants, moist heat, and, on occasion, antidepressant drugs and psychotherapy.

3. **Chronic daily headache**

a. **Etiology.** Patients with migraine or tension headache can develop chronic daily headaches spontaneously or as a result of excessive use of analgesics or ergotamines.

b. **Therapy.** Treatment consists of **withdrawal from excessive medications. Intravenous DHE** 45 given for 2–3 days can help break the headache cycle. **Prophylactic migraine agents** can help prevent a headache recurrence.

4. **Cluster headache**

a. **Clinical features.** Cluster headaches are severe periorbital headaches, 30–90 minutes in duration, that occur once or several times daily over a period of several weeks or months. The unilateral pain may be accompanied by ipsilateral lacrimation, conjunctival injection, nasal congestion, and Horner's syndrome. The typical patient is a middle-aged man. Patients with cluster headaches often pace, as opposed to migraineurs, who seek quiet, dark places. The pain may be severe enough to provoke sufferers to attempt suicide!

b. **Therapy**

(1) **Abortive and symptomatic treatment** of single headaches includes the administration of 100% oxygen, ergotamines, analgesics, or sumatriptan.

(2) **Abortive treatment for a cluster** of headaches usually consists of a short course of corticosteroids.

(3) **Prophylactic agents** may include lithium and calcium channel blockers.

5. **Temporal (giant cell) arteritis** (see also Chapter 11 XII D 1)

a. **Clinical features.** Patients older than the age of 50 years who complain of a headache centered about one temple or located in the occipital area should be evaluated for giant cell arteritis. Associated symptoms include visual disturbances, jaw claudication, fever, arthralgias and myalgias, and weight loss. Polymyalgia rheumatica (PMR) is also present in approximately 50% of patients with giant cell arteritis.

b. **Diagnosis.** The erythrocyte sedimentation rate is typically greater than 40 mm/hour, and the C-reactive protein level is elevated. Biopsy of the temporal arteries confirms the diagnosis.

c. **Therapy. Corticosteroid treatment** can bring rapid relief but must be maintained for many months.

6. **Benign (idiopathic) intracranial hypertension (pseudotumor cerebri)** has no known cause but is associated with obesity, pregnancy, oral contraceptives, SLE, cranial venous sinus thrombosis, and a host of other conditions.

a. **Clinical features.** The development of a relatively constant, generalized headache in patients with a clear sensorium, papilledema, and an otherwise normal neurologic examination is suggestive of benign intracranial hypertension. Visual obscurations can occur, and visual loss is the most serious complication.

    b. **Diagnosis.** The diagnosis is suggested by a CT or MRI scan, showing normal or small ventricles. The diagnosis can be confirmed by finding an elevated CSF opening pressure and an otherwise normal CSF analysis.

    c. **Therapy**

      (1) Visual acuity and fields should be monitored.

      (2) **Serial LPs** can relieve the syndrome.

      (3) **Corticosteroids, acetazolamide,** or **furosemide** may be administered.

      (4) Refractory disease has been managed with **lumboperitoneal shunting of CSF** or **optic nerve sheath fenestration.**

7. **Trigeminal neuralgia (tic douloureux)** is a syndrome that most often is idiopathic but has been associated with MS, neoplasia, and purported vascular "loops" that impinge on the trigeminal nerve.

    a. **Clinical features.** Lightning-quick, severe facial pains occur in the distribution of the trigeminal nerve in the setting of an otherwise normal exam. The pains are classically brought on by various stimuli such as light touch, chewing, cold substances, or wind.

    b. **Therapy. Carbamazepine** remains the first-line treatment, **but alternative treatments include baclofen, gabapentin, surgery to remove the vascular loops,** and **stereotactic radiation therapy.**

8. **Indomethacin-responsive headaches** are characterized by severe, unilateral pains that may be relieved by treatment with indomethacin.

    a. **Chronic paroxysmal hemicrania** is characterized by painful, multiple attacks (up to 40 daily) that last from 2 minutes to 2 hours with nocturnal awakenings and associated autonomic features. Women are more affected than men. Alcohol can precipitate the attacks.

    b. **Episodic paroxysmal hemicrania** is characterized by painful, multiple attacks (6–30 daily) that last up to 30 minutes and are associated with nocturnal awakenings and other autonomic features. Remissions lasting months to years can occur.

9. **Low-pressure headaches** are characterized by headaches that substantially worsen when patients are upright and improve when supine.

    a. **Etiology.** Postural headaches typically occur after an LP but can develop spontaneously as a result of dural tears.

    b. **Diagnosis.** MRI may show generalized dural enhancement, low-lying cerebellar tonsils, and a "kinked" brainstem.

    c. **Therapy.** Treatment consists of a **blood patch** (injection of autologous blood into the lumbar epidural space) or repair of the dural tear.

V   WEAKNESS

Many disorders can cause weakness. To pinpoint the causative disorder, the physician must first determine which part of the nervous system is diseased.

A **Anatomic and functional approach**   Weakness can result from dysfunction at various points in the central nervous system (CNS) or peripheral nervous system (PNS). Specific localization depends upon recognition of the pattern of weakness and associated findings.

1. **CNS disorders.** Dysfunction of the pyramidal tracks or upper motor neurons is classically associated with "upper motor neuron signs" and "pyramidal weakness."

    a. Upper motor neuron signs consist of increased reflexes, upgoing toes, and increased tone (spasticity).

    b. Pyramidal weakness refers to a pattern in which the extensors are weaker than the flexors in the upper extremity, and the flexors are weaker than the extensors in the lower extremity.

2. **PNS disorders.** Dysfunction of the motor unit (lower motor neurons and the muscle fibers they innervate) is associated with "lower motor neuron signs" and "site-specific weakness."

    a. Lower motor neuron signs refer to reduced or absent reflexes, downgoing or mute toes, and decreased tone, as well as atrophy and fasciculations (involuntary muscle twitches).

    b. Site-specific weakness refers to the specific patterns associated with pathology along the various sites of the motor unit.

      (i) Lower motor neuron disease such as polio may produce weakness at various sites.

      (ii) Nerve root disease will produce weakness in a "myotomal" pattern akin to the dermatomal sensory loss.

      (iii) Disorders of the neuromuscular junction generally produce proximal weakness.

      (iv) Disorders of muscle (myopathies) also produce proximal weakness.

B **Specific patterns of CNS pathology by anatomic location** (each pattern should be associated with upper motor neuron signs and pyramidal weakness)

1. **Cortical** (precentral gyrus) lesions may be distinguished by associated changes on mental status examination.
   a. Small lesions may be associated with monoplegia and possible sensory loss in same area.
   b. Large hemispheric lesions (e.g., middle cerebral artery stroke) produce hemiparesis, hemisensory loss, and homonymous hemianopia. Aphasia is commonly seen with left-sided lesions while neglect may be seen with right-sided lesions.

2. **Subcortical lesions** (in the deep white matter or posterior limb of the internal capsule) classically produce a hemiparesis with the pattern of face = arm = leg, with possible hemisensory loss but no visual changes and only rare mental status changes.

3. **Midbrain** lesions (in the cerebral peduncles) are rarely seen in isolation but may cause a subcortical pattern of weakness (face = arm = leg) with associated third nerve dysfunction or marked tremor.

4. **Pontine** lesions produce a subcortical pattern of weakness (face = arm = leg), possible hemisensory loss, and possible cranial nerve defects.

5. **Medullary** lesions are rarely seen in isolation; vascular lesions usually cause a contralateral hemiparesis sparing the face, ipsilateral tongue deviation, and contralateral loss of vibration and proprioception (medial medullary syndrome).

6. **Spinal cord** lesions (involving the corticospinal tracts) cause ipsilateral weakness below the level of the lesion.

C **Specific patterns of PNS pathology** by anatomic location (each pattern may have some lower motor neuron signs but "site-specific" weakness)

1. **Motor neuron diseases** (diseases of the anterior horn cell such as amyotrophic lateral sclerosis [ALS]) are pure motor disturbances with severe generalized weakness, wasting, hyporeflexia, and fasciculations.

2. **Radiculopathies** (nerve root disorders) produce weakness and sensory loss in the distribution of a nerve root ("myotomal" weakness and "dermatomal" sensory loss, respectively), as well as radicular or shooting pain.

3. **Plexopathies** (e.g., brachial, lumbar, or sacral) produce weakness, numbness, hyporeflexia, and pain in an entire limb.

4. **Neuropathies** generally produce distal numbness, weakness, and reflex loss.

5. **Neuromuscular junction disorders** such as myasthenia gravis are pure motor disorders characterized by proximal weakness.

6. **Myopathies** (disorders of muscle) are pure motor syndromes usually characterized by proximal weakness, with hyporeflexia only in very weak muscles.

VI   DISEQUILIBRIUM AND DIZZINESS

A **Ataxia** (gait instability) can be caused by cerebellar dysfunction or disorders of the motor or sensory system.

1. **Cerebellar dysfunction.** In addition to clumsiness and limb or truncal instability, as manifested by incoordination and impaired stance and gait, patients may exhibit hypotonia and ocular dysmetria.
   a. **Acute cerebellar dysfunction** (e.g., stroke, MS, neoplasia) typically manifests with unilateral findings.
   b. Causes of relatively symmetric **subacute** or **chronic cerebellar dysfunction** include alcoholic cerebellar degeneration; drug intoxication (e.g., phenytoin); cerebellar or spinocerebellar degenerations; and paraneoplastic, immune-mediated degeneration.

2. **Motor or sensory disorders.** Patients with strength in the 2/5–4/5 grade range (see Table 12–3) may appear clumsy, as may patients with a sensory neuropathy, dorsal root ganglion disease, posterior column dysfunction, or parietal lobe disease (parietal ataxia).

B **Dizziness**

1. **Approach to the patient**

   a. **History.** It is imperative to obtain a thorough history. By paying special attention to associated symptoms, the physician may be able to identify pathology of the inner ear, eighth cranial nerve, or CNS as the cause of the dizziness.

   b. **Physical examination.** The physician uses several screening techniques to search for evidence of structural disease.

      (1) **Nystagmus** is present in many patients who have vertigo. The nystagmus can be observed spontaneously (when the patient gazes straight ahead, laterally, or vertically), or it may be elicited by using Frenzel lenses to block visual fixation, by having the patient shake his or her head during ophthalmoscopy, or by covering the contralateral eye during ophthalmoscopy (to decrease visual fixation).

         (a) **Horizontal or vertical nystagmus** is characterized by a slow eye drift and a rapid shift in the opposite direction.

         (b) **Torsional nystagmus** is characterized by a slow clockwise or counterclockwise rotation and a rapid movement in the opposite direction.

         (c) The direction of nystagmus refers to the direction of the fast component of eye movement. Nystagmus is away from the affected ear (i.e., slow phase of eye movement is toward the side of the lesion). It is often of a mixed horizontal and torsional type.

      (2) **Gaze mechanisms** should be tested, including **saccadic speed** and **accuracy** and the integrity of **smooth pursuits.** The presence of **ocular dysmetria** and **visual acuity** while shaking the head should be noted. **Suppression of the vestibulo-ocular reflex** (which may be tested by asking the patient to fixate on a target moving synchronously with the head) should be noted as well. The **head thrust maneuver** may demonstrate abnormal corrective saccades.

      (3) **The physician should check for the presence of benign paroxysmal positional vertigo (BPPV)** by performing the Nylen–Bárány maneuver (i.e., by hyperextending the patient's neck and rotating the patient's head laterally as the patient is rapidly moved from a seated to a supine position). Rotary nystagmus with a linear component that appears after a several-second latency period suggests BPPV.

      (4) Vertigo that worsens when pressure is applied to the tragus may suggest a perilymphatic fistula.

2. **Selected causes of dizziness**

   a. **Labyrinthitis (vestibular neuronitis)** is an inflammatory condition of the inner ear characterized by the acute onset of a spinning sensation (vertigo), exacerbated by movement, and associated with nausea and vomiting. The condition is usually believed to be viral or bacterial in origin.

   b. **Ménière's disease** is characterized by episodic vertigo accompanied by nystagmus, tinnitus, fluctuating hearing loss, and aural discomfort.

   c. **BPPV** occurs when the patient moves his or her head (e.g., by rolling over in bed, looking up, or standing up). This condition is usually idiopathic in nature but can be caused by trauma, viral or ischemic injury, or drug toxicity. A unique physical therapy technique that can be used to decrease symptoms of BPPV has been developed.

   d. **Drug-induced vestibulopathy** can be caused by gentamicin, streptomycin, furosemide, and cisplatin.

   e. **Eighth cranial nerve disease** can be associated with hearing loss. Causes include acoustic neuroma, metastatic disease, vasculitis, and basilar meningitis associated with infectious and inflammatory processes.

   f. **Lateral medullary syndrome (Wallenberg's syndrome)** is due to occlusion of the vertebral or posterior inferior cerebellar artery.

      (1) Patients often feel that the external world is "tilting" and complain of feeling propelled toward one side (usually the side of the lesion).

    (2) Physical examination can indicate nystagmus (often horizontal–torsional and away from the lesion), ipsilateral ataxia, ipsilateral Horner's syndrome (characterized by ptosis, miosis, and anhidrosis), and ipsilateral facial sensory impairment with contralateral body sensory loss.

   g. Cerebellar disease can be caused by stroke, tumor, infection, or degenerative and inflammatory disease (Online XVIII H). Paraneoplastic cerebellar degeneration is associated with anti-Yo antibodies (leading to Purkinje cell loss) and anti-Ri (antineuronal) antibodies. Physical examination indicates ataxia and postural instability and many types of nystagmus. Opsoclonus is associated with anti-Ri antibodies.

   h. Brainstem lesions are typically associated with cranial nerve, motor, sensory, and cerebellar dysfunction.

   i. Other causes of dizziness include postural hypotension, hyperventilation, hypoglycemia, hypothyroidism, epilepsy, migraine, psychiatric disorders (e.g., depression, anxiety, and somatization disorders), and multisensory impairment (i.e., poor vision and positional sense).

3. Therapy

   a. Dizziness may be relieved by **treating the underlying disease.** If the underlying disease is unknown or otherwise untreatable, **acute symptomatic therapy** includes the use of meclizine, prochlorperazine, promethazine, topical scopolamine, and diazepam.

   b. Vestibular and gait exercises may help habituate the vestibular pathways to the abnormal influences of the disease.

   c. Chronic, poorly defined causes of dizziness can be managed by withdrawing the patient from drugs that affect the vestibular system. This action may allow a better reevaluation of the patient. Treatment with a **low dose** of a **benzodiazepine** and **vestibular and gait exercises** may be effective.

VII   PAIN SYNDROMES

Pain can arise from various structures within the body, including viscera, bones, muscles, connective tissue, and nerves. Neuropathic pain can have a variety of qualities, including burning, shooting, aching, or stabbing. In addition to the quality of the pain, location, severity, and ameliorating and exacerbating factors are all important characteristics in assisting with making a diagnosis. The time course is particularly important for determining the etiology of the pain.

A **Pain originating from the lower back**

1. Etiology

   a. Diagnostic considerations include local muscular strain, traumatic conditions of the spine, degenerative and inflammatory arthritides, neoplastic and infectious processes, and nerve root irritation.

   b. Neurologic dysfunction commonly develops from impingement on nerve roots by disk material, bony overgrowth, or thickened ligaments.

2. Disorders associated with low back pain

   a. Sciatica denotes a syndrome of sharp pain radiating from the low back to the buttock, down the back of the thigh to the calf, and, at times, over the bottom or top of the foot. Sciatica is commonly associated with disk herniation but can result from other conditions that irritate nerve root L4, L5, or S1.

     (1) Clinical features. Myotomal weakness, dermatomal numbness, reduced, deep tendon reflexes, and pain that increases with straight-leg raising or when the patient coughs or has a bowel movement are characteristic features of a lumbar radiculopathy.

     (2) Diagnosis. Persistent symptoms and neurologic deficits warrant in-depth investigation, which commonly includes the use of lumbosacral x-rays, lumbar MRI, and EMG. CT myelography may be indicated for better definition of the bony anatomy or when patients cannot undergo MRI testing.

     (3) Therapy. Acute low back pain should be evaluated carefully. Treatment should be directed at the underlying disorder if possible.

       (a) Unless tumor or infection is the likely cause for sciatica, initial therapy should include avoidance of strenuous activity and treatment with **NSAIDs.** If the patient shows signs of a **cauda equina syndrome** (i.e., a flaccid bladder, rectal dysfunction, and bilateral leg weakness), **emergency surgery** is usually required.

     (b) Long-term therapy may be appropriate. As the acute syndrome remits, a regimen of **back-strengthening exercises** and **weight loss** (if applicable) can be helpful. Surgery (e.g., **laminectomy**) may be necessary to relieve persistent symptoms.

  b. Lumbar stenosis is another common condition resulting in low back pain. Patients often have a congenitally small lumbar canal. Over time, bony and ligamentous overgrowth and disk protrusions may further encroach on the neural and vascular contents of the canal and foramina.

    (1) Clinical features. Patients develop pain and, occasionally, numbness and **weakness** with **ambulation** and **prolonged standing,** but they are relatively comfortable at rest. The neurologic examination of resting patients is often quite normal.

    (2) Therapy. It is necessary to differentiate pain caused by lumbar stenosis from that caused by vascular insufficiency. If symptoms are severe, **decompression surgery** is often pursued for the former.

B Pain originating from the neck

1. Etiology. Neck pain is often due to trauma (e.g., "whiplash"). Degenerative and inflammatory bone and disk disease can lead to nerve root irritation and is also a common source of neck pain. Local infection should be considered for acute symptoms; a neoplasm may be the culprit when subacute symptoms exist.

2. Disorders associated with neck pain

  a. Cervical radiculopathy. Pain can radiate in a dermatomal pattern with a parallel loss of sensation. Weakness may be in a myotomal distribution with a corresponding loss of deep tendon reflexes.

  b. Arthritis. The cervical radiculopathy associated with cervical arthritis (spondylosis) can be treated with physical therapy, **NSAIDs, and muscle relaxants, but surgery** may be warranted in some instances.

C Selected pain syndromes

1. Herpes zoster

  a. Acute syndrome. "Shingles" is a painful condition caused by the activation of a latent herpes zoster infection, which affects the nerves that supply the skin. Although shingles is most common in the elderly, it can occur in immunosuppressed patients as well.

    (1) Clinical features. The rash, characterized by painful vesicles on an erythematous base, may be preceded by discomfort. The pain often abates when the skin lesions heal but may persist and lead to postherpetic neuralgia.

    (2) Therapy

      (a) Corticosteroids may lessen the risk of postherpetic neuralgia in nonimmunosuppressed patients older than 60 years.

      (b) Famciclovir decreases the duration of postherpetic neuralgia in **immunocompetent patients.**

      (c) Acyclovir should be given to **immunosuppressed patients** to hasten recovery.

      (d) Analgesics, tricyclic antidepressants, gabapentin, and **topiramate** treat pain during the acute phase of the illness.

  b. Chronic syndrome

    (1) Once the vesicles have healed, residual discomfort can be managed with gabapentin, topical lidocaine, pregabalin, and capsaicin ointment.

    (2) Tricyclic antidepressants, carbamazepine and other anticonvulsant medications, vapocoolant spray, transcutaneous electrical nerve stimulation, and, occasionally, surgical intervention may be effective.

2. Complex regional pain syndrome (reflex sympathetic dystrophy; sympathetic maintained pain).

D Chronic pain syndromes

Nonmalignant pain syndromes, when chronic, can be especially difficult to evaluate and manage.

1. Care should be taken to assess patients fully for remedial problems (e.g., lumbar stenosis). An **interdisciplinary team approach** is best.

2. Use of **antidepressants** and **supportive psychotherapy,** coupled with **attempts to improve the patient's functional status,** can be beneficial. In selected instances, **chronic opiate** therapy can be beneficial.

VIII STROKE

A stroke can be defined as an acute neurologic deficit on a vascular basis. Stroke is a major health concern, representing a significant cause of long-term disability.

A Introduction

1. Strokes can be divided into broadly **ischemic** and **hemorrhagic processes.** Asymptomatic lesions in either category can predispose patients to future disease.

2. **Optimal management** requires precise diagnosis.

   a. **General principles of management** of symptomatic patients include monitoring for signs of clinical deterioration, ensuring adequate oxygenation, maintaining euvolemia, avoiding extremes of blood pressure without excessively lowering high blood pressure, treating infection and fever, and using normal saline (rather than glucose solutions) for intravenous hydration. Efforts should be made to prevent deep venous thrombosis and decubiti, avoid aspiration, maintain nutrition, and attend to bowel and bladder function.

   b. **Rehabilitation** of patients with persistent neurologic defects is important.

      (1) Multidisciplinary therapy involving physical, occupational, and speech therapy can be pursued on an inpatient or outpatient basis.

      (2) Depression occurs frequently and may be treated medically.

B Ischemic stroke

1. **Introduction**

   a. **Etiology.** Causes include cardiogenic emboli, extracranial and intracranial large-artery disease, small-artery disease, and various systemic and hematologic disorders.

   b. **Clinical signs**

      (1) Impaired carotid territory circulation produces symptoms of contralateral weakness and sensory loss, aphasia or neglect, and ipsilateral transient monocular blindness (amaurosis fugax). Typically, the weakness or numbness is greatest in the face and the arm and is less pronounced in the leg.

      (2) A diagnosis of vertebrobasilar disease is fairly certain if there is transient binocular blindness or other bilateral visual disturbances, diplopia, ataxia, quadriparesis, or vertigo associated with other neurologic symptoms.

   c. **Therapy.** New treatments for acute ischemic stroke are under investigation, driven by the evidence that there is at least a 3- to 6-hour "therapeutic window" during which intervention may lessen brain damage.

      (1) **Thrombolytic agents** may be administered with an acceptable incidence of hemorrhagic infarction and intraparenchymal hematoma. A randomized, double-blind trial of intravenous recombinant **tissue plasminogen activator (t-PA)** administered no more than 3 hours after the onset of an acute ischemic stroke at a dose of 0.9 mg/kg (with 10% of the dose given as a bolus and the remainder infused over 1 hour) resulted in an improved clinical outcome at 3 months in patients treated with the active drug. Patients treated with t-PA were more likely to sustain a symptomatic intracerebral hemorrhage during the first 36 hours; however, there was no significant difference in mortality between treated and untreated patients.

         (a) Treatment with t-PA appears to be beneficial for patients with small- or large-artery occlusive disease or cardioembolic stroke. Because there is such a narrow window of opportunity for the administration of t-PA, rare patients destined to have a transient ischemic attack [see VIII B 2] will be inadvertently treated.

         (b) Patients to be treated with t-PA must meet strict criteria to minimize the risk of hemorrhagic complications. In addition, no anticoagulants or antiplatelet agents should be administered for 24 hours after t-PA treatment, and blood pressure elevations should be treated. **Contraindications** include the following:

(i) A rapidly improving neurologic deficit or minor symptoms

(ii) A baseline CT scan showing evidence of intracranial hemorrhage

(iii) A systolic blood pressure >185 mm Hg or a diastolic blood pressure >110 mm Hg

(iv) A medication-induced or disease-related coagulopathy

(v) A history of hemorrhagic stoke, recent surgery, or another invasive procedure

(2) Although not yet "standard of care," there is increasing experience with intra-arterial thrombolysis and several mechanical approaches to intra-arterial clot lysis for patients acutely presenting with large-artery thromboembolic occlusions. A variety of imaging techniques, including CT and MR perfusion scans, MR diffusion, and CT or MR angiography, may assist in patient selection.

2. **Transient ischemic attacks (TIAs)** are short-lived neurologic deficits, typically lasting minutes. A recent recommendation is that the maximal duration of a TIA be revised downward to 1 hour, in contrast to the classic definition of up to 24 hours. Symptoms are attributable to ischemia in the carotid or vertebrobasilar arterial distributions. The distinction between a TIA and a stroke is arbitrary, and even a brief symptomatic episode of cerebral ischemia, in conjunction with an abnormal diffusion-weighted imaging (DWI) scan, might be construed as representing a stroke. Both warrant complete evaluation to determine the underlying pathophysiology and decrease the risk of subsequent ischemic events.

a. **Etiology.** Although TIAs often result from atherosclerotic large-vessel disease, other diagnostic possibilities deserve consideration, including cardiogenic emboli, aortic arch atherothrombotic emboli, other large-artery disorders such as dissection and fibromuscular dysplasia, small-artery disease, hematologic disorders, and migraine. Other disease entities such as seizures, tumors, subdural hematomas, and MS sometimes masquerade as a TIA.

b. **Evaluation.** Diagnostic studies should include a CBC, syphilis serology, a coagulation profile, and a CT scan or MRI. A transthoracic or transesophageal echocardiogram and 24-hour ambulatory electrocardiography (ECG) monitoring may be indicated.

(1) A duplex examination of the extracranial carotid artery territory is often informative.

(2) TCD studies, MRA, and CTA can provide insight into the extracranial and intracranial arterial circulation.

(3) Conventional interventional angiography is the definitive test to outline the vascular anatomy.

(4) Patients with an unrevealing cardiac evaluation who are thought to have an embolus may benefit from a transesophageal echocardiogram.

(5) If clinical suspicion exists, an LP can be used to evaluate the possibility of CNS inflammation.

c. **Therapy.** If atherosclerosis is suspected as the cause of transient cerebral ischemia, control of risk factors for atherosclerosis is essential [see Chapter 2 III A 2]. An evaluation for coronary artery disease is also appropriate.

(1) **Extracranial carotid artery disease.** Carotid endarterectomy is superior to medical therapy in the prevention of ischemic stroke in patients experiencing a TIA ipsilateral to an angiographically demonstrated 50%–99% stenosis at the internal carotid artery origin.

(a) Patients with less severe stenosis should be treated with aspirin. Clopidogrel or aspirin combined with slow-release dipyridamole is also effective in preventing stroke.

(b) Risk factor management pertinent to atherosclerosis is appropriate.

(2) **Intracranial large-artery disease.** A TIA can result from large-artery stenosis or occlusion. Recent evidence suggests that aspirin therapy is safer than, and as effective as, anticoagulation therapy for symptomatic intracranial large-artery stenosis.

(3) **Other causes of TIA.** Therapy should be directed at the appropriate pathophysiologic process. For instance, anticoagulants are frequently used in patients with a source of cardiogenic emboli.

3. **Cardiogenic embolic stroke**

a. **Etiology.** The most common cause of embolic stroke is nonvalvular atrial fibrillation.

(1) Other conditions associated with cardiogenic emboli include recent myocardial infarction (MI), an akinetic ventricular segment, dilated cardiomyopathy, a prosthetic heart

valve, infective and nonbacterial thrombotic endocarditis, left heart myxoma, left atrial spontaneous contrast echo, and atrial septal aneurysm.

(2) A patent foramen ovale (PFO) or atrial septal defect predisposes patients to paradoxical emboli, especially if there is a documented venous thrombosis. Patients younger than 55 years of age with a PFO and an associated atrial septal aneurysm may be at particularly high risk for embolic stroke.

(3) Other cardiac conditions, such as mitral valve prolapse or a hypokinetic ventricular segment, are rarely associated with a cardiogenic embolus.

b. Diagnosis. The diagnosis is most certain if there is an abrupt onset of neurologic dysfunction, an underlying cardiac condition known to predispose to emboli, strokes in multiple vascular territories, hemorrhagic arterial infarction, systemic emboli, an absence of concurrent conditions known to cause stroke, and angiography demonstrating (potentially transient) vessel occlusions in the absence of an intrinsic vasculopathy. Patients who have a cardiac embolism rarely present with all of these conditions.

c. Therapy. An ischemic infarction caused by a cardiogenic embolus may develop into a hemorrhagic infarction, especially if reperfusion occurs or the infarction is large. Therefore, care must be taken to lessen the risk of parenchymal hemorrhage in acutely ill patients while simultaneously taking measures to protect them from another embolic stroke.

(1) If the patient has had a relatively small ischemic embolic infarction, a CT scan should be obtained. If no blood is present, a continuous infusion of heparin is administered. A partial thromboplastin time (PTT) greater than twice the control value should be avoided to minimize the risk of hemorrhagic conversion of the ischemic infarction and clinical worsening.

(2) If the patient has had a large ischemic embolic infarction, anticoagulation therapy should be withheld for 5–7 days. If the patient is recovering and a subsequent CT scan reveals no blood, heparin may be administered.

(3) Subsequent treatment with oral anticoagulants depends on the underlying disease process and the patient's general condition.

4. Large-artery disease

a. Aortic arch atheromas or **thrombi.** These thrombi, which are visualized by transesophageal echocardiography, can embolize to the cerebral circulation and cause stroke. Optimal management is yet to be defined but usually involves antiplatelet or anticoagulation therapy, with the latter being used for mobile, pedunculated thrombi.

b. Asymptomatic cervical bruit and carotid stenosis. The combination of an internal carotid artery bruit and atherosclerosis at the internal carotid artery origin is a marker for coronary artery disease, as well as for cerebrovascular disease. Approximately 2% of these patients will have an ischemic stroke each year. Patients with a hemodynamically significant or progressive stenosis are at increased risk for cerebral infarction.

(1) **Etiology.** A midcervical bruit can be caused by a hyperdynamic circulation (e.g., as in anemia, pregnancy, and thyrotoxicosis), an external carotid artery stenosis, an internal carotid artery stenosis, or a venous hum.

(2) **Diagnosis.** Noninvasive vascular testing [see I C 3 d] is helpful in determining whether the bruit originates from atherosclerotic internal carotid artery disease and whether the lesion is hemodynamically significant. Angiography is usually used if the patient is a surgical candidate.

(3) **Therapy**

(a) **Control of risk factors for atherosclerosis** [see Chapter 2 III A 2]. Antiplatelet therapy (aspirin, clopidogrel, or aspirin combined with slow-release dipyridamole) is often prescribed, and a careful coronary artery evaluation is warranted.

(b) **Medical treatment.** Patients with less than a 50% internal carotid artery stenosis should be managed medically.

(c) **Carotid endarterectomy**

(i) Patients with a 50%–99% stenosis who undergo **carotid endarterectomy** have less risk of ipsilateral stroke than patients managed medically if surgery can be achieved with less than 3% risk of complications.

(ii) **Prophylactic carotid endarterectomy** for unilateral, slightly or moderately stenotic, asymptomatic internal carotid artery disease before major cardiac or vascular surgery is **usually inadvisable.**

c. **Ischemic infarction.** An understanding of neuroanatomy is essential to localize the compromised area of the brain and to correlate this information with a likely site of vascular disease.

(1) **Etiology**

(a) **Large-artery occlusive disease** can cause ischemic infarction, either by being a source of artery-to-artery emboli or by causing hypoperfusion distal to a hemodynamically significant vascular stenosis. Large-artery disease can involve the extracranial or intracranial portions of the cerebrovascular circulation.

(b) Vascular conditions other than atherosclerosis (e.g., **arterial dissection, arteritis, Takayasu's syndrome, fibromuscular dysplasia,** and **radiation-induced vasculopathy**) should be considered.

(2) **Diagnosis.** Diagnostic studies are pursued to define the vascular anatomy. CTA, MRA, carotid duplex, TCD, and conventional angiography can be used. The scope of testing is determined, in part, by the clinical condition of the patient and whether carotid endarterectomy or antithrombotic therapy is a primary therapeutic consideration. The more accurate the definition of the underlying cause of the infarction, the more precise is the determination of prognosis and treatment.

(3) **Therapy**

(a) **Extracranial carotid artery disease.** If the patient has sustained a minor infarction with a functional recovery and has a 50%–99% atherosclerotic stenosis of the ipsilateral origin of the internal carotid artery, carotid endarterectomy is superior to medical therapy for prevention of subsequent stroke. If the stenosis is less than 50%, therapy with antiplatelet drugs is appropriate.

(b) **Intracranial large-artery disease**

(i) If the infarction is caused by a severe stenosis or occlusion of a large intracranial artery, recent evidence suggests that aspirin therapy is safer than, and equally effective as, anticoagulation therapy.

(ii) Some physicians use anticoagulation agents if the patient has new symptoms.

5. **Small-artery disease.** The infarctions resulting from small-artery disease typically are deep in the hemispheres or the pontomesencephalic region and are known as **lacunae.** The lesions are less than or equal to 15 mm in diameter.

a. **Etiology.** The underlying vascular lesion is usually hypertension-associated lipohyalinosis. Diabetes mellitus is also associated with lacunar infarcts. A small atheromatous plaque blocking the ostium of an arteriole may, on occasion, be the cause of some occlusions, as may infectious or sterile inflammation, cardiogenic emboli, and large-artery occlusive disease.

b. **Diagnosis**

(1) Ischemic events from small-artery disease cause stereotypic syndromes such as pure motor or sensory stroke, sensorimotor stroke, clumsy hand–dysarthria syndrome, and ataxic hemiparesis.

(2) Patients should be screened for the possibility of cardiogenic emboli, large-artery occlusive disease, and hematologic and inflammatory disorders [see VIII B] if they are not hypertensive or if their history, examination, or routine diagnostic tests suggest a cause other than hypertension.

c. **Therapy** is directed at controlling hypertension. If another condition is defined as the cause of the infarction, appropriate intervention should be pursued. Antiplatelet therapy may be administered to decrease the likelihood of subsequent ischemic stroke.

6. **Hematologic and systemic conditions.** These disturbances are associated with ischemic infarction.

a. **Associated conditions.** Sickle cell disease, hyperviscosity associated with polycythemia and paraproteinemias, and hypercoagulability are conditions associated with ischemic stroke.

b. **Etiology.** Hypercoagulability is associated with antiphospholipid antibodies (including anticardiolipins and the lupus anticoagulant syndrome), hyperhomocysteinemia, deficiency of proteins C and S, activated protein C resistance, antithrombin III deficiency, malignancy, nephrotic syndrome, and pregnancy, as well as several other conditions.

7. **The young ischemic stroke patient.** Patients younger than 45 years of age who present with stroke are often diagnostic challenges. The potential etiologies are vast and include, but are not limited to, the following conditions:

   a. Drug (especially cocaine) and alcohol abuse

   b. Hypercoagulable states

   c. Cardiogenic emboli

   d. Migraine

   e. Vasculitis and other rare arterial lesions

   f. CNS infection, including HIV-associated conditions

   g. Cancer

   h. Disorders of homocysteine metabolism

   i. Familial conditions (e.g., neurofibromatosis [NF], von Hippel–Lindau disease)

   j. Pregnancy and the postpartum state

8. **The deteriorating ischemic stroke patient**

   a. **Pathophysiology**

      (1) The patient's condition may deteriorate as a result of progressive occlusion of arteries from clot propagation or artery-to-artery emboli or because of subsequent cardiogenic emboli. Deterioration also may result from excessive lowering of blood pressure or inadequate anticoagulation therapy.

      (2) Hemorrhagic infarction or a parenchymal hematoma can occur spontaneously or as a result of thrombolytic or anticoagulation therapy.

      (3) If heparin is being used as treatment, the possibility of heparin-induced thrombosis (with associated thrombocytopenia) should be considered.

      (4) Cerebral edema can develop, causing shifting of brain structures and an increase in the ICP.

   b. **Approach to the patient.** Ideally, continuing efforts should be made to define the pathophysiology of the stroke.

      (1) The blood pressure and degree of hydration should be checked.

      (2) A CT scan should be obtained to define mass effect and hemorrhagic complications.

      (3) A hematocrit, platelet count, and clotting profile should be obtained as appropriate.

   c. **Therapy.** Patients should be confined to bed, and extremes of blood pressure should be avoided.

      (1) Appropriate hydration should be maintained with normal saline, and increases in ICP should be treated, as necessary.

      (2) Consideration can be given to novel, interventional neuroradiologic techniques such as intra-arterial thrombolysis and angioplasty, depending on the degree of neurologic impairment, the time course of the illness, and the availability of resources.

C Hemorrhagic disorders

1. **Subarachnoid hemorrhage**

   a. **Etiology.** The most common causes of SAH are **trauma** and **ruptured berry aneurysms.**

      (1) Other causes include coagulopathies, mycotic aneurysm, arteriovenous malformation, vasculitis, and sympathomimetic drugs.

      (2) **Aneurysms** may be familial and can be associated with polycystic kidney disease, coarctation of the aorta, fibromuscular dysplasia, Moyamoya disease, polyarteritis nodosa, pseudoxanthoma elasticum, and Marfan and Ehlers–Danlos syndromes.

   b. **Diagnosis**

      (1) **Clinical signs.** A patient who has a ruptured berry aneurysm typically complains of "the worst headache of my life," but examination may reveal few objective findings. Other patients can present with meningismus, altered mental status, and focal neurologic findings. A partial third nerve palsy with pupillary dilation is suggestive of a posterior communicating artery aneurysm.

      (2) **Diagnostic studies.** A **CT scan** reveals the presence of subarachnoid blood in most patients (Figure 12–3). If the index of suspicion for an SAH is high but a CT scan is unrevealing, an LP provides the proper diagnosis. Conventional interventional angiography is necessary to characterize the aneurysm.

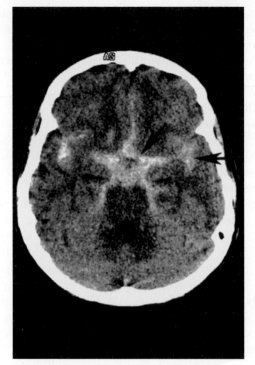

FIGURE 12–3 A nonenhanced computed tomography (CT) scan demonstrating a subarachnoid hemorrhage (SAH). Note the blood in the basal cisterns and the Sylvian fissures.

    c. Therapy. Treatment of aneurysmal SAH is aimed at **controlling complications,** which include rebleeding, vasospasm leading to delayed ischemic stroke, hyponatremia, acute or chronic hydrocephalus, intraparenchymal and intraventricular hematoma, and cardiac arrhythmias. Unfortunately, the mortality rate from aneurysmal rupture approaches 50%, although recent studies suggest improved outcomes. Interventional neuroradiologic techniques are playing a larger role in the management of aneurysms.

      (1) Rebleeding most frequently occurs in the first 48 hours after aneurysmal rupture. **Early intervention** to isolate the aneurysm should be performed when possible to eliminate the threat of rebleeding. Surgical "clipping" or endovascular therapy, which involves placing thrombogenic "coils" in the aneurysm, can be used to isolate the aneurysm.

      (2) The course of **vasospasm** can be followed with TCD and CTA and treated accordingly.

        (a) The development of ischemic stroke from vasospasm is less likely when **nimodipine,** a calcium channel blocker that may inhibit vasoconstriction or provide neuronal protection from ischemia, is administered.

        (b) Prophylaxis against symptomatic vasospasm also includes maintaining patients in a euvolemic state and avoiding hypotension.

        (c) If the aneurysm has been isolated from the circulatory system, symptomatic vasospasm may be treated with **hypervolemic therapy,** coupled with a moderate increase in blood pressure.

        (d) Refractory vasospasm may be amenable to angioplasty or selective intra-arterial papaverine or calcium antagonist infusion.

      (3) Symptomatic hydrocephalus can be treated with a ventricular drain, repeated LPs, or ventriculoperitoneal shunting, as dictated by clinical circumstances.

2. Intraparenchymal hematoma

    a. Diagnostic considerations. Chronic hypertension is often, but not invariably, associated with hemorrhage in the region of the putamen, thalamus, cerebellum, and pons.

      (1) An intraparenchymal hemorrhage that is not accompanied by a history of hypertension should prompt a search for an underlying cause of bleeding (e.g., coagulopathy, aneurysm, arteriovenous malformation, or tumor), particularly if the hemorrhage is not located in a region of the brain typically associated with hypertensive bleeding.

(2) In elderly patients, lobar hematomas, especially if multiple, may be indicative of amyloid angiopathy. The *APOE4* allele may be a risk factor for amyloid angiopathy and amyloid angiopathy–related hemorrhage.

(3) Coagulopathies (especially when induced by thrombolytic therapy) and the use of drugs such as cocaine and sympathomimetics are associated with intraparenchymal hematoma.

b. Diagnosis

(1) Clinical signs

(a) A **large putaminal hematoma** causes impaired consciousness, contralateral hemiparesis and sensory loss, and gaze preference to the side of the hemorrhage.

(b) Thalamic hemorrhage can lead to impaired consciousness, contralateral weakness and sensory loss, diminished vertical gaze, and small, poorly reactive pupils (i.e., Parinaud's syndrome).

(c) Patients with **cerebellar hemorrhage** may present with dizziness, impaired gait and stance, and limb ataxia. If the hematoma is large, impaired consciousness, cranial nerve palsies (including eye movement abnormalities), and weakness can develop.

(d) The classic signs of **pontine hemorrhage** include coma, pinpoint reactive pupils, impaired lateral ocular motility, and quadriplegia with decerebrate posturing. Small pontine hemorrhages cause more-restricted pontine syndromes.

(2) Diagnostic studies. A CT scan is central to diagnosis. A coagulation profile and drug toxicology screen should be performed. Angiography may be appropriate in normotensive patients and in those with hemorrhage at atypical sites to screen for vascular malformations.

c. Therapy

(1) Taking measures to lower the elevated ICP associated with parenchymal hematoma can improve outcome.

(2) With cerebellar hematomas, surgical resection is a lifesaving measure. Surgical resection of hematomas at other sites is receiving increasing attention.

(3) A coagulopathy should be treated appropriately.

3. Arteriovenous malformation. Headaches, seizures, and intraparenchymal hemorrhages or, occasionally, SAHs may result. Therapeutic intervention may incorporate multiple modalities, including surgery, interventional radiology with embolization, and stereotactic radiosurgery.

IX   **SEIZURES AND EPILEPSY**

A seizure can be defined as a clinical event associated with abnormal, excessive electrical activity in the brain. Manifestations of seizures include impairment or loss of consciousness and sensory, motor, or behavioral abnormalities. The term **epilepsy** describes a syndrome characterized by recurrent unprovoked seizures.

A **Classification**   Optimal management of seizure patients depends on proper classification of the seizure type. Seizures can be categorized as **generalized** or **partial (focal)**.

1. Generalized seizures usually involve loss of consciousness.

a. Generalized convulsive seizures consist of tonic, clonic, or tonic–clonic (grand mal) motor activity. **Postictal obtundation** and **confusion** commonly last minutes and, occasionally, hours after a seizure. The EEG often shows generalized spikes or spikes and slow waves.

b. Absence seizures are characterized by brief staring spells without a postictal state. Typically, the EEG demonstrates generalized 3-Hz spike-wave discharges.

2. Simple partial (focal) seizures are not accompanied by an impairment of consciousness and are restricted to one part of the body

a. Simple partial seizures can be characterized as being sensory, motor, or autonomic. Simple motor seizures present with clonic movements of a limb, simple sensory seizures present with no outwardly visible signs but only as sensory phenomena to the patient (akin to hallucinations), and simple autonomic seizures present as paroxysmal sweating, flushing, or tachycardia.

b. The EEG may show a focal rhythmic discharge at the onset of a simple partial seizure, but, occasionally, no abnormal activity is detected during the seizure. Between seizures focal spikes may be seen.

3. **Complex partial (focal) seizures** are often characterized by an **aura** followed by **impaired awareness.** The EEG often shows interictal spikes or spikes with associated slow waves in the temporal or frontotemporal areas and ictal focal rhythmic discharges. Generalized motor seizures may develop secondarily.

   a. The **aura** may involve **hallucinations** (e.g., olfactory, visual, auditory, or gustatory) and complex **illusions** (e.g., of having experienced a new event or of never having experienced a commonplace event). However, patients frequently do not recall their aura.

   b. Nausea or vomiting, focal sensory perceptions, and focal tonic or clonic activity may accompany a complex seizure.

   c. After the aura, there may be an episode of impaired consciousness, lasting seconds to several minutes, during which time automatisms may be observed. Return to baseline cognitive abilities can take several minutes.

4. Status epilepticus is defined as an episode of repeated or ongoing seizure activity with impaired arousal lasting at least 30 minutes. Status epilepticus may involve both **convulsive** (generalized tonic–clonic activity) and **nonconvulsive** (absence or complex partial) seizures.

   a. Patients experiencing convulsive seizures are at risk for hypoxia, aspiration, acidosis, hypotension, hyperthermia, myoglobinuria, hypoglycemia, and multiple physical injuries.

   b. Patients experiencing nonconvulsive seizures can appear delirious. A fluctuating mental status and subtle automatisms or myoclonic jerks are clues to the diagnosis, and the EEG is confirmatory.

B **Etiology** Table 12–6 outlines some of the many causes of seizures. Several seizure types have a defined genetic basis: autosomal dominant frontal lobe epilepsy (neuronal nicotinic acetylcholine receptor mutation) and autosomal dominant temporal lobe epilepsy with auditory features.

C **Diagnosis**

1. **Patient history** and **physical examination** can aid in the determination of whether a seizure or some other transient event was responsible for the patient's symptoms.

   a. A **family history of epilepsy** or a **history of febrile convulsions** is relevant.

   b. An **accurate description of the event by an observer** is helpful in defining the problem.

   c. **Urinary incontinence, back pain** (from a vertebral compression fracture), **myalgias,** and **oral lacerations** are clues to proper diagnosis.

   d. **Fever, fatigue, stress, alcohol withdrawal, medications,** and **menses** can provoke seizures.

2. **Differential diagnosis.** Other conditions that may produce sudden loss of consciousness are discussed in II A. Psychogenic seizures should be considered if patients exhibit nonstereotypic events, have an unexpected resistance to antiepileptic drugs, or have a psychiatric disorder.

TABLE 12–6   Selected Causes of Seizures

Idiopathic	Infection
Genetic predisposition	Meningitis, abscess, and encephalitis
Mesial temporal sclerosis	Degenerative diseases
Metabolic abnormalities	Alzheimer's disease
Hyponatremia	Trauma
Hypoglycemia or hyperglycemia	Eclampsia
Hypocalcemia	Drugs
Hypomagnesemia	Theophylline
Uremia	Lidocaine
Vascular disease and stroke	Cocaine
Infarction, especially cortical	Drug and substance withdrawal
Vascular malformation	Anticonvulsant medications
Vasculitis	Benzodiazepines
Inflammatory causes	Alcohol
Systemic lupus erythematosus	Psychogenic causes
Neoplasia	
Metastatic and primary brain tumors	

3. **Diagnostic studies**
    a. The **EEG** is central to the evaluation of seizure patients. The best technique for fully characterizing a seizure disorder is continuous video EEG monitoring, but this is not usually used as an initial diagnostic test. A normal EEG does not exclude the diagnosis of epilepsy since the sensitivity of a single routine EEG is only 50%.
    b. An **MRI** scan is the most useful modality for detecting lesions that may cause seizures.
    c. **SPECT** and **positron emission tomography (PET)** can provide additional information to help localize a seizure focus.
    d. **Laboratory studies** are indicated to evaluate potential metabolic or toxic causes, including glucose, sodium, calcium, blood urea nitrogen (BUN), creatinine (Cr), liver function tests (LFTs), and toxin screen.

D **Therapy**

1. **General considerations.** If a seizure is the suspected diagnosis, decisions about therapy depend on the underlying cause.
    a. Correction of hyponatremia, hypoglycemia, or drug intoxication may be all that is necessary.
    b. Patients with a neurologic condition known to be associated with recurrent seizures often require medication.
    c. Anticonvulsant therapy is often not initiated in patients with a single, unprovoked seizure in the setting of a normal exam and normal imaging.

2. **Medical therapy**
    a. **General principles.** An attempt is usually made to prevent subsequent seizures by using a **single agent,** to limit toxic effects. The drug should be administered in **progressive doses** until seizure control has been achieved or until drug toxicity occurs. Only if monotherapy fails should a second drug be added. If control is then obtained, the first agent might be carefully withdrawn.
    b. **Specific agents.** The choice of medication should be based on the seizure type, bearing in mind possible contraindications and side effects.
        (1) Typically, generalized convulsive, simple partial, and complex partial seizures are treated with carbamazepine, phenytoin, valproic acid, topiramate, levetiracetam, lamotrigine, or zonisamide.
        (2) Ethosuximide or valproic acid is used for absence seizures.
        (3) Valproic acid is particularly effective for treating myoclonic epilepsy.
        (4) **Lamotrigine, gabapentin, tiagabine, oxcarbazepine,** and **topiramate** are adjunctive medications for the treatment of patients with refractory partial seizures.

3. **Surgical therapy.** Patients refractory to medical therapy may be candidates for surgery. **Temporal lobe resection, ablation of a cortical seizure focus,** and **corpus callosum sectioning** can reduce seizure frequency in some patients who meet specific criteria. Alternatively, **vagus nerve stimulation** may help control seizures.

4. **Control of status epilepticus.** Generalized convulsive status epilepticus is a life-threatening condition; therefore, management of convulsive status epilepticus requires making certain that the airway is unobstructed and maintaining adequate oxygenation, blood pressure, and hydration. Definition of the underlying problem is essential.
    a. **Glucose** and **thiamine** should be administered after blood samples for glucose, electrolytes, renal function, anticonvulsant drug levels, and toxicology have been obtained.
    b. Often, **intravenous diazepam** or **lorazepam** (at a dose of 0.1 mg/kg) is given to stop the convulsions. Lorazepam carries less risk of respiratory depression or arrest and remains effective for longer periods.
    c. Administration of a benzodiazepine is followed by administration of **phenytoin, fosphenytoin,** or **phenobarbital (all at doses of 20 mg/kg).**
    d. If convulsions continue after loading doses of phenytoin or fosphenytoin or phenobarbital have been administered, intravenous **midazolam, propofol,** or **pentobarbital** can be given in a carefully supervised setting, with continuous EEG monitoring, until the seizure discharges are eliminated from the EEG.
    e. Diminished cardiac output, bradycardia, and hypotension often limit the dose of intravenous anticonvulsants. **Fluid resuscitation** and **vasopressors** may be used.

5. **Psychosocial issues.** The following issues are important to consider when managing epilepsy.
   a. Patients may be depressed, have behavioral disturbances, and often require vocational support services. Frequently, community support services are available.
   b. Review of the patient's **driving status** and work and play environment is necessary.
   c. Family and friends need to be counseled as to how to manage a convulsion.
   d. Women of childbearing age should be counseled about issues relating to pregnancy.
   e. Pregnant women should be maintained on monotherapy at the lowest effective dose, given that seizures may harm the fetus and the risk of birth defects increases with polypharmacy.

X MOVEMENT DISORDERS

Movement disorders are conditions involving abnormalities of motor control as opposed to strength. These conditions generally result from disturbances within the basal ganglia, cerebellum, and substantia nigra. Movement disorders can generally be divided into hypokinetic disorders in which patients have difficulty initiating movements (e.g. Parkinson's disease and parkinsonism) and hyperkinetic disorders, whereby patients exhibit involuntary movements.

A Parkinson's disease

1. **Pathogenesis**
   a. Parkinson's disease is characterized by a degeneration of cells in the substantia nigra, which causes a deficiency of dopamine (a neurotransmitter) in the CNS, leading to a series of changes in motor control pathways. The mechanism behind the degeneration of these cells is unknown, although hypotheses center about free radical damage and impaired mitochondrial oxidative function.

   b, c. Genetics

2. **Diagnosis**
   a. **Clinical symptoms and signs**
      (1) Parkinson's disease patients often complain of "slowing down"; they have trouble dressing, arising from a seated position, climbing or descending stairs, writing, and turning over in bed.
      (2) On examination, **rigidity** and **akinesia** or **bradykinesia** are present, and a 3-Hz **resting tremor** and **postural instability** are often evident. Signs are often asymmetric early in the disease.
      (3) Cognitive impairment develops in more than 50% of patients over time.
   b. **Differential diagnosis.** The diagnosis is a clinical determination, although, at times, testing to exclude other entities presenting as parkinsonism is indicated.
      (1) Sometimes **serial observations** are necessary to determine whether the parkinsonian state is the harbinger of another neurologic illness; this is of special concern in patients who do not have the **characteristic "pill rolling"** or **resting tremor** of **Parkinson's disease** or fail to respond to levodopa therapy.
      (2) Conditions that may produce parkinsonian symptoms similar to those found in patients with Parkinson's disease include NPH, multiple strokes, hypothyroidism, drug effects [e.g., neuroleptics (dopamine-blocking agents), metoclopramide, diltiazem, and reserpine], Wilson's disease, anoxic encephalopathy, and intoxication (e.g., by carbon monoxide, manganese, or 1-methyl-4-phenyl-1,2,3,6-tetrahydropyridine [MPTP]).
      (3) Rare neurologic disorders that may have parkinsonian features are summarized in Online Table 12–7.

3. **Therapy.** Parkinson's disease is a progressive disease. Therefore, management protocols vary depending on the patient's symptoms and the extent of functional impairment.
   a. **Early therapy.** Several medications are available to treat Parkinson's disease.
      (1) **Carbidopa/levodopa combinations** are the mainstay of treatment for Parkinson's disease. This treatment should begin when the disease impairs the patient's functional status. A sustained-release formulation of carbidopa/levodopa is available and provides a more uniform clinical response than conventional dosing.

        (a) **Levodopa** is converted to dopamine by the presynaptic neuron and therefore increases the amount of neurotransmitter available to the postsynaptic dopamine receptor.

        (b) **Carbidopa** blocks systemic conversion of levodopa to dopamine, thereby decreasing the undesirable systemic effects of levodopa.

   (2) **Dopamine agonists** are increasingly being used at initial therapy, especially in younger patients. They may have some neuroprotective benefits. Drugs include **pramipexole, ropinirole, pergolide,** and **bromocriptine.**

   (3) **Anticholinergics,** which improve the cholinergic–dopaminergic balance in the basal ganglia, are particularly helpful in treating tremor. However, they may contribute to cognitive impairment.

   (4) **Amantadine,** which increases the availability of dopamine to the postsynaptic neuron, can be effective early in the course of the disease or as an adjunctive therapy later in the disease course to help "smooth out" motor function.

b. Advanced therapy. In the later stages of the disease, therapy is directed at optimizing the patient's functional status and avoiding adverse effects of medication.

   (1) **Dopamine agonists.** If the therapeutic response to carbidopa/levodopa therapy is inadequate, or if the patient cannot tolerate the medication, **pramipexole, ropinirole, pergolide,** or **bromocriptine** may be administered.

        (a) These drugs are **direct postsynaptic dopamine-receptor agonists.**

        (b) A combination of carbidopa/levodopa and a dopamine agonist seems to be particularly effective and is often well tolerated. Dopamine agonists help decrease motor fluctuations when used in conjunction with carbidopa/levodopa.

   (2) **Management with disease progression.** Management of Parkinson's disease becomes increasingly difficult as the disease progresses. **"Wearing off"** effects, **dyskinesias,** and wide, random swings in patient mobility (**"on-off" phenomena**) develop. A sustained-release form of carbidopa/levodopa (alone or in combination with a dopamine agonist) can be used. **Catechol *O*-methyltransferase inhibitors,** which increase the synaptic availability of levodopa by blocking its degradation, also can be used to manage unstable patients.

c. Ancillary therapy

   (1) Other therapeutic maneuvers include the **strategic reduction of medication** if patients are experiencing dyskinesia and **judicious use of psychotropic agents** to treat the various untoward behavioral consequences of Parkinson's disease (e.g., insomnia, hallucinations, agitation).

   (2) **Dietary manipulations** that **redistribute** or **limit protein** intake during the day may improve the efficacy of levodopa.

   (3) **Physical therapy** and an **exercise program** help optimize mobility.

   (4) **Deep brain stimulation** offers a new therapeutic option for refractory Parkinson's disease patients.

   (5) The role of surgical implants of dopamine-containing cells for the treatment of Parkinson's disease remains experimental.

B **Hyperkinetic disorders**

1. Tremor

a. Benign essential tremor (ET) is characterized by a posture-related 5- to 9-Hz oscillation of the hands and forearms that impairs performance of fine motor tasks.

   (1) **ET** is often familial and may be accompanied by **titubation (head tremor).**

   (2) Consumption of alcohol may temporarily suppress the tremor; stress, caffeine, or sleep deprivation may exacerbate the condition.

   (3) **β-Adrenergic blocking agents** and **primidone** are effective treatments.

b. An **action (kinetic) tremor** is evident when patients reach for objects; there may be a relatively mild accompanying postural and intention component. Treatment with **clonazepam** may be useful.

2. Chorea describes **rapid, "dance-like" limb** and **facial movements that may make the patient appear "fidgety."** Causes include hyperthyroidism, drugs (e.g., birth control pills and levodopa), Sydenham's chorea, pregnancy, SLE, antiphospholipid syndrome, stroke, porphyria, Wilson's disease, Lyme disease, Huntington's disease, and neuroacanthocytosis.

3. **Athetosis** generally refers to **involuntary, slow, writhing, "snake-like" limb movements.** Causes include Wilson's disease, Huntington's disease, anoxic encephalopathy, trauma, birth control pills, and several rare hereditary disorders.

4. **Dystonia** describes **slow, writhing, sustained,** and **involuntary contractions of the proximal limb, trunk,** and **neck musculature.** Dystonia is associated with Wilson's disease, Parkinson's disease, Huntington's disease, trauma, neuronal storage disorders, encephalitis, drugs (e.g., neuroleptics, levodopa), and other rare hereditary conditions.

   a, b. Genetics

   c. Focal dystonias such as writer's cramp, blepharospasm, spastic dysphonia, and torticollis can occur. Treatment with local botulinum toxin infiltration can be beneficial.

   d. Some patients with dystonia may exhibit chorea and athetosis.

5. **Hemiballismus** describes **wild, flinging, principally proximal movements** of the **arms** or **legs.** It is often caused by infarcts in the subthalamic nucleus. Haloperidol can decrease the involuntary movements.

6. **Blepharospasm,** or involuntary forced eye closure, can occur in isolation or as part of a more widespread disorder such as Parkinson's disease, stroke, or Meige's syndrome (orofacial dystonia). Blepharospasm can be of such severity as to cause functional blindness.

   a. Many drugs have been tried in an attempt to control the problem with modest effect.

   b. Administration of botulinum toxin about the eyes can provide relief by decreasing neuromuscular transmissions.

7. **Neuroleptic-associated movement disorders** represent a spectrum of disorders related to the acute or chronic administration of neuroleptic medications (although for selected conditions, other drugs are implicated as well).

   a. **Acute dystonia** typically occurs shortly after the first few doses of a neuroleptic agent.

      (1) **Clinical signs** include uncontrollable face, neck, tongue, and eye muscle (oculogyric crisis) spasms.

      (2) **Therapy** consists of the administration of anticholinergics or diphenhydramine.

   b. **Parkinsonism** can develop with neuroleptic use. Therapy consists of decreasing the dose of the neuroleptic agent, changing to another neuroleptic drug, administering an anticholinergic agent, or using amantadine, a carbidopa/levodopa preparation, or an "atypical" neuroleptic such as clozapine, risperidone, or olanzapine.

   c. **Tardive dyskinesia** is characterized by almost constant writhing movements of the mouth and tongue, possibly accompanied by blepharospasm, respiratory grunts, choreoathetosis, and truncal hyperactivity. Ill-fitting dentures or an edentulous state can cause mouthing movements that are mistaken for tardive dyskinesia.

      (1) Tardive dyskinesia is usually an adverse side effect of long-term use of neuroleptic agents; occasionally other drugs such as amphetamines, antihistamines (including metoclopramide), and carbamazepine are causally implicated.

      (2) If a medication is implicated as the cause of the problem, the offending agent should be discontinued if possible. Clonazepam, reserpine, tetrabenazine, and other drugs have been used to treat tardive dyskinesia with variable success. Use of an "atypical" neuroleptic such as clozapine is another option.

   d. **Other neuroleptic-associated movement disorders** include tardive dystonia, akathisia (motor restlessness), and the rabbit syndrome (rhythmic lip movements).

   e. **Neuroleptic malignant syndrome (NMS)** is an idiosyncratic reaction to neuroleptic agents. It can also occur in Parkinson's disease patients after the abrupt discontinuation of antiparkinsonian medications. Dopamine receptor blockade is thought to be the cause of NMS.

      (1) **Clinical signs** include altered mentation, high fever, rigidity, autonomic instability, high creatine kinase (CK) levels, and myoglobinuria.

      (2) **Therapy** for this potentially lethal condition includes hydration, cooling blankets, antipyretics, dantrolene, and levodopa/carbidopa preparations or bromocriptine, although the use of antiparkinsonian drugs is controversial.

8. **Meige's syndrome (orofacial dystonia)**

9. **Hemifacial spasm**

10. **Tics**

XI **DEMYELINATING DISEASES**

A **Multiple sclerosis (MS)** is characterized by multiple foci of CNS demyelination that produce clinical manifestations "separated in time and space." Patients either experience clinical remissions (often followed by relapses) or chronic, progressive symptoms.

1. **Pathophysiology.** Although the cause of MS remains unknown, a predominant theory contends that MS is an immunologic disorder associated with CNS immunoglobulin production and alteration of T and B lymphocytes. The **pathologic hallmark** of MS is inflammation associated with areas of **demyelination scattered about CNS white matter.** Recent findings have also documented **axonal disruption.**

2. **Diagnosis**
   a. **Clinical signs**
      (1) The diagnosis is most certain if neurologic problems occur over an extended period and involve several white matter pathways. MRI findings can be used as evidence of disease dissemination over time and anatomic space.
      (2) Several patterns emerge that are suggestive of MS, including **optic neuritis** (a sign of which is the Marcus Gunn pupil or afferent pupillary defect) and **internuclear ophthalmoplegia,** either in isolation or in association with corticospinal tract or cerebellar signs. Long-term follow-up indicates that 74% of women and 34% of men who present with isolated optic neuritis ultimately develop MS.
      (3) Neurologic signs that can be localized to a single discrete area in the CNS such as the brainstem or craniocervical junction should suggest an alternate diagnosis such as a tumor or arteriovenous malformation.
   b. **Differential diagnosis.** There is no specific diagnostic marker for MS; the physician needs to exclude other conditions that can masquerade as MS. Among these disorders are somatization disorder, SLE, brainstem or spinal vascular malformation, Sjögren's syndrome, Lyme disease, HIV infection, vitamin B_{12} deficiency, brainstem neoplasm, vasculitis, sarcoidosis, and adrenomyeloleukodystrophy.
   c. **Diagnostic studies**
      (1) **MRI** is an excellent technique for visualizing white matter lesions. Although its diagnostic specificity is poor, the contrast agent **gadolinium–diethylenetriamine penta-acetic acid (DTPA)** indicates areas of breakdown of the blood–brain barrier. Serial MRI studies show white matter lesions that may come and go without clinical manifestations.
      (2) **Examination of the CSF** can indicate a sterile inflammation with a mild protein elevation; modest, predominantly mononuclear pleocytosis; an elevated IgG index; oligoclonal bands; and increased myelin basic protein. Only occasionally do all of these abnormalities occur in a single patient.
      (3) **Visual, brainstem auditory,** and **somatosensory EPs** and **central motor conduction studies** can demonstrate clinically silent disruption of white matter tracts.

3. **Therapy.** There is no cure for MS.
   a. **Corticosteroid therapy** may hasten maximal recovery from an acute exacerbation. If optic neuritis is treated, high doses of intravenous corticosteroids (e.g., methylprednisolone) are preferable to lower, oral doses of prednisone
   b. **Interferon-β** (IFN-β) therapy decreases the frequency of relapses, especially moderate and severe attacks. As judged by serial MRI studies, disease activity is lessened with IFN-β treatment.
   c. **Glatiramer acetate** also decreases the frequency of relapses, especially for patients with mild disease.
   d. Otherwise, treatment is directed at **symptoms.**
      (1) **Modafinil, amantadine,** and **pemoline** can improve **fatigue.**
      (2) **Baclofen, tizanidine,** and **diazepam** improve **spasticity.**
      (3) A **variety of agents** may help **urologic dysfunction,** depending on the specific problem.
   e. Patients with severe disease may respond to immunosuppressive therapy.

B **Central pontine myelinolysis**

1. **Etiology.** Demyelination of the pons and deep cerebral white matter has been associated with the **excessively rapid correction** of **severe hyponatremia.** Central pontine myelinolysis has been seen in alcoholics, in malnourished patients, and in patients taking diuretics.

2. **Diagnosis.** Patients develop **impaired arousal, quadriparesis,** and **pseudobulbar signs. MRI** or **CT scan** confirms the diagnosis.

3. **Therapy** consists of supportive measures. Hyponatremia should be corrected **slowly,** and hypernatremia should be avoided.

XII MYELOPATHY AND OTHER SPINAL CORD DISORDERS

A **Definition** Myelopathy refers to a disorder of the spinal cord. Specific syndromes occur in relation to the various motor and sensory tracts affected by the different disease processes (Figure 12–4).

B **Etiology** Selected causes of myelopathy are listed in 🔗 Online Table 12–8.

C **Clinical signs** Disease affecting the spinal cord can present with principally **"long tract signs"** or a combination of long tract signs and **local radicular features.**

1. **Long tract motor signs** result from the disruption of descending corticospinal tracts and consist of **weakness, spasticity,** and **hyperreflexia.**

2. **Impaired sensation** results from disordered function of ascending spinothalamic (pain and temperature) and dorsal column pathways (vibration and proprioception) (see Figure 12–4).

3. **Bowel, bladder, and erectile function may be compromised.**

4. **Local radicular symptoms and signs** include radiating pain, weakness, and **sensory loss** and are referable to one or several myotomes and dermatomes. These findings help define the rostral–caudal extent of a lesion (Figure 12–5).

D **Selected conditions**

1. **Syringomyelia (syrinx)**
   a. **Definition.** Syringomyelia is a condition of unknown cause resulting in **cavitation of the spinal cord.** Syringomyelia can occur in isolation or in association with a **Chiari malformation** (i.e., descent of the cerebellar tonsils into the cervical spinal canal).
   b. **Diagnosis**
      (1) **Signs of lower motor neuron dysfunction** develop on a segmental basis and are accompanied by **upper motor neuron signs** caudal to the cavity.
      (2) **Segmental loss of pain and temperature appreciation** results from local disruption of the crossing spinothalamic fibers by the cavity (syrinx). Impaired ascending dorsal column sensibility occasionally occurs caudal to the cavity.
      (3) **MRI** of the spine is the **optimal diagnostic test** (🔗 Online Figure 12–6).

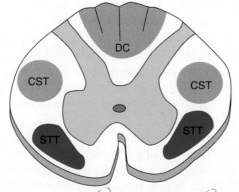

FIGURE 12–4 Cross section of the spinal cord at C1. *CST,* corticospinal tract; *DC,* dorsal column; *STT,* spinothalamic tract.

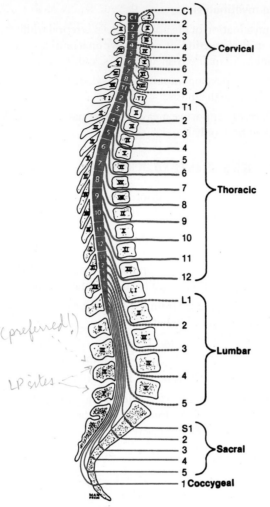

(preferred!)

LP sites

① C_{1-8}
T_{1-12}
L_{1-5}
S_{1-5}
coccyx

FIGURE 12–5 Topographic relationship among nerve roots, spinal cord segments, and the bodies and spinous processes of the vertebrae, which are indicated by Roman numerals.

  c. **Therapy. Surgery** is occasionally indicated to decompress the fluid-filled spinal cord cavity and to perform a biopsy of the wall to evaluate the possibility of a cavitary neoplasm. **Otherwise, treatment is supportive.**

2. **Transverse myelitis.** Inflammation of the spinal cord can cause an acute myelopathy.

  a. **Etiology.** Although many cases of segmental transverse inflammation are idiopathic, MS, SLE, and various infectious agents may cause transverse myelitis.

  b. **Diagnosis.** Patients may experience localized back or radicular pain, followed by prickling or burning sensations and progressive weakness in the legs. Bowel and bladder disturbances are usually present.

  c. **Therapy. Corticosteroid treatment** is often advocated but is of unproven value.

3. The **Brown-Séquard syndrome** is caused by a lesion of one side of the spinal cord at a discrete level. There is caudal ipsilateral upper motor neuron weakness, upper motor neuron signs, and loss of proprioception and vibratory sensation, as well as contralateral loss of pain and temperature sensation.

4. **Anterior spinal artery occlusion**

  a. **Etiology.** Blockage of a radicular artery to the spinal cord can cause an ischemic infarction.

    (1) many cases, the **artery of Adamkiewicz,** a branch of the aorta supplying the anterior two thirds of the lumbar spinal cord, is compromised.

    (2) Thrombosis can be caused by aortic dissection, local atherosclerosis, vasculitis, and hyperviscosity.

    b. Diagnosis. Patients present with flaccid, hyporeflexic paraplegia, impaired lower extremity pain and temperature sensation, and compromised bladder and bowel function. However, position and vibration senses are usually preserved.

    c. Therapy consists of treatment of the disease responsible for the spinal cord infarction.

XIII   NEUROPATHY

A Classification   Neuropathies may be classified by:

1. **Course** (acute, subacute, or chronic)
2. **Type of symptoms and signs** (sensory, motor, autonomic, or any combination of the three)
3. **Presence of pain** (hyperesthesia or dysesthesia)
4. **Distribution** (generalized, focal, or multifocal)
5. **NCS/EMG features** (axonal or demyelinating)

B Etiology   Selected causes of neuropathy are listed in Tables 12–9A and 12–9B.

TABLE 12–9A   Selected Types and Causes of Neuropathy

Neuropathy	Causes		
	ACUTE	**SUBACUTE OR CHRONIC**	**CHRONIC**
Sensory neuropathy		Diabetes mellitus	Toxins
		Uremia	Vitamin B_6 intoxication
		Alcohol abuse	Sjögren's syndrome*
		Deficiencies	Paraneoplastic (anti-Hu antibody)*
		Vitamins B_1, B_6, B_{12}, niacin	Paraproteinemia
		HIV	Cryoglobulinemia
		Hereditary neuropathies	Amyloidosis
		Drugs	Leprosy
		Vinca alkaloids	
		Cisplatin	
		Phenytoin	
		2′,3′-Dideoxycytidine	
Motor neuropathy	Guillain–Barré syndrome	CIDP	
	Diabetes mellitus (proximal ischemic neuropathy)	Lead intoxication	
		Multifocal motor neuropathy	
	Critical illness polyneuropathy	Antibodies to GM_1	
	Porphyria	Charcot–Marie–Tooth disease	
Sensorimotor neuropathy		Diabetes mellitus	CIDP/DADS
		Uremia	Charcot–Marie–Tooth disease
		Critical illness polyneuropathy	Other hereditary neuropathies
		Vasculitis	Metachromatic leukodystrophy
		Hypothyroidism	Refsum's disease
		Lyme disease	Adrenomyeloneuropathy
		Paraproteinemia†	Lipoprotein deficiencies
		Cryoglobulinemia	Sarcoidosis
		Paraneoplastic	
		Drugs	
		Toxins	
Autonomic neuropathy	Guillain–Barré syndrome	Diabetes mellitus	HIV
	Porphyria	Amyloidosis	Vincristine
		Familial dysautonomia	

HIV, human immunodeficiency virus; CIDP, chronic inflammatory demyelinating polyneuropathy; DADS, distal acquired demyelinating symmetric neuropathy.

*Also, sensory neuronopathy.

†Including myelin-associated glycoprotein (MAG) antibody and monoclonal gammopathy.

TABLE 12–9B Selected Types and Causes of Neuropathy Classified by Other Features	
Neuropathy	**Causes**
Dysesthetic neuropathy	Diabetes mellitus Alcohol abuse Human immunodeficiency virus 2′,3′-Dideoxycytidine Vasculitis
Axonal neuropathy	Diabetes mellitus Uremia Drugs and toxins Critical illness polyneuropathy Vasculitis Paraproteinemia Cryoglobulinemia Vitamin B_{12} deficiency Hereditary neuropathies
Demyelinating neuropathy	Guillain–Barré syndrome Chronic inflammatory demyelinating polyneuropathy Paraproteinemia* Hereditary neuropathies
Multifocal (mononeuritis multiplex) neuropathy	Diabetes mellitus Vasculitis Lyme disease Leprosy Sarcoidosis Hereditary liability to pressure palsy Malignant infiltrates

*Including myelin-associated glycoprotein (MAG) antibody and monoclonal gammopathy.

C Therapy   Control of the underlying disease process is critical.

1. If impaired sensation renders the patient prone to injury, protective measures should be taken.
2. Weakness (e.g., wrist or foot drops) calls for appropriate support braces and physical therapy.
3. Autonomic insufficiency is difficult to manage; orthostatic hypotension can be treated with agents that expand blood volume (e.g., fludrocortisone) and increase vascular tone (e.g., midodrine).
4. For pain a number of medications have been used, including anesthetic agents such as topical lidocaine, antidepressants such as tricyclic antidepressants and duloxetine, and antiepileptic drugs such as carbamazepine, phenytoin, and gabapentin.

D Selected syndromes

1. **Compression neuropathies**
   a. **Pathophysiology**
      (1) Nerve damage can result from repeated wear against firm surfaces such as bone or fibrous tissue, resulting in motor and sensory deficits in the distribution of the affected nerve.
      (2) Common sites of nerve compression include the **median nerve** at the wrist (carpal tunnel), the **ulnar nerve** at the elbow, and the **peroneal nerve** at the fibular head.
   b. **Etiology. Carpal tunnel syndrome** can result from repetitive wrist movements, trauma, carpal tunnel stenosis, arthritides (rheumatoid arthritis and crystal-induced synovitis), diabetes mellitus, myxedema, pregnancy, birth control pills, acromegaly, and infiltrative processes such as amyloidosis.
   c. **Diagnosis.** A positive Tinel's sign (eliciting paresthesias by percussing the nerve at the site of compression) may be seen clinically. NCS may reveal evidence of focal demyelination. If compression is severe, evidence of axonal injury may appear (e.g., muscle wasting, denervation on the EMG).
   d. **Therapy. Treatment of underlying conditions** is important. Splinting often alleviates the condition, especially if aggravating maneuvers can be eliminated. Local corticosteroid injections may be beneficial. **Surgical decompression** of the nerve is necessary at times.

2. **Guillain–Barré syndrome**
   a. **Definition and etiology.** Guillain–Barré syndrome is a demyelinating, predominately motor polyneuropathy that usually occurs in otherwise healthy individuals. The illness can follow a nonspecific viral syndrome or be associated with HIV infection, *Campylobacter jejuni* infection, hepatitis, infectious mononucleosis, *Mycoplasma pneumoniae* infection, vaccination, surgery, lymphoma, or SLE.
   b. **Diagnosis**
      (1) **Clinical signs**
         (a) Classically, patients present with progressive weakness and areflexia. Progression of the disease should not extend beyond 4–6 weeks.
         (b) **Generalized paralysis** can develop gradually or relatively acutely, impeding respiratory function.
         (c) Relatively minor sensory signs and symptoms occur, but patients often complain of painful extremities.
         (d) The **autonomic nervous system** is often involved, leading to **cardiac arrhythmias** and **wide swings in blood pressure.**
      (2) **Diagnostic studies**
         (a) Examination of the CSF generally shows an elevated protein and fewer than 50 mononuclear cells/mm^3 (**cytoalbuminemic dissociation**).
         (b) The motor nerve conduction velocities are typically slowed.
         (c) Serum studies should include a Lyme titer and serum protein electrophoresis (SPEP) to exclude Lyme disease and a paraproteinemia, respectively.
   c. **Therapy**
      (1) **Plasmapheresis** can shorten the length of time that patients are dependent on a respirator and unable to ambulate. Criteria to initiate plasmapheresis include the inability to walk or rapid progression of the disease.
      (2) **Intravenous immunoglobulin treatment** has been shown to be equally efficacious and is better tolerated than plasmapheresis.
3. **Diabetic neuropathy** [see also Chapter 10 IV A 7 d]. Diabetes mellitus causes several neuropathic syndromes. The nerve injury may be secondary to chronic ischemia (related to microvascular disease) that leads to axonal damage.
   a. **Types**
      (1) A predominantly sensory, distal, symmetric, small-fiber polyneuropathy can be dysesthetic and involve pain and temperature modalities more than vibration and position senses.
      (2) A predominantly sensory, distal, symmetric, large-fiber polyneuropathy may occur, affecting vibration and position modalities.
      (3) A sensorimotor neuropathy can develop.
      (4) An autonomic neuropathy or a mononeuropathy or mononeuritis multiplex can occur.
      (5) Proximal diabetic neuropathy (i.e., diabetic amyotrophy) typically involves injury to the lumbar plexus and is characterized by weakness, numbness, and pain in the thigh region.
   b. **Therapy.** As a group, patients with better blood glucose control have a less severe polyneuropathy. However, in individual patients, symptoms usually do not respond to tighter blood glucose control.
4. **Chronic inflammatory demyelinating polyneuropathy (CIDP)** is a more persistent, progressive disease with clinical features similar to those of Guillain–Barré syndrome. The condition can be idiopathic or associated with a monoclonal gammopathy.
   a. **Diagnosis.** NCS indicate slowing of the conduction velocities, and the CSF total protein is elevated, similar to that seen in Guillain–Barré (**cytoalbuminemic dissociation**).
   b. **Therapy.** CIDP is responsive to corticosteroid therapy, plasmapheresis, intravenous immunoglobulin administration, and various immunosuppressant drugs such as cyclophosphamide.

XIV DISORDERS OF THE NEUROMUSCULAR JUNCTION

A Myasthenia gravis

1. **Etiology.** Antibodies directed against the acetylcholine receptor on the muscle membrane cause an increased rate of receptor destruction and a functional disconnection between the nerve and muscle.

2. Diagnosis

a. Clinical signs. Patients are often young women or older men who complain of double vision, difficulty swallowing and speaking, and limb weakness and fatigue. On examination, one may see ptosis, eye movement abnormalities, and proximal weakness. A thymoma is present in 10%–25% of patients.

b. Diagnostic studies

(1) Administration of **intravenous edrophonium** (a short-acting cholinesterase inhibitor) usually produces a transient improvement in strength in patients suffering from myasthenia gravis. Patients with respiratory compromise or excessive oral secretions should not be given edrophonium because they may be unable to compensate for the increase in secretions that occurs after administration of this agent.

(2) Repetitive nerve stimulation studies can demonstrate a decremental response of the compound muscle action potential.

(3) Acetylcholine receptor antibodies can be detected in the blood of 80%–90% of patients.

(4) A **thoracic CT** or **MRI scan** shows a thymoma, if present.

3. Therapy

a. Cholinesterase inhibitors (e.g., pyridostigmine) are the mainstay of initial therapy.

b. Thymectomy can often lead to improvement but has never been definitely studied in a randomized, double-blind clinical trial; the presence of a thymoma is a definite indication for surgery.

c. Corticosteroids, steroid-sparing agents, intravenous immunoglobulin, and **plasmapheresis** are effective in patients with refractory disease.

B Eaton–Lambert myasthenic syndrome

1. Pathophysiology. This syndrome results when antibodies directed against the calcium channels on the presynaptic membrane of the neuromuscular junction interfere with the calcium-mediated release of acetylcholine vesicles in response to nerve stimulation. This syndrome is often associated with an underlying malignancy, especially **small cell carcinoma of the lung,** and autoimmune diseases.

2. Diagnosis

a. Clinical signs. Patients complain of weakness and fatigue, have diminished deep tendon reflexes, and may have impaired autonomic function, leading to dry mouth and poor visual accommodation. Unlike myasthenia, strength improves with activity, and ptosis and facial weakness are generally absent.

b. Diagnostic studies. Repetitive nerve stimulation studies at fast rates show an incremental response of the compound muscle action potential.

3. Therapy. Diaminopyridine, plasmapheresis, intravenous immunoglobulin, or immunosuppressive therapy may be helpful.

XV DISORDERS OF MUSCLE

A Muscular dystrophies

1. Types of muscular dystrophies

a. Duchenne muscular dystrophy (DMD) is an X-linked recessive disorder caused by mutations in the dystrophin gene. The normal gene product, dystrophin, is a membrane-associated cytoskeletal protein that is absent in this condition.

(1) Patients experience progressive muscle weakness that begins proximally and becomes generalized.

(2) Prednisone slows progression of weakness.

(3) Death usually occurs in the third decade of life, often as a result of pneumonia, respiratory failure, or heart failure.

b. Becker's muscular dystrophy (BMD) is similar to DMD but less severe. BMD patients harbor mutations that lead to dystrophin that is reduced in quality or quantity. Patients with BMD have a **more benign course than those with DMD, with a 50%** survival rate beyond age 50 years.

    c. Myotonic muscular dystrophy is an autosomal dominant disorder due to a CTG expansion in a gene on chromosome 19 that leads to aberrant RNA splicing of a chloride channel transcript. The severity of disease generally worsens with successive generations, and the CTG repeats increase proportionately (a phenomenon known as "anticipation").

        (1) Clinical signs include a characteristic muscle myotonia (i.e., muscle cramps in response to contraction or percussion), distal weakness, cataracts, frontal balding, impaired intellect, hypersomnia, testicular atrophy, cardiomyopathy, and cardiac conduction defects.

        (2) Death typically occurs in the fifth or sixth decade as a result of respiratory compromise or cardiac arrhythmias.

    d. Facioscapulohumeral muscular dystrophy is an autosomal dominant disorder characterized by progressive weakness of the face, neck, upper torso, and proximal arms. The responsible gene is located on chromosome 4.

    e. Limb-girdle muscular dystrophy is actually a group of autosomal dominant and recessive disorders characterized by progressive proximal muscle weakness.

        (1) The disorder represents a group of conditions with different genes a but similar phenotype.

        (2) Patients may have defects in their dystrophin-associated proteins (e.g., members of the dystrophin–glycoprotein complex), other membrane-associated proteins, or components of the contractile apparatus.

2. Diagnosis. Patients typically have an **elevated serum CK level. EMG** demonstrates a "myopathic" pattern (i.e., brief, small-amplitude muscle potentials). A **muscle biopsy** is often informative, but **genetic studies** are definitive, if available.

B **Acquired myopathies**

1. Etiology. Muscle disease can be caused by inflammatory, toxic, or metabolic processes (Table 12–10).

2. Diagnosis

    a. Clinical signs. A patient history and examination may provide clues to the diagnosis.

        (1) Weakness is usually proximal and symmetric. Disease onset can be acute, subacute, or chronic.

        (2) Swallowing and breathing can be compromised, and myoglobinuria may result from rapid muscle destruction, leading to renal insufficiency.

    b. Diagnostic studies. The serum CK should be markedly elevated with toxic or inflammatory processes but normal with metabolic disorders. The EMG should reveal a "myopathic" pattern of small, short motor units. A muscle biopsy is often informative if not diagnostic.

3. Selected syndromes

    a. Steroid myopathy is usually caused by chronic corticosteroid therapy and is associated with proximal muscle weakness and wasting. The serum CK level is normal, the EMG is usually unremarkable, but a muscle biopsy may show atrophy of the type II muscle fibers.

TABLE 12–10 Selected Causes of Acquired Myopathy	
Polymyositis	Endocrine disorders
Idiopathic	Hypothyroidism
Associated with other connective tissue	Hyperthyroidism
diseases, infectious agents (including human	Cushing's disease and iatrogenic corticosteroid
immunodeficiency virus), and drugs	administration
Dermatomyositis	Addison's disease
Associated with malignancy	Acromegaly
Inclusion body myositis	Drugs (e.g., "statins," ε-aminocaproic acid,
Electrolyte disorders	procainamide, zidovudine, phencyclidine,
Hypokalemia	ʟ-tryptophan)
Hyperkalemia	
Hypercalcemia	
Hypomagnesemia	
Hypophosphatemia	

b. With **polymyositis,** the associated infiltration of lymphocytes destroys muscle fiber [see Chapter 11 X A, C].

c. Inclusion body myositis is an inflammatory myopathy characterized by distal and proximal weakness and a resistance to corticosteroid therapy. Patients classically demonstrate significant weakness in their wrist and finger flexors.

    (1) Diagnosis. Muscle biopsy demonstrates inflammation and inclusion bodies (including "rimmed vacuoles") that contain amyloid. Cytotoxic T (Tc) cells are active against a muscle antigen.

    (2) Therapy. There is **no accepted treatment.**

d. Polymyalgia rheumatica (PMR) is not a myopathy but can masquerade as one.

    (1) Clinical signs

        (a) Patients often appear weak, but the major symptom is **painful (tender, aching,** and **stiff) muscles.**

        (b) Activities such as ascending stairs may be difficult to perform. On formal strength testing, patients may appear slightly weak, presumably because the pain prevents maximal effort. It has been found that if the pain can be relieved, strength is preserved.

        (c) Temporal (giant cell) arteritis is present in 15%–20% of patients.

    (2) Diagnostic studies. The erythrocyte sedimentation rate usually is significantly elevated but may be normal. The serum CK level is normal, and the EMG is unremarkable. Muscle histology is normal; biopsy is usually not performed.

    (3) Therapy. NSAID or corticosteroid therapy should bring about a rapid resolution of symptoms.

C **Nondystrophic myotonias (channelopathies)** are characterized by prolonged muscle relaxation after voluntary contraction or mechanical stimulation.

    1. Clinical signs. Online Table 12–11 summarizes the clinical features of the nondystrophic myotonias.

    2. Therapy. Treatment includes the use of quinine, phenytoin, and mexiletene.

D **Metabolic myopathies** (inherited) include disorders of carbohydrate and lipid metabolism. Diagnosis relies on demonstration of the responsible enzymatic defect. Treatment generally consists of dietary modification but in rare cases includes enzyme replacement (e.g., Pompe's disease).

E **Myoglobinuria** can be caused by crush injuries, vascular occlusions, infection, toxins, drugs, metabolic myopathies, hyperthermia, and severe inflammation.

    1. Diagnosis is aided by documenting a markedly elevated serum CK level and urinary myoglobin. The latter can be suspected on the basis of dark (brownish) urine and a positive dipstick for blood in the absence of RBCs in the urine.

    2. Therapy should be directed at the underlying cause. Patients must be kept vigorously hydrated to prevent kidney damage.

F **Acute quadriplegic myopathy** can develop as a complication of critical illness and the systemic inflammatory response syndrome. There is an association with the use of corticosteroids and nondepolarizing neuromuscular blocking agents. Treatment is supportive.

XVI   INFECTION

A **Meningitis, encephalitis, and neurologic complaints associated with HIV infection** are discussed in Chapter 9.

B **Brain abscess**

    1. Etiology. An abscess can occur after neurosurgery or penetrating head trauma, in association with otitis media, sinus infections, or poor oral hygiene, in patients with a bacteremia, and in individuals with a pulmonary arteriovenous malformation or cardiac right-to-left shunt.

    2. Diagnosis

      a. Clinical signs. Patients may present with headache, seizures, an altered mental status, and focal deficits, but the exam may be very unimpressive.

    b. Diagnostic studies. CT or **MRI scanning** can easily demonstrate a ring-enhancing lesion, although differentiation from a tumor can be difficult.

  3. Therapy. Empiric treatment should be directed against aerobic and microaerophilic gram-positive streptococci and anaerobes, including *Bacteroides fragilis.*

    a. Antibiotic therapy often includes penicillin, chloramphenicol, metronidazole, and cefotaxime or trimethoprim–sulfamethoxazole. The clinical setting can help define the most likely pathogen.

    b. Therapy is monitored by serial brain imaging techniques.

    c. Often, **surgical excision** of the abscess **can be avoided,** but **stereotactic biopsy and drainage** is often required to guide therapy.

C A **spinal epidural abscess** is usually caused by hematogenous seeding of an infective organism and is characterized by local pain and tenderness, fever, and neurologic signs and symptoms appropriate to the site of the infection.

  1. Diagnosis can be aided by **spinal MRI** or **CT scans** and **myelography.**

  2. Surgical drainage is indicated along with **antibiotic therapy.**

D Neurosyphilis

  1. Stages and clinical signs

    a. Asymptomatic disease. CSF abnormalities may be the only sign of infection.

    b. Acute syphilitic meningitis usually develops within 2 years of primary infection. Headache, meningismus, hydrocephalus, and cranial nerve palsies can occur.

    c. Cerebrovascular (meningovascular) syphilis manifests months to years after primary infection. Affected patients present with ischemic strokes (often associated with headache) and behavioral abnormalities.

    d. General paresis develops one to two decades after primary infection and is characterized by a progressive dementia.

    e. Tabes dorsalis also manifests 10–20 years after primary infection with "lightning pains" in the limbs, paresthesias, bladder dysfunction, gait instability, Argyll Robertson pupils (i.e., impaired pupillary light reaction with preserved pupillary constriction to accommodation, perhaps as a result of a midbrain tegmental lesion), areflexia (especially at the ankles), and loss of position and vibration sensation.

  2. Diagnostic studies. Patients with HIV infection are at particular risk for neurosyphilis.

    a. Almost all patients with neurosyphilis have a **reactive serum fluorescent treponemal antibody (FTA-ABS) test.** Patients with a nonreactive CSF FTA-ABS test do not have neurosyphilis.

    b. The CSF VDRL test is often reactive in neurosyphilis, but a nonreactive CSF VDRL test is found in 25%–75% of patients with neurologic disease years removed from the primary infection.

    c. Other CSF findings include a predominantly mononuclear pleocytosis and an elevated protein and IgG index.

  3. Therapy. High-dose penicillin is the treatment of choice for neurosyphilis. Patients with concurrent HIV infection develop neurosyphilis earlier and may be more resistant to therapy than immunocompetent patients.

XVII PRIMARY CENTRAL NERVOUS SYSTEM TUMORS

Although primary brain tumors are relatively uncommon, they seem to be increasing in incidence.

A Astrocytic neoplasms

  1. Astrocytomas are neoplasms with slight hypercellularity and pleomorphism. **Anaplastic astrocytomas** are characterized as having moderate cellularity and pleomorphism and some vascular proliferation.

    a. Clinical signs. Patients with astrocytomas and anaplastic astrocytomas typically present with focal hemispheric neurologic dysfunction, convulsions, or headache.

    b. Therapy. Anaplastic astrocytomas can be treated with **surgery** and **radiotherapy. Chemotherapy** may be helpful.

   c. **Prognosis.** Outcome is inversely related to the patient's age and the presence of tumor necrosis. The survival rate after 2 years is 38%–50%. Other predictors of outcome include the patient's functional status and the amount of residual tumor after initial surgery.

  2. **Glioblastoma multiforme** is a high-grade glioma with moderate-to-marked hypercellularity, pleomorphism, and necrosis; vascular proliferation may be present.

   a. **Clinical signs.** Clinical features are similar to those of less aggressive tumors. CT or MRI scans typically show an enhancing, irregular mass (Online Figure 12–7).

   b. **Therapy.** Treatment includes **corticosteroid therapy** (for edema reduction), **surgical debulking, radiation therapy,** and **chemotherapy,** systemically or locally administered.

   c. **Prognosis.** The prognosis of glioblastoma multiforme is **poor,** with a survival rate of 10% after 24 months.

B **Oligodendrogliomas**

  1. **Clinical signs.** Patients with these infiltrating tumors commonly present with headache and convulsions; focal neurologic deficits can develop. Imaging may show evidence of hemorrhage or calcification.

  2. **Therapy.** Anaplastic oligodendrogliomas seem to be responsive to **radiation therapy** and **chemotherapy. Surgery** is the mainstay of treatment.

  3. **Prognosis.** The overall median length of survival is 53 months.

C **Meningiomas** are tumors that arise from the meninges and slowly enlarge, causing mass effect that displaces normal structures. Angioblastic meningiomas are locally invasive.

  1. **Clinical signs.** Headache, seizures, and focal neurologic signs can occur.

  2. **Therapy.** Treatment is **surgical resection; radiation therapy** can be used for invasive tumors.

  3. **Prognosis.** If the entire tumor can be surgically resected, the majority of patients do well. If the entire tumor cannot be removed, the patient may experience recurrence of symptoms.

D **Schwannomas** of the eighth cranial nerve (acoustic neuromas) typically arise from the vestibular component of the nerve. They can enlarge and displace structures around the cerebellopontine angle.

  1. **Clinical signs.** Patients develop dizziness, hearing loss, and tinnitus. A diminished corneal reflex may be a sign of trigeminal or facial nerve compromise by the enlarging mass.

  2. **Diagnostic studies.** Diagnosis is best made with an enhanced MRI.

  3. **Therapy.** Treatment options include **surgical resection** or **stereotactic radiation therapy.**

  4. **Prognosis.** Small tumors can be surgically cured. If residual tumor remains, recurrent symptoms can develop, usually years later.

E **Primary CNS lymphoma** is increasing in incidence, especially in immunocompromised patients. Occasionally, primary CNS lymphoma presents as meningeal lymphomatosis.

  1. **Diagnostic studies. Imaging studies** show one or more intensely enhancing lesions, typically in a periventricular distribution. The diagnosis can be established with stereotactic biopsy.

  2. **Therapy.** Although initial treatment with corticosteroids can lead to a rapid decrease in the size of the mass, ultimate survival depends on radiation therapy and chemotherapy.

  3. **Prognosis.** The development of multimodality treatment protocols has extended patient survival for years, especially in immunocompetent patients.

 XVIII **HEREDITARY DISORDERS**

A **Wilson's disease (hepatolenticular degeneration)**

B **Neurofibromatosis (NF)**

C **von Hippel–Lindau disease**

D Osler–Weber–Rendu disease (hereditary hemorrhagic telangiectasia)

E Tuberous sclerosis

F Down syndrome (trisomy 21)

G Huntington's disease

H Cerebellar atrophies

I Peroxisome disorders

J Mitochondrial disorders

XIX TOXIC AND METABOLIC DISORDERS

A **Vitamin B$_{12}$ deficiency**   This vitamin deficiency results in subacute combined degeneration (SCD).

1. **Pathophysiology.** Deficiency of vitamin B$_{12}$ leads to demyelination and dysfunction of various tracts of the spinal cord (dorsal columns and corticospinal tracts).

2. **Diagnosis**
   a. **Clinical signs.** Neurologic manifestations include cognitive impairment, diminished proprioception and vibratory sensation, upper motor neuron signs (hyperreflexia and upgoing toes), with stiff gait and a sensory neuropathy.
   b. **Diagnosis.** Patients typically have anemia, macrocytosis, and a low vitamin B$_{12}$ level. However, neurologic disease can occur without anemia or macrocytosis. If the diagnosis remains suspect in a patient with a normal or marginally decreased serum vitamin B$_{12}$ level, an elevated serum methylmalonic acid and total homocysteine can confirm the presence of vitamin B$_{12}$ deficiency.

3. **Therapy.** Treatment is administration of **cobalamin** either parenterally or orally.

B Acute intermittent porphyria

C **Complications of alcohol abuse**   Alcohol may affect the nervous system by itself (i.e., alcohol intoxication, addiction, or withdrawal) or in tandem with a nutritional deficiency.

1. **Complications from intoxication, addiction, and withdrawal**
   a. **Acute alcohol intoxication** causes delirium and incoordination.
      (1) Severe intoxication can lead to metabolic coma with respiratory depression.
      (2) Alcoholic **"blackouts"** are characterized by the inability to form new memories in spite of preservation of consciousness.
   b. **Alcohol withdrawal** causes early symptoms of tremulousness and hallucinosis. Delirium tremens is seen during late withdrawal from alcohol. Benzodiazepines may be used to treat alcohol withdrawal symptoms.
   c. **Alcohol-related seizures ("rum fits")** are brief, generalized tonic–clonic convulsions that frequently occur in clusters.
      (1) Alcohol-related seizures are thought to occur primarily within 48 hours following cessation of chronic alcohol intake.
      (2) Typically, patients are alert shortly after the seizure. They do not have seizure discharges on an interictal EEG.
      (3) **Therapy** should be directed at the underlying alcohol abuse. Anticonvulsant medications are not indicated for typical alcohol-related seizures.
   d. Alcohol abuse is associated with **cerebral atrophy** and **cognitive impairments** and may **predispose patients to stroke.**
   e. Alcoholic patients may develop a **myopathy** that is acute or chronic and predominantly affects the proximal muscles. **Rhabdomyolysis** can complicate the acute disorder.

2. **Complications related to nutritional deficiencies**
   a. **Wernicke's encephalopathy** is seen in malnourished alcoholic patients who have a **thiamine deficiency.**
      (1) **Clinical signs.** Patients typically exhibit aspects of the classic triad of encephalopathy, eye movement abnormalities, and ataxia.
      (2) **Diagnosis** is clinical.
      (3) **Therapy.** High-dose parenteral thiamine administration should ameliorate the acute illness.
   b. **Korsakoff's psychosis** is a chronic encephalopathy that is seen in alcoholic patients with protracted thiamine deficiency.
      (1) **Clinical signs.** Features include retrograde and anterograde memory deficits, apathy, and impaired problem-solving abilities.
      (2) **Therapy.** Unfortunately, patients may not improve with abstinence from alcohol or thiamine administration.
   c. **Sensory neuropathy** is caused by alcohol and often leads to dysesthesias. Although this axonal neuropathy is probably related to concurrent malnutrition, alcohol itself may be toxic to nerves.
   d. **Cerebellar degeneration** may occur in alcoholics. The anterior and superior vermis are particularly affected. Patients have difficulty with gait and stance; nystagmus and arm ataxia are not prominent.

D **Drug abuse**

1. Use of **cocaine** or **"crack"** can result in seizures, ischemic stroke, subarachnoid and intraparenchymal hemorrhage, and rhabdomyolysis. Hemorrhagic strokes may be associated with an underlying vascular lesion; definition of the vascular anatomy is usually indicated to search for an aneurysm or arteriovenous malformation.

2. Use of **heroin** can cause a metabolic coma. Miosis is a characteristic finding in heroin users. Heroin has been associated with rhabdomyolysis, chronic myopathy, transverse myelitis, and peripheral neuropathies.

3. Ingestion of **phencyclidine (PCP)** can cause a wide range of neurologic disturbances ranging from acute psychosis to coma. Nystagmus, miosis, ataxia, myoclonus, dystonic posturing, generalized rigidity, dyskinesias, and seizures can occur.

4. Ingestion of **"ecstasy"** (an amphetamine analog) can cause delirium, hyperthermia, and rhabdomyolysis. This drug selectively damages serotoninergic neurons.

XX SLEEP DISORDERS

A **Narcolepsy** is characterized by hypersomnia with short latency periods for the onset of daytime sleep and the early development of rapid eye movement (REM) sleep. Patients awaken refreshed from sleep attacks.

1. **Etiology.** Narcolepsy has been associated with a number of genes, including one on chromosome 6. The vast majority of patients have antigens for HLA-DR2 and HLA-DQB1.

2. **Clinical signs.** Features include **cataplexy** (i.e., transient episodes of diminished muscle tone), **sleep paralysis,** and **vivid dreams** at the beginning and end of sleep.

3. **Therapy.** CNS stimulants, including methylphenidate, pemoline, and modafinil are the mainstays of treatment to diminish the hypersomnia. Protriptyline and imipramine have been used to treat the associated cataplexy.

B **Sleep apnea** may be attributed to obstructive causes (e.g., obesity, a small oropharynx), nonobstructive (CNS) causes, or both.

1. **Clinical signs.** Patients have daytime hypersomnia and can develop nocturnal hypoxia, pulmonary hypertension, and cardiac arrhythmias.

2. **Therapy.** The first-line treatment for obstructive sleep apnea consists of utilizing continuous positive airway pressure (CPAP) machines or oral appliances. In refractory cases, surgical interventions such as uvulopalatopharyngoplasty (UPPP), tracheostomy, and various minimally invasive surgical techniques for the tongue and throat have been advocated.

C **Periodic leg movements in sleep** involve flexor contractions in the legs. Patients may also experience restless legs syndrome while awake.

1. **Clinical signs.** Patients are momentarily aroused during the night, leading to poor sleep quality and daytime hypersomnia.

2. **Therapy.** Treatment options include carbidopa/levodopa combinations, dopamine agonists, gabapentin, opiates, and clonazepam.

XXI TRAUMA

A **Brain injury**

1. A **concussion** is a momentary disruption of brain function following head injury that results in a brief loss of consciousness.
   a. **Clinical signs.** After awakening, patients complain of headache, impaired memory, poor concentration, blurred vision, tinnitus, dizziness, and nausea.
   b. **Duration of symptoms.** Symptoms can persist for days or weeks as the **postconcussion syndrome. Posttraumatic migraine** can develop but may be alleviated by medications traditionally used to treat migraines.

2. **Severe head trauma** can cause brain contusions, epidural and subdural hematoma, penetrating brain injuries, SAH, and CSF leaks.
   a. **Clinical signs.** Progressive mental status changes leading to coma and focal neurologic signs can develop.
   b. **Diagnostic studies.** Emergent CT scanning can help delineate the extent of the problem.
   c. **Therapy.** Control of ICP and neurosurgical evaluation are indicated as appropriate.

3. A **subdural hematoma** can result from acute head trauma. Patients present with an altered mental status and focal neurologic findings (e.g., hemiparesis). In some instances a subdural hematoma may result from minor head trauma, such that patients present with subtle subacute or chronic behavioral changes and mild focal deficits. At times, no history of trauma is elicited; this is especially true in elderly patients.
   a. **Diagnostic studies.** A CT scan is very helpful in documenting the presence of a subdural hematoma (Online Figure 12–8).
   b. **Therapy.** Neurosurgical intervention is usually indicated for an acute subdural hematoma; a chronic subdural hematoma may not require surgery.

B **Spinal cord injury** can result in an acute paraparesis or quadriparesis. Central cord syndrome, which can follow hyperextension of the cervical cord, consists of "segmental" loss of pain and temperature sensation in the arms or upper trunk in conjunction with signs of a myelopathy (e.g., hyperreflexia and spasticity in the legs).

1. **Diagnostic studies.** Because the vertebral column may not be stable, patients should be immobilized while a radiographic assessment is made.

2. **Therapy.** High-dose methylprednisolone therapy given within 8 hours of injury can improve outcome.

Study Questions

1. A 70-year-old man, a retired professor, complains of weakness and fatigue. Any physical activity is an effort, and he cannot find a comfortable position at rest. He has lost 5 pounds over the past month. Physical examination is normal. Which of the following diagnoses is most likely?

- A Amyotrophic lateral sclerosis
- B Hypokalemia
- C Temporal (giant cell) arteritis
- D Polymyalgia rheumatica
- E Polymyositis

2. A 29-year-old woman suddenly develops a left hemiparesis. The patient experienced a deep venous thrombosis in her right leg 3 years ago. Which of the following conditions is the most likely cause of this patient's deficit?

- A Nonvalvular atrial fibrillation
- B Lupus anticoagulant
- C Mitral valve prolapse
- D Multiple sclerosis
- E Astrocytoma

3. An assembly-line worker complains of awakening at night with right-hand discomfort that resolves after several minutes. After 3 weeks of continuing symptoms, he seeks medical advice. Examination discloses mild weakness of thumb abduction and diminished pain sensibility on the palmar aspect of the thumb and index finger. Which of the following diagnoses is most likely?

- A Carpal tunnel syndrome
- B Cervical radiculopathy
- C Reflex sympathetic dystrophy
- D Tendinitis
- E Left middle cerebral artery ischemic attacks

4. A 73-year-old woman presents with a 6-month history of deteriorating gait and low back discomfort, which is exacerbated by walking. Examination is unremarkable except for hypoactive muscle stretch reflexes in the legs. Radiographs of the lumbosacral area show the expected degenerative changes associated with a woman of her age. Which of the following diagnoses is most likely?

- A Acute lumbar disk herniation
- B Lumbar stenosis
- C Myopathy
- D Normal-pressure hydrocephalus
- E Cervical stenosis

5. A 45-year-old right-handed man complains that he has had difficulty holding and using a writing instrument for the past year. He notes the development of right-hand and forearm spasms only when writing. Physical examination is unremarkable. Which of the following diagnoses is most likely?

- A Parkinson's disease
- B Focal dystonia
- C Carpal tunnel syndrome
- D Cervical radiculopathy
- E Benign essential tremor

6. A 24-year-old construction worker with a 2-year history of low back pain complains of an acute onset of bilateral leg weakness and incontinence. Which of the following treatments would be the best management tactic?

- A Administration of nonsteroidal anti-inflammatory drugs
- B Emergency surgery

C Strict bed rest
D Lumbar traction
E Back exercises

7. A 32-year-old man presents with repetitive generalized motor convulsions that continue for 35 minutes until 2 mg of lorazepam are administered intravenously. The next course of action should be to administer which of the following?

A Phenytoin intravenously
B Carbamazepine orally
C Pentobarbital intravenously
D Ethosuximide orally
E Diazepam rectally

8. A 78-year-old woman complains of experiencing headaches and progressive confusion for the past month. She has a left hemianopia and cannot dress herself. A computed tomography scan demonstrates a large, irregularly enhancing mass in the right parietal lobe. There is no obvious systemic disease. Which of the following diagnoses is most likely?

A Brain abscess
B Glioblastoma multiforme
C Meningioma
D Metastasis
E Central nervous system lymphoma

9. A 63-year-old woman develops intermittent dizziness. Examination shows a diminished right corneal reflex and mild hearing loss in the right ear. Which of the following diagnoses is most likely?

A Cerebellopontine angle tumor
B Benign paroxysmal positional vertigo *(BPPV)*
C Lateral medullary syndrome
D Ménière's disease
E Pontine infarction *(Not assoc ē hearing loss!)*

10. A previously vigorous 80-year-old woman collapses when getting out of bed. Examination of her legs indicates bilateral weakness, loss of pain and temperature sensation, and areflexia but normal proprioception and vibratory sensation. Her bladder is distended. The remainder of the examination is unremarkable. Which of the following diagnoses is most likely?

A Guillain–Barré syndrome
B Anterior cerebral artery occlusion
C Cauda equina syndrome
D Anterior spinal artery occlusion
E Thoracic spinal cord compression

11. A 70-year-old man reports that over the last 4 months he has had progressive difficulty walking. Examination indicates generalized weakness in the arms and legs and the absence of muscle stretch reflexes. Motor nerve conduction velocities are slowed. Which of the following diagnoses is most likely?

A Guillain–Barré syndrome
B Lead poisoning
C Chronic inflammatory demyelinating polyneuropathy
D Amyotrophic lateral sclerosis
E Polymyositis

12. A 56-year-old man presents with a 2-year history of impotence and not feeling "right." Examination reveals masked facies, bradykinesia, rigidity, mild ataxia, and postural hypotension. The diagnosis is which of the following?

A Parkinson's disease
B Subacute combined degeneration *(SCD)*

C) Multiple systems atrophy (Shy-Drager syndrome)
D) Spinocerebellar degeneration
E) Vitamin E deficiency

13. A patient with a subarachnoid hemorrhage caused by a right anterior communicating artery aneurysm undergoes successful surgery 2 days after the hemorrhage. Seven days later, right arm weakness develops. Which of the following diagnoses is most likely?

A) Hydrocephalus
B) Meningitis
C) Repeat hemorrhage
D) Vasospasm
E) Hyponatremia

14. A 17-year-old high school varsity diver develops a headache, dizziness, left-sided arm and leg clumsiness, and loss of pain and temperature sensation on the left face and right body after a practice session. Which of the following diagnoses is most likely?

A) Benign paroxysmal positional vertigo
B) Multiple sclerosis
C) Vertebral artery dissection
D) Astrocytoma
E) Labyrinthitis
F) Migraine with aura

15. A 26-year-old woman presents with recurrent throbbing headaches accompanied by nausea, emesis, photophobia, and phonophobia. She has been treating herself with acetaminophen and ice packs to her forehead. A reasonable therapeutic intervention to reduce the frequency of the headaches might be to prescribe:

A) Baclofen
B) Amitriptyline (TCA) → ppx med
C) Indomethacin
D) Corticosteroids
E) Sumatriptan → abortive med

16. A 76-year-old woman has been experiencing left temporal headaches for the prior 3 weeks. Over the prior 2 days she has had several brief episodes of cloudy vision in her left eye. On questioning, she notes a 5-pound weight loss over the last 2 weeks, which she attributes to discomfort when chewing. Therapy should be initiated with:

A) Baclofen
B) Amitriptyline
C) Indomethacin
D) Corticosteroids
E) Sumatriptan

17. A 57-year-old man has a 2-month history of severe, daily headaches that involve the right periorbital area. The headaches typically last 60–90 minutes and occur once or twice daily. Over-the-counter medications have not provided relief. Chiropractic manipulation did not help. The patient is desperate for relief because he cannot work during the headache episodes. A reasonable treatment strategy is to initiate:

A) Baclofen
B) Amitriptyline
C) Indomethacin
D) Corticosteroids
E) Gabapentin

18. A 53-year-old woman with the sudden onset of "the worst headache of her life" presents to the emergency department. She has a history of migraine but states that the current headache is not like her usual headaches. Results of her physical examination are unremarkable. Which of the following is the initial preferred diagnostic test?

- A Angiogram
- B Computed tomography scan
- C Transcranial Doppler
- D Magnetic resonance imaging
- E Magnetic resonance angiography

19. A 78-year-old man with a history of type 1 (insulin-dependent) diabetes mellitus, hypertension, hypercholesterolemia, and remote smoking presents with the acute onset of aphasia. On examination, he has trouble expressing himself and has mild right facial and arm weakness. There is a left carotid bruit. The most definitive strategy for secondary stroke prevention will likely be:

- A Acute heparin administration followed by warfarin
- B Extracranial intracranial bypass surgery
- C Warfarin and aspirin combined therapy
- D Carotid endarterectomy
- E Aspirin monotherapy

20. A 32-year-old woman who is 1 week postpartum presents with progressive headache and confusion. On examination she is afebrile with a blood pressure of 110/65 mm Hg. Papilledema is noted. The most likely diagnosis is:

- A Pseudotumor cerebri
- B Pituitary apoplexy
- C Bacterial meningitis
- D Sagittal sinus thrombosis
- E Eclampsia

21. A 67-year-old woman with a history of hypertension, diabetes mellitus, and smoking presents to the emergency department at 8:30 AM with a mild expressive aphasia, right facial weakness, and mild right arm weakness. She had awakened at 7:00 AM and was speaking to her husband when her speech suddenly became difficult and weakness was noted. Her husband called 911, and she was transported to the hospital, where her blood pressure was 165/85 mm Hg. The preferred treatment is:

- A Aspirin
- B Heparin
- C Warfarin
- D Recombinant tissue-type plasminogen activator (rt-PA)
- E Clopidogrel

22. A 62-year-old woman has a 2-month history of mild but progressive confusion. She occasionally has difficulty in following a conversation. On the morning of presentation to the hospital, she developed 30 seconds of right face and arm twitching, followed by increased confusion. Examination shows difficulties in speech comprehension and a subtle right homonymous hemianopia. A brain CT scan shows a 2- to 3-cm ill-defined region of low density in the left parietal lobe that does not enhance with IV contrast. The most likely diagnosis is:

- A Multiple sclerosis
- B Stroke
- C Astrocytoma
- D Abscess
- E Metastasis

Answers and Explanations

1. The answer is D [IV B 5 a; XV B 3 d (1), (2)]. Polymyalgia rheumatica (PMR) is characterized by muscle discomfort, and patients often present with vague complaints, as in this case. By definition, the results of the neuromuscular examination are normal.

Amyotrophic lateral sclerosis can cause fatigue and diminished activity, but discomfort is less frequently a complaint. In addition, the exam should be abnormal in some respects. Hypokalemia can cause muscle weakness, but discomfort is not a typical feature. Temporal (giant cell) arteritis can occur with PMR, but this patient has no complaint of headache or symptoms referable to vision. Polymyositis can cause muscle discomfort, but there should be accompanying weakness. The serum creatine kinase level is often elevated.

2. The answer is B [VIII B 6 b]. The lupus anticoagulant (an antiphospholipid antibody) is associated with peripheral venous thrombosis and ischemic (arterial) stroke. In patients with a history of deep venous thrombosis, the possibility of a paradoxical embolus causing a stroke (via a right-to-left cardiac shunt) should also be considered.

Nonvalvular atrial fibrillation is a common cause of stroke in the elderly, but there is no reason to suspect a rhythm disturbance in this patient. Mitral valve prolapse has been associated with cardiogenic emboli and stroke. However, a search for other causes of stroke should always be made because mitral valve prolapse is a relatively common entity and the association with stroke is weak. Multiple sclerosis and an astrocytoma can cause neurologic deficits in young patients; however, these conditions are not associated with deep venous thrombosis unless the patient is immobilized. These diagnoses should be considered in the evaluation of patients with hemiparesis, but the patient's history can often serve as a clue to guide diagnostic thinking.

3. The answer is A [XIII D 1 a, b]. People such as assembly-line workers and typists are particularly prone to carpal tunnel syndrome because their daily activities require repetitive wrist movements, which may, in time, compress the median nerve, causing neuropathy. Awakening at night with hand discomfort is a common complaint, and the findings on examination support the diagnosis.

A cervical radiculopathy can cause some of these findings. However, the history is more suggestive of carpal tunnel syndrome. Patients with a cervical radiculopathy often have a concurrent carpal tunnel syndrome and vice versa. The history and examination are not supportive of a diagnosis of tendinitis or reflex sympathetic dystrophy. Transient ischemic attacks rarely cause discomfort and are not associated with neurologic deficits after 24 hours have elapsed.

4. The answer is B [VII A 2 b]. Lumbar stenosis is caused by degenerative changes in the lumbosacral spine, often in association with a congenitally small lumbosacral intraspinal space. The history is often that of vague low back discomfort associated with subtle findings on examination referable to impingement on motor and sensory roots. Diagnosis can be made by the characteristic finding of an "hourglass" appearance on magnetic resonance imaging scans.

An acute disk herniation is characterized by low back discomfort and pain extending in a radicular fashion down one or both legs. Examination is often consistent with impingement on a single sensory or motor nerve root. A myopathy can cause an impaired gait, low back pain because of weakness, and hypoactive muscle stretch reflexes, typically at the knees. However, this condition is much less common than lumbar stenosis and therefore is not the most likely diagnosis. Normal-pressure hydrocephalus causes an apractic gait (i.e., difficulty in walking in spite of an intact motor, sensory, and cerebellar examination), cognitive impairment, and urinary incontinence. The clinical picture is not consistent with this diagnosis. Cervical stenosis can cause a myelopathy and resultant gait problem. Because the patient does not exhibit signs of a myelopathy, this diagnosis is unlikely.

5. The answer is B [X B 1; X B 4; XIII D 1 a, b]. Writer's cramp is a focal dystonia of unknown cause. Patients develop symptoms of cramps or spasms with altered hand and arm posture when attempting the specific task of writing. Examination of the patient is otherwise normal.

Micrographia is a symptom of Parkinson's disease but is usually accompanied by signs of rigidity, bradykinesia, and tremor. Carpal tunnel syndrome is caused by pressure on the median nerve as it enters the hand via the carpal tunnel. Median nerve dysfunction leads to hand weakness and loss of sensation, which can affect writing, but usually not cramping in the forearm muscles. A cervical radiculopathy can lead to hand numbness, weakness, and hyporeflexia but not usually cramping that is task specific. The exact distribution of findings depends on the nerve roots involved. A benign essential tremor is characterized by a limb tremor but not cramps. Carpal tunnel syndrome, cervical radiculopathy, and benign essential tremor are all unlikely, given the patient's normal exam at presentation.

6. The answer is B [VII A 2 a (2), (3)]. The patient probably has an acute disk herniation causing a cauda equina syndrome, an indication for emergency surgery. Surgery should be considered as an elective intervention for those patients with sciatica, nondisabling neurologic deficits, and disk herniation (as demonstrated by appropriate imaging techniques) who fail to respond to 6 weeks of conservative management.

Nonsteroidal anti-inflammatory drugs can be helpful in the treatment of acute, and possibly chronic, low back pain; however, they are not indicated as primary therapy for patients with acute, severe neurologic disability. Avoidance of strenuous activity is very helpful for the treatment of acute back pain, but that therapy is not appropriate for this patient. Lumbar traction is probably not effective for the treatment of low back pain. Patients typically cannot exercise during the first few days of acute back pain. However, as the acute pain subsides, an exercise program may help prevent future problems.

7. The answer is A [IX D 2 b (1), (2), 4 b, c]. Administration of intravenous lorazepam should be followed by the administration of phenytoin (or fosphenytoin) to control status epilepticus because the duration of action of lorazepam is limited. Therefore, unless there is a contraindication, the patient should receive a loading dose of phenytoin (or fosphenytoin) intravenously.

Carbamazepine is an effective anticonvulsant, but it cannot be given intravenously or intramuscularly. Therefore, a therapeutic level cannot be rapidly achieved, given a drug half-life of 8–12 hours. Intravenous pentobarbital can be used to control repetitive seizures. However, because the patient is not currently convulsing, induction of barbiturate coma is not indicated. Ethosuximide is indicated for the treatment of absence but not generalized tonic–clonic seizures. Rectal diazepam is used to abort seizures temporarily, especially in children.

8. The answer is B [XVII A 2]. A large, irregularly enhancing central nervous system (CNS) mass in an elderly patient without systemic cancer is highly suggestive of a glioblastoma multiforme. However, a biopsy is necessary before a definitive diagnosis can be made.

The patient has no predisposing condition for a brain abscess such as poor dentition or intravenous drug abuse. A meningioma can occur in the parietal area and distort the brain; however, a "convexity" meningioma is typically a homogeneously enhancing lesion. In the absence of systemic cancer, a brain metastasis is an unlikely cause of the patient's problem. However, without a biopsy, the diagnosis of metastatic disease cannot be excluded. CNS lymphoma typically manifests as a homogeneously enhancing mass lesion. Patients with human immunodeficiency virus infection and other immunocompromised patients are prone to CNS lymphoma; in other populations, CNS lymphoma is rare.

9. The answer is A [XVII D 1–3]. A cerebellopontine angle tumor such as a schwannoma can cause intermittent dizziness. The tumor can arise from the eighth cranial nerve, thereby also affecting hearing, and can affect the trigeminal or facial nerves, thereby causing impairment of the corneal reflex.

Benign paroxysmal positional vertigo causes intermittent brief dizziness that is dependent on postural changes. Nystagmus is characteristic, but there are no other neurologic deficits. A lateral medullary syndrome usually causes constant dizziness that is exacerbated with movement, but hearing is usually normal. Ménière's disease causes intermittent dizziness and hearing loss, but the corneal reflex is not diminished. A pontine infarction does not cause intermittent symptoms and rarely causes hearing loss.

10. The answer is D [XII D 4 b]. Thrombosis of the caudal anterior spinal artery leads to a flaccid paraplegia, loss of pain and temperature sensation, and bowel and bladder dysfunction. The blood supply to the caudal spinal cord arises from the aorta via the lumbar artery of Adamkiewicz. The perfusion territory of the anterior spinal artery involves the anterior horn cells, corticospinal tracts, and the pain and temperature pathways (spinothalamic tracts) but not the dorsal columns (which are responsible for proprioception and vibratory sensation).

In the Guillain–Barré syndrome, which rarely develops suddenly, loss of temperature and pain sensation can occur but rarely without a concurrent loss of position and vibration sense. Sensory loss is usually less severe than motor loss. Generalized areflexia is common. An anterior cerebral artery thrombosis, especially when bilateral, causes leg weakness, but sensory loss, when present, involves all modalities. Upper motor neuron signs should be present in the legs. A cauda equina syndrome [VII A 2 (3) a] can cause a flaccid paraplegia, but all sensory modalities should be compromised. Thoracic spinal cord compression is often associated with back pain, leg weakness, and sphincter dysfunction, but again all sensory modalities should be affected.

11. The answer is C [XIII D 4; Tables 12–9A and 12–9B]. Chronic inflammatory demyelinating polyneuropathy (CIDP) is characterized by progressive weakness that occurs over an extended time (e.g., >8 weeks), absent muscle stretch reflexes, and slowed motor nerve conduction velocities.

Guillain–Barré syndrome rarely causes progressive weakness beyond 8 weeks. The clinical features of Guillain–Barré syndrome and CIDP are often similar. Lead poisoning can cause a motor neuropathy in children but only rarely in adults. Patients often present with distal weakness, including a classic wrist drop. Amyotrophic lateral sclerosis causes progressive weakness, but motor conduction velocities are usually normal, and deep tendon reflexes are often hyperactive. Polymyositis causes progressive proximal (greater than distal) weakness and is not associated with impaired motor conduction velocities. Muscle stretch reflexes are often preserved in proportion to the muscle strength.

12. The answer is C [VI A 1 b; X A 2 a (2); XIX A 2 a; ⊕ Online Table 12–7]. The signs and symptoms are most consistent with multiple systems atrophy (Shy–Drager syndrome).

The early appearance of autonomic dysfunction (impotence and postural hypotension) and ataxia favors the diagnosis of Shy–Drager syndrome over Parkinson's disease. Subacute combined degeneration due to vitamin B_{12} deficiency does not produce Parkinsonian features. Spinocerebellar degeneration is characterized by cerebellar dysfunction and an accompanying upper motor neuron syndrome. Extrapyramidal and autonomic dysfunctions are not prominent features. Vitamin E deficiency can masquerade as spinocerebellar degeneration.

13. The answer is D [VIII C 1 c (2)]. Vasospasm can develop several days after an aneurysmal subarachnoid hemorrhage (SAH). Patients present with progressive weakness and alterations in consciousness. Early in the course, a computed tomography scan may not reveal an ischemic infarction.

Hydrocephalus can occur immediately after an SAH or weeks to months later. Symptoms are typically nonfocal, and, if the hydrocephalus develops acutely, it is often accompanied by a depressed level of consciousness. Bacterial meningitis can develop after a craniotomy. Typically, there is fever and impaired arousal. Focal signs can develop but are rarely the presenting feature. Although a repeat hemorrhage can occur after clipping of an aneurysm if the aneurysm is not completely isolated from the circulation, it is unusual for this to happen and present with a focal deficit, as opposed to depressed consciousness. Hyponatremia, which can develop after SAH, can cause an altered sensorium and seizures but not unilateral weakness.

14. The answer is C [VI B 2 f]. The patient has manifestations of a lateral medullary syndrome. In a young patient who has subjected himself to strenuous neck movements the most likely etiology is vertebral artery dissection.

Benign paroxysmal positional vertigo causes sudden episodes of dizziness, typically with changes in head position. However, there are no associated neurologic signs other than nystagmus or possibly hearing loss. Multiple sclerosis (MS) can cause dizziness and clumsiness. However, the constellation of findings in this patient, which is referable to a single site within the brain, make the diagnosis of MS less likely. An astrocytoma can cause dizziness, unsteadiness, and often headache. The onset is typically insidious and the symptoms progressive. Labyrinthitis causes severe vertigo. Patients find it difficult to move about and prefer to remain still. Gait instability can occur because of the profound dizziness in the absence of cerebellar deficits. There are no neurologic signs other than nystagmus and possibly unilateral hearing loss. Migraine with aura is associated with headache and focal neurologic symptoms and signs. Unless patients have a history similar to that described, they should be evaluated for alternative diagnoses such as arterial dissection.

15. The answer is B [IV B 1 d (1), (3) (a)]. Migraine headaches respond well to treatment with tricyclic antidepressants such as amitriptyline. This patient has been unresponsive to over-the-counter acetaminophen. Assuming she is having frequent headaches that are interfering with her lifestyle, it is reasonable to begin treatment with a prophylactic migraine medication.

Baclofen is not effective for migraine. Indomethacin is not commonly prescribed for migraine; although it may benefit an acute headache episode, it is not considered a prophylactic medication. Similarly, corticosteroids can be helpful in the treatment of a severe, acute migraine headache but are not used for migraine prophylaxis. Sumatriptan is an effective abortive agent for migraine but it is not indicated as a prophylactic medication.

16. The answer is D [IV B 5 c]. This patient likely has giant cell (temporal) arteritis. The treatment of choice for giant cell arteritis is corticosteroids. An erythrocyte sedimentation rate and C-reactive protein assay should be obtained before beginning corticosteroid therapy. Although awaiting a temporal artery biopsy should not delay initiation of therapy in patients with visuals symptoms, a biopsy should be obtained urgently (within days) of beginning treatment in order to confirm the diagnosis.

Neither baclofen, amitriptyline, indomethacin, nor sumatriptan is indicated for giant cell arteritis.

17. The answer is D [IV B 4 b (2)]. The patient's history is suggestive of cluster headaches. Cluster headaches can be extremely debilitating to patients and even push some individuals to attempting suicide. Oxygen can be used as an abortive agent, but corticosteroids are effective at breaking a cluster of headaches. Baclofen is used as a second-line agent for trigeminal neuralgia but not cluster headaches. Similarly, amitriptyline is used as a prophylactic agent for migraine but not in cluster headaches. Indomethacin is the drug of choice for a variant of cluster headaches known as chronic paroxysmal hemicrania. Gabapentin is used in certain neuropathic pain syndromes such as postherpetic neuralgia but is not a first-line agent for cluster headaches.

18. The answer is B [VIII C 1 b (2); IV A 3 b]. The history is highly suggestive of subarachnoid hemorrhage (SAH). A brain computed tomography (CT) scan is the best test to screen for intracranial hemorrhage and should be emergently obtained to document subarachnoid blood. If the scan is normal and the history is suggestive of SAH, the woman should undergo a lumbar puncture to assess for blood before the physician concludes that she does not have a SAH.

A conventional angiogram is necessary to evaluate for an aneurysm, but is not used to diagnose a SAH. Similarly, a magnetic resonance angiogram is less invasive than a conventional angiogram but has the same indications (but lower sensitivity). Transcranial Doppler studies can detect cerebral artery vasospasm as a complication of SAH, but they are not used to diagnose SAH. Brain magnetic resonance imaging is not as sensitive as brain CT for the detection of SAH and therefore is not considered the procedure of choice.

19. The answer is D [VIII B 4 c (1) (a), (3) (a)]. The patient has a nondisabling stroke. His risk factor profile and the presence of an ipsilateral bruit suggest that the most likely cause of his stroke may be left internal carotid artery stenosis. The definitive intervention to prevent subsequent stroke is carotid endarterectomy.

Acute heparin administration and subsequent warfarin therapy have not been demonstrated to be effective for secondary stroke prevention in this setting. Likewise, there is no role for extracranial–intracranial bypass surgery. A combination of warfarin and aspirin has not been shown to be more effective than carotid endarterectomy for secondary stroke prevention in patients with high-grade stenosis. Although aspirin is appropriate therapy for secondary stroke prevention for stroke due to arterial disease, treatment with aspirin should not preclude carotid endarterectomy in patients with appreciable stenosis. Aspirin should be administered after carotid endarterectomy to decrease the risk of postoperative stroke.

20. The answer is D [IV B 6]. The patient's presentation suggests sagittal sinus thrombosis. Although this condition is associated with the hypercoagulable state of pregnancy, further testing is indicated to evaluate the possibility of an underlying chronic hypercoagulable condition.

Pseudotumor cerebri (idiopathic intracranial hypertension) can present in association with pregnancy, and although it is characterized by headache and papilledema, confusion is not characteristic.

Pituitary apoplexy can occur postpartum. It is characterized by headache and visual dysfunction. Papilledema and confusion are not common sequelae of pituitary apoplexy.

Although bacterial meningitis causes headache, confusion, and papilledema, patients are typically febrile.

Eclampsia can cause headache and confusion as well as papilledema. However, the patient's normal blood pressure is evidence against this diagnosis. In addition, there is no mention of proteinuria or seizures in the patient's history.

21. The answer is D [VIII B 1 c (1)]. The patient has had the acute onset of a neurologic deficit consistent with a stroke. She is presenting for medical care within 3 hours of symptom onset. No contraindications to intravenous thrombolytic therapy with recombinant tissue-type plasminogen activator (rt-PA) is mentioned. The patient should have an emergent brain CT scan, and if no alternate diagnoses are suggested (tumor, subdural hematoma, etc.), intravenous rt-PA should be administered.

Aspirin is standard of care if the patient had presented more than 3–4.5 hours after symptom onset. There is little evidence that heparin or warfarin therapy is beneficial in this setting, and there is an increased incidence of bleeding with these anticoagulants. Clopidogrel is a therapeutic alternative for secondary stroke prevention, but its use should not take precedence over the administration of rt-PA.

If rt-PA is administered, aspirin administration should be delayed 24 hours. In addition, if low-dose heparin is administered for deep venous thrombosis prophylaxis, its use should also be delayed for 24 hours before rt-PA use.

22. The answer is C [XVII A 1 a]. The patient presents with a 2-month history of progressive neurologic deficits. The CT scan shows an area of low density, and there is no mention of mass effect. The most likely diagnosis is an astrocytoma, which may not have much in the way of mass effect or enhancement on CT scan.

The progressive history is against a stroke. Multiple sclerosis rarely presents in this age group and would not be expected to cause a large area of decreased density on CT scan. An abscess or metastasis would have substantial mass effect and enhancement on CT scan.

chapter 13

Dermatologic Disorders

CORINNE ERICKSON · MARCIA DRISCOLL

I   STRUCTURE AND FUNCTION OF SKIN

(Online Figure 13–1)

(Online Figure 13–2)

II   DERMATOLOGIC DIAGNOSIS

A **General considerations**   The foundation of dermatologic diagnosis relies on physical examination of the skin to first identify the morphology of the primary skin lesion(s). Based on morphology, a differential diagnosis is generated, and a final diagnosis is determined by using the dermatologic history and appropriate laboratory studies.

B **Examination of the skin**

1. **Inspection** of the skin defines morphology, color, distribution, and configuration.
   a. **Morphology.** Primary lesions of the skin are classified based on morphology (Table 13–1).
   b. **Distribution.** The location and extent of the primary eruption are important characteristics in defining the disease process.
      (1) Localized: involvement of limited areas of the skin
      (2) Diffuse: widespread involvement of the skin
      (3) Bilateral: symmetric involvement
      (4) Dermatomal: involvement limited to skin over a dermatome (e.g., herpes zoster)
      (5) Acral: involvement of the skin of the distal extremities
   c. **Configuration** (Online Figures 13–3 through 13–6). Several features of primary lesions are important in defining the disease process.
      (1) Number (single vs. multiple)
      (2) Spatial relationship (i.e., grouped)
      (3) Shape (i.e., annular, linear, serpiginous, and polycyclic)
2. **Palpation** determines the texture, consistency, and depth of lesions, as well as the temperature, tenderness, and quality of erythema (i.e., blanchable).

C **Dermatologic history**

1. **History of the eruption.** The essential historical qualifiers for any cutaneous eruption include the following:
   a. Onset and progression
   b. Duration and course
   c. Symptoms
   d. Treatment and response
2. **Medical history.** A history of medical problems focused on cutaneous findings, including allergies, should be elicited.
3. **Medication history.** A detailed medication history is vital, especially when evaluating eruptions that may be triggered by medications. The medication history should include prescription and over-the-counter (OTC) medications, vitamins, eye drops, and herbal supplements.

TABLE 13–1   Terms Used in the Morphologic Description of Skin Lesions

Term	Description	Appearance
Papule	Small, solid, elevated lesion; papules are generally <1 cm in diameter	Papule
Plaque	Broad-based papule that occupies a relatively large surface area in comparison with its height above skin level, >1 cm	
Macule	Flat lesion of variable size and shape that differs from surrounding skin because of its color, <1 cm	Macule
Patch	Description of very large macules or a thin but large plaque, >1 cm	
Nodule	Palpable, firm, round-to-spheroid lesion with a depth of involvement greater than that of a papule	Nodule
Cyst	Epithelial-lined sac that contains liquid or semisolid material (fluid, cells, and cell products)	
Vesicle	Fluid-filled, elevated lesion <1 cm in diameter	Bulla / Vesicle
Bulla	Large vesicle (>1 cm)	Bulla / Vesicle
Pustule	Raised lesion that contains purulent exudate (i.e., pus)	Pustule
Wheal	Flat-topped papule or plaque that is characteristically evanescent, disappearing within hours (i.e., hive)	Wheal
Erosion	Circumscribed, superficial depression caused by loss of all or portion of viable epidermis	Ulcer / Erosion / Fissure
Ulcer	Deep depression resulting from destruction of epidermis and at least upper (papillary) dermis	Ulcer / Erosion / Fissure

TABLE 13–1   Terms Used in the Morphologic Description of Skin Lesions (*Continued*)

Term	Description	Appearance
Fissure	Linear crack in skin	Ulcer Erosion Fissure
Furuncle	Deep necrotizing form of folliculitis with pus accumulation; several furuncles may coalesce to form a **carbuncle**	
Abscess	Localized accumulation of purulent material so deep in dermis or subcutaneous tissue that pus is usually not visible on the surface of the skin	
Sinus	Tract leading from suppurative cavity to skin surface or between cystic or abscess cavities	
Atrophy	Epidermal atrophy: thinning of epidermis associated with decrease in number of epidermal cells Dermal atrophy: usually manifested as depression of skin; results from decrease in dermal connective tissue	Atrophy
Sclerosis	Circumscribed or diffuse hardening or induration in skin	
Scaling	Abnormal shedding or accumulation of stratum corneum in perceptible flakes	Scale
Papulosquamous	Eruptions consisting of scaling papules	
Crusts	Hardened deposits of dried serum, blood, or purulent exudate	Crust
Excoriations	Superficial excavations of epidermis that may be linear or punctate and result from scratching	Excoriations
Lichenification	Thickening of the epidermis resulting from chronic scratching	Lichenification
Poikiloderma	Combination of atrophy, telangiectasia, and pigmentary changes (hyperpigmentation and hypopigmentation)	

4. **Social history.** A detailed social history often provides diagnostic clues for cutaneous findings. The social history should focus on skin care (habits and products used), occupation, home environment, sexually transmitted diseases, and travel.

5. **Family history.** A family history is important in assessing skin disease predisposition and susceptibility, particularly for allergy, skin cancer, psoriasis, and rheumatic disease.

D **Dermatology laboratory tests**

1. **Direct microscopic examination.** Preparations of skin scrapings from scaling and blistering eruptions can provide important diagnostic information.
   a. **Potassium hydroxide (KOH) preparation.** KOH digests cellular material and facilitates the visualization of fungal hyphae, yeast forms, and scabies mites.
   b. **Tzanck smear.** Giemsa- or Wright-stained scrapings from herpetic vesicles reveal multinucleated giant cells.
   c. **Gram stain.** Gram-positive and gram-negative bacteria may be identified.
   d. **Darkfield microscopy.** Visualization of spirochetes (*Treponema pallidum*) from preparations of primary chancre and secondary lesions is diagnostic of syphilis.
   e. **Scabies preparation.** A #15 scalpel blade is dipped in mineral oil, and a drop of oil is placed on the area of skin to be scraped. The sample is obtained then transferred to a glass slide, covered with a drop of mineral oil, and examined under 10× for evidence of mites, eggs, or scybala.

2. **Skin cultures.** Bacterial, viral, and fungal cultures can be obtained from skin swabs or skin biopsies.

3. **Patch testing.** This method is used for identifying compounds responsible for allergic contact dermatitis. Common and suspected compounds are placed on the skin under occlusion (i.e., patch) for 48–72 hours. Induction of cutaneous inflammation at specific patch sites identifies sensitizing agents.

4. **Phototesting and photopatch testing**
   a. **Phototesting** uses specialized light sources that deliver specific ranges and quantities of ultraviolet (UV) light to document photosensitivity in individuals with suspected photosensitivity.
   b. **Photopatch testing** combines patch testing and phototesting to identify photosensitizing compounds, which produce a photosensitivity reaction when exposed to UV light. Suspected photosensitizing compounds are patch tested with and without UV exposure.

5. **Skin biopsy** provides tissue for histopathologic evaluation.
   a. **Biopsy techniques**
      (1) **Punch biopsy** is a commonly used technique to obtain 2- to 8-mm cylindrical skin samples.
      (2) **Tangential (shave) biopsy** is a rapid technique used to obtain superficial skin samples.
      (3) **Incisional biopsy** is used to obtain large or deep (including panniculus) skin samples.
      (4) **Excisional biopsy** is used to obtain an entire lesion (e.g., suspicious pigmented lesion) for histologic review.
   b. **Examination of biopsy tissue**
      (1) **Light microscopy** is used to evaluate routine (hematoxylin and eosin) and special (e.g., periodic acid–Schiff) stains, as well as immunohistochemical (monoclonal antibody) stains.
      (2) **Immunofluorescent microscopy** is used for the identification of immunoreactants (e.g., autoimmune antibodies).
      (3) **Electron microscopy** is used for specialized studies that require visualization of subcellular structures.

III DERMATOLOGIC THERAPY

A **General considerations** Topical therapies are frequently used in treating dermatologic diseases and often provide alternatives to systemic therapies. The chief advantages of topical therapies may include higher efficacy and limited systemic toxicities, whereas the selection of topical therapies and systemic therapies for dermatologic diseases is guided by basic clinical management principles.

1. Therapeutic goals should be defined.
   a. Is therapy intended to cure or ameliorate (control) the disease?
   b. Is therapy intended to be short term or long term?

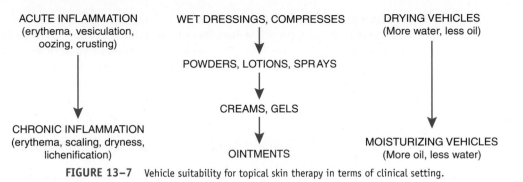

FIGURE 13–7 Vehicle suitability for topical skin therapy in terms of clinical setting.

2. Therapy should maximize the benefit-to-risk ratio and minimize toxicity.

3. Patient compliance should be considered and promoted.

4. Cost-effectiveness should be evaluated as part of therapeutic decision making.

B **Topical therapy**

1. Two variables are involved in the selection of topical therapy. Both the medication and the vehicle to be used must be appropriate for the specific disorder being treated.

2. Generally, acute inflammation is treated with aqueous drying vehicles, and chronic inflammation is treated with more lubricating and moisturizing preparations (Figure 13–7).

3. Vehicle choice may be influenced by body site. For example, lotions, solutions, and sprays are more effective in hairy areas (e.g., scalp).

4. Water, oil, and particulate composition of a vehicle determine its characteristics.
    a. Ointments are emulsions of water, predominately in oil, and thus more moisturizing.
    b. Creams are emulsions of oil, predominately in water, and thus less moisturizing than ointments.
    c. Gels are semisolid emulsions of alcohol or acetone in an organic polymer (agar, gelatin).
    d. Lotions are powders in a water base.
    e. Solutions, sprays, and aerosols have a base of water, alcohol, or propylene glycol and tend to have more of a drying effect.

5. Topical corticosteroids are prescribed for a variety of inflammatory and pruritic conditions.
    a. Potency. Halogenated corticosteroids have the greatest potency. Potency of topical corticosteroids is measured by vasoconstrictive capacity and may be categorized as low, medium, or high (Online Table 13–2).
    b. Use
       (1) High-potency topical corticosteroids (e.g., clobetasol) are used for the short-term treatment of acute and severe inflammatory eruptions.
       (2) Mid- to low-potency topical steroids (e.g., triamcinolone) are used for treatment of mild-to-moderate inflammatory eruptions and for maintenance therapy or prolonged therapy.
       (3) Low-potency topical steroids (e.g., hydrocortisone) are the only steroids to be prescribed for the face and intertriginous areas (skin folds of the axillae, inframammary region, abdominal pannus, and groin) because of the increased risk of local side effects in these areas.
       (4) In general, prolonged use of topical steroids should be avoided. Tachyphylaxis and side effects are associated with prolonged topical steroid use. If prolonged topical steroid therapy is required, tapering to steroids of a lower potency is advised.
       (5) Occlusion is an important adjuvant to topical therapy and increases absorption by increasing hydration and temperature. Materials such as plastic (Saran) wrap, gloves, and shower caps can be used as occlusive dressings.
       (6) Twice-daily application is generally recommended because of patient compliance. Individuals are more likely to treat their skin in the morning and evening when dressing and undressing. No compelling clinical data demonstrate an increase in efficacy with a frequency of application of more than twice-daily application.
       (7) See Online Table 13–2 for complete steroid potency listing.

    c. Dispensing

        (1) Prescribing the appropriate quantity of topical steroids is important for both compliance and safety. 🖱 Online Table 13–3 presents guidelines for prescribing topical steroids.

        (2) Most creams, ointments, and gels are commercially available in small (15 or 30 g) or large (45 or 60 g) tubes.

        (3) Most solutions and lotions are commercially available in small (30 mL) or large (60 mL) bottles.

    d. Complications

        (1) Local side effects occur with prolonged use, especially on intertriginous areas and on the face (🖱 Online Table 13–4).

        (2) Systemic side effects may result from systemic absorption. Systemic absorption may result in hypothalamus–pituitary–adrenal (HPA)–axis suppression. Risk factors for HPA-axis suppression include impaired barrier function, increased surface area of treated skin, high potency, use of occlusion, and prolonged use.

6. Topical antibiotics are useful agents for the treatment of secondary bacterial infection of superficial wounds and burns and for the treatment of primary superficial skin infections (e.g., impetigo). Prescription agents include mupirocin cream or ointment, silver sulfadiazine cream, and retapamulin ointment (Altabax). Nonprescription agents include Bacitracin, Polysporin (polymyxin B sulfate, bacitracin zinc), and Neosporin (neomycin sulfate, polymyxin B sulfate, bacitracin zinc).

7. Topical antifungals are prescribed for the treatment of superficial yeast (e.g., candidiasis) and fungal (e.g., dermatophyte) infections of the skin. Generally, the topical agent is available as a cream, but other formulations include powder, lacquer (for nails), spray, gel, solution, vaginal suppository, and oral troche. Topical antifungal agents are listed in 🖱 Online Table 13–5.

8. Topical antivirals are often prescribed for human papilloma virus (HPV). Imiquimod (5% cream) has been approved for the treatment of external genital warts. It is an immune-response modifier that induces cytokines, including interferon-α (IFN-α), at the treatment site. Podofilox (0.05% topical solution) can also be prescribed for external genital warts.

C **Systemic therapy**

1. **Systemic corticosteroids** are an available option in dermatologic therapy for severe inflammatory diseases of the skin that are not amenable to topical steroid therapy.

    a. **Prednisone** is the oral steroid of choice of the oral agents used for treatment of dermatologic diseases.

    b. There are a variety of treatment regimens. For suppression of most inflammatory dermatoses in adults, an initial starting oral dose of 40–60 mg/day of prednisone is commonly used. For acute conditions, the prednisone is tapered over 10–20 days. If the course of therapy for suppression is too short, a flare and exacerbation may occur when prednisone is discontinued.

    c. Once the disease has been controlled with daily prednisone therapy, it is appropriate to change to an alternate-day dose, which will maintain disease control with less HPA-axis suppression. This decreases the frequency of most side effects except cataracts, osteoporosis, and osteonecrosis.

2. Oral antihistamines are often used to treat pruritus associated with a wide range of skin diseases, particularly those that are mediated by type I histamine-mediated immune responses (e.g., urticaria).

    a. Competitive antagonists for histamine H_1 receptors are commonly prescribed. These agents are metabolized in the liver. The shorter-acting agents last 3–6 hours, and the longer-acting agents last 12–24 hours.

    b. Complications of antihistamines include anticholinergic side effects (e.g., glaucoma, constipation, and xerostomia) and sedation. The longer-acting antihistamines produce less sedation.

    c. In recalcitrant cases of pruritus, H_2 antagonists are added in combination with H_1 antihistamines. H_1- and H_2-receptor blockade also may be achieved with the use of doxepin, a tricyclic antidepressant with strong H_1 and H_2 antihistamine blocking effects. Both H_1 and H_2 antihistamines are available in prescription and nonprescription form (🖱 Online Table 13–6).

IV   **ACNE AND ROSACEA**

A   **Acne vulgaris**

1. **Definition.** Acne vulgaris is a common disorder of the **pilosebaceous unit** (hair follicle and sebaceous glands), located primarily on the face and trunk. It is manifested by follicular comedones with or without inflammatory papules, pustules, and nodules.

2. **Epidemiology.** Acne vulgaris affects 85%–100% of individuals to some degree during their lifetime.

3. **Etiology**
   a. The obstruction of sebaceous follicles is due to excessive sebum production by sebaceous glands in combination with excessive desquamation of the follicular epithelium.
   b. Inflammatory changes are linked to the presence of *Propionibacterium acnes,* a resident, lipophilic anaerobe. *P. acnes* proliferates in the microenvironment created by excess sebum and desquamated follicular cells. This bacterium produces chemotactic factors and proinflammatory mediators that contribute to inflammation.

4. **Pathophysiology**
   a. Acne may begin in the prepubertal period, when increasing amounts of adrenal androgens (dehydroepiandrosterone sulfate [DHEAS]) stimulate sebaceous gland hyperplasia and increased sebum production.
   b. Abnormal follicular differentiation is coupled with this phenomenon, resulting in the development of the primary acne lesions, noninflammatory open and closed comedones ("blackheads" and "whiteheads," respectively).
   c. Dermal inflammation and follicular rupture can lead to acne scarring.

5. **Clinical features** (Online Figure 13–8)
   a. Sites of involvement include the **face** and **upper trunk.**
   b. **Noninflammatory (comedonal) acne** is dominated by open or closed comedones without inflammatory lesions.
   c. Mild **inflammatory acne** is characterized by inflammatory papules and comedones.
   d. Moderate inflammatory acne is characterized by comedones, inflammatory papules, and pustules.
   e. **Nodulocystic acne** is characterized by comedones, inflammatory papules/pustules, and inflammatory nodules (>5 mm). Scarring is often evident.

6. **Diagnosis.** The diagnosis of acne vulgaris is clinical.

7. **Therapy.** Treatment is directed toward the pathogenic factors involved, including follicular dyskeratinization, excess sebum production, hormonal influences, and *P. acnes.* The severity of the acne determines the type and level of therapy.
   a. **Topical therapy**
      (1) **Topical retinoids** are comedolytic and anti-inflammatory. The most commonly prescribed topical retinoids include adapalene, tazarotene, and tretinoin. They are usually used in combination with other treatments. Patients are advised to apply these in small amounts at bedtime.
      (2) **Topical antibiotics** target *P. acnes.* Commonly prescribed topical antibiotics include erythromycin and clindamycin.
      (3) **Benzoyl peroxide** has antimicrobial properties against *P. acnes.* Benzoyl peroxide is the active ingredient in many over-the-counter topical skin care products; it is available in a variety of formulations, including soaps, washes, lotions, creams, and gels. In addition, it is available by prescription. Benzoyl peroxide is often combined with topical antibiotics to improve efficacy and reduce antibiotic resistance.
   b. **Systemic therapy**
      (1) **Oral antibiotics.** Lipophilic antibiotics are most effective against *P. acnes.* Tetracycline, doxycycline, and minocycline are commonly prescribed for inflammatory acne.
      (2) **Isotretinoin.** This systemic retinoid is highly effective in treating severe and nodulocystic acne that is recalcitrant to oral antibiotic and topical therapies. It causes normalization of epidermal differentiation, depresses sebum production, is anti-inflammatory, and reduces levels of *P. acnes* in the skin. Informed consent with contraception counseling and baseline

laboratory tests (including serum pregnancy test) are mandatory before the initiation of therapy and throughout treatment. **Mandatory participation in the iPLEDGE program is required for prescribers and patients receiving isotretinoin.**

(3) **Hormonal therapy.** This alternative to systemic antibiotics and isotretinoin in women with persistent acne involves treatment with estrogen or an antiandrogen. Oral contraceptives may be effective. Combination oral contraceptive pills (norgestimate–ethinyl estradiol) containing low levels of progestational compounds are preferred. Yaz (drospirenone/ethinyl estradiol) also has U.S. Food and Drug Administration (FDA) approval for the treatment of acne. Spironolactone, which reduces androgen production, may be used alone or in combination with an oral contraceptive.

B **Rosacea**

1. **Definition.** Rosacea is a disorder of the blood vessels and sebaceous glands of the face characterized by erythema, telangiectasia, flushing, and an inflammatory papulopustular eruption resembling acne.

2. **Epidemiology.** Rosacea is a common disorder that affects approximately 14 million adults in the United States. It is seen more frequently in fair-skinned individuals of European and Celtic descent.

3. **Etiology.** The precise etiology of rosacea is unknown. Clinical signs and symptoms result from the interaction of genetic susceptibility with environmental triggers (UV radiation and temperature changes) and dietary triggers (hot drinks, alcohol, and spicy foods).

4. **Pathophysiology**
   a. Vascular lability results in intermittent facial flushing, leading to persistent redness and telangiectasias that affect the central face and occasionally the eyes.
   b. The pathogenesis of the sebaceous hyperplasia and the inflammatory papules and pustules is unclear. Mites of the genus *Demodex* (indigenous to human hair follicles) appear in greater numbers, but their etiologic role has not been established.

5. **Clinical features** (Online Figure 13–9)
   a. Flushing, erythema, and telangiectasia can occur over the cheeks, forehead, and chin.
   b. Inflammatory papules and pustules involve the nose, forehead, and the cheeks, with an absence of comedones and scarring.
   c. Rhinophyma is a prominence of sebaceous glands of the nose that produces thickened skin and disfigurement in extreme cases.
   d. Ocular rosacea produces ocular signs that may include conjunctival injection, edema, chalazion, and episcleritis.

6. **Diagnosis.** The diagnosis is clinical. Overlapping features of acne vulgaris may sometimes be present, and it may be difficult to differentiate acne vulgaris and rosacea.

7. **Therapy.** Avoidance of environmental and dietary triggers is an important strategy to reduce signs and symptoms.
   a. **Topical antibiotics** (e.g., topical metronidazole, azelaic acid) may be prescribed for mild disease.
   b. **Systemic antibiotics** (e.g., tetracycline, doxycycline, and minocycline) are usually effective in treating acneiform lesions but have limited effectiveness in treating the facial erythema.
   c. **Retinoids** (e.g., isotretinoin) are prescribed as a one-time course (similar to acne therapy) and may be an effective treatment for severe cases. Alternatively, long-term, low-dose isotretinoin can be used.

V AUTOIMMUNE BLISTERING DISEASES: PEMPHIGUS AND BULLOUS PEMPHIGOID

A **General considerations**

1. Autoimmune blistering diseases are characterized by blistering of the skin and mucous membranes associated with the deposition of autoantibodies.

2. Localization of autoantibodies to epitopes in the epidermis, basement membrane zone, or dermis defines the specific clinical features, histopathology, and direct immunofluorescent staining pattern (Online Table 13–7).

TABLE 13–8	Comparison of Autoimmune Blistering Diseases	
Bullous Pemphigoid	**Pemphigus Vulgaris**	**Paraneoplastic Pemphigoid**
Average age at onset, 65 years	Average age at onset, <35 years	Ages vary
Tense bullae	Flaccid bullae	Varied bullae
Rarely involves mucous membrane	Often involves mucous membranes	Often involves mucous membranes

3. Most autoimmune blistering diseases are idiopathic but may be associated with medications, such as pemphigus [see V B] and linear immunoglobulin A (IgA) dermatosis [see XII E 14], pregnancy (herpes gestationis; see 🖭 Online Table 13–7), autoimmune disease (bullous lupus erythematosus; Table 13–8), or malignancy (paraneoplastic pemphigus).

4. Two of the most commonly encountered forms of autoimmune blistering diseases are pemphigus and bullous pemphigoid. Paraneoplastic pemphigoid is rarely seen.

B **Pemphigus**

1. **Epidemiology.** The incidence of pemphigus varies from 1 per 1,000,000 to 50 per 1,000,000 population, depending on the type of pemphigus and ethnicity. The onset of pemphigus is typically young to mid adulthood (<35 years of age), and both sexes are affected equally (see Table 13–8).

2. **Etiology.** Pemphigus is an immune-mediated disease associated with the production of IgG autoantibodies that target intraepidermal epitopes. The precise cause of autoantibody production is unknown. Certain drugs may trigger pemphigus in some individuals. Exacerbating drugs include penicillamine and captopril.

3. **Pathophysiology.** Pemphigus is mediated by IgG targeting of desmoglein, a transmembrane glycoprotein component of desmosomes. Desmosomes are responsible for intercellular adhesion of keratinocytes, and their binding by pemphigus autoantibodies results in separation of keratinocytes (acantholysis) and production of intraepidermal blisters.
   a. **Pemphigus vulgaris** develops from IgG targeting of desmoglein 3 (on keratinocytes of mucous membranes and skin) and desmoglein 1 (on keratinocytes of skin). Blistering results from splitting through the suprabasal portion of the epidermis.
   b. **Pemphigus foliaceus** develops from IgG targeting desmoglein 1, resulting in more superficial blistering within the subcorneal portion of the epidermis.

4. **Clinical features**
   a. **Pemphigus vulgaris** is characterized by dysphagia secondary to oral lesions (90% of cases) (🖭 Online Figure 13–10). Skin blisters are distributed predominately on the trunk and scalp. They are flaccid and break easily (see Table 13–8). Both Nikolsky's sign (separation of normal epidermis from the basal layer with light rubbing) and Asboe-Hansen's sign (extension of the blister into normal skin with light pressure on lateral edge) are positive.
   b. **Pemphigus foliaceus** is characterized by more crusted or denuded lesions (due to the superficial nature of the blistering) with involvement of the face, scalp, and trunk. Oral involvement is rare.

5. **Diagnosis.** Inspection of the skin and identification of primary lesions provide a clinical diagnosis. **Skin biopsy** is required to confirm the clinical impression.
   a. **Histology** shows intraepidermal acantholysis at the suprabasal (pemphigus vulgaris) or subcorneal (pemphigus foliaceus) level.
   b. **Direct immunofluorescence (DIF)** of perilesional skin biopsy specimens shows IgG deposition throughout the intercellular spaces between keratinocytes.
   c. **Indirect immunofluorescence (IIF)** detects circulating IgG autoantibodies in the patient's serum. Serum titer levels usually mirror disease activity.

6. **Therapy**
   a. **Systemic corticosteroids** are used to provide rapid control of the blistering process.
   b. **Immunosuppressants** are used in combination with corticosteroids and as steroid-sparing agents for long-term control and maintenance. These agents include azathioprine, mycophenolate mofetil, cyclophosphamide, methotrexate, cyclosporine, intravenous immune globulin (IVIG), and antibiotics.

C **Bullous pemphigoid**

1. **Epidemiology.** The exact incidence of bullous pemphigoid in the United States is unknown. The reported incidence in Europe is 6.6 cases per million annually. The average age at onset is 65 years.

2. **Etiology.** Bullous pemphigoid is an immune-mediated disease associated with the production of IgG autoantibodies that target basement membrane epitopes. The precise cause of autoantibody production is unknown. Bullous pemphigoid has been reported to be precipitated by photo-therapy, radiation therapy, and exposure to certain medications. Drugs that exacerbate bullous pemphigoid include furosemide, nonsteroidal anti-inflammatory drugs (NSAIDs), captopril, penicillamine, and antibiotics.

3. **Pathophysiology.** The IgG autoantibodies of bullous pemphigoid target desmoplakin 1 (bullous pemphigoid antigen 1) and collagen XVII (bullous pemphigoid antigen 2), which are intracellular and transmembrane components, respectively, of hemidesmosomes. Hemidesmosomes are responsible for the adhesion of basal keratinocytes with the basement membrane. The binding of antibodies at the basement membrane activates complement and attracts inflammatory cells to release proteases, leading to subepidermal blister formation. (See 🔊 online Section I on structure and function.)

4. **Clinical features**
   a. Tense bullae, with or without erythema, usually involve the trunk and flexural areas of the skin (🔊 Online Figure 13–11) (see Table 13–8).
   b. Mucosal involvement rarely occurs.
   c. Persistent urticarial lesions subsequently develop bullae.

5. **Diagnosis**
   a. **Clinical inspection** of the skin and identification of primary lesions yield a clinical diagnosis. Skin biopsy for histology and DIF are required to confirm the clinical impression.
      (1) **Histology** shows subepidermal split with an intact epidermis as the blister roof. Eosinophils often predominate in the dermal infiltrate.
      (2) **DIF** reveals linear IgG and C3 deposition along the dermal–epidermal junction (DEJ). Bullous pemphigoid can be differentiated from other subepidermal autoimmune blistering diseases by incubating the skin biopsy sample in 1 mole/L salt before performing DIF. This process induces cleavage through the lamina lucida. DIF on salt-split skin shows IgG on the blister roof (epidermal side of split skin).
   b. **IIF** can detect circulating IgG autoantibodies in the serum of most patients. However, titer levels do not correlate with disease activity.

6. **Therapy.** Mild cases may be controlled with antibiotics and topical steroids. Moderate and severe cases require systemic corticosteroids and steroid-sparing immunosuppressants, such as those used to treat pemphigus.

D **Paraneoplastic pemphigus**

1. **Definition.** Paraneoplastic pemphigus is an autoimmune blistering disease characterized by severe mucosal involvement and association with an underlying malignancy.

2. **Epidemiology.** Paraneoplastic pemphigus is rare. Since its first description in 1990, only 60+ cases have been reported.

3. **Etiology.** The most common malignancy associated with paraneoplastic pemphigus is non-Hodgkin's lymphoma.

4. **Pathophysiology.** An immune response to tumor antigens is thought to generate autoantibodies that attack the skin.

5. **Clinical features**
   a. Painful oral mucosal erosions that usually present as mucositis with crusting are the dominant clinical feature.
   b. Mucosal membranes of the eyes, nose, pharynx, tonsils, and genitalia may be affected.
   c. Cutaneous eruption is typically polymorphous. Combinations of blisters, ulcerations, erythematous macules and papules, scaly plaques, urticarial plaques, diffuse erythroderma, and erosions have been reported.

6. **Diagnosis:** Skin biopsy and DIF confirm the diagnosis.

7. **Therapy:** Symptomatic relief and treatment of superinfection, if present, are necessary.
   a. Immunosuppressive agents are often ineffective.
   b. Treatment of underlying malignancy may not result in skin clearing.

VI   CUTANEOUS REACTION PATTERNS

Each dermatologic diagnosis included in this section represents a specific cutaneous reaction that can develop in response to multiple causes. The clinical diagnosis of each of these cutaneous reaction patterns requires a thorough investigation into the underlying cause that may vary from case to case.

A   Erythema multiforme

1. **Epidemiology.** The true incidence of erythema multiforme in the United States is unknown.
   a. **Erythema multiforme minor** (less severe form) may account for up to 1% of dermatology office visits.
   b. **Erythema multiforme major** (more severe form) occurs at an incidence of 0.6 to 8.0 cases per million per year.

2. **Etiology.** Approximately 50% of cases are idiopathic; no underlying cause is identified.
   a. **Infection.** The most common causes of erythema multiforme are infectious (viral, bacterial, and fungal). Herpes simplex virus (HSV) is the most common infectious etiology, followed by *Mycoplasma pneumoniae*. Recurrent erythema multiforme (minor or major) can accompany recurrent HSV infection.
   b. **Drug reaction.** The major precipitants for erythema multiforme major are medications, especially anticonvulsants, NSAIDs, and antibiotics.

3. **Pathophysiology.** Erythema multiforme is an acute hypersensitivity reaction to a variety of stimuli. It is a cytotoxic immunologic reaction resulting in epidermal keratinocyte necrosis associated with a dense lymphocytic infiltrate within the dermis. Immune complex deposition is nonspecific. Subepidermal bullae formation occurs in severe forms.

4. **Clinical features.** Based on the severity of features and the extent of mucous membrane involvement, erythema multiforme may be categorized into minor and major forms.
   a. **Erythema multiforme minor. Iris** or **target lesions** are erythematous macules or papules with concentric red borders and central purpura or vesicles (Online Figure 13–12). Erythema multiforme tends to be symmetric and have an acral distribution, with lesions involving the palms and soles. Lesions may involve extremities and face and coalesce and become generalized. Mild oral cavity blistering may be seen in up to 25% of cases. Resolution usually occurs within 2 weeks.
   b. **Erythema multiforme major (Stevens–Johnson syndrome).** Skin findings are similar to those of erythema multiforme minor but are more severe: <10% of skin area is involved. Mouth, lips, and bulbar conjunctivae are most commonly affected, with mucous membranes severely affected. Oral bullae break easily and create erosions that readily become secondarily infected, often causing pain and bloody, crusted lips.
   c. **Toxic epidermal necrolysis.** Skin lesions are similar to erythema multiforme but involve >10% of total skin surface area. IVIG can be used as treatment. Despite treatment, mortality is high.

5. **Diagnosis.** Clinical inspection of the skin and identification of primary skin lesions yields a clinical diagnosis. Skin biopsy confirms the clinical impression. Evaluation of the underlying cause should accompany a clinical diagnosis.

6. **Therapy.** Treatment of the underlying cause and withdrawal of any offending drugs is the first management step. Supportive care and symptomatic relief of painful and secondarily infected mucocutaneous lesions is initiated. Use of systemic corticosteroids is controversial.

B   Lichen planus

1. **Epidemiology.** The incidence is estimated at 1% of new patient office visits in the United States.

2. **Etiology.** The exact etiology of lichen planus is unknown. Most cases are idiopathic. A positive family history in a few cases suggests a genetic predisposition. Associated liver disease, including hepatitis C infection, chronic active hepatitis, and primary biliary cirrhosis, as well as autoimmune disorders such as ulcerative colitis, dermatomyositis, and myasthenia gravis, may occur. Medications may cause a skin eruption similar to lichen planus (lichenoid drug reaction).

3. **Pathophysiology.** Lichen planus is a cell-mediated immunologic reaction targeting the epidermal keratinocytes. A dense lymphocytic infiltrate at the DEJ (lichenoid infiltrate) participates in the destruction of basal keratinocytes (basal vacuolization). Immunogenetic predisposition may play a role in the pathogenesis. Human leukocyte antigen DR1 (HLA-DR1) and HLA-DR10 are associated with idiopathic lichen planus, and HLA-B7 is associated with familial cases.

4. **Clinical features** (Online Figure 13–13). Most idiopathic cases are self-limiting, lasting 6–18 months. Other cases can be chronic and recurrent, particularly oral lichen planus.
   a. Polygonal papules are violaceous (purple), pruritic, and flat topped (lichenoid), usually covered with fine scales. Lesions vary in size from 1 mm to greater than 1 cm in diameter.
   b. The distribution of lesions typically involves flexor surfaces of the upper extremities (wrists), genitalia, and mucous membranes. Nails and scalp may also be involved.
   c. Oral lesions involve the tongue and buccal mucosa and may be asymptomatic plaques displaying a white reticular pattern (Wickham striae). Erosive lesions are painful.
   d. Nail dystrophy with nail plate thinning and ridging may be seen in 10% of cases. Nail matrix involvement may lead to scarring of the nail bed (pterygium formation).
   e. Scalp involvement (lichen planopilaris) is seen more often in women and produces follicular inflammation, often resulting in scarring alopecia.
   f. Lesions resolve with residual postinflammatory hyperpigmentation.

5. **Diagnosis.** Clinical inspection of the skin and identification of primary skin lesions provides a clinical diagnosis. Skin biopsy confirms the clinical impression. Evaluation of the underlying cause and associated disorders should accompany a clinical diagnosis.

6. **Therapy.** Treatment of an identifiable underlying cause and **withdrawal of any offending drugs** are the first management steps. **Antihistamines** and topical steroids are effective in mild, self-limiting cases. **Systemic corticosteroids** are used acutely to suppress more severe cases. Long-term control of chronic cases may require phototherapy or **steroid-sparing immunosuppressants. Topical and systemic retinoids**, as well as **topical and systemic cyclosporine**, have been shown to be active in some cases.

C **Urticaria** (hives) is a common cutaneous reaction pattern requiring investigation into its underlying etiology (Online Figure 13–14). It is covered in detail in Chapter 8 IV.

D **Pyoderma gangrenosum**

1. **Epidemiology.** The incidence of pyoderma gangrenosum in the United States is estimated at approximately 1 per 100,000 people each year.

2. **Etiology.** Pyoderma gangrenosum is an ulcerative skin disorder of unknown etiology. Several diseases are commonly associated with pyoderma gangrenosum (Table 13–9). No underlying disease association is present in 50% of cases.

3. **Pathophysiology.** The pathophysiology of pyoderma gangrenosum is poorly understood. It appears to be an immune-mediated reaction involving an intense and destructive neutrophilic

---

TABLE 13–9   Diseases Associated with Pyoderma Gangrenosum

Inflammatory bowel disease: ulcerative colitis or Crohn's disease
Polyarthritis (usually symmetric; either seronegative or seropositive)
Hematologic diseases
Myeloid leukemias
Immunoglobulin A monoclonal gammopathy
Myelomas (immunoglobulin A type, predominantly)
Hepatic diseases: hepatitis and primary biliary cirrhosis
Collagen vascular diseases: lupus erythematosus and Sjögren's syndrome

infiltrate within the dermis. The dermal inflammatory reaction causes purulent ulceration. Immunocomplex deposition is nonspecific.

4. **Clinical features** (Online Figure 13–15)
   a. Initial presentation may be erythematous to violaceous painful nodules that quickly ulcerate.
   b. Deep and purulent ulcers with highly inflammatory and tender borders develop.
   c. Ulcer margins are typically undermined. Violaceous borders overhang the ulcer bed.
   d. The lower extremities are typically affected. Variants may affect other areas.
   e. **Pathergy**—the development of new lesions or aggravation of existing ones after trauma—may occur.

5. **Diagnosis.** Pyoderma gangrenosum is a clinicopathologic diagnosis of exclusion and is made after other causes of cutaneous ulcerations have been ruled out. There is no specific laboratory test, and the histopathology is only suggestive, not diagnostic. A **skin biopsy** with tissue sent for histology and cultures is required to establish a diagnosis. Appropriate laboratory studies, imaging studies, and diagnostic procedures (e.g., colonoscopy or bone marrow biopsy) should be ordered to identify any associated diseases (see Table 13–9).

6. **Differential diagnosis**
   a. Bacterial infection (*Pseudomonas* or anaerobic [clostridial] infections)
   b. Atypical mycobacterial infection
   c. Deep fungal infection (North American blastomycosis)
   d. Amebiasis
   e. Bromoderma and iododerma
   f. Rheumatoid vasculitis
   g. Brown recluse spider bite
   h. Wegener's granulomatosis

7. **Therapy.** Effective treatment of the associated underlying disease most often results in control of pyoderma gangrenosum.
   a. Local wound care and dressings are aimed at gentle cleansing of the ulcer base.
   b. **Surgical debridement** or surgical therapy (skin grafting) is **contraindicated.**
   c. Intralesional corticosteroid injections into new nodules or the borders of small ulcers may be effective as an early intervention.
   d. Systemic corticosteroids are often required to gain rapid control of the destructive skin changes. High doses of oral prednisone and intravenous pulsed methylprednisolone are effective. Other systemic therapies include cyclosporine, tacrolimus, mycophenolate mofetil, azathioprine, cyclophosphamide, chlorambucil, dapsone, thalidomide, and intravenous immunoglobulin.

E **Erythema nodosum**

1. **Epidemiology.** The incidence is unknown. Erythema nodosum occurs more frequently in young adults and in women.

2. **Etiology.** This immune-mediated reaction may occur in association with systemic disease (Table 13–10) or **adverse drug reaction** (most commonly oral contraceptives), or it may be **idiopathic.**

3. **Pathophysiology.** Erythema nodosum appears to be delayed-type hypersensitivity reaction targeting the subcutaneous fat (panniculus). A lymphohistiocytic infiltrate develops, resulting in nonsuppurative inflammatory nodules. No circulating immunocomplexes have been found.

TABLE 13–10 Systemic Diseases Associated with Erythema Nodosum

Bacterial infections (streptococcal infections; most common bacterial cause)
Fungal infections (coccidioidomycosis; most common fungal infection)
Pregnancy
Sarcoidosis
Inflammatory bowel disease
Hodgkin's disease and lymphoma
Behçet's disease

4. **Clinical features** (Online Figure 13–16)
   a. A prodrome of flu-like symptoms, including fever and arthralgia, may occur.
   b. Lesions begin as poorly defined red, tender nodules that are 2–6 cm in diameter.
   c. Lesions are typically distributed over the anterior lower leg but may appear on any surface.
   d. Individual lesions develop over 2 weeks, with gradual softening and a bruise-like appearance. The overlying skin usually desquamates. Leg pain and ankle swelling may persist for weeks.
   e. Thirty percent of idiopathic cases may last more than 6 months.

5. **Diagnosis.** Clinical inspection of the skin and identification of primary skin lesions provides a clinical diagnosis. An incisional skin biopsy with adequate sampling of the subcutaneous fat confirms the clinical impression and is reserved for diagnostically difficult cases. Evaluation of an underlying cause and associated disorders should accompany the clinical diagnosis.

6. **Therapy.** Treatment of an identifiable underlying cause and withdrawal of any offending drugs is the first management step. In idiopathic or self-limited cases, symptomatic relief with NSAIDs, compression dressings, and leg elevation is usually satisfactory. In persistent cases, systemic agents such as colchicine and liquid supersaturated potassium iodide have proven effective.

VII   DERMATITIS

A **General considerations**   The term *dermatitis* can be defined as inflammation of the skin. It is often used as a general term to describe skin findings, such as "rash"; however, it also is used in the diagnoses of specific cutaneous diseases. Three of the most prevalent dermatitides are described in this section.

B **Atopic dermatitis**

1. **Definitions**
   a. **Atopic dermatitis** (atopic eczema or eczema) refers to the chronic, relapsing cutaneous manifestations generated from pruritus and scratching, associated with an underlying allergic predisposition (atopy).
   b. **Atopy** is a hereditary predisposition toward developing hypersensitivity reactions, associated with elevated serum immunoglobulin E (IgE) levels, including asthma, allergic rhinitis, and atopic dermatitis.

2. **Epidemiology.** Atopic dermatitis affects as much as 12% of the U.S. population.

3. **Etiology.** The precise etiology is unknown. There is a clear familial pattern of inheritance for atopic dermatitis and for all forms of atopy. Studies suggest an autosomal dominant inheritance pattern with variable penetrance. Genetic susceptibility interacts with various environmental and dietary triggers.

4. **Clinical features** (Online Figure 13–17)
   a. Atopic dermatitis is primarily manifested in infancy and childhood. Approximately one third of the cases persist, to some degree, into adulthood.
   b. The **flexor areas of the arms, legs, and neck** are primarily involved in children and adults. Severe cases may result in generalized erythroderma.
   c. Lesions often become secondarily infected with bacteria from scratching and are characterized by yellow crusting with impetigo.
   d. Hand and foot dermatitis may be the only manifestation of atopic dermatitis in adults with a history of atopy. Findings include erythema, scaling or peeling, and fissuring of the palms, soles, and fingers.

6. **Diagnosis.** Atopic dermatitis is a clinical diagnosis. Serum IgE levels are usually elevated. A skin biopsy may be helpful in confirming the clinical diagnosis and ruling out other disorders.

7. **Therapy**
   a. **Prevention** is effective in reducing acute exacerbations and complications.
      (1) Exacerbating triggers should be identified and avoided.
      (2) Good skin care maintenance should be practiced.
         (a) Daily bathing should be recommended in lukewarm water, with mild, moisturizing soaps.
         (b) Use of moisturizers after bathing is recommended.

b. **Topical treatments**
  (1) **Topical corticosteroids.** Medium- to high-potency topical steroids that can be tapered to low-potency topical corticosteroids are the best treatment for acute exacerbations.
  (2) **Topical macrolide immunosuppressants.** Pimecrolimus cream and tacrolimus ointment have been approved for the treatment of atopic dermatitis. These calcineurin inhibitors that are similar to cyclosporine are effective steroid-sparing therapies for the treatment of acute flares of atopic dermatitis.
  (3) **Lubricants.** The skin should be moisturized with emollients during treatment of acute flares as well as during maintenance therapy.
c. **Systemic treatments**
  (1) **Systemic corticosteroids.** A short course of oral prednisone for treatment of acute and severe flares may be helpful in gaining rapid control.
  (2) **Oral antibiotics.** Antibiotics are prescribed to treat secondary infections when present.
  (3) **Antihistamines.** The pruritus of atopic dermatitis is not directly mediated by histamine, but H_1 and H_2 histamine blockade may be effective in recalcitrant cases. The sedative effects of antihistamines taken at bedtime may provide relief from scratching during sleep and thus reduce a perpetuating factor.

C **Allergic contact dermatitis**

1. **Definitions**
   a. **Allergic contact dermatitis** is inflammation of the skin induced by a delayed-type hypersensitivity (allergy) reaction to a specific allergen that contacts the skin.
   b. Irritant contact dermatitis is cutaneous inflammation induced by the direct contact and toxic effects of chemicals contacting the skin. Occupational dermatitis refers to allergic contact dermatitis or irritant contact dermatitis that occurs in the workplace.
2. **Epidemiology.** The incidence of both allergic and irritant contact dermatitis has been estimated to be 13.6 cases per 1000 population in the United States. Surveys indicate that contact dermatitis is one of the most frequent dermatologic diagnoses and represents between 5% and 9% of dermatology office visits. Occupational dermatitis represents up to 20% of all reported occupational diseases in the United States.
3. **Etiology.** Cutaneous contact with a specific allergen results in allergic contact dermatitis in susceptible individuals. Approximately 3000 chemical compounds have been documented as specific causes of allergic contact dermatitis. Online Table 13–11 lists some common chemicals.
4. **Pathophysiology.** Small molecules (haptens, <500 daltons) bind carrier proteins on epidermal antigen-presenting cells (Langerhans cells). Langerhans cells process antigenic molecules and present them to $CD4^+$ T lymphocytes (helper T cells), which stimulate secretion of inflammatory mediators. Langerhans cells migrate from the epidermis to the regional draining lymph nodes and stimulate proliferation and activation of antigen-specific T cells. Expanded numbers of antigen-specific T cells circulate into the skin and amplify the inflammatory reaction. Initial sensitization may be acute or chronic. Usually 10–14 days pass after an initial acute exposure to a strong contact allergen before an individual becomes sensitized. Some initial exposures may not result in clinically apparent allergic contact dermatitis. Once an individual is sensitized to a chemical, allergic contact dermatitis develops within hours to several days of reexposure.
5. **Clinical features** (Online Figure 13–18)
   a. Acute disease is characterized by pruritic papules and vesicles on an erythematous base.
   b. Acute exposures result in cutaneous inflammation and pruritus lasting 2–3 weeks.
   c. The distribution tends to be asymmetric and depends on the nature of the contact. Linear or geometric configurations often are present.
   d. Chronic allergic contact dermatitis, caused by chronic exposure to allergen, may produce lichenified, pruritic plaques.
   e. Occasionally, allergic contact dermatitis may generalize and produce a diffuse exfoliative erythroderma.
6. **Diagnosis.** The diagnosis is usually made on clinical grounds. **Skin biopsy** may support the clinical diagnosis in difficult cases. The initial site of dermatitis often provides the best clues

regarding the potential cause of disease. **Patch testing** is required to confirm the diagnosis and identify the external chemicals to which the person is allergic.

7. **Therapy.** Prevention is the mainstay of therapy. Identification of the offending agent and avoidance reduce risk for chronic or recurrent dermatitis.
   a. **Topical treatments**
      (1) High-potency **topical corticosteroid** creams are effective when prescribed for 2-week courses.
      (2) **Drying agents,** such as calamine lotion or cool compresses (with saline or aluminum acetate solution), are helpful in soothing and drying acute, localized vesicular eruptions.
      (3) Individuals with widespread vesicular eruptions may obtain relief from cool oatmeal baths.
   b. **Systemic treatments**
      (1) **Corticosteroids.** Severe or diffuse disease often requires treatment with a 2- to 3-week course of oral prednisone. Short (5-day) courses of Solu-Medrol "dose packs" are inadequate. When discontinued, they usually result in flaring of symptoms.
      (2) Oral H_1 **antihistamines** often are helpful in diminishing pruritus.

D **Seborrheic dermatitis**

1. **Definition.** Seborrheic dermatitis (seborrhea) is a chronic and recurrent papulosquamous disorder with a distinctive distribution involving the scalp and central face, chest, axillae, and groin.

2. **Epidemiology.** Seborrheic dermatitis is a common disorder.

3. **Etiology**
   a. The precise etiology is unknown. An aberrant immune response to endogenous yeast forms (*Pityrosporum ovale*) has been speculated.
   b. Triggers associated with flares include seasonal changes, trauma (e.g., scratching), emotional stress, and medications. Such medications, which may also induce seborrheic dermatitis, include psychotropic medications (e.g., chlorpromazine, haloperidol, and lithium), benzodiazepines, cimetidine, ethionamide, gold, IFN-α, methyldopa, and psoralen. In addition, Parkinson's disease and acquired immunodeficiency syndrome (AIDS) are associated with flares.

4. **Pathophysiology.** Cutaneous inflammation may result from normal levels of *P. ovale* releasing inflammatory free fatty acids. *P. ovale* is also able to activate the alternative complement pathway in affected individuals who have decreased humoral and cellular immune responses.

5. **Clinical features.** Seborrheic dermatitis affects adults but may be seen in infants (**cradle cap**).
   a. The scalp is usually involved in all cases. Disease may vary from mild, patchy scaling (dandruff) to widespread pruritic, erythematous, thick, adherent greasy scales.
   b. Disease usually moves from the scalp to the face, affecting the eyebrows and nasolabial folds (T-zone) (🔍 Online Figure 13–19). The chest, axillae, and groin also may be affected.
   c. A **seborrheic blepharitis** may occur, and rarely, a generalized exfoliative erythroderma may develop in severe cases.

6. **Diagnosis.** Seborrheic dermatitis is usually well recognized on clinical inspection and by history.

7. **Therapy.** Mild cases of scalp involvement (dandruff) respond to over-the-counter shampoos that contain salicylic acid, tar, selenium, sulfur, zinc, or ketoconazole.
   a. **Topical corticosteroids** are effective for short-term treatment of acute flares.
   b. **Topical antifungals** are effective for prolonged treatment of the skin.

VIII PSORIASIS

A **Definition**   Psoriasis is a chronic, relapsing skin disease that manifests as a papulosquamous eruption with variable clinical manifestations but typically occurs as inflammatory plaques with excessive white scaling in a predominately extensor distribution.

B **Epidemiology**   Psoriasis affects approximately 2%–3% of the U.S. population, or 6.4 million cases. Approximately 200,000 new cases occur annually. The median age at onset is 28 years.

C **Etiology**   Psoriasis appears to be an autoimmune disease with a genetic predisposition. It is mostly likely inherited as a polygenic, autosomal dominant disease with variable penetrance. The precise target of the immune response is unknown. HLA-B13, HLA-B17, HLA-BW57, and HLA-CW6 are most frequently associated with psoriasis. As many as one third of patients report that one family member is affected. Psoriasis tends to flare during winter months and improve in the summer months as a function of sun (UV) exposure. Drugs that exacerbate psoriasis include β-adrenergic blockers, lithium, and angiotensin-converting-enzyme inhibitors.

D **Pathophysiology**   Psoriasis is an immune-mediated disease associated with a mixed inflammatory dermal infiltrate that initiates and maintains an increase in the proliferation rate of epidermal keratinocytes in affected areas. The increased keratinocyte turnover rate produces epidermal thickening (**acanthosis**) and disruption of normal epidermal differentiation, resulting in scaling. Disease onset and flares often follow upper respiratory infections (e.g., streptococcal pharyngitis), suggesting that superantigen activation of pathogenic T lymphocytes or molecular mimicry of cutaneous antigens plays a role in pathogenesis.

E **Clinical features**
1. **Plaque-type psoriasis** occurs as raised erythematous plaques covered with a white scale (Online Figure 13–20). Scratching the scale may lead to punctate bleeding (the Auspitz sign).
2. The **distribution** of psoriatic lesions includes the **extensor surfaces** of the extremities (knees and elbows), scalp, and trunk (particularly the presacral area).
3. Psoriasis may affect the **nails** and cause pitting of the nail plates, yellow discoloration, and thickening and separation from the nail bed.
4. Lesions often develop at sites of cutaneous injury or trauma (Köebner phenomenon).
5. **Guttate (tear-shaped) psoriasis** is a clinical variant that develops rapidly, most often after a streptococcal upper respiratory infection. Multiple, small (<1 cm) psoriatic lesions are distributed on the trunk and extremities.
6. **Pustular psoriasis** is a typically severe clinical variant that presents with sterile pustules appearing within plaques or diffusely. A pustular psoriasis flare may be associated with hypocalcemia.
7. **Erythrodermic psoriasis** is a severe clinical variant that presents as a generalized erythema with extensive scaling and exfoliation.
8. **Psoriatic arthritis** of varying severity affects approximately 10% of psoriatic patients [see Chapter 11 IV B 3].

F **Diagnosis**   Psoriasis is usually well recognized on clinical inspection of the skin and usually distinguished from other papulosquamous eruptions. Skin biopsy confirms the clinical impression.

G **Therapy**   Treatment is tailored to the severity of psoriasis, which is usually estimated by the percentage of the body surface area involved. Topical therapies are used in mild cases, and phototherapy and systemic agents are used for moderate-to-severe cases.
1. **Topical agents** include keratolytic agents (salicylic acid), coal tar preparations, topical steroids, topical vitamin D_3 analogs (calcipotriene), and topical retinoids. **Phototherapy** with psoralen plus UV-A light (PUVA) or UV-B light is very effective in cases with generalized skin involvement.
2. **Systemic agents** include oral retinoids (acitretin), methotrexate (particularly for arthritis), cyclosporine, and biologic agents. Biologic agents include alefacept (a fusion protein that targets T lymphocyte antigen molecule CD2), etanercept (a fusion protein that targets tumor necrosis factor), infliximab (a monoclonal antibody that targets tumor necrosis factor), and ustekinumab (a monoclonal antibody that targets interleukin-12 [IL-12] and IL-23). **Systemic corticosteroids should be avoided** because of severe rebound flares on withdrawal.

IX   PITYRIASIS ROSEA

A **Definition**   Pityriasis rosea is a benign, self-limited **papulosquamous exanthem** with a distinctive distribution involving the **trunk.**

B **Epidemiology**   In children and young adults, the estimated incidence is 0.3%–3% of dermatology visits.

C **Etiology**   Pityriasis rosea appears to be an **infectious exanthem,** but no definitive etiologic agent has been identified. Case clusters among contacts have been reported. There appears to be a seasonal predilection to spring, autumn, and winter. The rate of recurrence is low (3%). Drug-induced pityriasis rosea associated with such agents as captopril, gold, and D-penicillamine has been described.

D **Pathophysiology**   An initial solitary lesion (**herald patch**) develops in 50%–90% of cases, followed by a secondary crop of lesions that appear over 2–21 days. Lesions spontaneously regress by 6 weeks.

E **Clinical features**   (Online Figure 13–21)

1. The **herald patch** typically measures 1–3 cm in diameter and usually is located on the trunk or proximal extremities. The patch is oval or round and is erythematous with fine, peripheral (collarette) scaling.

2. The **secondary eruption** is similar in appearance but ranges in size from 0.5 to 1.0 cm. The lesion is symmetric on the trunk and follows the lines of cleavage of the skin, producing a **"Christmas tree"** pattern on the back.

3. Lesions are usually asymptomatic but may be pruritic.

F **Diagnosis**   Pityriasis rosea is usually well recognized on clinical inspection of the skin and readily distinguished from other papulosquamous eruptions.

G **Therapy**   Pityriasis rosea is a self-limited disease, and no specific treatment is usually necessary. Topical steroids may be used to relieve pruritus. UV radiation therapy has been used to hasten the resolution of lesions.

X   SKIN CANCERS

A **Basal cell carcinoma**

1. **Definition.** Basal cell carcinoma is a neoplastic growth of the basal cell layer of epidermis.

2. **Epidemiology.** Basal cell carcinoma is the most common type of cancer in the United States. Approximately 1 million new cases occur each year.

3. **Etiology.** The multifactorial etiology includes genetic susceptibility and environmental exposure to UV light (sunlight).

4. **Pathophysiology**
   a. Neoplastic transformation of basal keratinocytes produces downward growth into underlying dermis and deeper tissues. Basal cell carcinoma is locally invasive without metastatic capacity.
   b. **Basal cell nevus syndrome** (Gorlin's syndrome) is a rare autosomal dominant syndrome with germline mutations in the *ptch* gene, resulting in increased basal cell carcinomas and developmental abnormalities of the skeletal system, genitourinary system, and central nervous system.

5. **Clinical features**
   a. A persistent skin lesion is usually in the 3- to 6-mm size range and on sun-exposed areas of the skin.
   b. Lesions are flesh colored to red, may be a plaque or a papule, and have a pearly or translucent quality (Online Figure 13–22). Telangiectasis may be present.
   c. Some lesions may be brown to black (pigmented basal cell carcinoma).
   d. The borders are rolled with central depressions, ulceration, or crusting (**rodent ulcer**).
   e. Lesions located on the central face and ears are at high risk for recurrence.
   f. Histologic variants include morpheaform basal cell carcinoma (scar-like quality and histologic fibrosis) and multicentric basal cell carcinoma (indistinct borders with histologic skip areas) and are at high risk for recurrence.

6. **Diagnosis.** The diagnosis is made by clinical inspection of skin and skin biopsy confirmation.

7. **Therapy**
   a. **Surgery.** The cure rate is 90%–99%, depending on the tumor site and surgical technique. Surgical techniques include technique excision, Mohs micrographic surgery, curettage with electrodesiccation, and cryosurgery.

   b. Radiation therapy. The 5-year cure rate is 90%–95% when treatment is executed properly. This treatment modality should be avoided in cases of recurrent basal cell carcinomas, large tumors, tumors in high-risk areas, and tumors with an aggressive growth pattern, due to higher failure rates.

   c. Topical therapy: Imiquimod and 5′-fluorouracil topical creams are FDA approved for the treatment of superficial basal cell carcinoma. The 5-year clearance rate has been reported to be 90%.

B **Squamous cell carcinoma**

1. **Definition.** Squamous cell carcinoma is a neoplastic growth of the suprabasal cell layer of epidermis.

2. **Epidemiology.** Squamous cell carcinoma is the second-most-common type of cancer in the United States. Approximately 400,000 new cases occur each year.

3. **Etiology.** The etiology is multifactorial and includes genetic susceptibility and environmental exposure to UV light (sunlight).

4. **Pathophysiology**

   a. Neoplastic transformation of suprabasal keratinocytes produces intraepidermal (in situ) foci leading to tumor invasion of underlying dermis and deeper tissues. UV-induced *p53* gene mutations are identified in precursor lesions (**actinic keratosis),** of which 0.1%–1.0% progress to squamous cell carcinoma in situ. Squamous cell carcinomas are locally invasive. Histopathology of lesions progresses from well differentiated to poorly differentiated. Metastatic progression to regional lymph nodes occurs in 1%–3% of cases.

   b. Xeroderma pigmentosum is an autosomal recessive syndrome with germline mutations in one of the xeroderma pigmentosum nucleotide excision repair genes (*XPA* through *XPG*), resulting in photosensitivity and early onset and increased frequency of skin cancers, predominately squamous cell carcinoma.

5. **Clinical features** (Online Figure 13–23)

   a. Persistent lesions usually are detected on sun-exposed areas of the skin.

   b. The red, scaling plaques have variable degrees of firmness. Actinic keratoses are superficial without a palpable component.

   c. Large lesions (>1 cm) may be nodular with ulceration or secondary crusting.

   d. A subset of these carcinomas are considered high risk for metastasis. Risk factors for metastasis include location on the lower lip or ear, histologic features such as poor differentiation, invasion more than 4 mm into the dermis, perineural invasion, occurrence in immunosuppressed patients, and development in burn sites.

6. **Diagnosis.** The diagnosis of squamous cell carcinoma is made by clinical inspection of skin and confirmed by skin biopsy.

7. **Therapy**

   a. Surgery. The cure rate is 90%–99% depending on the tumor site and surgical technique. Surgical techniques include excision, Mohs micrographic surgery, curettage with electrodesiccation, and cryosurgery.

   b. Radiation therapy. The cure rate for primary squamous cell carcinoma is 90%. Prophylactic postoperative radiation to the site may be indicated in high-risk lesions.

   c. Topical therapy. Both 5′-fluorouracil cream and imiquimod cream are approved for topical treatment of squamous cell carcinoma in situ.

C **Melanoma**

1. **Definition.** Melanoma is the neoplastic growth of melanocytes.

2. **Epidemiology**

   a. Incidence. Close to 60,000 new cases of melanoma occur each year in the United States.

   b. Risk factors

      (1) Genetic. Ten percent of cases of melanoma are familial; at least one relative is affected. From 1% to 3% of cases of melanoma are hereditary; two or more first-degree relatives are affected with melanoma and have a germline mutation in the *CDKN2A* gene.

(2) Previous melanoma. Patients who have had one melanoma have a 5% probability of a second primary melanoma.

(3) Environmental. The risk of melanoma increases with increased UV exposure, particularly with an increased number of severe sunburns in individuals younger than 20 years of age.

(4) Pigmentation. The following factors are associated with an increased risk of melanoma.

    (a) Fair complexion (readily sunburns and never tans, blue eyes, red or blonde hair)

    (b) Increased number of melanocytic nevi (moles) (>25)

    (c) Presence of **large melanocytic nevi** (>6 mm)

    (d) Presence of **atypical (dysplastic) nevi** (>5 mm with varying degrees of irregular clinical features [see X C 5]).

3. Etiology. The multifactorial etiology includes genetic susceptibility and environmental exposure to UV light (sunlight).

4. Pathophysiology. The initial stages of neoplastic transformation result in upward (pagetoid) growth of cytologically atypical melanocytes within epidermis (in situ). Tumor progression results in invasion of underlying dermis and deeper tissues. Regional lymph node metastasis usually precedes metastasis to distant sites, typically skin, lung, brain, and liver. In most cases, *BRAF* gene mutations are detected in early melanoma tumor progression.

5. Clinical features. The vast majority of cutaneous melanomas have unstable clinical features that change over time. Characteristic features may be remembered using the mnemonic "ABCD" (Online Figure 13–24):

a. Asymmetry: a deviation in the overall round-to-oval configuration

b. Border: an irregular circumference of the lesion. The indistinct margins may blend into the flesh-colored background.

c. Color: nonuniformity of pigmentation with variations in color, including black, blue, and red hues

d. Diameter: generally greater than 6 mm for detection

6. Diagnosis. The diagnosis of melanoma is made by clinical inspection of skin and confirmed by excisional biopsy.

7. Staging Refer to American Joint Committee on Cancer (AJCC) 2002 guidelines for full details (Online Table 13–12).

a. Four clinical stages are defined for melanoma.

    (1) Stage I: skin involvement with a primary tumor <2 mm in thickness without ulceration.

    (2) Stage II: skin involvement with a primary tumor >2 mm in thickness with or without ulceration.

    (3) Stage III: any tumor with lymph node involvement

    (4) Stage IV: metastatic disease to distant skin and viscera

b. Sentinel lymph node mapping and biopsy is a surgical staging procedure that identifies the most likely lymph node draining the primary tumor. This technique is most often used in melanoma cases with primary tumor >1 mm in thickness and no evidence of lymphadenopathy or distant metastasis.

8. Therapy

a. Surgery

    (1) Primary excision. Surgical excision of primary tumor with clear margins is primary therapy.

    (2) Nodal dissection. Elective node dissection is controversial. Some investigators attribute a prophylactic benefit to node dissection for lesions 1.50–3.99 mm in depth. Lymphadenectomy is indicated for patients in whom adenopathy develops in the absence of metastatic disease.

b. Chemotherapy is of little benefit and does not confer a survival benefit in patients with metastatic disease. Drugs with documented activity include dacarbazine, cisplatin, and the nitrosoureas.

    (1) Dacarbazine is considered the best single agent, with a 15% response rate. Neither tamoxifen nor IFN-α adds to the response seen with dacarbazine.

    (2) The **combination of dacarbazine, carmustine, cisplatin, and tamoxifen** has been reported to have a 50% response rate. However, randomized clinical trials have not confirmed this rate.

c. **Biologic response modifiers** have modest antitumor activity in patients with metastatic disease.

   (1) **IFN-α** has a 15%–20% response rate, primarily in soft tissue and lung metastases. Adjuvant IFN therapy may improve the disease-free and overall survival rates for stage III patients and those with nodal metastases that are resected.

   (2) **High-dose IL-2** has elicited long-term complete responses in a small proportion of patients with metastatic melanoma. In phase II clinical trials, chemotherapy plus IL-2 and IFN-α had high response rates, but randomized phase III clinical trials have not confirmed these results.

   (3) Other experimental procedures include **antitumor vaccines** and **monoclonal antibody therapy.**

9. **Prognosis.** The Breslow depth, which is the thickness of the melanoma (depth of invasion) measured in millimeters from the stratum corneum to the deepest penetration of the tumor, is thought to be the best prognostic indicator. Prognostic factors associated with increased risk for melanoma metastasis include the following:

   a. Primary tumor depth of invasion (>1 mm)
   b. Primary tumor mitotic rate ($1/mm^2$)
   c. Primary tumor ulceration
   d. Vascular or lymphatic invasion
   e. Age >65 years
   f. Primary tumor located on trunk or head and neck
   g. Male sex

10. **Prevention**

    a. **Primary prevention** for melanoma involves sun avoidance. Recommendations include the following:

       (1) Avoid mid-day sun (10:00 AM to 2:00 PM) and artificial tanning.
       (2) Seek shade when possible.
       (3) Use protective clothing (hats, long sleeves, and sunglasses).
       (4) Frequently apply sunscreen with a sun protection factor (SPF) of 30 or higher.

    b. **Secondary prevention** for melanoma involves early detection and surveillance. Recommendations include the following:

       (1) Perform regular, periodic skin self-examination.
       (2) Have a skin examination and screening by a dermatologist (high-risk patients).
       (3) Have a biopsy of clinically suspicious pigmented lesions.

D **Cutaneous T Cell lymphoma**

1. **Definition.** Cutaneous T-cell lymphoma (CTCL) constitutes a clonal proliferation of malignant T lymphocytes (T cells). CTCL begins as an indolent lymphoma involving the skin but may progress to involve lymph nodes, blood, and other visceral organs. CTCL has two clinical variants.

   a. **Mycosis fungoides** classically evolves slowly through progressive stages of cutaneous involvement from the patch and plaque stage (stages I–II), through the tumor or erythrodermic stage (stage III), with progression to extracutaneous involvement (stage IV).

   b. **Sézary's syndrome,** the more rapidly progressing variant, presents as stage IV disease with diffuse skin involvement (erythroderma), lymphadenopathy, and leukocytosis characterized by the presence of lymphocytes with an atypical cerebriform nuclear morphology. These lymphocytes are referred to as Sézary cells.

2. **Epidemiology.** An estimated 1000 new cases of CTCL occur each year in the United States.

3. **Etiology.** The etiology of CTCL is unknown. It appears to be an acquired disease with no known risk factors, case clustering, or genetic predisposition.

4. **Pathophysiology.** Infiltration of the skin is characterized by the presence of neoplastic T cells within the epidermis (epidermotropism) as single cells or in clusters (**Pautrier microabscess**). Immunophenotyping of the neoplastic T cells shows expression of CD4 (helper subset) antigen. The constellation of immunologic abnormalities associated with CTCL has been closely correlated to aberrant Th-2 cytokine expression and regulation.

5. Clinical features

a. Early onset of lesions typically involve a **"bathing trunk" distribution,** including sun-protected areas: buttocks, hips, axillae, and women's breasts (🖰 Online Figure 13–25).

b. Lesions progress from patch, to plaque, and to tumors or erythroderma, and they involve an increasing percentage of the skin surface area.

(1) **Patches** are red, scaling macules with variable size (1–15 cm), shapes (round, oval, or crescent), and configurations (serpiginous or annular).

(2) **Plaques** are red, variably infiltrated plaques that typically evolve from patches.

(3) **Tumors** are reddish to violaceous nodules (1–15 cm) that often superficially ulcerate.

(4) **Exfoliative erythroderma** is diffuse redness and exfoliative scaling often associated with hyperkeratosis of the palms and soles and lymphadenopathy.

6. Diagnosis. The diagnosis of CTCL is made by clinical inspection of skin and confirmed by skin biopsy. Because CTCL may be slow to evolve, several skin biopsies may be necessary to diagnose.

7. Therapy

a. **Skin-directed therapy.** These therapies are typically used in early stages with no evidence of extracutaneous involvement. They may be combined with systemic therapies in advanced stages.

(1) Topical chemotherapy may be effective. Mechlorethamine (nitrogen mustard) or carmustine is mixed into a topical vehicle (water or ointment) and applied directly on the skin.

(2) Topical retinoids are used. Bexarotene gel has been approved for topical use in CTCL.

(3) Phototherapy is useful in CTCL.

(4) Electron beam radiation therapy has been shown to be very effective in resolving CTCL.

b. **Systemic therapies** are typically used in cases of evident extracutaneous involvement (blood, lymph nodes, or visceral organs).

(1) Biologic response modifiers are often used as single agents or in combination.

(a) IFN-α

(b) Extracorporeal photopheresis

(c) Retinoids (bexarotene)

(d) IL-2 fusion toxin (denileukin diftitox; toxin fused to IL-2 to selectively expose toxin only to malignant cells)

(2) Drugs used in both single-agent and combination chemotherapy of T cell non-Hodgkin's lymphomas also are used to treat CTCL.

XI CUTANEOUS INFECTIONS AND INFESTATIONS

[A] **Bacterial skin infections** usually start in areas of trauma or impaired barrier function of the skin. *Staphylococcus aureus* and *Streptococcus pyogenes* are the predominant organisms that cause skin infection in healthy, nonimmunocompromised individuals.

1. Clinical presentations

a. **Impetigo** is a superficial, intraepidermal, highly contagious vesiculopustular, often oozing eruption. Lesions have golden crusts (🖰 Online Figure 13–26). Frequency is highest in children.

b. **Cellulitis** is an acute spreading infection of the dermis and subcutaneous tissue manifested by warmth, erythema, swelling, and tenderness. *S. pyogenes* infections are often associated with ascending lymphangitis (🖰 Online Figure 13–27).

c. **Furuncle** is a deep necrotizing form of folliculitis that occurs as a warm, tender, erythematous, fluctuant, purulent nodule centered on a hair follicle. Several furuncles may coalesce, forming a carbuncle.

d. **Abscess** is a localized accumulation of purulent material deep in the dermis or subcutaneous tissue. The pus is usually not visible on the surface of the skin.

2. Therapy

a. **Impetigo.** Compresses to dry the area are necessary. Topical antibiotics (e.g., mupirocin) are used against *Staphylococcus* and *Streptococcus*. Systemic antibiotics also may be effective.

b. **Cellulitis.** Systemic antibiotics are used against *Staphylococcus* and *Streptococcus*.

c. **Furuncles and abscesses.** Lesions should be drained, and systemic antibiotic therapy should be used.

B **Fungal skin infections**

1. **Clinical presentations**
   a. **Dermatophytoses.** Dermatophytes cause a superficial fungal infection of the dead keratin of skin, hair, and nails. *Epidermophyton, Microsporum,* and *Trichophyton* species infect humans. Infection is characterized by erythematous and scaling macules with active raised borders, often with central clearing (ringworm).
      (1) **Tinea capitis** is infection of scalp hair and produces alopecia.
      (2) **Tinea corporis** is infection of the trunk and extremities (Online Figure 13–28).
      (3) **Tinea manuum** and **tinea pedis** are infections of the palms, soles, and interdigital webs. The resultant web space maceration often is the site of entry for secondary bacterial cellulitis.
      (4) **Tinea cruris** is infection of the groin.
      (5) **Tinea barbae** is infection of the beard area and neck. Males are typically affected.
      (6) **Tinea faciale** is infection of the face.
      (7) **Tinea unguium (onychomycosis)** is infection of the nail and produces thickened, yellow nails.
   b. **Candidiasis.** This superficial yeast infection (*Candida albicans*) affects moist intertriginous areas. Superficial pustules rapidly rupture, producing confluent erythematous, moist erosions with scaling borders and satellite lesions on the periphery (Online Figure 13–29).
   c. **Tinea versicolor.** Endogenous yeast forms (***Malassezia furfur***) cause numerous, well-marginated, finely scaly, oval-to-round pink, hypopigmented or hyperpigmented macules scattered over the trunk (Online Figure 13–30).

2. **Diagnosis.** KOH preparations and fungal cultures of scales confirm the clinical diagnosis.
   a. **Dermatophytoses.** Long-branched hyphae are apparent on KOH examination.
   b. **Candidiasis.** Budding spores (pseudohyphae) are apparent on KOH examination.
   c. **Tinea versicolor.** Spores and short hyphae ("spaghetti and meatballs") are apparent on KOH examination.

3. **Therapy**
   a. **Dermatophytoses** are treated with topical antifungal agents. Tinea capitis requires oral griseofulvin. Onychomycosis responds best to oral agents (e.g., griseofulvin, itraconazole, and terbinafine).
   b. **Candidiasis** is treated with topical antifungal creams. Care should be taken to keep areas of involvement dry. Rarely is systemic therapy needed.
   c. **Tinea versicolor** is treated with topical agents. It also responds to single doses of oral keto-conazole.

C **Viral skin infections**

1. **Clinical presentations**
   a. **Herpes simplex virus (HSV)** infections cause a prodrome of pain preceding the appearance of grouped vesicles on an erythematous base. Typically, HSV type 1 causes herpes labialis (cold sores, fever blisters), and HSV type 2 causes genital herpes. HSV infections tend to be recurrent and may be exacerbated by stress, the menstrual cycle, and immunosuppression (Online Figure 13–31).
   b. **Herpes zoster** infections (shingles) cause a prodrome of pain radiating along a dermatome before an eruption of multiple erythematous vesicles, which have a dermatomal distribution. Herpes zoster infections, which are ultimately caused by **varicella-zoster virus (VZV),** represent the reactivation of latent varicella virus (chickenpox) from the dorsal ganglia of spinal and central nerves (Online Figure 13–32).
   c. **Verruca vulgaris (warts)** are caused by **human papilloma virus** (HPV) infection of the epidermis. Fleshed-colored verrucous papules typically occur on the extremities (Online Figure 13–33).
      (1) **Verruca plana (flat warts)** are 2- to 4-mm, flat-topped, flesh-colored papules that affect the face.
      (2) **Condyloma acuminata** are genital warts that tend to develop cauliflower-like macerated papules.

2. Diagnosis

a. Tzanck smear detects multinucleated giant cells of both HSV and VZV. Direct fluorescent antibody staining and culture of blisters identify HSV.

b. Skin biopsy confirms the clinical impression of warts if needed and identifies lesions of bowenoid papulosis.

3. Therapy

a. HSV and herpes zoster. Systemic antivirals (acyclovir, valacyclovir, and famciclovir) reduce viral shedding and time to heal.

b. Warts. Therapy includes a variety of modalities such as **topical salicylic acid preparations, trichloroacetic acid, cryotherapy, laser therapy, curettage and electrodesiccation, and intralesional bleomycin or IFN-α.** Additional topical therapies for genital warts include **podophyllin** and **imiquimod.**

D **Rickettsial diseases** Rickettsiae are pleomorphic bacteria that are obligate intracellular parasites. Transmitted to humans by ticks and mites, they cause acute systemic infections that may be accompanied by a rash.

1. Clinical presentations. Rocky Mountain spotted fever. Tick-borne *Rickettsia rickettsii* causes fever, myalgias, headache, and a petechial rash that typically begins around wrists and ankles or trunk. Involvement of the palms and soles may occur after the fifth day of symptoms.

2. Diagnosis. Serology confirms the diagnosis of rickettsial diseases. Skin biopsy specimens of petechial lesions show vasculitis.

3. Therapy. Rickettsial diseases are treated with antibiotic therapy and supportive therapy. Doxycycline is the drug of choice. Rickettsialpox is a self-limiting disease, and occasionally antibiotics may not be necessary.

E **Infestations**

1. Clinical presentations

a. Scabies. This intensely pruritic and highly contagious infestation of the epidermis is caused by the *Sarcoptes scabiei* mite. The mite burrows into the skin. The resultant 1- to 3-mm burrows, papules, vesicles, and secondary excoriations are concentrated in the web spaces of the fingers, flexor aspects of the wrists, antecubital fossa, axilla, areola and nipples, umbilicus, buttocks, and feet (Online Figure 13–34).

b. Pediculosis. This infestation of the skin with **lice (ectoparasites)** is caused by *Pediculus humanus capitis* **(head louse),** *Pediculus humanus corporis* **(body louse),** and *Pthirus pubis* **(pubic louse).** Pediculosis spreads from person to person by close physical contact or through fomites (e.g., combs, clothes, hats, or linens). All forms produce itching with 2- to 4-mm erythematous papules, excoriations, and often crusting. Lice and **nits (eggs attached to hairs)** are visible on clinical inspection (Online Figures 13–35A and 13–35B).

2. Diagnosis

a. Scabies. Diagnosis is confirmed with microscopic examination of skin scrapings from primary lesions showing scabies mites and eggs.

b. Pediculosis. Diagnosis is confirmed with microscopic examination of nits and lice.

3. Therapy

a. Scabies. Scabicides (e.g., **permethrin**) are prescribed for patients, household members, and close personal contacts. All bed linen and clothing should be washed in hot water. Symptomatic treatment may involve antihistamines.

b. Pediculosis. Pediculicides (**permethrin, pyrethrin, lindane shampoo or lotion**) are applied topically and should be reapplied in 7 days. All contacts should be treated. Bed linen, clothing, and other materials (e.g., combs) should be washed in hot water.

XII CUTANEOUS DRUG REACTIONS

A **Definition** A cutaneous drug reaction is an adverse drug reaction involving the skin that results from exposure to a medication by ingestion, topical application, injection, instillation, insertion, or inhalation.

TABLE 13–14 Drugs Frequently Associated with Cutaneous Reactions	
Drug	**Reaction Rate (per 1000)**
Trimethoprim–sulfamethoxazole	59
Ampicillin	52
Semisynthetic penicillins	36
Corticotropin	28
Erythromycin	23
Sulfisoxazole	17
Penicillin G	16
Gentamicin sulfate	16
Practolol	16
Cephalosporins	13
Quinidine	12

B **Epidemiology** As many as 5% of courses of drug therapy are complicated by adverse drug reactions. Approximately 30% of hospitalized medical patients develop at least one adverse drug reaction during the course of their hospitalization (3 million each year in the United States), and 2%–3% of these patients develop skin reactions (60,000–90,000 each year).

 C **Etiology and pathophysiology**

D **Clinical features**

1. Cutaneous drug reactions vary in their presentation and include a wide array of primary lesions and skin findings (Online Table 13–13).

2. Some drugs are associated with an increased frequency of a particular cutaneous reaction. However, a drug may cause urticaria in one person, vasculitis in another, and erythema multiforme in another.

3. Some medications produce cutaneous reactions with greater frequency (Table 13–14).

E **Types of cutaneous drug reactions** The various cutaneous drug reactions are frequently associated with a prototype drug (Online Table 13–15).

   1. **Morbilliform eruption** (Online Figure 13–36)

     a. This measles-like eruption is the most common type of cutaneous drug reaction.

     b. The primary lesion is a minute, erythematous macule that often fades with pressure. Lesions form larger areas of confluence, causing widespread and symmetric erythema.

   2. **Urticarial eruption**

     a. Urticaria is the second-most-common type of cutaneous drug reaction [see Chapter 8 IV].

     b. Drugs may cause urticaria by immunologic (IgE dependent or immune complex dependent) or nonimmunologic (direct histamine liberation) mechanisms.

   3. **Lichenoid eruption.** Drugs may cause lichen planus-like eruptions [see VI B]. Mucosal involvement is rare.

   4. **Vasculitis** (Online Figure 13–37).

     a. Vasculitis occurs as palpable purpura as a result of blood vessel damage and extravasations of erythrocytes into the dermis.

     b. Patients often present with vasculitis in dependent areas (e.g., legs).

     c. Allopurinol is the prototype causal drug. Thiazides and sulfonamides also may cause vasculitis.

   5. **Erythema multiforme** [see VI A]. Sulfonamides are the prototype causal drugs. Barbiturates, hydantoins, and thiazides also may cause erythema multiforme.

   6. **Exfoliative erythroderma** (Online Figure 13–38). Exfoliative erythroderma occurs as a generalized erythema with exfoliative scaling. Mucous membranes are usually spared.

   7. **Toxic epidermal necrolysis** (TEN) (Online Figure 13–39). TEN occurs as a fulminating, generalized sloughing of skin with complete necrosis of epidermis comparable to second-degree burn. Mucous membranes are severely affected. Mortality is high [see VI A 4 c].

8. **Pigmentary alterations.** These changes may occur in response to a medication through a variety of mechanisms.
    a. Increased melanin production often results in macular hyperpigmentation of the face termed **melasma** (🔊 Online Figure 13–40) and is often associated with oral contraceptive use.
    b. Deposition of pigmented materials results from heavy metals (e.g., silver nitrate).
    c. Deposition of lipofuscin results from amiodarone.

9. **Acneiform eruption** (🔊 Online Figure 13–41).
    a. Drug-induced acne has a rapid onset of acneiform lesions in a similar stage of development involving areas other than the face.
    b. Acneiform eruptions may occur at any age.

10. **Pustular eruption: acute generalized exanthematous pustulosis (AGEP)**
    a. **AGEP**
    b. Scarlatiniform erythema disseminates rapidly and is accompanied by >100 nonfollicular pustules. Typically occurs within 5 days of taking causative medication. Fever is universal.

11. **Erythema nodosum** [see VI E].

12. **Fixed drug eruption** (🔊 Online Figure 13–42).
    a. A fixed drug eruption produces a demarcated oval or circular erythema that heals with residual hyperpigmentation. Lesions tend to be solitary but may be multiple.
    b. Reexposure to the offending drug causes lesions to develop in the same location.

13. **Lupus-like syndrome** (🔊 Online Figure 13–43). The cutaneous findings of drug-induced lupus are usually indistinguishable from those of systemic lupus erythematosus.

14. **Photosensitivity eruptions** (🔊 Online Figure 13–44).
    a. Photosensitivity reactions require the presence of both light and the inciting drug.
    b. Specific wavelengths of light known as the "action spectrum" (285–425 nm) are required to initiate a photosensitive drug reaction.
    c. A **phototoxic reaction** (nonimmunologic) results from direct cellular injury when a drug is photoactivated by light.
    d. A **photoallergic reaction** (immune mediated) results when light interacts with a drug to produce an immunogenic intermediate or metabolite that stimulates an immune response.

15. **Drug-induced linear IgA dermatosis** (LAD) (🔊 Online Figure 13–45).
    a. The heterogeneous pruritic lesions include tense bullae. There is a predominately extensor distribution with mucosal involvement in approximately 70% of cases.
    b. DIF of skin biopsy specimens shows linear deposits of IgA along the basement membrane that are identical to those found in idiopathic cases of LAD of adult and childhood.
    c. IgA autoantibodies target collagen XVII (BPAG 2) and type VII collagen.

F **Diagnosis**   A cutaneous drug reaction should be suspected in any widespread rash of rapid onset.

1. It is critical to obtain a complete drug history.
    a. Ask specifically about tonics, laxatives, sedatives, tranquilizers, pain medications, vitamins, oral contraceptive pills, eye drops, inhalants, immunizations, and suppositories.
    b. In hospitalized patients, check the patient's chart for medication orders, including PRN (as-needed) medications, STAT (immediate) orders, anesthetics, and diagnostic agents (e.g., contrast media and radioactive tracers).

2. Determine which drug is the most likely causal agent.
    a. Drugs started within 1 week before the appearance of the eruption are most likely causal.
    b. Drugs with a high frequency of cutaneous reactions are most likely causal.
    c. Drugs commonly causing the morphologic pattern present clinically should be suspected.

3. A skin biopsy may assist in making a diagnosis. Although there is no single histologic finding diagnostic of a drug eruption, other causes of the eruption may be ruled out.

G **Therapy**

1. The causal drug should be discontinued if possible. Some clinical situations prevent discontinuation of the causal drug.

2. Topical or systemic corticosteroids (for relatively severe eruptions) may produce symptomatic relief.

3. Antihistamines may help relieve associated pruritus.

4. Topical care consists of soothing baths or compresses and appropriate dressings. When present, secondary infections should be treated.

XIII SELECTED CUTANEOUS MANIFESTATIONS OF SYSTEMIC DISEASES

A **General considerations** The skin is often affected by systemic diseases. Cutaneous manifestations of systemic diseases may develop concurrently as a disease progresses or may be one of the early signs and symptoms leading to an initial diagnosis. Recognition of associated cutaneous manifestations aids in the diagnosis and management of many systemic diseases.

B **Stasis dermatitis**

1. **Definition. Stasis dermatitis** is a common inflammatory skin disease that occurs on the lower extremities in individuals with chronic venous insufficiency. Stasis dermatitis is the earliest skin change associated with venous insufficiency and may lead to venous leg ulceration and fibrosis.

2. **Epidemiology.** The estimated prevalence of stasis dermatitis is approximately 6%–7% in individuals older than 50 years of age.

3. **Etiology.** Venous insufficiency is the underlying cause of the cutaneous changes seen in stasis dermatitis/lipodermatosclerosis.

4. **Pathophysiology**
   a. Decreased competency of the one-way valvular system in the deep venous plexus of the legs results in backflow of blood from the deep venous system to the superficial venous system, producing venous hypertension. The link between venous hypertension and cutaneous changes is not precisely understood.
   b. Venous hypertension produces increased flow rates and high oxygen tension, contrary to early theories that hypothesized that an incompetent venous system leads to pooling of blood and reduced blood flow and oxygen tension in dermal capillaries.
   c. Increased venous hydrostatic pressure increases permeability of the dermal microcirculation and results in the formation of fibrin cuffs around dermal capillaries. However, fibrin cuffs have not been found to decrease oxygen diffusion significantly.
   d. Venous hypertension has been shown to result in leukocyte trapping in the microcirculation that may result in the increased release of inflammatory mediators and leukocyte sludging that contribute to tissue ischemia.

5. **Clinical features** (Online Figure 13–46).
   a. Acute and chronic changes, including edema, varicosities, and diffuse red-brown discoloration representing dermal deposits of hemosiderin (from degraded, extravasated erythrocytes), may occur against a background of skin changes.
   b. Clinical changes occur bilaterally. The medial ankle is most frequently and severely involved.
   c. Early findings include erythematous scaling of a lower extremity.
   d. Exudative, weeping patches, and plaques may be associated with secondary infection.
   e. Ulceration may occur and generally tends to be medial with exudative bases. Healing results in scarring.
   f. Lichenification and hyperpigmentation may occur as a consequence of chronic scratching and rubbing. Induration, fibrosis, and scarring may result with constriction around the ankles, producing an inverted bowling pin appearance in the lower leg (lipodermatosclerosis).

6. **Diagnosis.** Clinical inspection and venous Doppler studies establish the diagnosis of stasis dermatitis/lipodermatosclerosis in the setting of venous insufficiency. Skin biopsies are rarely indicated but rule out other diagnoses, especially when ulceration is present.

7. **Therapy**
   a. Topical therapy is directed at the relief of signs and symptoms. Treatments include compresses for weeping lesions, local wound care for ulcerations, and short-term use of mid-potency topical corticosteroids for reducing symptomatic inflammation and itching.
   b. Obvious superficial infections (impetiginization) should be treated with topical mupirocin or a systemic antibiotic with activity against *Staphylococcus* and *Streptococcus* species.

    c. Maintenance therapy requires use of moisturizers to prevent dryness and breakdown of the skin.

    d. Compression stockings and elevation of legs at rest are important mainstays of maintenance and prevention. Arterial insufficiency is often present in patients with venous insufficiency; therefore, assessing the patient's peripheral arterial circulation with a Doppler study is advised before recommending compression therapy.

C Cutaneous sarcoidosis

1. **Definition.** Sarcoidosis is characterized by noncaseating epithelioid granulomas that primarily affect the lungs. The lymphatic (especially pulmonary lymph nodes), ophthalmic, nervous, musculoskeletal, hepatic, cardiac, renal, and endocrine systems are also affected. In addition, the skin is often affected, and recognition and evaluation of these skin lesions often aids in establishing the diagnosis.

2. **Epidemiology.** The incidence of sarcoidosis is 1–40 per 100,000 population in the United States. It is more prevalent among African Americans than among whites.

3. **Etiology.** The exact etiology of sarcoidosis has not been clearly defined. Immunogenetic susceptibility and environmental exposure influence disease expression. Etiologic agents may include infections, environmental agents, or autoantigens.

4. **Pathophysiology.** Impaired humoral and cellular responses have been documented in patients with sarcoidosis. Chronic antigen exposure may lead to a chronic Th1 cytokine–driven response, which results in granuloma formation.

5. **Clinical features** (Online Figure 13–47).
   a. Macular or papular sarcoidosis is the most common morphology in cutaneous sarcoidosis and is characterized by asymptomatic red-brown macules and papules often involving the face, periorbital, nasolabial folds, or extensor surfaces.
   b. **Lupus pernio** is the most distinctive of sarcoid skin lesions and is characterized by reddish to violaceous indurated plaques and nodules that usually affect the nostrils, cheeks, ears, and lips. This is associated with an increased risk of pulmonary sarcoidosis.
   c. Plaque sarcoidosis is characterized by round-to-oval, red-brown to violaceous infiltrated plaques, which are often distributed symmetrically and have an annular appearance. The center of the plaques may be atrophic or scaly.
   d. Subcutaneous nodular sarcoidosis (Darier–Roussy sarcoidosis) is characterized by nontender, firm, flesh-colored or violaceous 0.5- to 2-cm nodules that are commonly found on the extremities or on the trunk.
   e. Scars from previous trauma may become infiltrated and tender with a reddish or violaceous color.
   f. Erythema nodosum is a hypersensitivity reaction that may develop in the setting of sarcoidosis. It is often associated with hilar lymphadenopathy, anterior uveitis, or polyarthritis (Löfgren's syndrome). This indicates a good prognosis.

6. **Diagnosis.** Clinical inspection and skin biopsy demonstrating diagnostic noncaseating granulomas are the basis of diagnosis. Additional skin biopsy specimens should be sent for special stains and cultures to rule out infectious causes of granuloma formation, including mycobacterial and deep fungal infections.

7. **Therapy.** Treatment of underlying manifestations is paramount.
   a. Topical or intralesional corticosteroids (triamcinolone acetonide) may be used to treat cutaneous lesions.
   b. To avoid scarring, systemic immunosuppressants are used for recalcitrant lesions that do not respond to intralesional corticosteroids. Immunosuppressants for cutaneous sarcoidosis include methotrexate, azathioprine, and chlorambucil. Other reportedly useful therapeutic agents include antimalarial drugs (hydroxychloroquine and chloroquine), cyclosporine, oral isotretinoin, allopurinol, and thalidomide.

D Dermatitis herpetiformis

1. **Definition.** Dermatitis herpetiformis is an autoimmune blistering skin disease associated with gluten-sensitive enteropathy (GSE, celiac disease).

2. **Epidemiology.** The estimated frequency of dermatitis herpetiformis in the United States is approximately 39 cases per 100,000 population.

3. **Etiology.** Deposits of IgA in the skin lead to pruritic blistering in patients with GSE.

4. **Pathophysiology**
   a. Pathogenesis is associated with the presence of GSE, an increased expression of HLA-A1, HLA-B8, HLA-DR3, and HLA-DQ2 haplotypes, and granular deposition of IgA at the DEJ of the skin.
   b. Susceptible individuals, as determined by HLA haplotype, may develop a cell-mediated immune response resulting in T cell activation in the small bowel mucosa exacerbated by a sensitivity to gluten, a protein present in barley, rye, and wheat but not in rice.
   c. Cutaneous inflammation is predominated by a dermal infiltrate of neutrophils with microabscess formation and progression to subepidermal vesicle formation through the lamina lucida of the basement membrane zone. DIF shows a granular deposition of IgA.

5. **Clinical features**
   a. Skin lesions are extremely pruritic groups of erythematous vesicles, most frequently located on extensor surfaces.
   b. Lesions often are pustular or crusted from excoriation.

6. **Diagnosis.** Skin biopsy and DIF confirm the diagnosis.

7. **Therapy.** Dapsone and sulfapyridine are the primary drugs used in treatment. Relief of symptoms may be seen within 24–48 hours of the start of therapy. Patients may choose to control the skin disease with a gluten-free diet.

E Calciphylaxis

1. **Definition.** Calciphylaxis is the phenomenon of vascular calcification and skin necrosis in end-stage renal disease (ESRD).

2. **Epidemiology.** Calciphylaxis is extremely rare in the general population, affecting 1%–4% of patients with ESRD.

3. **Etiology.** The precise etiology is uncertain, but hypercalcemia, hyperphosphatemia, elevated calcium phosphate products, and secondary hyperparathyroidism associated with ESRD are contributing factors. In the absence of renal disease, there are case reports of occurrence of calciphylaxis in association with primary hyperparathyroidism, cirrhosis, and rheumatoid arthritis.

4. **Pathophysiology**
   a. The pathogenesis is poorly defined. Vascular calcification is a constant finding and may sensitize the vascular microenvironment to hypercoagulability or promote intimal hyperplasia and vascular occlusion.
   b. Alternatively, extensive endothelial calcification and intimal hyperplasia, which are known to compromise the luminal size of vessels in calciphylaxis, may result in vascular occlusion. These mechanisms remain hypothetical and have not yet been proven to lead to calciphylaxis.

5. **Clinical features**
   a. Early lesions of calciphylaxis develop suddenly and progress rapidly as nonspecific violaceous mottling or as erythematous papules, plaques, or nodules.
   b. Lesions progress with a stellate purpuric configuration with central necrosis and are extremely painful and tender.
   c. Lesions may be singular or numerous.
   d. Lesions may occur either distally on the lower legs or proximally in areas of body fat, such as the lower abdomen, thighs, and buttocks.

6. **Diagnosis.** The diagnosis is confirmed by incisional skin biopsy with adequate sampling of the subcutaneous tissue. Laboratory studies evaluating renal, endocrine, and coagulation status should be ordered.

7. **Therapy.** Local treatment involves wound care with debridement to avoid wound infection and sepsis. Hyperbaric oxygen therapy may be useful.

F **Porphyria cutanea tarda**

1. **Definition.** Porphyria cutanea tarda (PCT) is a photosensitive blistering disorder that results from a hereditary or acquired deficiency in the activity of the hepatic heme synthetic enzyme uroporphyrinogen decarboxylase (URO-D).

2. **Epidemiology.** The exact incidence of PCT in the United States is not known but is estimated to be approximately 3 per 100,000 people. PCT is the most common type of porphyria.

3. **Etiology.** Germline mutations in the gene encoding URO-D are detected in individuals affected with familial forms of PCT. Clinical expression of both the familial and acquired forms often requires exposure to hepatotoxic agents or conditions, including ethanol, estrogens, excess iron stores, hepatitis C virus, and human immunodeficiency virus (HIV).

4. **Pathophysiology.** Reduced hepatic URO-D activity results in overproduction of uroporphyrin (URO) and coproporphyrin (COPRO). Both URO and COPRO are water soluble and are excreted in elevated levels in the urine. In addition, they are photoactive molecules and absorb energy from visible light and produce a phototoxic reaction that results in increased mechanical fragility of the skin after sunlight exposure.

5. **Clinical features** (🔴 Online Figure 13–48).
   a. Fragility of sun-exposed skin after mechanical trauma is the most common finding. This leads to erosions and tense bullae on the dorsal aspects of the hands, forearms, and face.
   b. Healing of crusted erosions and blisters leaves scars, milia (tiny subepidermal keratinous cysts), and hyperpigmented and hypopigmented atrophic patches.
   c. Hypertrichosis and hyperpigmentation are often visible over the temporal and malar facial areas.
   d. Scleroderma-like changes may occur over the preauricular face, neck, chest, and the back. These sclerodermoid plaques can develop dystrophic calcification.
   e. A urine sample is often grossly discolored with a tea- or wine-colored tint.

6. **Diagnosis**
   a. The diagnosis is confirmed by a history of photosensitivity, characteristic skin findings, a skin biopsy for histology and DIF (which is negative for immunoreactants), and elevated URO and COPRO levels in a 24-hour urine collection.
   b. Any underlying etiology or associated disorder should be evaluated with laboratory studies, including hematologic and iron profiles, liver function tests, and screening for hepatitis and HIV.

7. **Therapy**
   a. Exacerbating factors should be eliminated or minimized. Such measures include avoidance of sunlight, elimination of alcohol, and discontinuation of estrogen when possible.
   b. Therapeutic phlebotomy is often successful in reducing excess iron stores in tissue, which is followed by improvement of deregulated heme synthesis due to URO-D inhibition. One unit of whole blood is removed weekly every 2–3 weeks, as tolerated by the patient.
   c. When phlebotomy is contraindicated, low doses of chloroquine phosphate or hydroxychloroquine sulfate may be prescribed. These drugs displace hepatic iron stores. Large doses can cause severe hepatotoxicity.

Study Questions

1. A middle-aged man who has recently begun taking captopril and hydrochlorothiazide for hypertension develops an itchy rash in sun-exposed areas. What is the most likely cutaneous diagnosis?

- (A) Urticaria
- (B) Erythema multiforme
- (C) Photosensitivity reaction
- (D) Erythema nodosum
- (E) Vasculitis

2. An adolescent girl presents with a 1-year history of acne that she has been treating with over-the-counter medications. Examination shows comedones and an occasional inflammatory papule on the face. She inquires about isotretinoin and would like to know whether it would be appropriate for her acne. You inform her that isotretinoin is indicated for the treatment of which of the following types of acne?

- (A) Comedonal acne
- (B) Mild inflammatory acne
- (C) Moderate inflammatory acne
- (D) Nodulocystic acne
- (E) Steroid acne

3. A young man presents with widespread acute allergic contact dermatitis to poison ivy. Which of the following formulations is likely to be the most therapeutically effective?

- (A) Low-potency corticosteroid cream
- (B) High-potency corticosteroid cream
- (C) Mid- to high-potency corticosteroid ointment
- (D) Short burst of systemic steroids
- (E) Three-week systemic steroid taper

4. A young woman develops an acute flare of plaque-type psoriasis on her trunk and extremities. Which of the following formulations is likely to be the most therapeutically effective?

- (A) Low-potency corticosteroid cream
- (B) High-potency corticosteroid cream
- (C) Mid- to high-potency corticosteroid solution
- (D) Mid- to high-potency corticosteroid ointment
- (E) Systemic corticosteroid treatment

5. A middle-aged man develops an acute flare of scalp psoriasis. Which of the following formulations is likely to be the most therapeutically effective?

- (A) Low-potency corticosteroid cream
- (B) High-potency corticosteroid cream
- (C) Mid- to high-potency corticosteroid solution
- (D) Mid- to high-potency corticosteroid ointment
- (E) Systemic corticosteroid treatment

6. A middle-aged woman develops an acute flare of seborrheic dermatitis affecting the nasolabial folds of her face. Which of the following formulations is likely to be the most therapeutically effective?

- (A) Low-potency corticosteroid cream
- (B) High-potency corticosteroid cream
- (C) Mid- to high-potency corticosteroid solution
- (D) Mid- to high-potency corticosteroid ointment
- (E) Systemic corticosteroid treatment

7. A 40-year-old woman develops painful ulcers in her mouth followed by a blistering eruption on the trunk. Examination shows erosions on the soft palate and pharynx as well as 0.5- to 1.5-cm crusted superficial erosions and flaccid bullae on the trunk. Skin biopsy reveals epidermal acantholysis and IgG intercellular staining. What is the most likely diagnosis?

[A] Bullous pemphigoid
[B] Pemphigus vulgaris
[C] Paraneoplastic pemphigus
[D] Erythema multiforme
[E] Porphyria cutanea tarda

8. A 35-year-old woman with a history of Crohn's disease develops a painful nodule on her lower leg that soon ulcerates. Examination shows an extremely tender, deep, 8 × 10–cm ulceration with a purulent base and erythematous undermined borders. What is the most likely diagnosis?

[A] Erythema nodosum
[B] Stasis dermatitis
[C] Pyoderma gangrenosum
[D] Vasculitis
[E] Calciphylaxis

9. A middle-aged man presents with a red rash on the abdomen. Examination shows a 5-cm erythematous scaling plaque with central clearing. A potassium hydroxide preparation from a scraping of the scales shows branched hyphae. What is the most accurate diagnosis?

[A] Candidiasis
[B] Tinea versicolor
[C] Herpes simplex
[D] Tinea capitis
[E] Tinea corporis

10. An elderly woman with Parkinson's disease presents with a red scaling rash on the face that has waxed and waned for several months. Examination shows mild erythema with greasy scales predominantly over the eyebrows and nasolabial folds with extension onto the malar surfaces of the face. What is the most likely diagnosis?

[A] Psoriasis
[B] Tinea versicolor
[C] Lupus erythematosus
[D] Seborrheic dermatitis
[E] Allergic contact dermatitis

11. A 55-year-old man presents with a chronic rash over the buttocks and hips that has been unresponsive to topical steroids. It has recently started to itch. Examination shows 6- to 12-cm erythematous, scaling plaques in a "bathing trunk" distribution. Potassium hydroxide preparation is negative for evidence of a fungal infection. A skin biopsy indicates an atypical lymphocytic infiltrate with evidence of epidermotropism and Pautrier microabscess formation. What is the most likely diagnosis?

[A] Impetigo
[B] Psoriasis
[C] Cutaneous T cell lymphoma (mycosis fungoides)
[D] Tinea corporis
[E] Atopic dermatitis

12. A 48-year-old woman with a fair complexion presents with a 4-mm pearly papule with a central crust located on the medial canthus of the right eye. A skin biopsy shows a well-circumscribed basal cell carcinoma. Which of the following clinical features makes the risk of recurrence of basal cell carcinoma high?

[A] Size of the lesion
[B] Fair complexion

C Histologic features
D Location of the lesion
E Gender

13. A 65-year-old man with a fair complexion presents with a 9-mm hyperkeratotic, erythematous plaque on the left jaw and no regional lymphadenopathy. A skin biopsy shows a poorly differentiated squamous cell carcinoma of skin with evidence of perineural invasion. Which of the following clinical features makes the risk of metastasis in squamous cell carcinoma high?

A Size of the lesion
B Fair complexion
C Histologic features
D Location of the lesion
E Gender

14. A middle-aged woman presents with an itchy eruption over her arms and trunk several days after gardening. Skin examination shows the changes seen in the ⊘ online photo. What is the mostly likely diagnosis?

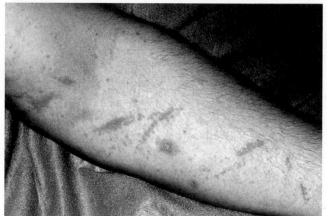

A Allergic contact dermatitis
B Herpes simplex infection
C Bullous pemphigoid
D Atopic dermatitis
E Vasculitis

15. An elderly man presents with a blistering eruption over the left thoracic back, flank, and chest. It developed shortly after he began to experience intense burning and pain in the affected areas. Examination shows grouped vesicles on an erythematous base in a dermatomal distribution over the left torso. A Tzanck smear from one of the vesicles shows the findings shown in the ⊘ online photo. What is the mostly likely diagnosis?

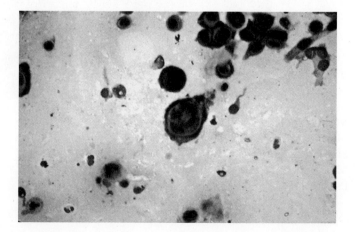

A Scabies mite infestation
B Pemphigus vulgaris associated with acantholytic cells
C Herpes zoster associated with multinucleated giant cells
D Herpes simplex associated with multinucleated giant cells
E Impetigo associated with gram-positive cocci

16. A middle-aged woman complains of severe sunburn 1 day after going to the beach and 2 days after initiating a course of oral sulfamethoxazole–trimethoprim for a bladder infection. Skin examination shows changes shown in the 🖱 online photo. What is the mostly likely diagnosis?

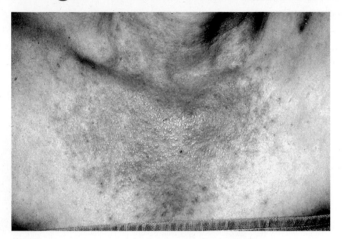

A Lichen planus
B Atopic dermatitis
C Seborrheic dermatitis
D Psoriasis
E Photosensitivity reaction

17. A middle-aged woman notes an asymptomatic dark area on her trunk several weeks after taking over-the-counter laxatives for constipation. Skin examination shows the changes shown in the 🖱 online photo. What is the mostly likely diagnosis?

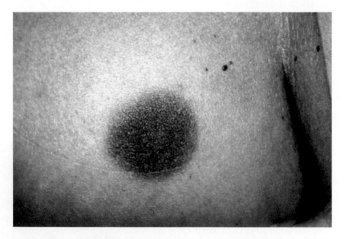

A Melasma
B Melanocytic nevus (mole)
C Fixed drug eruption
D Melanoma
E Psoriasis

18. A pregnant woman develops painful nodules on her legs. Skin examination shows the changes shown in the 🖱 online photo. What is the mostly likely diagnosis?

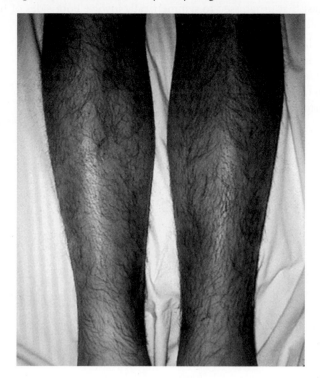

  A Stasis dermatitis
  B Cellulitis
  C Vasculitis
  D Erythema nodosum
  E Erythema multiforme

19. What histologic characteristic of the lesion pictured in the 🖱 online photo is the best prognostic indicator for this patient?

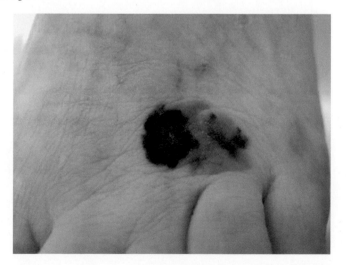

  A Ulceration
  B Mitoses per high-powered field
  C Degree of inflammatory infiltrate
  D Breslow depth
  E Perineural invasion

20. A 26-year-old man comes to your office complaining of an itchy rash on his back that developed over the last 2 weeks. He reports that the rash initially started as a small, scaly, raised, oval-shaped lesion on his chest that progressed to symmetrically involve both sides of his back in a "Christmas tree" like pattern. Which of the following is the most appropriate next step?

A Initiate topical antifungal treatment
B Initiate topical steroid treatment
C Initiate systemic steroid treatment
D No treatment for self-limited condition
E Perform skin biopsy

Answers and Explanations

1. The answer is C [XII E 14]. Hydrochlorothiazide is associated with a high frequency of photosensitivity. Captopril, an angiotensin-converting-enzyme inhibitor, is associated with a high frequency of papulosquamous skin reactions. The clinical findings do not support the diagnoses of urticaria, erythema multiforme, erythema nodosum, or vasculitis.

2. The answer is D [IV A 7 b (2)]. Isotretinoin is only indicated for the treatment of severe and recalcitrant nodulocystic acne. This agent should not be prescribed for milder forms of acne. Steroid acne responds to the discontinuation of systemic steroids and topical tretinoin.

3–6. The answers are: 3—B [III 📖 Online Table 13–5], **4—D** [III 📖 Online Table 13–5], **5—C** [III 📖 Online Table 13–5], **6—A** [III 📖 Online Table 13–5]. Both the potency and the vehicle of a topical corticosteroid must be appropriate for the specific clinical setting. High-potency topical steroids are used for the short-term treatment of acute and severe inflammatory eruptions. A cream has drying effects, and a high-potency steroid cream is well suited for treatment of a vesicular allergic contact dermatitis. An ointment has moisturizing effects, and a mid- to high-potency steroid ointment is highly effective for treating dry, scaly psoriatic plagues. Solutions and lotions are the vehicle of choice for the scalp; therefore, a mid- to high-potency steroid solution is effective for treating a flare of scalp psoriasis. Low-potency topical steroids are the only steroids used on the face. The drying effects of a cream are desirable for a greasy, scaling flare of seborrheic dermatitis in this location. Systemic corticosteroids are not necessary except in more severe and widespread dermatologic cases.

7. The answer is B [V B]. Pemphigus vulgaris typically affects middle-aged individuals and often presents with dysphagia and oral involvement. Bullae are flaccid, and direct immunofluorescence shows IgG intercellular staining. Conversely, bullous pemphigoid rarely involves oral mucosa and usually presents with tense bullae with linear IgG and C3 along the dermal–epidermal junction. Paraneoplastic pemphigus is characterized by severe oral involvement and heterogeneous skin lesions with histologic and direct immunofluorescent features of both pemphigus and pemphigoid. Erythema multiforme usually is characterized by target-like lesions on the palms and soles and distinct histopathology. Porphyria cutanea tarda is characterized by photosensitivity and tense bullae in a photodistribution and is associated with elevated urinary porphyrins.

8. The answer is C [VI D]. The clinical findings of a deep purulent and painful ulcer are typical of pyoderma gangrenosum, which often is associated with inflammatory bowel disease. Erythema nodosum is not an ulcerative process. Stasis dermatitis may be ulcerative but not to the extent of pyoderma gangrenosum. Palpable purpura is the hallmark of vasculitis (severe cases may result in ulceration). Calciphylaxis produces necrotic skin lesions.

9. The answer is E [XI B]. Dermatophyte infection of the body (tinea corporis) typically produces annular lesions that, on potassium hydroxide (KOH) preparation, show branched hyphae. Candidiasis produces pustules that form coalescent areas of erythema, typically in intertriginous areas, and KOH examination shows budding spores. Tinea versicolor produces confluent, scaling macules on the trunk, and KOH examination shows spores and nonbranched hyphae. Herpes simplex is a blistering eruption, and a Tzanck smear shows multinucleated giant cells. Tinea capitis is a dermatophyte infection that affects the scalp.

10. The answer is D [VII D]. Greasy scales along the T-zone of the face are typical of seborrheic dermatitis. Flares of seborrheic dermatitis are seen in patients with Parkinson's disease. Psoriasis and tinea versicolor rarely affect the face. Lupus erythematosus is characterized by a more prominent malar erythema and does not significantly involve the eyebrows and nasolabial fold. Allergic contact dermatitis is typically characterized by linear features to its configuration.

11. The answer is C [X D]. A papulosquamous eruption in a bathing trunk distribution can be seen with cutaneous T cell lymphoma, tinea corporis, or possibly psoriasis. The skin biopsy shows diagnostic changes with atypical lymphocytes infiltrating the epidermis (epidermotropism) and forming clusters within the epidermis (Pautrier microabscess). Impetigo typically has golden crusts as a predominant feature. Atopic dermatitis predominantly affects flexor areas.

12. The answer is D [X A]. The location of a basal cell carcinoma on the medial canthus of the eye determines where a lesion is at high risk for recurrence. The central face (eyes and nose) and ears are high-risk areas for recurrence of basal cell carcinoma. A fair complexion is associated with an increased incidence of basal cell carcinoma, both high- and low-risk lesions, and is not a clinical feature specific for high-risk basal cell carcinoma. Histologic features such as fibrosis (morpheaform basal cell carcinoma) and skip areas (multicentric basal cell carcinoma) are associated with high risk of recurrence for basal cell carcinoma. Gender is not a factor in determining the risk of basal cell carcinoma.

13. The answer is C [X B]. Two histologic features of a squamous cell carcinoma that are associated with high risk for metastasis are poor differentiation and perineural invasion. Other factors such as location on the lower lip and size greater than 1 cm also contribute to metastasis. In this patient, the lesion is on the left jaw, and it is just less than 1 cm in diameter. Gender and complexion do not increase the risk for metastasis.

14. The answer is A [VII C]. The photo demonstrates erythematous macules and vesicles in a distinctive linear configuration. Such a configuration is typical of a contact dermatitis. Grouped vesicles, typical of herpes simplex infection, are not seen. Tense bullae, typical of bullous pemphigoid, is not present. Flexor involvement, typical of atopic dermatitis, is not seen. There is no evidence of palpable purpura, typical of vasculitis.

15. The answer is C [XI C 1 a]. The photo demonstrates a Tzanck smear (stained with Giemsa stain) of scraping from blisters showing multinucleated giant cells. Multinucleated giant cells can be seen on Tzanck smears of herpes zoster and herpes simplex. The patient has a typical presentation of herpes zoster because of the clinical history of neuritic pain associated with blistering in a dermatomal distribution. Scabies can be visualized with scraping of web-space burrows from patients with scabies. Acantholytic cells can be visualized when scraping blisters of pemphigus vulgaris. A Gram stain of impetigo reveals gram-positive cocci of *Staphylococcus* or *Streptococcus* species.

16. The answer is E [XII E 14]. The photo demonstrates an erythematous maculopapular eruption with a sharp and discrete border, outlining the V of the neck, indicative of a photodistribution. The history indicates that the patient was started on sulfamethoxazole, which has a high frequency of photosensitive reactions. The distribution and clinical features seen in the figure are not typical of lichen planus, atopic dermatitis, seborrheic dermatitis, or psoriasis.

17. The answer is C [XII E 12]. The photo demonstrates a well-circumscribed, slate gray, hyperpigmented area typical of a fixed drug eruption. Phenolphthalein, a common ingredient of over-the-counter laxatives, is associated with a high frequency of fixed drug eruptions. Melasma is hyperpigmentation, typically on the face. The history and slate gray color are not typical of a melanocytic nevus. The lesion is well circumscribed with no features of asymmetry or pigment irregularity that can be seen in melanoma. Psoriasis does not produce pigmented lesions.

18. The answer is D [VI E]. The photo demonstrates inflammatory nodules on the lower extremity, which is typical of erythema nodosum. Pregnancy is associated with erythema nodosum. Stasis dermatitis is characterized by confluent changes about the ankles. Cellulitis typically affects one extremity with confluent erythema. Vasculitis is characterized by palpable purpura. Erythema multiforme is characterized by target lesions distributed peripherally.

19. The answer is D [X C 9]. The patient has a lesion that is consistent with melanoma. Although all the factors listed affect the prognosis of patients with melanoma, the best prognostic indicator is the thickness of the melanoma (i.e., depth of invasion) from the stratum corneum to the deepest penetration of the tumor, also known as the Breslow depth.

20. The answer is D [IX G]. The patient has a rash that is consistent with pityriasis rosea. Reassurance that the condition is self-limited is the most appropriate next step. Topical antifungals, steroids, or systemic steroid treatment are not warranted at this time. Skin biopsy is not indicated at this time either.

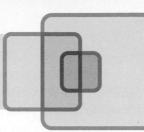

Case Studies in Clinical Decision Making

CASE 1

Healthy 62-Year-Old Man with Painful Knee

A 62-year-old man comes to your office for evaluation of a painful left knee. He notes that he has always been physically active and likes to run 3 miles two or three times per week. In the last few months, he has noted an aching of his left knee particularly the day after a vigorous run. He denies any swelling, redness, systemic symptoms, or any other affected joints. He finds that a few doses of ibuprofen relieve his symptoms. He does not have a regular internist and would like to establish care with you. He has had no major medical problems. Of note, his father died of a myocardial infarction in his late 70s and had several colonic polyps removed. His mother is still living and has diabetes and mild hypertension but is otherwise well. His review of systems is noncontributory. He did smoke cigarettes for a few years in his 20s, but none since that time. He is a social drinker and engages in no high-risk behavior.

QUESTION

- *What components of the physical examination are essential to perform in this patient?*

DISCUSSION

Preventive health care continues from birth through late adulthood. This male patient is in his early 60s and has not had regular internal medicine care. Key parts of the physical examination include assessment of his risk for major morbidity and mortality, including cardiovascular disease and malignancy. Therefore, one should perform a careful assessment of his blood pressure and cardiovascular system, including cardiac and pulmonary examinations, palpation of peripheral pulses, and auscultation for carotid and abdominal bruits. You should record his height and weight, calculating his body mass index (BMI). An easy to use online calculator is available at http://www.nhlbisupport.com/bmi/. The patient should have a digital rectal examination to assess his prostate and identify any rectal masses.

> You determine his blood pressure to be 138/88 mm Hg, pulse 72, and BMI 26.5. The remainder of his full physical examination is normal. Specifically, his knee has full range of motion without any effusion, redness, palpable tenderness, crepitus, or laxity. After discussion with the patient, you determine that his knee symptoms are likely due to overuse or mild osteoarthritis. You refer him to a physical therapist who specializes in sports injuries to work with the patient on his muscle balance, core strength, and alignment. You suggest that he can continue using ibuprofen as needed, and that if the physical therapy is not helpful, you will order further testing to look for bony or ligamentous damage. The patient then turns to what is probably his main concern—is there anything else he should be doing to remain healthy and active?

QUESTION

- *What other tests should you perform to assess the patient's risk for future diseases and maintain his good health?*

639

DISCUSSION

Preventive health in a man in his 60s includes a variety of screening tests. Those suggested by various national organizations such as the U.S. Preventive Services Task Force (USPSTF) include the following:

1. **Cancer screening:** Performing a digital rectal examination, ordering a screening colonoscopy, and giving the patient a set of stool cards to check for occult blood are appropriate in this patient. His father had colonic polyps, placing the patient at risk for polyps and possibly colorectal cancer. Screening for prostate cancer with a serum prostate-specific antigen (PSA) is controversial. Current guidelines recommend discussing the potential risks and benefits of the PSA test, particularly the potential for false-positive and false-negative results. There is no clear evidence that a routine chest x-ray, computer tomography (CT) scan, or sputum cytology is an effective screening tool for lung cancer.

2. **Cardiovascular health:** You have already determined his blood pressure. A fasting lipid profile should be obtained. He does have a history of smoking, and when he reaches the age of 65 years he should undergo an abdominal sonogram to screen for aortic aneurysm. Screening for coronary artery disease, carotid stenosis, or peripheral vascular disease is not recommended for asymptomatic individuals.

3. **Other medical conditions:** The patient's mother has diabetes. Even if there was no family history of diabetes, the America Diabetes Association recommends that all adults be screened for diabetes with a random or fasting glucose. If the patient was still actively smoking, you would discuss a plan for smoking cessation. In addition, the patient should be screened for symptoms of depression, particularly when staff-assisted depression support is readily available.

4. **Immunizations:** At the age of 60 years, the patient should receive an annual influenza vaccination in the fall. Tdap (tetanus, diphtheria, and pertussis) should be given once as a booster to adults, followed by Td every 10 years. Vaccination against herpes zoster should be given once at age 60 years. Pneumococcal vaccine will be recommended for this patient at age 65 years.

   The patient is amenable to your recommendations for a screening colonoscopy and immunization with Tdap and to prevent herpes zoster.

QUESTIONS

☐ *What recommendations do you have for the management of his borderline blood pressure readings and BMI of 26.5?*

☐ *Are there other laboratory studies that you would like to order?*

DISCUSSION

The patient's blood pressure reading is in the prehypertension range. It is important to evaluate for end-organ damage by checking renal function with a basic metabolic panel and a urinalysis and evaluating his electrocardiogram. If these are normal, no medications are indicated at this time. However, the patient should make an effort to lose weight so that his BMI decreases below 25.0, modestly restrict sodium intake, and limit alcohol consumption. He already exercises extensively and should be encouraged to continue this routine. Depending on his lab results and his future blood pressure readings, he may be a candidate for aspirin prophylaxis. The use of aspirin must be weighed against the potential risks and his 10-year risk of an adverse cardiovascular event.

CASE 2

Syncope

A 64-year-old man is walking around a shopping mall with his wife when he suddenly loses consciousness and falls to the ground. An ambulance brings him to the emergency department. On arrival to the hospital, the man is awake and alert and complaining only of pain in his right elbow, which he apparently injured when he fell. He is placed on a cardiac monitor, and blood is drawn for laboratory work, which includes a complete blood count (CBC) and electrolyte, glucose, calcium, and cardiac enzyme studies.

QUESTIONS

☐ *What is the definition of syncope?*

☐ *What are some of the causes of a sudden loss of consciousness?*

DISCUSSION

Syncope is a sudden, temporary loss of consciousness caused by a lack of cerebral perfusion. The causes of sudden loss of consciousness can be divided into three major categories—cardiovascular, neurologic, and metabolic.

Cardiovascular syncope occurs when the cardiovascular system fails to maintain adequate blood pressure for cerebral perfusion. Inadequate stroke volume, inadequate heart rate, or inadequate total peripheral resistance all could be causes of cardiovascular syncope. Impairment in stroke volume sufficient enough to cause syncope may be seen in ischemia and myocardial infarction (MI), dehydration or hemorrhage, or as a result of tachyarrhythmias, which impair ventricular filling. Mitral, aortic, or idiopathic hypertrophic subaortic stenosis, atrial myxoma, and pulmonary embolism also may cause syncope by obstructing cardiac inflow or outflow. Severe bradycardia (i.e., heart rate <40 bpm), such as occurs in heart block and sick sinus syndrome, may cause syncope. In some circumstances, cardiac output is adequate, but total peripheral resistance is reduced, leading to a decrease in blood pressure. Autonomic dysfunction or the use of vasodilators may reduce total peripheral resistance to the extent that syncope results. A common manifestation of syncope induced by reduced total peripheral resistance is the "vasovagal faint," which affects approximately 50% of the population at some point during the course of a lifetime.

Head trauma, stroke, or cerebrovascular disease may all cause loss of consciousness. Sudden increases in intracranial pressure (ICP) can compromise cerebral perfusion and cause a loss of consciousness, even in the setting of normal systemic blood pressure. A classic example is a colloid cyst of the third ventricle that acts as a ball valve and causes sudden obstructive hydrocephalus. Only rarely do disorders of the cerebrovascular system compromise perfusion to such an extent as to cause syncope. Therefore, syncope should not be viewed as a usual manifestation of a transient ischemic attack (TIA). Rarely, patients with compromise of distal basilar artery circulation experience a sudden loss of consciousness because of impaired perfusion of the ascending reticular activating system.

Seizures are commonly considered in the differential diagnosis of syncope. However, seizures in adults rarely cause a loss of consciousness that is not associated with repetitive motor activity. It should be noted that some patients with syncope attributable to cardiac or circulatory failure have some generalized involuntary motor activity resulting from impaired cerebral perfusion, but this motor activity does not represent a primary convulsive event.

Finally, impaired delivery of essential nutrients to the brain (e.g., as a result of hypoglycemia or hypoxia) can cause a sudden loss of consciousness. However, metabolic disturbances usually worsen gradually and cause obtundation before loss of consciousness; therefore, the true definition of syncope is not generally met.

> **Additional history indicates that the fall was not preceded by an aura and that the patient remained continent during the episode. He awoke spontaneously and was not confused on awakening. The patient has had several previous episodes of light-headedness during exertion but says he never lost consciousness during those episodes. The patient does not recall anything unusual about the day before his syncopal episode, except that he experienced mild angina that was immediately relieved by a single sublingual nitroglycerin tablet.**

QUESTIONS

☐ *What is significant about the onset and recovery of this syncopal episode?*

☐ *Based on the foregoing limited history, what process do you most suspect as a cause of this patient's syncope?*

DISCUSSION

The abrupt onset of loss of consciousness is characteristic of a cardiac cause. There were no warning symptoms to suggest the aura of a seizure; no discrete neurologic symptoms characteristic of a TIA; and no diaphoresis, nausea, and wooziness such as would be associated with a vasovagal or hypoglycemic episode. That the patient remained continent during the event supports a cardiac or vasovagal cause, but this information is probably not very helpful in decision making; the continence of a patient during a seizure is more likely related to whether the patient's bladder is full at the time of the event. The lack of confusion on awakening argues against a seizure episode, although patients with atonic seizures can very rapidly regain normal cognition. Patients with a complex partial seizure do have a period of confusion often lasting several minutes. An important question to ask the patient's wife is whether her husband displayed any involuntary motor activity while unconscious. If he remained limp, this would argue strongly against the event being a seizure.

The patient's history of several prior episodes of light-headedness during exertion suggests an underlying abnormality of the cardiovascular system. In particular, this history in an older patient should direct attention to the heart. Two facts reinforce this impression: (1) the patient apparently has a history of angina and (2) he has been taking nitroglycerin.

In summary, a cardiac cause of syncope is highly likely in this patient because of the abrupt onset of the loss of consciousness and the history of angina. The most likely cardiac causes of syncope, given this history, include ischemia, ventricular tachyarrhythmia, or left ventricular outflow tract obstruction. Autonomic dysfunction or volume depletion is less likely.

The patient's medical history is significant because of sporadic bouts of angina, for which he takes nitroglycerin, which he borrows from his wife. The angina has not recently increased in frequency or intensity. The patient has had a heart murmur for many years but has been told that it is not significant. He takes no regular medications. His father died of a heart attack at age 60, and his mother had a mild stroke at 70 but did not die until 10 years later.

QUESTION

▢ *What is the significance of the patient's angina, family history, and heart murmur?*

DISCUSSION

The patient's angina suggests the possibility of coronary artery disease, and further evaluation by either stress testing or cardiac catheterization is warranted to assess the degree and severity of atherosclerosis.

The significance of the family history is not very helpful. Although a "heart attack" at age 60 in the patient's father does suggest premature coronary disease, many patients who are labeled as heart attack victims have not truly sustained an MI. The patient's mother's stroke at age 70 might represent athero-sclerotic disease (at a relatively advanced age) or a hemorrhagic event. Certainly, the patient's history raises the possibility that atherosclerosis of the coronary or cerebral arterial circulation is causing the patient's symptoms. Although stroke or TIA due to large artery occlusive disease rarely is a cause of syncope, some patients with bilateral severe internal carotid artery stenosis may have syncopal events. The significance of the murmur is unclear from the history alone, but it suggests that underlying structural cardiac disease could be contributing to the patient's symptoms.

Although it is very likely that this patient has suffered syncope from a cardiovascular cause, the additional information does not help sway our clinical judgment one way or the other. It adds some "soft" features suggestive of coronary artery or valvular heart disease, which might in turn be responsible for a cardiac arrhythmia leading to syncope. However, this additional history is also entirely consistent with the absence of significant heart disease.

Physical examination shows a well-developed, well-nourished white man in no acute distress. His vital signs include a pulse of 88 bpm, respiratory rate of 14 breaths/minute, blood pressure of 108/74 mm Hg, and a temperature of 37.2°C. The patient's skin is warm and dry, his pupils are equal and reactive to light and accommodation, and his lungs are clear. Cardiac examination indicates a normal S_1, a soft S_2, and an S_4. He has a harsh, late-peaking systolic ejection murmur that is loudest in the aortic area and radiates to both carotids, which demonstrate delayed upstroke and low volume. There are no carotid bruits, and there is no jugular venous distention. Examination of the abdomen and extremities shows no abnormalities, with the exception of a bruise on the right elbow. Neurologic examination is completely within normal limits.

QUESTIONS

▢ *Which of these signs and symptoms are significant?*

▢ *How does this physical examination influence the differential diagnosis?*

▢ *What studies would you like to obtain?*

DISCUSSION

The patient's appearance does not suggest a systemic illness. Obtaining supine and upright blood pressure and pulse determinations is important in light of the patient's relatively low blood pressure. The patient does have a slightly high pulse, which suggests dehydration. That his skin is dry also raises the possibility of dehydration, as well as autonomic failure with resultant postural hypotension. His preserved pupillary accommodation attests to preservation of parasympathetic nervous function but leaves open the possibility of sympathetic nervous system failure. The harsh, late-peaking, systolic ejection murmur, the delayed and reduced carotid upstrokes, and the soft S_2 are highly suggestive of aortic stenosis, an important cause of syncope. The lack of carotid bruits must be considered within the context of a loud precordial murmur that is already radiating into the neck; critical carotid stenoses can be missed because of masking sounds (as in this patient). Patients with preocclusive stenosis at the internal carotid artery origin may not have enough forceful perfusion to generate an audible bruit.

The information from the examination directs attention to the heart. Of particular concern is the possibility of structural heart disease as a cause of impaired aortic area outflow. Given the patient's history, consideration also should be given to the possibility of associated coronary artery disease and, less likely, carotid artery disease.

Usually the next studies that are ordered in patients suspected of having cardiac disease are the electrocardiogram (ECG) and the chest radiograph. However, in this case neither is likely to be very informative. The ECG may show evidence of left ventricular hypertrophy, but some patients with severe aortic stenosis fail to demonstrate this finding. Thus, a negative ECG should not dissuade one from the diagnosis. Typically, the chest radiograph in aortic stenosis shows a normal-sized heart, sometimes with a boot-shaped configuration indicative of concentric left ventricular hypertrophy. Again, this finding is not specific.

The most important study to be ordered at this time is an echocardiogram with Doppler evaluation of the aortic valve. The echocardiogram demonstrates the concentric left ventricular hypertrophy typical of aortic stenosis. Furthermore, it demonstrates severe restriction of the aortic valve leaflets. Both of these findings are consistent with the diagnosis but do not help quantify the severity of the disease. However, Doppler evaluation of the aortic valve can quantify the transvalvular aortic gradient precisely. In most cases the echo Doppler study is adequate to confirm the diagnosis and to arrive at a decision regarding surgery. Because this patient is in the coronary disease age group and because of the history of angina, cardiac catheterization to confirm the aortic valve gradient and to define the coronary anatomy with coronary arteriograms should also be performed.

An ECG shows left ventricular hypertrophy but no evidence of past or present ischemia. A chest radiograph is within normal limits, and a radiograph of the right elbow is also normal. Laboratory values are noncontributory. The patient is sent for an echocardiogram with Doppler examination. The echocardiogram shows a calcified aortic value and left ventricular hypertrophy, both consistent with calcific aortic stenosis. The aortic valve gradient is 70 mm Hg. The patient is admitted to the hospital for a cardiac catheterization and probable aortic valve replacement because only 50% of patients with aortic stenosis who have syncope achieve a 3-year survival if left untreated.

QUESTIONS

- *What are some of the causes of aortic stenosis?*
- *What is the pathophysiology underlying the physical signs and symptoms that characterize aortic stenosis?*

DISCUSSION

Causes of aortic stenosis include congenital, rheumatic, and calcific conditions. In this patient's age group, calcific aortic stenosis is of particular concern. There is no evidence of a dynamic subvalvular left ventricular outflow tract obstruction, as may be seen with hypertrophic cardiomyopathy.

In aortic stenosis, the heart muscles force blood through a stenotic valve, which results in pressure overload on the left ventricle and subsequent concentric left ventricular hypertrophy. The clinical triad of angina, syncope, and heart failure is typical. The angina is the result of impaired blood flow limiting oxygen to the enlarged myocardium. The syncope can be caused by a decrease in the heart's ability to increase cardiac output across the stenotic valve. Syncope also can occur because of arrhythmias resulting from calcification within the cardiac conduction system. The patient's low systemic blood pressure is a consequence of his impaired cardiac output. The diminished S_2 is the result of impaired valve motion from the aortic disease. The S_4 is a result of decreased left ventricular compliance.

This case illustrates that, with an appropriate history and physical examination, clues to the cause of a patient's syncope can be defined. Further evaluation can then be tailored to the patient. However, a cause for syncope is not readily evident in many patients. In these situations, a review of the patient's history may be informative. For example, did the syncope occur after a meal or during straining at defecation? In the patient with recurrent syncope, a Holter monitor to examine for arrhythmias, a stress test to try to induce the arrhythmia responsible for the syncope, autonomic testing to examine the integrity of postural reflexes, and an echocardiogram to search for underlying cardiac pathology may be warranted. If arrhythmias are the suspected cause, electrophysiologic stimulation in selected cases may provoke the causative arrhythmia. If occlusive cerebrovascular disease is suspected, a carotid duplex examination, magnetic resonance angiography (MRA), transcranial Doppler studies, or interventional angiography should be considered. If a neurologic etiology is suspected, an electroencephalogram (EEG) to look for seizure activity and magnetic resonance imaging (MRI) to look for structural brain abnormalities are warranted.

CASE 3A

Shortness of Breath in a Young Woman

A 38-year-old African American woman comes to the emergency department with a chief complaint of shortness of breath on exertion that has progressively worsened in the last 6 months. Her symptoms have become so severe that she now has difficulty in eating secondary to extreme dyspnea, and this has resulted in a 27-pound weight loss. She also notes a severe cough productive of white sputum but denies fevers, chills, or night sweats. Before the onset of symptoms (about 6 months ago), she was in good health.

QUESTIONS

- *What are your immediate concerns in this patient?*
- *How does the onset of symptoms help formulate a differential diagnosis?*
- *What are the most likely diagnostic considerations?*

DISCUSSION

On initial evaluation of this patient in the emergency department, care must be taken to ensure that she has an adequate airway. Her vital signs must also be assessed, with specific attention to respiratory rate, heart rate, and temperature. Supplemental oxygen should be provided to ensure an oxygen saturation of greater than 94%. Blood should be drawn for arterial blood gas analysis, complete blood count (CBC), and chemistries. A chest radiograph (posteroanterior and lateral views) and electrocardiogram (ECG) also should be ordered.

The causes of shortness of breath in this age group can include acute and chronic infections; cardiac malformations, including valvular dysfunction; anemia; and chronic lung disease, including interstitial lung disease. In general, cardiac causes are easy to exclude in two situations: (1) when the patient has no history of heart problems at birth (i.e., congenital) or in early childhood, and (2) when the cardiac examination is normal. In addition, anemia can be excluded when there is no history of continuing heavy menstrual blood loss or gastrointestinal hemorrhage.

The duration of this patient's symptoms makes an acute infection very unlikely and suggests a chronic infection or one of the interstitial lung diseases. However, the lack of a persistent fever, chills, or recurrent night sweats makes chronic infection less probable, although acquired immunodeficiency syndrome (AIDS)–related infections such as *Pneumocystis carinii* pneumonia (PCP) can present with a paucity of constitutional symptoms. Furthermore, this patient is at particular demographic risk for the development of sarcoidosis, a chronic granulomatous disorder of unknown cause that commonly affects young African American women.

Other diagnostic considerations include pulmonary lymphangioleiomyomatosis, hypersensitivity pneumonitis, eosinophilic granuloma, idiopathic pulmonary fibrosis, and interstitial lung disease secondary to connective tissue disorders or vasculitis. Pulmonary lymphangioleiomyomatosis, a disorder characterized by proliferation of atypical smooth muscle cells, leads to parenchymal lung disease, pleural effusions, hemoptysis, and pneumothorax; however, it is exceedingly rare. Hypersensitivity pneumonitis also can occur in younger individuals after exposure to a variety of occupational and environmental triggers. Although it is usually self-limited, it can become chronic. Eosinophilic granuloma, a rare disorder, is characterized by abnormal proliferation of histiocytes, leading to infiltrative lung disease in the third and fourth decades of life. This condition, which occurs predominantly in smokers, is almost exclusively a disease of whites. Idiopathic pulmonary fibrosis often causes insidious, progressive respiratory impairment, but it is uncommon in patients younger than 40 years old. Pulmonary manifestations of vasculitis or connective tissue disorders, however, are most common in younger patients.

> Three months before the woman entered the hospital, she had to stop working because of severe exercise limitation. She has no history of occupational exposure to dusts or chemicals. A married woman, she has been in a monogamous relationship for many years. A test for human immunodeficiency virus (HIV) 3 months ago was negative. She is a Jehovah's Witness, denies use of tobacco or illicit drugs, and has lived in an urban neighborhood all her life. She denies skin rash, chest pain, or arthralgias but admits to seeing "spots before her eyes" and having occasional nausea and vomiting.

QUESTIONS

- *How does the patient's social and occupational history assist in narrowing the differential diagnosis?*
- *What is the significance of the patient's complaints?*

DISCUSSION

The social and family history contributes more to ruling out other causes of chronic lung disease than establishing a definitive diagnosis. Specifically, sarcoidosis is more common among nonsmokers, in contrast to eosinophilic granuloma, which is almost exclusively a disease of smokers. Furthermore, the patient's monogamous relationship, opposition to blood transfusion on religious grounds, and abstinence from intravenous drug use, as well as the negative HIV test, put her at a much lower risk for PCP infection, which usually occurs in patients with well-established HIV disease. The absence of a significant travel history also helps eliminate chronic fungal infection as a diagnostic possibility. Another pertinent negative factor is the lack of any significant environmental or occupational exposures, which makes hypersensitivity pneumonitis less likely. However, this condition cannot be excluded completely because certain exposures are quite subtle or temporally remote; they can be missed without a rigorous exposure history.

A careful review of systems is critical to evaluate for disorders that can affect multiple organ systems. Ocular involvement can lead to photophobia, tearing, pain, and loss of vision. Gastrointestinal involvement can result in dysphagia, abdominal pain, jaundice, and nausea and vomiting. Infiltration of other organ systems can lead to skin rashes, syncope, irregular heart rhythm, chest pain, poor urine output, joint pain, and lymph node enlargement. Disorders that are particularly prone to manifest in multiple organ systems include the connective tissue disorders such as systemic lupus erythematosus (SLE) and scleroderma, as well as the vasculitides, including Wegener's granulomatosis. In addition, sarcoidosis may occur in almost any organ system of the body.

> On examination, the woman is in mild distress secondary to dyspnea. Her pulse is 104 bpm, her respiratory rate is 28 breaths/minute, her temperature is 35.8°C, and her blood pressure is 140/80 mm Hg. Her mucous membranes are dry. There is jugular venous distention with no significant adenopathy. She is not using accessory muscles of respiration, and lung examination shows coarse breath sounds bilaterally without wheezing, rales, dullness to percussion, or egophony. Cardiac examination indicates tachycardia, with a 2/6 systolic murmur at the left sternal border and an S_3 at the right sternal border. There is no hepatosplenomegaly. The extremities show 1+ pitting edema without clubbing, and there is no skin rash. Neurologic examination is unremarkable.

QUESTION

- *What is the significance of the findings on physical examination?*

DISCUSSION

Although many patients with interstitial lung disease present with clinically silent pulmonary involvement, some exhibit advanced lung scarring. Physical findings, which are often absent early in the disease, become apparent only when advanced pulmonary hypertension and cor pulmonale have developed. These findings include the presence of a tricuspid regurgitation murmur, a right-sided S_3, a right ventricular or sternal heave, and congestion of the liver and lower extremities. In addition, patients with interstitial lung disease generally present with inspiratory rales, or crackles. However, these are less likely to be heard in patients with sarcoidosis or other granulomatous interstitial lung diseases. In addition, a careful search for any extrapulmonary manifestations should be undertaken.

The patient's initial laboratory findings include a pH of 7.44, a $PaCO_2$ of 36.2 mm Hg, and a PaO_2 of 52 mm Hg on room air. Blood urea nitrogen (BUN), creatinine, serum calcium, and serum albumin are normal. Chest radiographs (posteroanterior and lateral views) show bilateral reticulonodular interstitial infiltrates, with widening of the right paratracheal region and fullness of both hila, suggestive of mediastinal lymphadenopathy. Minimal cardiomegaly is also noted. An ECG shows normal sinus rhythm with right atrial enlargement. Spirometry and lung volume analysis obtained shortly thereafter indicate a forced vital capacity (FVC) of 1.25 L (43% of predicted), a forced expiratory volume in 1 second (FEV_1) of 1.02 L (43% of predicted), and an FEV_1/FVC ratio of 82%. The total lung capacity (TLC) is 1.26 L (44%), and the diffusing capacity (D_LCO) is 7.3 mL/min/mm Hg (29% predicted).

QUESTIONS

☐ *What is the significance of the radiographic findings?*

☐ *How would you interpret the pulmonary function tests?*

☐ *What further tests should be performed to help make the diagnosis?*

DISCUSSION

The radiographic findings confirm the presence of interstitial lung disease; in fact, they are quite suggestive of pulmonary sarcoidosis. Intrathoracic lymphadenopathy, which occurs in 75%–90% of patients with sarcoidosis, is usually present in the bronchopulmonary, tracheobronchial, and paratracheal chains. This contrasts with lymphangioleiomyomatosis, hypersensitivity pneumonitis, connective tissue disorders, and vasculitis, in which intrathoracic lymphadenopathy is distinctly uncommon. The lung parenchyma also may be involved in sarcoidosis; affected patients usually demonstrate bilateral reticulonodular infiltrates, although a wide variety of other parenchymal abnormalities, including bullous changes, alveolar infiltrates, peripheral nodules, and fibrosis or "honeycombing," may be present.

The International Congress on Sarcoidosis has proposed the following radiographic classification of the disease: stage 0, absence of abnormalities; stage 1, lymph node enlargement without parenchymal abnormalities; stage 2, lymph node enlargement and diffuse parenchymal disease; stage 3, diffuse parenchymal disease without adenopathy; and stage 4, pulmonary fibrosis. The findings in this patient would be consistent with stage 2 disease.

The pulmonary function tests indicate a markedly reduced TLC, which is suggestive of severe restrictive lung disease with a significant impairment in the D_LCO and resting arterial hypoxemia. These findings correlate with the radiographic abnormalities just described and indicate an extensive parenchymal process. However, other diffuse interstitial processes can produce similar physiologic derangements, limiting the specificity of the test results. Of note, airflow obstruction resulting from granulomatous infiltration of the airways may be evident in some patients but is absent in this patient who has a normal FEV_1/FVC ratio.

Making a definitive diagnosis of sarcoidosis can be challenging. Tissue diagnosis, which is often pursued, may be falsely positive, especially if lymph node or liver biopsy is performed. When radiographic evidence of parenchymal disease is present, as in this patient, bronchoscopy with transbronchial biopsy is preferred; the sensitivity of this method is 85%–90%. In certain patients, some noninvasive studies may be useful. These include the serum angiotensin-converting-enzyme (ACE) level, percentage of lymphocytes in bronchoalveolar lavage (BAL) fluid, and gallium lung scanning.

The patient undergoes fiberoptic bronchoscopy and transbronchial lung biopsy. Review of the pathologic specimens indicates the presence of multiple noncaseating granulomas. Stains and cultures for acid-fast bacilli and fungi are negative. The serum ACE level is elevated at 111 U/L (range: 8–52). The echocardiogram is significant for a severely dilated right ventricle with preserved left ventricular function and an estimated pulmonary artery systolic pressure of 90 mm Hg. Moderate tricuspid regurgitation is present.

QUESTIONS

☐ *What is the significance of the pathologic findings and the elevated serum ACE level?*

☐ *How do you interpret the results of echocardiography?*

☐ *What treatment options are available?*

DISCUSSION

The presence of noncaseating granulomas in the correct clinical scenario is virtually pathognomonic for sarcoidosis. However, similar granulomas may occur in a wide variety of other diseases, including tuberculosis, fungal infection, malignancy, berylliosis, and foreign-body reaction. Although the ACE level supports the diagnosis, it is relatively nonspecific and may be elevated in patients with tuberculosis, histoplasmosis, leprosy, and HIV infection. Nevertheless, the ACE level may be a useful marker of disease activity. It has been shown that a progressive decrease in the ACE level may reflect spontaneous remission of disease or response to therapy.

The results of echocardiography are consistent with the presence of severe pulmonary hypertension and cor pulmonale. These are expected sequelae of severe, diffuse parenchymal involvement and chronic hypoxemia. The presence of such extensive disease in vital organs such as the lungs and heart (and the eyes or central nervous system [CNS]) mandates the institution of definitive therapy. In patients with asymptomatic disease or involvement of nonvital organs, therapy may be withheld and patients closely followed. The rationale behind this approach is the observation that 30%–50% of cases spontaneously remit in a period of up to 3 years, with an additional 20%–30% of cases remaining relatively stable over the same period.

The most successful therapy for sarcoidosis has been the administration of systemic corticosteroids such as prednisone at a dose of 20–60 mg by mouth daily. If patients respond, the treatment is continued at the lowest possible dose to maintain remission of disease for a period of several weeks or months before stopping. Occasionally, disease recurs with tapering of the steroid dose, and an upward adjustment is required. Unfortunately, the use of steroids can lead to multiple untoward effects, including the development of osteoporosis, cataracts, diabetes, hypertension, psychiatric disturbances, and immunosuppression. Although there has been much effort to develop alternative treatment regimens, including chloroquine and methotrexate, these have met with very limited success.

CASE 3B

Dyspnea

A 58-year-old man calls an ambulance complaining that he "cannot get enough air" and that he is "suffocating." When the paramedics arrive, they find that the man is alert and oriented but that he cannot speak more than one or two words at a time because of shortness of breath. On the way to the emergency department, the paramedics insert an intravenous line and administer fluids. They also give the man oxygen at a rate of 15 L/minute via mask.

QUESTIONS

- *How would you define dyspnea?*
- *What are your immediate concerns about this patient?*
- *What are some of the mechanisms that produce dyspnea?*

DISCUSSION

From his complaints and physical appearance, this man appears to be suffering from symptoms of dyspnea, a condition that is defined as any uncomfortable awareness of breathing. It involves both the perception of an abnormal sensation and a reaction to that perception. Dyspnea has many causes, most of which are cardiac or pulmonary in origin.

The overriding concern in a patient with dyspnea is to rule out the possibility of serious cardiac or pulmonary causes of the symptoms. Evaluation should begin with a check of vital signs, including blood pressure, pulse, respiratory rate, and temperature, to begin to narrow the list of potential major cardiac or pulmonary causes of dyspnea. Conditions that are associated with symptoms of dyspnea include pulmonary vascular disease (e.g., pulmonary embolism, pulmonary hypertension secondary to chronic obstructive pulmonary disease [COPD]), interstitial lung disease, asthma, neuromuscular disease, chest wall disease, and congestive heart failure (CHF), including that caused by the various types of heart disease, including valvular disease, hypertension, cardiomyopathy, and pulmonary edema. Although chest pain would be a more common presenting symptom of myocardial infarction (MI) than dyspnea would be, MI should be considered and ruled out with cardiac enzyme studies and an electrocardiogram (ECG).

Another concern in this case (i.e., a new patient without a known cause of dyspnea) is the administration of oxygen at a high flow rate (i.e., 15 L/minute), which may be the wrong approach if this man has obstructive pulmonary disease with carbon dioxide retention. Delivery of inspired oxygen at a high concentration can worsen carbon dioxide retention.

On arrival at the emergency department, the man is still short of breath and breathing at a rate of 28 respirations/minute. His other vital signs show a pulse of 110 bpm, a blood pressure of 150/85 mm Hg, and a temperature of 38.1°C. Initial history reveals that 6 days ago the patient developed an upper respiratory infection with rhinorrhea and a cough productive of thick yellow sputum. He has been short of breath for the last few days, but his symptoms worsened in the last several hours. He notes that he is more short of breath with minimal exertion and often begins to cough as a result of any effort. He denies chest pain or tightness.

The patient's past medical history is significant because of two previous hospital admissions for similar episodes. He also has a history of hypertension, for which he is supposed to take a mild diuretic once a day; however, he ran out of the drug and has not yet refilled his prescription. He uses an inhaler as needed but denies other medications or drug allergies. The patient says that he has smoked two packs of cigarettes per day for 30 years and that he drinks three to four beers per night. He is not married and recently lost his job in construction because he tires too easily.

QUESTIONS

- *How do these descriptions of the patient's symptoms help you in thinking about your differential diagnosis?*
- *How can you differentiate between cardiac and pulmonary causes of dyspnea?*

DISCUSSION

The subsequent history is more suggestive of an acute illness superimposed on an underlying chronic process (e.g., chronic lung disease with CHF or upper respiratory infection exacerbation) than of an acute process (e.g., acute MI, pulmonary embolism). The differential diagnosis at this point includes obstructive pulmonary disease, asthma, CHF, infection, and a tumor (a possibility in a patient with COPD and a history of cigarette smoking). The physician should also keep in mind the possibility of work-related exposures such as asbestos, asthma sensitizers, and other occupational pulmonary toxins. Although the chronicity of symptoms points more toward a chronic than an acute process, the possibility of an acute MI should still be ruled out. Recurrent pulmonary embolism also is a possibility at this point, and ventilation–perfusion scanning with lower-extremity Doppler studies may be indicated.

Physical examination shows a well-developed, slightly overweight, white man in moderate respiratory distress with vital signs as noted above. His skin is moist without cyanosis, his neck shows mildly dilated jugular veins, his lungs reveal a prolonged expiratory phase with expiratory wheezes in all lung fields and poor respiratory effort, and examination of his heart reveals a prominent S_3 but no murmurs. Examination of his abdomen is unremarkable, revealing a slightly enlarged liver, and his extremities show 2+ peripheral edema.

QUESTIONS

- *What do these physical signs suggest?*
- *What disease process would be at the top of your differential diagnosis now?*
- *What laboratory tests or studies would you like to obtain?*

DISCUSSION

The expiratory wheezing and increased respiratory effort noted on physical examination of this patient suggest the presence of obstructive lung disease. In addition, there is an S_3 gallop and peripheral edema. The S_3 and dilated jugular veins suggest left-sided heart failure, and the enlarged liver and peripheral edema suggest right-sided heart failure. The wheezes may be associated with either obstructive lung disease or CHF. At this point, it is essential to differentiate cardiac from pulmonary causes of this man's distress to plan an effective treatment. A chest radiograph along with an ECG, cardiac enzyme studies, and a complete blood count (CBC) with differential would help determine whether the patient has either or both underlying conditions.

The emergency department physician calls for the patient's old records, orders some laboratory tests (including arterial blood gas studies on oxygen, a CBC, a serum electrolyte panel, a cardiac enzyme analysis, a sputum culture, a "stat" ECG, and a portable radiograph). The ECG suggests some right axis deviation and sinus tachycardia but no ischemic changes. The results of the arterial blood gas studies are returned promptly and show a pH of 7.44, a PaO_2 of 81 mm Hg, a $PaCO_2$ of 50 mm Hg, and an O_2 saturation of 95% on 3 L FiO_2 by nasal cannula.

QUESTION

☐ *What sort of pattern do the arterial blood gas findings suggest?*

DISCUSSION

The arterial blood gas findings represent adequate oxygenation (normal PaO_2 = 80 mm Hg or above) with mild hypercarbia (normal $PaCO_2$ = 40 mm Hg) and a normal pH. The normal pH suggests a chronic process.

The patient's chest radiograph suggests a mild prominence of the pulmonary vascular markings. Otherwise, there are no radiographic changes.

QUESTION

☐ *Which diagnoses are less likely because of these radiographic results?*

DISCUSSION

The radiographic findings make the possibility of postobstructive pneumonitis, tumor, or pneumonia much less likely and are more compatible with a COPD exacerbation with some mild CHF. There is no mass to suggest a tumor, and there are no infiltrates to suggest pneumonia.

Because the patient continues to have respiratory distress and is very uncomfortable without the oxygen, he is admitted to the hospital. His old records reveal that his previous admissions were for exacerbations of bronchitis. He is started on fluids, oxygen, diuretics, and a broad-spectrum antibiotic.

QUESTIONS

☐ *What are your goals for therapy for this patient?*

☐ *How can you prevent similar episodes from happening again?*

DISCUSSION

The goals for this patient are to control the exacerbation of his bronchitis with antibiotics and bronchodilators and to return him to baseline respiratory status. Peak flow measurements should be obtained before and after bronchodilators are administered, and the possibility of using corticosteroids along with the routine bronchodilator therapeutic regimen should be entertained. The possibility of underlying heart disease also should be addressed. An echocardiogram would be indicated at this time to determine if there is any cardiac functional abnormality. The most likely diagnosis here is chronic bronchitis exacerbated by an upper respiratory infection without pneumonia, with an underlying possibility of mild CHF. Future prophylaxis should include immunization against influenza as well as pneumococcal vaccine. In addition, the possibility of entering a pulmonary rehabilitation program should be discussed with the patient.

CASE 4

Deep Venous Thrombosis

A 28-year-old man consults his primary physician because of a sudden onset of shortness of breath and right pleuritic chest pain, having returned 3 days before the onset of symptoms from a business trip to Tokyo. He has been in excellent health all his life and takes no medications. His medical history is negative, with the exception of tonsillectomy at age 10 years without bleeding complications and an appendectomy at age 18 years, which was followed 10 days later by an episode of right calf tenderness and swelling that resolved spontaneously without specific therapy. Family history indicated that his father died suddenly at age 35 years of a "heart attack," and his sister died suddenly of unknown cause at age 25 years postpartum. On physical examination, he is a physically fit–appearing man complaining of right-sided chest discomfort on deep inspiration and moderate distress with shortness of breath. Vital signs showed blood pressure (BP) 110/60 mm Hg, pulse 114 bpm, respirations 24 breaths/minute, and temperature 37.5°C. Examination of the heart indicates a summation gallop at the apex with a prominent P2 at the base. Auscultation of the lungs discloses a pleural friction rub heard in the right axilla. The remainder of the physical examination is negative, with the exception of tenderness on palpation of the left calf, with pain elicited by dorsiflexion of the left foot. Subtle, but definite slight edema was present in the left ankle.

QUESTIONS

- *What is your differential diagnosis and the most likely explanation for his symptoms?*
- *What initial diagnostic studies should be carried out immediately to confirm the diagnosis?*

DISCUSSION

A chest x-ray was obtained, which showed no abnormality. An electrocardiogram (ECG) showed sinus tachycardia with clockwise rotation and right-axis deviation. An arterial blood sample was obtained, which showed the following results: partial pressure of oxygen in the arterial blood (PaO_2) = 63 mm Hg, partial pressure of carbon dioxide in the arterial blood ($PaCO_2$) = 31 mm Hg, pH is 7.49, and arterial oxygen saturation is 87%.

QUESTIONS

- *How do you interpret these findings?*
- *What diagnostic studies should be done next?*
- *Would you consider instituting any form of therapy based on the results at this point?*
- *Would you consider obtaining any further diagnostic studies before instituting therapy?*

DISCUSSION

The normal chest x-ray essentially excludes pneumonia or other pulmonary parenchymal pathology as the cause for the patient's symptoms. The ECG showed only nonspecific findings but is consistent with abnormalities observed in pulmonary embolic disease. The arterial blood gas studies show evidence of oxygen desaturation, mild respiratory alkalosis, and an abnormal alveolar–arterial gradient that, in the absence of pulmonary parenchymal disease, strongly suggests a ventilation/perfusion (V/Q) abnormality such as is observed in acute pulmonary embolism (PE).

The correct diagnostic procedure is a V/Q lung scan or spiral computed tomography (CT) scanning of the chest. However, before sending the patient to the radiology department, it would be appropriate to institute heparin therapy immediately based on a presumptive working diagnosis of PE because the next embolus, if massive, might be fatal. However, before instituting heparin therapy, it would be desirable to obtain satisfactorily collected blood samples for preliminary investigation of a thrombophilic state because the results from such a workup are difficult or impossible to interpret after anticoagulant therapy has been instituted. Even in the face of acute venous thromboembolic disease, some of the coagulation-based studies are not subject to definitive interpretation and therefore should also be repeated at a later date when the patient is asymptomatic and not receiving anticoagulant therapy. At this point in the workup, venous blood samples can be obtained and properly stored for the following determinations pending the results of the V/Q scan:

> Protein C
> Protein S
> Prothrombin 20210
> Factor V Leiden
> Lupus anticoagulant/anticardiolipin antibodies
> Antithrombin III
> Homocysteine

Of these studies, homocysteine, anticardiolipin antibodies, and genetic testing for prothrombin 20210 and factor V Leiden will not be affected by the acute event or anticoagulant medicines. In addition, a baseline prothrombin time and partial thromboplastin time (PTT) should be obtained before the institution of anticoagulant therapy.

The spiral CT scan of the chest showed a large PE in the right middle lobe. Alternatively, a V/Q scan can be used to estimate the probability of a PE in the setting of contrast dye allergy. Consideration also could be given to carrying out Doppler ultrasonography to investigate the possibility of deep venous thrombosis (DVT) as the source of a PE, although if the results of the V/Q scan or spiral CT definitively establish a diagnosis of PE, further investigation for DVT is unnecessary. The D-dimer test is most useful in a patient with a low pretest probability for having thromboembolic disease; if it is within normal limits, it virtually excludes the possibility of PE.

QUESTION

☐ *Having established a diagnosis of pulmonary thromboembolism, what further therapy should you institute?*

DISCUSSION

Administration of heparin therapy followed by the initiation of therapy with an oral anticoagulant such as warfarin should be instituted. Heparin should be maintained for at least 5 days and warfarin for a variable time thereafter (see later discussion).

QUESTIONS

☐ *What is the rationale for concurrent administration of heparin and oral anticoagulants?*

☐ *How are these two therapies monitored?*

DISCUSSION

The rationale for concurrent administration of heparin and oral anticoagulants is the following: Heparin induces immediate anticoagulation by enhancing the activity of endogenous antithrombin III, whereas vitamin K antagonists such as Coumadin (which inhibit the synthesis of factors II, VII, IX, and X, prothrombin, protein C, and protein S) require approximately 4–6 days to become fully effective based on the half-lives of the vitamin K–dependent proteins. However, by decreasing the synthesis of protein C and protein S, Coumadin actually can initially enhance the propensity to thrombosis, resulting in "Coumadin-induced skin necrosis" unless given simultaneously with heparin. Abrupt discontinuation of heparin therapy without coverage by oral anticoagulants can decrease the concentration of antithrombin III and is associated with a high relapse rate of thrombosis. Unfractionated heparin is monitored by the PTT, whereas warfarin therapy is monitored by the prothrombin time (PT)/international normalized ratio (INR). Recently, the use of low–molecular-weight forms of heparin (LMWH) in place of standard heparin has increased. LMWH can be dosed on a weight basis with no need to monitor PTT, which is a big advantage.

QUESTIONS

☐ *Why is follow-up so important in the management of this patient?*

☐ *What should be the objective of follow-up management?*

DISCUSSION

This patient developed DVT and PE at a young age, has a prior personal history suggestive of thromboembolism, and has a strong family history suggestive of PE in first-degree relatives. Therefore, he is a likely candidate for diagnosis of an inherited thrombophilia, such as deficiency of protein C, protein S, antithrombin III, the prothrombin 20210 polymorphism, or factor V Leiden. Studies to investigate these possibilities should be confirmed either using the aforementioned initially obtained specimens or after a 6- to 12-month period of treatment with oral anticoagulants, followed by a 1- to 2-week period off oral anticoagulants to reestablish a normal level of these proteins. If deficiencies of one or more of these proteins are established, consideration should be given to long-term prophylaxis with oral anticoagulants.

The patient was treated with LMWH and did well. Initial hypercoagulable state workup indicated factor V Leiden heterozygous state by genetic testing. The epidemiology of this thrombotic event fits nicely into the current thinking, according to which "multiple hits" are responsible for most events. In this case, his genetic susceptibility (factor V Leiden) combined with unusual venous stasis (prolonged plane ride) triggered a thromboembolic complication. Other triggering events include general anesthesia for more than 1 hour, immobilization by casting of the leg, and pregnancy and the postpartum state. This patient is currently on long-term Coumadin and requires indefinite anticoagulation because he has an underlying genetic hypercoagulable state and has experienced multiple thrombotic events.

Breast Lump

A 41-year-old premenopausal white woman goes to her physician after discovering a lump in her left breast while doing a breast self-examination in the shower. She had thought in the past that she might have felt something in the same location, but now feels that the lump has gotten larger.

QUESTION

☐ *What additional historical information would you like to have from this patient?*

DISCUSSION

Eighty percent of women with breast lumps find the lump while performing a breast self-examination. As part of this patient's history, the physician should ask the patient about her risk factors for breast cancer. The physician should also ask the following questions: How long has the patient has been aware of the lump? What was its original size? When did it increase in size, and by how much? It also might help to know whether the mass changed in size in conjunction with the patient's menstrual period because benign disease can regress after the menstrual cycle. If the mass is not clinically suspicious, it might be appropriate to reevaluate the patient after her next menstrual cycle when the flow ends—if the mass persists, further workup with an ultrasound and diagnostic mammogram is necessary. If the mass is solid and suspicious on ultrasound, a core biopsy is needed to rule out malignancy. Did the patient experience any discharge from the nipples? If so, was it bloody or clear? The presence of breast edema, discoloration, or pain is important to ascertain. Finally, the patient should be asked whether she has had any mammograms in the past.

> Further history reveals that the patient first discovered the lump in the upper outer quadrant of her left breast about 4 months ago, but she did not seek medical attention because she has always had large, "lumpy," fibrocystic breasts. The patient's menstrual period does not seem to have affected the presence of the lump in any way. She has not experienced nipple discharge, breast edema or discoloration, or pain.
>
> The patient has no previous medical or surgical history and takes no medications. One of her paternal cousins died of breast cancer at age 45 years, but none of her other female relatives have had any cancers. Both of her parents are alive; her father has hypertension and coronary artery disease. The patient, who has experienced no symptoms of menopause, first began to menstruate at age 12 years and has had regular periods lasting 4 days on a 30-day cycle. She was pregnant three times at age 29, 33, and 36 years, and she has one 5-year-old daughter, with the first and second pregnancies having ended in miscarriage. She uses a diaphragm for birth control. Although the patient had a baseline mammogram at age 35 years, she has not had one since then, and she has not seen a gynecologist for more than 1 year.

QUESTIONS

☐ *What risk factors does this patient have for developing breast cancer?*

☐ *What diseases might be included in your differential diagnosis at this point?*

DISCUSSION

The most important risk factors for breast cancer are family history—maternal and/or paternal history of breast cancer, male breast cancer or ovarian cancer (especially if the patient has a first-degree relative who developed premenopausal breast cancer), a history of fibrocystic disease, a history of previous breast biopsies, early onset of menarche, late onset of menopause, a first pregnancy after the age of 30 years, and use of hormone replacement therapy by a postmenopausal patient. A patient's lack of risk factors for breast cancer should not dissuade the physician from performing the necessary procedures to rule out malignancy. Although most breast cancers are found in the upper outer quadrant, location should not change the physician's approach to excluding malignancy.

A young, premenopausal woman with a breast lump could have a benign mass such as a fibroadenoma or a cyst. Breast lumps are benign in 80% of cases, but malignancy must be ruled out. If the lump is indeed malignant, the patient has a higher chance of lymph node metastasis and micrometastatic disease as the tumor increases in size.

Physical examination shows a well-developed, thin, white woman who is slightly anxious but in no acute distress. The physical examination is normal except for the presence of a 2-cm mass in the upper, outer quadrant of the left breast. The mass appears firm and somewhat mobile. There is no obvious asymmetry between breasts, skin dimpling, or redness. No axillary nodes are palpable, and there are no masses in the right breast.

QUESTION

☐ *What would you do next to evaluate this patient?*

DISCUSSION

All patients with a definable mass should have an ultrasound and a mammogram; because this patient has not had a mammogram in 6 years, having one now would probably be especially worthwhile. A breast lump is visible on a mammogram alone in 20% of cases. However, mammograms are often difficult to interpret in premenopausal patients or postmenopausal patients taking estrogen replacement therapy, which may increase the breast tissue density on mammogram; dense (mammographically white) normal glandular breast tissue may obscure tumor masses of similar density. When a woman goes through menopause, the breast tissue may eventually become less dense mammographically; however, this process is not immediate and, in fact, can take several years. Due to the increase in the fat composition of the breast tissue in postmenopausal women, the mammogram has more of a gray background and is easier to interpret. The gray serves as an ideal background for identification of new breast abnormalities, which appear whiter in contrast to the normal breast tissue. A negative mammogram does not necessarily imply that a patient's mass is not cancerous.

In addition to having a mammogram, this patient should be referred for an ultrasound of the breast, which can determine whether the mass is solid or cystic. If the mass is cystic (simple cyst) a needle aspiration of the cyst should be performed to evaluate for the presence of fluid. If the mass disappears with aspiration of the fluid, then it is most likely a benign cyst (assuming the cytology is negative). Less than 1% of patients in whom the mass totally disappears have malignant cells seen on cyst aspiration. A cystic lesion seen on ultrasound examination should be the same size as the palpable mass. If there are internal echoes within the cyst, then a solid lesion cannot be ruled out, and carcinoma is still a possibility. In this case, a needle biopsy is then recommended to obtain tissue for pathologic evaluation.

If the mass is solid on breast ultrasound, the contents of the needle should be placed on a slide and submitted for cytology. Even if the cytology is benign, a malignant lesion still cannot be ruled out, and a core needle biopsy to obtain more tissue for diagnosis should be performed. The majority of patients with suspicious breast lumps can undergo a core needle biopsy under ultrasound or mammographic guidance (stereotactic biopsy). Very few patients with suspicious breast masses will need an excisional surgical biopsy to diagnose their breast cancer.

Attempted fine-needle aspiration does not produce any fluid. A mammogram shows a well-defined 2.2-cm density in the left upper, outer quadrant. No other densities or calcifications are noted. An ultrasound of the density confirms a solid mass 2.2 cm in diameter, which corresponds with the mammographic density.

The suspicious mammogram, coupled with the enlarging, palpable mass and the failure to aspirate fluid, led the physician to recommend that the patient undergo an ultrasound-guided biopsy of the lesion. The patient was referred to a radiology facility for an ultrasound-guided core needle biopsy of the suspicious lesion. The pathology report confirmed an infiltrating ductal carcinoma, grade 3, estrogen receptor positive (90%), progesterone receptor positive (50%), and Her2/*neu* positive (+3) by immunohistochemical (IHC) stains.

QUESTIONS

☐ *How would you stage this patient's cancer?*

☐ *What would be your preferred mode of treatment?*

☐ *What is the patient's prognosis?*

DISCUSSION

This patient would be classified as having clinical stage II disease because the tumor measures between 2 and 5 cm in diameter and there are no fixed nodes or distant metastases. Most patients with stage I or

II breast cancer can undergo lumpectomy (breast conservation surgery) and sentinel lymph node biopsy with further axillary lymph node dissection only if the sentinel lymph node is positive for metastases. Radiation therapy to the whole breast is given to all patients who have breast conservation therapy. The cure rates associated with this mode of treatment are equivalent to those for a modified radical mastectomy, if the patient meets certain criteria. Because this patient does not have multicentric disease in the breast, defined as two separate masses in two different quadrants of the breast, or a tumor greater than 5 cm in diameter, she is an optimal candidate for breast conservation therapy with lumpectomy, sentinel lymph node biopsy, and whole-breast radiation therapy. Breast MRI can be considered for further workup of both breasts before lumpectomy surgery, to rule out mammographically occult multicentricity of her breast cancer and also to rule out contralateral breast lesions.

Before the decision is made to perform a lumpectomy and sentinel lymph node biopsy, the patient should be seen by a radiation therapist. If the radiation therapist feels that the patient is not an optimal candidate for whole-breast radiation after lumpectomy, then a modified radical mastectomy is warranted. If the patient chooses to have a modified radical mastectomy, she has the option of undergoing breast reconstruction surgery at the time of the mastectomy or at some future time.

Adjuvant hormonal therapy, chemotherapy, and radiation therapy (i.e., radiation therapy for purposes other than breast conservation) also may play a role in treating patients with breast cancer. Adjuvant chemotherapy is almost always given before adjuvant radiation therapy.

Patients who present with large breast tumors (>5 cm in diameter) or with unresectable tumors may need neoadjuvant chemotherapy, which means that the chemotherapy is given first to shrink the tumor and then is followed by surgery and radiation therapy. Because the majority of breast tumors respond to neoadjuvant chemotherapy, this approach can be very valuable, as it allows the surgeon to completely resect the tumor.

Prognosis varies widely in breast cancer patients. Approximately 50% of patients with operable breast cancer develop recurrent disease unless they receive adjuvant chemotherapy or hormone therapy. Prognostic factors include tumor size, axillary node status, the histopathology of the tumor, hormone receptor status (estrogen and progesterone), the S-phase fraction and DNA index, and oncogene expression (Her2/*neu*). Most young premenopausal women with stage II breast cancer receive adjuvant chemotherapy and hormonal therapy, in addition to surgery and radiation therapy, if the tumor is estrogen and/or progesterone receptor positive. Women with Her2/*neu*-positive breast cancer also receive trastuzumab, a monoclonal antibody against Her2/*neu*, in conjunction with chemotherapy and then as maintenance for a total of 52 weeks.

CASE 6

Gastrointestinal Bleeding

A 54-year-old white man presents to his general practitioner's office complaining of fatigue. He says that he tires easily and often feels light-headed and short of breath after climbing a single flight of steps or taking a short walk. He says that he is having difficulty at work because he is "just not himself."

QUESTIONS

▢ *What are some possible causes of generalized fatigue and weakness?*

▢ *What other questions would you like to ask this patient?*

DISCUSSION

Fatigue and weakness are common complaints that can be psychogenic or physical in origin. It is important to differentiate between these broad etiologic categories. Psychogenic causes consist of anxiety states and depression. Physical causes include infectious disease, metabolic disorders, blood dyscrasias, renal disease, liver disease, chronic pulmonary disease, chronic cardiovascular disease, neoplastic diseases, and neuromuscular disease.

To narrow the diagnostic possibilities for this patient's fatigue and weakness, additional history should be obtained. The patient should be questioned about whether he has experienced weight loss, fever, chills, chest pain, paroxysmal nocturnal dyspnea, orthopnea, pedal edema, abdominal pain, changes in bowel habits, melena, hematochezia, polyuria, polydipsia, polyphagia, intolerance to heat or cold, or insomnia. A positive answer to these questions often, although not always, indicates a physical or organic cause of fatigue and weakness.

Further history indicates that the patient's symptoms started about 2 months ago and have steadily worsened. He claims he was in excellent health until this time; in fact, he has not had a routine physical examination in approximately 2 years because he has felt healthy. The patient takes no medications, except for the occasional use of acetaminophen or laxatives. He is an executive in a publishing company who smokes approximately half a pack of cigarettes per day and drinks a martini or two at lunch. He has no significant family history, except that an estranged older brother died after an abdominal operation for an unknown cause.

The patient denies chest pain or palpitations but has occasional shortness of breath and dyspnea on exertion, as described previously. He has had no loss of appetite and even jokes that he can eat even on days when he is a bit "irregular." When asked about his constipation, he notes that he sometimes has difficulty passing his stool, but the stool is of normal consistency. He reports that his stools have seemed a bit darker lately, but he thought it might be due to laxatives he took for constipation; he has not noticed any bright red blood in the stool and denies hematemesis, nausea, vomiting, or diarrhea.

QUESTION

▢ *Which of these signs and symptoms concern you?*

DISCUSSION

This patient's history raises several points of concern. His symptoms began 2 months ago, meaning that they are chronic complaints, and they have steadily worsened—an ominous sign. Acute complaints could be attributed to an acute viral or self-limited illness. Symptoms that have been present for a long time (2–3 years or more) suggest a chronic nonprogressive illness such as irritable bowel syndrome.

However, in a patient who was previously symptom free and in excellent health, a 2-month history of symptoms that have steadily worsened would suggest a new and potentially serious change that could be compatible with inflammatory bowel disease, infectious states (e.g., giardiasis), or malignant disease involving the gastrointestinal tract, particularly the colon.

The absence of medications would eliminate the possibility that a side effect of a drug (e.g., an antihypertensive agent) is responsible for the fatigue and shortness of breath. Smoking is clearly associated with numerous malignancies, including bronchogenic and pancreatic carcinoma, in addition to its known cardiovascular and pulmonary effects. The family history of an abdominal operation for an unknown cause raises the possibility of colon cancer, which has a twofold to threefold increased incidence in first-degree relatives. Dyspnea on exertion could signify a cardiovascular cause but also could be associated with anemia. The "abnormally dark stools" might be indicative of melena, which would suggest that the upper gastrointestinal tract (above the ligament of Treitz) is the most likely source of bleeding, whereas dark red or maroon-colored stools typically indicate blood emanating from the right colon.

Physical examination shows a well-developed, overweight white man with a somewhat rapid respiratory rate (i.e., 20 respirations/minute). Other vital signs show a pulse of 94 bpm, a blood pressure of 110/60 mm Hg, and a normal temperature. The patient's skin is pale, as are his mucous membranes. His lungs are clear on auscultation, and his heart rhythm is regular, with normal first and second heart sounds (S_1 and S_2) and no third or fourth heart sound (S_3 or S_4). His abdomen is soft, without tenderness or obvious masses. His extremities show no cyanosis or edema; he has prolonged capillary refill. His rectal examination shows no palpable masses, but a dark, heme-positive stool is noted.

QUESTIONS

▢ *Based on this physical examination, what do you suspect is the cause of this man's fatigue?*

▢ *What are some of the causes of melena?*

▢ *What disorders produce hematochezia?*

▢ *How would you proceed in working up the heme-positive stool?*

DISCUSSION

Physical examination shows an individual whose skin and mucous membranes are pale and who has heme-positive stool. These signs suggest that the patient has gastrointestinal bleeding and is most likely anemic, possibly the reason he is feeling fatigued.

Melena is the passage of dark, tarry stools due to the presence of blood altered by intestinal juices. It is most commonly caused by upper gastrointestinal bleeding (e.g., duodenal ulcer disease, gastric ulcer disease, upper gastrointestinal malignancy, hemorrhagic gastritis, erosive esophagitis, esophageal varices or Mallory–Weiss tears, or vascular ectasia of the stomach). In an individual who is not acutely ill, peptic ulcer disease would be the most common cause; esophageal varices or a Mallory–Weiss tear of the distal esophagus would be unlikely.

Hematochezia is the passage of blood from the rectum, which varies in color from dark red or maroon (from bleeding in the right colon) to bright red (as a result of bleeding from a more distal colonic source or the anal ring itself). Hematochezia may be caused by colonic diverticulosis and angiodysplasia, hemorrhoids, fissures, colon polyps, colon carcinoma, ulcerative colitis, infectious dysentery (especially *Shigella*, *Campylobacter*, and amebic colitis), and ischemic colitis. Occasionally, an upper gastrointestinal source (e.g., brisk bleeding from a peptic ulcer) could lead to the passage of bright red blood from the rectum. Generally, this occurrence is seen in a patient who is hemodynamically unstable and would be identified by the finding of blood on the passage of a nasogastric tube into the stomach.

The initial workup for heme-positive stool depends on the patient's history and physical examination. If the history and examination are suggestive of an upper gastrointestinal source, initial evaluation should include upper endoscopy. However, in most cases of occult gastrointestinal bleeding when a lower gastrointestinal source is expected, colonoscopy is indicated. If this study is unrevealing, an upper gastrointestinal source should be pursued, followed by an evaluation of the small bowel if no source is found. Upper gastrointestinal endoscopy is the best initial first study. If no upper gastrointestinal source is identified, small bowel enteroscopy, small bowel follow-through, or wireless capsule endoscopy is indicated.

A nasogastric tube is inserted but does not reveal any evidence of blood. The physician has an anoscope in his office, but anoscopy does not show any obvious lesions. In-office hemoglobin and hematocrit tests give values of 9.4 g/dL and 36%, respectively. The physician decides to refer the patient to a gastroenterologist for further workup of the gastrointestinal bleeding.

QUESTIONS

☐ *Why does the physician first look for evidence of upper gastrointestinal bleeding?*

☐ *What are the most common causes of lower gastrointestinal bleeding in this age group?*

DISCUSSION

The patient's description suggested dark stool, but the history and physical exam could not clearly identify melena. Therefore, an upper gastrointestinal source was sought by the passage of a nasogastric tube. In approximately 75%–80% of cases, an upper gastrointestinal bleeding source can be identified by blood in the nasogastric tube. Occasionally, bleeding from a duodenal ulcer will not reflux into the stomach and result in a gastric aspirate that is negative for blood.

In this patient's age group, the two most common causes of massive lower gastrointestinal bleeding are diverticulosis and angiodysplasia, while colonic polyp or malignancy should be suspected for chronic low-grade bleeding. The differential diagnosis would also include those conditions known to cause hematochezia, as discussed earlier. A bleeding diathesis caused by a primary hematologic source such as leukemia, thrombocytopenia, hemophilia, or disseminated intravascular coagulation (DIC) should also be considered but are less likely.

The gastroenterologist sees the patient immediately, and some laboratory tests are performed. A complete blood count (CBC) shows a white blood cell (WBC) count of 7.2/mm³, a platelet count of 525,000/mm³, and hemoglobin and hematocrit consistent with the previous values. Red blood cell (RBC) indices show a mean corpuscular volume (MCV) of 70 μm³ and a mean corpuscular hemoglobin (MCH) of 25 pg. Serum iron and transferrin are decreased. Prothrombin time (PT) and partial thromboplastin (PTT) are normal, as are electrolyte, blood urea nitrogen (BUN), and creatinine levels.

QUESTIONS

☐ *What type of anemia do these values suggest?*

☐ *Which of the previously mentioned differential diagnoses can be ruled out by the laboratory values?*

- *What conditions are the highest on your differential?*
- *What are your immediate management plans?*

DISCUSSION

The laboratory findings suggest a microcytic, hypochromic anemia. The MCV of 70 mm^3 and the MCH of 25 pg are compatible with this diagnosis. The differential diagnosis of this type of anemia includes iron deficiency caused by poor intake, lack of absorption, or chronic blood loss. An elevated platelet count is often seen in patients with this condition. The usual source of chronic occult blood loss is from the gastrointestinal tract. Iron chelation therapy for lead intoxication also may cause this type of anemia. Congenital anemia such as thalassemia is also associated with hypochromic, microcytic anemia. Iron-deficiency states are characterized by a low serum iron, a high total iron-binding capacity, and a low ferritin level.

The normal PT and PTT make a bleeding diathesis unlikely. Anemia of chronic renal insufficiency would be ruled out by the normal BUN and creatinine levels.

The most likely causes of this patient's problems are those involving chronic gastrointestinal blood loss (i.e., colonic polyp, colonic neoplasm, or angiodysplasia). Of particular concern is colonic neoplasm, in light of the patient's recent history of a change in bowel habits (constipation).

Immediate management goals include correcting hypovolemia if present, monitoring serial hemoglobin and hematocrit values to be certain that the patient does not have ongoing bleeding, arresting any active hemorrhage, and preventing recurrent hemorrhage.

The gastroenterologist arranges for a colonoscopy. During the colonoscopy, five hemorrhagic-appearing polyps are noted in the descending portion of the colon. The polyps are 1–2 cm in size, and most are pedunculated. These lesions are removed by snare cautery and sent to pathology for evaluation.

QUESTIONS

- *What other procedures could have been used to investigate this problem?*
- *Why was colonoscopy useful in this case?*
- *What would have prevented colonoscopy from being a useful diagnostic tool?*

DISCUSSION

If bleeding were active and profuse, a technetium-labeled RBC scan, angiography, or both could locate a bleeding source, especially if the blood loss exceeded 0.2–1.0 mL/min. In this patient's situation, colonoscopy is the test of choice because it can be both diagnostic and therapeutic if a colonic lesion is discovered.

Furthermore, colonoscopy was useful because there was no active bleeding to limit total examination of the colonic mucosa. However, if the bowel lumen had been coated with blood, a small polyp or arteriovenous malformation could have been missed. In addition, if hemodynamic instability makes the patient a poor candidate for adequate sedation, a thorough evaluation of the colon may not be possible.

Pathology indicates villous adenomatous polyps with no foci of carcinoma. The patient is reassured, treated with iron supplements, and told to return in 1 year for a follow-up colonoscopy. If unremarkable, a repeat colonoscopy at 3–5 years would be indicated.

QUESTIONS

- *What factors about polyps increase the risk of adenocarcinoma?*
- *What would the treatment have been if foci of malignant cells had been found?*

DISCUSSION

Adenomatous and villous adenomatous polyps are considered precursors for adenocarcinoma. The risk of adenocarcinoma in patients with colonic polyps increases in proportion to the amount of villous tissue present in the polyp. Polyps that are sessile or greater than 2 cm in diameter also carry an increased risk for developing into carcinoma. Management of a malignant focus in a colonic polyp depends on the type of polyp. If a polyp is pedunculated on a long stalk and the malignant cells have not invaded the stalk, the patient could be cured by simple colonoscopic polypectomy. However, if the malignant cells have invaded the stalk, or if the polyp is sessile and the malignant cells reach the margins of resection, the patient would require a segmental colonic resection. In either case, follow-up colonoscopy is indicated on a periodic basis in patients who have adenomatous colonic polyps or if a malignancy is identified in any such lesions.

Newly Discovered Renal Failure

A 62-year-old man visits his physician for a routine physical examination. He mentions that he has to get out of bed to urinate more frequently than he used to (two to three times each night) and that he has difficulty initiating and maintaining a urinary stream. In addition, he states that he has experienced mild shortness of breath on walking two to three flights of stairs and that his regular biweekly workouts at the gym have been much more difficult for him lately.

Physical examination shows moderate pallor, a blood pressure of 150/105 mm Hg, a pulse of 80 bpm, and a respiratory rate of 18 breaths/minute. There is trace pedal edema. Examination of the chest and heart shows no abnormalities. Examination of the abdomen shows slight fullness in the lower abdomen but neither tenderness nor pain.

Laboratory work is obtained, including a complete blood count (CBC), electrolyte, glucose, calcium, and renal studies. The results of these studies are as follows: blood urea nitrogen (BUN), 88 mg/dL; creatinine, 6.4 mg/dL; sodium, 137 mEq/L; potassium, 5.9 mEq/L; chloride, 112 mEq/L; bicarbonate, 16 mEq/L; hemoglobin, 8.7 g/dL.

QUESTIONS

☐ *What is the first determination you should make with respect to this patient?*

☐ *What additional information might help you make this determination?*

☐ *What is the most likely cause of this patient's renal insufficiency? Does the patient's altered electrolyte and acid–base metabolism support this diagnosis?*

DISCUSSION

The determination of onset of renal failure is crucial to determine the proper therapeutic approach. Acute kidney injury implies the potential for reversibility, and therefore every effort must be made to identify any ongoing injurious agents that adversely affect the kidney. In addition, acute support through some form of renal replacement therapy may be required until renal recovery can occur. Conversely, the presence of chronic renal failure suggests that the patient has sustained irreversible injury. The patient must then be treated in a way to prevent further loss of kidney function. Chronic renal replacement therapy, either through dialysis support or through transplantation, may be necessary.

The determination of chronicity of renal failure can be difficult. In patients with acute kidney injury, a clear precipitating event (e.g., sepsis, shock, exposure to nephrotoxic agents such as gentamicin or intravenous contrast) usually can be identified. The determination of the onset of chronic disease is more problematic. The time of initiation of subtle symptoms consistent with renal failure (e.g., pruritus) may be helpful in determining the onset of the disease. Renal ultrasound provides information about kidney size, which typically is reduced in chronic kidney disease and normal in acute injury. Exceptions include diabetic nephropathy and amyloidosis, which may be associated with normal or enlarged kidneys, and polycystic kidney disease, which may be associated with extremely large kidneys despite coexistent renal failure. Chronic kidney disease is typically associated with secondary hyperparathyroidism; subperiosteal resorption is typically seen radiographically. In addition, generalized bone demineralization, loss of bone mass at the acromi–oclavicular joint, or mottling of the skull may be important findings. Anemia is typically seen in chronic kidney disease because erythropoietin levels are reduced as kidney mass is reduced. However, anemia may develop rather rapidly, and occasionally, severe anemia is seen in both acute and chronic renal failure; it likely explains the dyspnea in this patient.

This patient most likely has acute renal insufficiency as a result of chronic obstructive uropathy. This conclusion stems from the history of difficulty voiding; the presence of bladder fullness on physical examination; and the findings of renal failure, hyperkalemia, and metabolic acidosis. Other common causes of acute kidney injury in the ambulatory setting include toxic nephropathy from medication use and acute glomerulonephritis. In men, the most common cause of chronic obstructive nephropathy is prostatic hypertrophy, but bladder cancer or prostatic cancer is possible as well. The patient has hyperchloremic hypobicarbonatemia with associated hyperkalemia. This constellation of findings is common in patients with chronic kidney disease, particularly in association with obstructive uropathy. The hypobicarbonatemia suggests metabolic acidosis but also could be caused by chronic respiratory alkalosis.

The presence of renal insufficiency makes metabolic acidosis the most likely cause of the hypobicarbonatemia in this patient. The high chloride level reflects the fact that electrical neutrality must be maintained by body fluids, and as bicarbonate levels fall, preferential chloride reabsorption with sodium occurs in the renal tubules. Because the kidney is unable to generate new bicarbonate, bicarbonate levels fall. A reduced bicarbonate level is typical of all forms of renal failure.

The increase in serum potassium is an important indication of obstructive uropathy. Potassium is secreted in the distal nephron but requires adequate amounts of aldosterone as well as a normally responsive distal tubule potassium transport system for normal excretion. Chronic obstructive uropathy is associated with impairment of potassium excretion, occasionally secondary to reduced aldosterone levels but more typically due to a direct tubular abnormality. Correction of the underlying obstructive process leads to a normalization of potassium excretion and a return of serum potassium levels to the normal range.

> **Renal ultrasound is performed and confirms the diagnosis of obstructive uropathy. A Foley catheter is put in place.**

QUESTION

- *What clinical problem should be anticipated after relief of obstruction?*

DISCUSSION

On relief of obstruction, it is typical for patients with obstructive uropathy to undergo a striking diuresis. The source of the diuresis is a combination of excretion of previously retained solutes and fluids as well as a mild residual tubular defect in sodium and water conservation. This massive diuresis typically remits once the patient's BUN and creatinine have leveled off.

Dialysis, either by hemodialysis or peritoneal dialysis, may be necessary in patients with renal insufficiency secondary to obstructive uropathy, but attempts should always be made to correct the obstructive uropathy before initiating hemodialysis. The decision to perform dialysis must be made on an individual basis and defies simple categorization. Hemodialysis is indicated in patients with pericarditis. Congestive heart failure also may be an indication for dialysis therapy to achieve fluid removal. Institution of dialysis should not be made on the basis of the absolute BUN level alone, although most clinicians believe that the BUN should be maintained below 150 mg/dL.

CASE 8

Recurrent Sinopulmonary Infections in a Child

A change to 2 (more likely age of presentation for XLA)-year-old boy is brought to your office for routine follow-up. It is noted that the child has another ear infection. On reviewing his chart, you note that the child has had numerous ear infections, several sinus infections, and three episodes of documented pneumonia. None of these infections has required hospitalization. The child has always responded well to antibiotics.

QUESTIONS

- *What physical examination findings would make the practitioner question whether this child was immunologically normal?*
- *What is the normal number of infections for a child of this age?*
- *What are other diseases that could be causing the recurrent infections?*

DISCUSSION

The child presented here has a common problem: recurrent sinopulmonary infections. The difference between a child who is having multiple infections and one who has immune deficiency is sometimes subtle. It is normal for a child of this age to have anywhere between 8 and 12 upper respiratory infections per year. Most of these would occur during the winter months.

If a child is presently in day care, then that number of infections can be higher. In addition, it is sometimes very difficult to distinguish between a viral otitis media and a bacterial one; this can lead to an overuse of antibiotics.

Several clinical signs may indicate that the child may have an immune deficiency and not just a normal number of infections, including absence of lymphoid tissue. This is seen in X-linked agammaglobulinemia (XLA). Therefore, the child with XLA will have virtually no tonsillar or adenoidal tissue. When the examiner tries to palpate for lymph nodes, they will not be easily found. Furthermore, children with this disease commonly have very severe ear infections, and the otoscopic examination may show scarred and deformed tympanic membranes which is very different from what is found in most children with recurrent ear infections. Pyogenic encapsulated bacteria such as *Streptococcus pneumonia*, *Haemophilus influenzae*, *Staphylococcus aureus*, and *Pseudomonas* species usually cause these infections. With all of these organisms, antibodies are important for opsonization and killing of the bacteria. Finally, if the child had many episodes of pneumonia, they may have chronic scarring in the chest, but that is an unusual finding and would not be identified by physical examination but rather by radiologic studies. Another important physical finding to look for in a child with recurrent sinopulmonary infections is nasal polyps and clubbing of the nail beds. If found, cystic fibrosis evaluation (sweat chloride) should be considered.

The differential diagnosis for this child also includes anatomic abnormalities of the upper airway, gastroesophageal reflux, and potentially even atopy as the cause of recurrent otitis media and sinusitis.

Other types of immune deficiencies also can cause recurrent infections. The most common would be a severe combined immune deficiency, but such children almost always present before 1 year of life. Other immune deficiencies also can present at this age and would need to be evaluated (e.g., Common Variable Immunodeficiency (CVID), Complement Deficiency and Wiskott–Aldrich).

> **On careful examination, you note that the child has very scarred tympanic membranes. You also note that he has very small tonsils. In addition, you also review the chart carefully and note that this child has received antibiotics since the age of 1, almost on a monthly basis.**

QUESTION

- *What immunologic and radiologic studies would be indicated?*

DISCUSSION

The serologic evaluation would center on the child's immunoglobulins and antibody function. This could be done either in a stepwise fashion or as a comprehensive examination. The first step would involve measuring the quantitative IgG, IgM, and IgA. Other tests that could be done would involve functional antibodies to the vaccines that the child has received to evaluate the child's ability to mount an antibody response (tetanus, hemophilus influenza (Hib) and pneumococcal antibodies). A CH50 should be sent to assess the complement system and a complete blood count with differential to look for anemia and cytopenia. If there is evidence of lymphopenia on CBC and/or if the immunoglobulins are abnormal, then T and B cell subsets by flow cytometry to identify whether mature B cells are present (low in XLA) or if T cell subsets are low (seen in SCID and in 50% of CVID patients). The radiologic studies that could be performed would include a chest x-ray, looking for scarring from previous pneumonias, a lateral neck film to evaluate adenoidal tissue, and possibly a modified barium swallow to identify whether the child has gastroesophageal reflux.

> **The laboratory values are available and indicate that the child does have X-linked agammaglobulinemia: IgG levels of 150 mg/dL (normal = 600–1500 mg/dL), undetectable antibody titers to diphtheria and tetanus, normal T cell indices, and no detected mature B cells (CD19+). The child is referred to a pediatric immunologist, and infusions of intravenous gammaglobulin (IVIG) are started.**

QUESTIONS

- *Should the child receive other medications in addition to the intravenous (IV) gamma-globulin?*
- *Does the child need immunizations now that he is receiving gamma-globulin?*

DISCUSSION

Children with XLA require close follow-up by an immunologist. IVIG will help to prevent severe systemic infections, but may not prevent otitis media and sinusitis. If infections occur, these patients require aggressive antibiotic treatment.

Immunizations are not only unnecessary but in some cases contraindicated in this child. The child with XLA has no ability to generate an antibody response; therefore, immunizations will not be helpful. In fact, immunizations with live viruses such as live polio vaccine and measles mumps rubella vaccine can be detrimental. It was this population that was the impetus for the change from using a live polio virus to the killed vaccine that is currently in use.

The child is doing well, and the family is concerned about other issues they need to face. They are worried that even with the replacement therapy, his immune system is not normal.

QUESTIONS

- *Are there other infections and other manifestations that merit concern?*
- *Are these children susceptible to other infections?*

DISCUSSION

These children, before the advent of IV gamma-globulin, would commonly succumb to echovirus or Coxsackie virus infections. They would develop a chronic meningoencephalitis that would be insidious and have progressive neurologic symptoms. These infections would go on to be quite debilitating, if not fatal. These children less commonly are susceptible to a variety of other ailments, including protein-losing enteropathy, malabsorption, neutropenia, alopecia totalis, and amyloidosis. They also may have an autoimmune seronegative arthritis that is not related to an infection. The arthritis usually affects the large joints, causing hydrarthrosis and limited range of movement without joint pain or destruction.

These children handle most other infections quite well. They are not more susceptible to herpes infection or tuberculosis. When they do have these infections, they are no more serious than infections that occur in any normal patient and are self-limited. *Pneumocystis carinii* has been observed in a few patients with XLA, but those are usually extremely debilitated patients.

CASE 9

HIV Infection

A 37-year-old man who was diagnosed with human immunodeficiency virus type 1 (HIV-1) infection 4 years ago has experienced good overall health for 3 years despite a falling CD4 count. Although he was strongly encouraged to continue to take antiretroviral drugs, he stopped because of intolerable side effects. Fourteen months ago, he developed headaches and mild confusion at a time when his CD4 count was 94 cells/mm^3. Imaging studies and spinal fluid analysis confirmed the diagnosis of cryptococcal meningitis, and the patient responded well to antifungal therapy. He also consented to take antiretroviral drugs again.

QUESTIONS

- *What is the value of the CD4 count in monitoring patients who are infected with HIV-1?*
- *What are the major neurologic problems encountered in people with HIV-1 infection?*

DISCUSSION

When levels of circulating CD4 cells drop below certain thresholds, various interventions such as infection prophylaxis or antiretroviral therapy should be offered to the patient. (For example, when the CD4 count drops to less than 200 cells/mm^3, prophylaxis for *Pneumocystis carinii* pneumonia [PCP] should be initiated.) The CD4 count can be performed in many hospital and reference laboratories. The "viral load," as measured by quantitating the amount of viral nucleic acid in the blood, is primarily a measure of the rate of the disease's progression and of its response to drug therapy.

It is very common for patients infected by HIV-1 to experience a long period of clinical latency. Active viral replication occurs during all phases of the disease, but symptoms usually do not become apparent until there has been a substantial reduction in host immune function. Intervention with antiretroviral drugs can prevent, delay, or reverse this immune deterioration. Evaluation of clinical parameters (e.g., weight loss, decreasing functional capacity, development of one or more specific problems) and laboratory tests (e.g., enumeration of CD4 cells or quantitation of viral RNA) indicates the stage of HIV disease.

Several neurologic infections can complicate HIV-1 infection; the two most common conditions are cryptococcal meningitis and toxoplasmic encephalitis. Both of these infections occur relatively late in the course of HIV-1 infection, at a time when there are clinical or laboratory clues of strikingly diminished cellular immunity. Patients with cryptococcal infection commonly present with a chronic meningitis characterized by headache and diffuse, often mild neurologic symptoms. Patients with toxoplasmosis more often present with focal neurologic findings or seizures. Dementia secondary to HIV-1 infection is also common late in the course of the disease. Less common neurologic complications include progressive multifocal leukoencephalopathy, central nervous system (CNS) lymphoma, neurosyphilis, *Listeria* meningitis, herpes simplex encephalitis, and cytomegalovirus (CMV) encephalitis.

> **The patient was able to return to work as a financial planner 14 months ago, and he seemed to be tolerating his medications. His drug regimen consisted of trimethoprim–sulfamethoxazole 3 days a week; isoniazid daily; fluconazole; and zidovudine, lamivudine, and lopinavir/ritonavir.**
>
> **During this office visit, the patient says he is less peppy than usual after a bout of gastrointestinal illness consisting of watery diarrhea and crampy abdominal pain. He thinks he may have had some fevers over the last 2 weeks, but he has not taken his temperature.**

QUESTIONS

- *What is the purpose of each of the medications the patient is currently taking?*
- *What is the differential diagnosis of watery diarrhea in advanced HIV infection?*
- *What diagnostic tests can be done to determine the cause of watery diarrhea?*
- *Of what significance is fever in individuals with advanced HIV infection?*

DISCUSSION

This patient is receiving a number of medications that are common to patients with HIV infection. Zidovudine, lamivudine, and lopinavir/ritonavir are four of the growing list of antiretroviral drugs available for direct suppression of HIV. Trimethoprim–sulfamethoxazole is used to prevent *P. carinii* infection, but it is also partly effective in preventing symptomatic toxoplasmosis and in reducing the number of bacterial infections. The fluconazole is given to prevent a recurrence of the patient's previously documented cryptococcal meningitis. Because the rate of symptomatic recurrence of cryptococcal meningitis is high, fluconazole should be given until the patient's immune function improves substantially. The isoniazid is used to prevent tuberculosis in a patient who has already been infected (i.e., one who tested positive using the purified protein derivative [PPD] test). There is no accepted indication for monotherapy in patients with active tuberculosis.

Watery diarrhea is a common complication of HIV infection. Many cases are self-limited, and no specific etiology is determined. However, a wide variety of pathogens have been associated with this syndrome. The most common and perhaps the hardest to treat is *Cryptosporidium parvum*. Other protozoans that can cause diarrhea of this nature are *Giardia intestinalis*, microsporidia, and *Isospora belli*. Common bacterial agents of watery diarrhea include *Escherichia coli*, *Salmonella*, and *Campylobacter*. When a patient is undergoing or has recently completed a course of antibacterial therapy, diarrhea secondary to the toxin produced by *Clostridium difficile* should always be considered.

Diagnostic tests for watery diarrhea should be ordered when the diarrhea is persistent or extremely symptomatic. Usually, stool specimens are sent for microscopic assessment of protozoa (some laboratories call this test the ova and parasites test). The laboratory should be notified that cryptosporidia and other unusual protozoa are being sought. Stool cultures should also be sent. If a patient is currently undergoing or has just completed a course of antibacterial therapy, toxin tests for *C. difficile* should be ordered as well. If these noninvasive tests do not yield a result, further evaluation could entail endoscopic studies of the lower gastrointestinal tract or aspiration of the upper intestinal contents. A definitive diagnosis can be elusive if the first few stool tests are negative.

Fever is a very nonspecific problem in patients with advanced HIV infection. The development of new fever should prompt a careful history and physical evaluation. In addition to the large spectrum of infections that can produce a fever, a number of noninfectious processes such as malignancies and drug reactions should be considered. If the patient history, physical examination, chest radiographs, and routine laboratory tests do not suggest an organ-specific abnormality, disseminated infections such as *Mycobacterium avium-intracellulare* (MAI), histoplasmosis, CMV, and HIV itself should be considered as causes of the fever.

On examination, the patient looks alert but pale. His temperature is 38°C, but otherwise, his vital signs are normal. The patient has lost 6 pounds since his last visit, 6 weeks earlier. Otherwise, there are no focal abnormalities. Laboratory testing shows a hemoglobin of 9.0 g/dL and a white blood cell (WBC) count of 3400 cells/mm^3 with a normal differential. The mean corpuscular volume (MCV) is 99 μm^3, and the serum vitamin B$_{12}$ level is at the lower limit of normal. The patient's CD4 count is 32 cells/mm^3. Chemistries show mild elevation of aspartate aminotransferase (AST) and alanine aminotransferase (ALT).

QUESTIONS

▢ *What is the differential diagnosis of the macrocytic anemia?*

▢ *What is the significance of the weight loss?*

▢ *Why has this patient not responded to antiretroviral therapy?*

DISCUSSION

Macrocytic anemia is fairly common in patients with advanced HIV infection. Although nutritional deficiencies should be considered as potential causes of macrocytic anemia, the disorder is far more commonly associated with drug therapy—zidovudine or the antimetabolites of trimethoprim–sulfamethoxazole can cause macrocytic anemia. In many cases, the anemia is mild and only bears watching, but sometimes patients are given leucovorin (folinic acid) to combat the folate depletion brought on by zidovudine or trimethoprim–sulfamethoxazole. The serum levels of vitamin B$_{12}$ can be depressed in patients with acquired immunodeficiency syndrome (AIDS), but there is rarely a response to injections of vitamin B$_{12}$.

Weight loss is a sign of active disease associated with HIV infection. In many patients, no obvious malabsorption, infection, or malignancy is present to account for weight loss, so efforts are directed at increasing the lean body weight. Nutritional supplements and hormonal manipulations are the most common interventions. Many infections are associated with weight loss, but in the absence of malabsorption or organ dysfunction, disseminated infections should be considered first.

The patient may not have responded to antiretroviral agents for several reasons. First, he may not have fully adhered to the treatment regimen; this noncompliance can result in both incomplete viral suppression and early emergence of resistant viral strains. Second, he may have been infected with a strain of HIV-1 that was already resistant to one or more of the antiretroviral drugs. Third, his initial viral load may have been so high that even perfect medication habits and a drug-susceptible viral strain will not have lowered his viral load sufficiently to allow for good immune reconstitution. Although a change in medications can help some of these patients, it is now clear that some individuals will not respond optimally to antiretroviral therapy despite all efforts. At this point, laboratory tests can help confirm which antiretrovirals might be expected to work. Resistance tests (akin to bacterial tests for susceptibility or resistance) can be ordered. They are expensive and often difficult to interpret, but they can be extremely helpful in fashioning an effective treatment schedule. A review of medications with an emphasis on the importance of full adherence would be necessary with the next change of medications.

Blood cultures for mycobacteria are reported as positive 2 weeks later. The patient's fever has persisted, and he has lost 3 more pounds. He still has no localizing complaints. Repeat complete blood count (CBC) and chemistry tests show no change.

QUESTION

▢ *What is the most likely explanation for the positive blood cultures?*

DISCUSSION

Most likely, the positive blood cultures represent infection with *M. avium-intracellulare* rather than *Mycobacterium tuberculosis*. Disseminated tuberculosis without any organ involvement is rare, and it is even rarer to find positive blood cultures for *M. tuberculosis* at all (except in patients with overwhelming, possibly terminal, tuberculosis). In addition, it would be even more unusual (although not impossible) for cultures to be positive when the patient is on prophylactic isoniazid therapy.

M. avium-intracellulare is a commonly occurring late complication of HIV infection, which is not at all susceptible to isoniazid. MAI would most likely account for the weight loss seen in this patient. Patients with MAI infection have infiltration of many organs (with very little tissue reaction), with frequent high titers of mycobacteria in the blood and bone marrow. Many affected patients experience a partial or complete reversal of weight loss when the bacterial infection is brought under control.

> The patient is started on therapy with three oral agents: ofloxacin, clarithromycin, and ethambutol. A gradual reduction in fever occurs, and he is able to return to work full-time. His weight stabilizes, and he is comfortable except for intermittent nausea from the large number of pills that he takes daily. Laboratory tests show that his viral isolate is treatable with didanosine, emtricitabine, and tenofovir, which can be given on a once-a-day schedule.

QUESTION

- *What is the patient's prognosis?*
- *Could this infection have been prevented?*

DISCUSSION

MAI infection may be controlled but is essentially never cured in people with AIDS unless their immune dysfunction is reversed. Although MAI infection is rarely the direct cause of death in such individuals, mycobacteremia is a predictor of earlier mortality and increased morbidity. Treatment of mycobacteremia can benefit those people who tolerate the therapy and who are not moribund at its inception. Prevention of MAI infection is possible with the use of drugs in the macrolide and rifamycin classes. Rifamycins have significant interactions with many anti–HIV-1 medications and should be used cautiously. Macrolides such as azithromycin and clarithromycin can be used as prophylaxis in patients at risk ($<$75 CD4+ cells/mm^3). These provide significant although not complete protection from MAI infection. The simplification of his treatment might help him to maintain good adherence to treatment.

CASE 10

Coma in a Diabetic Patient

A 20-year-old college student is rushed to the emergency department by ambulance after being found comatose by her roommate in her dormitory room. She is known to have type 1 (insulin-dependent) diabetes mellitus that has been well controlled by diet and insulin.

QUESTIONS

- *What are your immediate concerns about this patient?*
- *What are possible mechanisms of coma in a diabetic patient?*
- *What is at the top of your differential diagnosis?*

DISCUSSION

When the patient first arrives in the emergency department, an adequate airway should be ensured, vital signs should be measured to assess circulatory status, intravenous access should be established, and blood should be drawn for chemistries, arterial blood gas measurements, and a fingerstick glucose determination. Then additional information should be obtained from the patient's friend.

The causes of coma that are directly related to diabetes are diabetic ketoacidosis, hypoglycemia, and hyperosmolar nonketotic coma. The latter occurs mainly in elderly patients with type 2 (non–insulin-dependent) diabetes, so the first diagnostic impressions when this patient arrives in the emergency department are diabetic ketoacidosis and hypoglycemia.

Diabetic ketoacidosis occurs when there is a severe insulin deficiency, which causes an inability to utilize glucose and leads to hyperglycemia, ketosis, and acidosis. Hypoglycemia in a diabetic patient is usually the result of an imbalance between the factors that lower the blood glucose level—primarily administered insulin, oral hypoglycemic agents (in patients with type 2 diabetes), and exercise—and the factors that raise the blood glucose level, namely food ingestion and hepatic output of glucose. Diabetic ketoacidosis and hypoglycemia should be ruled out before serious consideration is given to other causes of coma such as drug overdose, seizures, stroke, or meningitis.

> The roommate recalls that the patient has been complaining of an "upset stomach" for 2 days, with some nausea, anorexia, mild diarrhea, and increasing abdominal pain. She seemed a bit groggy that morning and did not go to classes. Because she was unable to eat breakfast, she did not

take her morning insulin dose. The roommate returned from class at 3:00 pm and found the patient lying in bed, breathing deeply and unresponsive to questions.

QUESTIONS

▢ *What risk factors does this patient have for the development of diabetic ketoacidosis?*

▢ *What is the significance of each of the patient's complaints?*

DISCUSSION

The apparently gradual onset over a period of hours, the preceding illness, and the omission of an insulin dose strongly suggest diabetic ketoacidosis rather than hypoglycemia as the most likely diagnosis. Illnesses such as upper respiratory infection or gastroenteritis may increase the need for insulin because of stress-related increases in catecholamines, cortisol, and glucagon; omitting insulin doses because of the illness makes matters worse. The gastrointestinal symptoms at the onset of illness suggest that gastroenteritis was the precipitating event, although the increasing abdominal pain could have been caused also by the developing ketoacidosis.

Why does abdominal pain sometimes occur in diabetic ketoacidosis? Gastric distention may be a factor, and it is known that ketosis from other causes such as starvation may lead to gastrointestinal symptoms such as anorexia, nausea, and vomiting. However, the precise cause of abdominal pain in diabetic ketoacidosis is not known. The grogginess that the patient experienced earlier in the day suggests that the process leading to mental obtundation had already started. The symptoms of diabetic ketoacidosis are typically gradual in onset (over several hours), whereas the mental changes of hypoglycemia commonly have a relatively sudden onset, which is usually preceded by adrenergic symptoms such as sweating, tremor, and palpitations.

On examination, the patient is unresponsive, with dry skin and mucous membranes and rapid, deep respirations. Her blood pressure is 100/60 mm Hg supine, falling to 80/50 mm Hg when the head of the bed is raised. The neck veins are collapsed when the patient is lying supine. Her pulse rate is 110 bpm, her respiratory rate is 24 breaths/minute, and her temperature is 37°C. She winces when moderate pressure is applied to her abdomen. The deep tendon reflexes are hypoactive.

QUESTIONS

▢ *Do these physical findings aid in differentiating between diabetic ketoacidosis and hypoglycemia?*

▢ *What is the significance of the patient's respiratory pattern?*

DISCUSSION

These physical findings are highly suggestive of diabetic ketoacidosis. Insufficient insulin action makes glucose unavailable to the tissues, and the liver responds by producing ketones as an alternative fuel. The rising blood levels of glucose and ketones cause an osmotic diuresis, producing dehydration and intravascular volume depletion, with orthostatic hypotension. The osmotic diuresis leads to urinary losses of potassium (vomiting increases its loss) and other electrolytes; hypokalemia causes muscle weakness and decreased reflexes and respiratory paralysis if severe. Abdominal pain and tenderness, perhaps caused by the ketosis, may be severe. The rapid, deep respirations, called Kussmaul's respirations, are caused by stimulation of the respiratory center by acidosis. This leads to respiratory alkalosis, which partially offsets the metabolic acidosis.

Blood glucose by fingerstick, determined soon after the patient's arrival in the emergency department, is found to be greater than 400 mg/dL. Urine dipstick testing is strongly positive for glucose and ketones. Treatment is started with an intravenous infusion of normal saline solution at a rate of 1000 mL/hour.

QUESTIONS

▢ *What is the rationale behind ordering these laboratory tests?*

▢ *What initial steps should be taken at this point to manage this patient's condition?*

DISCUSSION

The elevated blood and urine glucose levels and urine ketone levels confirm the diagnosis of diabetic ketoacidosis. The first priority in treatment is fluid replacement, which can be started while the initial laboratory results are awaited. An infusion of normal saline (1 L/hour for the first 2 hours) should be given if intravascular volume depletion is severe, as indicated by the orthostatic hypotension and decreased central venous pressure (decreased neck vein filling). Once the diagnosis of diabetic ketoacidosis is confirmed, insulin therapy should be started.

Intravenous infusion of regular insulin is started at a rate of 5 U/hour (0.1 U/kg per hour). Initial laboratory results include the following serum findings: glucose level of 520 mg/dL, sodium level of 132 mEq/L, potassium level of 3.3 mEq/L, and normal phosphate, calcium, and chloride levels. Blood urea nitrogen (BUN) and creatinine are slightly elevated, as is serum amylase. The white blood cell (WBC) count is 14,500/mm³. Arterial blood gas analysis indicates a pH of 7.20, bicarbonate of 8 mEq/L, and a pattern consistent with high-anion-gap metabolic acidosis.

QUESTIONS

☐ *How do these laboratory values affect your differential diagnosis?*

☐ *What is the significance of the elevated amylase?*

☐ *What is the significance of the leukocytosis?*

☐ *What processes are included in your differential diagnosis for high-anion-gap acidosis?*

DISCUSSION

These laboratory findings are typical of moderately severe diabetic ketoacidosis. The metabolic acidosis is caused by the hepatic production of ketone bodies, which must be buffered by bicarbonate. Sodium tends to be low because of the osmotic effect of hyperglycemia, which increases extracellular water, thereby diluting serum sodium. Potassium, although initially high because of movement out of cells, falls to low levels as urinary losses occur. Although serum phosphate may be normal initially, large urinary losses often lead to depletion of total body phosphate, which should be replaced. The BUN and creatinine tend to be slightly increased because of the effect of volume depletion on renal function.

Serum amylase often is increased, but this usually is attributed to transient leakage from the salivary glands as well as the pancreas and does not usually indicate pancreatitis.

Leukocytosis is common in diabetic ketoacidosis. If infection is not present, the increased WBC count may be attributed to dehydration or to the increased glucocorticoid activity and catecholamine secretion that can occur in response to stress.

The high anion gap is caused by the presence of an unmeasured anion, in this case ketone bodies. Other important causes of high-anion-gap acidosis include renal failure, alcoholic ketoacidosis, lactic acidosis, and toxic substances such as salicylates, ethylene glycol, and methanol.

After 6 hours of treatment, the patient is awake, breathing comfortably at a rate of 18 respirations per minute, and able to respond to questions. The serum glucose level is 210 mg/dL, the arterial blood pH is 7.34, and the serum bicarbonate level is 14 mEq/L. Urine ketones are now only weakly positive.

QUESTIONS

☐ *What other types of acute care might this patient require?*

☐ *What are some of the potential complications of diabetic ketoacidosis?*

DISCUSSION

Because insulin therapy is still needed to treat the resolving ketosis and acidosis, glucose should now be added to the intravenous fluids to prevent hypoglycemia. Potassium and phosphate should be replaced as indicated by blood values.

Despite of careful treatment, patients with diabetic ketoacidosis have a mortality rate of 5%–10%. Death may be caused by overwhelming infection, by irreversible shock, or by arterial thrombosis causing myocardial infarction or stroke. Cerebral edema is a rare complication that occasionally occurs in children who appear to be responding well to treatment and may cause death. A more rapid decrease in glucose levels in blood than in the cerebrospinal fluid (CSF) causes fluid to enter the relatively hyperosmolar CSF compartment, leading to increased intracranial pressure and cerebral edema.

Polyarthritis

A 65-year-old woman presents to your office with a several-week history of pain and stiffness in her shoulders, hips, and hands. This began 2 weeks after visiting her grandchildren. Within a few weeks, she noted swelling in her hands and feet in addition to generalized stiffness lasting most of the morning. She had a low-grade fever but denied any chills, sweats, or weight loss. She had no associated headache, jaw claudication, or visual changes. She denied photosensitivity, oral ulcers, sicca symptoms, Raynaud's, serositis, history of miscarriages, or blood clots. She does have a family history of psoriasis.

QUESTIONS

- ☐ *Based on her history, what type of arthritis is this: inflammatory or noninflammatory?*
- ☐ *How does the pattern of joint involvement help in determining the type of arthritis?*
- ☐ *What is your differential diagnosis?*

DISCUSSION

The patient's history of morning stiffness lasting more than 1 hour suggests that inflammatory arthritis is the cause of her symptoms. At this juncture, the arthritis has been present only for a few weeks; therefore, infectious etiologies must be considered. She does have a low-grade fever, but rarely does a bacterial arthritis present in a polyarticular fashion such as this unless the patient is critically ill or has a history of intravenous drug use. Viral infections may present in this manner with a new-onset inflammatory arthritis. Of particular concern in this patient would be parvovirus B19 infection, as she has been exposed to young children. Parvovirus B19 infection, or Fifth's disease, is endemic among school-aged children. Children typically present with a rash on their cheeks, giving them a "slapped cheek" appearance, in conjunction with a low-grade fever and mild constitutional symptoms. Adults infected with parvovirus B19 may develop a flu-like illness and mild maculopapular rash on the extremities, with arthralgias and arthritis seen in approximately 20% of patients. The arthritis is symmetric and can be confused with rheumatoid arthritis (RA).

Young to middle-aged adult women are at highest risk for the arthropathy. Diagnostic testing soon after the onset of symptoms is helpful in making this diagnosis. A positive IgM antibody suggests active infection. A positive IgG antibody is consistent with prior exposure, but it is not helpful in the diagnosis, given the high prevalence of seroconversion in the general population. Although the presence of fever raises the index of suspicion for an infectious process, many patients with noninfectious inflammatory arthritis can have low-grade fevers.

Other concerns in this patient, given her age, include a paraneoplastic syndrome or polymyalgia rheumatica (PMR), especially in light of the proximal shoulder and pelvic girdle involvement. PMR may rarely have an associated inflammatory arthritis of the peripheral joints. Rheumatoid arthritis, systemic lupus erythematosus, scleroderma, and polymyositis all may present with an inflammatory symmetric polyarthritis. Psoriatic arthritis, although usually presenting in an asymmetric oligoarticular fashion, may present with a symmetric pattern of joint involvement, as can a crystalline arthritis such as gout (particularly in elderly women).

On examination, the patient is in obvious discomfort related to her joints. Her temperature is 38°C. She has a small, slightly raised erythematous scaly rash in her hairline and around her ears and in her umbilicus. No nail pits are present. There are no other mucocutaneous lesions. The temporal arteries have good pulsations and are nontender. There is no adenopathy. The cardiopulmonary and abdominal examinations are normal. The musculoskeletal examination is notable for limitation of motion of her shoulders secondary to pain and stiffness. She has obvious synovitis (synovial thickening with tenderness) of her bilateral wrists, metacarpophalangeal (MCP) joints, proximal interphalangeal (PIP) joints, ankles, and metatarsophalangeal (MTP) joints. There are no "sausage digits," and there is no evidence of an enthesopathy. She had mild warmth in both of her knees with moderate joint effusions. There was no sclerodactyly, muscle atrophy, or weakness.

QUESTIONS

- ☐ *How do the findings on physical examination guide your differential diagnosis?*
- ☐ *What information should you seek from diagnostic tests at this time?*

DISCUSSION

The examination confirms the presence of a symmetric inflammatory polyarthritis. Thus, the differential includes RA, systemic lupus erythematosus (SLE), polymyalgia rheumatica, and, less likely infectious, psoriatic and crystalline arthritis. The patient has a rash that has the appearance of psoriasis. Psoriatic arthritis develops in only 5% of patients with psoriasis. The risk of psoriatic arthritis increases with a family history of spondyloarthropathy or extensive nail pitting. There are five different patterns of psoriatic arthritis [see Chapter 11, IV B 3 d (2)]. It is possible that this patient has a pseudorheumatoid pattern of psoriatic arthritis. The differential diagnosis still includes viral illness such as parvovirus B19, rheumatoid arthritis, SLE, and malignancy. It is now unlikely based on the physical examination that the patient has scleroderma or an inflammatory myopathy. At this point, a complete blood count (CBC) and a comprehensive metabolic profile will help eliminate other systemic illnesses, such as a viral hepatitis and malignancy. Systemic measures of inflammation, such as an erythrocyte sedimentation rate (ESR) or C-reactive protein (CRP), are nonspecific indicators of inflammation and are not helpful in the diagnosis but may be helpful in assessing response to treatment. Parvovirus serology should be evaluated, given her exposure to children. A rheumatoid factor (RF), anti–cyclic citrullinated peptide (anti-CCP), and an antinuclear antibody (ANA) may be helpful in the diagnosis, given the symmetric presentation of her arthritis. It is important to keep in mind that 15% of patients with RA have a negative RF. A synovial fluid analysis would be helpful in assessing the degree of synovial inflammation and to evaluate the presence of crystals.

> The test results come back as follows: hemoglobin is 10.5 g/dL, the white blood cell (WBC) count is 8300/μL, and the platelet count is 500,000/μL. The Westergren erythrocyte sedimentation rate is 78 mm/hour. A comprehensive metabolic profile is normal. The RF is positive at 349 IU/mL, and anti-CCP is 80 IU/mL. The ANA is positive at 1:80 speckled. Parvovirus antibody IgG and IgM are negative. The x-rays of her hands and wrist show mild periarticular osteopenia around her MCPs. No erosions are seen. Synovial fluid analysis indicates 18,000 WBCs with 80% polymorphonuclear cells (PMNs) and 20% lymphs. No crystals were seen.

QUESTIONS

- *What is the diagnosis?*
- *What additional diagnostic tests are appropriate to confirm the diagnosis?*
- *What therapeutic approach is most appropriate now?*

DISCUSSION

At this point, RA is the most likely diagnosis, given the morning stiffness, symmetric joint involvement, the presence of the serum RF, inflammatory synovial fluid, and the radiographic feature of periarticular osteopenia. There is no evidence of an associated malignancy, and PMR and psoriatic arthritis are less likely, given the positive RF. Parvovirus has been excluded based on negative serologies. The patient must have arthritis for a period of 6 weeks to definitively diagnose RA, to ensure that other viral or self-limited entities are not contributing to the patient's arthritis. In the meantime, the patient is started on nonsteroidal anti-inflammatory drug (NSAID) therapy and returns in 4 weeks.

> On return 4 weeks later, the patient still has morning stiffness lasting most of the day. Her examination is notable for the presence of aggressive synovitis in her wrists, MCPs, PIPs, knee, ankle, and metatarsophalangeal joints. The results of the tests are reviewed with the patient, and therapeutic approach is outlined.

QUESTIONS

- *What therapies should be considered at this juncture?*
- *Should steroids be given?*

DISCUSSION

Now that it is clear that the arthritis has been present for 6 weeks, it is important that a disease-modifying antirheumatic drug (DMARD) be started immediately, as erosions occur early in the disease course. The gold standard in the treatment of RA is methotrexate. Before starting methotrexate, a baseline hepatitis screen and chest x-ray should be done. In addition, it is becoming standard practice to obtain a test for tuberculosis (purified protein derivative [PPD]) because if the methotrexate is ineffective, an anti–tumor necrosis factor (TNF) agent may be considered. There have been documented cases of reactivation of tuberculosis during anti-TNF therapy. While on the methotrexate, the patient must abstain from alcohol and have laboratory work every 6–8 weeks to monitor for toxicity. A short course of low-dose steroids may be helpful in controlling some of the symptoms while waiting for a DMARD to work, but a long-term course of steroids has no role in halting the progression of disease and is fraught with many potential side effects and long-term complications. The patient elects to start methotrexate therapy. Folic acid 1 mg daily is prescribed to diminish the likelihood of stomatitis.

Acute Low Back Pain

A 35-year-old man presents to the emergency department with a 2-day history of severe low back pain. The pain is worse when he sits up and better when he lies flat on his back. He claims to be well, although he recently experienced polyarthralgias, chills, and sweating. He reports that he was hospitalized for some form of hepatitis 2 years ago; he says it resolved uneventfully and he does not know what caused it. He denies alcohol or drug abuse.

QUESTIONS

- *What are your immediate concerns about this patient's low back pain?*
- *What conditions might cause referred back pain?*
- *What additional information do you want to know about the pain?*

DISCUSSION

The history of chills and sweats makes one consider an infectious process more seriously than other possible causes of this low back pain. The man describes the pain as severe, which makes it more worrisome. The fact that the pain is worse when sitting upright and better with recumbency is not particularly helpful in suggesting a specific, potentially serious cause of this back complaint.

Pain that is insidious in onset, associated with prolonged morning stiffness, relieved by exercise, and worsened by rest suggests underlying inflammatory back pain, typically the sacroiliitis of the spondyloarthropathies. In contrast, mechanical low back pain often is sudden in onset, worsened by exercise, and improved by rest. Pain that is ripping or tearing and perhaps associated with abdominal complaints is typical of an expanding abdominal aortic aneurysm. Pain associated with bladder or bowel incontinence and saddle anesthesia suggests a midline lumbar disk herniation with cauda equina compression; pain associated with leg sensory or motor complaints suggests lateral disk herniation and spinal nerve compression; and pain associated with gastrointestinal or genitourinary complaints suggests a need to investigate an intra-abdominal source as the cause. Constitutional complaints such as fever and chills make an infection more likely. Pain increasing with recumbency (the opposite of this patient's complaint) suggests a possible tumor; midline pain suggests a tumor, an infection, or a compression fracture.

Ninety percent of low back pain is caused by self-limited biomechanical or strain problems, but it is important to look for features that make an acute medical condition more likely. There is important information still to be obtained about the nature of this patient's back pain.

On initial examination, the patient is writhing in discomfort and asking for intramuscular narcotics. His temperature is 38.3°C, and prominent needle tracks are observed on his hands and legs. Diffuse tenderness and guarding are noted on abdominal examination. Marked tenderness is noted over the entire low back paraspinal region, and prominent percussion tenderness is noted over several lumbar and sacral vertebrae. The patient cooperates poorly with strength testing, but deep tendon reflexes and sensation are intact and anal wink and perianal sensations are normal. The patient complains of hamstring tenderness when either leg is raised in a straightened, extended position.

QUESTIONS

- *How do the findings on physical examination help you in thinking about your differential diagnosis?*
- *What information should you seek from laboratory tests and procedures at this time?*

DISCUSSION

Several findings on physical examination place self-limited musculoskeletal pain far down the differential diagnosis list. For one thing, it is known that the patient is likely abusing intravenous drugs, even though he denied this in the history. Narcotic drug-seeking behavior makes the physical examination more difficult to interpret because exaggerated responses to physical examination maneuvers are common in drug-abusing patients. In addition, the patient has a fever and prominent findings on abdominal and back palpation as well as on spinal percussion. Intravenous drug abuse and fever make an infectious process (e.g., epidural abscess, paraspinal or perirectal collection, septic sacroiliitis) much more likely. No specific evidence for an aortic aneurysm exists on abdominal examination, and there is no neurologic evidence for cauda equina compression or discogenic nerve compression. No evidence has been presented for a potential referred source of pain such as a penetrating duodenal ulcer (gastrointestinal source) or a renal infection or stone (genitourinary source). There is no evidence of a spondyloarthropathy.

A complete blood count (CBC) might help with evaluation of an infectious process, particularly if leukocytosis is present. Amylase would be increased with pancreatitis and bowel emergencies (e.g., small bowel obstruction). The erythrocyte sedimentation rate is nonspecific, but significant elevation also might suggest an infection, particularly osteomyelitis. Urinalysis is important for discovering a potential genitourinary infection. Three sets of paired blood cultures should be obtained because bacterial endocarditis can present with musculoskeletal complaints, and any bacterial process in the low back might be associated with bacteremia. Plain radiographs of the low back and sacroiliac joints quite likely might be normal, although patients with discitis can have intervertebral narrowing and vertebral end-plate destruction; those with sacroiliitis can have sacroiliac joint erosions and sclerosis. A magnetic resonance imaging (MRI) is the best imaging modality for evaluating soft-tissue or intraspinal collections, particularly to rule out an epidural abscess.

The test results come back as follows: hemoglobin is 11.3 g/dL, the white blood cell (WBC) count is 15,000/μL, and the platelet count is 500,000/μL. The Westergren erythrocyte sedimentation rate is 100 mm/hour. Chemistries indicate only an elevated alkaline phosphatase; amylase is normal. Urinalysis is negative. Chest radiograph, lumbar spine radiograph, and pelvic radiographs are unrevealing.

Several hours later, the patient continues to require high doses of intramuscular narcotic for pain control and still complains of severe low back pain. He says that he is having difficulty walking to the bathroom because of leg weakness. His maximum temperature is 38.9°C. Physical examination indicates continuing poor cooperation with strength testing, but he appears to be severely weak (3/5 on muscle strength testing) in all lower extremity muscle groups. He also has decreased sensation to pinprick from the toes to the navel and prominent increased deep tendon reflexes in the lower extremities, with four beats of clonus bilaterally.

QUESTIONS

▢ *What is the most likely diagnosis at this point?*

▢ *What additional diagnostic tests are appropriate to confirm a diagnosis?*

▢ *What therapeutic approach is most appropriate now?*

DISCUSSION

The neurologic findings (leg weakness, abdominal sensory level, increased reflexes, and clonus) suggest spinal cord compression with features of an upper motor neuron lesion. When the history of intravenous drug abuse, fever, low back pain, and progressive neurologic deficit is added, the differential diagnosis narrows markedly. The patient's sensory level to about T12 suggests that the cord compression is occurring at this level, probably from an epidural abscess. Conditions such as transverse myelitis or an ischemic myelopathy at T12 cord level or a midline herniated thoracic disk are still possible, but these diagnoses are less likely to explain the fever or to be associated with intravenous drug abuse. Given the high index of suspicion for infection, empiric antibiotic administration should be strongly considered.

The best procedure for confirming a diagnosis is an MRI scan. This test will best discriminate between an intrinsic cord lesion (e.g., transverse myelitis) and an extrinsic compression (e.g., due to an abscess or herniated disk). The test should be done emergently because early surgical intervention is critical to preservation of lower extremity function.

The emergency MRI scan shows an epidural abscess at T12, and surgical débridement is carried out immediately. *Staphylococcus aureus* grows from one set of the blood cultures and the abscess.

QUESTION

▢ *What remaining treatment modalities should be used now?*

DISCUSSION

The patient should be treated for 4–6 weeks with antibiotics effective against *S. aureus,* initially intravenously. He should be carefully watched for features of bacterial endocarditis, despite the fact that only one blood culture was positive. Furthermore, the patient should receive intensive physical therapy once the acute pain subsides so that he can recover lower extremity strength and the ability to walk.

CASE 12

Severe Headache

A 62-year-old woman calls your office because of a severe headache that came on suddenly 1 hour ago. Her medical history is significant for headaches associated with menses, which ceased 12 years ago, and one or two throbbing headaches annually since menopause. She has hypertension controlled with an angiotensin-converting-enzyme (ACE) inhibitor and beta-blocker and dyslipidemia treated with a statin, and she smokes one-half pack per day in spite of repeated urgings to stop smoking.

QUESTIONS

▢ *What are some possible causes of headache?*

▢ *What other questions would you like to ask this patient?*

DISCUSSION

The causes of headache are numerous. In a patient with headaches, it is useful to characterize each type of headache and develop a working hypothesis as to the cause of each headache. In this patient, there are potentially three types of headache: perimenstrual headaches, postmenopausal headaches, and the severe headache prompting her to seek medical attention at this time.

Head pain is caused by disorders of the head or neck, including neurologic disorders. Problems as diverse as giant cell arteritis, acute glaucoma, sinusitis, dental abscess, temporomandibular joint dysfunction, trigeminal neuralgia, or cervical arthritis can cause head discomfort. Intracranial causes of headache include central nervous system (CNS) mass lesions such as primary or metastatic tumors, abscesses, hydrocephalus, meningitis, superior sagittal sinus thrombosis, subarachnoid hemorrhage, and migraine.

One approach to the differential diagnosis of headache is to distinguish acute, life-threatening disorders such as meningitis and subarachnoid hemorrhage from chronic conditions such as migraine. Furthermore, it is helpful to differentiate conditions that require specific, urgent intervention such as giant cell arteritis or acute glaucoma from more chronic disorders such as migraine or cervical arthritis.

Further history shows that the patient's perimenstrual headaches were characterized by holocephalic throbbing discomfort that started 1–2 days before menses and lasted 2–3 days. She graded the headache pain as 7/10. There was occasional nausea and photophobia. The patient found relief with nonsteroidal anti-inflammatory medications. Her postmenopausal headaches occurred every 3–4 months and again were holocephalic and throbbing but only lasted a few hours or an entire day. The pain was 4–6/10 and was relieved with the same medications she had used for her perimenstrual headaches.

The patient denies any visual symptoms, including diplopia, jaw claudication, nasal drainage, dental pain, jaw "clicking," facial pain, or neck discomfort. She denied weakness or numbness in any limb and did not think she had a fever.

The patient states that she has never had a headache like her current one, which is holocephalic and graded as 9–10/10. The pain is constant, and she has nausea and photophobia. She was gardening when the headache suddenly began, and she had momentarily collapsed to her knees. A dose of naproxen brought no relief.

QUESTIONS

☐ *What are your diagnostic considerations?*

☐ *What do you advise the patient to do?*

DISCUSSION

The patient's symptoms are not similar to her prior headache history, which are consistent with migraine. There are no symptoms to suggest local ocular, sinus, dental, or musculoskeletal sources of pain. Of concern is the sudden onset of severe, atypical head pain. It is not clear from the patient's history whether the collapse was due to brief weakness, loss of consciousness, or both. The collapse, accompanied by nausea, suggests a neurologic problem such as a stroke syndrome (vertebrobasilar disease, intracranial hemorrhage) or increased intracranial pressure (hydrocephalus, sagittal sinus thrombosis, subarachnoid hemorrhage [SAH]). Her lack of focal neurologic symptoms is not supportive of vertebrobasilar disease or an intracerebral hematoma. The rapid onset of symptoms is not consistent with the presentation of sagittal sinus thrombosis.

Subarachnoid hemorrhage presents as "the worst headache of my life." The headache is typically of sudden onset, holocephalic, and severe and can be accompanied by nausea and brief loss of consciousness, probably reflecting a transient increase in intracranial pressure. Photophobia can occur, as can emesis. Typically there are no immediate focal neurologic symptoms or signs, although diplopia can reflect damage to the oculomotor nerve from the mass effect of a posterior communicating artery aneurysm. Smoking is a risk factor for SAH.

Because of your concern about SAH, you advise the patient to call 911 and have an ambulance transport her to the hospital. You contact the hospital to inform them about the patient's arrival and your diagnostic suspicion.

QUESTIONS

☐ *To which aspects of the physical examination should the emergency department physicians be particularly alert?*

☐ *What diagnostic tests are most essential to the patient's evaluation?*

DISCUSSION

Patients presenting with SAH frequently are quite hypertensive because of elevated catecholamine levels and increased intracranial pressure. Although patients with SAH can have a low-grade fever, elevated temperature should raise concern for an infectious process rather than SAH. If a patient has impaired consciousness, there should be concern about airway protection, and intubation should be considered.

The emergency department physician should examine the head and neck for the causes of headache referred to previously. Although evidence of meningeal irritation, such as Kernig's and Brudzinski's signs, should be looked for in patients with a possible SAH, these signs are frequently absent early in the clinical course.

A critical determinant of outcome after SAH is the patient's level of consciousness on presentation, with progressively impaired arousal being associated with a worse prognosis. An oculomotor palsy in an alert patient is particularly suggestive of a posterior communicating artery aneurysm, and an abducens palsy suggests increased intracranial pressure (a "false localizing sign"). Alert or obtunded patients with SAH rarely have other focal neurologic signs such as a hemiparesis.

The best initial test for the diagnosis of SAH is the presence of subarachnoid blood on a brain computed tomography (CT) scan. If blood is present, there is no need to perform a lumbar puncture. A modest proportion of alert patients with SAH have an unremarkable CT scan; in these individuals, a lumbar puncture is indicated to document the presence of bleeding.

Clotting studies (platelet count, prothrombin time, and activated partial thrombin time) are appropriate to screen for a bleeding diathesis. A serum sodium should be obtained because SAH patients are prone to disturbances in sodium concentration. An electrocardiogram may show findings such as peaked T waves or arrhythmias, which may represent catecholamine-associated cardiac effects.

The patient's blood pressure is 185/95 mm Hg; she is afebrile. She has no neck rigidity and a normal head and neck examination. She is alert and cognitively intact. Her neurologic examination is normal.

A brain CT scan shows subarachnoid blood with mild dilation of the ventricles. Clotting studies, serum sodium concentration, and the ECG are normal.

QUESTIONS

☐ *What are the next management steps?*

☐ *At this time, to what complications should the patient's physicians be alert?*

DISCUSSION

Patients with SAH should be placed in an intensive care unit. There should be frequent neurologic evaluations. Extremes of blood pressure should be avoided. It is helpful to consider the following relationship: cerebral perfusion pressure = mean arterial pressure – intracranial pressure. A cerebral perfusion pressure of 70–80 mm Hg is desirable. In an alert patient who presumably does not have a critical elevation of intracranial pressure, a mean blood pressure of approximately 90–100 mm Hg can be targeted. Labetalol is a particularly effective antihypertensive agent in this setting because it does not cause an elevation in intracranial pressure.

Hydration with normal saline is appropriate so as to maintain a euvolemic state. Mild sedation and analgesia for headache should be considered, and agents to prevent straining with bowel movements can be prescribed.

Nimodipine, a calcium channel antagonist, decreases the incidence of delayed ischemic deficits secondary to cerebral vasospasm. Unfortunately, it can cause excessive hypotension, which can exacerbate cerebral ischemia if not adequately treated.

Neurosurgical and radiologic consultation should be obtained, and urgent four-vessel angiography is necessary to document all aneurysms that the patient may have.

Complications at this time include the development of hydrocephalus attributable to disruption of cerebrospinal fluid flow patterns by subarachnoid (or intraventricular) blood, aneurysmal rebleeding, and hyponatremia. A decreased serum sodium level can be caused by overhydration, the syndrome of inappropriate secretion of antidiuretic hormone, and cerebral salt wasting. These complications can cause diminished consciousness, seizures, and, occasionally, focal neurologic signs.

> **The patient's blood pressure is successfully controlled with labetalol. Nimodipine is well tolerated. A cerebral angiogram indicates a single anterior communicating artery aneurysm measuring 10 mm in its largest diameter. The patient remains alert and cognitively intact. The patient, family, and physician team discuss treatment options to prevent rebleeding, including surgical "clipping" or endovascular "coiling" of the aneurysm. The patient decides on surgical intervention, which is performed on the second hospital day.**

QUESTIONS

☐ *At this time, to what complications should the patient's physicians be alert?*

☐ *What management strategies should be pursued?*

DISCUSSION

An operative complication of anterior communicating artery aneurysm surgery is cognitive dysfunction because of injury to basal forebrain structures. After surgery, patients are still at risk for hydrocephalus and hyponatremia. With successful isolation of the aneurysm from the cerebral circulation, the risk of rebleeding should be nil. Of concern at this time is the development of delayed ischemic neurologic deficits due to cerebral vasospasm. This complication is thought to be attributable to the effects of subarachnoid blood on the intracranial arteries; there is vasoconstriction with associated histologic findings of intimal hyperplasia and smooth muscle proliferation. Patients can develop impaired consciousness and focal neurologic deficits.

Serial transcranial Doppler (TCD) studies can show increasing blood flow velocities, which can be a harbinger of subsequent clinically significant cerebral vasospasm. Medical management to prevent symptomatic vasospasm and symptomatic cerebral ischemia includes nimodipine and "triple H therapy": hemodilution, hypertension, and hypervolemia. Optimal oxygen transportation occurs at hematocrits in the 30–35 range. Elevation of the mean arterial blood pressure by 10%–20%, together with hypervolemia, can prevent or treat cerebral ischemia caused by vasospasm.

> **The patient is cognitively intact after surgery. Blood pressure and serum sodium levels are in an acceptable range. However, serial TCD studies show a progressive elevation of blood flow velocities in the middle and anterior cerebral arteries. Triple H therapy is begun. On the third postoperative**

day, the patient becomes obtunded, and a mild right hemiparesis develops despite optimal medical management. A brain CT scan shows a left frontal ischemic infarction; there is no evidence of new hemorrhage.

QUESTIONS

- What is the probable cause of the patient's new stroke?
- What management options might be considered?

DISCUSSION

The patient has sustained an ischemic infarction caused by cerebral vasospasm. A cerebral angiogram should be obtained to define the extent of the vasospasm. Interventional neuroradiologic approaches to the treatment of medically refractory symptomatic vasospasm include angioplasty and intra-arterial infusion of papaverine.

The patient is taken to the angiography suite. Images demonstrate diffuse vasospasm, worse in the left middle cerebral artery. Angioplasty is performed and successfully dilates the left middle cerebral artery. Several papaverine infusions are directed at the distal branches of the anterior and middle cerebral arteries.

Over the next several days, the patient has a progressive decline in consciousness and develops a left hemiparesis. Repeat CT scans show multiple areas of ischemic infarction. A repeat angiogram shows severe diffuse vasospasm.

Two weeks after her SAH, the patient has lost all evidence of brain function and is declared brain dead.

COMMENT

Despite many advances in neurologic intensive care, aneurysmal SAH remains a disease with a mortality rate approaching 40%–50%. Patients are at risk for many complications, and although they may appear quite intact on presentation, their clinical course can be perilous.

CASE 13

Oral Erosions and a Rash

A 29-year-old African American man presents to the emergency department with the chief complaint of painful mouth erosions that have developed over 3 days. The initial symptom was a burning sensation of the left upper lip. Then tender sores developed on the gums and progressed to involve the entire mouth. Swallowing has become difficult because of increased secretions and pain. A rash has erupted on the patient's arms and legs within the last day.

Before the onset of symptoms, the patient was in good health. He has no ongoing or past medical problems. He takes no medications, vitamins, or herbal supplements. He has no known allergies and has no history of atopy. He works as a security officer and denies participating in any activities that pose a high risk for human immunodeficiency virus (HIV) infection. There is no family history of autoimmune disease or cancer. Review of systems is remarkable for a headache.

QUESTION

- What is the differential diagnosis based on the history of oral erosions and a rash?

DISCUSSION

The differential diagnosis of oral erosions includes infectious causes. Herpes simplex virus (HSV) infection produces localized blistering and secondary erosions that may affect the gingiva, buccal mucosa, and palate. It is also the most common infectious etiology of erythema multiforme. Hand-foot-and-mouth disease (a coxsackievirus infection) produces blistering and erosions of the palate, buccal mucosa, gingiva, and tongue, as well as blisters on the hands and feet. Autoimmune blistering diseases such as pemphigus vulgaris and paraneoplastic pemphigus involve the oral mucosa and skin. An adverse reaction to a systemic medication can affect the mucous membranes. Erythema multiforme major and toxic epidermal necrolysis are the most severe forms of an adverse drug reaction. An allergic contact dermatitis to oral hygiene products (e.g., toothpaste, mouthwash) can produce inflammatory changes and erosions of the oral mucosa. Lichen planus is associated with erosive oral lesions. Systemic disorders such as inflammatory bowel disease, systemic lupus erythematosus, and Behçet's disease may involve the oral mucosa and cause erosive lesions.

> The patient appears to be in mild distress and has a temperature of 99.8F (37.28C). Physical examination of the skin shows grouped erythematous vesicles and pustules on the left upper lip. The vermilion border is crusted with dried blood, and the anterior gingiva, buccal mucosa, and soft palate are bright red and eroded with serous exudate. The arms and legs show 0.5- to 1.0-cm erythematous round macules without scaling. The dorsum of the hands, the palms, and the soles have 1-cm, erythematous, target-like macules with a central violaceous hue. There is shotty submental and cervical lymphadenopathy.

QUESTION

☐ *What tests would you perform to narrow the differential diagnosis?*

DISCUSSION

Samples for a Tzanck smear and HSV antibody test should be taken from the grouped vesiculopustules of the left upper lip to identify the presence of HSV. The upper lip and oral mucosa should be swabbed, and bacterial and viral cultures should be obtained to confirm an infectious etiology. A skin biopsy from the buccal mucosa and one of the target-like lesions should be obtained to confirm the diagnosis and rule out other causes of oral erosions, such as pemphigus vulgaris.

> The Tzanck smear reveals multinucleated giant cells. Subsequent results demonstrate positive HSV type 1 cultures for the lip and skin biopsies of the buccal mucosa and hand characterized by histologic changes consistent with erythema multiforme.

QUESTIONS

☐ *What acute treatment should you provide?*

☐ *What are the long-term treatment issues?*

DISCUSSION

To reduce viral shedding and increase healing time, oral antiviral therapy should be initiated at appropriate doses for primary HSV infection. For oral pain relief, a topical anesthetic, such as viscous lidocaine, should be provided with instructions for the patient to swish and spit out up to four times a day. A short, 10- to 14-day course of oral prednisone may provide additional relief of acute inflammation of the erythema multiforme reaction; however, use of corticosteroids in erythema multiforme remains controversial.

The associated constitutional symptoms (headache and low-grade fever), lymphadenopathy, and no history of HSV indicate that the infection is primary and that the patient is at risk for recurrent episodes. The patient should be educated regarding the natural history of herpes labialis, its infectivity, and the signs and symptoms of recurrence. Because of the severe nature of the patient's reaction to his initial eruption, he should be provided with a prescription for an oral antiviral agent with the instructions to initiate therapy at the first symptoms of recurrence. If the patient develops frequent eruptions such that the episodic antiviral therapy proves to be ineffective in suppressing erythema multiforme, then ongoing prophylactic doses of antiviral agents should be used for long-term suppression.

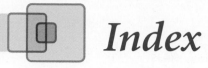

Index

Note: Page numbers followed by an "f" denote figures; those followed by a "t"
denote tables and those followed by a " 🌐" denote complete text available online.

A

Abatacept, for rheumatoid arthritis, 488t
Abciximab, 31, 32
Abdominal aortic aneurysm, 3, 262
Abdominal pain, diagnostic entities for, 13, 15
Abdominal vasculature diseases, 262–263
Abnormal fibrinogens, 132
Abnormal intestinal motility, 226
Abnormal plasminogens, 132
Abnormalities in blood coagulation, 369
Abscess, 622
Absolute erythrocytosis, 121, 122
Absolute neutrophil count (ANC), 212
Acarbose, for oral antihyperglycemic agents, 451t
ACE inhibitors, 33, 329
Acetaminophen, 10, 367, 506
   liver disease, 253t
Achalasia, 218, 264
Acid
   carbonic, 317
   nonvolatile, 318, 319
Acid-base metabolism, normal, 🌐
Acid-base metabolism disorders, 315–320
   metabolic acidosis, 317–319
   metabolic alkalosis, 319–320
   respiratory acidosis, 315–316
   respiratory alkalosis, 316–317
Acidemia
   acute kidney injury, 276, 277, 279
   respiratory acidosis, 315, 316
Acidosis, 314
   metabolic, 317–319
   respiratory, 315–316
Acitretin, for psoriasis, 617
Acne vulgaris, 607–608, 🌐f
Acneiform eruption, 626, 🌐f
Acquired aldosterone deficiency, 314
Acquired coagulation disorders, 129–131
Acquired immunodeficiency syndrome (AIDS), 135
Acquired myopathies, 585–586
Acquired or hereditary angioedema (HAE), 346
Acquired sideroblastic anemias, 116
Acromegaly
   clinical features, 418–419
   diagnosis, 419
   etiology, 418
   therapy, 419
Acromegaly, 42
ACTH deficiency, 420
Actinic keratosis, 619
Actinomycetes, 385
Action (kinetic) tremor, 576
Activated protein C resistance, 132
Active relaxation, abnormalities in, 18
Acute aortic insufficiency, 38, 39
Acute appendicitis, 235, 272
Acute chest syndrome, 120
Acute cholecystitis, 246–247
Acute conduction system abnormalities, 33
Acute coronary syndrome (ACS), 29
Acute DIC, 205
Acute disk herniation, 596
Acute dystonia, 577

Acute eosinophilic pneumonia (AEP), 109
Acute fatty liver, 259
Acute gastritis, 220
Acute generalized exanthematous pustulosis (AGEP), 626
Acute gouty arthritis, 499
Acute hyponatremia, 306
Acute intermittent porphyria, 🌐
Acute interstitial nephritis, 297–298
Acute interstitial pneumonitis (AIP), 101
Acute kidney injury (AKI), 274–278
   causes of, 275t
   clinical course, 276, 277f
   clinical features of, 274–275
   diagnosis of, 275–276
   therapy, 277–278
Acute leukemias
   classification and epidemiology, 137–138
   clinical features, 138
   diagnosis, 138
   prognosis, 139
   therapy, 138–139
Acute low back pain
   case study on, 669–671
Acute lymphocytic leukemia (ALL), 137, 🌐
Acute mediastinitis, 96
Acute meningitis, 373
   classification, 374
   clinical features, 374
   etiology
      aseptic meningitis, 374
      bacterial meningitis, 374, 374t
   therapy, 374
      aseptic meningitis, 375
      bacterial meningitis, 374–375
Acute mesenteric ischemia, 262–263
Acute myelogenous leukemia (AML), 137, 138, 🌐
Acute nonlymphocytic leukemia (ANLL), 138
Acute pancreatitis, 243–244
Acute pericarditis
   clinical features, 46
   diagnosis, 46–47
   etiology, 46
   therapy, 47
Acute pyelonephritis, symptoms of, 385
Acute quadriplegic myopathy, 586
Acute renal disease, 303
Acute respiratory distress syndrome (ARDS), 83–84, 101, 244
   clinical course, 83–84
   clinical features, 83–84
   definition, 83
   diagnosis, 83–84
   etiology, 83
   pathology, 83
   pathophysiology, 83
   therapy, 84
Acute respiratory failure
   classification, 82
   definition, 81
   pathophysiology, 82
   therapy, 82–83
Acute rheumatic fever (ARF), 536–537
Acute syphilitic meningitis, 587